LEGAL MEDICINE

PATHOLOGY AND TOXICOLOGY

LEGAL MEDICINE
PATHOLOGY AND TOXICOLOGY

by

THOMAS A. GONZALES, M.D.

Chief Medical Examiner of the City of New York (Retired); Professor of Forensic Medicine, New York University Post-Graduate Medical School; Lecturer on Criminologic Medicine, New York Police Academy

MORGAN VANCE, M.D.

Deputy Chief Medical Examiner of the City of New York; Associate Professor of Forensic Medicine, New York University Post-Graduate Medical School; Lecturer in Forensic Medicine, College of Physicians and Surgeons, Columbia University; Lecturer on Criminologic Medicine, New York Police Academy

MILTON HELPERN, M.D.

Chief Medical Examiner of the City of New York; Associate Professor of Forensic Medicine, New York University Post-Graduate Medical School; Lecturer in Legal Medicine, Cornell University Medical College; Lecturer on Criminologic Medicine, New York Police Academy

and

CHARLES J. UMBERGER, PH.D.

Toxicologist, Office of the Chief Medical Examiner of the City of New York; Assistant Professor of Forensic Toxicology, New York University Post-Graduate Medical School

Introduction by
HARRISON S. MARTLAND

SECOND EDITION

APPLETON-CENTURY-CROFTS, INC.

NEW YORK

To the Memory of

CHARLES NORRIS

First Chief Medical Examiner

of

the City of New York

PREFACE

In preparing the second edition the authors were confronted with such an accumulation of new material that they found it necessary to enlarge the scope of the book. The method of presentation is still based on the division of the subject into legal medicine and toxicology. The principal changes are a more detailed description of the various subjects, and the addition of new original photographs to illustrate the characteristic conditions and typical pathologic lesions encountered in medicolegal cases.

For the pathologist who must determine the cause of death by autopsy and sometimes decide whether the deceased died of a trauma or a natural disease condition, a knowledge of medicolegal pathology is a matter of importance. Accordingly the first forty chapters are devoted for the most part to this subject. Four chapters (6, 7, 8, 36) are concerned with the role played by traumatic lesions and natural disease processes in causing death, especially when there is an association of these two factors in the same case.

Statistical data compiled from the Annual Reports of the Office of the Chief Medical Examiner in the City of New York from 1918 to 1951 have been incorporated in the different chapters indicating the frequency of deaths from natural causes from the different types of trauma, especially their subdivisions into accidental, suicidal or homicidal varieties. It was considered that such an arrangement of material helped to round-out the overall conception of medicolegal conditions as they are encountered in a large metropolitan center like New York City.

Much new material has been introduced to elaborate the old text. Entirely new subject matter has been added, such as the autopsy findings in embalmed bodies in Chapter 5; cardiac contusions in Chapter 11; traumatic cerebral edema in Chapter 12; injuries incurred in sport in Chapter 14; the Rh-Hr groups in Chapter 27; pathologic lesions in poison cases in Chapter 29; uranium compounds in Chapter 31; the more recent organic drugs in Chapter 35; and operative and postoperative deaths in Chapter 38.

Subjects considered a part of medical jurisprudence such as the corpus delicti, the responsibility of the physician to the government, malpractice, insanity, confidential communications, dying declarations and insurance claims are again presented, but at greater length and in more detail. The authors are grateful to Mr. Rowland H. Long, General Counsel of the Massachusetts Mutual Life Insurance Company, for his advice and help in preparing this material.

The authors are indebted to Alexander S. Wiener, the serologist in the Office of the Chief Medical Examiner in the City of New York, for his advice and assistance in rewriting Chapter 27 on the *Human Blood Groups*, especially the Rh-Hr section and other recent discoveries.

An entirely new discussion dealing with the analytic phase of toxicology is presented, subdivided on the basis of the classification of poisons which is determined, in turn, by the analytic methods for their detection. The material, representing data and unpublished experimental work compiled over a period of some fifteen years, has been obtained and organized primarily from the files of the Microchemical-Physical Laboratory. The technical divisions of the Office of the Chief Medical Examiner in the City of New York comprise the Forensic Pathology Laboratory, the Bacteriology-Serology Laboratory, the Chemical Laboratory, and the Microchemical-Physical Laboratory. When the Microchemical-Physical Laboratory was instituted, one of its functions was the application and adaptation of all physical and analytic methods, new and old, for the detection of new pharmaceuticals. Emphasis from the start has been on the qualitative analysis of poisons as unknowns, without regard to history or autopsy findings, and the text is presented this way. Following the text as described could require more sample material than is usually available and more labor than might be practical in routine laboratory operations. We assume the analyst has sufficient working knowledge to take those shortcuts inherent in any analytic process; the material has not been written or intended for the untrained or inexperienced person.

Chapter 42 follows conventional, straightforward procedures for the analysis of gaseous poisons in air and their detection in tissue and body fluids. In Chapter 43, the mechanics of spectrographic analysis are omitted. The text is concerned primarily with the interpretation of spectrographic plates in the qualitative analysis of the general unknown type of case, based on observations of normal and toxic levels of metals in human tissues. Methods for the preparation of test samples and specific qualitative and quantitative procedures for individual metals most likely to be encountered are also described. Methods of analysis for the inorganic, nonmetallic poisons discussed in Chapter 44 are adaptations of existing schemes of analysis in inorganic qualitative chemistry, applied to the special problems of toxicology. In Chapter 45, which is concerned with steam distillation and the isolation and identification of volatile compounds, part of the material is taken from the process for the routine examination for volatile poisons as used in the Chemical Laboratory of the Medical Examiner's Office. Chapter 46 is a discussion of ethyl alcohol and the problems pertaining to its analysis and the physiologic significance of the chemical values. Whereas the material in the other chapters is relatively complete, Chapter 47 is the introduction to and partial analysis for the nonvolatile organic compounds. Infrared and ultraviolet spectrophotometry, as well as other specialized procedures which should be integral parts of the analyses, have not been included. The special chemical and physical properties of individual compounds from which final confirmation is made must be obtained from the literature. The material was developed from the point of view of analysis for an unknown. Consequently organization was based on the reactions, and compounds, with few exceptions, are not discussed individually. The reactions for each compound are summarized in the Appendix although they are not tabulated in the Index.

The authors are particularly indebted to Grace Adams Khan of the Microchemical-Physical Laboratory who was instrumental in the preparation of the analytic toxicology section, and to D. Alan Eagleson who, while a Dazian Fellow in Forensic Toxicology in the New York University Post-Graduate Medical School, did much to develop methods and to check and complete existing procedures. Leo Dal Cortivo, biochemist, Hospital for Special Surgery, helped develop organic methods and cross-checked data on color reactions. The authors also wish to thank associates of the medical examiner's laboratories: L. Goldbaum for the quantitative determination of metals and work on the identification of the acid extraction group; A. Stolman for work on color reaction in nonaqueous solutions; M. Feldstein for work on the identification of barbiturates; A. Ames and H. Siegel for work on alcohol and volatile compounds; and H. Schwartz for work on the recovery of organic compounds from tissue. The authors are also indebted to A. O. Gettler and his students for their work from the Chemical Laboratory of the Chief Medical Examiner.

The authors also desire to thank the publisher for aid and encouragement in the preparation of this volume.

THOMAS A. GONZALES
MORGAN VANCE
MILTON HELPERN
CHARLES J. UMBERGER

CONTENTS

INTRODUCTION

This book is one of the few authoritative works on legal medicine and toxicology in this country. Condensed in a single volume, suitable for everyday reference, is the knowledge of a group of experts based upon the medical investigation of violent, sudden and suspicious deaths in the medical examiner's office of the second largest city in the world. This work aptly confirms the opinion of Littlejohn that "There is only one path to the mastery of forensic medicine, and that is, an extensive practical experience acquired by a daily whole-time application and study of the medical problems which are presented by the crimes of a large community."

Told in their own language and profusely illustrated, the contents represent cases actually observed and investigated by the authors. They show that forensic medicine is a practical science which rests upon correct and accurate interpretation of fact; a science upon which the life and happiness of the individual and the safety of the community often rests.

All recent advances in legal medicine have been given due consideration. In civil life as well as in military life, the character and types of weapon have changed, and industrial advances have also brought forth new occupational hazards and poisons. Many developments in toxicology, especially micro-analysis, have been necessary to cope with this progress. Further, the great incidence of automobile injuries, the accidents associated with aviation, and the threat of chemical warfare have created situations which require considerable additions to the subject matter of any work on legal medicine.

The volume is especially valuable to those of us who are trying to improve the status of legal medicine and toxicology. In attempting to obtain proper support for such work we are constantly confronted with the statements of those who call attention to the vast material and excellent type of work performed in the continental medicolegal institutes. The authors clearly show what has been and what is being done in America.

While it is true that adequate physical equipment and competent personnel of an institution make for careful work in the actual performance of the medicolegal autopsy, experience has shown that in many instances a careful analysis of details at the scene of the crime by the medical officer, in conjunction with the police, is as important as the actual autopsy. The Medical Examiner's Act of the City of New York specifically requires that a medical examiner observe and take charge of the body at the scene of the crime. The practical application of this system is well described in this book.

The number of investigations made by the Office of the Chief Medical Examiner of the City of New York far exceeds that of any similar institute in the world. In the City of New York about 81,000 deaths occur annually; of these, some 20,000 must be investigated by the medical examiner's office. This office issues approximately twenty per cent of all death certificates. Few people realize the vast amount of work such investigations necessitate. The toxicological work done under the auspices of this office is enormous; materials from over 2,000 human bodies are analyzed annually for the presence of poisons.

In the discussion of the various poisons this book gives in complete detail the symptoms, lethal doses and autopsy findings, and in addition, the directions for collecting and transporting the proper organs to the toxicologist for analysis. Unlike most previous works on the subject, details of analysis for, and identification of, the various poisons have been confined to three separate chapters instead of the usual procedure of giving such details at the end of the discussion of each poison. In these chapters the system of routine toxicological examination employed in the toxicological laboratory of the Office of the Chief Medical Examiner under the supervision of Dr. Alexander O. Gettler is clearly described.

This book reflects the knowledge gained by the authors at the autopsy tables of the City Mortuary located in the Department of Laboratories at Bellevue Hospital. For many years they have performed the necropsies on almost all the cases which come under the jurisdiction of the Medical Examiner's Office of the Borough of Manhattan.

All the authors were close associates of Dr. Charles Norris, the first Chief Medical Examiner of the City of New York whose foresight, patience, honesty and ceaseless effort developed his office into one of the outstanding agencies of its kind.

It would have been a great source of pride to their Chief to know that his pupils have dedicated this work in his honor. Dr. Norris would have derived great satisfaction had he lived to know that this group of his followers forms one of the most prominent teaching organizations in this country to which the student may turn for expert instruction in forensic medicine. His pupils man the staff of the Department of Forensic Medicine at the New York University College of Medicine—a department which he conceived and organized in 1934. The authors also teach forensic medicine at the College of Physicians and Surgeons of Columbia University and at the Cornell University Medical College, as well as at other schools in the City of New York.

This book so completely and thoroughly covers the subjects of legal medicine and toxicology that it should become the handbook and daily guide for the coroner, the coroner's physician, the county physician, the medical examiner, the toxicologist and the pathologist. Further, any laboratory assistant or technician who, in an official or semi-official capacity, may be called upon to aid in the investigation of the so-called coroner's case, will find the work invaluable.

But the value of the book does not end here. The text should serve as a guide for teaching and for reference in the police schools and crime laboratories. It will be of aid to the police, homicide squads, detectives and photographers in the scientific detection of crime and in the apprehension and conviction of the criminal.

Finally, the surgeon, the internist, especially the cardiologist, as well as the members of the legal profession, criminologists, and those who are interested in the occupational hazards and poisons of present-day industry should find a wealth of material and detailed instruction in this work.

HARRISON S. MARTLAND

LEGAL MEDICINE

PATHOLOGY AND TOXICOLOGY

1

The Medical Examiner and the Coroner

Definition of Terms. The practice of using the terms legal medicine and medical jurisprudence interchangeably has led to considerable confusion as to their correct meaning. Actually they denote essentially different subjects which, however, are closely related. Medical jurisprudence is that part of the law which is concerned with the regulations governing the professional practice of the doctor of medicine. Portions of this subject which are important to the physician will be discussed in subsequent sections. Legal or forensic medicine is that part of medical science which is employed by the legal authorities for the solution of legal problems. Theoretically all branches of medicine may be included in this definition, for the law has used them all when need has arisen, and any doctor who testifies in court in his professional capacity can be considered a practitioner of legal medicine. The term, however, is usually restricted to that specialized branch of medical knowledge used by physicians officially employed by the local government of a community when they investigate suspicious and violent deaths, or cases involving nonfatal injury such as rapes, sexual offenses or abortions which may subsequently come before the courts. In the United States the medical investigation of fatal cases is done most often by an elected official of the county known as the coroner. In a few states, however, similar functions are performed by a physician known as the medical examiner who is an appointed officer of the county or municipal government.

THE CORONER

The office of the coroner originated in the early days of English history, probably a few decades before the Norman Conquest. Originally the coroner was appointed by the King to represent the Crown as its magistrate in a certain district. The first incumbents of this office were men in high station, usually of noble blood, and the office enjoyed high prestige. The duty of the coroner was to see that the interests of the Crown were given due recognition, especially in transactions involving money, such as the discovery of treasure or the investigation of crimes punishable by fines.

The statute of Edward IV (4 Ed. I. *stiled de officio coronatoris*) stated specifically that the coroners in every county were to be the conservators of the peace and were to be chosen according to the rules contained in the statutes concerning their election. When a coroner was informed of any death from felony or misadventure, or of treasure unlawfully buried in the earth, or of a case of rape, or of a jail break, or of similar disturbances of the peace, he issued a mandate to the sheriff to summon to him the people in the adjacent townships to inquire about the truth of the matter. If the problem concerned a corpse which had apparently died a violent death, the coroner and jurors selected by him viewed the dead body and proceeded to make an investigation and inquest into the circumstances of death; at the end of the proceedings they decided by what means and why the deceased came to an untimely end. If enough evidence was produced at the inquest to charge

1

a person with the crime of felonious homicide, the sheriff would be directed to seize the lands and the coroner to confiscate the chattels of the accused for the Crown. In like manner, if a person suspected of a crime became a fugitive, whether guilty or not, the coroner was empowered to declare him an outlaw and to seize his goods and chattels. Even in cases of misadventure, if a domestic animal or a moveable object was instrumental in causing the death of a person, it was forfeited to the king under the name of a deodand; similarly, the property of a suicide was confiscated. These few specimens of the statute will be sufficient to indicate the activities of the early coroners.

As the centuries passed and the social conditions of England changed, the status of the coroner declined both in the rank of the individual selected to fill that office and in the prestige accorded the office itself. The important duties were gradually stripped from him until his principal function was to hold inquests on all cases of death of a violent or suspicious nature. The duties of the coroner in present-day England have been somewhat modified from those of his medieval prototype but not altered in any essential particular. When colonies of Englishmen began to settle in other parts of the world, the institution of coroner was transferred there and at this day is found in the British Commonwealths and in most states of the American Union.

In the United States the coroner is typically a county official elected by popular vote for a term of office which varies from two to four years; in order to continue in office he must be re-elected at the end of that period. In most communities previous knowledge of law or medicine is not considered essential for a coroner, and the only qualification is that the candidate should be eligible for a place on the ticket of the predominant political party. In some states, as in Louisiana, the coroner when possible must be a graduate of a medical school and licensed to practice in that state.

The duties of the coroner are principally the investigation of all cases of suspicious or violent death which have occurred in his county. The laws defining his authority over deaths of this sort vary in the different states and are often phrased in vague language, but the tendency is to limit the cases under his jurisdiction to deaths which have presumably resulted from external causes. In some communities other duties may be assigned to the coroner, such as the examination of allegedly psychopathic individuals, responsibility for the health of persons in the jails, or the assumption of duties usually assigned to a sheriff.

When the coroner is notified of a death which requires his official attention, he follows a routine which varies with the individual community. Usually either he or his representative visits the body at the scene of death and decides whether or not the circumstances warrant an extensive investigation. If he considers that the case is not a suspicious one he may release the remains to the next of kin without further formality; in this case a physician appointed by him may issue the death certificate, or that duty may be assumed by another organization, as, for example, in Cook County, Illinois, where it is performed by the Registrar of the Health Department. If an autopsy is required the coroner is empowered to perform it, if he is a physician, or to delegate a physician to perform it. If poisoning is suspected the coroner usually has the authority to make provision for all necessary chemical analyses on the organs of the deceased.

If the case is a suspicious one, an inquest is conducted in order to determine the way in which the deceased met his death. In some localities a jury is selected and taken to view the body in company with the coroner; in other places this visit is not considered essential. The coroner then convenes his court over which he presides as judge with the jury in attendance and proceeds to take the testimony of witnesses under oath. Most of the time he conducts the examination of the witnesses himself but on occasion he may allow attorneys representing interested parties to ask questions. Medical testimony may be taken or the report of the autopsy may be read into the record, but the coroner usually has the right to disregard such evidence at his discretion. At the end of the hearing the coroner may deliver a charge to the jury and allow them to bring in a verdict on how death occurred: by natural causes, misadventure, suicide or homicide. In some cases he may direct the jury to bring in a certain verdict without allowing them to vote. As a result of testimony given in his court the coroner can order the arrest of any person or persons implicated in a homicide, in which case he must transmit the findings of his court to the higher authorities. In some jurisdictions the coroner conducts his court like a magistrate without a jury.

The coroner system in practice has shown itself to be entirely inadequate for the duties it must perform. The incumbent of such an office labors under such heavy disadvantages that even with the best intentions he is hampered in his work. The laws which regulate his duties lack precision, especially in defining the kinds of cases which come under his jurisdiction. In performing a necessary autopsy he is exposed continually to the possibility of a liability suit brought by relatives of the deceased who may question the legality of the autopsy. Like most minor elected officials he is vulnerable to pressure from politicians, an influence which rarely works for disinterested ends. He is usually crippled by lack of funds so that there is little chance for him to improve his organization.

The basic theory behind the coroner system is fallacious: that a local magistrate without special qualifications in law or medicine can conduct a judicial investigation successfully for the purpose of determining the cause of death. The determination of the cause of death is purely a medical problem, and it is only in comparatively recent times that the coroner has sought medical aid for this purpose. Generally his medical representatives have not always been competent and there is nothing in the existing statutes which will ensure that his physicians will be the ones best qualified for their duties. The coroner system is entirely unsuitable for the complexities of present-day civilization and needs to be replaced by a more workable type of medicolegal organization.

THE MEDICAL EXAMINER

The first suggestions of the medical examiner system are to be found in the *archiatri populares* of the Roman Empire, who were official physicians appointed for certain districts principally to treat the indigent sick. There is not any record to indicate that these physicians had any medicolegal functions. The *archiatri* are principally significant as an indication that the governing powers had begun to realize that medical knowledge was worthy of employment by the state.

Town physicians similar to the *archiatri* were a regular institution in the European cities of the Middle Ages; they served the community as medical practitioners, army surgeons, police doctors and medicolegal experts. The statute laws of some of the northern Italian republics in the thirteenth to the sixteenth centuries specified the qualifications a physician must possess to be employed as an expert in legal medicine. One such law stipulated that the incumbent should be 30 years of age, a resident for 20 years in the district where he was to serve, politically reliable and competently trained in the legal branch of the profession. The statutes generally required the official expert to visit a dead or wounded individual as soon as possible, to examine his injuries and to make a written report in which the physician is to express his opinion on whether or not the lesions were mortal. The examination consisted of a visual inspection of the wounds; autopsies at that period were not officially recognized. In some laws there was the stipulation that at least two experts should participate in the same examination in order to avoid error as much as possible. The experts were called in to investigate suspected cases of poisoning, to examine psychopathic individuals and to give testimony in criminal and civil trials. Here the true beginnings of the European medicolegal systems made their appearance, for here the state recognized the value of medical knowledge for certain processes of law.

The Bamberg Code appeared in 1507 and the *Constitutio criminalis Carolina* enacted by the Emperor Charles V appeared in 1530; both increased the importance of legal medicine by their insistence that medical testimony was an essential part of the proof in trials involving questions of infanticide, abortion, poisoning, fatal wounds and other forms of bodily injury. The statute did not specify that autopsies were to be performed on the bodies of the victims in cases of this type. In 1562 a judicial autopsy was performed in Paris by Ambroïse Paré, and around the end of the sixteenth century the autopsy in medicolegal cases began to be generally practiced. With the increasing complexity of European civilization in the nineteenth century, the different governments were forced to improve the administration of forensic medicine, and this resulted in the establishment of the great medicolegal institutes all over the continent in the large centers of population.

The system in the European cities allots to the police and the judicial authorities the duty of investigating the circumstances of all deaths reported to them, and if there is any suspicion or appearance of criminal violence, the body is sent to the medicolegal institute for autopsy. Cases of death which do not belong to this category are usually disposed of through some other channel. Except on special occasions the medicolegal experts are rarely called in to investigate the scene where the body was found. They are principally concerned in performing the autopsy and such chemical and microscopic examinations as may be necessary to establish the cause of death. In addition the medicolegal institutes are occupied with a number of heterogeneous activities which include: (1) interpretation of laws regulating the practice of medicine or of laws requiring medical knowledge for their interpretation; (2) psychiatric examination of individuals involved in court trials in which mental sanity is a point at issue; (3) examination of persons whose claims for state insurance are open to controversy; (4) alcohol determinations on the blood and urine of persons involved in traffic accidents; (5) blood group determinations on the principals in paternity cases; and (6) performance of police laboratory examinations. Such divergent pursuits are a heritage from the days when medicolegal science was much simpler and the experts gladly assumed any scientific task which might be allotted to them by the legal authorities. At the present time these duties present quite a problem in administration, and many of them could be transferred to other laboratories and organizations which could perform them more efficiently. Everything considered, however, the European institutes have functioned satisfactorily, though they are open to criticism on matters which will be discussed later.

The present method of medicolegal investigation in Scotland deserves a brief description as it is derived from the system used in France and has no connection with the coroner system of England. Each district in Scotland is served by an official called the procurator-fiscal who in addition to being the prosecutor has the duty of investigating all cases of death which have occurred without the attendance of a physician, or unexpectedly, or by violent means or under suspicious circumstances. This official has the power to call in the police and to direct their investigation, and he has the authority to summon witnesses before him in order to obtain the facts. If the case seems to him to be homicidal, he is empowered to call in two physicians to examine the body; and he can order an autopsy after he has obtained the authorization of the sheriff in the district. When his report is complete, it is sent with the autopsy findings to the higher legal authorities in the Crown Office of Scotland for final disposal.

The medical examiner systems in the United States are based upon the same principles as those underlying the European institutes, though somewhat modified in the process of adaptation to conditions in this country. The American organizations have two advantages over the European: (1) the American medical examiners concentrate their efforts on the investigation of deaths which have occurred as a result of violence or under suspicious circumstances and are consequently not harried by the unrelated activities embraced by the European institutes; (2) the American systems, unlike the European, prescribe the visit of the examining physician to the scene where the body was found. This greatly reduces the chance of losing important items of medical evidence which otherwise might be overlooked.

The first medical examiner system was established in Massachusetts where it was adopted in 1877, after the abolition of the coroner's office. Similarly, in New York City, the Office of the Chief Medical Examiner was established by a law passed by the state legislature in 1915 and began to function in 1918. Today the medical examiner system also exists in the states of Maine, Maryland, New Hampshire, Rhode Island and Virginia and in some of the counties of New York and New Jersey. The original Massachusetts and New York City organizations are the prototypes of the other medical examiner systems in the United States: Massachusetts has been the model for the systems in the New England states; and the medical examiner offices in Essex County, New Jersey, and Nassau and Westchester Counties, New York, and in the states of Maryland and Virginia have been patterned after that of New York City. It is probable that the future development of the system in the United States will follow the practice of the offices in New York City or in Massachusetts. As these differ from each other in some essential particulars it is desirable to describe them in more detail.

The medical examiners in Massachusetts are appointed for terms of seven years by the governor with the advice and consent of the council, according to the formula that they shall be "able and discreet men learned in the science of medicine." In their respective districts they investigate all deaths which are supposed to have occurred from violence, and they perform autopsies "upon being authorized in writing by the district attorney, mayor or selectmen of the district." After he has investigated the circumstances of death the medical examiner may issue his death certificate merely after an external examination of the body, and he performs an autopsy when the district attorney decides that the nature of the case is such that this procedure is warranted. Provision is also made for all necessary chemical examinations.

The original Massachusetts medical examiner system labors under several disadvantages: the first is that a medical examiner and his assistant are appointed for a district and work under conditions which do not allow them contact with other examiners so that mutual aid and criticism are generally lacking. The second disadvantage is inherent in the appointment of the medical examiner by the governor of the state. The governor is given considerable freedom in selecting the physician to fill this office and is not constrained by law to choose the best qualified person. The most serious criticism can be directed against that part of the law which places in the district attorney the power to determine whether or not an autopsy shall be performed in any particular case. Such officials do not always realize that certain types of homicide may masquerade as natural deaths and be totally overlooked unless an autopsy is performed. The refusal of a district attorney to allow an autopsy on a case of this type would seriously hamper the medical investigation and thus create difficulties for his own prosecution. This same criticism can be urged with equal force against the medicolegal systems in Scotland and on the continent of Europe which place similar discretionary powers in the hands of the legal authorities.

Recently the powers of the medical examiners in Massachusetts have been extended. Chapter 38 of the General Laws of the Commonwealth of Massachusetts (as amended by Chapter 632 of Acts and Resolves of 1945) gives the medical examiners discretionary authority to perform autopsies, similar to the provisions in the New York Law.

The Office of the Chief Medical Examiner in New York City is organized in a somewhat different fashion.* The head of the office called the Chief Medical Examiner, is appointed by the mayor from the classified lists compiled by the Municipal Civil Service on the basis of a competitive examination. He is authorized to make appointments of qualified deputy and assistant medical examiners and other employees from the classified civil service lists as may be provided pursuant to law. The law states that the chief medical examiner is to be a skilled pathologist and microscopist, and that his deputy and assistant medical examiners are to have the same qualifications. The distinctive feature of this office is that it functions as an organization with a responsible head having general charge of the way in which it performs its duties.

It is required by statute that the Office of the Chief Medical Examiner shall be open day and night with a clerk always present. When calls are received from the police or from physicians or hospitals notifying the office of a case of death which requires its attention, the clerk relays the information to the medical examiner on duty. He visits the scene of death and makes his investigation independently of other agencies. He inquires into the circumstances of death, takes the names of witnesses and examines the body at the scene. He then writes out a report of his investigation and files the record in the Office of the Chief Medical Examiner.

Deaths with which the medical examiner is especially concerned are those which have occurred "as the result of criminal violence, or by a casualty, or by suicide, or suddenly when in apparent health, or when unattended by a physician, or in prison, or in any suspicious or unusual manner." If the medical examiner is convinced from his examination of the body and of the circumstances that the cause of death can be ascertained beyond a reasonable doubt and that the death is not a suspicious one, he may issue a certificate of death based upon his investigation of the circumstances and the external examination of the remains and release the body to the relatives. However, if he believes that an autopsy is necessary, he or another medical examiner performs the autopsy. The autopsy findings are recorded in detail and together with

* See Appendix for the law providing for the establishment and operation of the Office of Chief Medical Examiner in New York City.

other data on the case are filed in the records in the central office. Whenever necessary, chemical, microscopic, serologic and bacteriologic examinations are performed on the organs or secretions of the deceased in the appropriate laboratories which are part of the organization.

The chief medical examiner or his assistants have the power to subpoena witnesses and take testimony under oath concerning any matter within the jurisdiction of the office. Such hearings are solely for the purpose of obtaining information about the circumstances of death to enable the medical examiner to qualify and classify properly the death which he is investigating. The medical examiner does not have any judicial functions similar to the coroner, nor has he any official authority to order the arrest of any person. In New York City the judicial powers of the coroner have been transferred to the magistrate's court.

The records in the Office of the Chief Medical Examiner are an indispensable part of the government of the city. Reports of the findings in homicidal and suspicious deaths are sent regularly to the district attorney as they are necessary for his work as prosecutor. The case records are also subpoenaed in civil court actions and workmen's compensation hearings.

The medical examiner system of New York City has worked satisfactorily not only in the metropolis but also in Essex County, New Jersey, Nassau and Westchester Counties, New York, and more recently in the states of Maryland and Virginia. Although the system is not perfect by any means, it gives more satisfactory results than any so far devised. It possesses the advantages of an organization which has a responsible commander who allows his subordinates freedom and discretion in their investigations. The fact that the individual medical examiner is responsible for determining the cause of death and issuing the death certificate tends to make him especially careful in carrying out his investigations and less likely to overlook deaths of a suspicious nature.

REFERENCES

American Medical Association. Report of the Committee to Study the Relationship of Medicine to Law.

Baas, J. H. Outlines of the History of Medicine, translated by H. E. Handerson, New York, J. H. Vail Co., 1889.

Bohne, G. Die Gerichtliche Medizin im italienischen Statutarrecht des 13–16 Jahrhunderts, Vrtljsehr. f. gerichtl. Med., 61:66, 238, 1921.

Ford, R. The medical examiner and the practicing physician, New England J. Med., 239:1001, 1948.

Herzog, A. W. Medical Jurisprudence, Indianapolis, The Bobbs-Merrill Co., 1931.

Landé, K. E. Forensic medicine in Europe, New England J. Med., 218:826, 1936.

Leary, T. The Massachusetts Medicolegal System, New York, The Rockefeller Foundation, Division of Medical Education, 1928, p. 297.

Littlejohn, H. H. Department of Forensic Medicine, University of Edinburgh, New York, The Rockefeller Foundation, Division of Medical Education, 1928, p. 187.

Moritz, A. R. Legal medicine in Europe, Am. J. M. Jurisp., 2:73, 1939.

Schultz, O. T. Possibilities and Need for Development of Legal Medicine in the United States, National Research Council, Bull. No. 87, October, 1932.

———— and Morgan, E. M. The Coroner and the Medical Examiner, National Research Council, Bull. No. 64, July, 1928.

Vance, B. M. A critical review of the medical examiner system, Am. J. M. Jurisp., 2:243, 1939.

———— Fundamental characteristics of different medicolegal systems in the United States, New York State J. Med., 44:2472, 1944.

Webster, R. W. Legal Medicine and Toxicology, Philadelphia, W. B. Saunders Co., 1930.

Weinmann, G. H. Compendium of the Statute Laws of the Coroners and Medical Examiners in the United States, National Research Council, Bull. No. 83, August, 1931.

2

Investigation at the Scene of Death

The medical examiner or coroner's physician must determine by his investigation whether death in any given case is due to natural causes or to trauma. If it is the result of trauma, he must decide whether it occurred accidentally or was inflicted with suicidal purpose or with homicidal intent. In this task the examination of the scene where the body was found is a matter of considerable importance. The following account is a description of the method of investigation employed by the Office of the Chief Medical Examiner in the City of New York.

PROCEDURE

As soon as the medical examiner is notified of a death requiring his attention, he proceeds promptly to the scene and takes charge of the body as required by law. If the case is a homicide, or a suspected one, he usually finds members of the police department in charge and their different specialists conducting their own line of investigation, such as examining different objects and surfaces for fingerprints, photographing the body and the premises or searching for weapons. It is advisable in many instances for the medical examiner to delay his investigations until the police have finished their work as a matter of cooperation with that department and in order not to disturb any clues.

The way in which the medical examiner conducts his investigation will depend largely on circumstances. As soon as possible he should note on his report the time of his arrival at the scene and the nature and location of the premises. If the proper persons are present, the body of the deceased should be identified to him by a relative or friend whose name, relationship to the dead person and address are duly recorded on the report. The police officers who were the first to arrive at the scene also identify the body to the medical examiner and their names, titles, shield numbers and precinct are entered on the record. The significance of these identifications in the establishing of the corpus delicti will be discussed later. If the requisite information can be obtained, the data which are necessary for the death certificate may be compiled.

It is important for the medical examiner to obtain all possible information about the circumstances of death from the police and other persons. Some victims may die or be killed in the presence of witnesses, in which case the manner and time of death is easily ascertained. In other instances a body is found dead, and it may not be easy to determine just how, when and where death occurred. Usually the place where the corpse is found is the scene of death, but it is always possible that the body was brought there from some other location in order to confuse the police investigation. It must be remembered that the scene of death is not always the place where the fatal injuries were received, for some traumatic injuries of the head, chest and abdomen are not immediately disabling, and the victim may move himself from the place of occurrence a long distance to the place where death supervened (Fig. 2-1).

The time of death must be established as accurately as possible. In cases in which the body was found dead, the medical examiner must be informed of the date and hour when this discovery was made and also the date and hour when the deceased was last known to have been alive. If these two times are correct, death must have occurred in the interval between them, but without further investigation it would be hopeless to determine even approximately the moment of death. The first observations of the examiner should be made on the body with reference to the signs of

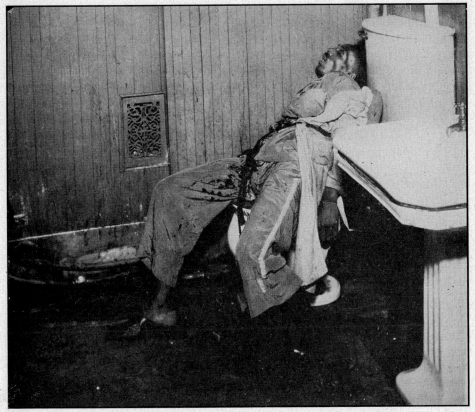

Fig. 2-1. Scene of Homicidal Death, Fatal Stabbing Having Occurred Elsewhere.

Victim, after having been stabbed through the heart while on the street, ran up two flights of stairs into his apartment and locked himself in the bathroom where he died.

death that are present, for it is at this time that these findings are most significant as indicators of the interval which has elapsed since death; many hours later when the autopsy is performed, the signs may have been so altered that they will not yield the desired information. The corpse should be examined at the scene as early as possible to see if it is warm, partly chilled or thoroughly cold. If it is warm and lax the inference would be that death took place only a short time before, while if cold and stiff, the signs would suggest that a longer interval had elapsed since death. The nature and distribution of the postmortem lividity, the presence or absence of rigor mortis, bacterial decomposition, mummification and similar postmortem changes must be carefully recorded on the report. All these findings must be considered along with such factors as the temperature of the surroundings, the clothing, the position and nutrition of the body and other influences which may accelerate or retard the development of the various signs of death. Observations should also be made on any other objects on the premises which may be of value in establishing the postmortem interval, as, for example, dates on mail and newspapers, the condition of food on the table and similar phenomena. If the medical examiner is called upon to give his opinion concerning the postmortem interval, he must take all the available facts into consideration and give a cautious and properly qualified answer so as not to mislead the police by a false assumption of accuracy. However, if the interval since death can be reliably determined, it would be very helpful for the police, for it gives them a basis on which they can check the alibis of various suspects.

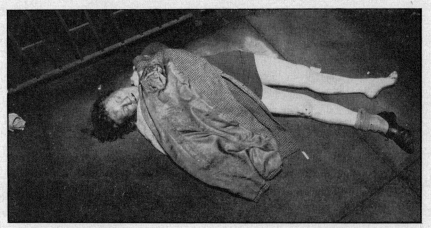

Courtesy Police Dept., City of New York

Fig. 2-2. Body Removed from Scene of Homicidal Death.

Dead body as found on sidewalk where it was deposited by perpetrator who carried it down from tenement flat during the darkness of the dim-out. Victim had been strangled 24 hours before and body had lain face down until disposal. Note lividity of face and pale pressure areas and anterior lividity on lower extremities indicating original prone position of the body.

The position of the body and its relation to the surroundings must be carefully observed. Photographs such as those taken by the police photographers are valuable in preserving a visual record of the scene, and they may be supplemented by a diagrammatic drawing made by the medical examiner for his record. He must also dictate or write up his observations. These should include a description of the body, its location on the premises, its position, the clothing on the corpse and its condition, the different injuries present, the distribution and condition of any blood that has been shed, the character of any suspected weapons, the presence of any outstanding marks on the body which may serve for identification and any other detail which may be pertinent. These matters will be considered more specifically and at greater length later.

It is important for the medical examiner to find out from the police whether the body is still in its original position or whether it has been shifted since its discovery. In some cases an ambulance surgeon may have attempted resuscitation of the victim, and the medical examiner should be informed of this if he is to evaluate the significance of any disturbances which may have been caused by these procedures, such as disarrangement of clothing, use of tourniquets, application of surgical dressing to wounds and other factors. The distribution of the postmortem lividity on the body may give an important clue as to whether or not the body was shifted after death (Fig. 2-2).

Injuries and wounds on the body must be described at the scene with enough thoroughness to meet the exigencies of the individual case. With bullet wounds it is frequently desirable to link the entrance wounds with their proper exits as it may enable the detectives to locate the bullets at the scene. In some instances bullets may lodge just under the skin and may be removed by a small incision. Early possession of a bullet may help the police considerably as it enables them to compare the

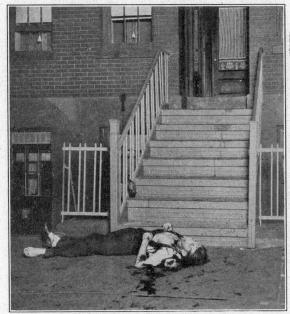

Courtesy Police Dept., City of New York

Fig. 2-3. Blood at Scene of Homicidal Stabbing.

Note blood streaming down from upper steps of tenement house stoop where stabbing occurred, and on sidewalk alongside victim. Left slipper caught in railing.

missile with a suspected gun or with any discharged cartridge shells. Any stabbing instruments or blunt instruments found on the premises should be compared with injuries found on the corpse. The examiner must distinguish genuine traumatic lesions from adventitious marks resulting from postmortem decomposition or from the ravages of insects or animals. The different types of injury will receive full consideration in later pages.

Suspected lethal weapons should be sent to the laboratory to be examined for traces of blood, hairs and pieces of tissues. Hairs found in the victim's hands should also be sent to the laboratory. In abortion cases, tissue fragments found in waste pails or on any instruments should be taken for histologic examination and blood-stained articles or free blood should be retained for grouping. Seminal stains discovered on the person and clothing of the deceased in fatal cases of rape should be preserved for a microscopic examination or if possible for a group determination. In cases of poisoning the vessel containing the poison should be transported to the toxicologist. All these subjects will be given due consideration under their proper headings. The chief concern in sending a specimen to the laboratory is to make certain that the specimen is properly identified to the laboratory specialist so that his examination can be connected with the crime.

Blood stains at the scene deserve special consideration because they may furnish valuable clues to incidents which occurred during the crime. For example, in some bullet wounds and stab wounds there may be a distinct trail of blood in the form of large crenated drops on the floor or blood-stained smears on the wall, which indicate the movements of the deceased from where he was wounded to where he finally collapsed. Figures 2-3 and 2-4 are graphic depictions of the information furnished by the examination of the blood stains at the scene of death.

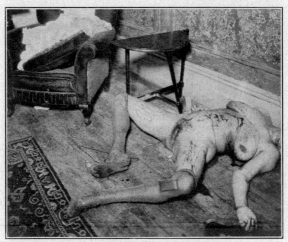

Courtesy Police Dept., City of New York

Fig. 2-4. Homicidal Stabbing.

Vertical streams of blood on abdomen and thighs indicate that deceased was standing when stabbed through right breast and chest. Body was limp and warm when examined at scene by medical examiner shortly after crime was discovered.

After the investigation of the scene of death, it may be possible to form an opinion as to whether death was caused by homicidal, suicidal or accidental means or resulted from natural causes. This subject will be discussed briefly here, since it will be considered in more detail under the different forms of trauma.

HOMICIDES

It is the safest plan to consider any fatal injury as possibly homicidal unless the investigation proves otherwise. Multiple bullet wounds (Chapter 16) and multiple stab wounds (Chapter 15) are usually homicidal, especially if they are located in the back or in a part of the body where the deceased could not easily have wounded himself by his own efforts. Typical homicidal blunt force injuries are illustrated in Chapters 9 through 14. The cases of manual strangulation, ligature strangulation, smothering and drowning illustrated in Chapters 17 and 18 are also indicative of homicide. Other types of injury are not so easily diagnosed and can only be identified as homicides after an investigation of the circumstances of the case and sometimes not until the autopsy has been performed. It is especially important for the police to discover the possible motive for the crime.

If cases of suicide are investigated thoroughly, indications will appear that the deceased had a definite intention of taking his life. A suicide note in which such a purpose is declared may be found or the history of a previous attempt at self-destruction may be elicited. Any suicide note found at the scene by the medical examiner should be added to the file of the case as important evidence. There is, of course, the rare possibility that the suicide note is a falsified document meant to cover up a homicide.

Occasionally a suicide will try two or more methods before he finally succeeds. For example, one person drank an ounce of tincture of iodine and then jumped out of a fifth story window. In another case an individual attempted to stab himself in the head and following this to cut his throat; when these methods were not successful he hanged himself from a gas pipe which broke under the weight of his body. Death resulted from illuminating gas poisoning (Chapter 19). Some cases of suicide have cut their wrists and throats in an attempt to bleed to death and later have drowned themselves or flung themselves from a high window (Chapter 15). Multiple self-inflicted stab and incised wounds are not infrequently encountered (Chapter 15).

The theory of suicide is favored if signs are present indicating that the deceased had made preparation to make his death certain, as in cases of illuminating gas poisoning in which he has attached the open end of a gas tube near his nostrils or mouth or has closed the cracks in the doors and window by cloth and paper. In such instances the possibility that the death is homicidal and that the scene has been manufactured to suggest suicide must be considered, unless the deceased has locked himself in the room in a fashion to preclude this possibility.

Cases which are obviously suicidal are illustrated as follows: gunshot wounds (Chapter 16), stab wounds (Chapter 15), hanging (Chapter 17) and drowning (Chapter 18). Other cases such as falls from a height, some deaths from drowning, carbon monoxide asphyxiations and different types of poisoning are not so easily recognized as suicidal and require an investigation of the circumstances and the discovery of a possible motive for self-destruction before excluding homicide or accident. Sometimes questioning by the investigator at the time that the body was found may reveal such motives for suicide as loss of money, disappointment in love, fear of disgrace, psychopathic tendencies of different kinds or dread of the ravages of an incurable disease.

The motive for suicide may not be apparent or certifiable in every instance because of the circumstances, but it may become evident when the autopsy is performed. In one such instance, the deceased, a white man of 80 years, committed suicide by drinking a solution of mercuric chloride. The autopsy disclosed not only the gastrointestinal lesions characteristic of the poison but also a sizeable carcinoma of the stomach. In another case the victim, a white man of 62 years, committed suicide by means of illuminating gas; the autopsy revealed an epithelioma of the esophagus with liver and regional lymph node metastases. Lesions of this type, if they are sufficiently developed to evoke clinical signs and symptoms, may well furnish the sufferer with a motive for suicide. Similarly, a pregnancy found in an unmarried woman may be an important clue if the other evidence in the case indicated that she took her own life.

Occasionally a rapidly fulminating infectious disease such as a primary pneumonia may cause a toxic delirium and precipitate a suicidal attempt on the part of the victim. In one case a 50 year old white man died of multiple injuries after jumping from a bridge; at autopsy there was found a widespread lobular pneumonia due to the hemolytic streptococcus. In another case a soldier was found dead in a hotel bedroom with a few shallow cuts on his left wrist but no evidence of loss of blood; the autopsy disclosed a marked lobar pneumonia which not only caused death but even induced the unsuccessful attempt at suicide. In many suicidal cases in younger women, the uterus is found in the menstrual stage, for at this period depressive tendencies are most apt to manifest themselves.

The following case illustrates how investigation at the scene may help to diagnose a suicidal death which was not obviously such at first glance. The body of a young colored woman was found at the foot of a long flight of stairs, lying on her back, with the legs flexed under her body and her head resting on the right hand corner of the lowest step. The blade of a long jackknife was stuck in her chest, penetrating one of the interspaces, the pericardium and the heart and causing death by intrapericardial hemorrhage (Fig. 2-5). On the landing of the stairs

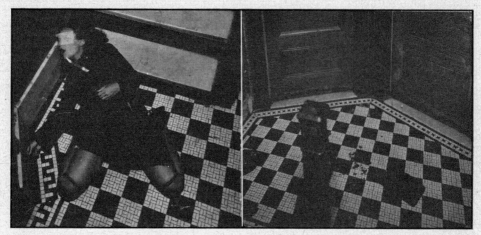

Courtesy Police Dept., City of New York

Fig. 2-5. Suicidal Stabbing at First Suspicious of Homicide.

Left. Undisturbed dead body as found in tenement hallway by police and medical examiner. Knife handle and part of blade protruding from fatal stab wound.

Right. Landing at top of stairs where deceased stabbed herself. Note drops of blood and pocketbook on the tile floor. Deceased came out of apartment door on right.

above, a number of drops of blood were spattered in an area about 18 inches square, and the pocketbook of the deceased lay close by. The investigation disclosed that the knife was the property of the deceased and had been purchased only the day prior to her death. It was also learned that the deceased had, just prior to her death, been visiting her estranged husband whose apartment opened onto the landing at the head of the stairs. Evidently failing to patch up their differences, she emerged onto the landing and was seen to stagger and slump to her knees. The witness who saw this ran for assistance, but when she returned the deceased was at the foot of the stairs, having either slid or staggered to the place where she was found. What probably happened was that the deceased, when she emerged onto the landing, had brandished the knife, probably with the intention of only wounding herself to arouse the sympathy of her husband, but in her emotion had inadvertently driven it too far into her chest. The track of the stab wound was a short one and could have been self-inflicted with only a slight degree of violence. Later it was found that the deceased had been despondent over her marital troubles and had threatened to commit suicide. All the factors in the case were more in favor of suicide than of any other interpretation.

ACCIDENTS

Accidental deaths can be diagnosed only by correlating the circumstances with the results obtained at autopsy. The following case illustrates how necessary the investigation of the scene is in those instances in which witnesses of the actual occurrence were lacking.

A man 55 years of age was found dead in his room, fully dressed, lying face down in a pool of blood. There was a laceration of the left eyebrow but no other sign of injury externally. The room was a narrow one containing two cots; one cot stood against one wall, while a second cot parallel with the first stood under a mantelpiece on the opposite wall. A few drops of blood were present on the bedclothes of the cot under the mantelpiece; and drops of blood led across the room to the other cot, the bedclothes of which were stained with blood, rather deeply at one spot near the pillow. The deceased was lying between the two cots, his head on the floor. A close examination of the mantelpiece disclosed a short, greasy area on its sharp edge, to which were attached a few short hairs similar to those in the left eyebrow of the deceased. While the autopsy did not disclose any further injury, it did show that the deceased had a moderately severe arteriosclerosis of the kidney vessels, an enlarged heart and an appreciable quantity of alcohol in the brain. The hemorrhage noted at the scene of death was due to a severe nasal bleeding. The final judgment was that the deceased, in a tipsy condition, had fallen over the cot under the mantelpiece, lacerating his left eyebrow, and upon this began to bleed from the nose, partly as the result of trauma and partly as the result of high blood pressure. He staggered away, collapsed against the cot on the opposite side of the room and finally slumped to the floor. Death was due to the accidentally induced epistaxis combined with a severe arteriosclerotic nephrosclerosis and a moderately severe grade of acute alcoholism.

Accidental deaths are most likely to be caused by generalized blunt force, drowning, burns, electric injuries, asphyxiation by certain gases and some types of poisoning. It is quite unusual to find accidental instances of bullet wounds, stab wounds, blunt instrument injuries or cases of strangulation; these are mostly homicidal or suicidal. An accidental stabbing in which the deceased was transfixed by falling on a long, heavy, pointed fragment of mirror glass is shown in Figure 15-19.

Some cases are recognizable as accidental even when the actual occurrence was not witnessed. For example, if a woman is found in a back yard dead of multiple fractures, tangled in a clothesline with pieces of wet wash, and an open window is observed four floors above in her apartment, the evidence would strongly suggest an accidental fall from the window while hanging out the clothes, provided there is nothing to suggest a suicidal or homicidal interpretation. Many cases of trauma of the accidental type are associated with acute alcoholism, inasmuch as intoxicated individuals are liable to stumble into misadventures of all sorts. It must be remembered, however, that acute alcoholism is also encountered frequently in homicidal or suicidal deaths.

NATURAL CAUSES OF DEATH

Persons suffering from a natural disease condition may die suddenly in the presence of witnesses or they may be found dead under various conditions. Many of these cases have a previous medical history which may strongly suggest the cause of death while others occasionally die without previously complaining of any symptoms worthy of note. In all such instances death from external causes cannot be ruled out except by an autopsy, for conditions like cyanide poisoning or a slow cerebral compression from an epidural hemorrhage complicating a skull fracture may cause death in a way that respectively suggests coronary artery disease or spontaneous cerebral hemorrhage.

Fatal traumatic shock caused by severe injury in the absence of external signs of trauma may be mistaken for the signs of cardiac collapse. In a recent case a watchman who fell down an elevator shaft sustained fatal injuries without immediate loss of consciousness or inability to walk, but with rapid onset of shock. He did not reveal the accident to his associates when they discovered him at the bottom of the shaft, so that when he climbed unassisted out of the pit and suddenly died in their presence, they believed that he had suffered a heart attack; they reported the case as such to the police and medical examiner. The autopsy revealed a heart without any serious pathologic lesions, multiple rib fractures, a dislocated shoulder, lacerations of the mesentery and a fracture of the lower lumbar spine. The fact that an individual dies apparently of a natural disease condition in the presence of bona fide witnesses does not preclude the possibility of violent death.

Further discussion of natural causes of death and their relation to trauma will be found in Chapter 6.

REFERENCES

Helpern, M.   The postmortem examination in cases of suspected homicide, Ann. Int. Med., 24:666, 1946; J. Crim. Law & Criminol., 36:485, 1946.
———— The postmortem examination in homicides, Am. J. M. Jurisp., 1:165, 1938.
Vance, B. M.   The work of a medical examiner's office, Am. J. M. Jurisp., 1:95, 1938.

3

Identification

Identification is the recognition of an individual as determined by characteristics which distinguish that individual from all others. A knowledge of this subject is obviously of the greatest medicolegal importance. Identification and the identity of an individual are matters that are of considerable concern to the courts and must be established by proof in practically every type of civil and criminal court action. One of the principal parts of the examination of the dead body by the medical examiner is the description and enumeration of physical characteristics which may help to identify it.

The subject of identification may be conveniently subdivided into identification of the living and identification of the dead.

IDENTIFICATION OF THE LIVING

Civil Cases. It is occasionally necessary to establish the identification of a living person in civil court actions concerned with such problems as marriage, inheritance, insurance claims or liability for torts.* In many cases this is easily accomplished by introducing official records and other incontestable proofs, but if these are lacking an attempt is made to confirm or disprove identity by the testimony of witnesses, handwriting, and photographs or descriptions given by relatives or friends concerning the bodily characteristics and distinguishing marks possessed by the person in question. None of these methods can be regarded as infallible though some are less open to objection than others.

There are plenty of examples to indicate that a witness claiming to recognize a certain individual as the same one whom he saw for less than a minute at a certain locality on a certain hour and date is likely to make an erroneous identification. Observation under these conditions is likely to be faulty, and observers are more than usually open to suggestions of the imagination. The degree of reliability of this kind of testimony depends a great deal on the circumstances of each case, especially on how well known the one identified is to the person making the identification and on how dependable the identifier can be considered for the qualities of honesty and accuracy.

Handwriting, though characteristic for the individual, especially if it is written rapidly, may be disguised or forged and must be used with caution in determining the identity of a person. In doubtful cases the specimens of handwriting should be passed upon by an expert. Photographs have only a limited value as a means of identification and will be discussed presently.

Descriptions of a person given by his relatives and friends are not dependable and in the past have led to many erroneous identifications. Resemblances between individuals who are not related are sometimes striking, and it is easy to see how one

---

* Tort is a legal term denoting a private or civil wrong against such rights of an individual as his life, property, personal freedom or reputation, but excluding a wrongful act classified as a breach of contract.

might be mistaken for the other. When the identifying witnesses have not seen the person they are identifying for a number of years the chances of error are much increased. The unreliability of any identification based on the recollection of the physical traits of the person in question by friends and relatives is shown in the famous case of Sir Roger Tichborne who supposedly perished at sea in 1854. Some time afterward a man claiming to be the missing baronet appeared and was accepted as the heir to the Tichborne baronetcy and estates by the mother of Sir Roger, the family solicitor and 17 servants of the family. Eventually, however, discrepancies between the mental and physical traits of the claimant and those which were known to be characteristic of the real Sir Roger were noticed and the fraud was disclosed.

Criminal Cases. The identification of an individual for the purposes of a criminal court action is an important duty of the police department. Formerly the Bertillon system of anthropometric measurements, supplemented by a detailed description of all the features of the body including special marks and scars, was used by many police systems of the world as a method of identification. The measurements included the anteroposterior diameters of the head and trunk, the span of the outstretched arms, the lengths of the left middle finger, left little finger, left forearm and left foot, the length and breadth of the right ear, and the color of the left iris. A complete Bertillon description would give an accurate word picture of a person so that his likeness could be reconstructed from the chart. This method, however, has been discontinued and other, less complicated systems have displaced it.

Whenever a first offender is arrested, tried and convicted, the Police Department of New York City prepares his identification chart and stores it among their records. This file consists of pedigree, photographs and fingerprints of the prisoner.

The pedigree of the prisoner includes a description of his person in addition to data concerned with the crime. The form of pedigree employed in New York City states only the name of the prisoner, his alias, residence, the crime charged, color of skin, age, height, build, color of hair, color of eyes, complexion, presence or absence of mustache, birthplace, occupation, date of arrest, name of arresting officer, precinct and remarks concerning the type of crime committed.

The photographs consist of a front view of the head and a profile view of the right side of the head. Considerable care is used in preparing these pictures, and the position of the head, the distance of the camera from the subject, and the background are determined according to definite rules which aim to standardize the photographs and to reproduce the characteristic features as clearly as possible. As a sole means of identification, photographs are not always reliable, and they may be a source of error even when they are inspected by experts. The physiognomy of a person may be modified by changes in his hair growth, by injuries, by advancing years, by cosmetic surgery and by other factors. Many regard the ear as the best criterion for identification, as it retains its characteristics with less variation than any other feature.

The fingerprints are also taken according to a standard routine. The palmar surfaces of the tips of the fingers are stained to the first distal joint with ink and then rolled on glazed paper from without inward in such a way as to obtain an impression of the whole tip. Each finger is treated separately in the same way, and the 10 impressions are placed in the space set aside for them. The finger tips of each hand are then placed on the paper simultaneously without motion, so as to obtain a record of the impressions as they are likely to be laid on a surface naturally. The impressions of the two thumbs are then taken simultaneously (Fig. 3-1). The prints are then filed with the photographs and the pedigree and constitute the record of the prisoner.

This type of identification chart has served the New York City Police Department quite as well as more complicated forms. The pedigree might be lengthened

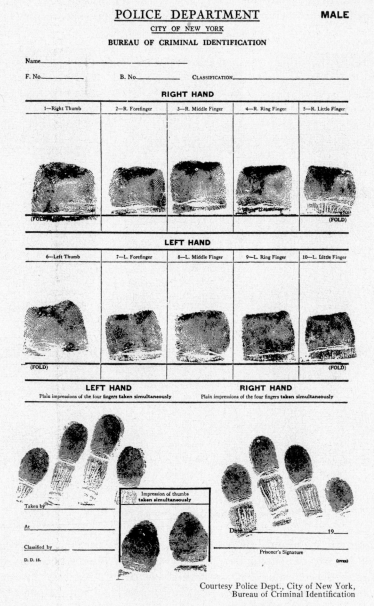

Courtesy Police Dept., City of New York,
Bureau of Criminal Identification

Fig. 3-1. Specimen Fingerprint Record.

so as to include many bodily characters and abnormalities which will be discussed under identification of the dead, but inasmuch as the fingerprint patterns are distinctive and permanent in individuals and will identify them positively, there is no need to increase the complexity of the chart. The patterns of finger impressions are classified as loops, whorls, arches and composite forms, as shown in Figure 3-2, and are capable of almost infinite variation so that it has been estimated that there is one chance in 64 billion of two persons presenting identical fingerprints. For fuller description of this subject and the other routine methods of police identification, the reader is referred to Webster, to Kuhne and to Söderman and O'Connell.

The difficulty of identifying a person arrested for a crime in a city like New York depends upon whether or not the prisoner has a previous record. If he is an

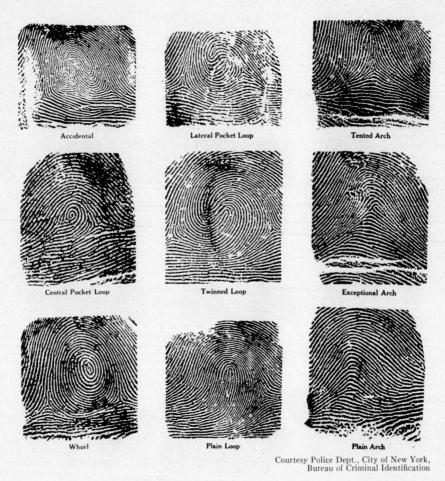

Accidental	Lateral Pocket Loop	Tented Arch
Central Pocket Loop	Twinned Loop	Exceptional Arch
Whorl	Plain Loop	Plain Arch

Courtesy Police Dept., City of New York,
Bureau of Criminal Identification

Fig. 3-2. Standard Fingerprint Patterns.

old offender, the problem is much simplified, as the prisoner may be recognized at the time of his arrest or later in the police line-up, and all that is necessary is to refer to the files. If the individual has not been convicted of a felony or of certain misdemeanors, his record will not be present in the files. However, the police may send the classification of his fingerprints by telegraphic code to the Federal Bureau of Investigation and to the Department of Correction in New York State in hope that records of them exist in these bureaus. Without an identification chart it is more difficult to establish a person's identity, especially in a large center of population. The individual under arrest may give a false name or he may carry with him false identification papers, and it would be far from easy to discover his true name unless he was recognized by someone who knew him. Even then the same objections exist which have been mentioned in civil court cases concerning identifying witnesses, since there is always the chance that the identifier has been misled by a fortuitous resemblance or is naturally deficient in his powers of observation.

POLICE DEPARTMENT
CITY OF NEW YORK
REPORT OF   MISSING / UNIDENTIFIED   PERSON

Det. District_____ Sqd._____
Case No._____
M. P. Bur. No._____
Date of This Report_____

SURNAME	FIRST NAME, INITIALS		NATIVITY	SEX	AGE	COLOR
ADDRESS		LAST SEEN AT		DATE AND TIME SEEN		A.M. P.M.
PROBABLE DESTINATION		CAUSE OF ABSENCE		DATE AND TIME REPORTED		A.M P.M

PHYSICAL NOTE PECULIARITIES	CLOTHING—GIVE COLOR, FABRIC, STYLE, LABEL, WHERE POSSIBLE	STRIKE OUT IRRELEVANT WORDS	MISCELLANEOUS INFORMATION	
HEIGHT FT. IN.	HEADGEAR		OCCUPATION OR SCHOOL	
WEIGHT	OVER OR TOP COAT		EVER FINGERPRINTED? WHERE AND WHEN?	
BUILD	SUIT OR DRESS			
COMPLEXION	JACKET OR SWEATER		LAUNDRY MARKS	DRY CLEANER MARKS
HAIR	TROUSERS OR SKIRT		PHOTO RECEIVED	PREVIOUSLY MISSING?
EYES	SHIRT OR BLOUSE	VEST	PUBLICITY DESIRED?	SOCIAL SECURITY NO.
GLASSES, TYPE	TIE OR FUR PIECE	SCARF	PRELIMINARY INVESTIGATION	
MUSTACHE–BEARD	HOSE	GLOVES	DESK OFFICER	
TEETH	SHOES		TELEGRAPH BUREAU	
	HANDBAG		BUREAU OF INFORMATION	
SCARS	LUGGAGE		OTHERS	
	JEWELRY WORN			
DEFORMITIES				
	MONEY CARRIED		NOTIFICATION TO MISSING PERSONS BUR. BY	
TATTOO MARKS	CHARACTERISTICS, HABITS, MANNERISMS		RECEIVED AT MISSING PERSONS BUREAU BY	
			ASSIGNED	SQUAD
CONDITION PHYSICAL MENTAL			ASSIGNED	M. P BUR
REPORTED BY		ADDRESS	TELEPHONE NO.	RELATIONSHIP
REMARKS				

_____ Signature of Assigned Detective.   D.D.13   _____ Commanding Officer

If a person is reported missing from his proper surroundings by his friends or relatives, the Bureau of Missing Persons of the Police Department is given the duty of locating the absent individual and determining whether he is alive or dead. The detective assigned obtains a description of the missing person from relatives, as to sex, age, race, height, weight and other distinguishing features, and especially notes the time, place and circumstances under which he was last seen. Attempts are made to trace his movements and at the same time a watch is kept on all nameless individuals admitted to hospitals and on all unidentified bodies brought to city mortuaries. Many of the people reported missing are finally located by the investigations of the Bureau.

Cases of amnesia occasionally confront the police as a problem in identity and may be difficult to solve. The victim is often unable to furnish his name or give clues which would connect him with his former life. Unless he is recognized by a friend or found to correspond to the description of a person reported missing, his identity may be hard to discover.

Other organizations beside police departments compile similar identification charts, as, for example, the Federal Bureau of Identification, the Army and Navy of the United States, the Coast Guard, the Federal, State, and Municipal Civil Service. Some organizations employ systems in which the method of identification is applied to a special purpose. Thus many maternity hospitals take the footprints of all infants born under their auspices in order to avoid the error of assigning the wrong infant to the mother. In the newborn infant the footprint can be used as a reliable means of identification though later in life it is less satisfactory than fingerprints.

The question has often arisen whether or not a governmental bureau of identification should be established in which the charts of the entire population would be filed. The Federal Bureau of Investigation has a civilian fingerprint file in which any person in the United States is privileged to put his fingerprints on record, but as this is voluntary the file contains only a fraction of the people. It is not the intention of the authors to discuss the practicability of establishing an identification bureau of nation-wide scope, as that is a project for the future. If it happened to be in existence, however, it would offer advantages in determining the identity of individuals who are classified as unknown or who travel under a false name.

IDENTIFICATION OF THE DEAD

It is necessary for the police and medical examiner to determine the identity of all dead persons who are found in their jurisdiction, and the procedure for establishing identification is pursued in all cases in which the name of the body is not known. Occasionally this routine investigation is carried out even when the dead individual has a name, especially when his remains are unclaimed, because he may have been passing himself off under an alias.

Police Investigation. When an unknown body is found in New York City, it is searched by the police department to see if the clothing contains letters, bank books or other documents which may give a clue to the name and address of the individual. In many instances the personal belongings indicate the identity of the deceased. Then steps are taken to notify the relatives and friends of his death so that someone can view the body and identify it. If the identification is made without hesitation by individuals who satisfy the police of their responsibility, it is accepted and the name duly entered on the records.

If this preliminary search is fruitless the remains are sent to the city mortuary where a police officer, attached to the Bureau of Missing Persons, examines the clothing and the body, takes measurements of its height and weight, and notes the apparent age, sex, color of the skin, dental pattern, fractures, scars, missing parts and other distinguishing marks. In addition, fingerprints are taken of all fingers on both hands and sent to the Headquarters Division of the Police Department and in certain instances to other jurisdictions for comparison with their files. If these methods fail to establish an identification in two weeks, the corpse is photographed, front view and side view, and the photographs are put in the files. They are preserved for reference in the event that relatives of the deceased might come forward at some future time, searching for him as a missing person. After these precautions are taken, the body is interred in the city cemetery. If an identification is made subsequently, the remains can be reclaimed by the relatives and buried elsewhere. This same procedure is also carried out on unclaimed bodies which have a name, before their burial in the city cemetery, in order to avoid error if a claim should be made for them later.

Medical Examiner Investigation. The medical examiner is concerned with the proper identification of unknown dead persons because all bodies of this type come under his jurisdiction. He is responsible for their correct identification, and his own examination should parallel and supplement the work of the police officer from the Missing Persons Bureau. Accordingly, before the performance of an autopsy the medical examiner makes a routine examination of the remains in which he carefully notes and describes physical characteristics and special features which might be valuable in identifying the body.

The examination must be carried out according to a systematic plan, and the first part should be devoted to indicating the general type of the body. The important points are: the race; the sex; the apparent age as estimated from the general appearance of the body; the height measured from the bottom of the heels to the top of the crown; the weight of the nude body measured on the scale; the natural hue of the skin as determined by the race of the individual; a brief description of the stature mentioning specifically the size and length of the bones, the state of the muscles and the state of the nutrition.

The *height and weight* of dead infants, children and adolescents are important as part of the data which will enable the examiner to estimate the age of the body; but in order to avoid error they must be correlated with other observations such as the stage of development in the teeth and the presence or absence of ossification centers in the bones. The size of different individuals varies so much during growth, especially after the first postnatal year, that a reliable table of heights and weights is difficult to compile. At birth the average full-term infant is 20 inches in height and weighs about six to seven and a half pounds. According to Sydney Smith, the infant gains about a pound a month during the first year, and its height at the end of the year is about 29½ inches. In Table 3-1, the figures adapted from Sydney Smith represent the increase in height and weight from 1 to 18 years in males. The corresponding measurements for females are slightly smaller.

In Table 3-1, the figures compiled by Bakwin and Bakwin give the average heights and weights of infants and older children as a result of measurements made on a large number of individuals in New York City. In male infants at the end of the first 12 months, the average height is 30¾ inches and the average weight is 23¾ pounds. The corresponding measurements for female infants are slightly smaller. In older children, the average heights for boys and girls show insignificant differences up to 14 years, at which age the average for boys is 66 inches and for girls, 64 inches. Up to 11 years the weight averages for both sexes do not differ greatly, but from 11 to 14 years inclusive the average weight of girls exceeds that of boys. The height and weight averages for both infants and older children are greater than those compiled by Sydney Smith. Bakwin and Bakwin state that their tables, prepared from data on children who were receiving the best available care, apply to white children.

Table 3-1. Average Heights and Weights in Older Children (Males)

	ADAPTED FROM SYDNEY SMITH		ADAPTED FROM BAKWIN AND BAKWIN *	
Age (years)	Height (inches)	Weight (lbs.)	Height (inches)	Weight (lbs.)
1	29½	18½	30¼	23¾
2	32½	32½	35	29½
3	35	34	40	33½
4	37	36	42½	38½
5	40	40	45	42
6	43	44½	47	49
7	46	49¾	50	55
8	47	55	52½	62
9	49¾	60½	54½	70
10	51¾	67½	56½	76
11	53½	72	58½	83
12	55	76¾	60	90
13	57	82½	63	98
14	59¼	92	66	115
15	62¼	102		
16	64¼	119		
17	66½	131		
18	67	137		

* According to Bakwin and Bakwin the average heights and weights for girls from 11 to 14 years are as follows: 11 years, height 59 inches, weight 86 pounds; 12 years, height 61 inches, weight 96 pounds; 13 years, height 63 inches, weight 106 pounds; 14 years, height 64 inches, weight 117 pounds.

These measurement data are principally useful as an indication of the general rate of growth in infants and older children and must be applied with considerable caution in the solution of a specific problem which may confront the examiner.

The *hair* on different parts of the body should be carefully described. On the scalp the significant qualities are its abundance, texture, length, distribution, whether kinky, curly or straight, degree of baldness, whether uncut or recently barbered, color, presence or absence of gray hairs, whether dyed or bleached and any other noteworthy characteristics. The color, type and abundance of hair growth at the eyebrows, eyelashes, and nasal and ear orifices should be mentioned. On the lips, chin and jaws, the distribution of the hair growth should be described and its type, color, degree of coarseness and profusion noted, and a record made of whether the face is clean shaven, unshaven or what combination of mustache and beard is present. The hairs on the trunk, extremities, axillae and pubis should receive the same attention, especially in regard to sparsity or profusion, distribution and color. The hair characteristics will be described in greater length in another chapter.

The *eyes* must be examined and the color of the irides determined. Any abnormalities such as absence of the eyeball, glass eyes, deformities of the eyeball, opacities of the cornea and lens must be recorded.

The *nose, mouth, ears and chin* should receive a brief description, though their characters will be demonstrated more satisfactorily in photographs. Scars on the face are important for identification and should be measured and described accurately. The lobes of the ears, especially in females, should be examined closely for the small perforations which are made for earrings.

Description of the *teeth* is important and under certain conditions may be used as a means of identification if the sex, race, age, height, weight and general appear-

ance of the individual sought corresponds to that of the body which is being examined. If the teeth of the unknown corpse show the result of such dental operations
as extractions, fitting of dentures, permanent bridge work, fitting of crowns and
filling of cavities, they will present a set of artificial but individual characteristics. If
the charts of the operating dentist are available they can be compared with the teeth
of the deceased and the proposed identification disproved or established by the results of this comparison. The medical examiner should note all missing teeth, record
all dental work and describe such findings as irregularity of the teeth, all unfilled
cavities, abnormalities and pigmentation of the enamel, abnormalities of the gums
and other features worthy of mention. A convenient method of graphically register-
ing such examinations is by the use of a dental diagram. In a few cases a postmortem
roentgen ray photograph of the jaws is desirable if it is important to show conditions
deep in the bones as, for example, alveolar abscesses or unerupted teeth. Changes
which occur in the teeth during infancy and childhood and are valuable for indicating age will be discussed later.

Old *amputations,* old *fractures* and *deformities of the bones* either from injuries
or disease should be carefully described. The best way of recording such lesions is
by an ordinary photograph or by a roentgen ray photograph which can often demonstrate the true nature of the lesion more conveniently than actual dissection. In the
bodies of infants, children and adolescents the roentgen ray photograph will bring
out the centers of ossification, the presence or absence of fusion between adjacent
segments, or other processes which might give a clue to the age of the individual. In
an elderly person they might demonstrate the senile osteoporosis and the various
sclerotic changes due to age. In addition such pictures have the advantage of furnishing a permanent record of the case. The changes in the bones which are important for determining the age will be discussed at greater length on pages 42-46.

Abnormal conditions on the skin must be described. Among these may be mentioned pigmentations like argyria and jaundice, eruptions like psoriasis or acne, or
small nodules such as birth marks, angiomas, warts, wens, pigmented moles and
similar growths. The nodules may be quite important if they occur on the face or
other part of the body where they would intrude themselves on the notice of friends
or relatives.

Tattoo marks are designs imprinted in the skin by a needle which carries in such
dyes as cinnabar, indigo, Prussian blue, cobalt and India ink. The technic varies,
but the most permanent pictures are made when the dye is carried into the dermis.
Tattoo marks may serve to identify an individual, especially in cases in which he has
had his name or initials tattooed on the skin. Most of the marks are found on the
arms and forearms but may be present on other parts of the body (Fig. 3-3). Tattoo
marks fade with age and occasionally disappear in periods varying from 30 to 60
years. Some of the more superficial marks can be removed by corrosives, but usually
a scar remains after any such attempt.

The *feet and hands* deserve attention especially in regard to callus formations,
old amputations of the digits, deformities of the nails and other lesions due to injuries and disease. The character of calluses on the hands may furnish a clue to
the occupation of the deceased.

It is important occasionally to consider the *scars* on a body in connection with
identification, especially if they are the result of old injuries. The following facts
in connection with their formation are worthy of note:

If the original wound was a clean-cut incision, it may heal rapidly by primary intention without leaving any obviously visible scar on the skin. On the other hand if healing is secondary and slow with the formation of much granulation tissue, a scar will be formed. The extent and permanence of the scar will depend to a great degree on the amount of granulation tissue originally present during healing. After healing has taken place the color of the cicatrix is at first red because of the number of blood vessels in it, but during the next four to six weeks these vessels shrink and the scar becomes pale. After this the color is at first slightly brown, but in the course of a few months or years the scar becomes firm, white and glistening. The changes

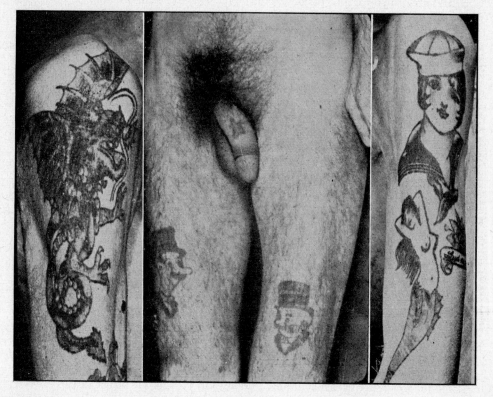

Fig. 3-3. Bizarre and Erotic Tattoos.

which occur after healing are too variable in their development to serve as criteria for estimating the age of the lesion.

Scars may be characteristic of the type of injury which produced them. The scars of bullet wounds, for example, are circular depressions in the skin slightly smaller than the original hole. It is important from the standpoint of differential diagnosis to find an exit scar or the internal scar of an old bullet tract or an encapsulated bullet. Stab wounds due to a knife blade leave ovoid or elliptical scars, some of which are depressed below the level of the skin while others are elevated because of keloid formation. If the original penetration is caused by the blade of an ice pick, the resulting scar will be small and circular.

Incised wounds may cause long tape-like scars, more or less depressed below the surface of the skin, and their probable origin can be indicated only by their location, direction and extent. Old wounds of homicidal and suicidal attempts usually leave scars on the face, neck and extremities, and less often on other parts of the body.

Attempted suicidal cuts of the throat may heal as deeply depressed horizontal cicatrices on the front part of the neck, firmly attached to the larynx. The scars due to old operations occur at the customary sites for these operations, and often show dot-like suture scars in pairs juxtaposed at regular intervals along their length so that they are easily recognized.

Severe lacerations of the skin due to blunt force leave large depressed irregular scars. Some of these are associated with healed fractures and are attached firmly to the bone.

In cases of burns, if the original lesion was a blister, it may persist after healing as a flat white scar. If the burn was associated with loss of tissue, a broad and wrinkled cicatrix with a tendency to contraction and distortion is produced. A hyperplastic growth known as a keloid may occur in the scar and form a large mass, especially in the Negro race. Similar scars are produced by severe burns from corrosive chemicals.

The authors have also seen wrinkled cicatrices of the deep burn type covered by skin epithelium which developed over huge decubital ulcers of the sacral regions in two cases of stab wounds partially severing the dorsal spinal cord.

Vaccination scars are circular, flat, slightly pitted scars which are located usually on the outer surface of the arm or thigh. Multiple vaccination scars are apt to be encountered on persons born in European countries.

Contusions and abrasions usually heal without leaving scars unless they are large and become infected.

The hypodermic scars of drug addicts are circular and pitted like deep vaccination marks and are the result of small abscesses caused by the needle injection. Many of them are colored blue or green as a result of the introduction into the subcutaneous tissues of soot or other substances with the narcotic solution which has usually come out of a dirty spoon or syringe. They may be found in large numbers over the thighs, arms, forearms and lower abdomen. Similar pigmented linear scars are observed over the superficial veins in the antecubital fossae and the anterior surface of the forearm in drug addicts who inject the narcotic solution directly into the veins (Fig. 34-2).

Many skin diseases like acne, smallpox, syphilis and others may leave multiple scars on the skin which are easily identified.

Criteria of Identification. The medical examiner and the detective from the Bureau of Missing Persons between them compile the following data suitable for identification: the description of the clothing, personal property and personal characteristics of the deceased; the fingerprints and the routine photographs. The physical features are valuable as confirmatory signs but cannot be accepted as conclusive unless substantiated by other evidence. The fingerprints are certain criteria of identification only if the deceased has his prints on file somewhere so that a comparison can be made. The teeth may help to identify an individual, especially in cases in which dental work is present and the corresponding dental charts are available. The photographs are valuable confirmatory evidence, but unless used with care may lead to error. Their chief use is to serve as a convenient reference file to be consulted by people who visit the city mortuary seeking missing relatives.

The unreliability of photographs as a means of identification was illustrated by a woman who visited the Bureau of Missing Persons at the city mortuary and looked over the photographs of unnamed or unclaimed dead individuals in hopes of finding her estranged husband whom she had not seen for several years. She claimed that one set of photographs represented her husband

and persisted in her identification even when it was pointed out that the deceased in the pictures was known by a different name and had initials of that name tattooed on his right forearm. All doubts were eventually resolved when her real husband died and was duly identified under his proper name. Her error was explainable by the fact that the two men had similar features, were clean shaven and had the same kind of hair growth and bald spot on the scalp.

Occasionally people claim the wrong body either mistakenly or rarely with the deliberate purpose of committing fraud. To avoid all the confusion and waste of time which must follow such a false identification, it is best that the medical examiner or the detective question the claimants at length before they are shown the body and elicit from them such pertinent information as their relationship to the person whom they are seeking, when and where he was last seen alive, in what condition his affairs were and similar facts. The claimants should describe the clothing and person of the missing individual to the best of their ability and if possible furnish a photograph of their relative or friend for the purposes of comparison. Occasionally the description of body characteristics and clothing is published in the newspapers or broadcast by the Bureau of Missing Persons, and a person bent on fraud may have obtained the essential facts about the description from the press or radio. Questioning of the claimants may elicit facts which indicate an irreconcilable discrepancy between the description given by them and the true characterization of the body. If there is any chance that the identification is correct, the remains should be viewed and the different items checked in detail. In doubtful cases the fingerprints and dental records of the deceased may help in solving the problem, if there are any records to which they may be compared. In any event the identification should not be accepted if there is any doubt as to its genuineness.

The Corpus Delicti. If death was the result of criminal violence, the law requires other formalities of identification to be observed in addition to the routine investigation, in order to prove the corpus delicti or the body of evidence which indicates the crime of homicide. The term includes not only the body of the victim, though that is the most essential part of the evidence, but also any other facts which are conclusive of death by foul play. Any object or part of a weapon found in the body and responsible for death is a part of the corpus delicti, as for example a bullet or a broken knife blade. Clothing worn by the deceased at the time that the final injury occurred is also a part of the corpus delicti if it shows marks caused by the lethal weapons. Drawings or photographs of the deceased showing the fatal injuries belong in the same category. The medical examiner finding such evidence should mark it for identification in order that he may introduce it in court if necessary.

The corpus delicti can be proved if the medical examiner and other witnesses establish the fact that a certain individual is dead, that death was the result of criminal violence and that it occurred at a certain place and time under certain circumstances. Unless there is convincing proof of these points, the case against the accused cannot be substantiated. The fact of death and the cause of death are part of the direct testimony of the physician, from knowledge which he has gained from the autopsy. The identity of the deceased is established by a relative or close friend who sees the remains in the presence of the medical examiner and states that the body is that of a certain person. The connection with the scene and the circumstances of death are obtained by having a police officer identify the corpse as that of the same person he saw at a certain place and time, under the given circumstances. In this way the evidence is prepared which establishes the principal part of the corpus delicti, namely, the identity of the dead body and the fact that death was the result of violence, inflicted in a certain way at a certain time and place. The actual circumstances which occurred at the time of the crime must be furnished by other witnesses.

The medical examiner during his testimony at a homicide trial must mention the various identifications made to him and then proceed to give the results of the autopsy. During his testimony he must state what materials he retained for toxicologic examination and give the date and place at which he identified them to the toxicologists, if it is at all necessary to introduce the toxicologic examination as evidence (pages 704 and 705). The bullets, knife blades or any part of a blunt

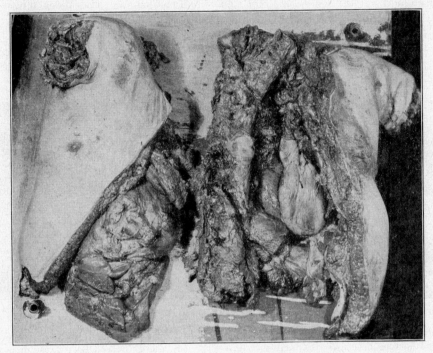

Fig. 3-4. Unidentified Dismembered Human Remains.

Halves of upper part of torso found in sewer manhole. The left half contains the heart. Cause of death not determinable.

instrument found in the body are identified by the medical examiner and are admitted among the exhibits connected with the corpus delicti. The clothing of the deceased, if previously examined by the witness and properly marked for identification, can be also included in the evidence. In the same way drawings and photographs can be introduced as part of the corpus delicti if they are identified by the person who prepared them.

Identification of Unrecognizable Remains. The hardest problem of identification occurs when the body is presented in such a state that it is not recognizable. This is seen in cases of: (1) extensive postmortem decomposition, especially in bodies long submerged; (2) extensive burning, as in a conflagration or furnace, or as in chemical destruction of the body by strong acids or alkalis; (3) mutilation of the body either by a human assailant or by such fortuitous means as bomb explosions, subway trains, machinery or postmortem ravages of animals.

The identification may be facilitated by the nature of the surroundings and the circumstances under which the body was found. Thus if the remains were found in a room or house known to be occupied by a certain individual and the personal property and general characteristics of the corpse corresponded with that person, there would be a strong presumption of identity from these facts alone. In other cases an individual of a certain type may be reported missing by his relatives and if a body is found which answers to the same description, the detectives are at least given a suggestion as to which line of investigation they should pursue. Many of these remains, regardless of how unpromising they may seem as subjects for identification, are nevertheless traced to their proper identity because there was some clue which could be used as a guide to the right solution. There are other cases, however, in which the body fragments are not characteristic and since the circumstances do not furnish any revealing clues, an identification cannot be made. Figures 3-4 and 3-5 are illustrations of two cases in which the dismembered, mutilated remains were not identified and the cause of death not determinable.

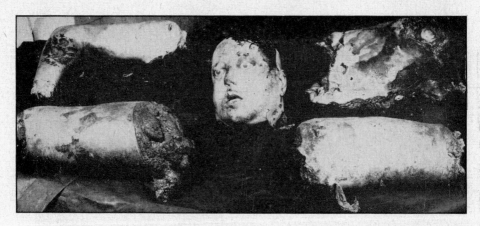

Fig. 3-5. Unidentified Human Remains Dismembered Prior to Disposal in Water.

Head, thighs, right shoulder, right arm and tattooed forearm found within a 24 hour period floating in various parts of Upper New York Bay and Gravesend Bay. Cause of death not determinable. Compare with Figure 3-8.

BODIES CHANGED BY POSTMORTEM DECOMPOSITION. Gaseous decomposition causes a marked discoloration of the skin and swelling of the body from the accumulation of gas in the tissues and cavities, so that the natural likeness is distorted. In addition, if the body is exposed in the air, it may be eaten by insects or various animals; and if it is in the water, it may be devoured by marine animals, lose flesh from the macerating action and friction of the water or be dismembered by the action of propellers on steamboats. While such remains are unrecognizable as far as their physical appearance is concerned, often clues are found which solve the problem of identification satisfactorily. In one case the body had reached the state of decomposition at which the skin of the palmar surfaces could be detached, and fingerprints taken from the shells of finger skin as illustrated in Figure 3-6 were clear enough to identify the body. In another instance the corpse had been submerged for a long time and had lost much of its flesh, but its apparent age and height corresponded with that of a certain person who had been drowned in those waters some months previously; the aid of the missing man's dentist was sought and a comparison of his dental records with the plates and fillings in the teeth of the body showed an exact correspondence, thus establishing identity.

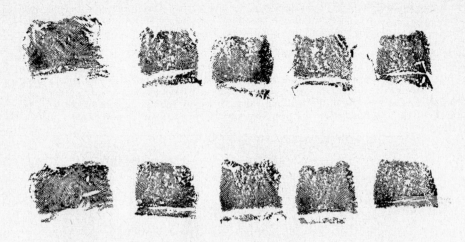

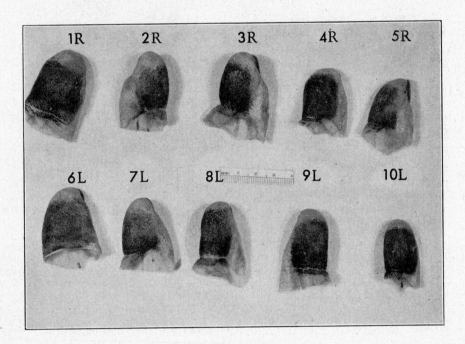

Fig. 3-6. Identification of Decomposed Drowned Body by Fingerprints.

Top. Fingerprints obtained with shells of skin shown below. Upper row, right hand; lower row, left hand. From left to right: thumb, index finger, middle finger, ring finger, little finger.

Bottom. Shells of macerated skin detached from fingers of an unrecognizable decomposed, drowned body from which prints shown above were made. The body illustrated in Figures 4-25 through 27 was also identified in this way. (Preparation of finger tips and prints by Detective John Aievoli, Missing Persons Bureau, Police Dept., City of New York.)

A similar case occurred in which a female body was recovered from the water in such an advanced state of decomposition that it was unrecognizable; it was identified by a peculiar irregularity of the upper teeth and the dental work. These corresponded with the dental chart of a woman known to have committed suicide about 11 months previously. Figure 3-7 shows a photograph of the deceased taken during life and another taken of the body after it had been submerged for 11 months.

Another case was that of a female body recovered from the waters around New York City. A wire was twisted around the neck, and the body had been so long submerged that most of the flesh was removed from the face and hands. Strangely enough the lobe of the left ear was comparatively intact and showed a depressed scar of pin-sized caliber on the outer surface but

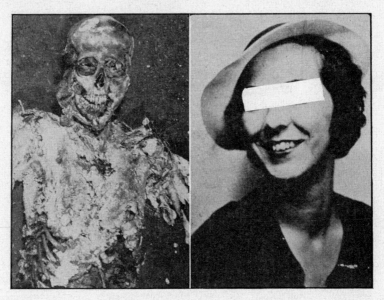

Fig. 3-7. Identification after Advanced Decomposition from Prolonged Submersion.

Disappearance of distal parts of extremities and soft tissue from head and torso of body submerged in North River for 11 months after suicidal drowning. Identification by dental chart. Irregularity of upper incisor teeth evident in photographs of cadaver and of deceased during life.

no mark on the inner surface. The body was suspected of being that of a woman who had been murdered about six months previously. The identification was made when relatives of the deceased appeared, for they described the height and missing teeth of the remains accurately and in addition mentioned the small scar on the lobe of the left ear. This was explained as an attempt to pierce that ear for earrings in childhood; because of the pain the deceased stopped the operation before it was completed, hence the peculiar mark on the ear.

BODIES DAMAGED BY FIRE OR CORROSIVE CHEMICALS. Bodies burned in a conflagration and converted into an unrecognizable carbonaceous mass are often identified by the fact that the fire occurred in their own home, and also by such additional help as the postmortem examination of the remains can reveal. In tenement conflagrations in New York City, especially when a number of persons perish, the fire department is careful to note on the identification tag the floor and room in which the body was found. By a careful examination of these bodies and a patient check of their characteristics with the different claimants, it is possible to identify most of them correctly.

Rarely individuals who perpetrate a homicide may dispose of the body by thrusting it into a furnace in toto or in segments after dismembering it piecemeal. In some of the cases the fire may consume practically everything except a few bones and teeth which might be difficult to use for identification unless characteristic dental work is present. The difficulty of establishing the corpus delicti under such circumstances is sometimes not easily surmountable.

Dr. Charles H. Hochman and the late Dr. Louis A. Lefkowitz, medical examiners in the borough of the Bronx, New York City, investigated a crime of this type in which the body of a strangled 10 year old girl was burned in a furnace by her assailant who was the janitor of the building where the crime occurred. All that remained were five barrels of ashes which were carefully sifted by the medical examiners and police and found to contain, in addition to a metal belt buckle belonging to the victim, about 100 fragments of incinerated bone and teeth. The seven identifiable tooth fragments were submitted by the district attorney to the late Dr. Moses Diamond, a dentist at the Columbia University Dental College, who established that the fragments were parts of human permanent incisor, cuspid, premolar and first molar teeth, from the same person and consistent with the victim's age of 10 years, 4 months. In addition the maxillary first premolar tooth revealed a rare hereditary groove on the lingual side of its buccal root identical with that on a corresponding tooth of the mother. The findings were sufficient to identify the scant incinerated remains in the ashes as those of the slain girl. The defendant, who had confessed to the crime, was convicted of murder in the first degree. The validity of the corpus delicti was upheld by the New York State Court of Appeals.

The corrosive acids and alkalis have been used even more rarely for the purpose of destroying the remains after a homicide. They remove the soft parts rapidly and eventually may destroy the bones and teeth. Unless such insoluble objects as gold fillings in the teeth or gold jewelry were present on the body at the time of the destruction, a satisfactory identification would be difficult.

BODIES DAMAGED BY MUTILATION. Mutilation of the body may occur in several ways. It may be caused by the ravages of animals post mortem, or by dismemberment by moving vehicles like subway trains or by machinery, or by bomb explosions which may obliterate the individual except for a few tags of human flesh. The perpetrator of a crime sometimes resorts to mutilation in order to render the remains unrecognizable or divides the body into segments so that it can be disposed of more readily. This has even been done in nonhomicidal cases in which the deceased died of natural causes or of noncriminal violence. Fearful that he would be suspected of murder or believing in his own mind that he had caused the death by felonious means, the mutilator dismembered the body to dispose of it clandestinely and so avoid the notice of the police and other authorities.

One case seen by the authors was a minor example of mutilation intended to conceal the identity of the victim. A trunk evidently of recent purchase was brought into a Railway Express office and booked for a distant city. The agent noted at the time that it was relatively heavy for its size, but became interested enough to summon the police only when he saw a red fluid seeping from one of its corners. The detectives opened it to find the body of a small man with red hair and well preserved features carefully folded up inside. The autopsy disclosed that the victim had died of a bullet wound of the skull and brain; in addition, the palmar surface of each finger tip had been painstakingly cut away and a skin area two inches square, presumably the site of a tattoo mark, had been dissected from the right forearm. The findings suggested that the deceased had a criminal record which was confirmed and the identification made by consulting the photographic files of the police department. In the meantime the trunk was traced to the store where it had been purchased and eventually the assailant was located and apprehended.

Another case seen by the authors was a mutilation with the intent to cut the body into segments of such size that it would be conveniently disposed of in various parts of the city. The torso was discovered partly immersed in a swamp in Long Island City, minus its legs which had been amputated at the hips but with head, neck, chest, abdomen and arms intact. The body was that of a young white woman in the early twenties with fair skin, lusterless blond hair, a distinct down on her cheeks and ears pierced for earrings. Her height was estimated at about 5 feet, 2 inches. The legs were discovered later in another part of New York City and could be fitted to the torso. This body was never identified, but not for want of claimants, for five separate men insisted that the remains were those of their wives who had deserted them some time before. All of the women in question were found to be very much alive. In this case all the clues and examinations were in vain because they failed to direct the investigation toward a likely identification.

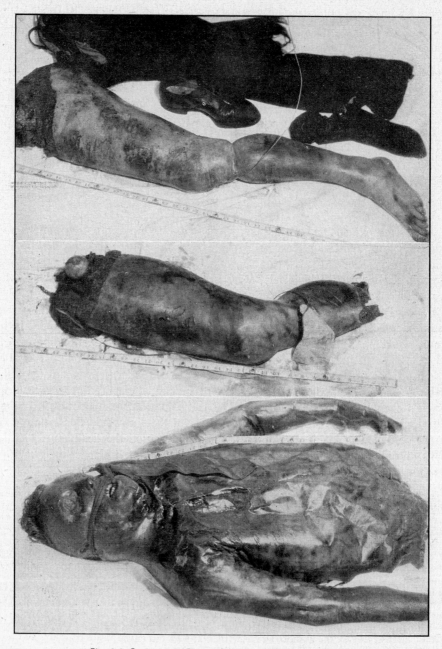

Fig. 3-8. Postmortem Dismemberment by Propeller Blades.

Torso and extremities found floating several miles apart in Hudson and East Rivers. Identification by clothing on left lower extremity. Deceased committed suicide by jumping off ferry boat one week before body parts were found. Identification clarified circumstances of death and dismemberment.

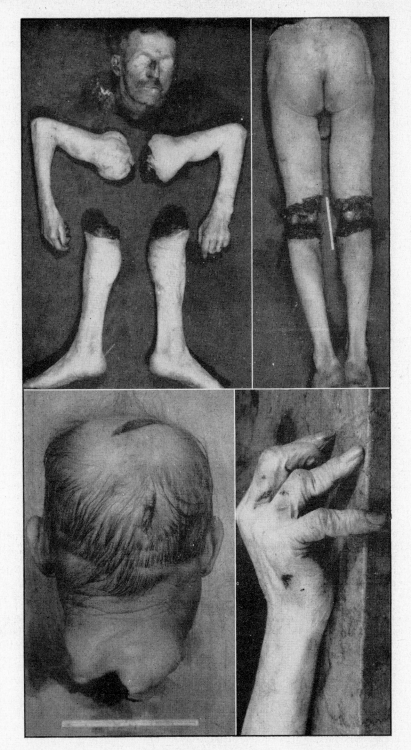

Fig. 3-9. Dismemberment after Homicide.

The four extremities were found in a wooden box; the head, wrapped in paper, was recovered nearby and later the hips and thighs in one piece. Note blunt weapon defense wounds on right hand and scalp wounds; the skull and larynx were found fractured.

Cases of mutilation should always be studied from the standpoint of how the body was sectioned and whether the operator displayed any knowledge of anatomy in dividing it into segments. He might, for example, cut through the joints with a knife or he might saw through bones or chop through them with a cleaver. The physician examining such remains should be cautious about expressing his opinion concerning the skill or lack of skill of the operator, especially if postmortem decomposition is present. If the remains are found floating in a body of water traversed by steamships, the possibility should be considered that the mutilation was caused by the action of a propeller and not by a human assailant. In propeller injuries the extremities and members are cut off at one stroke with much shattering of bones, or the body is mangled by repeated blows of the blades. The systematic dismemberment such as would be the case if the sectioning was done by a human assailant is generally absent. There are cases, however, in which the mechanical postmortem dismemberment of a submerged body is difficult to distinguish from that performed by a human agent.

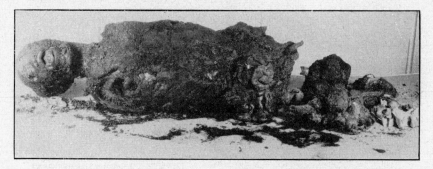

Fig. 3-10. Disposal of Body after Homicide by Dismemberment and Incineration.

Note charred segments of thigh, extensive incineration of head and dismembered torso. Depressed comminuted skull fracture found in occipital region. Absence of carbon monoxide from blood confirmed that death occurred before body was burned. Identification by teeth. Perpetrator confessed bludgeoning victim to death and dismembering body in his home, then incinerating parts in bonfire in vacant lot.

The case illustrated in Figure 3-8 is an example of postmortem dismemberment probably produced by propeller blades. The deceased was observed to jump from a ferryboat into the Hudson River obviously with suicidal intent. One week later the torso, swollen from decomposition, was removed from the same river; and shortly after this the lower extremities, also decomposed, were found several miles away, one in the East River, the other in the Hudson. The clothing on the left lower extremity yielded laundry and cleaning marks which led to the identification of the body and the solution of the case.

Figure 3-9 illustrates the dismemberment of a body by the perpetrator of a homicide. The four extremities were the first recovered, then the head and finally the hips and thighs; the upper part of the trunk was never found. The symmetric and systematic division of the remains into sections indicates that the work was done by a human operator with instruments. The identity of the deceased was finally established from the head. Further examination revealed that death was caused by fractures of the skull and larynx, and the presence of scalp lacerations and blunt force defense injuries on the right hand pointed to a homicidal assault.

The body shown in Figure 3-10 was partially incinerated in a bonfire in a vacant lot. It was also dismembered and autopsy revealed that death had resulted from a depressed skull fracture. Identification was established by examination of the teeth. The perpetrator confessed to the killing, dismemberment and incineration of the body.

The Ruxton case in Scotland, reported by Glaister and Brash in 1937, is a good example of identifications made on two mutilated bodies of persons slain in the same homicide. The perpetrator of the crime killed his wife and a maid servant, dismembered the bodies and even stripped the skin from the faces to render them unrecognizable. The separate segments of the two bodies were scattered in various places around the town of Moffat in order to complicate the researches of the police. A number of the pieces were collected, however, including the two skulls, and all were painstakingly joined in an attempt at reconstruction. Though many parts were missing, enough were found to enable the investigators to determine the heights and the physical statures of the two victims. One was a woman with large bones and pronounced features, the other was smaller and had less prominent features. Fortunately the police found photographs of both victims taken during life. The skull

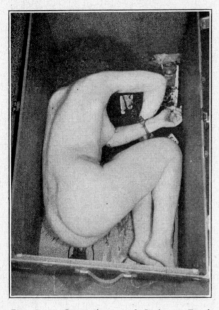

Fig. 3-11. Concealment of Body in Trunk after Murder.

After having been handcuffed and stabbed to death by husband, body of deceased was placed in trunk in bedroom. Crime was discovered by lover who narrowly escaped similar fate at hands of husband.

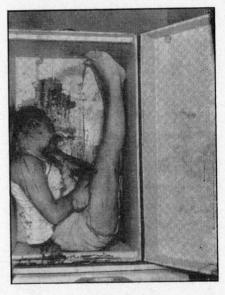

Fig. 3-12. Disposal of Body in Trunk after Murder.

Body of victim placed in trunk which was dumped in street. Death from blunt weapon head injuries. Note ease with which limp body can be folded into trunk for disposal without dismemberment.

of each deceased was photographed in the same position as that assumed in the photographs of the living persons, and prints were made bringing all the pictures to the same scale. It was possible then to superimpose the skull onto the corresponding face and to demonstrate that the bony structure fitted into the contours of that particular head. The evidence was sufficient to establish the identity of the two women.

Attempts at Disposal of Unmutilated Bodies. Occasionally an attempt is made to conceal a homicide and dispose of the body without further mutilation or dismemberment by placing it inside a large trunk which can be disposed of in various ways. The trunk with the body may be stored in the basement of a house where it may not arouse interest until the odors of putrefaction become noticeable, or it may be carried off and dumped in some secluded area or shipped by express to some distant destination. If suspicions were not aroused, it would be easy to conceal a murdered body in a trunk, have it delivered into an outside state room on a passenger ship and dispose of it by dumping it through a conveniently located porthole into the ocean. It is remarkable how easily an adult body can be folded into an average size trunk if the adjustment is made prior to the onset of rigor mortis. In some cases which were discovered, identification of the body and determination of the cause of death were made without too much trouble. Examples of homicide in which the dead body was placed in a trunk for concealment are shown in Figures 3-11 and 3-12. Occasionally the body of a newborn infant in a case of infanticide or of a newborn fetus in a concealed stillbirth is disposed of by placing it in a small suitcase and depositing it in the parcel room of a public place like a railway station (page 601).

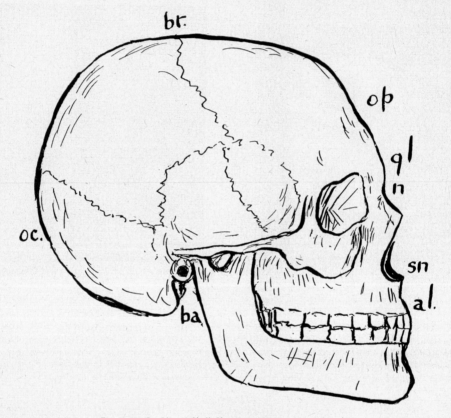

Fig. 3-13. Profile of Skull Showing Anatomic Landmarks.

al, alveolar process; ba, basion; br, bregma; gl, glabella; n, nasion; oc, occipital point; op, ophryon; sn, subnasal point.

Examination of Unidentifiable Remains. If the remains are of such a nature that a clue to their identity is not forthcoming, they should be examined with a view to determining the race, sex, age and probable height and weight of the person to whom they belong. The parts can be preserved by embalming and immersion in formalin.

RACE. If some of the skin and hair, especially the scalp hair, is well preserved it may be possible to distinguish the race of the individual. The white race has pale or slightly pigmented skin with straight to curled blond to dark brown hair, eyes of various shades of blue to dark brown, relatively hairy body and moderate development of the axillary sweat glands. The Chinese, American Indians, Japanese and similar peoples have a pigmented skin of yellowish brown to reddish brown, long coarse straight black hair, dark brown eyes, comparatively slight growth of body hair, and slight axillary sweat gland development. The Negro and allied races have dark brown skin, kinky black hair, dark brown eyes, comparatively slight growth of body hair and marked axillary sweat gland development. If the individual under consideration is hybrid, the determination of race may not be easy.

The best method of investigation in the event that only bones are present is to take different measurements of the skull and pelvis. The length, breadth, height and circumference of the cranial cavity are recorded; and the degree of projection of the jaws, the form of the nasal aperture and the form of the orbits are determined. The pelvic dimensions measured are those of the true pelvis.

Skull. The circumference of the cranium is the circumference of a horizontal plane passing through the ophryon and the occipital point (Fig. 3-13). The length of the cranium is measured between the glabella and the occipital point. The breadth is the greatest diameter across the skull above the mastoid bones. The height is the measurement from the basion to the bregma.

The *breadth index* is the proportion of the breadth as compared with the length,

or $\dfrac{\text{breadth of skull} \times 100}{\text{length of skull}}$

The *height index* is the proportion of the height as compared with the length,

or $\dfrac{\text{height of skull} \times 100}{\text{length of skull}}$

The *orbital index* is the length of the orbit as compared with its breadth, or

$\dfrac{\text{breadth of orbit} \times 100}{\text{length of orbit}}$

The *gnathic index* is the measurement from the basion to the nasal bones, multiplied by 100, divided by the measurement from the basion to the alveolar process.

The *nasal index* is the height of the nasal aperture as compared with its width,

or $\dfrac{\text{width of nasal aperture} \times 100}{\text{height}}$

Pelvis. The *pelvic index* is the anteroposterior diameter of the pelvis as compared with the transverse diameter.

Table 3-2. Anthropometric Table from Quain Compiled by Ewing

	CRANIAL CAPACITY	BREADTH INDEX	HEIGHT INDEX	ORBITAL INDEX	GNATHIC INDEX	NASAL INDEX	PELVIC INDEX
English	1,480 ml.	76 Meso-cephalic	71	88 Mesoseme	96 Ortho-gnathous	46 Lepto-rhine	80 Platy-pellic
Chinese	1,430 ml.	79 Meso-cephalic	75	90 Megaseme	99 Meso-gnathous	50 Meso-rhine	
Negro	1,350 ml.	73 Dolicho-cephalic	72		104 Pro-gnathous	55 Platy-rhine	93 Meso-pellic
Australian	1,300 ml.	71 Dolicho-cephalic	71	81 Microseme	104 Pro-gnathous	57 Platy-rhine	97 Dolicho-pellic

Table 3-2 is to be used as a guide to the typical characteristics of the skulls and pelves of the main subdivisions of the human race but should not be applied too literally when investigating a specific specimen, since the bones may belong to an atypical individual or a person of mixed blood. Of the bones, the skull presents the best criterion for distinguishing the races, while the pelvis is less reliable for this purpose.

A graphic and practical procedure is to articulate the skull with the lower jaw-bone and then cover them with modeling clay. It is possible at times to mold the outside layer into a fair likeness of the deceased, which may help to identify his race. This procedure is most efficiently employed when the modeler can be guided by a photograph of the suspected individual. If a reasonable likeness to the person in the photograph can be obtained from the moulage of the skull, at least a possibility of identity is established. Without some authentic representation of the deceased there would not be any assurance that the result of the modeling would bear any resemblance to the original person, for many features such as the curve of the nose, the shape of the ear and the amount of subcutaneous fat in the face, all of which are important in producing distinctive facial characters, cannot be determined from a mere inspection of the skull.

SEX. The sex of the individual can be identified if the sexual organs or the breasts are well preserved. The problem is more difficult if fragments of the body are present which are not particularly diagnostic. In general the female has less hair on the trunk, has more delicate extremities, more subcutaneous fat and less musculature. Her bones are smaller, lighter, with thinner shafts and relatively wider medullary spaces than the male. The cranial cavity is smaller and the bony ridges are less prominent; the lower jaw is narrower, the chin less projecting and the face as a whole smaller in proportion to the cranium than in the male. The female thorax is shorter and more rounded, the sternum is relatively shorter and the hands and feet are relatively smaller than in the male.

The pelves of the sexes, however, show more marked differences than any other bones. The ilia of the female are more nearly vertical, and the false pelvis is somewhat narrower than in the male pelvis. In the female the inlet of the true pelvis is ovoid, its breadth and capacity are greater, the height of the pelvis is less, the sacrum is broader and projects less into the opening; while in the male the opening is cordiform because of the projection of the sacral promontory into the inlet, the capacity of the true pelvis is less and the bones are thicker. In the female pelvis the depth of the symphysis pubis is less, the subpubic arch is wider and there is more space between the ischial tuberosities than in the male; in the female the greater sciatic notch has a gradual curve while in the male the curve is shorter; in the female the obturator foramen has a triangular shape and in the male the foramen is ovoid; the preauricular notch is deeper in the female but shallow or absent in the male pelvis.

Enough data may be obtained from the study of the bones to form an opinion as to the sex of the remains. In some cases, however, the evidence may not be complete enough to warrant a definite diagnosis.

AGE. It may be possible to estimate the age of a person from an examination of his remains even when much of the body is destroyed. This is accomplished by correlating all the available data in the case with conditions which are normally present in the individual at the different stages of life.

Changes occur in the skin and its appendages during growth and decline, but they are of such a nature that they are not useful as accurate criteria of age. During the period from infancy to the end of puberty the layers of the epidermis, dermis and subcutaneous fat increase in thickness and the sweat and sebaceous glands increase in size. Microscopically there is an increase in the size of the individual fat cells as well as an increase in their number. During adult life the changes are slight, except for atrophy of these different layers in old age and a loss of elasticity in the skin due to decrease of elastic fibers in the dermis. Mention should be made of the increased development of the sweat glands in the axilla, which are not present in infancy and childhood but appear during puberty about the time that the sexual organs are reaching maturity.

The changes in the scalp hairs may furnish a general indication of the age, but they cannot be relied upon as they present such great individual variations. The hairs during infancy and childhood gradually increase in size and amount of pigmentation up to the latter half of puberty; about the fourth decade the hair becomes gray through a gradual and progressive loss of pigment. This subject will be discussed more fully in Chapter 28.

The internal viscera gradually increase in size during the first 20 years of life but after maturity show little alteration until old age sets in, when they undergo a variable amount of atrophy. The changes in size are observable in the cellular constituents of the organs on microscopic examination, especially in the glandular organs or the muscular tissues. They are not, however, of any value in the determination of age inasmuch as they are affected by many other factors like malnutrition, chronic disease processes and similar conditions.

The male and female sexual organs undergo a rapid development and variation in structure at the time of puberty, manifested microscopically in the male by the appearance of spermatogenesis in the testes and in the female by changes in the breasts, ovaries and uterus occasioned by the onset of menstruation.

The aorta increases in caliber and in the thickness of its wall during the first two decades, and at maturity the average circumference of the ascending portion is from 5 to 6 cm. After this stage the aorta distends gradually until the corresponding measurement for middle age and senility is 7 to 9 cm., even in individuals whose heart and blood vessels are free of pathologic lesions. However, these changes are so variable and so modified in many persons by hypertension or arteriosclerotic changes in the vessel wall that they cannot be trusted as criteria for age determination.

The distribution of the red bone marrow is normally altered during childhood and adolescence. In the first six years of life all the bones contain red marrow, but in the seventh year fatty marrow makes its appearance and in the fourteenth year is visible to the naked eye. In adult life the flat bones such as the ribs, vertebrae, sternum, pelvis and skull contain red marrow, while in the long bones yellow fatty marrow has replaced the red, first in the shaft and then in the epiphyses. Such replacement takes place earlier in the distal bones of the extremities such as the tibia before it is fully developed in the proximal bones such as the femur. Of course if the individual is suffering from a severe chronic anemia or a leukemia which causes hyperplasia of the bone marrow, evaluation of the marrow distribution in relation to age is impossible.

The best criterion of age determination in infancy and childhood is the skeleton and in particular the centers of ossification in the various bones. This process follows a regular course in the body. In the second and third months of fetal life centers of ossification form in the shafts of the long bones of the extremities, the clavicle, lower jaw and vertebral column. At the time of birth the shafts of the long bones are ossified completely and there is enough development in the cranial, facial, spinal, pelvic and chest bones to support the body tissues. The process, however, is not complete, as many small tuberosities, bones and epiphyses receive their centers of ossification after birth. Thus in the first year after birth such centers appear at stated intervals in the tarsus and carpus and are convenient criteria for estimating the age. In adolescence the developing bone in the epiphyses fuses with the shaft of the long bones at different periods, and the presence or absence of cartilage between shaft and epiphysis may be helpful in determining how old the individual actually is.

TIME OF APPEARANCE AND FUSION OF OSSIFICATION CENTERS

The sequence of the growth and fusion of the ossification centers furnishes an important guide for the estimation of the age of a body. In this respect, it is more practical and less confusing to narrate systematically the chronologic development of each individual bone rather than to catalogue the changes in the entire skeleton for each separate year of its development. In the following description taken from *Spalteholz' Hand Atlas of Human Anatomy,* the periods expressed in weeks and months refer to prenatal development; the postnatal development of the bones is given in years.

SKULL BONES

Occipital Bone. Ossification centers or nuclei appear in the lower and upper squamous portions in the sixth and seventh weeks, in the basilar portion in the tenth week and in the lateral portions in the eighth week. At birth, the bone consists of four pieces; the squamous part unites with the lateral parts in the first to the fourth year; the lateral pieces with the basilar portion in the third to the sixth year.

Sphenoid Bone. This bone develops from seven pairs of nuclei which appear from the end of the second month to shortly after the end of the third month. At birth the bone consists of three parts: the centrally located body and lesser wings; and the greater wings, each of which is united with a pterygoid portion. These three parts grow together during the first year. At birth the sphenoidal sinus is pinhead in size; it begins to grow at the beginning of the fourth year and in the ninth to the tenth year has grown into the body of the sphenoid. The union of the basilar portion of the sphenoid and occipital bones occurs about the twentieth year.

Temporal Bones. The temporal bone at birth consists of three parts: the squamous, whose ossification center appeared at the end of the second month; the tympanic, whose center appeared at the middle of the third month; and petrous, whose ossification began in the fifth month. The petrous bone encloses the labyrinth in the sixth month. The upper end of the styloid process ossifies shortly before birth, the lower and shortly after birth; they unite in middle life. The tympanic ossicles ossify in the second half of the fifth month. The mastoid process of the temporal bone develops as an outgrowth from the squamous and the petrous portions and is not well developed until adult life. The mastoid cells appear at puberty.

Frontal Bone. A center of ossification appears on each side at the end of the second month. Frontal sinuses appear at the end of the first year and are completely developed at puberty. The two halves of the frontal bone unite after the third year.

Parietal Bones. Two centers of ossification develop in each at the end of the second month.

Ethmoid Bone. The center for the papyraceous portion appears at the end of the fifth month; that for the crista galli and perpendicular lamina at the end of the first year. Ossification is not complete until the sixteenth year.

Nasal Bones. Ossification centers appear at the end of the second month.

Palatine and Zygomatic Bones. Centers of ossification are developed in the eighth week.

Mandible. An ossification center for the ramus and body appears on each side in the seventh week. The two halves of the jaw unite in the first or second year.

Fontanelles. They are six in number and lie in the angles of the parietal bones. The anterior is the largest and closes after the first half of the second year. The other fontanelles, the posterior, the two sphenoidal and the two mastoidal, close during the first half year.

Hyoid Bone. There are five ossification centers; those for the body and greater horns appear at the end of fetal life; those for the lesser horns only after birth. The greater horns unite with the body in middle life.

BONES OF THE TRUNK

Vertebrae (in general). Each vertebra has three ossification centers, one for the body, and one for each half of the neural arch. The nuclei of the arches develop in the eighth week, the nucleus for the body soon after. At birth the three vertebral nuclei are separated by cartilage. The arch nuclei fuse in the first year. Bony union of the arch and body nuclei begins in the dorsal spine from the third to the sixth year. At puberty, there are thin epiphyses on the upper and lower surfaces of the body of each vertebra and also on the apices of the transverse and spinous processes. These do not fuse with the main nuclei until the twentieth year.

Atlas. Two symmetrical nuclei appear on either side in the eighth week for ossification of the posterior arch and lateral masses. They unite in the third to the fifth year. A nucleus appears in the anterior arch in the first year and fuses with the other two nuclei in the fifth to the ninth year.

Epistropheus (Axis). The lower part of the body and the two halves of the neural arch each receives a nucleus in the eighth week. A double nucleus which soon fuses appears in the upper part of the body and base of the dens (odontoid process) in the fourth to fifth month. This part of the dens unites with the body and the lateral parts in the fourth to the sixth year, and then the two latter fuse with each other. A special nucleus appears in the tip of the dens in the second year which unites with the main mass in the twelfth year. An epiphysis forms at the caudal end of the body. A small cartilaginous disk remains inside the bone at the junction of the dens and body until old age.

Seventh Cervical Vertebra. A special nucleus may appear in the second to the fifth month, in the ventral portion of the transverse process, which unites with the body after birth; it may not unite and then may give rise to a movable cervical rib.

Lumbar Vertebrae. The mammillary processes of the twelfth thoracic, the five lumbar and the first sacral vertebrae have special epiphysial nuclei which appear at puberty or later and fuse with the rest of the vertebra after the eighteenth year.

Sacrum. Like other vertebrae, each sacral vertebra develops from three main centers of ossification. The nuclei for the bodies of the first to the third appear at the end of the third month, for the fourth and fifth about the fifth to the eighth month. The lateral nuclei for the upper vertebrae appear in the fifth or the sixth month. Nuclei also appear on each side of the bodies of the first, second or third sacral vertebrae in the fifth to the seventh month forming the lateral parts which bear the auricular surfaces. They fuse with the body and arch nuclei in the second to the fifth year after which the body and arch nuclei unite. The lateral nuclei fuse with each other from the seventh to the fifteenth year. Two epiphysial plates for each body appear about the fifteenth year, and two for each lateral border of the sacrum appear between the eighteenth and the twentieth year. The five sacral vertebrae are separated by cartilage until puberty when the lateral portions grow together, after which fusion of epiphyses and bodies takes place and ossification of the intervertebral disks occurs. The process extends from below upward, and at about the twenty-fifth year the sacrum becomes a single bone; at this time the lateral epiphysial plates also fuse with it.

Coccyx. Each vertebra ossifies from one nucleus, the first in the first year; while the lower four ossify later, some not before puberty. The lower three vertebrae usually unite about the thirtieth year.

Ribs. Centers of ossification appear at the end of the second month. They extend from the angles into the heads. The division into bony and cartilaginous portions is evident in the fourth month. At puberty, one epiphysial nucleus appears at each head and two at the tubercles; these fuse with the body of the rib after the twentieth year.

Sternum. The centers of ossification are multiple and variable as to place and time of occurrence. A nucleus usually appears in the manubrium about the third to the sixth month. Paired and unpaired nuclei occur in the body, fusing from the sixth to the twenty-fifth year. An epiphysial nucleus near the clavicular incisura fuses with the manubrium from the twenty-fifth to the twenty-eighth. A center of ossification may appear in the xiphoid in the sixth year and fuse later in life with the body.

BONES OF THE UPPER EXTREMITY

Scapula. The main center of ossification appears in the eighth week and forms the body, spine and base of the glenoid cavity. A nucleus appears in the coracoid process in the first year of life, fusing with the main mass at puberty. In the tenth to the twelfth year, the subcoracoid nucleus occurs in the base of the coracoid process and the upper edge of the glenoid fossa and this fuses with the main mass about the eighteenth year. Epiphysial centers appear in the acromion process in the fifteenth to the eighteenth year, fusing with the spine about the twentieth year; in the superior lateral part of the coracoid process, in the surface of the glenoid cavity, and on the inferior angle in the sixteenth to the eighteenth years; on the vertebral border in the eighteenth to the twentieth years. In the eighteenth to the twenty-fourth years these epiphyses unite in the order given with the body of the scapular.

Clavicle. A center of ossification develops in the shaft at the end of the sixth week. This is the first ossification center to appear in the body. The epiphysial center at the sternal end occurs in the eighteenth to the twentieth year and unites with the shaft in the twentieth to the twenty-fifth year.

Humerus. The nucleus of the shaft appears in the sixth to the seventh week. At the proximal end, an epiphysial nucleus appears for the head in the first to the second year and sometimes before birth; a nucleus appears in the greater tubercle in the first to the third year, and in the lesser tubercle in the third to the fifth year; these coalesce in the fourth to the sixth year and unite with the shaft in the sixteenth to the twenty-fifth year. At the distal end, an epiphysial nucleus appears in the capitulum in the first to the third year; in the medial epicondyle in the fifth to the ninth year; in the trochlea in the eighth to the sixteenth year; in the lateral epicondyle in the eleventh to the eighteenth year; the three lateral nuclei first unite with each other and then with the shaft in the sixteenth to the seventeenth year; the medial epicondyle unites with the shaft in the eighteenth year.

Radius. The ossification center of the shaft occurs in the seventh week; the distal epiphysial nucleus between the eighth embryonal month and the third year, uniting with the shaft in the twenty-first to the twenty-fifth year; the proximal epiphysial nucleus between the fourth and the ninth year, uniting with the shaft in the seventeenth to the twentieth year.

Ulna. The center of ossification of the shaft appears in the seventh week, a few days after that of the radius. The distal epiphysial nucleus appears in the sixth to the ninth year, uniting with the shaft in the eighteenth to the twenty-fourth year. The proximal epiphysial nucleus appears in the olecranon in the eighth to the fourteenth year, uniting with the shaft in the seventeenth year.

Carpal Bones. The nuclei in the os capitatum (os magnum) and os hamatum (unciform) appear in the first year; in the os triquetrum (cuneiform) in the second to the third year; in the os lunatum (semilunar) in the third to the fifth year; in the os naviculare (scaphoid), multangulum majus (trapezium) and multangulum minus (trapezoid) in the fourth to the sixth year; in the os pisiforme in the ninth to the thirteenth year.

Metacarpal Bones. The ossification center for each shaft appears in the ninth week. The distal epiphysial nuclei appear in the second to the fifth metacarpals from the second to the third year; the proximal epiphysial nucleus for the first metacarpal appears in the third year. The epiphyses unite with the shafts about the fifteenth to the twentieth year.

Phalanges. In the first row, the diaphysial nuclei appear in the ninth week and the proximal epiphysial nuclei in the first to the third year.

In the second row, the diaphysial nuclei appear in the eleventh to the twelfth week, and the proximal epiphysial nuclei in the second to the third year.

In the third row, the shaft nuclei appear in the seventh to the eighth week and the proximal epiphysial nuclei in the second to the third year.

The epiphyses unite with the diaphyses between the eighteenth and the twentieth years.

Sesamoid Bones. These usually ossify between the thirteenth and fourteenth years or sometimes later.

BONES OF THE LOWER EXTREMITY

Hip Bone (Os Coxae). An ossification center for the ilium appears in the eighth week; for the ischium in the fourth month; for the pubis in the fourth to the fifth month. These three nuclei form the acetabulum where they remain separated from each other until puberty with a Y-shaped cartilage in between. The nucleus between the ilium and the pubis unites in the ninth to the twelfth year, forming the os acetabuli which unites with the os pubis at the time of puberty. The inferior rami of the pubis and ischium unite between the seventh and eighth years. The three main parts unite with each other and the acetabular nuclei about the twentieth year.

The epiphysial nuclei appear after puberty; one along the iliac crest, which unites with the rest of the bone between the twentieth and twenty-fifth years; a second at the ischial tuberosity, which unites between the seventeenth and the twenty-fourth years; the third at the spine of the ischium, which unites between the eighteenth and the twentieth years. An epiphysial nucleus in the symphysial surface of the pubis appears in the eighteenth to the twentieth year, and unites after the twentieth year.

Femur. The ossification center of the shaft appears in the seventh week. The nucleus for the distal epiphysis appears in the ninth month shortly before birth, uniting with the shaft about the twentieth to the twenty-fourth year. Three proximal epiphysial nuclei of the head appear in the first year and unite with the shaft in the eighteenth to the nineteenth year. The greater trochanter nucleus appears in the third to the fourth year and unites with the shaft in the eighteenth year. The nucleus for the lesser trochanter appears in the eleventh to the fourteenth year and unites with the shaft in the seventeenth year.

Patella. The ossification center appears in the third to the fifth year.

Tibia. The shaft nucleus appears in the seventh week of fetal life. The proximal epiphysial nucleus appears shortly before birth and unites with the shaft in the nineteenth to the twenty-fourth year. The nucleus of the distal epiphysis appears in the second year and unites with the shaft in the sixteenth to the nineteenth year.

Fibula. The ossification center for the shaft appears about the fifty-fifth day. The distal epiphysial nucleus appears about the second year and unites with the shaft from the twentieth to the twenty-second year. The proximal epiphysial nucleus appears from the third to the fifth year and unites with the shaft between the twenty-second and the twenty-fourth year.

Tarsal Bones. The calcaneus or os calcis shows an ossification center in the sixth fetal month; in the seventh to the tenth year, a posterior epiphysial nucleus appears and unites with the bone in the thirteenth to the twentieth year.

The ossification center for the talus, or the astragalus, appears in the sixth to the seventh fetal month. The nucleus for the cuboid appears shortly before or after a full term birth. The nucleus for the third cuneiform appears in the first year; that for the first cuneiform in the second to the fourth year; that for the second cuneiform in the third to the fourth year; and that for the navicular in the fourth to the fifth year.

Metatarsal Bones. The centers of ossification for the diaphyses appear in the eighth to the tenth week. The proximal epiphysial nucleus for the first metatarsal and the distal epiphysial nuclei for the second to the fifth metatarsals appear from the third to the eighth year and unite with the shaft from the fourteenth to the twenty-first year.

Phalanges. First row: The shaft nuclei appear in the third fetal month and the proximal epiphysial nuclei in the third year.

Second row: The shaft nuclei appear in the fourth to the tenth fetal month and the proximal epiphysial nuclei in the third year.

Third row: The shaft nuclei appear in the ninth week and the proximal epiphysial nuclei in the fourth year.

The epiphyses unite with the shafts about the fourteenth to the twenty-first year.

Sesamoid. These bones in the big toe ossify in the twelfth to the fourteenth year.

It may not be easy to estimate the age of the body by the osseous changes after the thirtieth year, except in old age when senile changes occur. The bones tend to become more brittle, the fatty marrow more abundant, the cancellous tissue more rarefied, the medullary cavities large, the bone lighter and the compact osseous tissue denser. The sutures of the vault of the skull remain distinct until middle life when they tend to fuse, but there is wide individual variation in this process. The costal cartilages tend to ossify and the laryngeal cartilages show bone formation, but this change is not a constant one. The vertebral bodies become flattened anteriorly and a moderate kyphosis develops in senile individuals.

Krogman, on the basis of his own studies and those of T. W. Todd, emphasizes the importance of the changes in the pubic symphysis as a criterion in the estimation of the age of the skeleton from the end of the second decade. During the third decade, the ridges and grooves on the symphysial surface of the pubic bones, and the ossific nodules derived from patchy ossification centers in the adjoining symphysial cartilage and deposited on the symphysial surfaces of the bones, gradually disappear. During the same period and continuing into the fourth and fifth decades, the elongated oval outline and margins of these bony surfaces become more sharply delineated. In the fourth decade, the symphysial bony surfaces are fairly smooth. Their sharp delineation is maintained through the fifth decade, but in the sixth decade their continuity is gradually destroyed by secondary erosion.

Krogman also stresses the closure of the skull sutures as another criterion of age between the twenty-fifth and fiftieth years and points out that the process starts on the inner table but does not always extend through to the outer table and that therefore the extent of suture closure in the skull as an indication of age is only valid if the observations are made on the inner surface.

The condition of the lower jaw varies for the different periods of life. In the infant the body of the jaw is shallow, forming an obtuse angle with the ramus; the mental foramen is near the lower margin and the coronoid process projects above the condyle. In adult life the body becomes longer and larger and joins the ramus at a right angle, and the condyle grows and projects above the coronoid process. In old age the angle between the body and the ramus becomes obtuse, the alveolar margin atrophies because the teeth are lost, and the mental foramen opens near the alveolar border.

The most satisfactory method of investigating bones in an incomplete or mutilated body is to take roentgen ray photographs of the remains by which the ossification centers and the cartilaginous lines of epiphysial separation will be demonstrated with the least difficulty. In some instances it may be desirable to make a longitudinal section of a long bone with a saw as illustrated by the following case:

After a conflagration two bodies of the same stature, but so badly burned as to be unrecognizable, were found in the same room. One was a man of 45 years and the other was his son of 14 years, but it was impossible to distinguish them by external inspection. The difficulty was resolved by making a longitudinal section through the left humerus from each body with a saw. In one the bone was continuous between shaft and head thus indicating the father, and in the other there was a line of epiphysial cartilage between head and shaft which identified the son.

The facts obtained by examination of the bony skeleton must be judged with great caution, especially in later adult life when individual peculiarities may alter the rate of osseous changes. Various endocrine disturbances may hasten or delay the appearance of the primary or secondary ossification centers or the closure of the epiphyses, factors which may result in disproportion between the length of the bones of the extremities as compared to those of the trunk.

The teeth may give reliable information as to the age in childhood and youth; beyond adult life the changes are too uncertain to be of value.

The appearance of the *20 temporary teeth* is as follows:

6 to 8 months	lower central incisors
Eighth month	upper central incisors
8 to 10 months	upper lateral incisors
10 to 12 months	lower lateral incisors
12 to 14 months	first molars
18 to 20 months	canines
22 to 24 months	posterior molars

The *32 permanent teeth* erupt as follows:

Sixth year	first molars
Seventh year	middle incisors
Eighth year	lateral incisors
Ninth year	first bicuspids
Tenth year	second bicuspids
Eleventh to twelfth years	canines
Twelfth to fourteenth years	second molars
After the twenty-first year	the third molars or wisdom teeth

HEIGHT AND WEIGHT. If only partial remains of a body are available, it may be possible to guess the height and weight of the deceased from measurements of the fragments, but so variable are human proportions that close accuracy cannot always be expected. Many people have devised formulae for calculating the height from the dimensions of different bones, and while these may give a basis for estimation, the results obtained must always be regarded as an approximation and not as the accurate product of a mathematic formula.

If femur, humerus or radius is present, it is measured in centimeters from joint surface to joint surface with the cartilage in place; the tibia is measured from knee articulation minus the spine to the end of the internal malleolus. From these measurements the height of the dead body may be calculated by Pearson's formula as follows:

Height in centimeters equals:

MALE	FEMALE
81.231 plus 1.880 times length of femur	73.163 plus 1.945 times length of femur
70.714 plus 2.894 times length of humerus	72.046 plus 2.754 times length of humerus
78.807 plus 2.376 times length of tibia	75.369 plus 2.352 times length of tibia
86.465 plus 3.271 times length of radius	82.189 plus 3.343 times length of radius

To obtain the height of the living body, 1.5 cm. is subtracted from the final result for male bodies and 2 cm. for female bodies.

Other measurements that have been recommended for the estimation of the body length are the following:

With the arms extended laterally at right angles to the body, the distance from the tip of the right middle finger to that of the left middle finger equals the height.

Twice the length of one arm plus 12 inches for the clavicles and 1.5 inches for the sternum is approximately the height.

From the vertex of the skull to the symphysis pubis is one half of the height. This is not always true, as the vertex-symphysis measurement sometimes exceeds one half of the height by two inches.

From the sternal notch to the symphysis is about one third of the height.

From the base of the skull to the os coccyx is about 44 per cent of the height.

None of these formulae can be relied upon implicitly, because at best they are only guides for the purpose of obtaining some approximation of the height.

The estimation of the weight is even more problematic and cannot be obtained unless the remains yield some idea of the size of the bones, the muscular development and the adipose tissue of the deceased.

REFERENCES

Bakwin, H., and Bakwin, R. M.   Growth Standards for Children, Dept. of Pediat., New York University, and New York Infirmary for Women and Children.

Bertillon, A.   Identification of the Living, translated by R. W. Webster, from Peterson, Haines and Webster, Legal Medicine and Toxicology, Philadelphia, W. B. Saunders Co., 1923, Vol. 1, pp. 63-131.

Boyd, W.   A Textbook of Pathology, Philadelphia, Lea & Febiger, 1940.

Eastman, N. J.   William's Obstetrics, 10th ed., New York, Appleton-Century-Crofts, Inc., 1950.

Ewing, J.   Identity, from Peterson, Haines and Webster, Legal Medicine and Toxicology, Philadelphia, W. B. Saunders Co., 1923, Vol. 1, pp. 123-174.

Glaister, J., and Brash, J. C.   Medico-legal Aspects of the Ruxton Case, Baltimore, William Wood & Co., 1937.

Krogman, W. M.   The Human Skeleton in Legal Medicine, in Symposium on Medicolegal Problems, series 2, S. A. Levinson, Ed., Philadelphia, J. B. Lippincott Co., 1949, pp. 1-92.

Kuhne, F.   Finger Print Instructor, New York, Munn & Co., 1935.

Quain, J.   Elements of Anatomy, 11th ed., New York, Longmans, Green & Co., 1915.

Ronchese, F.   Occupational Marks, New York, Grune and Stratton, 1948.

Smith, S.   Forensic Medicine, London, J. and A. Churchill, 1940.

Södermann, H., and O'Connell, J. J.   Modern Criminal Investigation, 4th ed., New York, Funk & Wagnalls Co., 1952.

Spalteholz, W.   Hand Atlas of Human Anatomy, 7th ed., translated by L. Barker, Philadelphia, J. B. Lippincott Co., 1943.

Webster, R. W.   Legal Medicine and Toxicology, Philadelphia, W. B. Saunders Co., 1930.

4

The Signs of Death

Answers to the following questions must be obtained in every case of death which is the subject of an official investigation. These questions are:

1. Is the body dead?
2. How long has the body been dead?
3. What is the cause of death?

The present chapter deals with the methods of establishing the fact that the body is dead and of estimating the postmortem interval or the length of time that has elapsed since death. This is done by considering the signs of death which are present in the individual case and evaluating their significance. The cause of death will be discussed in Chapter 5.

It is important to define the terms life and death in order to understand the meaning of the different signs of death. Life can be considered as the sum total of the vital processes by which the physical integrity of the body is maintained. In death these processes cease, and life becomes extinct; since the factors protecting the body no longer operate, its disintegration then begins.

The preservation of animal life depends on the smooth functioning of the oxygen cycle, that is, the breathing in of oxygen and its use by the system. Four sets of organs are concerned with this function: (1) The vital centers in the medulla initiate the respiratory movements. (2) The lungs appropriate oxygen from the inspired air, transfer it to the red blood cells in the pulmonary capillaries and at the same time receive carbon dioxide and other waste products from the blood plasma for excretion in the expired air. (3) The blood conveys the oxygen-containing erythrocytes from the lungs to the tissues. There the tissue cells appropriate the oxygen and transfer the carbon dioxide and the waste products to the blood plasma. The nonoxygenated red cells and the waste material in the plasma are carried by the blood to the lungs. (4) The heart and blood vessels propel and conduct the blood from the lungs to the tissues and from the tissues to the lungs.

EARLY POSTMORTEM CHANGES

As long as the oxygen cycle is maintained the individual lives. The cells remain healthy, food and water are ingested and absorbed, metabolism is normal, excretion continues and locomotion is possible. The physiologic chemical processes are maintained in a balanced state, the various intracellular and extracellular enzymes are neutralized by antagonistic ferments and any autodestruction of the body is held in check. During life, damage inflicted on the organism by the outer world is repaired and invasion of putrefactive microorganisms successfully repelled.

When death occurs, the oxygen cycle is stopped. Highly organized tissues like the central nervous system perish rapidly, so that the body becomes motionless and insensible; similarly, the respiratory movements are discontinued, the heart ceases to beat and the blood to flow. The individual as an organism is extinguished and life is no longer possible, though some tissues and cells may preserve an independent existence a short time after death. During the first two hours post mortem the intestinal musculature may display active peristalsis, some of the skeletal muscles may contract under mechanical and electric stimuli, and in rare instances the heart may beat faintly in an abortive fashion. The spermatozoa live for a longer period. The authors have seen cases in which spermatozoa removed from the male urethra 24 hours post mortem were alive and motile. All these structures die eventually because the disintegration of the body creates conditions incompatible with their existence.

The postmortem alterations in the chemistry of the organism may release the destructive action of certain enzymes in the cells and organs by eliminating antagonistic enzymes that normally hold them in check. As a result, autolytic processes may be noted in several tissues within 24 hours after death. In the parenchymatous cells of the kidneys the autolytic processes may be demonstrated microscopically by the appearance of granules in the cytoplasm or the loss of staining properties in the nuclei. More striking examples of such postmortem changes are represented by the maceration of fetuses which have died in utero, by the zones of softening in the hyperplastic thymus of infants, by the softening in the brain of the newborn child, by the softening between cortex and medulla in the suprarenal capsule and by the disintegration in the pancreas, stomach and esophagus. The pancreas when acted upon after death by its own ferments shows areas of autolysis and fatty acid formation not attended by inflammatory reaction. The stomach and esophagus present different grades of postmortem digestion by the gastric juice, especially conspicuous in cases which have died as a result of an intracranial lesion. In the early stages of the process there is simple erosion of the mucous membrane; the formation of acid hematin in the submucous veins causes these vessels to stand out as a brown or black network. In the late stages there are irregularly shaped, reactionless, ovoid or circular perforations of the fundus of the stomach or of the esophagus which may allow the stomach contents to enter the abdomen or chest cavities and cause a certain amount of discoloration and postmortem digestion of the serous surfaces. These changes must be distinguished from actual pathologic lesions. Such differentiation is usually not difficult because the disintegration referable to the autolysis is not accompanied by any intravital reaction. At the same time the changes must not be confused with the postmortem results of bacterial decomposition in the same tissues, a condition which will be described later.

Postmortem changes also occur in the blood of the heart and larger blood vessels; they are especially noticeable in the right side of the heart and the pulmonary artery. These changes vary, depending on the conditions in the individual case. If a person is dying slowly of an acute infectious disease, or in any other condition in which the fibrinogen content of the blood is increased and the sedimentation rate of the erythrocytes is accelerated, a clot begins to form in the heart in the later agonal stages as the circulation fails. The red blood cells sink to the dependent portions of the cardiac cavities and the white cells and platelets float on top. When the process is completed a few hours after death, the upper part of the clot will be pale yellow in color or of the chicken-fat type and the lower portion will be a dark, currant-jelly red in color. In suddenly fatal conditions in which the blood does not usually contain an excess of fibrinogen and the sedimentation rate is not increased, the blood in the heart may be fluid; if the fibrinogen is in excess without any increase in the sedimentation rate, the heart will contain currant-jelly clots.

EXTERNAL SIGNS OF DEATH

The most useful signs of death are those which can be detected by external examination of the body. They are the ones which the medical examiner elicits in his investigation of the body at the scene, and it is upon these signs that he relies to determine the presence of death and to estimate the approximate lapse of time since death. These signs are as follows:

1. Loss of movement
2. Stoppage of the heart and respiration
3. Loss of body heat
4. Postmortem lividity
5. Rigor mortis
6. Signs of death in the eyes
7. Postmortem decomposition: putrefaction, mummification, adipocere formation
8. Later destruction of the body in air, water, earth

1. **Loss of Movement.** The earliest sign of death in a body is the loss of movement in its parts, as determined by visual inspection. While it is a convenient criterion for determining that life is absent, it can lead to error if precautions are not taken. Some varieties of death due to external causes, as for example submersion or corrosive poisoning, are associated with severe shock; and the victim may be so depressed that the ability to move appears definitely lost even before life is extinct. Wrong diagnoses have been made on cases of this type because the investigator has not made his observations with sufficient care. In order to avoid a needless mistake other signs of death should be demonstrated to substantiate the diagnosis.

2. **Stoppage of the Heart and Respiration.** The stopping of the heart and respiratory movements is the first indication that the oxygen cycle has been interrupted. It is the only reliable sign of death in the early postmortem stages, and when it can be demonstrated beyond any doubt the individual can be pronounced dead with certainty. The best way to elicit this sign is to listen carefully with the stethoscope over the precordial area where the heart beat can be recognized readily and similarly, over the larynx where the faintest breath sound can be heard. The chance of error is slight with this test, and a wrong diagnosis is rarely made.

Many writings on legal medicine are concerned with the conditions which presumably simulate death. In insane patients there are states of depression which are said to produce a death-like appearance: one, known as catalepsy, is characterized by a sudden onset of coma, muscles which are rigid but still react to the electric current, a low body temperature, insensibility to touch and slight but demonstrable heart and respiratory movements; another known as trance, is characterized by a comatose state, pallid skin, flaccid muscles with lost reflexes and feeble heart and respiratory action. On superficial inspection such conditions may convey the impression that the individual is dead, but signs of life would be revealed if the victim were properly examined.

A sudden fainting spell or syncope simulates death for a fraction of a minute, but the person so stricken quickly recovers and solves the problem for the examiner. In cases of profound shock from physical violence, burns, electricity, exposure to cold, submersion, corrosive poisoning or profound coma from alcohol, chloral hydrate, opium, barbiturates or similar conditions, the vital centers may be so depressed and the cardiac and respiratory movements so weakened that they may be overlooked on casual examination. The use of a little care in these cases will eliminate the chance of a wrong diagnosis.

The greatest danger of erroneously pronouncing dead a person in a state of profound shock occurs when the doctor is compelled to examine the patient under unfavorable circumstances, as in a cramped space or without sufficient light. An example of such an error is the case of a young woman who drank lysol® with suicidal intent. She was in such a state of collapse that a doctor, examining her under unsatisfactory conditions, failed to detect the feeble cardiac and respiratory movements and diagnosed her as dead. The case was referred to the medical examiner who, arriving after two hours, found the victim still alive. She died several hours later in the hospital.

Many methods for the determination of death in the early postmortem stages have been recommended but are of doubtful value. These include: holding a mirror before the mouth and nose of the allegedly dead person and watching for any condensation of moisture on its surface as a sign of breathing; holding a feather before the nose so that if the victim breathes the feather will be agitated; placing a glass partly full of mercury on the chest and watching the surface of the liquid, which will ripple with the least respiratory movement. Some recommend that the examiner drop melted sealing wax on the breast of the deceased. If the blood is flowing in the blood vessels, an inflammatory edema will develop about the wax. In doubtful cases, others suggest cutting the radial artery; if blood pulsates from the cut end, the circulation still persists. Another test is the injection of a dilute alkaline solution of fluorescin into the subcutaneous tissues. If life is present the sclera of the eyeball will turn green in a few minutes, but if the body is dead no such change will occur. These tests should be discarded in favor of the stethoscopic examination.

3. **Loss of Body Heat.** When life is extinct, heat production in the body stops and its temperature is lowered gradually to that of the surroundings. The rate with which the heat is lost is not uniform and varies with the circumstances. The more exposed parts like the hands and face cool in from a few minutes to four hours depending on the temperature of the environment. The skin nearest the trunk, especially where the body is clad, may retain part of its warmth for from 6 to 12 hours. The internal organs may be still warm long after the surface of the body has been cooled. In general, small or emaciated individuals lose their warmth rapidly in cold surroundings, especially if they are nude. Large obese cadavers lying fully clad in a warm room lose heat slowly. Beyond such general rules the examiner cannot rely on heat loss in the body as a criterion for estimating the postmortem interval. He can form his opinion only by evaluating all the different factors which might influence this phenomenon in the individual case.

If the corpse is exposed to a source of heat for a few hours shortly after death, the temperature of the flesh will be raised and not lowered. This is illustrated by the case of a woman who was strangled and exposed on a roof from sunrise to 10 A.M.; when she was examined at that time her entire body was definitely warm to the touch and yet rigor mortis was complete. Four and a half hours' exposure to the rays of the sun was sufficient to raise the surface temperature in spite of the coolness of the surrounding atmosphere. Later when the body was removed to a cool compartment in the morgue, its temperature was lowered because it was separated from the source of heat.

Another apparent exception to postmortem cooling is encountered occasionally in deaths from acute infectious diseases like lobar pneumonia or typhoid fever. In such cases a postmortem rise of temperature occurs which lasts a few hours and gradually subsides to that of the surroundings.

A body in zero weather may undergo freezing and become stony hard from the formation of ice in the cavities and blood vessels. The ice inside the skull may expand to such an extent that some of the sutures of the skull like the sagittal or coronal may separate and thus simulate an antemortem fracture. The postmortem separation is not accompanied, however, by the signs of vital reaction which would occur in the case of a fracture. The freezing process varies in rapidity from a few hours to several days, depending on circumstances. If the body is thoroughly frozen it will be preserved fairly well, but if the cold affects only the surface tissues and fails to reach the viscera, decomposition may take place in the internal parts of the cadaver. After a frozen body has been thawed, it tends to undergo comparatively rapid decomposition.

4. **Postmortem Suggillations or Lividity.** Postmortem suggillations are the purplish red or purplish blue discolorations which appear under the skin of the dependent parts of the body after death. They are caused by the stoppage of the circulation, the stagnation of the blood in the blood vessels and its tendency to sink by the force of gravity. The blood flows into the finer subcutaneous vessels, engorging them and giving a red and blue tinge to the livid area on the under surface of the corpse. In contrast the upper portions of the body, drained of blood, are pale.

The *position of the corpse* determines the site of the lividity. In most cases of death the body lies on its back so that the blood settles posteriorly, appearing first in the neck and shoulders and then spreading over the entire back (Fig. 4-1). At points like the buttocks and shoulder blades the skin may be compressed by a supporting surface so that the blood cannot flow into the subcutaneous vessels and as a result such areas are pale. Occasionally when the blood volume is large, the pressure of gravity may cause a postmortem rupture of some of the smaller blood vessels, producing a minute circular hemorrhage known as a Tardieu spot. These lesions are found most frequently in the loose connective tissues of the neck and shoulders.

If the body is lying in the prone position, face down, the suggillations appear in the loose connective tissues in front, the color of the lividity is intense and Tardieu spots are common (Fig. 4-2). Sometimes the congestion is so great that minute blood vessels are ruptured in the nose, and an appreciable flow of blood will occur from the nasal orifice.

The *location of the lividity* indicates in many instances the position of the body during the postmortem interval. If the deceased has been lying on one side, the blood will settle on that side. If the corpse has been suspended in the upright position, suggillations and Tardieu spots will appear in the lower extremities (Fig. 4-3). In some instances it is possible to detect from the distribution of the lividity that the position of the body has been changed since death (Fig. 2-2). For example, if a cadaver has been lying in the prone position for four hours post mortem and is then turned over to the supine position, suggillations will be found on the front and back indicating the shift in position after death. On the other hand if the shift is made before the suggillations appear in the first position, the blood will gravitate to the new location and will not indicate the original position of the body.

The lividity makes its appearance from about 20 minutes to an hour after death in plethoric individuals, and from about one to four hours in anemic persons; it is usually complete in about 12 hours. It is difficult to estimate the postmortem interval from a consideration of the postmortem lividity alone.

The color of the lividity has considerable diagnostic significance. Oxyhemoglobin appears in the subcutaneous blood as a red flush and reduced hemoglobin as a plum color or a bluish violet discoloration (Fig. 4-1 and 4-5). Occasionally in some bodies the lividity may show a reddish tinge side by side with lividity showing a bluish tinge. This is due in all probabilty to varying proportions of oxyhemoglobin and reduced hemoglobin in these different areas. Some believe that in a few bodies

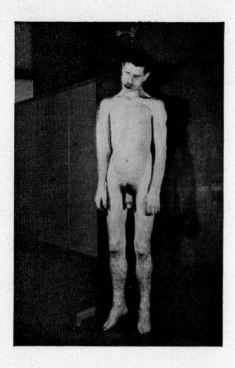

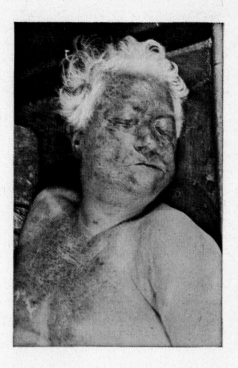

Fig. 4-1. Vertical dependent lividity of lower extremities and hands. Suicidal hanging. Note also greenish postmortem discoloration of abdomen.

Fig. 4-2. Intense indigo blue dependent postural lividity with discrete and confluent postmortem hemorrhages. Natural death. Body found slumped forward in chair.

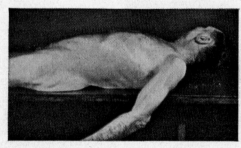

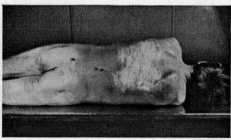

Fig. 4-3. Cherry red carboxyhemoglobin lividity. Suicidal inhalation of illuminating gas. Body found lying on left side. Blood 70 per cent saturated with carbon monoxide.

Fig. 4-4. Plum colored ordinary lividity of back. Note pale areas on buttocks and chest due to pressure of weight of body. Death from heart disease. Body found in supine position.

Varieties of Postmortem Lividity

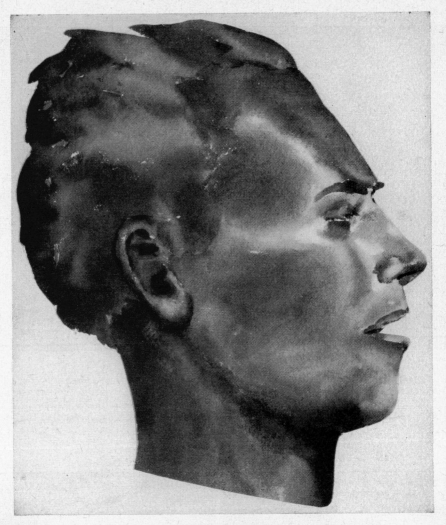

Fig. 4-5. Plum Colored Postmortem Lividity of Reduced Hemoglobin; Postural Asphyxia in a Fatal
Case of Acute Alcoholism.

oxidation of some of the hemoglobin occurs after death from oxygen in the air
which may penetrate the skin, but this has not been satisfactorily proved. It is
possible that in the early postmortem interval reduced hemoglobin may be formed
from oxyhemoglobin present in the blood at the time of death by some of the tissues
which, still alive, extract the oxygen from the adjacent red blood cells. Asphyxial
deaths usually show an intense bluish violet and purplish lividity referable to the
large amounts of reduced hemoglobin in the blood (Fig. 4-5). The light red suggillations in recently drowned cases are due partly to the lack of engorgement of the
subcutaneous blood vessels as a result of their contraction from immersion of the
body in cold water and partly to the presence of oxyhemoglobin. In carbon monoxide
poisoning the suggillations have a distinct cherry red color due to the formation of
carboxyhemoglobin (Figs. 4-4 and 4-6). In poisoning by potassium chlorate (Fig.
4-7) or nitrobenzene the hemoglobin is changed to methemoglobin, the lividity has
a brownish violet color, and the blood has a coffee or chocolate brown tinge.

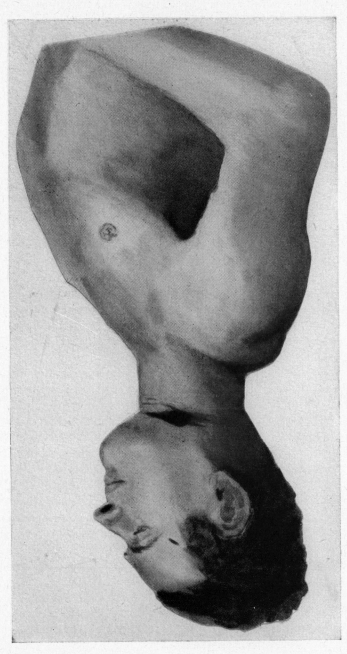

Fig. 4-6. Postmortem Lividity; Carboxyhemoglobin.

Carbon monoxide poisoning. Same case as illustrated in Figure 15-26 on page 363. The deceased had first unsuccessfully attempted to cut his throat and stab himself through the scalp. He then tried to hang himself with his belt which broke. In falling, his head struck and broke off a protruding gas jet.

Changes in postmortem lividity also occur when putrefaction sets in. In the early stages there is some hemolysis of the blood, diffusion of blood-stained fluid from the engorged vessels into the surrounding tissues and collections of similar fluid in the chest or abdominal cavities. As bacterial decomposition progresses the postmortem lividity becomes dusky in color and turns brown and green before finally disappearing with the destruction of the blood. In mummification the lividity may turn brown to black with the desiccation of the body, but if the blood is scant the change may be inconspicuous.

Some suggillations are similar in external appearance to an antemortem contusion or ecchymosis, but if decomposition has not begun a distinction between the two is possible. If the suspected area is incised, the suggillations will show blood in the blood vessels but none in the surrounding tissues, while a bruise or ecchymosis will show extravasation of blood into the subcutaneous tissues. When decomposition occurs, diffusion of hemolyzed blood takes place into the subcutaneous tissues spontaneously and may resemble and be difficult to differentiate from an ecchymosis. For the same reason small contusions tend to grow larger because of postmortem hemolysis and diffusion.

Postmortem lividity also occurs in the internal organs. If the body has been lying in the supine position, the kidneys, spine, cerebellum and posterior portions of the lungs may be engorged with blood. In the prone position the anterior portion of the lungs, the liver and the gastrointestinal tract are usually congested; bacterial decomposition under such conditions is apt to develop rapidly because the engorged intestinal vessels are brought into close contact with anaerobic bacteria in the lumen of the intestines, and the stage is set for a rapid invasion and growth of these organisms through the blood vessels of the body.

5. **Rigor Mortis.** Rigor mortis, the stiffness which develops in the muscles of the body after death, depends upon postmortem chemical changes affecting the glycogen and other constituents of the muscle cytoplasm. For a short time after death the reaction of the muscle protoplasm is slightly alkaline, and as long as this condition endures the skeletal muscles remain flexible. In most cases the reaction changes from alkaline to acid from two to six hours post mortem because of the conversion of glycogen and other substances to sarcolactic and phosphoric acids. Rigidity then begins to develop in the muscles of the face, jaw, upper extremities, trunk and lower extremities, appearing in about the sequence mentioned; the process is completed in about two to six hours. Occasionally because of some peculiarity in the individual case the rigor may start in other muscles and develop in somewhat different order. The muscles become not only stiffened but also shortened and the intensity of the process is said to be proportional to the amount of glycogen originally present in the muscle. In the stage of complete rigor it is difficult to change the position of the limbs because of the stiffness. This stiffness endures from 12 to 48 hours, or until the muscle protoplasm becomes alkaline again from other chemical changes. The rigor then passes off gradually in the same order in which it appeared, that is, in the face, jaw, neck, arms, legs and trunk.

Different conditions alter the onset, persistence and disappearance of rigor mortis. In most cases in which a person dies quietly without undergoing muscular exertion the muscles are relaxed, the jaw may drop open, and the stiffening develops gradually in the manner just described. On the other hand if muscular activity has occurred just prior to death the process is accelerated; thus individuals who have died in convulsions from strychnine poisoning have shown complete rigidity in the

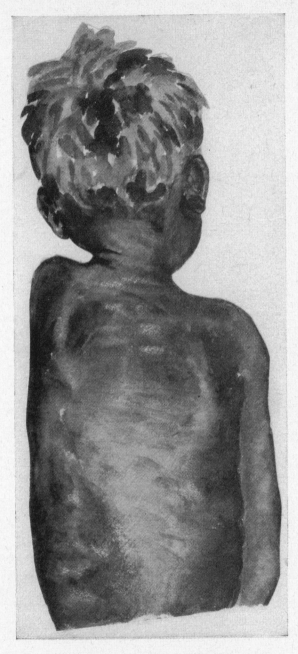

Fig. 4-7. Postmortem Lividity; Methemoglobinemia Due to
Poisoning by Potassium Chlorate.

first hour after death. Cases of instantaneous rigor mortis have been described in which the entire body became rigid immediately after the person died, and the phenomenon has been attributed to intense muscular action and exertion prior to death.* In general, individuals with powerful muscles develop postmortem rigor slowly and retain it for a long time. Those with poorly developed musculature, such as infants or emaciated persons, become rigid rapidly and lose their rigidity rapidly. Heat speeds the onset of rigor and accelerates its dissolution. Cold tends to hasten the onset but to retard the dissolution of the rigidity, so that the stiffness is retained for days or even weeks. In such cases it may be impossible to distinguish true rigor mortis from stiffness attributable to freezing or mummification.

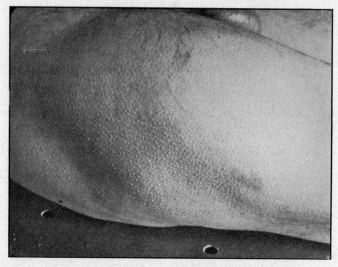

Fig. 4-8. Cutis Anserina, Goose Flesh, Conspicuously Developed on Thigh.

This results from contraction of the arrectores pilorum muscles before or immediately after death, followed by rigor mortis. It occurs if the body is chilled at the time of death as in most drownings.

Rigor mortis also affects the smooth muscles of the internal organs; the most striking changes occur in the heart, the myocardium consistently developing postmortem rigidity soon after death. However, the authors have seen two rare cases in which the muscles of the auricle contracted spasmodically hours after death, though the ventricular muscle did not respond; in one of these cases the skeletal muscles showed rigor mortis at the time that the myocardium was contracting.

Rarely, if the uterus is in labor at the moment of death, with an open os uteri, the postmortem contraction may cause the uterus to contract and expel the fetus. This phenomenon is comparable to the activity of the heart and intestines after death and is not rigor mortis. In many cases of submersion the arrectores pilorum, the muscles attached to the hair follicles, contract and then develop rigor mortis; the rough cutis anserina or goose flesh so produced persists (Fig. 4-8). This condition is encountered occasionally in death from other causes, especially if the body has been chilled.

---

* The term cadaveric spasm has been applied in some textbooks of forensic medicine to conditions which, according to the description in the text, resemble instantaneous rigor mortis. At the same time it is claimed that cadaveric spasm does not possess any resemblance to rigor mortis. The reason for making this distinction is not given.

The different phenomena connected with rigor mortis are sometimes helpful in estimating the postmortem interval. The usual regularity of the way in which muscle rigidity develops has led many authorities to put much reliance on the state of rigor mortis in a body as a basis for such estimations. One authority quoted by Herzog declares that if rigidity is found in the torso and arms but not in the legs, death probably occurred less than 12 hours before; and if the legs are stiff but not the torso and arms, it is probable that the body has been dead three days. Any estimations of this sort must be made with caution. The authors saw a case of cerebral malaria which showed postmortem rigidity in the lower extremities but had lost it in the jaw, upper extremities and trunk when the body was examined four days after death. The onset and dissolution of rigor mortis are subject to so many variations, however, that the different stages of the process rarely can be used as definite criteria for determining the time of death.

The following case is a good example of a medicolegal problem in which the stage of rigor mortis in a corpse was a point of importance. The deceased, a white man of 60 years, was found dead at 6 A.M. in his sleeping car berth by the porter, who declared that "his arm was stiff" at that time. At 8 A.M. the body was examined by a physician who discovered that complete rigor mortis was present. The deceased was known to have gone to bed at 9 P.M. the evening before and not to have left his berth after retiring which was unusual because he suffered from an enlarged prostate and was accustomed to empty his bladder several times during a night. Although an autopsy was not done, the circumstances seemed to indicate that he died of natural causes. The question at issue was whether the deceased had died before or after midnight, for at that time a life insurance policy covering him became null and void. In this case it was not possible to fix the time of death definitely by the state of the rigor mortis, though the other circumstances suggested that he had died before 12 P.M.

It is important to remember that before rigor mortis develops the body can be moved to any posture and be fixed by the rigor in that posture. As a consequence, the position of the cadaver at the time of examination is not necessarily the same as its position at the time of death. It is also true that when postmortem rigidity is developing the extremities can be moved and the rigor, temporarily overcome, develops later to fix the extremities in their new posture. If the rigor is fully developed and is overcome by force, the stiffness is broken up permanently and the rigid muscles may show postmortem ruptures.

6. **Postmortem Eye Changes.** The changes in the eye furnish important confirmatory signs of death. The cornea immediately after death is glistening but a few hours later is covered by a thin opaque film of dried secretion. If the eyelids are open for any length of time after death, the exposed sclera may turn a reddish brown from drying.

Occasionally rigor mortis may affect the ciliary muscles of the irides unequally so that one pupil is larger than the other. If different segments of the same iris are unequally affected, the pupils may be irregularly ovoid in place of circular, or may assume an eccentric position in the iris. The changes which occur in the eyes from postmortem putrefaction and mummification will be considered under those headings.

7. **Postmortem Decomposition.** Postmortem decomposition is the process which attacks the integrity of the dead body and causes its destruction. It may take the form of putrefaction, mummification or a combination of both. Another type, adipocere formation, is less frequently encountered.

PUTREFACTION. This process occurs post mortem when the putrefactive bacteria enter the blood vessels through the intestinal tract or, less often, through an external skin wound. Because the protective agencies of the body are absent, the bacteria spread through the blood vessels, using the proteins and carbohydrates of the blood as culture media. The chief destructive bacterial agent is *Clostridium welchii,* which causes marked hemolysis, liquefaction of postmortem clots and of fresh thrombi and emboli, disintegration of tissues and gas formation in the blood vessels and tissue spaces; it may invade the body soon after death or several days later. According to Sydney Smith, *Escherichia coli* and *Proteus vulgaris* are also found in the blood in the early postmortem stages, while two days later *Bacillus mesentericus* and *Micrococcus albus* are fairly prevalent. Other bacteria may be present in the blood and organs of the cadaver either as a result of postmortem invasion or as a consequence of pathogenic or agonal bacteremia.

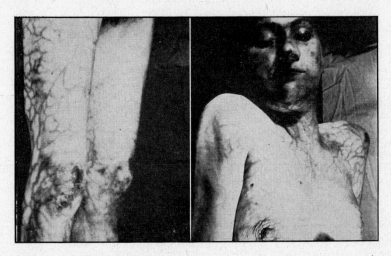

Fig. 4-9. Postmortem Staining and Visualization of Superficial Veins by Putrefactive Hemolysis. Suicidal Drowning in Hudson River. Body Submerged 30 Hours in July.

In a cool environment or when the body has been subjected to some degree of refrigeration a common external sign of bacterial decomposition appearing from about 24 to 48 hours post mortem is a dark green discoloration of the abdomen over the cecal or sigmoid regions (Fig. 4-3). This color results from the presence in the nearby tissues of sulfmethemoglobin and iron sulfide, produced by the action, on a hemoglobin derivative, of the hydrogen sulfide formed in the large intestine. The same greenish discoloration is often seen on the under surface of the liver where that organ is in contact with the transverse colon.

The gas-forming bacteria may invade the stomach and intestinal walls, frequently forming gas blebs in the submucous layer which project as small multilocular cysts of varying size into the lumen of the viscus. They then invade the blood vessels and spread through the blood, turning it dark from hemolysis and filling it with a large number of fine gas bubbles; later the gas distends the blood vessels and forces the blood which is not destroyed toward the periphery of the body. The wall of the vessel is stained a dirty crimson, changing to brown or green as the blood becomes further decomposed. The staining and visualization of the normally invisible subcutaneous veins by postmortem hemolysis is evident in Figure 4-9, the effect resembling that produced by an infrared photograph of the normal skin. The organs and tissues are invaded and discolored red, brown or black by the blood pigment; the aorta and the mucous membrane of the trachea are the first to show this change. Gas bubbles form in the solid viscera, and gas distends the abdominal and chest cavities.

When *Clostridium welchii* starts to grow in one of the parenchymatous organs, the cytoplasm of the cells disintegrates, the nuclei are destroyed by lysis or rhexis, the tissues take the stain poorly and the cells become disconnected so that there is loss of structural detail. Microscopically the bacteria form characteristic clumps in a tissue space and generate about themselves a bubble of gas, small at first but

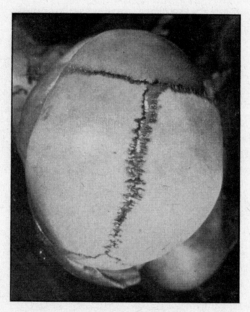

Fig. 4-10. Postmortem Separation of Sutures of Child's Skull Due to Pressure of Putrefactive Gases within Brain.

Six year old boy; accidental drowning; body submerged one week in early autumn.

soon increasing in size. These lesions first appear in the liver as small, opaque, yellowish gray, dendritic figures in the parenchyma; when the bubbles develop, the organ has a honey-combed, vesicular appearance. The chemical processes in this stage are those of reduction, the complicated proteins and carbohydrates being split into the simpler compounds of amino acids, leucine, tyrosine, ammonia, carbon dioxide, hydrogen sulfide and methane. Early in the process the gases are sometimes noninflammable, especially if the largest component is carbon dioxide, but as the decomposition progresses hydrogen sulfide is formed and, if present in large enough quantity, can be ignited to burn with a blue flame.

The end result of bacterial decomposition is the final destruction of the body. This may be effected by bacterial action alone but is often accomplished in conjunction with other mechanisms. In the later stages the organs are markedly discolored and, if sufficient moisture is present to prevent mummification, are converted into mushy, semifluid masses. The fat in the body disintegrates and becomes liquid and rancid. By this time all the complicated constituents of protoplasm have been reduced, and the chemical processes which follow are those of oxidation with the formation of phosphoric and sulfuric acids. The destructive action of the gas bacillus converts the brain into a pultaceous green-gray mass in which some of the architectural landmarks can at first be made out and then transforms it into a thick, putrescent fluid. The parenchymatous organs like the liver, kidneys, spleen and pancreas are soon destroyed; but the heart, lungs, voluntary muscle and smooth muscle tissue are affected more slowly. The uterus, prostate, fibrous tissues and bones resist the ravages of decomposition more successfully than the other structures. The bones are preserved the longest. The skeleton and teeth may endure for many years, especially if buried. Fairly intact skeletal remains of adults and

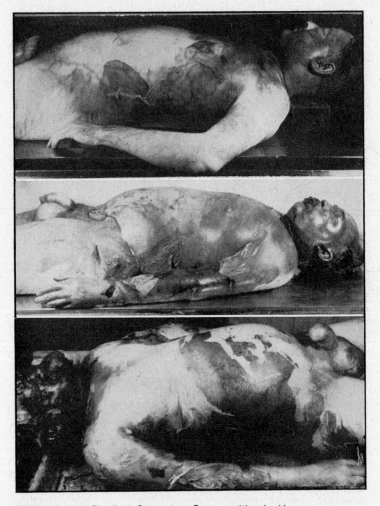

Fig. 4-11. Postmortem Decomposition in Air.

Top. Rapid decomposition with gas formation and discoloration in tissues of head and trunk, staining of superficial veins and separation of epidermis. Body dead 36 hours in bed in warm hotel room. Death from alcoholism; middle-aged white man.

Middle. Advanced putrefaction changes. Obliteration of features, protrusion of tongue and pressure on truss pad by gas in tissues. Body dead in hotel room two days in June. Death from alcoholism; 50 year old white man.

Bottom. Advanced putrefaction. In addition to marked gaseous distension of tissues and separation of the epidermis, decomposed liquefied fat has soaked through the skin of the abdomen to produce large yellowish stained areas (appearing brown in photograph) which on drying have a parchment-like texture. Elderly white man, dead from natural causes one week in a closed room.

children were unearthed during excavation for the foundation of an office building in the center of New York. The site had been an old graveyard abandoned 120 years before. The presence of the putrefactive gases within the brain and cranial cavity, may produce a separation of the sutures of the skull of a young child (Fig. 4-10).

The appearance of the body during bacterial decomposition varies with the circumstances attending the individual case and can be best described in connection with the medium in which it is decomposing; the changes due to putrefaction vary somewhat, depending on whether the remains are exposed in the air, floating in the water or buried in the earth. Regardless of the medium, however, the bodies exhibit in common such phenomena as general distention of the body cavities, tissues and blood vessels with gas, causing a ballooning of the face, neck, trunk, scrotum and penis (Fig. 4-11); and a red, green, brown or black discoloration of the skin, mucous membranes and irides caused by hemolysis and the action of hydrogen sulfide on the blood pigment. The gas in the body cavities exerts a marked internal pressure, causing the eyes to bulge, the tongue to project between the teeth, the lips to protrude in a frog-like fashion, blood to exude from the nose, stomach contents from the mouth and fecal material from the anus. This pressure may cause a postmortem expulsion of the fetus from the pregnant uterus followed by an eversion of the uterus. The gas formation in the blood vessels may force fluid, air or liquid fat between the epidermis and the dermis to produce a big blister which may rupture. The skin epithelium and the hair and nails may be easily separated from the dermis by disintegration at the roots. When the nutrient material is used up, the formation of gas ceases and the swelling gradually subsides; the gas leaves the tissues, usually by escaping as a result of damage to the structure or by drainage through a postmortem wound.

A curious effect of advanced postmortem decomposition is the formation of small miliary granules or plaques, 1 to 3 mm. in diameter, on the serous and endothelial surfaces of the body, such as the pleura, peritoneum, pericardium and endocardium (Fig. 4-12). Morphologically these areas resemble grayish white colonies of bacteria growing on the surface of an agar slant or plate. In a case described by Puchowski the plaques were found to consist of calcium phosphate, calcium carbonates, traces of fat, endothelial cells and bacteria. In cases seen by the authors large bacilli have been the main constituent of such plaques, growing in colonies on the endothelial surfaces with a local production of acid compounds; calcium from the body fluids combines with the acid and is deposited in the colony. The chief medicolegal significance of this finding is that these calcified areas formed after death are sometimes mistaken for inflammatory processes or the effects of a poison.

External conditions either accelerate or retard the rate of bacterial decomposition. A body in a moist warm climate will decompose rapidly because the body temperature is retained longer and the growth of putrefactive bacteria is favored. Similarly an obese, plethoric cadaver will undergo bacterial decomposition readily because the excess of fat slows the dissipation of the heat of the body and the excess of blood furnishes favorable growth conditions for the putrefactive organisms. If death is due to septicemia, *Clostridium welchii* may invade the body soon after death and form gas while the skin is still warm. Any condition which causes engorgement of the intestinal blood vessels will facilitate postmortem bacterial invasion, so that when a corpse is lying prone or in any other posture favoring such congestion it will decompose readily; a body in the supine position is not likely to develop

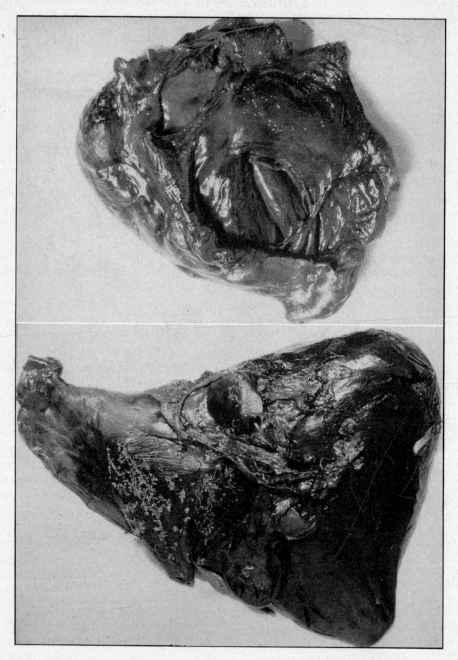

Fig. 4-12. Postmortem Miliary Plaques on Endocardium and Serous Surfaces.

These minute white plaques or granules are formed during advanced putrefaction and are composed of colonies of bacteria and calcium salts. Note location on endocardium of auricle (top) and on serosa on under surface of liver (bottom). They should not be mistaken for an inflammatory process.

intestinal congestion and does not usually decompose with the same readiness. A corpse in the nude condition expands easily with the gas formation and allows a rapid spread of bacteria through the blood vessels so that putrefactive changes are correspondingly rapid. A mutilated body will decompose more rapidly than one

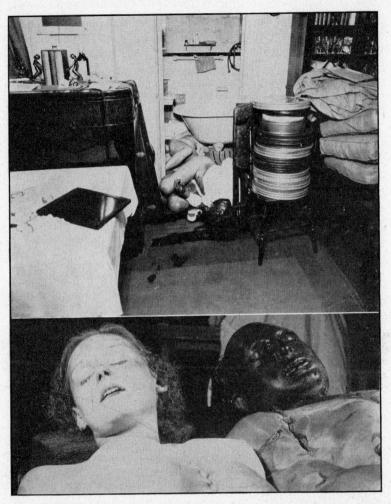

Fig. 4-13. Variations in Postmortem Decomposition in Two Bodies Dead Approximately the Same Length of Time.

Death resulted from slow poisoning by carbon monoxide generated by incomplete combustion in a defective gas-fueled refrigerator. The woman died on the cool tiled bathroom floor, the man with his head on a thick warm carpet, as shown in upper photograph. Postmortem interval about 60 hours. Both subjects white. Lower photograph reveals advanced putrefaction in man, none in woman.

which is intact because the external wounds provide the bacteria with additional points of entrance. In many cases limbs which have been amputated from a body shortly after death will not show as severe a grade of decomposition as the trunk because fewer bacteria have invaded the separated extremity.

The conditions which retard postmortem decomposition are those which hinder the growth of putrefactive bacteria and their spread through the blood vessels. Thus extreme cold is likely to inhibit bacterial putrefaction, especially in an exsanguinated body or in a poorly nourished cadaver which cools rapidly because of the scant amount of blood and fat present. The bodies of newborn infants which have not been fed and are not supplied with the ordinary bacterial flora will generally decompose at a slower rate than the remains of adults. A corpse which is undergoing mummification is not likely to develop extensive gaseous transformation as the drying of the tissues inhibits the invasion and the dissemination of the microorganisms. Similarly a body subjected to external pressure from clothing or from burial in earth or a coffin will not decompose as readily as a nude body because the external pressure prevents full expansion of the tissues and free passage of organisms through the blood.

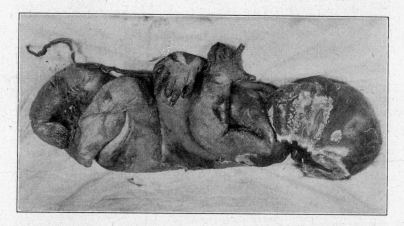

Fig. 4-14. Putrefaction. Mummification and Growth of Mold.

Newborn infant found in bedroom closet three months after death. Strangulation by ligature was suspected but this could not be established with certainty at necropsy. Note growth of mold on face and mummification of fingers and legs.

Any estimation of the postmortem interval based on the degree of postmortem decomposition must necessarily be an approximation. Since varying external conditions will speed or retard the process, it is difficult to select criteria which can be used as a basis for judgment. Not infrequently two or more bodies undergoing bacterial decomposition simultaneously in the same place and apparently exposed to identical external conditions will show different stages of the process (Fig. 4-13). The difficulties of arriving at some approximation of the postmortem interval by a consideration of the extent of the decomposition are hard to overcome.

MUMMIFICATION. Mummification, the desiccation or shriveling of the cadaver from the evaporation of water, is most likely to occur when the body is in dry surroundings like a sandy soil or a cool dry place like a cemetery vault. In ordinary surroundings it is usually preceded or accompanied by, and continues after, putrefaction (Figs. 4-14 and 4-15). The process begins in the exposed portions of the body like the face, hands and feet and then extends to the entire body, including the internal organs. As they are affected the parts become shriveled, shrunken and brown, showing all stages from a light brown to a black depending on whether the tissues are anemic or congested. As the skin contracts some of the fat cells in the subcutaneous tissues are broken and the liquid oil is forced into the dermis which becomes more or less translucent. The eyeball loses its rotundity and becomes flaccid. The internal organs become shrunken, hard, dark brown and black. The entire body contracts in thickness, loses weight and becomes stiff and brittle. If the mummified corpse is not protected, it will crumble gradually into dust from the impact of the outer world; but if it is protected it may be preserved for years. The process takes from 1 to 12 months to become complete, depending on the size of

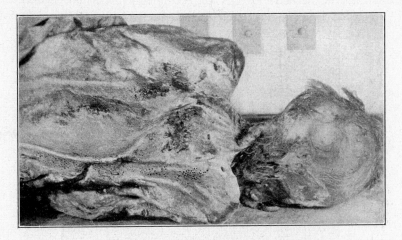

Fig. 4-15. Putrefaction Followed by Mummification.

Perforations made by maggots visible on skin of the back which has since become leathery and mummified. Empty pupa cases were also present. Body of a 65 year old man found in tenement six weeks after death from natural causes.

the body. It is not a satisfactory criterion by which one can measure the postmortem interval unless the examiner has had experience with the process of mummification in that particular district or in the particular circumstances under consideration.

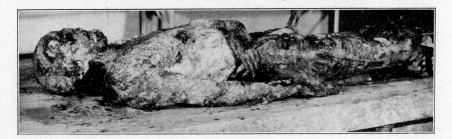

Fig. 4-16. Adipocere Formation on Chest and Upper Extremity in Decomposed Body.

The body was found wrapped in a burlap bag in a sewer. Postmortem interval was uncertain. The deceased was unidentified. The death was due to a bullet wound of the head.

ADIPOCERE. Adipocere, the formation of a dirty yellowish white waxy material in the outer layer of subcutaneous fat, occurs whenever a body has been submerged in water or wet soil for such a long time that it has lost the protecting epidermis and dermis (Figs. 4-16 and 4-17). It is produced by the postmortem decomposition of the fat into the fatty acids. According to one theory these acids combine with calcium and ammonium radicals to form insoluble soaps. Sydney Smith has made certain observations which have led him to believe that adipocere formation is a hydrogenation process in which an unsaturated fatty acid is converted to a saturated one. Adipocere has a rancid odor, floats in water, and dissolves in ether and alcohol; with dilute copper sulfate it gives a light greenish blue color, typical of Benda's reaction for fatty acids.

Adipocere is formed first in the subcutaneous tissues and later in the adipose tissues elsewhere in the body. It does not occur naturally in the viscera or in the nonfatty tissues such as the muscles, but it has been experimentally produced in a

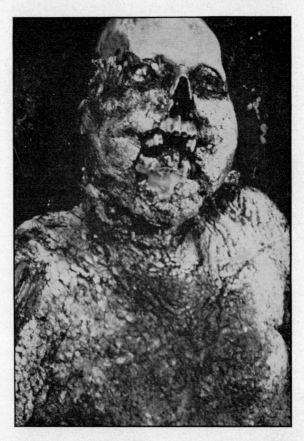

Fig. 4-17. Adipocere Formation After Six Months Submersion in Brackish Water of Hudson River. Note Detachment of Altered Soft Tissues from Top of Head and Jaws.

fatty liver. Adipocere is often associated with bacterial decomposition and according to the observations of Sydney Smith persists when the muscles and viscera have disappeared through putrefaction. It has been estimated that adipocere formation becomes complete in adult bodies in from a year to a year and a half, and in full term newborn infants in from about six to seven weeks; it does not occur in a fetus of less than seven months' gestation because the composition of the fat at that stage is not suitable for its development.

8. **Later Destruction of the Body.** The process of destruction continues until the body is obliterated. The speed with which this occurs depends on whether the body is decaying in the air, in the water or under the earth. The process, more rapid in the air than in the other two media, is expressed by the old formula of Casper, which states that one week in the air is equivalent to two weeks in the water or to eight weeks in the soil.

AIR. The decomposition in the air is caused by bacterial invasion, or by mummification, or by a combination of both. In rare instances other combinations are possible. Strassmann describes the case of a body partially submerged in a marsh with the result that the submerged portion showed adipocere formation and the part exposed to the air, mummification.

The way in which bacterial decomposition develops in the air depends on the postmortem position of the body. If it is lying prone, the blood gravitates to the head, neck and chest; the first signs of swelling and discoloration from gas formation are likely to appear in these regions. If it is lying in the supine position, especially if the head and chest are slightly raised, the gaseous distention and discoloration are most likely to appear in the lower abdomen and upper thighs. In either case the process extends to the entire body, developing as has already been described.

The characteristic features of bacterial decomposition in the air can be ascribed to the relative rapidity of the process and to the fact that the decomposing body is rarely disturbed by the surrounding medium, unless it is openly exposed to inclement weather. The only serious destruction likely to occur is from attacks by animals, birds or insects. The bacteria spread quickly through the blood vessels and into the tissue spaces, and a large amount of gas is rapidly formed. In the early stages the skin may be ballooned out and pale without discoloration, or the superficial veins of the neck, chest, abdomen and thighs may appear as a subcutaneous network stained reddish brown or greenish brown by the hemolyzed blood diffusing through the vessel walls. The pressure of the gas inside the vascular system may rupture some of the smaller subcutaneous vessels and cause in the fatty tissues a postmortem hemorrhage similar to a bruise. The increase of pressure in the body also causes bleeding from the nasal orifices by rupturing vessels in the nose or forcing blood out of the lungs.

Sometimes decomposition is so rapid that blood is quickly destroyed, the skin has a dull greenish gray appearance and the vessels and tissues are filled with gas. In places the gas may be forced out between dermis and epidermis forming large gaseous blisters on the surface; the outer skin layer over these areas may dry and become parchment-like. As the decomposition continues, the internal pressure may rupture some of the subcutaneous fat cells so that liquid fat is released; this may be forced through the dermis, causing an oily translucent patch in the skin (Fig. 4-11c), or it may raise the epidermis, producing a surface bleb filled with oil. When the bacterial invasion is comparatively slow and less blood destroyed, serum, either light yellow or blood stained, may exude into the subcutaneous tissues or cause a blister formation on the surface of the skin. All these different types of blisters tend to remain intact unless the corpse is disturbed, but if for any reason they rupture the denuded area dries and forms a reddish brown leathery patch which contrasts with the green and black discolorations of the intact skin. In the late postmortem stages exudation of fluid may occur in the pleural cavities and seems to be proportional to the amount of fluid present in the decomposing blood, though it is rarely as profuse as in the decomposing drowned cases.

Combinations of putrefaction and mummification frequently occur in cases in which the bacterial invasion and spread is slow. The hands, feet and features of the face may be shriveled and dark while the chest and abdomen are swollen from the formation of gas. On some of these bodies, especially if they are confined in a closet or covered by bedclothes, a growth of mold may be present on those parts which retain a certain amount of moisture, as for example the face, groin, scrotum, penis, perineum and axillae (Fig. 4-14).

If a decomposing body is not disturbed, it is conceivable that the processes of bacterial change and mummification would accomplish its destruction slowly but eventually. In the air the postmortem ravages of animals and insects hasten the process. Blowflies, for example, lay their eggs in any dead body that can be reached by them during the warm weather; the eggs are deposited around such openings as the nose, mouth, eyes, ear canals, anal and genital regions like minute white

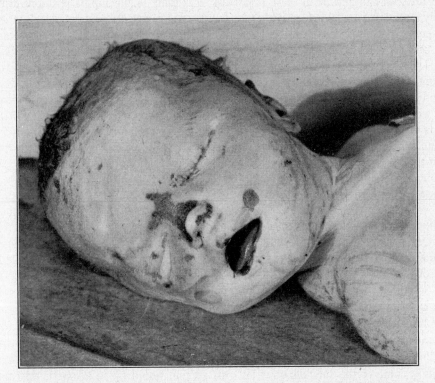

Fig. 4-18. Postmortem Destruction of Skin of Nose and Cheeks by Ants, Abandoned Infant.

stacks of cigars. In from 8 to 14 hours the eggs develop into larvae which burrow into the flesh, excavating large crateriform cavities in these areas. They eat rapidly and if present in sufficient numbers will remove all tissues except the bones in a few days. In the early stages of their invasion the maggots excrete a proteolytic ferment and cause a dirty gray slough to appear on the skin. Sometimes they burrow through the skin causing small perforations which give the impression of a sieve (Fig. 4-15). The stage of the larval development may give some clue to the length of time which has elapsed since death. For example, the eggs of the blowfly are changed into larvae in from 8 to 14 hours and from larvae into pupae after 9 to 12 days; after 12 more days the pupae develop into adult flies. The larvae and pupae of other types of flies develop in similar fashion but in accordance with their own time schedule. In any event if a large number of pupae are present it is reasonably certain that the corpse has been exposed for two weeks or more. For fuller information the reader is referred to the work of Smith and Glaister.

Beetles occasionally lay their eggs in cadavers and their larvae consume the flesh but not so rapidly as fly larvae. Cockroaches may feed to a certain extent on the dead body. Human remains exposed in the open may be attacked by ants which, biting off small pieces of flesh from the soft parts, leave brown serpiginous erosions (Fig. 4-18). The tropical varieties of ants are very efficient in removing flesh from the skeleton.

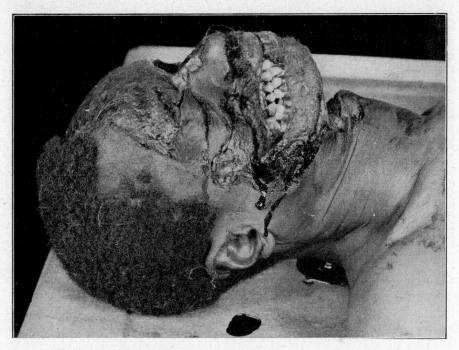

Fig. 4-19. Postmortem Destruction of Soft Tissues of Face and Neck by Rats.

Rats occasionally eat exposed portions of the face and hands where the skin is thin, leaving a characteristic gnawed surface (Figs. 4-19 and 4-20). Birds such as crows and buzzards may peck and tear at exposed cadavers, and the carnivora such as dogs and wolves may devour portions of the flesh. As a rule the marks which they inflict are characteristic and easily identified by the experienced observer.

The following illustrates the anthropophagic nature of dogs under certain circumstances. An elderly woman lived alone with two fox terriers as companions. After she had been missed for nine days, the police entered her apartment and found her remains partly eaten by the dogs. The skull was detached from the body and denuded of its flesh. Through a big hole in the upper part of the trunk near the neck the dogs had entered and devoured most of the internal viscera. Some of the brain still remained in the skull and on chemical examination gave the test for alcohol. The deceased had probably died as the result of ethyl alcohol poisoning and natural causes. After she died the dogs, not receiving any food, fed on the body of their mistress (Fig. 4-21). Another similar case in which after death the flesh from the lower extremity was eaten by dogs is shown in Figure 4-22.

WATER. If a dead body is submerged for any length of time in the water, it undergoes bacterial decomposition, becomes distended with gas and floats on the surface. As a large body of water is a restless medium and the body floating therein is subjected to a continual disturbance, postmortem changes characteristic of these conditions are noted. For example, since most submerged cadavers float face down with the head lower than the trunk, gaseous distention and postmortem discoloration

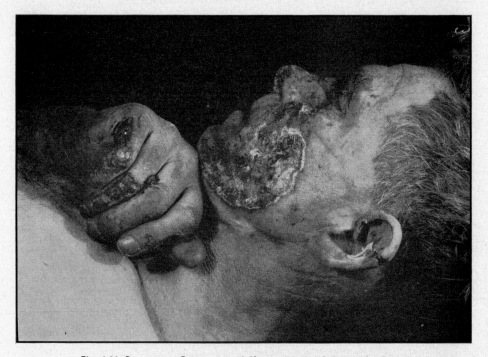

Fig. 4-20. Postmortem Destruction of Skin on Face and Fingers by Rats.

Note shallow defect with scalloped border resembling antemortem ulceration. Compare with Figure 4-19.

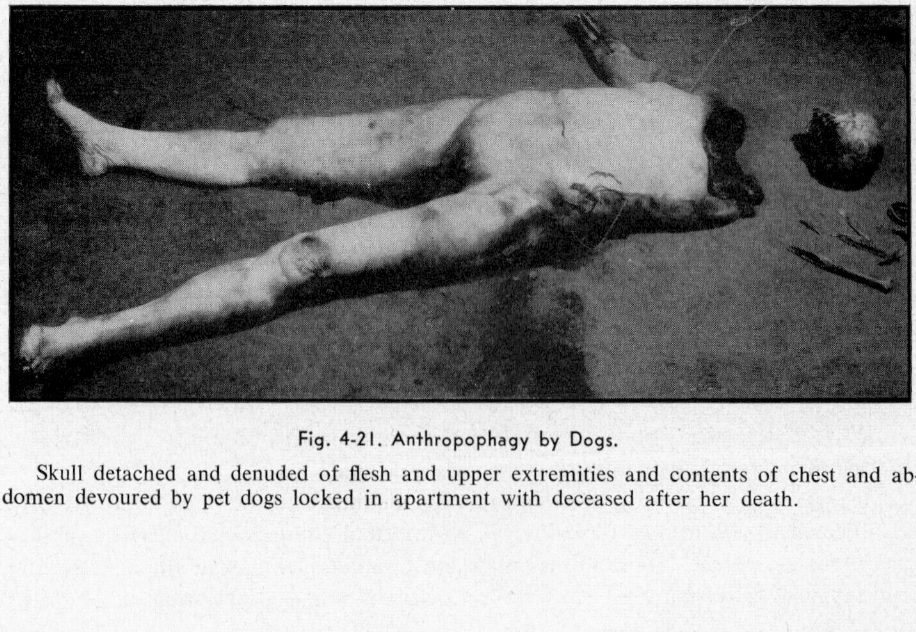

Fig. 4-21. Anthropophagy by Dogs.

Skull detached and denuded of flesh and upper extremities and contents of chest and abdomen devoured by pet dogs locked in apartment with deceased after her death.

consequently occur in that part of the body first. The skin has a pronounced greenish color, but by the constant disturbance in the water the epidermis is removed, leaving slimy, macerated raw areas. After the body is removed from the water, these areas become dry, brown and parchment-like. The epidermis of the hands and feet be-

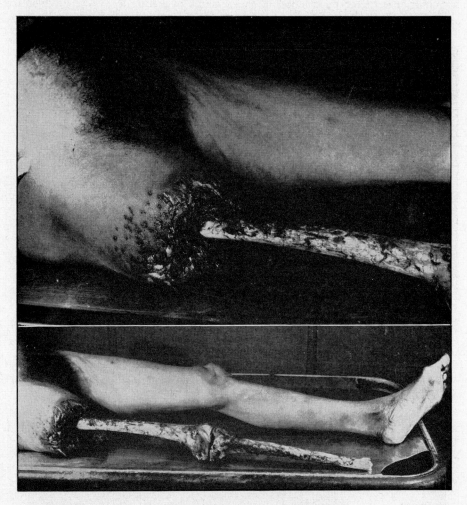

Fig. 4-22. Canine Anthropophagy after Homicide.

The deceased was stabbed through the chest and the dead body lay on a sofa with the right lower extremity hanging down. A pet dog, locked in the same room, devoured the right lower extremity as shown. Note teeth marks on the skin of the remaining portion of thigh in upper close-up photograph.

comes swollen, bleached and wrinkled after immersion (Figs. 4-23, 4-24, 18-17) and when the decomposition has reached a certain stage may be removed as a cast of the extremity (Figs. 4-25, 4-26, 4-27). The changes in the epidermis are more constant than the general rate of decomposition and may be used by an experienced observer to determine approximately the length of time that the body has been submerged. After several weeks in the water, macerated flesh may be stripped from the hands, forearms, legs, feet and face by the action of currents or the contact with floating objects (Fig. 4-28). If submersion has endured for a sufficient length of time, especially near a sewer, adipocere formation may occur. The internal findings in decomposing submerged bodies will be discussed in Chapter 18.

Bodies exposed to running water in a stream may collect a slimy growth of algae on the surface. Fish and crustacea and water rats in the vicinity of a sewer may contribute to the destruction of the remains by eating away the flesh of the ears, eyelids and lips, leaving gnawed areas (Fig. 4-29). Occasionally the ravages

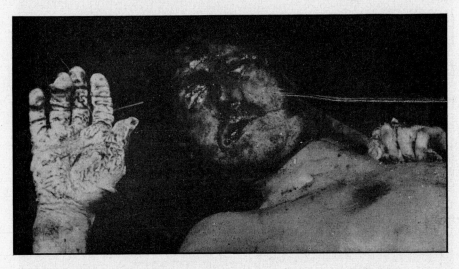

Fig. 4-23. Sodden, Bleached, Partly Detached Skin of Hands of Floater.
Decomposed body recovered from Hudson River after one week's submersion early in June.

are extensive. In the case of a man whose body was submerged for two weeks in June off the Long Island coast, the skeleton alone remained; fish and crustacea had eaten away the soft parts and the viscera. The rapid destruction of a submerged body in warm August weather is illustrated in Figure 4-30. The body of the 12 year old white boy was recovered from the Hudson River 12 days after

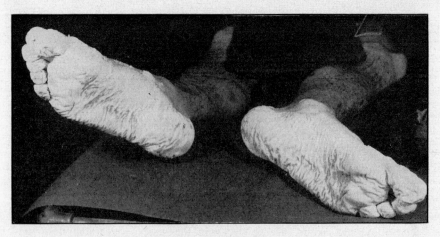

Fig. 4-24. Sodden, Bleached Feet of Floater.
Feet were covered with shoes and socks. Same case as Figure 4-23.

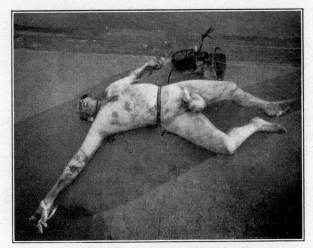

Fig. 4-25. Putrefaction in a Submerged Body, a Floater.

The deceased was shot twice through the head, after which the body, weighted down by 150 pounds of granite block, steel elevator cable, and packing wire was dumped in the river. Putrefactive gases produced in the tissues floated the body and its heavy anchor to the surface. See Figures 4-26 and 4-27.

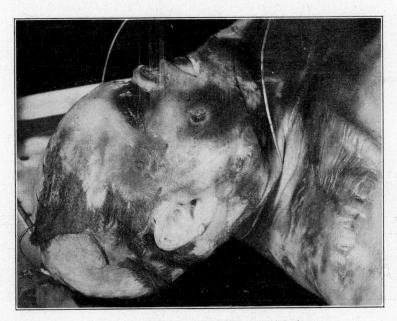

Fig. 4-26. Putrefaction in a Submerged Body.

Same case as in Figure 4-25. Postmortem decomposition has distorted the appearance of the body and facies but has not obliterated a large bullet wound on the right cheek and a smaller one posterior to the angle of the jaw.

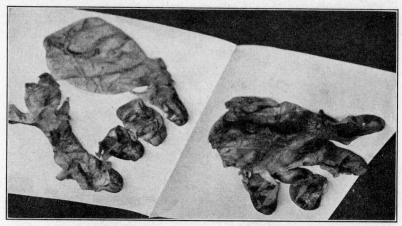

Fig. 4-27. Same Case as in Figure 4-25.

Identification of the deceased was made by the Police Department from fingerprints obtained with these shells of loosened skin peeled from the fingers. See Figure 3-6.

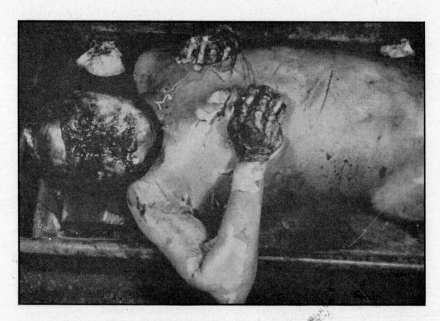

Fig. 4-28. Postmortem Decomposition Due to Prolonged Submersion.

Body recovered in April, 10 weeks after suicidal drowning in Hudson River. Identification by laundry marks on clothing and by appendectomy scar. Note loss of soft tissues of face and parts of fingers from macerating action of water.

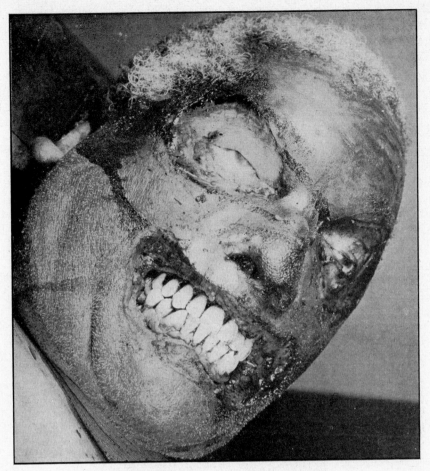

Fig. 4-29. Postmortem Mutilation of Face of Submerged Body.

Soft tissues around eyes and mouth eaten by water rats. Body submerged three days in Hudson River near sewer opening.

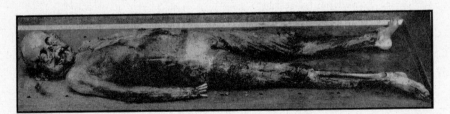

Fig. 4-30. Rapid Destruction of Submerged Body in Summer.

Body of 12 year old white boy recovered from river in mid-summer, 12 days after accidental drowning. Note almost complete skeletonization of head, loss of fingers and of soft tissues from legs, exposed bones of hands and relatively good preservation of feet protected by shoes.

accidental drowning. Most of the soft tissues had disappeared from the head and the teeth had loosened and dropped out of their sockets. The bones of the hands were exposed.

EARTH. The process of disintegration is slow after burial in earth because the temperature is low, the body usually clothed and not disturbed. Various combinations of mummification and bacterial decomposition occur. In the early stages mold may grow on the parts not mummified and extract water from the body, thus aiding

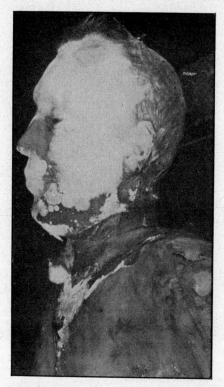

Fig. 4-31. Growth of White Mold on Interred Body.

Body of 47 year old white man, buried four months, from September to January, exhumed on insistence of relative who suspected foul play although autopsy in hospital had shown death was caused by bacterial endocarditis.

the mummification and delaying the decomposition of the underlying and internal tissues (Fig. 4-31). The ravages of fly and beetle larvae sometimes occur and accelerate the destruction.

Destruction of the body by fire and chemicals will be discussed in subsequent chapters.

CONDITIONS PRESERVING THE BODY

Embalming is a process applied to the body for the purpose of preservation. It consists in removing the contents of the gastrointestinal tract, the bladder and the blood vessels by a trocar and suction apparatus through a puncture wound of the abdomen, and then in injecting the vascular system with embalming fluid containing formaldehyde among other constituents. By this process the proteins are coagulated, the tissues are fixed, the different organs are bleached and hardened and the blood is converted into a brownish mass. The process stiffens the body, obscures many pathologic conditions and makes diagnosis difficult at autopsy.

The result of embalming depends on how soon the process is started after death and how thoroughly the remains are injected with the embalming fluid. If the preservative is introduced long after death and does not permeate the tissues, the body will exhibit a mixture of bacterial decomposition and mummification and will disintegrate in a few months. On the other hand if the injection is made shortly after death and performed efficiently, postmortem decomposition is inhibited. The remains can be preserved indefinitely if they are kept moist with an antiseptic solution; but if they are put into a grave they will mummify and slowly disintegrate.

Some conditions which occur in nature favor the preservation of the dead body. A hot dry climate in desert country predisposes to mummification; and if the body is not disturbed it will keep intact for centuries. Similarly, if it is frozen soon after death and kept in that state, it will remain in good preservation for decades. After they are thawed out such bodies decompose rapidly.

Bodies which have been in water or soil containing antiseptic substances sometimes become impregnated with these materials and do not decompose. As an example, well preserved human remains were recovered from a salt well at Salzburg where they had been reposing for 40 years. The salt had infiltrated all the tissues and had prevented postmortem decomposition from taking place. Some poisons are said to inhibit decomposition and retard bacterial changes, among which may be mentioned arsenic, zinc chloride, antimony and phosphorus.

Human remains in excellent states of preservation have been found from time to time in the bogs of different European countries. In 1873 in a peat bog at Omagh, the waters of which were reputed to contain numerous antiseptic substances, a body was discovered with the skin and its appendages well preserved and tanned, but the bones and viscera were not found; it was estimated that the body had been in the bog for about 100 years. In the bogs on the European continent similar human remains have been encountered, apparently preserved by various acids present in the water. The skin, nails and hair were well kept but tanned a deep brown; the bones and teeth retained their contours but were discolored and decalcified; the muscles and fat were not present and most of the internal viscera were destroyed; part of the clothing was intact and helped occasionally to identify the period when the body was submerged, in some instances, a matter of centuries.

ESTIMATION OF THE POSTMORTEM INTERVAL

As already noted, the signs of death develop at different intervals and vary widely under diverse circumstances. It is not always possible to tell with any degree of certainty from an examination of the body just how long an individual has been dead. The most that can be done is to consider the circumstances and calculate their effect on the development of the different signs of death. For example, it is important to know the temperature of the surroundings and whether or not the body is clothed before the investigator can use the loss of body temperature as a criterion for estimating the postmortem interval. Specific rules cannot be formulated on this subject for the guidance of an examining physician.

The scene of death may yield an important clue which will be helpful in estimating the postmortem interval. Such items as the dates on mail or newspapers, the degree of coagulation of milk in a milk bottle or the state of food on a table may be valuable indications of the time that has elapsed. The condition of the parasites on a dead body not infrequently give information of considerable moment; for example, lice on a cadaver live from three to six days, and if they are all dead, it is fair to assume that death had taken place more than six days prior to the time of the examination.

A remarkable example of advanced postmortem decomposition that went undiscovered for 11 months is shown in Figure 4-32. The putrefied, mummified, partly pulverized and skeletonized body of an old man was found in bed where death had occurred from natural causes 11 months before. The death certificate issued by the physician at that time was found on the

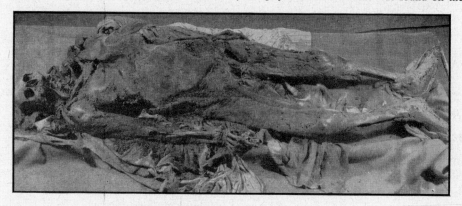

Fig. 4-32. Advanced Postmortem Decomposition in Unburied Body.

Mummified, partly skeletonized, putrefied body of an old man found in bed where death occurred from natural causes 11 months before.

dresser in the room where the body lay. The widow who kept the body at home continued to collect old age pension checks made out to the deceased during the entire time.

If the body is found in the open, the condition of the surroundings may furnish significant clues. For example, in the spring and summer grass and other plants under the body may lose their chlorophyll after eight days and appear pale; and

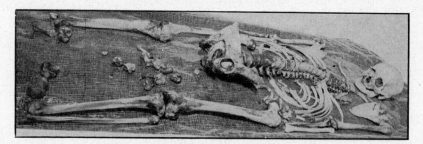

Fig. 4-33. Rapid Skeletonization of Body Exposed Outdoors in Warm Weather.

The remains of a 65 year old man, skeletonized by the ravages of insects and animals, found in a gully in October, three months after his disappearance. Identification was established through the clothing and laundry marks.

certain insects which seek dark places may congregate under the cadaver. In the winter time the condition of the clothing and of the ground under the body may help to establish its position in that neighborhood in relation to the most recent rainstorm and snowfall.

The unusual rapidity with which a body exposed outdoors in warm weather to the ravages of insects and animals can be completely skeletonized is illustrated

in Figure 4-33. The remains, including some dried scalp tissue and hair, clothed
in trousers, underwear and shirt were found in a gully on a farm colony for old
people on Staten Island and identified as those of a 65 year old inmate who was
afflicted with Parkinson's disease and had wandered off and disappeared three
months before.

The conditions found in the gastrointestinal and urinary tracts at autopsy sometimes furnish the investigator with a hint concerning the time of death. For example,
a body is found dead in bed; the circumstances and signs of death fail to disclose

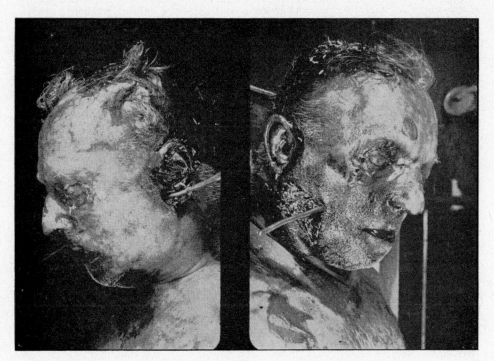

Fig. 4-34. Spurious Character of Apparent Postmortem Growth of Hair.

The body was discovered several days after death, considerably decomposed and infested
with maggots. A probe is inserted through a fatal bullet track in the head. The left side of
the face was on a pillow, the right side uncovered and exposed to the air. Note apparent
growth of gray hair on right side due to drying, and the smooth shaven appearance on the
undried out left side.

the postmortem interval with any degree of certainty. If the autopsy shows an empty
stomach, a rectum distended with feces and a bladder full of urine, such facts suggest that death occurred in the early morning before the hour of rising.

When the circumstances of death cannot be ascertained, the condition of the
food in the stomach and upper small intestine of the deceased may furnish information concerning the interval of time which has elapsed between the last meal and
the time of death. In the earlier stages of digestion, the stomach usually contains
gross particles of masticated food which later are converted into a mushy chyme.
In about two to four hours on the average, the chyme is emptied gradually from the
stomach into the duodenum where it is digested further; then it is transferred to
the upper end of the jejunum where some of its components are absorbed, especially fat which entering the chyle vessels gives them the appearance of being injected
with milky fluid. The duration of the digestive process varies within wide limits,

depending on the amount and character of the food ingested, the activity of the gastric juice and the physical condition of the deceased; in many instances when a person is suffering from severe cerebral concussion, undigested food may be present in the stomach after a period of coma of more than 24 hours. The findings in the upper gastrointestinal tract must be interpreted with caution and must be correlated with other important information concerning the death of the victim before an attempt is made to determine the duration of the digestive process in his stomach and intestines. Undigested food in the stomach at the time of death will remain recognizable for many weeks post mortem and has been helpful in identifying the badly decomposed remains of persons whenever information has been obtainable in reference to the last meal of the deceased.

The condition of the beard may help to establish a relationship between the time of death and the last shave of the deceased. Hair grows about 0.5 mm. a day during life but does not grow after death, contrary to popular folklore on the subject. The observations on the state of the beard must be made during the first 24 hours post mortem because after this the skin shrinks and the hairs may project more above the surface of the chin at 48 hours post mortem than at the time of death.

An interesting case illustrating that the apparent growth of hair is spurious and not real was encountered recently. The deceased, a white man of late middle age, had been shot dead through the head. The body was not discovered until several days later at which time considerable postmortem decomposition including infestation with fly maggots was evident. The left side of the face was on a pillow; the right side was uncovered and exposed to the air. As a result considerable drying had occurred on the right side which revealed an apparent short thick growth of gray beard hair. The spurious character of this apparent growth was shown by the smooth clean shaven appearance of the left side of the face which had been in contact with the pillow and thus protected from drying out (Fig. 4-34).

REFERENCES

Ewing, J. The Signs of Death, in Peterson, Haines and Webster, Legal Medicine and Toxicology, Philadelphia, W. B. Saunders Co., 1923, Vol. 1, pp. 175-209.

Gabriel, M. Die bisherigen Ergebnisse der Moorleichenforschung, Deutsche Ztschr. f. d. ges. gerichtl. Med., 15:226, 1930.

Herzog, A. Medical Jurisprudence, Indianapolis, The Bobbs-Merrill Co., 1931.

Koenig. Berl. klin. Wchnschr., 27:1212, Dec. 22, 1890.

Lancet, June 7, 1873, p. 817.

Merkel, H. Über Todeszeitbestimmungen an menschlichen Leichen, Deutsche Ztschr. f. d. ges. gerichtl. Med., 15:285, 1930.

Puchowski, P. Diagnostische Schwierigkeiten bei einen auf Vergiftung verdächtigen Falle, bedingt durch ungewöhnliche Fäulnisveränderungen, Deutsche Ztschr. f. d. ges. gerichtl. Med., 15:532, 1930.

Puppe, G. Atlas und Grundriss der gerichtlichen Medizin, J. F. Lehmann, 1908.

Reese, J. J. Textbook of Medical Jurisprudence and Toxicology, 8th ed., revised by D. H. McCarthy, Philadelphia, P. Blakiston's Son & Co., 1911.

Smith, S. Forensic Medicine, London, J. and A. Churchill, 1940.

———— and Glaister, J. Recent Advances in Forensic Medicine, 2nd ed., Philadelphia, P. Blakiston's Son & Co., 1939.

Strassmann, F. Lehrbuch des gerichtlichten Medizin, Berlin, Ferd. Enke, 1931.

Webster, R. W. Legal Medicine and Toxicology, Philadelphia, W. B. Saunders Co., 1930.

Williams, H. A. Human paleopathology, Arch. Path., 7:839, 1929.

5

The Medicolegal Autopsy:
Determination of the Cause of Death

THE MEDICOLEGAL AUTOPSY

The next investigation meriting consideration because of its importance in a medicolegal case is the autopsy. It differs in one fundamental particular from the autopsy performed on the body of a person who, under medical care, died of a natural disease condition and whose relatives have permitted this type of examination. In a consent autopsy, since a clinical history is usually present and the cause of death suspected, if not generally known, by the clinicians, the chief duty of the pathologist is to describe and study the pathologic conditions revealed by his dissection. In a medicolegal autopsy the medical examiner, in addition, must determine the cause of death, often without any clinical history or clue to guide him except the lesions of trauma or disease which he discovers post mortem. The correct appraisal of these lesions, as to whether they were innocuous or dangerous to life, is the duty of the medical examiner. When he has completed the autopsy and has received reports of all laboratory investigations, he must give his opinion concerning the conditions which were responsible for the death of the individual.

The cause of death is sometimes difficult to determine. To solve this problem it is necessary, in addition to performing an autopsy, to obtain all the information possible about the circumstances of the case. The testimony of relatives, of medical attendants and of bystanders may be important, especially with regard to the manner of death and the clinical manifestations which preceded it. An investigation of the scene of death is necessary, especially if there is any suspicion of foul play. In any doubtful case a complete autopsy should be performed, supplemented by histologic, microscopic, chemical, bacteriologic and serologic examinations. The difficulties of determining the cause of death will be discussed more fully later in this chapter.

The technic employed in performing the autopsy will now be described, and the various laboratory examinations used as aids in this investigtion will be considered.

Apparatus. The first requisites for an autopsy are proper equipment and tools. A table, three feet in height, broad enough to hold the organs after their removal, with running water and an adequate system of drainage, is necessary. The drains should be protected by wire mesh of sufficient fineness to prevent the loss of bullets and other small objects. There should be a large scale for weighing the body, smaller scales for weighing the organs, a measuring tape, short rulers and a 2 liter graduated container for measuring fluids.

The tools may be of any variety that can be used for the performance of the dissection. The types which are preferred in the Office of the Chief Medical Examiner of New York are as follows:

KNIVES. A large, curved, full-bellied knife with a slightly rounded point, used for the dissection of soft parts and for the section of brains.

A short knife with a straight, flat, but strong blade and a moderately sharp point, much like a knife used for paring potatoes. This is used for cutting costal cartilages, disarticulating joints or similar operations.

Scissors. A large pair of blunt, pointed scissors and an enterotome which is a pair of scissors with one projecting end covered by a blunt knob.

A small pair of scissors with one blunt end, to be used for opening small blood vessels or ducts.

Saw. The ordinary hand saw employed by a carpenter to be used for removing the skull cap or sawing bones in general.

Chisel. A chisel with a thin, but strong, flat blade, necessary for prying off the skull cap and for entering the spinal canal.

Hammer. A moderately heavy hammer or mallet to be used for driving in the chisel.

Forceps. A small pair of forceps for grasping tissue.

Costatomes and Bone Cutters. Surgical style.

Probes. A fine probe for exploring small ducts. A straight metal sound one-quarter inch in diameter for exploring bullet tracts. A curved urethral sound.

Any other instruments can be used as desired. Those just enumerated are sufficient for performing a comprehensive autopsy and have the advantage of being few in number.

Photographic equipment should also be available. This should include a sturdy view camera mounted on a heavy tripod capable of taking a 4 by 5, or 5 by 7 inch picture, and suitable lamps that can be moved about for the best illumination. In addition to photographs in black and white, color photographs can be taken at the same time with a 35 mm. camera fitted with a sliding focusing attachment. Such color transparencies are very valuable for recording wounds, lividities, corrosions and postmortem decomposition. They are easy to take and inexpensive.

Apparatus for photographing and developing roentgen ray films is a necessary part of the equipment at autopsy. Such films are useful in locating bullets in homicidal shootings and in demonstrating old fractures, bony deformities, ossification centers and other features necessary for identification.

Technic. The first part of the autopsy consists of the external examination and the second part, the dissection of the body. In performing the autopsy any technic which will serve the purpose is permissible, as long as it is compatible with a systematic and comprehensive examination of the body. The following scheme has been found useful in the autopsy work at the City Mortuary, New York City, principally because it can be varied to meet the unusual case. It is similar in many respects to that described in Delafield and Prudden, *Textbook of Pathology,* and other textbooks.

During the dissection the pathologist should dictate the findings to a stenographer who takes them in shorthand and later transcribes them into a regular typewritten protocol.

External Examination. First the body is weighed in the nude. Then the height of the body is measured from the top of the head to the bottom of the heels.

General Description. This includes sex, age, color, race, bony frame, deformities, stature, muscular development, nutrition, color of skin, presence of skin diseases, hair distribution on body, scars, tattoo marks, operation scars, moles, lymph node enlargements and any other points the pathologist may deem important.

Signs of Death. Absence of body heat, color and distribution of postmortem lividity, presence or absence of rigor mortis, signs of decomposition, postmortem lesions and similar signs.

Regional Description. The following scheme is useful:

Head. Scalp, hair (color, texture, length, bald spots and so forth).

Eyebrows.

Eyes: color of iris, presence of opacities like arcus senilis or cataract, condition of conjunctiva, presence of glass eyes, petechiae.

Ears: size, deformities and other characteristics.

Nose: size, shape and deformities.

Mouth: general condition, including state of teeth.

Teeth. In cases in which a record of the teeth is especially important, a form diagram of both jaws, indicating the definite abnormalities in each separate tooth, will give the most accurate record.

Extremities. All abnormalities should be described, as old fractures, amputations, scars, abnormalities of nails or calluses.

Trunk. Same as extremities. The presence or absence of hernias should be noted.

Genital Organs. Condition of penis in male and vaginal outlet in female.

Wounds. External wounds and other injuries should be placed in a section by themselves. They should be systematically arranged, taking up each section of the body in turn. The form, location, depth and nature of the various injuries should be given with accurate measurements. This matter will be discussed later under the headings of the various types of trauma.

A satisfactory method of recording wounds and other abnormalities is by means of drawings or diagrams, in which the lesions can be sketched in their proper form and proportions. Photography in black and white and in color should also be employed for this purpose.

Internal Examination. THE TRUNK. The incision should start a short distance below the suprasternal notch and run in the midline to just above the symphysis

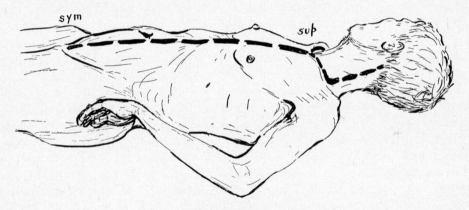

Fig. 5-1. Autopsy Incisions on Trunk.

Incisions indicated by dashed line: sym, symphysis pubis; sup, suprasternal notch. Routine incision is from sup to sym. Lines on side of neck indicate incisions for exposing neck organs.

pubis. Near the midpoint of the abdomen the cut is directed to the left of the navel (Fig. 5-1). The skin and the muscles are dissected away from the ribs on either side by rapid knife strokes. The recti muscles of the abdomen are divided about two inches above the symphysis by incising them from the peritoneal side. The abdomen is exposed adequately by this procedure and a description is made, noting the thickness of the panniculus, the condition of the recti muscles, the amount of fat in mesentery and omentum, whether or not fluid is present and if an abdominal inflammation is present. The abnormalities and position of the abdominal organs are described and, in addition, adhesions, old operations, pathologic processes, injuries and the height of diaphragm in relation to the ribs are noted. If blood, pus or any other fluid is present its quantity is measured.

The small intestine is separated from the mesentery by cutting it close to its insertion with a sawing motion of the knife. After this the large intestine is freed from its attachments. Both large and small intestines still joined to each other are removed, the upper and lower ends are tied and the intestines are set aside.

The chest is opened by severing the costal cartilages at their junctions with the ribs and then disarticulating the sternoclavicular joint on each side. The sternum is separated from the diaphragm and anterior mediastinum by dissection. The sternal plate with the costal cartilages is removed from the front of the chest. The sternoclavicular joint is disarticulated by cutting downward from the top of the joint and then cutting outward at right angles; these joints and the first costal cartilages are not cut until the pleural cavities are inspected, for fear of contaminating them with blood from severed innominate vessels. In this examination all abnormalities are noted and the parietal and visceral pleuras are described. Any blood, pus or fluid contained in the chest is measured.

The pericardium is opened and the outside of the heart is examined. Any blood, pus or fluid present in the pericardium is measured. All abnormalities are noted and recorded.

The procedure of opening the heart is started with the organ in situ. At this point specimens of blood should be collected from one of the cardiac chambers if chemical, serologic or bacteriologic examination of the blood is desired. In cases of drowning, blood is drawn from the right and left side of the heart for the determination of the sodium chloride content of the blood in each circulation. This process is described in greater detail on page 487.

The first incision into the heart starts at the apex of the right ventricle and extends up its anterior surface alongside the interventricular furrow into the pulmonary artery. The purpose of this is to see whether a pulmonary embolus is blocking the pulmonary artery. The contents of the right ventricle, right auricle and inferior vena cava are described, as to whether they are composed of fluid blood, currant jelly clot or chicken fat clot. Some antemortem emboli may be dislodged from the pulmonary artery by postmortem manipulation and be found in the right heart. Large emboli may be present in the right auricle and drop out of the inferior vena cava when it is cut across. An incision is made in the posterior lateral wall of the left ventricle, parallel with the interventricular septum, and the contents of the left side of the heart described in the same way.

The heart is removed by severing the larger vessels near the pericardial reflexion. The right side of the heart is opened by slitting the right auricle, between the inferior and the superior venae cavae, and then extending the incision through the tricuspid orifice down the posterior wall of the right auricle and ventricle to the apex until it joins the incision already made in situ. The left side of the heart is opened by severing the left auricle between the two sets of pulmonary veins. An incision is carried down through the mitral orifice along the posterior lateral wall of the left auricle and ventricle to the apex; from this point it is carried close to the anterior interventricular furrow up the left ventricle through the aortic valves into the aorta. The incision should pass between the pulmonary artery and the appendages of the left auricle and should not injure the anterior leaflet of the mitral valve.

After the heart is opened the chambers and the valves can be examined. Any peculiarities of the endocardium, valves, the papillary muscles, chordae tendineae or the myocardium should be menitoned. Any special hypertrophy of the different chambers, any abnormal openings like a foramen ovale or a perforate interventricular septum, any hemorrhages under the endocardium or in the myocardium and, in fact, any condition which seems of importance ought to be recorded.

The coronary vessels are examined by slitting them with the fine pair of scissors or by making serial cross incisions down the course of the vessels about 4 to 5 mm. apart. This latter method enables one to demonstrate the narrowing of the vessel and any antemortem thrombus in its lumen. The condition of the arteries should be described and any obstruction of the lumen noted. The myocardium should be examined carefully and the muscles of the left ventricle incised in a plane parallel to the epicardial and endocardial surfaces; this incision will reveal infarction and fibrosis most clearly.

The aorta should also be examined and abnormalities mentioned. It is important to note whether there is any chronic aortitis with plaque formation which obstructs the mouths of the coronary arteries.

The heart should be weighed and measurements taken of the circumference of the valves and of the thickness of the right and left ventricles. These notations are helpful in completing the description of the heart and give the pathologist data by which he can appraise its abnormality.

In cases in which death was the result of a severe hemorrhage, the ventricles of the heart can be incised transversely midway between the apex and the base. The contraction of the muscles and the narrowing of the ventricular lumen are demonstrated plainly by this method.

When an examination of the thoracic duct is indicated the right lung is shifted to the left, so that the right side of the thoracic spine is exposed. The thoracic duct is located by making an incision between the aorta and the vena azygos major.

The lungs are removed by severing the bronchi and the vessels of the hilus. They are examined by opening with the scissors first the pulmonary veins, then the bronchi and lastly the pulmonary arteries. The contents of the bronchi are noted as to whether they contain blood or mucus. The parenchyma may then be sectioned with the knife. Pneumonic areas, injuries and other pathologic processes are described and measured. Each organ is weighed separately.

After the lungs have been removed, the approximate amount and character of the blood which has flowed into the chest cavity from the large blood vessels is noted. The presence of much yellow postmortem clot would suggest an infectious disease or a high fibrinogen content in the blood. Fluid dark red blood in large quantity would indicate a death by asphyxia or some other form of sudden death. In death by hemorrhage the blood would be scant. In cases in which the patient has been unconscious for a period of several days the blood would be dark and thick from dehydration.

Circumstances may cause the pathologist to modify his technic of examining the chest organs. In cases of multiple bullet wounds involving both heart and lungs, it is best sometimes to remove these organs together with the vascular and tracheal attachments intact so that the wounds through the viscera can be traced more easily.

Cases of pneumothorax are demonstrated before the chest wall is penetrated. A pocket is dissected on the affected side between the chest wall and the skin and is filled with water. A costal interspace is perforated with the knife under water, and if air under pressure is present, it will bubble out of the opening through the water.

If air embolism is suspected the technic of opening the chest and the abdomen is modified so that the presence of air in the circulation can be demonstrated. The abdomen and the chest are exposed, care being taken not to injure the viscera and blood vessels in these cavities. Accordingly, the sternoclavicular joints and the cartilages of the first two ribs are not disturbed for fear of cutting the vessels in the upper chest. The pericardium is cut and the heart exposed. The abdomen and the pericardial sac are flooded with water. Air embolism is demonstrated in the abdominal vessels by puncturing the inferior vena cava under water, whereupon bubbles of air will escape from the submerged vein. In the same way the chambers of the heart can be punctured under water to show the presence of air in the cavities. The presence of air in the right ventricle will cause the heart to float, requiring forcible submersion to carry out the test.

The spleen is removed by severing the hilus. It is weighed and sectioned, and the character of parenchyma, follicles and septa noted. Injuries and pathologic conditions are described.

The liver is removed by itself or it is taken out attached to the stomach and the duodenum. The latter method is used whenever it is desirable to inspect the bile ducts. The pathologist cuts away the diaphragm on each side, strips the esophagus from its bed, and by going behind duodenum, pancreas and liver, separates the entire group of organs. The esophagus is opened on the left side by the enterotome, which also slits the stomach along its greater curvature and cuts the anterior surface of the duodenum. The contents of the stomach are described, the wall is examined and all abnormalities noted. The duodenum is treated in the same way.

After this the common bile duct is opened with the fine pair of scissors. It can be entered from the duodenum by means of a fine probe inserted into the papilla of Vater, or it can be entered by nicking the duct as it descends from the liver toward the pancreas. The portal vein and the hepatic artery can be explored at the same time.

The pancreas is examined and is sectioned as desired. All abnormalities should be noted. Mention should be made of areas of fat necrosis, if any are present.

Fat necrosis is demonstrated by adding a 20 per cent aqueous solution of copper sulfate to the suspected lesion. If fatty acids are present the necrotic area turns a bright greenish blue from the formation of copper oleate. This is known as Benda's reaction.

The liver is separated from the duodenum, weighed, measured and sectioned. The gallbladder is opened and described. The presence or absence of gallstones is stated.

Some livers contain a large deposit of hemosiderin which is demonstrated by Perle's reaction. A saturated solution of potassium ferrocyanide is poured upon the cut surface of the liver and then a 0.5 per cent solution of hydrochloric acid in 70 per cent alcohol is added. The presence of an iron-containing pigment is indicated by the development of a deep Prussian blue color.

If deposits of amyloid are to be tested for in organs like liver, spleen or kidneys, a solution of Gram's iodine is poured on the cut surface of the organ; any areas of amyloid which may be present will turn a dark mahogany brown in appearance. If this surface is moistened with dilute sulfuric acid, the color of the deposits changes to red, violet and finally blue, or the brown color may deepen in intensity.

The small intestines are slit by the enterotome near the mesenteric insertion. The large intestine is opened by the enterotome on its anterior surface. The character of the intestinal wall and the condition of the intestine are described.

Mention of the stomach contents and of the intestinal contents should be a routine procedure in every case. In most instances the information would not be significant, but occasionally it might be extremely important. In a homicide case in which the body of the deceased was partly destroyed by fire and decomposition, an identification was made by the contents of the stomach. The food in the stomach of the cadaver corresponded to the food which the deceased was known to have eaten at his last meal. The stomach contents, especially fruit and vegetable fragments, preserve their characteristics for months post mortem.

The adrenals are removed, examined and sectioned. The kidneys are shelled out of their bed with the ureters still in place but with the vessels severed. In some cases in which a thrombus of an artery or vein or an embolus of an artery is suspected, the vessels can be opened in situ prior to severance. After holding the kidney in alignment with its ureter a longitudinal incision is made from the lateral edge of the cortex into the hilum, exposing the pelvis. The ureters can be slit by the fine scissors as far as desired. The capsule is stripped from the kidneys and the cortex, external surface, pelvis and ureters described. If necessary, the kidneys may be removed attached by the ureters to the bladder and the pelvic organs. If there is no indication for this technic, the kidneys are severed from their attachments, stripped of all extraneous tissue and weighed, either separately or together.

The bladder, rectum and pelvic genitalia are separated by dissecting them away from the inside of the pelvis and removing as much of the pelvic outlet as seems desirable. In a case of rape the whole perineum from symphysis to os coccyx is removed. In the male the membranous urethra is cut usually, but occasionally it may be desirable to remove some of the penis and urethra by dissecting under the pubis and into the penile sheath. Care is taken to separate only the posterior portion of the penis and not to damage the organ too much, so that reconstruction will be possible.

The testes are examined by widening the spermatic canal just under the skin and forcing the testes upward through the openings. They are sectioned and described. The epididymides should be examined at the same time.

The bladder is opened from the fundus and the incision is carried into the urethra. The bladder wall and the amount and the character of the urine are described.

The prostate is sectioned and described. The seminal vesicles are exposed by incising the pelvic peritoneum and separating the bladder from the rectum. Their condition is noted.

The female genital organs are examined by removing the rectum or the bladder from the vaginal wall and slitting the vagina and the uterine cavity, anteriorly or posteriorly, up to the fundus. Two short incisions are made in the fundus, from the main longitudinal incision toward each cornu, in order to expose the endometrium. The ovaries are examined by sectioning them longitudinally with the knife. The tubes are examined by cutting cross sections at intervals. The dimensions of the uterus are recorded; and inflammation, signs of pregnancy or instrumentation are carefully noted. The condition of the ovarian veins is best examined prior to the removal of the kidneys and pelvic organs.

Wounds in the organs of the abdomen or pelvis must be described carefully and measured.

THE NECK. The organs of the neck are examined, in some instances by incising the trachea and the larynx in front and noting whether or not the air passages are obstructed. This method will suffice in cases of death due to natural causes or obvious injuries elsewhere in the body, but it is not applicable to cases of manual strangulation or lesions involving the neck organs. Here it is necessary to remove the air passages and associated structures like the thyroid gland and the thymic body. This is done by prolonging the incision around the base of the neck on each side or straight up to the chin. The organs are dissected away from the skin on the front and the sides and from the spine in the back. The attachments of the tongue to the lower jaw and of the throat to the bones of the palate and the pharynx are then severed. The entire contents of the neck can be removed then, en masse; the specimen should contain tongue, hyoid bone, soft palate, tonsils, pharynx, larynx, thyroid, thymus, muscles and vessels of the neck. The pharynx, esophagus, larynx and trachea can be opened from the posterior surface. The carotid arteries can be opened with the scissors. The thyroid gland and the thymic gland can be removed and weighed. The structures are described in detail and all abnormalities noted.

THE HEAD. The knife, saw and chisel are used to open the head. The first step is an incision in the scalp which starts behind one ear and is carried over the vertex of the scalp to the back of the opposite ear. If the head is bald on top the incision, for cosmetic reasons, can be carried posteriorly behind the bald patch (Fig. 5-2).

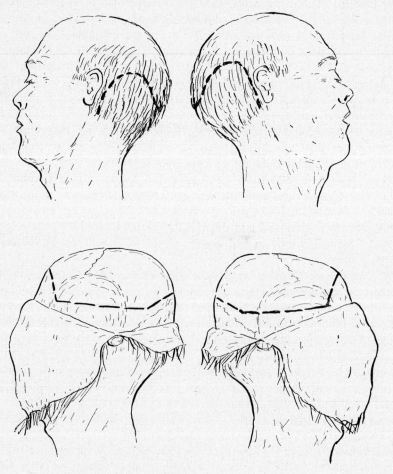

Fig. 5-2. Autopsy Incisions on Scalp and Skull.

The incisions are indicated by the dotted lines.

The scalp is then stripped from the skull by means of the chisel and knife until the top, front, back and sides of the cranial vault are exposed. The scalp, bone and temporal muscles are examined for injuries and other abnormalities. If a fracture of the skull is located on the vault it is traced as far as possible to the base, if necessary incising the temporal muscle in the process.

The top of the skull is removed by using the saw in a cut of six sections. One cut runs horizontally along the side of the skull, cutting the parietal bone at a level about one-half inch above the squamous portion of the temporal bone. It is made on both the right and left side. The front end of the cut should terminate in the lateral frontal region, and the posterior end should be located slightly behind and below the parietal boss on that side. From the front extremity of each lateral incision a cut is made which is directed forward and upward in such a way that the two meet in the midline about three inches in front of the coronal suture. From the posterior extremity of each lateral incision, two other cuts are directed backward and upward behind the parietal boss; these should meet in the midline just above the top of the lambdoidal suture (Fig. 5-2).

If it is desirable to keep the dura intact the saw should be used carefully and should not penetrate beyond the bone. The chisel is inserted, and with a few gentle taps of the mallet the calvarium is loosened and removed. The dura is exposed and the middle meningeal arteries are visible on its surface. Epidural and subdural hemorrhages can be discovered easily, and if any intracranial tension is present that fact will be evident. The superior longitudinal sinus is incised and its contents noted. If any intracranial hemorrhage is present the blood should be collected and measured.

The dura is incised parallel with the saw cut and the falx cerebri is cut in front. The brain is separated by cutting the vessels and nerves as they emerge from the skull, beginning with those in front and extending back to include the upper end of the spinal cord. The tentorium is severed carefully along the posterior border of the petrous bone, and the brain is removed.

The dura is then stripped from the base of the skull and a search is made for basal fractures. The dural venous sinuses should be opened with the fine pair of scissors. The bony cavities like the middle ear, mastoid, sphenoid and frontal sinus are opened from above by a sharp broad-bladed chisel. The pituitary and its fossa are examined.

The brain, after being weighed, can be sectioned by a number of methods, depending on the pathologic conditions present. The most useful routine method is to examine the outside of the brain and record all abnormalities on the surface, noting especially injuries, meningeal conditions, atrophy or flattening of convolutions or lesions of the circle of Willis. Then the brain is placed with its base on the table and a horizontal section is made through the organ about halfway between upper and lower surfaces. At this level the basal ganglia, lateral ventricles and white matter are exposed symmetrically by the section; and such lesions as cerebral hemorrhages or symmetrical areas of softening in the corpus striatum in carbon monoxide poisoning can be demonstrated to best advantage. This horizontal section produces a minimum of distortion of the brain tissue and allows the specimen to be fixed more satisfactorily if its preservation is required. The chief advantage of the method is that it enables the pathologist to expose a fatal lesion in the brain and determine the cause of death at the autopsy table, at the same time allowing preservation of the specimen for future use. Examples of this technic are shown in Figures 6-16, 6-25 and 33-1. The pons is incised transversely, just below the cerebral peduncles, and the cerebellum is cut horizontally or vertically as desired.

THE SPINAL CORD. The spinal cord is removed most easily from the back. An incision is made extending from the base of the skull to the sacral region, and the muscles are dissected away from the top of the spinal column. The laminae are sawed through the entire length of the spine on each side of the spinous process and are separated from the column by a little prying with the chisel. The spinal dura is exposed and is removed with the cord by severing the nerves from below up as they pass through the spinal foramina. When this process is complete the cord is separated at the foramen magnum. The cord usually is sectioned transversely and serially. If desirable it can be preserved for further investigation by fixing in 10 per cent formalin or Muller's fluid.

Fractures and luxations of the spine can be investigated satisfactorily by making a sagittal cut through the bodies of the vertebrae in situ either from the front of the spine in the case of a lumbar fracture, or from the rear in the case of a cervical fracture. The bones can be pried apart by the chisel and the extent of the fracture noted.

THE LOWER EXTREMITIES. The vessels of the lower extremities are examined best by longitudinal incisions made on the front or on the back of the leg, depending upon the part to be exposed. If the veins of the lower extremity are to be examined, a long incision on the back and the inner part of the thigh, extending from the popliteal space to the natal fold, will expose the vessels satisfactorily. If the head of the femur is to be examined an incision along the contour of the bone in front or back will allow the pathologist to reach the hip joint and disarticulate it. The knee can be exposed by incising the skin on the sides of the thigh and connecting them by a cross cut just under the patella. In a case of severe anemia the lower end of the femur is sawed upward in a longitudinal direction so as to expose the marrow cavity.

Injuries and other important lesions of the viscera can be depicted by drawings and photographs.

Laboratory Procedures. HISTOLOGIC TECHNIC. The tissues examined routinely under the microscope are lung, liver, pancreas, myocardium and coronary arteries, aorta, diaphragm, bronchus, adrenals, stomach, intestines, bladder, thyroid, thymus, especially in young people, testes and prostate in the male, uterus, tubes and ovaries in the female, pons or medulla with basilar artery, meninges, cortex of brain, basal nuclei of brain, bone and any other tissue which appears abnormal or is suspected of being abnormal. If an encephalitis or a poliomyelitis is suspected, tissue from different parts of the brain and cord is sectioned. In a case of rabies, tissue from the hippocampus and cerebellum may be sectioned. If the case is one of septic abortion, pieces of the uterus, ovary, mammary gland, ovarian veins and uterine veins are added.

The following method is a convenient routine procedure for preparing the tissues for histologic examination:

1. Fix the tissues in 10 per cent formalin, 24 to 48 hours.
2. Cut smaller pieces 2 mm. thick for sectioning.
3. Place in 80 per cent alcohol, 6 to 12 hours.
4. Place in acetone, 6 to 12 hours.
5. Place in clove oil until the tissue becomes clear.
6. Place in a thin solution of celloidin, made with equal parts of absolute alcohol and ether, 6 to 24 hours.
7. Place in a thick solution of celloidin, made with equal parts of absolute alcohol and ether, 6 to 24 hours.

After the specimens are embedded they are removed from the celloidin, mounted on section blocks and floated on a bath of chloroform. In two hours the chloroform will extract clove oil from the specimen and harden the celloidin so that it is ready to section. The sliding microtome is used to cut the sections, which are kept in 95 per cent alcohol. If preferred, the tissue can be prepared for section by the paraffin method.

The sections are stained by the following process:

1. Delafield's hematoxylin, 3 to 5 minutes.
2. Wash in water.
3. Decolorize rapidly until salmon pink in acid alcohol (5 per cent solution of hydro-chloric acid in 80 per cent alcohol).
4. Wash in water.
5. Dilute ammonia water, 0.5 per cent, 1 to 3 minutes until blue.
6. Wash in water.
7. Eosin, 1 per cent aqueous solution or 10 per cent alcoholic solution (95 per cent alcohol), 3 to 5 minutes.
8. Wash in 95 per cent alcohol, mount on slide and blot with blotting paper.
9. Add oil of thyme until clear, blot with blotting paper and mount in xylol balsam.

If the tissue is a piece of bone or a calcified coronary artery, it may be decalcified by the method recommended by Kolin. The tissue after fixation in the formaldehyde solution is allowed to stand at room temperature in a 5 per cent solution of glacial acetic acid in water, freshly prepared, until the pieces of tissue can be cut readily with a razor blade. This may require several weeks for pieces of dense bone; the process does not disturb the staining reaction of the tissue. The excess acetic acid is washed out in water and the segments for sectioning are subjected to the process outlined previously.

If the sections disclosed any pertinent facts connected with the cause of death, a report describing the microscopic appearance of the viscera should be made and attached to the autopsy protocol. Chorionic villi in the uterus, inflammatory areas in the meninges and the brain, trichinae in the muscles and neoplasms are the types of lesions generally discovered by the microscopic examination.

When fat embolism is suspected, frozen sections of formalin-fixed tissues are stained with a saturated solution of Sudan III in 70 per cent alcohol. The fat globules in the blood vessels of the different organs will be demonstrated plainly by this method. The section then is counter-stained in Delafield's hematoxylin, the fat appearing as bright red globules in the midst of bluish stained tissues. The same technic can be used to demonstrate fatty infiltration in the paren-chymatous cells of different organs. The Marchi method employing osmic acid will provide permanent preparations.

In degenerative processes in the brain or spinal cord, such as tabes dorsalis, injuries to the cord and similar lesions, the tissues are preserved in Müller's fluid (potassium dichromate 2.5 parts, sodium sulfate 1 part, water 100 parts). After two weeks' fixation the specimens are treated by the Marchi method, the Pal-Weigert stain or any other method which will demon-strate the degeneration of the tracts.

BACTERIOLOGIC EXAMINATION. Since many pathogenic microorganisms are diffi-cult to isolate, a well equipped bacteriologic laboratory, a supply of specially pre-pared media and the services of a competent bacteriologist are necessary. The more common bacteria, however, can be identified by relatively simple methods. Thus, as a routine measure, in a case of suspected septicemia, the spleen, heart's blood or any likely focus of infection is cultivated under sterile precautions.

The heart's blood is obtained by searing the unopened right ventricle in situ with a red hot spatula and perforating this area with a sterile pipet or a sterile syringe. A few milliliters of blood are withdrawn from the ventricle and mixed with melted nutrient agar (which has been cooled to 40° C.). The mixture is made in a sterile petri dish and is incubated for from 1 to 2 days. Colonies of an infecting organism grow in the blood agar.

The technic of cultivating the spleen is to sear the surface of the organ with a hot spatula, puncture the seared area with a sterile instrument and scrape out some of the unheated splenic pulp. Some of this is smeared on a blood-agar plate which is then placed in the incubator for from one to three days. Another portion of the splenic pulp is smeared directly on a glass slide and stained with Gram's stain.

When the colonies have developed upon the blood-agar plate, a few of them are smeared on a glass slide and stained with Gram's stain. The stained smear of the infected tissue is compared with the smear of the growth on the blood-agar, as a check against error through contamination.

The appearance of the colony on the blood-agar plate, combined with the results of the Gram stain, will enable the pathologist to recognize the more common septic invaders. The Gram stain, a valuable routine stain in bacteriologic work, is carried out as follows. The reagents are:

Aniline gentian violet (distilled water, 98 ml.; aniline oil, 2 ml. Filter, and to 75 ml. of the clear filtrate add 25 ml. of saturated alcoholic solution of gentian violet).

Gram's iodine (iodine, 1 gm.; potassium iodide, 2 gm.; distilled water, 300 ml.).

Carbolfuchsin (carbolic acid crystalline, 5 gm.; basic fuchsin, 1 gm.; 95 per cent alcohol, 10 ml.; distilled water, 100 ml. Dilute 1 to 20 with water for use as a counter stain).

Procedure. Fix in flame or with absolute methyl or ethyl alcohol. Stain in aniline gentian violet 3 minutes; wash in water. Gram's iodine, 2 minutes; wash in water. Decolorize in 95 per cent alcohol 1 minute. Dilute carbolfuchsin (1:20), 1 minute; wash and dry. Gram-positive organisms stain blue, gram-negative organisms, red.

Smears of pus from the urethra are stained with Gram's stain and the gonococci are demonstrated as gram-negative, biscuit-shaped diplococci in the polymorphonuclear leukocytes. Meningococci can be demonstrated in the pus from the meninges. The gonococci and meningococci must be cultivated on specially prepared media.

Inflammatory membranes in the throat are cultivated on a blood-agar plate and a Loeffler blood serum tube. The blood-agar colonies will demonstrate the presence of hemolytic streptococci. The Loeffler blood serum is incubated from 18 to 24 hours, and then a smear of the culture is stained about 3 minutes with Loeffler's alkaline-methylene blue (saturated alcoholic solution of methylene blue, 30 parts; an aqueous solution of 1:10,000 caustic potash, 100 parts). This method demonstrates the diphtheria bacillus with its characteristic metachromatic granules.

Secretions, exudates and tissues are smeared on a slide and stained for tubercle bacilli by the following method:

Ziehl-Neelsen carbolfuchsin, 5 minutes' steaming by heat.
Decolorize with acid alcohol, 2 minutes.
Counterstain with methylene blue.

The tubercle bacilli appear as long thin red rods against a blue field.

If the pathologist is dealing with a case of suspected typhoid fever, paratyphoid or dysentery, the most convenient method is to cultivate the infected material on a plate of Endo's medium or on nutrient agar containing basic fuchsin, sodium hyposulfite and lactose. When freshly prepared it is transparent pink in color. The infected material, whether splenic pulp, feces, urine or bile, is diluted with broth and then smeared upon the surface of the medium. After 24 hours' incubation the plate is examined. The colonies of bacteria which ferment lactose, such as the colon bacillus, are an opaque red, while those which do not ferment lactose, like the typhoid bacillus, form a small pearly white colony. The organism must be identified, however, by further cultivation on sugar media and by agglutination reactions with specific diagnostic sera.

Smears of brain cortex, spleen, and liver are stained sometimes with Giemsa's stain or Wright's stain to demonstrate malarial parasites. Negri bodies are searched for in the cells of the hippocampus when rabies is suspected. Smears of the bone marrow from the ribs are stained with Wright's stain in cases of blood dyscrasias.

Smears from chancres and mucous patches are examined fresh by the dark-field method or stained with Giemsa's or Fontana's stain to demonstrate spirochetes. The Levaditi method may be used on tissues.

The examination for spermatozoa will be discussed in Chapter 24.

It may be desirable in some cases in which a virus disease is suspected to save a piece of the brain or other appropriate tissue, depending on the suspected virus, for laboratory injections into animals. The tissue is collected under sterile precautions and preserved in 50 per cent sterile glycerine. The use of brain tissue would be indicated in cases of encephalitis and lung tissue in a disease like psittacosis.

Microscopic examination of feces for parasitic worms, ova and amebae is indicated in some cases. Cyst fluids are examined for echinococcus hooklets.

Chemical examinations for poisons are frequently necessary in medicolegal autopsies. The organs and materials which should be removed for this purpose and the technic of analysis will be discussed in detail in Chapters 37 through 42. When serologic examinations are indicated, the blood should be removed from the heart. Group determinations on blood and seminal fluid, important in some cases, will be dealt with in the chapter on blood groups.

The preservation of gross specimens is best accomplished by the Kaiserling method, which preserves much of the natural color. The technic is as follows:

(1) The specimen is trimmed and filled out with absorbent cotton to preserve its contours and cavities.

(2) It is then placed in a large volume of the fixing solution for two to seven days or longer, depending upon the nature and bulk of the specimen. The fixing solution is made of:

Formaldehyde (40 per cent)	200 ml.
Water	1,000 ml.
Potassium nitrate	15 gm.
Potassium acetate	30 gm.

(3) After thorough fixation the specimen is washed in running water and placed in fresh 80 to 95 per cent alcohol for one to six hours. The alcohol bath, to a great extent, will restore the original color to the specimen.

(4) After the color has been developed, the specimen is placed in a final preserving solution made of:

Potassium acetate	200 gm.
Glycerine	40 ml.
Water	2,000 ml.

In all laboratory examinations which might be introduced in court, care should be taken to extend the chain of identification from the autopsy table to every examiner and technician who is concerned with the tests. This will be discussed at length later.

THE EXAMINATION OF EXHUMED BODIES

Autopsies are performed on exhumed bodies for the following medicolegal purposes:

1. The prosecution of criminal cases such as homicides, suspected homicides disguised as suicides or other types of death, suspicious cases of poisoning and deaths as a result of criminal abortion, malpractice or negligence.

2. The determination of the cause of death in civil court cases such as accidental death claims, double indemnity insurance, workman's compensation claims, liability for malpractice, negligence or torts, survivorship and inheritance claims.

Two unusual examples of inheritance claims were encountered. In one a claim of inheritance was made by a 40 year old alleged illegitimate son, which finally resulted in an autopsy 3 years post mortem on the exhumed body of a spinster to determine whether or not she had ever borne a child. In another case the claims put forth in relation to an estate by the alleged children of a decedent forced an exhumation to substantiate the contention of the administrator that the intestate was castrated during infancy and incapable of begetting children. (State ex rel Meyer v Clifford 78 Wash. 555.)

The laws governing disinterments vary in different states. In some jurisdictions an exhumation for autopsy in a civil case requires in addition to written consent of the next of kin, a permit from the local health officer or the registrar of vital statistics. In other places the state health department is in control. Permits for the exhumation in criminal cases are issued by a justice of a court of record on request of the state attorney general, district attorney or other responsible official. In some localities the coroner is empowered to order an exhumation. In New York State the authority for granting permits for exhumations in both civil and criminal cases is vested in a Justice of the Supreme Court.

The exhumation in a criminal case is usually preceded by the complaint of an individual to the local district attorney that the death of his relative or friend was attended by foul play or suspicious circumstances. This official causes an investigation to be made and decides whether the evidence warrants an application to the court for disinterment and autopsy. In civil cases the exhumation for autopsy is requested by an interested party who later may become the plaintiff or defendant in a legal action arising out of the death; and the disinterment order is issued by an official who has the authority in that particular jurisdiction. In such cases written permission for exhumation and autopsy must be provided by or obtained from the next of kin of the deceased. Most insurance policy contracts providing indemnity for accidental death contain a clause giving the insurance company the right to demand an autopsy on the body of the deceased if a claim for accidental death benefits is made. In cases in which misrepresentation by the insured or suicide is suspected within the contestable period of two years after the issuance of the policy, the right to demand an autopsy from the next of kin is not provided in the contract.

After the necessary authorizations are obtained and arrangements made with the cemetery officials, the body is disinterred and delivered, usually by a licensed funeral director engaged for the purpose, for the examination and autopsy. The autopsy should be performed by an experienced pathologist familiar with the postmortem appearances in this type of case. In civil cases, it is customary for each of the parties with a legal interest in the results of the autopsy to have a pathologist present as a medical observer to represent them during the procedure. The pathologist responsible for the autopsy should provide a competent stenographer to whom he can dictate aloud all of the findings. The pathologists observing the autopsy should either indicate their agreement with the observations or express their disagreement or request that the autopsy record be amended to include additional information.

In suspected criminal cases, in which the exhumation and autopsy are carried out at the direction of the prosecuting attorney, after the body is disinterred and properly identified, the autopsy is performed by a pathologist designated by the district attorney. It is advisable in such cases to have another physician, preferably a pathologist, present as a witness to the procedure. In the event that there is no suspect or defendant prior to the autopsy, the question of a medical witness for the suspect or defendant does not arise. If there is a defendant or suspect, whether or not a medical witness is permitted to represent him at the autopsy is at the discretion of the prosecuting attorney.

Identification of the corpse in exhumation autopsies is as important as in any other medicolegal case. All the criteria discussed in the chapter on identification apply to the disinterred body. In addition the inscription borne by the name plate on the casket, the characteristics of the casket, the location of the burial plot and the grave number are duly recorded as aids to identification. If the funeral director who has charge of the exhumation is also the one who originally buried the body, he may identify the remains on the basis of his burial records. In cases where the features of the corpse are recognizable, any person who knew the deceased during life can view the body and make a formal identification.

The body is removed from the casket and divested of its clothing which should be examined and described, noting color, fabric, maker's labels, laundry and cleaners marks and other points of importance. If it is considered necessary for identification, finger prints may be taken and a chart made of the teeth. The body is measured and weighed. The weight of the body at the time of disinterment is less than its weight at the time of death, because of the loss of fluid post mortem by dehydration or other processes; this weight loss is dependent on so many variable factors that it is not practicable to use it for the purpose of calculating the weight of the corpse at the time of death.

Bodies Well Embalmed. The preservation of an exhumed body depends upon whether it has been well embalmed, whether the burial ground was dry or moist, and whether the disease or condition causing death favors postmortem putrefaction. The principle of the embalming process is to withdraw blood and other fluids, such as stomach and intestinal contents, urine and serous effusions, from the body by means of a large hollow needle called a trocar which is attached to a suction apparatus, and then to inject embalming fluid through the trocar into the body cavities or to inject it through a cannula into the vascular system and to drain the blood out of the blood vessels through a cannula introduced into another blood vessel. The chief constituent of embalming fluid is a solution of formaldehyde which causes coagulation of protein, hardening, shrinking and stiffening of the tissues and a bleaching of the muscles and parenchymatous organs. In a well-embalmed case, this process will extend to all parts of the body.

In the autopsy protocol on an exhumed embalmed body there must be a brief but sufficient description of any embalming incisions, trocar punctures or other marks which an embalmer might make on the body externally. The marks made by the trocar on the internal organs must also be described, especially if there is any question of antemortem traumatic injury in the case. The abdominal trocar puncture is usually found in the epigastrium as a circular hole about $\frac{3}{16}$ inch in diameter. Through this opening the trocar is directed in all directions puncturing and lacerating most of the organs and structures in the chest and abdomen. These postmortem punctures are characteristic, and in case of doubt may be distinguished from antemortem wounds by histologic examination which would demonstrate lack of intravital reaction. Embalmer's incisions are made over large blood vessels in the lower part of the neck in front, in the axilla and groin and are for the purpose of exposing the vessels so as to drain out blood and inject embalming fluid.

The embalming process, by removing blood and other material from the body, by producing numerous trocar punctures, and by the bleaching and hardening action of the embalming fluid, produces numerous artefacts and may make difficult the recognition and appraisal of pathologic changes. For example, large hemorrhages in the chest and abdomen may be removed by the trocar and thus interfere with the determination of the amount of blood loss. On the other hand, small hemorrhages in the fascial tissues or inhaled blood areas in the lung are not disturbed. In a well-embalmed body definite gross pathologic lesions like lobar pneumonia, coronary arteriosclerosis, cirrhosis of the liver and many neoplasms are easily recognizable; but some inflammatory lesions in the early stages like a suppurative leptomeningitis or a fibrinous pleuritis may be obscured by the embalming and be demonstrable only by histologic sections.

The hardening action of the embalming fluid may produce a number of artefacts which may be wrongly interpreted by the inexperienced observer. The voluntary muscles over the body may be stiffened by the action of the embalming fluid and may be mistaken for persistence of rigor mortis. The formaldehyde solution may have a coagulative action on the blood in the coronary, cerebral and pulmonary arteries and in some of the veins, producing reddish brown clots which resemble antemortem thrombi. In some instances the embalming fluid may produce discrete or diffuse hardened areas in the lung tissue which simulate, and have been mistaken for, pneumonic infiltration. All these artefacts can be detected by histologic examination which reveals their postmortem origin.

In medicolegal cases traumatic injuries like bullet wounds, stab wounds, blunt force injuries and other forms of trauma which leave definite, demonstrable lesions may be readily diagnosed in spite of the embalming. On the other hand cases of smothering, carbon dioxide asphyxiation, drowning and some cases of ligature strangulation, in which the diagnostic signs are not always obvious, may be difficult to identify in the exhumed body as their characteristic appearances may be obscured by the embalming process. In a case of submersion, use of the trocar and injection of the preservative fluids would make impossible the sodium chloride determinations in the blood from the right and left hearts and the examiner would have to rely upon evidence indicating that water had been inhaled into the bronchi, as for example the finding of minute algae, microscopic water animals or sand in the finer air tubes. Air embolism can not be demonstrated in embalmed bodies because of the disturbances created by the trocar punctures and the injection of fluid.

Embalming interferes with the detection and isolation of volatile poisons such as alcohol, paraldehyde, chloroform, cyanides and chloral hydrate. Many organic nonvolatile compounds are affected in the same way with the exception of strychnine and the barbiturates, which are more resistant to decomposition. Other poisons which can be recovered from embalmed bodies are the heavy metals and their salts, radioactive compounds and carbon monoxide. Even where the poison is detectable, the fluid injected into the body during embalming will dilute and diffuse the toxic substance so that quantitative estimation is made difficult. When a suspected poison case is exhumed, pieces of the sod from the burial plot, pieces of the casket and its trimmings, the wrappings and clothing from the body should be retained for chemical analysis. These precautions are important in case a claim is made that a poison found in the body came from the sources above mentioned. It is also essential to ascertain the composition of the embalming fluid used in a suspected case of poisoning for the same reason. In some states the composition of the embalming fluid is fixed by law.

The embalming process does not prevent the growth of molds (Fig. 4-31) on the exposed surfaces of the hands, the head, face and neck, and on moist portions of the body, the axillae and the external genitals. Most of these fungi belong to the genera *Aspergillus, Penicillium, Mucor* and others, and are colored white, yellow, green, blue and brown. As they grow they extract water from the adjacent tissues and when scraped from the skin leave a smooth dry or slightly moist surface. If they grow for a long period they produce a mummified appearance in the involved area but do not exert a destructive effect on the body. Occasionally molds are found in the internal viscera as an adventitious finding without producing any tissue reaction or more rarely as part of a pathologic fungus disease which is usually accompanied by a definite inflammation.

The larvae of the *Sarcophaga,* the blowfly and of the carrion beetles are inhibited by the embalming fluid so that the destructive effects of these scavengers are not frequently observed in well-preserved subjects. The larvae, pupae and adult forms of small dark-colored flies about the size of fruit flies are encountered occasionally and when the body is exposed to the air, the adult flies, after first showing great activity, rapidly disappear.

The well-embalmed body is preserved for a long time and even the internal organs remain in good condition and provide good material for histologic sectioning and staining. Sooner or later mummification sets in and the body dries and shrinks according to the description given on pages 66 and 67. The drying of the brain in a well-embalmed body causes it to separate from and shrink away from the anterior surface of the dura.

Bodies Poorly Embalmed. If the body has not been thoroughly embalmed, the changes which it undergoes are usually a combination of bacterial putrefaction and mummification. Mummification is usually evident on the exposed parts such as the hands, feet and features of the face; a growth of mold may also be present. Putrefaction is most often seen in parts not affected by the embalming fluid and is most evident on the abdomen and chest. There is a varying degree of swelling of the trunk, discoloration and desquamation of the skin, liquefaction of the subcutaneous fat which develops a rancid odor and other signs of slow disintegration. In some cases there may be partial destruction of the corpse by fly larvae or beetle larvae already mentioned, except where they are deterred by the embalming fluid. In cases in which the brain has not received embalming fluid it is found at autopsy as a putrescent mass.

Bodies Not Embalmed. The body not embalmed undergoes putrefaction, mummification or a combination of the two, depending upon the conditions in the body and in the grave. This process has been described on pages 69 and 70. If the coffin contains water the body may show adipocere formation on those parts submerged. If blowfly eggs or beetle eggs accompany the body into the coffin, the body may be stripped to a skeleton in a few months.

DETERMINATION OF THE CAUSE OF DEATH

In determining the underlying cause it is necessary to keep in mind that the actual production of death is due to some interference with the oxygen cycle, or rather with the functions of the organs which maintain the oxygen cycle. These organs are: (1) medullary centers; (2) blood; (3) respiratory organs; (4) circulatory system.

(1) When the medullary centers are damaged the respiratory movements cease and the oxygen cycle stops. A pure example of this type of interference is noted in cases of bulbar poliomyelitis.

(2) The oxygen cycle is damaged and death may occur whenever the blood loses its oxygen-carrying power, either through loss of red corpuscles as in a hemorrhage from a chronic duodenal ulcer or through degeneration of red blood cells as in severe anemia or by the formation of carboxyhemoglobin in carbon monoxide poisoning.

(3) The prevention of the oxygen interchange between the air in the alveoli and the red blood cells in the pulmonary capillaries results in asphyxia and is a fairly frequent cause of death. An example of this occurs in drowning.

(4) Death may be caused by the failure of the circulatory system to deliver sufficient blood to maintain the oxygen supply to the vital organs. An example of this type of death is noted in sudden cardiac collapse resulting from extensive coronary artery disease.

As Orth has explained, the interference with the oxygen cycle sets in motion a series of changes which finally ends with a paralysis of the vital centers in the medulla and a cessation of respiration and heart beat. In some deaths the cardiac muscle fails first and the respiratory movements continue for a few seconds after the heart beat has apparently ceased. In other cases, as in death from asphyxia or any other noxious action of the respiratory center, the heart may continue to beat for a few minutes after the respiratory movements have stopped.

The scheme of the oxygen cycle is a convenient way in which to present the pathologic physiology of death; but it cannot be used as a basis for a classification of the causes of death as now conceived in the terms of etiologic factors and pathologic entities. Most causes of death affect more than one of the component organs which are concerned with the oxygen cycle; for example, lobar pneumonia may produce a bacterial toxemia which paralyzes the respiratory center, damages the heart muscle and even affects the oxygen-carrying power of the blood; it may also cause some mechanical interference with respiration and a certain amount of asphyxia. It would be difficult to fit lobar pneumonia into any classification based on the oxygen cycle.

The classification of causes of death now used in vital statistics is based on etiologic factors and pathologic entities. It includes such general categories as infectious diseases, diseases of the central nervous system, circulatory system, respiratory system, digestive system, urinary system, genital system, skin, metabolic diseases, intoxications, poisons and traumas. The physician who fills out a death certificate should use terms which conform with such a classification, avoiding all terms which denote symptoms or symptom complexes and endeavoring to fit his diagnosis to a recognized pathologic condition. In some instances it is sufficient to mention the disease, for example, typhoid fever is in itself an adequate description of the cause of death. Other conditions may need qualification; for example, cirrhosis of the liver may necessitate the addition of "esophageal varices, spontaneous hemorrhage into the gastrointestinal tract" as a further explanation of the complication which produced death. For further discussion of the death certificate the reader is referred to Chapter 37.

A study of the yearly reports compiled by the Office of the Chief Medical Examiner in New York City indicates in a general way the main categories of the different causes of death and their relative frequency in the metropolis. The figures in Table 5-1 are yearly averages calculated on the basis of the 33-year period from 1918 to 1951; the total numbers of deaths in New York City are taken from the Department of Health Reports by calculating the yearly averages from 1918 to 1951 inclusive.

Table 5-1. Deaths in New York City

	YEARLY AVERAGE
Total number	76,513
Number investigated by the Office of the Chief Medical Examiner	15,699
Natural deaths	8,227
Violent deaths	5,594
Stillbirths	185
Abortions	85
No cases *	952

* Deaths reported as Medical Examiner's cases but rejected as such after investigation.

Table 5-1 indicates that the Office of the Chief Medical Examiner investigates from 19 to 20 per cent of all deaths in New York City. Further scrutiny of these figures reveals that violent deaths or deaths due to external causes (including abortions) comprise about 8 per cent of the total number of deaths while natural deaths are over 92 per cent of the total. Of the fatalities investigated by the Medical

Examiner, 60 per cent are due to disease conditions and about 40 per cent to external causes. The majority, but not all, of the natural deaths are sudden and unexpected and will be discussed in the next chapter. The statistics relating to the deaths from external causes will be considered in the separate chapters devoted to the different types of traumatic injury.

REFERENCES

Delafield, F., and Prudden, T. M. A Textbook of Pathology, Francis Carter Wood, Ed., New York, William Wood & Co., 1936.

Kolin, M. Technic for sectioning soft bones and hard tissues by celloidin and paraffin methods, Arch. Path., 33:86, 1942.

Mallory, F. B., and Wright, J. H. Pathological Technique, 8th ed., Philadelphia, W. B. Saunders Co., 1918.

Park, W. H., and Williams, A. W. Pathogenic Microorganisms, 11th ed., Philadelphia, Lea & Febiger, 1939.

Reports of the Office of the Chief Medical Examiner of the City of New York, 1918-1951.

Saphir, O. Autopsy Diagnosis and Technic, 2nd ed., New York, Paul B. Hœber, Inc., 1946.

Stitt, E. R., Clough, P. W., and Clough, M. C. Practical Bacteriology, Hematology and Animal Parasitology, 9th ed., New York, Blakiston Co., 1938.

Todd, J. C., and Sanford, A. H. Clinical Diagnosis by Laboratory Methods, Philadelphia, W. B. Saunders Co., 1931.

Weinmann, G. H. A Survey of the Law Concerning Dead Human Bodies, National Research Council, Bull. No. 73, 1929.

6

Unexpected and Sudden Natural Death

Many deaths from natural causes occur unexpectedly, suddenly or in an unusual manner, and are reported to the Office of the Chief Medical Examiner. According to the provisions of the Medical Examiner's Law, the Office shall investigate such cases as well as those which have died by violent means or under suspicious circumstances.

Emphasis should be placed on the unexpected character rather than the suddenness of these deaths occurring in apparently healthy people. In many instances the individual does not die instantaneously or immediately but may linger from a few minutes to over 24 hours after the onset of the illness. The expression natural death means that the exitus was caused entirely by disease and that traumatic injury or a poison did not play any part in bringing it about. It is sometimes difficult to draw a line of distinction between deaths due to natural causes and those which may have been remotely initiated by some external factor. Thus cirrhosis of the liver complicated by portal obstruction and a fatal hemorrhage from esophageal varices may be a sequel of an infectious hepatitis or of a syphilitic infection; but it may also result from chronic alcoholism or from acute or subacute liver necrosis produced by various poisons.

Circumstances Under Which Natural Deaths Occur. Natural deaths may be separated into two categories: (1) Those in which death has taken place in the presence of witnesses and under circumstances in which factors of physical and emotional strain may have played a role; thus it may have occurred during physical exertion while pushing a heavy object, while preparing for a journey, during sexual excitement or during an altercation. In other instances it may have occurred without any obvious precipitating factor. (2) Those in which the deceased is found dead under circumstances which are more or less suspicious; the body may be fully clothed as though the deceased had been engaged in some activity or lying in bed as though death had occurred during rest, sleep or adventure. The possibility that witnesses were present at the time of death and perhaps responsible for it has to be considered.

Factors That Determine the Performance of an Autopsy. In the routine medicolegal investigation of an unexpected and apparently natural death, the most important reason for the performance of an autopsy is to determine whether violence in any form has been in any way responsible; the circumstances under which death occurs are important in determining which cases shall be autopsied. In many instances the necropsy was performed because the circumstances were unusual, and it was found that the deceased who had died seemingly of a natural disease condition was actually killed by physical violence in spite of the absence of any external signs of injury. A good illustration of this type of case is that of the watchman, described on page 15. The age of the deceased, reliable medical information as to past health and the presence of witnesses at the time of death are also helpful in deciding the necessity for autopsy as part of the investigation.

Age is a consideration in deciding whether or not autopsy is to be done. Since sudden natural death is less frequent in younger persons, a suspicion of violent death is more likely to arise and the performance of a necropsy would then be indicated. In older persons sudden death is more frequent and more apt to take place under obviously nonsuspicious circumstances so that the investigation without autopsy is usually adequate. Objections to postmortem examination occur more often in such cases, and the medical examiner ordinarily finds it difficult to justify its arbitrary performance. Occasionally the relatives of the deceased desire to know the cause of an obviously natural death and the autopsy is performed at their request.

Another reason for the performance of an autopsy is that an insurance claim or a civil suit for damages based on an alleged accidental injury may be in preparation; the prospects of collecting benefits on such accidental deaths may prompt relatives to ask for this type of postmortem investigation to which they usually object when such considerations are not involved. Sometimes the existence of an insurance policy is concealed or denied for fear that an autopsy might disclose findings prejudicial to the beneficiary's interest. Finding the correct cause of death may discourage unnecessary and unwarranted litigation. Without autopsy there is too much room for speculation by misguided or interested medical experts.

Even when suspicion of foul play or trauma is absent the insurance claim may instigate the performance of an autopsy. If this reveals that death was caused by accidental injury, the beneficiary is entitled to the accidental-death benefit provisions of the policy. In other cases, in which violence was suspected because of the circumstances, death was found to have resulted from natural causes. There are other more difficult cases in which trauma and disease have combined to produce death. When payment on an insurance policy is contested because of fraudulent representation in the application, the autopsy findings may clarify the point at issue.

If the question of workmen's compensation should arise in connection with a death, it is to the interest of both the claimant and the insurance carrier to have the cause of death accurately determined. The lesions found at autopsy can be evaluated in their relationship to the alleged occupational accident and injury.

In the careful and complete performance of postmortem examinations the medical examiner contributes valuable data for the compilation of accurate vital statistics. He does this even though he is not concerned primarily with this problem as much as he is with the medical detection of violence. Of the large number of deaths occurring outside of hospitals, only those come to autopsy which are under the jurisdiction of the medical examiner. He may also function as a public health officer by recognizing and first calling attention to early fatalities in epidemic disease.

Lesions Causing Sudden Natural Death. The lesions which produce sudden and unexpected natural death for the most part belong in three categories. First, the largest group is made up of natural disease processes of slow or insidious development which damage a vital organ without evoking any striking symptoms until there is a sudden cessation of function. The most common example is sudden death from coronary artery disease. The second group comprises sudden and unexpected ruptures of blood vessels with the occurrence of fatal hemorrhage, as the bursting of an aortic aneurysm with hemorrhage into the pericardial sac, or of an aneurysm of the circle of Willis producing subarachnoid hemorrhage, or the rupture of an ectopic gestation with bleeding into the peritoneal cavity. The third group includes latent or overwhelming infectious diseases which develop without producing alarming or recognizable symptoms until death occurs, for example, ambulatory lobar pneumonia or bacterial endocarditis. More rarely a sudden shift in the position of a viscus may result in fatal shock, as when an ovarian cyst becomes twisted on its pedicle, or when there is a sudden obstruction of the bowel by volvulus or adhesions or by incarceration in a hernia, or obstruction of a duct such as the ureter or common bile duct by a calculus.

Recognition of the Cause of Death. Of the three main groups, vascular ruptures with hemorrhage are the easiest for the pathologist to recognize as the actual cause of death; infections are perhaps less obvious; chronic degenerative diseases or neoplasia are the most difficult to evaluate. In this last group there is always the possibility that the patient died of a rapidly developing condition due to trauma or disease which was not suspected clinically. For example, the autopsy may reveal a degree of coronary arteriosclerosis sufficient under some circumstances to cause death, but dissection of the neck may disclose that the deceased died from a fracture of the spine with an injury to the spinal cord, or from a foreign body impacted in the air passages, or from a lethal amount of poison as determined by chemical examination of the organs.

Any pathologist who has had wide autopsy experience is well acquainted with the fact that chronic disease processes ordinarily progress slowly, and that there may be little visible difference in the organs affected at a period long prior to death and at the moment when they play their role as a cause of death. A degree of coronary arteriosclerosis may be responsible for the sudden exitus of one patient while in another it is encountered fortuitously when the individual has died as a result of trauma, or poison, or from some other natural cause such as a cerebral hemorrhage. A complete autopsy is essential to exclude other conditions necessarily more immediate before ascribing death to the chronic disease in question.

A recent case will illustrate this point. The deceased, a middle-aged man who had been confined to jail, was found dead in his cell. There were no unusual external signs. The autopsy disclosed a rather severe grade of coronary arteriosclerosis and myocardial fibrosis sufficient to cause death under some circumstances. Dissection of the throat organs revealed a rolled up and crumpled necktie, apparently swallowed with suicidal intent, which was impacted in the pharynx so as to close the air passages. This obstruction was not visible through the mouth which was tightly closed by rigor mortis.

The determination of the cause of death is basically an interpretative process which includes (1) recognition of the pathologic changes found anatomically, bacteriologically and chemically, and (2) selection of the lesion or lesions which were fatal to the victim.

CLASSIFICATION AND STATISTICS OF CAUSES OF SUDDEN AND UNEXPECTED NATURAL DEATH

In the classification of causes of death it is practicable to group them on the basis of pathologic anatomy and etiology and to distribute them according to organ systems. Two thousand and thirty sudden natural deaths autopsied over a five and a half year period by the Office of the Chief Medical Examiner in the Borough of Manhattan, New York City, were analyzed by Helpern and Rabson. The results, grouped according to organ systems, were found to approximate those reported previously by Weyrich and by Lauren as shown in the Table 6-1.

Diseases of the circulatory apparatus (heart and aorta) lead with 44.9 per cent; the respiratory system follows with 23.1 per cent; the nervous system (brain and meninges) with 17.9 per cent; the digestive organs 6.5 per cent; urinary tract 1.9 per cent; genital tract 1.3 per cent; the combined digestive and urogenital group 9.7 per cent; a miscellaneous group totaled 4.4 per cent of which three-fifths were represented by malaria artificially transmitted among drug addicts.

The percentage distribution of all the natural deaths investigated by the Medical Examiner, including those which were not sudden and unexpected and those which were not autopsied,

Table 6-1. Sudden and Unexpected Natural Deaths.
Distribution According to Organ Systems.

	Helpern and Rabson 2,030 cases Jan., 1937- July, 1943 (per cent) 80.9 Male 19.1 Female	Weyrich 2,668 cases (per cent) 55.4 Male 44.6 Female	Lauren 403 cases * (per cent) 72.0 Male 28.0 Female
Heart and aorta	44.9	42	51
Respiratory system	23.1	23	12
Brain and meninges	17.9	9	15
Digestive and urogenital systems	9.7	13	9
Miscellaneous	4.4	13	12

From Helpern and Rabson, *New York State J. Med.*, 45:1199, 1945.

* Includes alcoholism; excludes children under 14.

differs somewhat from that obtained for the autopsied series. The classification compiled annually by the Medical Examiner conforms to the International List of Causes of Death which includes a subdivision of General Diseases not found practicable for the autopsied series.

The percentage distribution of the total of 8,525 natural deaths, 18 per cent of which were autopsied, for the year 1938 is as follows:

General diseases	9.7	Respiratory diseases	5.3
Circulatory diseases	68.9	Digestive diseases	2.8
Nervous system diseases	9.3	Urogenital diseases	1.8
	Miscellaneous diseases	2.2	

This larger group of unselected cases has a higher percentage of deaths from circulatory diseases than that found in the selected-autopsied group.

The further subdivision of the major categories of the 2,030 autopsied cases of sudden death in the Manhattan series according to pathologic anatomy and etiology is shown in Table 6-2.

Table 6-2. Analysis of 2,030 Autopsied Cases of Sudden and Unexpected Natural Death

ORGAN SYSTEM	SPECIFIC CAUSE	NUMBER	PERCENTAGE OF GROUP	PERCENTAGE OF TOTAL (2,030)
Heart and aorta, 912 cases, 44.9%	Coronary artery disease	617	67.7	30.4
	Syphilitic aortitis	107	11.7	5.3
	Valvular disease	83	9.2	4.1
	Cardiac hypertrophy	35	3.8	1.7
	Spontaneous rupture of aorta	25	2.7	1.2
	Others	45	4.9	2.2
Respiratory, 468 cases, 23.1%	Lobar pneumonia	176	37.6	8.7
	Bronchitis, bronchopneumonia	133	28.4	6.5
	Pulmonary tuberculosis	68	14.5	3.4
	Pulmonary embolism and infarction	31	6.7	1.6
	Others	60	12.8	2.9
Brain and meninges, 367 cases, 17.9%	Cerebral hemorrhage	110	30.4	5.4
	Subarachnoid hemorrhage	93	25.7	4.6
	Cerebellar hemorrhage	11	3.0	0.6
	Pontine hemorrhage	11	3.0	0.6
	Cerebral thrombosis and embolism	27	7.5	1.3
	Meningitis	38	10.6	1.9
	Brain tumor	29	8.0	1.4
	Others	43	11.8	2.1
Digestive and urogenital		198	—	9.7
Miscellaneous		90	—	4.4

From Helpern and Rabson, *New York State J. Med.*, 45:1198, 1945.

Two thirds of the deaths referable to the heart aorta were caused by coronary arteriosclerosis, its complications and sequelae. These represent 30.4 per cent of the total of 2,030 cases. This percentage would undoubtedly be higher if more of the older individuals who die suddenly could be autopsied. Syphilitic aortitis, complicated either by aneurysm, occlusion of coronary artery ostia or aortic valvular insufficiency, accounted for 11.7 per cent of the group or 5.3 per cent of the total. Nonsyphilitic valvular disease is next in frequency (9.2 per cent and 4.1 per cent); then cardiac hypertrophy unassociated with valvular defects and chiefly secondary to arterial hypertension (3.8 per cent and 1.7 per cent); spontaneous rupture of the aorta (2.7 per cent and 1.2 per cent); the other unlisted causes in this group, including congenital heart disease, total 4.9 per cent and 2.2 per cent respectively.

Lobar pneumonia held first place in the respiratory group and, next to coronary arteriosclerosis in frequency, comprised 8.7 per cent of the total of all autopsied sudden deaths. Next in frequency came bronchitis and bronchopneumonia (6.5 per cent), these deaths occurring chiefly in young infants; then pulmonary tuberculosis (3.4 per cent) and nontraumatic pulmonary embolism and infarction (1.6 per cent).

Among the deaths from diseases of the brain and meninges, spontaneous cerebral hemorrhage, chiefly into the basal ganglia from the lenticulostriate arteries in hypertensive and arteriosclerotic individuals, was most frequent, comprising a third of this group and 5.4 per cent of the entire series. Subarachnoid hemorrhage, in most cases from the rupture of a cerebral artery aneurysm, was almost as frequent with 4.6 per cent; included in this group are also some cases of intracerebral hemorrhage in locations other than the basal ganglia: localized subarachnoid hemorrhage overlying the insula and occasional subdural hemorrhage resulting from the rupture of demonstrable cerebral artery aneurysms. Cerebellar hemorrhage and pontile hemorrhage contributed 0.6 per cent each; cerebral thrombosis and embolism, 1.3 per cent; suppurative meningitis, 1.9 per cent, and brain tumors, 1.4 per cent.

The distribution of sudden and unexpected death by half decades according to organ systems in the New York series revealed the greatest incidence of occurrence between 45 and 54 years of age; this was 10 to 15 years later than the percentage peak of population, which was 35 to 39 years.

Sudden and unexpected natural deaths occurred four times more frequently among men than among women. A similar preponderance of the male sex is found in the incidence of violent deaths. Racial incidence was in proportion to population.

The study of the New York series did not include a small group of cases of apparently natural sudden death which after complete investigation and autopsy failed to reveal an adequate cause of death.

SUMMARY OF LESIONS CAUSING SUDDEN AND UNEXPECTED NATURAL DEATH

1. DISEASES OF THE HEART AND AORTA

   Occlusive Coronary Artery Disease

   Progressive coronary arteriosclerosis with narrowing and obliteration of lumen (Figs. 6-1 and 6-2) with or without associated myocardial damage such as fibrosis (most common (Fig. 6-3)) or old, recent or fresh infarction;

   Coronary arteriosclerosis complicated by old or recent coronary artery thrombosis (Fig. 6-2) (fresh coronary thrombosis not common), with or without associated old, recent or fresh myocardial infarction (Fig. 6-3), myocardial fibrosis, ventricular aneurysm (Fig. 6-4), rupture of fresh myocardial infarct or aneurysm producing intrapericardial hemorrhage and cardiac tamponade;

   Coronary artery embolism (rare) from mural thrombus or atheromatous plaque, or on aortic valve (Fig. 6-5);

   Stenosis of mouths of coronary arteries associated with chronic syphilitic aortitis (Fig. 6-6);

   Coronary atherosclerosis with hemorrhage into atheromatous plaque encroaching on lumen or leading to thrombosis; rupture of softened atheromatous plaque leading to thrombosis (mechanisms not frequently encountered as causes of sudden death);

   Spontaneous rupture and dissecting aneurysm with compression of lumen of coronary artery (very rare);

   Congenital anomalies of coronary arteries (rare).

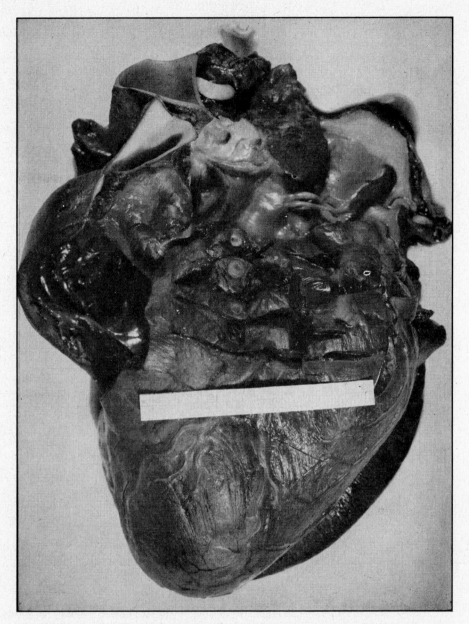

Fig. 6-1. Sudden Death from Segmental Occlusive Coronary Arteriosclerosis.

The heart, weighing 290 gm., of a 33 year old white man who died suddenly while at work after onset of precordial pain. No prior symptoms except mild indigestion the night before. Proximal segment of left coronary artery sectioned to show localized sclerotic occlusion 2 cm. from ostium. Note normal thickness of artery wall just below occluded segment.

Lesions of the Myocardium, Cardiac Valves, Endocardium and Pericardium

Acute or subacute toxic myocarditis following diphtheria, infections and trichinosis;

Tuberculosis or syphilis of the myocardium (rare);

Myocardial fibrosis following myocarditis;

Myocardial infarction with or without fibrosis or aneurysm, secondary to occlusive coronary disease; rupture of infarcted papillary muscle (Fig. 6-7);

Spontaneous rupture of myocardial infarct or aneurysm with hemopericardium (Fig. 6-4);

Spontaneous rupture of fatty heart (Fig. 6-8);

Left ventricular hypertrophy associated with chronic aortic valvular disease, especially aortic stenosis;

Left ventricular hypertrophy resulting from arterial hypertension either essential or secondary to renal disease;

Cor pulmonale: right ventricular hypertrophy associated with chronic pulmonary disease such as pneumoconiosis, emphysema or kyphoscoliosis;

Cardiac hypertrophy associated with hyperthyroidism;

Acute or subacute bacterial endocarditis;

Mitral stenosis, postrheumatic;

Aortic stenosis (Fig. 6-9), postrheumatic or sclerotic (Mönckeberg's sclerosis or sclerosis superimposed on congenital bicuspid aortic valve);

Aortic insufficiency, postrheumatic or secondary to syphilitic aortitis;

Mural thrombosis in auricles or ventricles with embolism, such as ball valve thrombus in left auricle closing orifice of stenotic mitral valve (Fig. 6-10), or thrombus in left ventricle associated with myocardial infarction or fibrosis causing cerebral artery embolism;

Pericarditis: septic, rheumatic or tuberculous.

Congenital Heart Disease

Lesions of the Aorta

Spontaneous rupture of ascending aorta (nonsyphilitic (Fig. 6-11)) with intrapericardial hemorrhage and cardiac tamponade; ruptures are complete or incomplete with formation of dissecting aneurysm and subsequent rupture of latter into pericardium but occasionally into pleural cavity; spontaneous rupture of aorta occasionally associated with coarctation of aorta, frequently with hypertension;

Syphilitic aortitis complicated by stenosis of mouths of coronary arteries, (Fig. 6-12); aortic insufficiency with left ventricular hypertrophy; aortic aneurysms (Fig. 6-13), single and multiple, with spontaneous rupture and hemorrhage into pericardial cavity, pleural cavity, bronchus, esophagus, externally through chest wall, subcutaneously into neck causing asphyxia by pressure on trachea (aneurysm of innominate artery);

Aneurysm of abdominal aorta secondary to atherosclerosis; rupture and hemorrhage into retroperitoneal tissues (Fig. 6-14);

Occlusive thrombosis of abdominal aorta secondary to atherosclerosis;

Mural thrombosis on atheromatous plaque with mesenteric embolism and infarction.

2. DISEASES OF THE RESPIRATORY SYSTEM

Lesions Causing Asphyxia

Septic or diphtheritic laryngitis (Fig. 6-15);

Acute laryngeal edema secondary to infection or to neoplasm of pharynx or larynx;

Bronchial asthma;

Pulmonary embolism secondary to static thrombosis or thrombophlebitis of deep veins of lower extremities or pelvis (Figs. 8-10 and 8-11);

Paradoxical embolism (Fig. 8-12).

Hemorrhage from Air Passages

Tuberculosis of lungs with cavitation;

Neoplasm of bronchus;

Bronchiectasis;

Lung abscess.

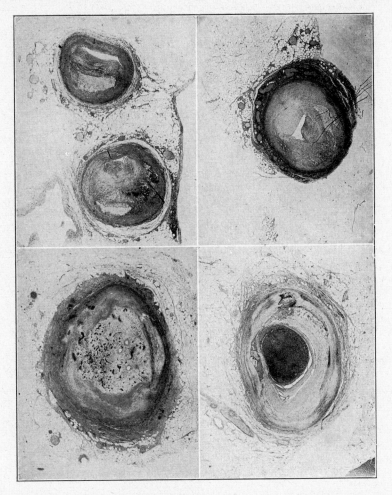

Fig. 6-2. Sudden Death Caused by Coronary Artery Disease. Cross Sections of Coronary Arteries, Low Magnification.

Top left. Advanced atherosclerosis of coronary arteries with almost complete obliteration of the lumen. No thrombosis. White man, 54 years of age.

Top right. Advanced atherosclerosis of a coronary artery with marked narrowing of the lumen. Note collateral circulation in adventitia. An adjacent sclerosed artery was occluded by an organized thrombus. The myocardium was extensively fibrosed. White man, 28 years of age.

Bottom left. Severe atherosclerosis of coronary artery completely occluded by an old organized and poorly canalized thrombus. White man, 67 years of age.

Bottom right. Severe atherosclerosis of right coronary artery with occlusion of lumen by a fresh thrombus. The left coronary artery was sclerosed and completely occluded by an old organized thrombus. White man, 60 years of age.

Sudden death from coronary artery disease is usually the result of a severe grade of atherosclerosis of the coronary arteries with narrowing of the lumen. The process may be extensive or localized to a part of one coronary artery. Thrombosis is not always found and when it is seen, the process is frequently an old one and the thrombus organized and canalized. Fresh thrombi are not common findings. When they are present the coronary arteries usually show severe sclerosis and old thrombosis.

Pneumothorax
    Spontaneous rupture of tuberculous cavern;
    Rupture of emphysematous bleb.

Pulmonary Infection
    Lobar pneumonia;
    Influenzal pneumonia;
    Tuberculosis;
    Bronchiectasis;
    Lung abscess;
    Parasitic cysts;
    Schistosomiasis;

3. DISEASES OF THE BRAIN AND MENINGES

Spontaneous cerebral hemorrhage usually associated with arteriosclerosis and hypertension and generally occurring in basal ganglia (internal capsule (Fig. 6-16)), less often in the pons (Fig. 6-17) and cerebellum (Fig. 6-18);

Spontaneous subarachnoid hemorrhage following rupture of a cerebral artery aneurysm usually on the circle of Willis (Figs. 6-19 and 6-20), or rupture of a hypoplastic cerebral artery;

Localized subarachnoid hemorrhage in fissure of Sylvius (Fig. 6-21), or intracerebral hemorrhage, elsewhere than in the basal ganglia or pons, from rupture of embedded aneurysms of the cerebral arteries;

Spontaneous subdural hemorrhage from rupture of a cerebral artery aneurysm;

Cerebral compression from bilateral chronic pachymeningitis interna hemorrhagica (Fig. 6-22);

Colloid cyst in third ventricle (Fig. 6-23);

Parasitic cyst in fourth ventricle (Fig. 6-24);

Brain abscess complicating otitis media (Fig. 6-25), or lung abscess;

Acute suppurative leptomeningitis;

Fulminating meningococcic infection without gross meningitis (Waterhouse—Friderichsen syndrome);

Acute polioencephalitis;

Syphilitic leptomeningitis and arteritis (Figs. 6-26 and 6-27);

General paresis;

Brain tumor (Figs. 6-28 and 6-29);

Epilepsy.

4. DISEASES OF THE DIGESTIVE TRACT AND UROGENITAL APPARATUS

Hemorrhage into Gastrointestinal Tract
    Ulcerating carcinoma of the tongue;
    Erosion of carcinoma of esophagus into the thoracic aorta;
    Chronic peptic ulcer, gastric or duodenal;
    Tuberculous ulcer of stomach (rare);
    Rupture of esophageal varices complicating cirrhosis of the liver.

Intra-abdominal Hemorrhage
    Spontaneous rupture of carcinoma or cavernoma of the liver;
    Rupture of ectopic pregnancy (Fig. 6-29);
    Spontaneous rupture of enlarged spleen in malaria or typhoid fever (Fig. 6-30).

Shock
    Intestinal obstruction caused by adhesions, volvulus, intussusception or incarceration of bowel in hernial sac;
    Gallstone in common duct;
    Acute pancreatitis;
    Twisting of pedicle of ovarian cyst or fibromyoma uteri.

Infection of Peritoneum
    Strangulated incarcerated hernia with rupture of intestine;

Perforation of peptic ulcer of stomach or duodenum (Fig. 6-31);

Perforation of intestinal carcinoma or typhoid or amebic ulcer of intestine;

Spontaneous rupture of bladder associated with prostatic hypertrophy or urethral stricture;

Phlegmonous gastritis.

Urogenital Lesions
   Chronic nephritis;
   Nephrolithiasis;
   Obstructive hydronephrosis and pyonephrosis;
   Tuberculosis of kidneys;
   Neoplasm of kidneys and bladder;

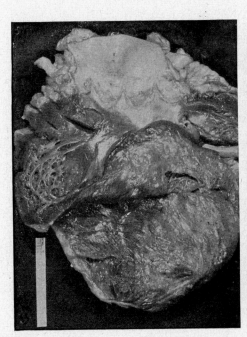 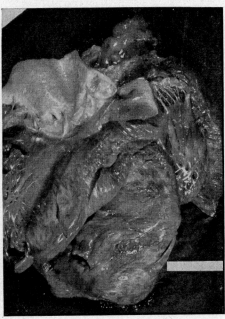

Fig. 6-3. Examples of Old and Fresh Myocardial Infarction Complicating Occlusive Coronary Artery Disease, Causing Sudden Death.

Left. Myocardial fibrosis representing replacement of old infarction of posterior wall of left ventricle; middle-aged white man.

Right. Massive fresh infarction of posterior wall of left ventricle; 51 year old white man.

Rupture of ectopic pregnancy;

Eclamptic toxemia of pregnancy;

Intra-uterine pregnancy or large fibromyoma uteri causing static thrombosis of pelvic veins and pulmonary embolism;

Severe anemia from prolonged, severe uterine hemorrhage caused by submucous fibromyomas;

Carcinoma of vulva eroding femoral vessels causing fatal hemorrhage.

5. MISCELLANEOUS
   Addison's disease;
   Pheochromocytoma of adrenal medulla causing hyperadrenalism (Fig. 6-32);
   Senile marasmus;
   Diabetes mellitus;
   Hemochromatosis;

Blood dyscrasias;

Status lymphaticus (Figs. 6-33 and 6-34);

Hyperthyroidism;

Malaria;

Severe spinal deformities;

Hemorrhage from varicose ulcer of leg;

Undetermined causes of death.

6. CHILDREN

Congenital anomalies;

Infectious diseases;

Convulsions with asphyxia;

Deficiency diseases such as rickets or scurvy;

Sudden natural deaths of infants in cribs and carriages in which the primary cause cannot be determined even after exhaustive autopsy.

DISEASES OF THE HEART AND AORTA

The percentage incidence and the various types of disease conditions in this group causing sudden and unexpected death have already been indicated. Not only does this category contribute the greatest number of all the cases but heart and aortic disease also cause sudden death to occur most rapidly, often instantaneously, in a way that is true of no other disease group. It is important to bear this in mind for not infrequently the victim of a fatal heart attack falls and sustains trivial or severe injury which has to be evaluated as a factor of lethal significance. When the injuries are slight, they contribute little if anything to the death and can be disregarded. Traumatic injury, unless it is very severe or extensive, does not kill instantaneously or rapidly.

The evaluation of the effect of any terminal injury should be made with the knowledge of how the same injury influences the individual when it occurs in the absence of natural disease. This extremely important medicolegal consideration has often been disregarded. Thus during a sudden fatal attack of heart disease, the deceased may have fallen from a standing position and sustained injury; because of the latter, the conclusion that death resulted from disease is erroneously disputed. Such a situation is encountered not infrequently in insurance claims for accidental death benefits, in compensation claims, in negligence actions and in criminal actions for alleged assault or homicide. It will help to clarify the confusion existent in the mind of a physician who is confronted with the responsibility of forming a valid opinion as to the cause of death in such cases if the conditions found at autopsy are evaluated in relation to the effects of trauma on the body.

Heart disease differs from the disease conditions of other organs in the sense that a heart which has once been affected by disease remains vulnerable and may cause sudden death, even though the active stage of the disease has healed. Obviously, active disease of the heart whether congenital, inflammatory, degenerative, hypertrophic or neoplastic is more apt to result in sudden death than is the heart with the so-called healed lesion. The healed heart, however, is not the equivalent of the normal organ and at any time may give out and stop more or less suddenly; the term healed when applied to the heart has not the same implication it has with other organs like the lung, kidney or liver. The ceaseless and variable activity of the heart may bring out an inadequacy of function caused not only by active disease but also by quiescent healed lesions. The damaged and repaired heart no longer possesses the same factor of safety in functional capacity when increased demands for activity are made on it. This does not imply that every heart which has been afflicted is in imminent danger of sudden or gradual failure but such an event can occur and must be anticipated. It is not infrequent in the experience of the medical examiner.

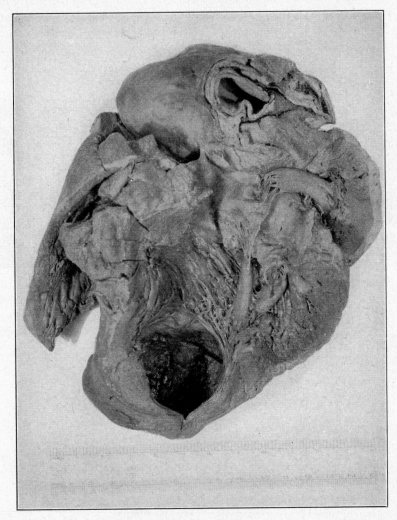

Fig. 6-4. Sudden Death: Spontaneous Rupture of a Cardiac Aneurysm; Hemopericardium. Extensive coronary arteriosclerosis, 60 year old white man.

Coronary Artery Disease. Roughly 67 per cent of all sudden deaths from heart disease are caused by arteriosclerosis of the coronary arteries. Extensive involvement of all the larger branches or an intense limited involvement of a large branch may gradually produce a partial or complete occlusion of the lumen so that in time the arteries are unable to deliver an adequate amount of blood to the myocardium; as a result of the coronary artery insufficiency the heart may suddenly stop.

In approximately 75 per cent of sudden deaths from coronary artery disease the lesion is a gradually progressive coronary arteriosclerosis without thrombosis but with marked luminal narrowing or complete occlusion of segments of one or both coronary arteries. In a few of these cases the sclerotic coronary arteries may also reveal old thrombotic occlusion or old hemorrhage into intimal atheromatous plaques. The intimal hemorrhages may raise the intima and narrow the lumen without thrombosis taking place. Luminal thrombosis and intimal hemorrhage are merely complications of the underlying atherosclerosis of the coronary arteries and rarely account for sudden death at the time they occur. They are more apt to enhance the progress of the sclerotic disease and to bring nearer the onset of the coronary

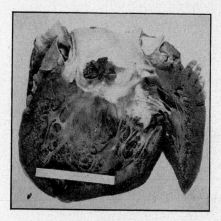

Fig. 6-5. Sudden Death Due to Coronary Artery Obstruction.

Large mural thrombus straddling commissure between right anterior and posterior valve cusps obstructing ostium of right coronary artery; 33 year old Negro; death shortly after onset of anginal symptoms.

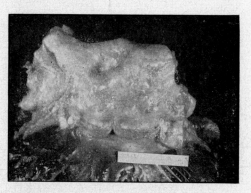

Fig. 6-6. Sudden Death Due to Complete Stenosis of Ostia of Coronary Arteries in Syphilitic Aortitis.

The deceased was a 48 year old Negro. This lesion is not as commonly encountered now as it formerly was.

insufficiency. Of the 75 per cent of cases in which nonthrombotic occlusive coronary sclerosis was the fatal lesion, 50 per cent revealed myocardial fibrosis; in 45 per cent fibrosis was absent and in 5 per cent there was myocardial infarction.

In only 25 per cent of the autopsied cases of sudden death from coronary artery disease were fresh thrombotic lesions encountered in the sclerotic coronary arteries; and in most of these, in addition to the advanced sclerosis, old thrombotic lesions and old subintimal hemorrhages were also noted. In some the basis for the thrombosis was the rupture of a softened atheromatous plaque as described by Leary; in other cases there was hemorrhage into an atheromatous plaque as described by Paterson. In other cases neither of these mechanisms could be demonstrated. In some instances the thrombus occluded a segment of a vessel proximal to a portion already partially or completely occluded by atherosclerosis or by an old thrombosis. In the 25 per cent group of cases with fresh thrombotic occlusion, fresh myocardial infarction was found in 75 per cent, about half of these with and half without antecedent fibrosis. In most of the thrombotic cases in which a myocardial infarct was encountered, the degree of occlusive coronary arteriosclerosis was sufficiently severe to produce prolonged ischemia of the myocardium and to contribute materially to the formation of the infarction, quite apart from any effects contributed by the thrombosis.

When a severe grade of coronary arteriosclerosis and insufficiency exists, transitory symptoms of angina pectoris may develop which are not associated with organic changes in the heart muscle. On the other hand, more serious effects may occur; the myocardium may undergo infarction or the heart may stop suddenly, even with minimal activity on the part of the patient. The same manifestations are more likely to develop in an aggravated form if the activity of such a heart is increased by physical exertion or emotional excitement. These factors add to the burden of the myocardium and necessitate an increased coronary blood flow, a demand which the diseased coronary arteries cannot supply. The influence of trauma on coronary arteriosclerosis is similar and will be discussed later.

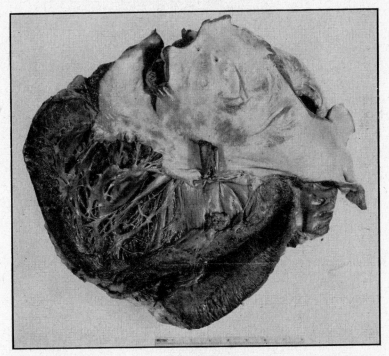

Fig. 6-7. Sudden Death from Myocardial Infarction with Rupture of Papillary Muscle Complicating Coronary Artery Disease.

Right coronary artery occluded; 60 year old white woman.

In evaluating the effect of exertion and emotion it is not too material whether the coronary arteriosclerosis has developed insidiously with progressive luminal narrowing or whether that process has been complicated by episodes of sudden intimal hemorrhage or luminal thrombosis which narrow the caliber of the vessel still more or even occlude it. There is no proof that exertion or emotion plays any necessary role in the production of intimal hemorrhage or coronary thrombosis; and there is no satisfactory evidence to indicate that these lesions arise otherwise than as spontaneous complications of coronary arteriosclerosis. The influence of exertion or emotion still operates in those cases in which coronary arteriosclerosis is complicated by luminal thrombosis or intimal hemorrhage, for these lesions merely add to the obstruction of the circulation through the coronary arteries and to the extent of the coronary insufficiency and render the heart even more susceptible to stress.

The more severe the lesions are in the coronary arteries or the myocardium, the less there is of cardiac reserve and the more effective will be the influence of any given exertion in the production of sudden death or in the development of a myocardial infarct. In severely damaged hearts a moderate amount of exertion or excitement may be sufficient to precipitate sudden death or myocardial infarction; in a heart in which the coronary arteries are only moderately sclerotic, the same

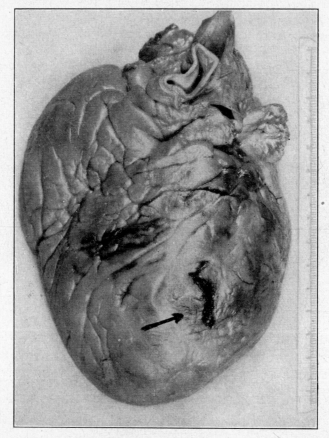

Fig. 6-8. Sudden Death: Spontaneous Rupture of Left Ventricle of Large Fatty Heart; Coronary Arteriosclerosis; Hemopericardium; 44 Year Old White Man.

effects are more apt to ensue after a very severe physical exertion. Occasionally even a normal heart with intact coronary circulation and myocardium may stop suddenly because of an unusual strain brought about by severe physical effort.

The authors have encountered such a case. A 17 year old boy swam 75 feet in an underwater race. After completing it, he was able to lift himself out of the pool only to collapse and die on the ledge. Autopsy revealed a dilated heart of normal weight without evidence of coronary, myocardial or valvular disease. In this case it was concluded that the combination of anoxia, severe physical exertion, increased heart action, and the inability of the coronary arteries to deliver normally oxygenated blood to the myocardium resulted in sudden cardiac failure.

Similarly, individuals suffering from a functional cardiac disturbance like an arrhythmia, for which an adequate anatomic basis cannot always be demonstrated at autopsy, may die suddenly during exertion or rest as a result of similar oxygen deficiency brought about by the functional disability.

In many sudden deaths from coronary artery disease, the symptoms by which the disease is usually recognized are absent or atypical; in other cases in which there are suggestive symptoms of angina pectoris, it may not be possible to detect objective clinical evidence of coronary disease even with the use of the electro-cardiograph. Death may take place with dramatic suddenness, without any prior warning and under the greatest variety of circumstances—during sleep, rest, ordinary activity, labor, sexual intercourse or under emotional or physical strain. Sud-

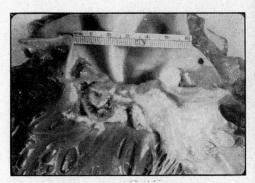

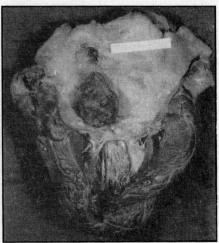

Fig. 6-9. Sudden Death Due to Aortic Stenosis.

Calcific aortic valvulitis with acquired bi-cuspid deformity of aortic valve; left ventricle hypertrophied; 37 year old white man who collapsed at work.

Fig. 6-10. Sudden Death Due to Blocking of Stenotic Mitral Valve by Pedunculated Mural Ball Valve Thrombus in Left Auricle.

Old rheumatic valvulitis; 48 year old white man.

den death is often the first and only symptom of an advanced occlusive coronary arteriosclerosis, with or without old or fresh thrombosis, with or without myocardial infarction. It may be precipitated by emotional or exertional stimuli which increase heart action; or the heart may suddenly stop even with complete rest because of inadequate coronary circulation. In addition some patients may experience acute heart failure on the basis of a myocardial insufficiency rather than as a result of coronary insufficiency. In some cases the coronary artery disease and the myocardial infarction are asymptomatic until such sequelae ensue as spontaneous rupture of the heart wall, hemopericardium and cardiac tamponade, aneurysm of the left ventricle with or without rupture, or mural thrombosis causing unexpected death from cerebral embolism.

It is surprising how much activity an individual may be capable of despite the presence of a fully developed massive myocardial infarct, as illustrated in the following case:

A middle-aged white man dropped dead while urinating in the lavatory of a railway station. He was returning to his home in the suburbs after attending a dinner during which he consumed a considerable amount of food and drink without apparent discomfort; he left the party in good spirits. When he collapsed his head struck the tiled floor and he sustained a fracture of the skull without any injury of the brain. Death in any event was instantaneous and too rapid to have been caused by the head injury. The autopsy disclosed lesions in the heart remarkable for their extent and severity. There were an advanced occlusive coronary arteriosclerosis with old and recent thrombosis and a large myocardial infarct of at least several days' duration. The stomach was filled with food and the brain contained a large amount of alcohol.

Occlusive coronary arteriosclerosis with its complications and sequelae is a common cause of sudden death in middle and old age and not rare as a cause of sudden death in young adults. In civil life few such deaths are encountered in the third decade; more occur in the fourth and a great many in the fifth and sixth decades and beyond. Curiously, sudden death from occlusive coronary arterio-

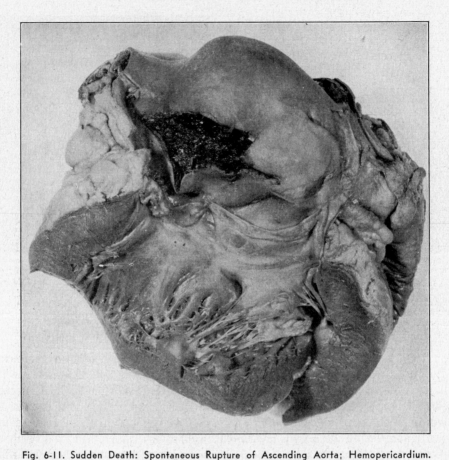

Fig. 6-11. Sudden Death: Spontaneous Rupture of Ascending Aorta; Hemopericardium.

Old healed tears are visible in the intima and media. Bicuspid aortic valve. White man, 30 years old.

sclerosis is encountered infrequently among women and among members of the Negro race. Coronary arteriosclerosis with its complications and sequelae is predominantly a disease of white men.

Although it is generally believed that coronary arteriosclerosis does not cause the heart to undergo hypertrophy, especially in cases uncomplicated by myocardial infarction or fibrosis, the analysis of a two year series by Rabson and Helpern revealed that 56 per cent of the hearts weighed more than 400 gm. and that more than half of these were heavier than 500 gm. Hypertrophy was observed in about three fourths of the fibrotic hearts. Whether or not hypertension existed in these cases could not be determined.

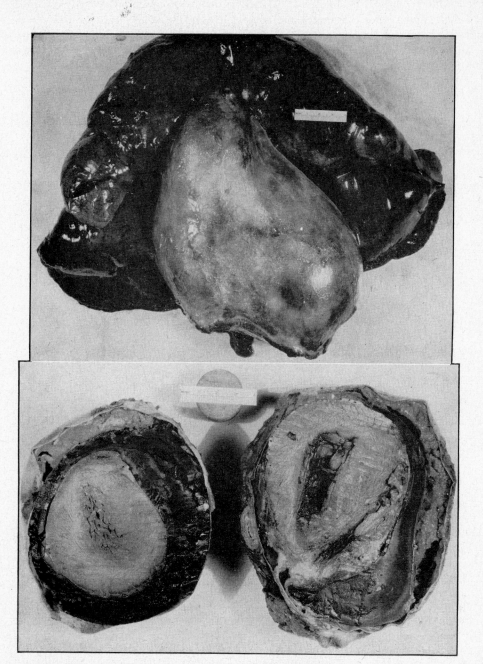

Fig. 6-12. Sudden Death: Hemopericardium with Cardiac Tamponade; Spontaneous Rupture of Ascending Aorta in 40 Year Old Negro.

Upper photograph reveals unopened pericardial sac distended by blood. The entire specimen was then hardened in formalin and sectioned crosswise to show tamponading of heart by blood in pericardial sac (lower photograph).

French and Dock analyzed 80 sudden deaths from coronary arteriosclerosis among young soldiers between the ages of 20 and 36 years. Ten per cent of the deaths occurred during sleep; 17 per cent of the fatal attacks began in the morning after rising and were associated with the usual activities before drill. Vigorous exertion appears to have preceded more than 33 per cent of the fatal attacks. Ninety-one

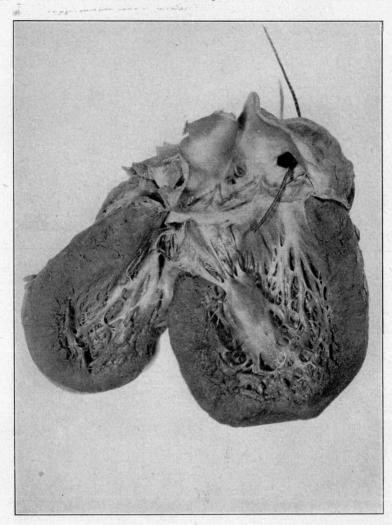

Fig. 6-13. Sudden Death: Spontaneous Rupture of Small Saccular Aneurysm of the Ascending Aorta; Hemopericardium; Syphilitic Aortitis; String Protruding from Mouth of Aneurysm and Perforation; Negro Male, 47 Years of Age.

per cent of the subjects were overweight. Coronary arteriosclerosis was the basis for the coronary occlusion in all cases; thrombosis was found in 36 per cent, myocardial infarction in 19 per cent and fibrosis in 59 per cent. The average heart weight was 365 gm., with three fourths of the weights between 300 and 440 gm. The pathologic lesions were similar to those observed in civil life by the medical examiner.

Sudden death may be caused by stenosis of the ostia of the coronary arteries as a result of syphilitic inflammation of the aorta. One or both coronary artery mouths may be completely or partially closed off with the length of the artery showing little if any change. Rarely syphilitic coronary arteritis with narrowing of the lumen may cause sudden death. Strassmann and Goldstein reported such a case and another has been observed by the authors. In this connection it is important to point out that round cell infiltration of the adventitia and the diseased intima is frequently observed in sclerotic coronary arteries. The thickening of the artery produced by syphilis is usually concentric in distribution, and the inflammatory cell infiltration is more intense.

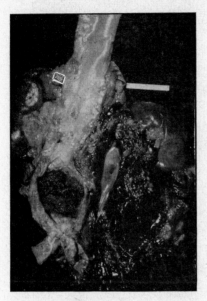

Fig. 6-14. Sudden Death: Rupture of Large Saccular Aneurysm of Abdominal Aorta with Massive Right-Sided Retroperitoneal Hemorrhage.

White man, 77 years old, found dead on floor in hotel room after a bout of venery.

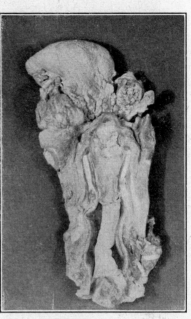

Fig. 6-15. Sudden Death: Laryngeal and Tracheal Diphtheria; Seven Year Old Negro Boy.

Note diphtheritic membrane lining larynx and extending down beyond bifurcation of trachea.

Rare anomalies of the coronary arteries may cause sudden death. Thus in the case of a white man in his middle twenties found dead, the autopsy disclosed a marked aneurysmal dilatation and tortuosity of both coronary arteries, the left arising from the pulmonary artery. The heart was moderately enlarged, the left ventricle dilated and the myocardium fibrotic. A lesion of another type was encountered by Dr. Eugene Clark in a robust, apparently healthy 22 year old man who dropped dead while exercising; the heart was normal in size but revealed a hypoplasia of the right coronary artery, the ostium of which was anomalously situated 1 cm. above the right posterior commissure; the anterior descending branch of the left coronary was also hypoplastic; the left circumflex branch was atheromatous and was apparently carrying the bulk of the circulatory load. There were several fibrous scars in the myocardium of the interventricular septum and at the apex. There were no other changes found on gross or microscopic examination.

A most unusual lesion of the coronary artery caused the unexpected death of a 38 year old white woman after some premonitory signs of angina pectoris. At autopsy the heart was found to be normal in size and the coronary arteries showed only a moderate amount of atheromatous change. There was a spontaneous rupture of the intima and media of the anterior descending branch of the left coronary artery about 2 cm. distal to its origin, which resulted in a dissecting hemorrhage between the media and the adventitia; this extended distally 6 cm. after which the hemorrhage re-entered the lumen, without escaping into the surrounding subepicardial tissues. Compression and complete occlusion of the lumen of the involved segment of the artery were produced by this tubular hemorrhage.

Acute occlusion of a coronary artery may occur from embolism into one of the larger branches. Such cases are extremely rare and usually result from the detachment of an elongated small mural thrombus which has formed on an atheromatous plaque above the ostium of the coronary artery. At times the thrombus

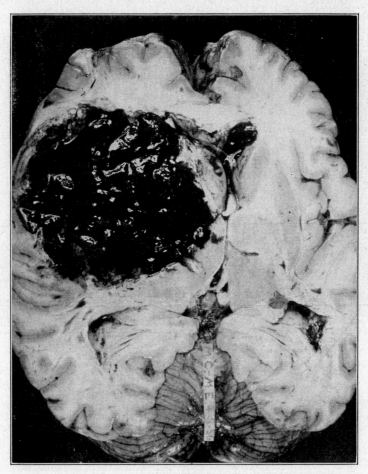

Fig. 6-16. Sudden Death: Spontaneous Cerebral Hemorrhage; Left Basal Ganglia; Cerebral Arteriosclerosis.

A common site for spontaneous cerebral hemorrhage.

may embolize into the lumen and remain attached to its site of origin, or it may block the ostium without entering it (Fig. 6-5). Multiple small coronary emboli have also been encountered in bacterial endocarditis of the aortic valves, but the primary condition is usually diagnosed during life and its embolic complication is rarely a factor in causing sudden death. Although coronary embolism is extremely rare it is diagnosed clinically too often by physicians who mistakenly attribute its source of origin to thrombi in the small veins of the lower extremities. The thrombi presumably travel to the right auricle, enter the left auricle via a patent foramen ovale and then lodge in the most convenient coronary artery. Theoretically such paradoxical embolism to the coronary arteries is possible, but it has never been encountered by the authors among thousands of autopsies nor are there authentic reports of such cases in the literature. A genuine case of paradoxical embolism, but not to the coronary arteries, and the special conditions under which this phenomenon takes place are described on page 179.

Myocardial Disease. Occasionally sudden death is caused by active toxic, acute or subacute myocarditis following focal infection elsewhere in the body as in a case of diphtheria, or as a septic infection of the heart muscle by pyogenic cocci

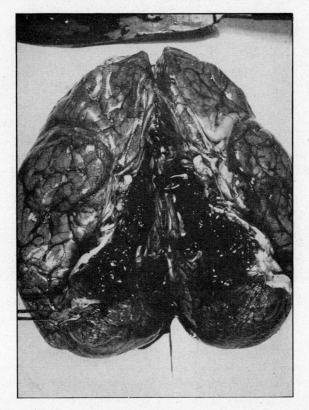

Fig. 6-17. Sudden Death: Massive Pontile Hemorrhage, Marked Cerebral Arteriosclerosis. Middle-aged white man. Pons sectioned sagittally.

as an accompaniment of a general septicemia; it may also occur during the fibrotic stage of a healed myocarditis. The acute or subacute stage of myocarditis may not present conspicuous gross pathologic changes and any flabbiness of the heart muscle which may be present may be overlooked, so that a microscopic examination may be necessary to demonstrate the lesion. Some cases of active myocarditis may be a manifestation of a general trichinosis and their true nature may be identified by microscopic examination of the diaphragm or other skeletal muscle. The fibrotic stage of a healed myocarditis is as a rule easily recognizable in the gross at autopsy.

An active rheumatic myocarditis will usually be accompanied by evidence of valvular inflammation and sometimes by active pericarditis. Rarely is disseminated tuberculosis of the myocardium responsible for sudden death. Gumma of the heart with or without rupture and hemopericardium is also rare. The authors recently encountered such a case in which a large aneurysm of the left ventricle at the apex ruptured to cause a hemopericardium. The gummatous inflammation was evident microscopically and serologic tests on the blood were strongly positive for syphilis. The patient had an incidental trichinosis.

Lipomatosis or excess fatty deposits in the heart with replacement and weakening of the myocardium are found in very obese persons and are usually associated with a definite grade of coronary arteriosclerosis. Sudden death may occur as a result of acute heart failure or from the spontaneous rupture of the weakened left ventricle producing a hemopericardium (Fig. 6-8). Similarly the spontaneous rup-

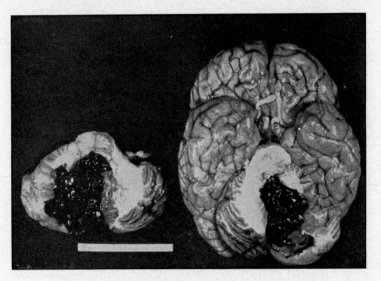

Fig. 6-18. Sudden Death. Spontaneous Cerebellar Hemorrhage, Cerebral Arteriosclerosis.
White woman, 50 years old, domestic. Onset of illness with vomiting spell.

ture of a fresh myocardial infarct may cause a hemopericardium and sudden death. In some instances of infarction a papillary muscle may rupture (Fig. 6-7) or the interventricular septum may perforate, followed rapidly by the death of the victim.

Hypertrophy of the heart from many causes may result in sudden fatal heart failure without the usual premonitory clinical signs of that condition. Perhaps the most commonly encountered cases are those in which there is left ventricular hypertrophy secondary either to primary essential hypertension of vascular origin or to the hypertension resulting from renal disease such as chronic glomerulonephritis, pyelonephritis, polycystic kidneys or to other causes. The coronary arteries show varying amounts of sclerosis but often the degree of narrowing is slight and the myocardium may show little if any fibrosis. Such hypertensive hearts range in size from about 500 to 800 gm. Death may occur suddenly without warning sometimes during inactivity, at other times during emotional or physical strain, or during or shortly after a verbal or physical altercation. Some of the individuals who die in this way are robust and physically active up to the time of death without premonitory symptoms of hypertensive disease. Sudden deaths from acute heart failure may be preceded by rapidly developing pulmonary edema. There may be important medicolegal implications in such sudden deaths especially if the deceased has also suffered some bodily injury. The nature and degree of the injury must be carefully evaluated in the light of the findings of the autopsy, which must be performed completely for proper interpretation.

In a case recently encountered by the authors a robust, middle-aged parking lot attendant who had never been ill, according to information obtained from his family, became involved in a heated argument leading to fisticuffs with the owner of an improperly parked automobile. During the fracas the attendant received a severe punch which broke his nose but did not cause him to lose consciousness. A few moments later he became short of breath, collapsed and

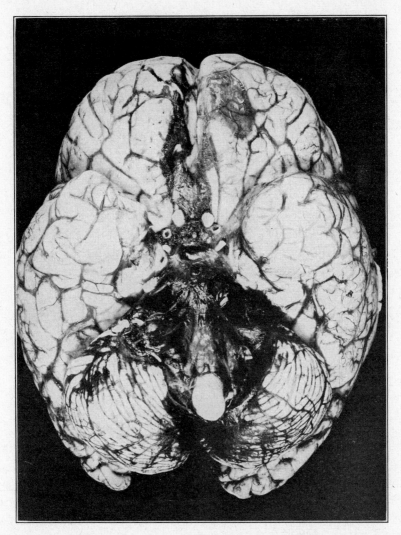

Fig. 6-19. Sudden Death: Spontaneous Hemorrhage into Right Frontal Lobe with Rupture into Ventricles and Extension to Subarachnoid Space; Rupture of Saccular Aneurysm (not visible) at Bifurcation of Right Anterior and Right Middle Cerebral Arteries; Brown Stain of an Old Subarachnoid Hemorrhage Visible on Under Surface of Left Frontal Lobe; White Woman, 22 Years of Age.

died. Autopsy revealed a large heart with a markedly hypertrophied left ventricle, marked pulmonary edema and congestion of the viscera. The injury was confined to the nose with a fracture between the cartilage and the nasal bones. The brain was not injured. The manner and time of death were characteristic of sudden death from heart disease. The injury in itself did not explain the death although it was felt to have contributed to it together with the emotional excitement and physical exertion. A charge of homicide could not be sustained against the assailant by the medical evidence although there was evidence for an assault charge. As is frequent in such cases, the relatives who knew the deceased to be in apparent health and of robust constitution would not believe the autopsy findings of heart disease nor accept the interpretation as to the cause of death.

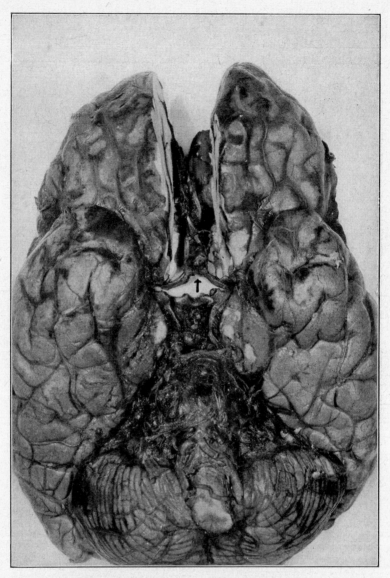

Fig. 6-20. Sudden Death: Spontaneous Subarachnoid Hemorrhage; Rupture of Saccular Aneurysm of Anterior Communicating Artery of Circle of Willis.

Medial portions of frontal lobes are cut away to expose the aneurysm. Arrow points to aneurysm. Negro woman, 29 years old. A considerable amount of the subarachnoid hemorrhage has been dissected away to expose the vessels in the circle of Willis.

Unsuspected thyrotoxicosis can cause the heart to hypertrophy as the result of overactivity due to excessive stimulation. Heart failure and death may be sudden in these cases.

Hypertrophy of the right ventricle or cor pulmonale may develop insidiously and cause sudden death. Any condition causing obstruction or hypertension of the pulmonary circuit may produce it. Thus it is encountered in various pneumoconioses, pulmonary emphysema associated with chronic inflammation of the bronchi, bronchiectasis, bronchial asthma and kyphoscoliosis, pulmonary fibrosis and obliterating endarteritis of the pulmonary vessels. It also occurs with pulmonary stenosis and after congenital defects of the interauricular and interventricular septa.

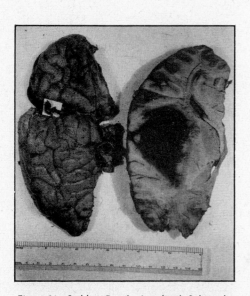

Fig. 6-21. Sudden Death. Localized Subarachnoid Hemorrhage Over Insula. Rupture of Saccular Aneurysm of Right Middle Cerebral Artery High Up in the Fissure of Sylvius.

White paper is inserted behind aneurysm. Middle-aged white man. The subarachnoid character of this type of hemorrhage is sometimes not recognized.

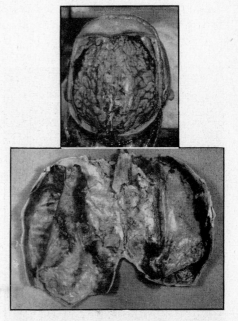

Fig. 6-22. Unexpected Death. Bilateral Chronic Subdural Hematoma with Satchel-like Compression of Cerebral Hemispheres; So-called Pachymeningitis Interna Hemorrhagica.

Note limiting membranes separating hematomas from surface of brain. Elderly white man. No definite history of trauma.

Valvular Disease. Left ventricular cardiac hypertrophy also develops as the result of valvular disease, especially after stenosis and insufficiency of the aortic valves. Aortic stenosis may follow rheumatic valvulitis or Mönckeberg's sclerosis of the aortic valves. Aortic insufficiency may be a sequel of rheumatic valvulitis or syphilitic aortitis with involvement and deformity of the aortic valves. Of the two conditions, stenosis and insufficiency, the former is more frequently encountered as a cause of left ventricular hypertrophy leading to sudden death. Such individuals may be robust and physically strong.

Other types of valvular disease, such as mitral stenosis in which hypertrophy and dilatation of the left auricle may occur, can cause sudden death. In mitral stenosis, especially when there has been auricular fibrillation, there is the possibility that a mural thrombus of the pedunculated ball valve type has formed in the left auricle and has impacted itself in or has otherwise closed off the narrowed valve orifice, causing sudden death (Fig. 6-10); or large emboli from thrombi in the auricle or on the valve may be transmitted to the brain resulting in unconsciousness, hemiplegia and death.

Aortic Disease. Syphilitic aortitis as a cause of sudden death has been mentioned in connection with two of its complications: stenosis of the ostia of one or both coronary arteries (Fig. 6-12), and insufficiency of the aortic valves resulting from separation of the valve cusps at the commissure and thickening, shrinkage and retraction of the cusps themselves from the extension of the syphilitic inflammation. Aortic insufficiency is not commonly encountered as a cause of sudden death; it is more apt to produce symptoms of cardiac decompensation gradually and to be diagnosed clinically. Sudden death is caused not infrequently by the

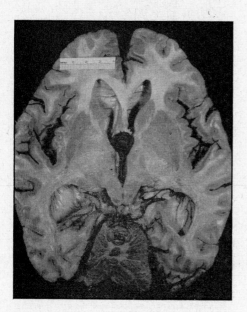

Fig. 6-23. Sudden Death. Colloid Cyst in Third Ventricle Obstructing Foramen of Monro. Moderate Internal Hydrocephalus.

White woman, 28 years old, died following headache of short duration.

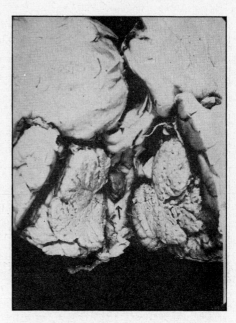

Fig. 6-24. Sudden Death. *Cysticercus cellulosae* (Larva of *Taenia solium,* the Pork Tapeworm) in the Fourth Ventricle of the Brain.

The arrow points to the parasitic cyst. A cysticercus may also lodge and develop in the third ventricle and cause unexpected death by blocking the ventricular system.

third complication of syphilitic aortitis, namely, aneurysm with rupture. Small saccular aneurysms of the ascending portion may not produce symptoms and may be clinically undetectable until sudden rupture and fatal hemopericardium occurs; larger aneurysms of the ascending aorta, the arch or the descending portion may also rupture with fatal hemorrhage. Depending upon the location of the aneurysm and the structures into which it erodes, hemorrhage may take place into the pericardial sac (Fig. 6-13), the trachea or bronchi, the pleural cavity, the esophagus, or even externally through the chest wall or at the base of the neck if the aneurysm happens to involve the innominate or the left common carotid artery.

Aneurysms of the abdominal aorta are not as common as those of the thoracic portion and are arteriosclerotic and not syphilitic in origin. They are usually saccular, fairly large and may rupture retroperitoneally (Fig. 6-14).

Spontaneous rupture of the ascending aorta may cause sudden death. Usually the hemorrhage occurs into the pericardial sac tamponading the heart (Fig. 6-11);

more rarely there is bleeding into the pleural cavity. The initial lesion is a rupture of the intima and media followed by a dissecting hemorrhage or so-called dissecting aneurysm of the entire aorta which may produce few or many clinical signs and symptoms. The end result is often a secondary rupture through the adventitia with a fatal pericardial or pleural hemorrhage. This type of aortic lesion is encountered

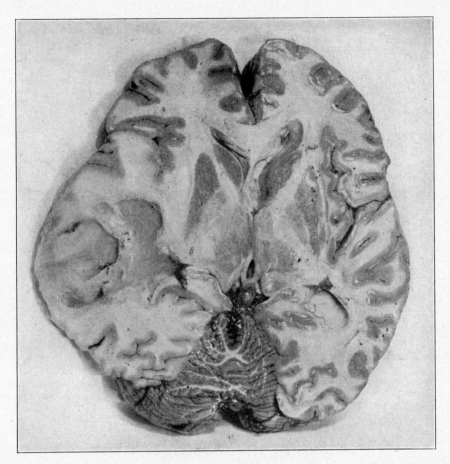

Fig. 6-25. Sudden Death: Brain Abscess of Left Temporal Lobe; Complication of Chronic Suppurative Otitis Media and Mastoiditis Not Suspected Clinically; White Man, 37 Years Old.

Brain sectioned horizontally.

from the third decade onward. The basis for the rupture and for the rapid dissection of the aorta by the extravasated blood is a mucinous degeneration of the medial coat of the aorta; it is not syphilitic or atherosclerotic in origin, but is more apt to occur in hypertensive individuals and occasionally is associated with coarctation of the aortic isthmus. In a number of cases the aorta reveals evidence of old incomplete tears in addition to the fresh fatal rupture (Fig. 6-11). Spontaneous rupture of the aorta is not encountered below the isthmus and is usually in the first part of the ascending portion. Traumatic ruptures, although they occur in the ascending as well as in the descending portions of the aorta, are characteristic and readily recognized for what they are, if for no other reason than their association with severe injuries to the other structures of the chest.

Occasionally sudden death of elderly persons is caused by occlusive thrombosis of the abdominal aorta secondary to a severe atherosclerosis. Instances have been encountered in young adults or middle-aged persons of mural thrombosis on otherwise harmless solitary atheromatous plaques in the ascending aorta, and these in rare instances have produced fatal coronary or cerebral embolism. Similar lesions of the thoracic aorta have resulted in mesenteric embolism and infarction of the intestines.

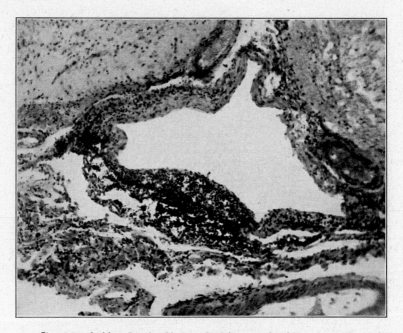

Fig. 6-26. Sudden Death. Chronic Syphilitic Basilar Leptomeningitis.

White man, 38 years of age. Death after slight trauma with symptoms suggesting brain injury. Note extensive round cell infiltration of leptomeninges. Section taken through pons. Low magnification.

DISEASES OF THE RESPIRATORY SYSTEM

Twenty-three and one-tenth per cent of the autopsied series of sudden natural deaths were caused by diseases of this organ system. Sudden death from hypertrophy of the right cardiac ventricle (*cor pulmonale*) secondary to chronic pulmonary disease has already been mentioned. Unexpected death may also result from *massive pulmonary embolism* due to detachment of large thrombi in the iliac or deep femoral veins. Noninfectious thrombosis can occur in the large veins of the pelvis and lower extremities usually as the result of stasis of blood flow in adult individuals confined to bed because of illness, surgical operation or traumatic injury. The development of such thrombi is favored by the presence of heart disease even in the absence of cardiac decompensation, by low-grade inflammation or degeneration of the vein walls, or by an increase of prothrombin in the blood. In most instances the thrombi are bland and appear to develop on the basis of the stasis of blood flow. Local factors such as pregnancy and large fibromyomata uteri may impede the venous return from the lower extremities and thus favor static thrombosis. In a few instances ambulatory individuals may develop such thrombi, but such cases are rare in the absence of thrombophlebitis. The process is often bilateral; and when search for the source of a massive pulmonary embolism is made at autopsy, both lower extremities should be examined and the iliac, deep femoral and popliteal veins should be explored. Pulmonary embolism sufficient to cause sudden death requires a thrombus of large size and these are mostly formed in the large veins of the pelvis and lower extremities. When such thrombi are freed from their attachments, they are transported through the inferior vena cava, the right side of the heart, and finally occlude the pulmonary artery causing acute asphyxia

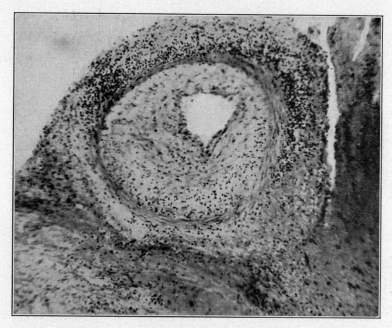

Fig. 6-27. Sudden Death: Spontaneous Subarachnoid Hemorrhage.

White man, 50 years old. Rupture of syphilitic aneurysm of cerebral artery. Syphilitic panarteritis of artery near aneurysm is shown in the photomicrograph.

(Figs. 8-10 and 8-11). Paradoxical embolism and the conditions required for its occurrence are discussed on page 179 (see Fig. 8-12).

Septic or *diphtheritic inflammation* of the throat may cause blocking of the air passages and a sudden fatal asphyxia (Fig. 6-15). *Laryngeal edema* from such causes as tumors of the pharynx, larynx and esophagus, septic infection of the pharynx, tonsils and larynx, and cellulitis of the neck can also cause asphyxia. An asphyxia characterized by prolonged expiratory dyspnea may produce death unexpectedly in *bronchial asthma* in which the obstruction to breathing is the result of a generalized muscular spasm of the smaller bronchi and of the presence of tenacious mucoid secretion in the large bronchi.

Fatal hemorrhage may arise from a *tuberculous cavity* in the lung or from a *bronchiectasis* or a *bronchial carcinoma*. In rare instances a tuberculous cavern or an emphysematous bleb may rupture into the pleural cavity and cause rapidly fatal *pneumothorax*.

Not infrequently various infections of the lungs, unrecognized during life, cause death unexpectedly from toxemia; of this group ambulatory *lobar pneumonia* is the most common example. Of the autopsied series of sudden deaths, 8.7 per cent were caused by this disease. In addition to being the second most common cause of sudden natural death, ambulatory, clinically unrecognized cases of lobar pneumonia may have other medicolegal implications; the patient may develop a toxic delirium and commit various antisocial acts of a homicidal or suicidal nature.

Occasionally influenzal or *viral pneumonia, tuberculosis, parasitic infections* of the lung, *chronic bronchitis* and *bronchiectasis* cause unexpected death evidently

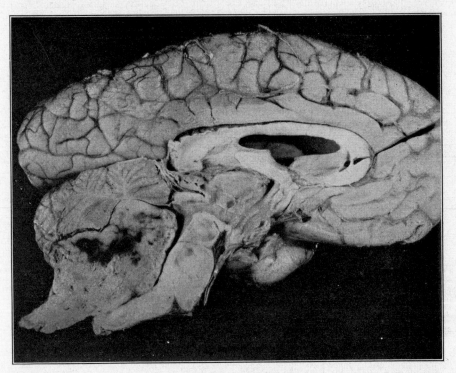

Fig. 6-28. Sudden Death: Brain Tumor (Ependymoma) of Fourth Ventricle Herniating into Foramen Magnum and Compressing Brain Stem.

Patient a 30 year old white woman who died shortly after chiropractic manipulation for pain in back of neck. Median sagittal section of brain.

from *toxemia. Bronchopneumonia* causes a certain number of sudden deaths in infants but in many cases where it is suspected it cannot be demonstrated by gross or microscopic examination.

DISEASES OF THE BRAIN AND MENINGES

Diseases of this organ system were responsible for 17.9 per cent of sudden and unexpected natural deaths in the autopsied series. A variety of important conditions is encountered in this group.

Spontaneous Cerebral Hemorrhage. This, a frequent cause of unexpected rapid death, was encountered in 5.4 per cent of the autopsied cases. The hemorrhage occurs most commonly in the basal ganglia (Fig. 6-16) from the rupture of a lenticulostriate artery; there is usually an underlying cerebral arteriosclerosis and arterial hypertension. This type of hemorrhage is the ordinary cerebral apoplexy. Death is usually not sudden but takes place after a variable period of coma during which a clinical diagnosis can usually be made. Such hemorrhage is encountered most frequently in late middle-aged or elderly persons. A number of such deaths occur in the absence of witnesses.

Clinically, spontaneous cerebral hemorrhage of this type has been mistaken for the traumatic variety of intracranial hemorrhage either because of a misleading history suggesting traumatic injury or because of the presence of superficial external

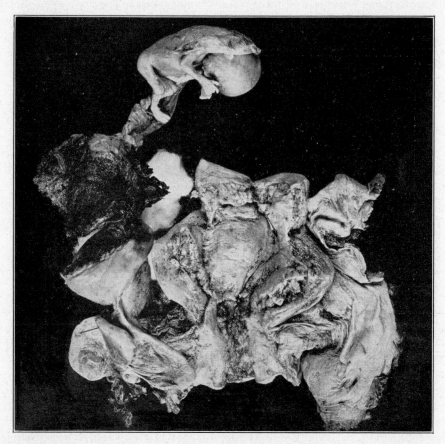

Fig. 6-29. Sudden Death: Rupture of Ectopic Tubal Pregnancy; Hemoperitoneum; Gestation About Three Months; Corpus Luteum in Right Ovary and Decidua Lining Uterus.

injuries of the head incident to the victim's falling unconscious when the hemorrhage occurred. On the other hand, cases of traumatic intracranial hemorrhage associated with fracture of the skull and even with unrecognized penetrating stab wounds of the skull and brain have been mistaken for the spontaneous variety because of the clinical signs, the absence of a history of traumatic injury and the absence of external signs of violence. An elevated blood pressure, both systolic and diastolic, can develop rapidly in cases of traumatic intracranial injury and its presence does not prove that an intracranial hemorrhage is necessarily spontaneous. Although the recognition at autopsy of a spontaneous cerebral hemorrhage arising in the basal ganglia or elsewhere should not be difficult for the trained pathologist, such hemorrhages have been erroneously designated as traumatic by inexperienced or careless observers unfamiliar with the characteristic locations and appearance of, and differences between, traumatic and spontaneous cerebral hemorrhages. Artefacts in the skull produced during the course of the autopsy have been mistaken for fractures, leading to further confusion and misinterpretation of the brain hemorrhage. Conversely, traumatic brain lacerations have been erroneously mistaken for the natural variety and associated fractures of the skull overlooked because the dura was not stripped from the base of the skull.

Spontaneous Pontine and Cerebellar Hemorrhages. These are encountered less commonly than the hemorrhages into the basal ganglia and they are also

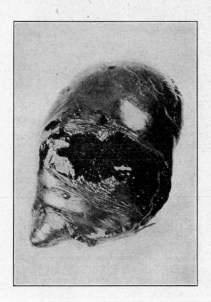

Fig. 6-30. Sudden Death: Spontaneous Rupture of Spleen; Typhoid Fever; Hemoperitoneum; White Male, 30 Years of Age.

A similar spontaneous rupture of a soft, engorged and friable spleen may take place in malaria.

usually complications of cerebral arteriosclerosis and arterial hypertension. Some cerebellar hemorrhages are the result of the rupture of an aneurysm of a cerebellar artery but in most cases an aneurysm cannot be demonstrated. Pontine hemorrhage and cerebellar hemorrhage each occurred in 0.6 per cent of the autopsied series of sudden natural deaths. The pontine variety of hemorrhage produces hyperpyrexia and the temperature may become elevated to 107° F. or higher. The pupils become constricted and the condition may be confused with morphine poisoning. In addition to the coma there are signs of bilateral pyramidal tract involvement. Death may occur fairly rapidly after the onset of the hemorrhage. At autopsy the hemorrhage in the pons is not visible until that structure is sectioned; a pontine hemorrhage has been overlooked because the pons was not opened, section of the cerebrum offering no clue to its presence. Not all pontine hemorrhages are of spontaneous origin. Traumatic hemorrhages in that part of the brain can occur but in association with other unmistakable evidence of traumatic intracranial injury.

Spontaneous hemorrhage into the cerebellum usually occurs in one of the hemispheres. It may cause death rapidly because of the location of that part of the brain beneath the tentorium, where any increase in pressure is exerted against the brain stem.

Spontaneous Subarachnoid Hemorrhage. Spontaneous subarachnoid hemorrhage is a common and important cause of sudden and unexpected natural death. Thus there were 95 deaths from this cause out of the total of 2,030 autopsied cases reported by Helpern and Rabson, representing 4.7 per cent of the total and 25.7

per cent of the disease of the brain and meninges. In the majority of the cases, the source of the subarachnoid hemorrhage was the rupture of an aneurysm of a cerebral artery, most often of the circle of Willis or its branches. The term berry aneurysm has been applied to these saccular dilatations of the cerebral arteries by Martland, who states that Eppinger used this descriptive term because the lesion was berry-like in size and color. Although these aneurysms have been designated as congenital, they are not found at birth but develop during life probably on the basis of a con-

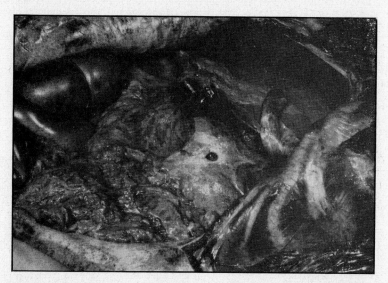

Fig. 6-31. Unexpected Death. Spontaneous Perforation of Chronic Duodenal Ulcer. Acute Suppurative Peritonitis.

White woman, 35 years old, died 24 hours after admission to the hospital for acute and chronic alcoholism. Perforated ulcer photographed in situ through autopsy incision.

genital weakness in the artery wall. Sometimes they are multiple and, as Forbus has pointed out, are situated at the bifurcation of the large branches of the circle of Willis. About three fourths of the ruptured aneurysms were found in the anterior portion of the circle of Willis on the anterior and middle cerebral arteries and on the anterior communicating artery. In the New York series saccular aneurysms as the source of hemorrhage were discovered in 64 out of 86 cases (74 per cent). Martland found a berry aneurysm as the source of fatal subarachnoid hemorrhage in a similar proportion of cases, 38 out of 54.

The most frequent anatomic variety of hemorrhage resulting from the rupture of a cerebral artery aneurysm is the diffuse type of subarachnoid hemorrhage. In this variety there is a rapid accumulation of blood on the undersurface of the brain with extension along the fissure of Sylvius and into the cisterna magna and fourth ventricle. Death is usually very rapid, presumably from medullary compression.

Examples of rapid, fatal, diffuse subarachnoid hemorrhage are illustrated in the following cases:

A sturdy Coast Guard chief petty officer, 26 years old, came home on week-end leave late Saturday afternoon. Before, during, and after dinner he drank several whiskey highballs. He and his wife retired about midnight. Shortly thereafter, during coitus, he made gurgling noises, and became unconscious. The wife rushed from the house to telephone for an ambulance. On her return, several minutes later, the man was dead. Autopsy revealed massive spontaneous subarachnoid hemorrhage arising from an easily identifiable aneurysm of the circle of Willis.

A 14 year old schoolboy was annoying the apartment house doorman by rollerskating in the lobby. When the lad refused to quit, the man slapped him across the face. The boy collapsed and died within a few minutes. At necropsy a large subarachnoid hemorrhage was found; the exact source of the bleeding could not be demonstrated. An aneurysm was not found, but there was an anomalous asymmetric development of the cerebral arteries, which were extremely delicate. There was no physical evidence of trauma. The doorman had been taken into custody but was released when the autopsy findings were disclosed.

A vigorous successful physician in his middle thirties, who had recently purchased a large amount of life insurance, was found dead by his wife in the morning 15 minutes after he had been heard talking to a patient on the telephone. There had been no prior history of illness and the medical examination at the time the policies were issued was negative. The death was certified by a private physician without autopsy as having resulted from coronary artery disease. The suddenness and other circumstances of the death, and the fact that the deceased had only recently become heavily insured, led to the suspicion that the death might not have been natural, but suicidal. Although the insurer did not have the right to demand an autopsy, the family, sensing suspicion, consented to autopsy which was performed about a month after death on the exhumed body. The cause of death was a spontaneous massive subarachnoid hemorrhage from the rupture of a very small aneurysm of a cerebral artery at the base of the brain.

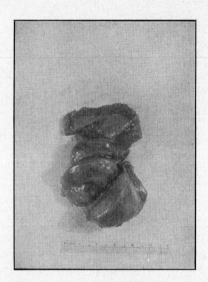 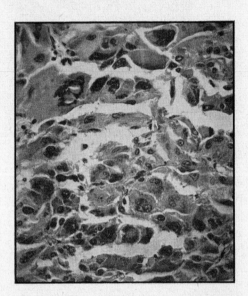

Fig. 6-32. Sudden Death One Hour After Onset of Severe Upper Abdominal Pain with Collapse. Pheochromocytoma of Right Adrenal Gland, Weighing 30 gm. and Containing 300 mg. of Adrenalin On Assay.

Left. Tumor in right adrenal gland.

Right. Photomicrograph of histologic section of tumor showing characteristic large irregular cells.

There is a less common form of subarachnoid hemorrhage following the rupture of an aneurysm of the middle cerebral artery high in the fissure of Sylvius. This results in a localized hematoma between the insula and the overlying brain. On casual examination, a section of the brain through such an area of hemorrhage suggests an intracerebral rather than a subarachnoid location (Fig. 6-21).

In a few instances a subarachnoid hemorrhage may distend and rupture the arachnoid so that the subdural space is filled with blood. Such subdural hemorrhage must not be confused with the traumatic variety. Helpern reported a case in which an aneurysm of the internal carotid artery ruptured directly into the subdural space and produced a pure subdural hemorrhage without any subarachnoid bleeding. Failure to search for and find the aneurysm in such a case may lead to the erroneous diagnosis of a traumatic subdural hemorrhage.

Aneurysms of the cerebral arteries during their development may embed themselves in the adjacent cerebral substance. Their subsequent rupture may give rise to an intracerebral hemorrhage with extension into the ventricles, followed by spread into the subarachnoid space (Fig. 6-19). At times the latter is uninvolved and remains free of hemorrhage. Such cases may bleed slowly; until the hemorrhage breaks into the ventricular system, the spinal fluid remains free of blood. Spontaneous intracerebral hemorrhage occurring at sites other than the basal ganglia is usually the result of the rupture of such an embedded aneurysm.

The following is an example of delayed death with confusing premonitory symptoms resulting from the slow rupture of an embedded cerebral artery aneurysm:

A 58 year old business executive, who was known to have hypertension but was otherwise well, developed a severe headache during a luncheon following a business meeting. He telephoned his physician and mentioned to him that he had never had such a severe headache before. His doctor advised him to come to his office immediately for an examination. Unaccompanied, the patient hailed a taxicab and gave the driver the address of the doctor's office which was in a professional building about a mile away. When the taxi arrived at its destination, the patient was conscious but disturbed and confused, and he was unable to state his doctor's name after entering the building, where he was not recognized by the attendant then on duty. Because of his excitement and mental confusion he was taken to the office of a psychiatrist on another floor in the same building. The psychiatrist diagnosed the patient's condition as alcoholism and instructed the taxi driver to take him home, which he did. By the time the cab arrived at the apartment house, the patient was stuporous. The driver called the superintendent of the house and told him the diagnosis that had been made by the psychiatrist. Believing the patient to be drunk, they half carried the now helpless man to his apartment where they laid him down on the floor in the belief that he would sleep off his "drunken condition." About two and a half hours had elapsed between the time the patient telephoned his doctor and the time that he was carried into his home. Several hours later, the superintendent looked in on the man, and, finding him now deeply unconscious, summoned a neighborhood doctor, who arrived shortly before the patient died. Not until after the patient's death did his own physician finally learn what had happened. The case was reported to the medical examiner's office for investigation, and because of the unusual circumstances an autopsy was performed. This revealed a ruptured saccular aneurysm, 6 mm. in size, of the circle of Willis located on the left anterior cerebral artery in the vicinity of the anterior communicating vessel; the aneurysm was embedded in the left frontal lobe. The rupture at first produced a localized intracerebral hemorrhage which in turn ruptured into the lateral ventricle and into the subarachnoid space. The premonitory symptoms of the rupture were first headache, then mental confusion and speech aphasia, and lastly unconsciousness.

In the examination of the brain at autopsy in cases of subarachnoid hemorrhage, the meninges should be stripped and the arteries exposed while the blood clot is still soft and easily washed away. In the medicolegal autopsy it is important to determine promptly the nature and source of the hemorrhage, especially in cases in which death has occurred during an altercation in which the alleged assailant has been arrested. A search for the aneurysm as the source of the hemorrhage should be made immediately and is best done on the fresh unfixed brain. The brain should not be put in formalin for hardening in the conventional way before it is completely and carefully dissected. The cerebral findings must be interpreted and correlated with those of the scalp, skull and the remainder of the body.

Of the 95 cases of subarachnoid hemorrhage, 73 were white and 22 were Negroes. Fifty-nine were men and 35 women. Since women make up about 20 per cent of the total number of medical examiner's cases and of the natural deaths, they are relatively more numerous in this group of cases.

Although it is generally believed that subarachnoid hemorrhage is predominately a disease of young persons, there is actually a wide age distribution of this condition. Only one case was observed under 5 years, one at 14 years and one at 19 years. The remainder ranged between 20 and 69 years; 12 in the third decade, 30 in the fourth, 30 in the fifth, 14 in the sixth, and 6 in the seventh. Thus fatal subarachnoid hemorrhage is relatively most common in adult life and middle age.

Of the 95 cases of subarachnoid hemorrhage, 17 were housewives; 12 laborers; 7 mechanics; 4 each were clerks, engineers, domestics, seamen; 2 each were janitors, stationary firemen and telephone operators; the occupation of the remainder was not recorded although about two-thirds were evidently laborers.

Death occurred at home in 43 instances, 10 of them in bed. In 8 cases the deceased died in bed but not at home, usually in a hotel or a rooming house. Fourteen subjects suffered their hemorrhage while walking in the street or park; 7 while doing arduous and 1 while doing sedentary work; 4 in public places and 4 while visiting friends. Information was obtained of the circumstances during which the disease manifested itself in only a small number of cases. An altercation was reported or suspected in 12 cases, 5 of these on the street. In these cases either no physical evidence of trauma or slight marks of traumatic injury were found, indicating that the trauma did not directly cause the hemorrhage. Of these 12 cases, a ruptured aneurysm was found in 3 subjects, its presence or absence was not stated in 2, in 7 an aneurysm could not be identified; in some, anomalies of the cerebral arteries were observed.

Acute alcoholism is not infrequently associated with fatal subarachnoid hemorrhage; it may be that the active hyperemia of the brain induced by alcohol is a factor in causing the aneurysm to rupture. Of the 43 cases in which alcohol determinations were made, 60 per cent revealed the presence of ethyl alcohol in amounts indicative of intoxication; a 4 plus (0.4 to 0.6 per cent) was found in 2 of these cases. With one exception all of the cases in which subarachnoid hemorrhage occurred during an altercation revealed amounts indicating intoxication (3 plus: 0.25 to 0.40 per cent). The brain was not chemically examined in the case of a 12 year old boy who collapsed and died of a subarachnoid hemorrhage following a slap in the face. In one case, methyl alcohol was found.

Death occurred within a few minutes after the onset of symptoms in 25 of the 95 cases; in less than half an hour in 6 cases, less than 1 hour in 6 cases, a few hours in 9 cases, and less than 6 hours in 8 cases. Fifty-seven cases (60 per cent) died within 6 hours. Nineteen lived several days and one survived 22 days. In Martland's series of 54 cases, 21 either were found dead or else died within 30 minutes after collapse. Thirty-three died more slowly: six lived 1 hour; six, 2 hours; five, 3 hours; three, 3 to 12 hours; four, 1 day; two, 2 days; two, 4 days; one, 5 days, and two, 6 days.

The characteristic syndrome of a spontaneous rupture of an artery of the circle of Willis with a subarachnoid hemorrhage consists of a severe headache which usually causes the patient to cry out with pain, vertigo, vomiting, followed rapidly by coma and convulsions. If death does not occur shortly, the patient may regain consciousness and other signs of meningeal irritation may be present. The spinal fluid is bloody and under increased pressure.

Saccular aneurysms of the cerebral arteries which give rise to most of the spontaneous subarachnoid hemorrhages are, as pointed out by Forbus, developmental in origin, the result of a combination of a congenital weakness of the vessel wall and the dynamics of blood flow. They occur most often at points of bifurcation of the larger arteries where this mechanism for their development is most effective. Their congenital origin is further indicated by the fact that they are not infrequently associated with malformations of the circle of Willis and also with other congenital anomalies such as polycystic kidneys, as in the cases described by O'Crowley and Martland.

In some instances the aneurysm forms on the basis of an atherosclerotic degeneration of the cerebral arteries. Such atherosclerotic aneurysms are encountered in older persons and usually involve the basilar artery as a fusiform dilatation or as a saccular formation at the distal end, projecting forward between the posterior communicating or posterior cerebral arteries. More rarely a cerebral artery aneurysm is associated with a syphilitic arteritis (Fig. 6-27).

Many cases among the 25 per cent in which the site of origin of the subarachnoid hemorrhage was not evident even after careful dissection showed arteries which were thin-walled, delicate, narrow in caliber and hypoplastic; such cerebral arteries were anomalously asymmetrical in distribution or were associated with evidences of status lymphaticus. Occasional fatal subarachnoid and intracerebral hemorrhages were observed in which the source of the bleeding was a mycotic aneurysm or infectious arteritis secondary to a bacterial endocarditis. In a few cases, a syphilitic arteritis without aneurysm formation of the cerebral arteries has been found accompanying spontaneous subarachnoid hemorrhage.

Multiple Cerebral Hemorrhages. Fatal cerebral hemorrhages, sometimes multiple, are occasionally encountered as a cause of unexpected death in persons suffering from undiagnosed chronic leukemia. A rare case of bilateral, almost symmetrical, hemorrhage disrupting both basal ganglia was observed in a 30 year old man suffering from Wilson's disease. The liver revealed a typical coarsely nodular cirrhosis (Fig. 6-35).

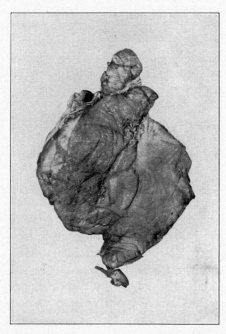

Fig. 6-33. Sudden Death: Status Thymicolymphaticus and Graves' Disease; Thymus 178 gm.; Negro Girl, 15 Years of Age, Who Died Suddenly Two Days after Rape.

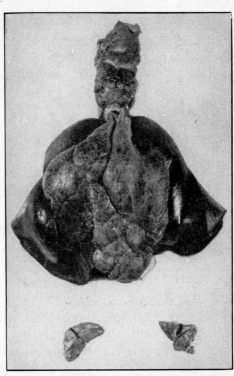

Fig. 6-34. Sudden Death. Status Thymicolymphaticus.

Autopsy revealed large thick thymus, weighing 77 gm., extending from neck to diaphragm with slight compression of trachea. Small thin adrenals. Petechial hemorrhages in thymus and beneath pleura. Chinese female infant, five months old, found dead in crib in unchanged position two hours after mother put her to sleep on left side. No other anatomical evidence of disease.

Pachymeningitis Interna Hemorrhagica. Insidiously developing and progressive bilateral pachymeningitis interna hemorrhagica may cause death by cerebral compression. In one such case both cerebral hemispheres were compressed symmetrically so that the top of the brain looked like an old-fashioned satchel (Fig. 6-26). Many of these chronic subdural hematomas arise spontaneously, especially when they are bilateral, though a few are probably traumatic in origin; most but not all of the unilateral hematomas are traumatic.

Cerebral Thrombosis and Embolism. Cerebral thrombosis is not a common cause of sudden natural death. It is more apt to occur in elderly persons suffering from advanced cerebral arteriosclerosis and as a complication during some other illness. In most cases the onset is gradual and the period of survival long enough to permit clinical diagnosis so that when death occurs the physician in attendance can certify the cause. Cerebral thrombosis usually involves the middle cerebral, basilar or vertebral arteries and produces cerebral infarction. Its extent and stage of development depend on the period of survival. Cerebral thrombosis and infarction are not infrequently encountered in elderly persons who have sustained injuries to various parts of the body not necessarily severe but sufficient to confine them to bed; these processes may complicate surgical operations. As in the case of spontaneous cerebral hemorrhage, the onset of a cerebral artery thrombosis may cause the individual to fall and sustain trivial injuries about the head; these may lead to a mistaken clinical diagnosis of traumatic intracranial hemorrhage and unnecessary craniotomy. A number of cases of suspected head injury were found at autopsy to be spontaneous cerebral thrombosis with infarction. The circumstances preceding the onset of symptoms may lead to the suspicion of foul play or accidental violence and in fatal cases necessitate investigation and autopsy by the medical examiner.

Spontaneous cerebral thrombosis and infarction in the presence of cerebral arteriosclerosis are not difficult to recognize at autopsy. In the absence of arteriosclerosis and in younger individuals, the finding of a cerebral artery occluded by a thrombus suggests the possibility that the process was embolic in origin. During the autopsy a careful search should be made for a mural thrombus either in the left auricle or ventricle or in the ascending portion and arch of the aorta. Such a thrombus might possibly be the source of embolism to the arteries of the brain. Silent myocardial infarction secondary to occlusive coronary arteriosclerosis may lead to persistent mural thrombosis in the left ventricle and a resultant fatal embolism to the brain. Similarly in mitral stenosis, a mural thrombosis in the left auricle may give rise to the same complication. The authors have encountered cases of unsuspected thrombosis of the aortic arch and of the common carotid arteries. These thromboses were the source of fatal embolism to the middle cerebral artery. The presence of multiple infarctions in the brain is suggestive of embolic occlusion of the cerebral arteries, but multiple cerebral thromboses can also occur. Embolic abscesses of brain can develop as the result of the discharge of septic emboli from the valves on the left side of the heart or from the thrombosed veins in the wall of a lung abscess. An embolic occlusion of a cerebral artery may also be derived from a mural thrombus formed over the site of a traumatic injury in the carotid arteries, the ascending aorta or the heart. Stab wounds and bullet wounds may initiate such a mural thrombosis. The thrombotic source in all cases of cerebral embolism should be determined and also whether or not the thrombosis was of spontaneous or traumatic origin.

Parasitic and Colloid Cysts. Cerebral compression of slow and insidious development may result from a parasitic infection, such as *Cysticercus cellulosae,* which blocks the flow of the cerebrospinal fluid through the fourth ventricle and produces a hydrocephalus (Fig. 6-24). Spontaneously developing colloid cysts of the third ventricle may result in a similar type of cerebral compression by blocking the foramen of Monro (Fig. 6-23).

Intracranial Neoplasms. Such tumors may increase in size slowly, causing atypical symptoms, until there is a sudden fatal onset of cerebral compression. Most of these tumors are primary gliomas (Figs. 6-28 and 6-36); a few are meningiomas which arise from the dura and press in the surface of the brain. The authors have seen a case of chordoma in a white woman of 35 years which developed insidiously in the arachnoid layer covering the basilar surface of the pons and compressing the basilar artery; death occurred suddenly during the injection of sodium morrhuate into varicose veins of the leg.

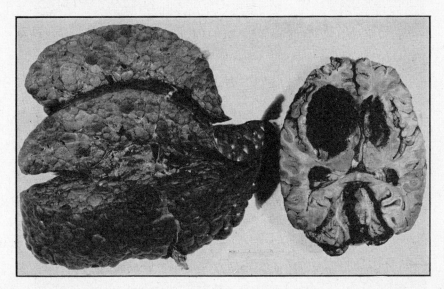

Fig. 6-35. Sudden Death: Spontaneous Bilateral Hemorrhage Disrupting Basal Ganglia. Typical Coarsely Nodular Cirrhosis of Liver.

Wilson's disease (hepatolenticular syndrome) in a 30 year old white man.

Occasionally metastatic tumors of the brain are a cause of unexpected death in persons who possess a silent primary growth elsewhere in the body such as a bronchial carcinoma, a malignant melanoma or a chorio-epithelioma.

The behavior disturbance associated with undiagnosed brain tumor may lead a person into situations of danger or may be the cause of fatal accidental injuries. In one case a white man was found dead on the subway tracks along which he had wandered some distance from the station. The autopsy disclosed gliomas in both frontal lobes which had produced a fatal cerebral compression. Had the body been struck by a train and the head demolished, it is unlikely that the true nature of the death would have been revealed.

Brain Abscess, Polioencephalitis and Meningitis. Brain abscess which is frequently a complication of a chronic otitis media and mastoiditis (Fig. 6-25) or is secondary to a clinically quiescent and unsuspected lung abscess, may develop insidiously and cause rapid death from cerebral compression. Acute polioencephalitis or encephalitis may be a cause of sudden or unexpected death. The intense congestion of the brain and spinal cord may suggest the nature of the lesion but the diagnosis can only be confirmed by histologic examination.

Fulminating meningococcic sepsis may cause rapid and unexpected death. In some of these cases the infection is so overwhelming that suppurative leptomeningitis, which is usually evident in more slowly developing cases, is absent. The meninges are intensely congested. Suggestive signs of this disease are cyanosis, extensive petechial and purpuric hemorrhages of the skin and conjunctivas and massive hemorrhages in both adrenal glands. In some cases the purpura was so

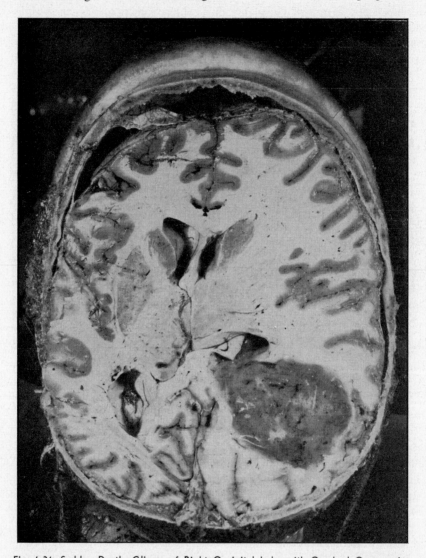

Fig. 6-36. Sudden Death: Glioma of Right Occipital Lobe with Cerebral Compression.

Brain photographed in situ after sectioning. A 15 year old boy who complained of pain in the throat. Sudden collapse and death in hospital yard after palliative treatment in clinic.

confluent as to be mistaken for bruises and to suggest that the deceased had been assaulted or maltreated. In other instances the rapid onset and intensity of the symptoms, often associated with vomiting, have led some to consider seriously the possibility of poisoning. The characteristic disease picture presented by fulminating meningococcic septicemia, characterized by petechiae and purpura, massive adrenal hemorrhage, rapid collapse and death, is also known as the Waterhouse-Friderichsen syndrome (Fig. 6-37). It is not infrequently encountered by the medical examiner.

Other cases of meningococcus septicemia without meningitis do not show adrenal hemorrhages but are accompanied by purpura and petechiae. The more common examples of meningococcic meningitis with or without skin rashes are less apt to come to the attention of the medical examiner. Martland has recently reported his findings in 19 fatal cases of the Waterhouse-Friderichsen syndrome; there were as many cases in adults as in children. The victims either were found dead or else died so rapidly after becoming ill as to warrant medicolegal investigation; in some of the cases prior to autopsy there was suspicion of poisoning, negligence and homicidal assault.

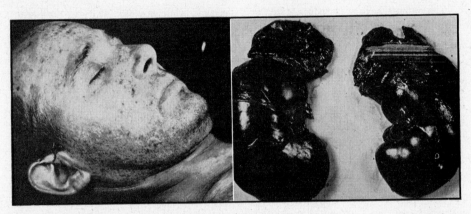

Fig. 6-37: Sudden Death: Fulminating Meningococcic Septicemia, Waterhouse Friderichsen Syndrome. White Man, 35 Years Old.

Left: purpuric rash on face, part of generalized eruption.
Right: massive bilateral adrenal hemorrhages.

Syphilitic Infection. Chronic syphilitic leptomeningitis is characterized by a round cell inflammatory infiltration in the pia arachnoid layer, best seen on the under surface of the pons and around the circle of Willis. It may be accompanied by a well developed syphilitic arteritis; thrombosis of some of the vessels may occur, and the brain may show an associated syphilitic encephalitis. The lesion may be a cause of unexpected death, sometimes under suspicious circumstances. A number of cases have occurred in which the victim has died during an altercation, without any or with only slight injury. Death may be preceded by neurologic symptoms suggesting an injury of the brain; in some cases craniotomy was performed erroneously because the symptoms were misinterpreted. At autopsy the lesion produced by syphilitic leptomeningitis, while not obvious in the gross, can readily be determined by histologic examination of the vessels and meninges at the base of the brain (Fig. 6-26).

Occasionally **general paresis** is found as a cause of sudden or unexpected death and the circumstances arising out of the peculiar behavior of the deceased may arouse suspicion of foul play. Thus the body of an adult Negro female was found on a cold day in winter lying in the park, partly concealed by the shrubbery near a stone wall. The body was lightly clad and the feet were bare; the shoes and stockings were found in the coat pocket of the deceased. Autopsy revealed a brain which was atrophied and firm with thickened meninges. The microscopic examination of the brain showed a chronic meningo-encephalitis; numerous spirochetes were found in the Levaditi preparations.

Epilepsy. Idiopathic epilepsy may be a cause of unexpected death if the victim becomes asphyxiated during the convulsive seizures. The autopsy usually does not reveal any structural alterations in the brain, and unless a history is obtained or the circumstances attending the death are known, the diagnosis of epilepsy cannot be made. Unfortunately many individuals regard the presence of epilepsy in their relatives as a disgrace and refuse to admit it to the medical examiner investigating the death. A certain number of natural deaths in young persons in which the autopsies are negative and the circumstances of death are not known are probably due to this disease.

The authors have seen such a case: a 15 year old white boy visiting New York with a school mate was found dead in bed in his hotel room. Although investigation of the circumstances suggested that death was due to natural causes and autopsy findings, histologic examination and negative toxicologic examination indicated that the deceased had died of asphyxia, they did not reveal the underlying cause. The only abnormality noted was that the cranium of the deceased was large and dolichocephalic, and the brain though normal in appearance weighed 2,400 gm., about 1,000 gm. over the average weight; the body was strongly built, 70 inches in height and 157 pounds in weight. After some difficulty a previous medical history of epileptic convulsions was obtained and death was finally explained as the result of asphyxia produced during a convulsion.

DISEASES OF THE DIGESTIVE TRACT AND UROGENITAL TRACT

Various lesions of the *digestive tract* by giving rise to severe hemorrhage may cause unexpected death. Fatal external bleeding has resulted from ulcerative carcinoma of the tongue. Massive hemorrhage into the gastrointestinal tract has occurred from an erosion of a carcinoma of the esophagus into the thoracic aorta, from a chronic gastric or duodenal ulcer, from a tuberculous ulcer of the stomach and from an esophageal varix complicating cirrhosis of the liver. Other lesions such as a spontaneous rupture of a carcinoma or a cavernoma of the liver, of an enlarged spleen in malaria or typhoid fever, of an aneurysm of the abdominal aorta or of a fallopian tube in an ectopic pregnancy may produce a fatal effusion of blood into the peritoneal cavity.

A rapidly fatal acute peritonitis may result from the spontaneous perforation of a peptic ulcer (Fig. 6-31), a typhoid ulcer of the intestine or an ulcerative carcinoma of the intestine. Sometimes the peritoneal infection may have its origin in an insidiously developing phlegmonous gastritis. Intestines incarcerated in a hernial sac may rupture spontaneously and be the cause of a fatal abdominal infection; the intestinal perforations found in these cases are very similar to the traumatic bursting ruptures of the intestine described on page 251.

The distended intestine proximal to an obstructing carcinoma of the large intestine may burst spontaneously with massive extravasation of feces into the peritoneal cavity and rapid death by shock. Sudden intestinal obstruction caused by adhesions or volvulus or a hernial sac may cause death by shock. Similarly, the sudden impaction of a gallstone in the common duct or an acute pancreatitis may cause rapid death by shock or toxemia.

Diseases of the *urogenital tract* such as a severe grade of nephritis, nephrolithiasis, renal tuberculosis or neoplasm, obstruction hydronephrosis or pyonephrosis may cause death unexpectedly, usually in uremia. Rarely spontaneous rupture of the urinary bladder, due to obstructive distention and weakening of the bladder wall from carcinoma, prostatic hypertrophy or urethral stricture, causes death by shock or peritonitis; these ruptures are similar to the traumatic ruptures of the bladder described on page 255. A few sudden deaths from shock result from the twisting of a pedunculated subserous fibromyoma of the uterus or of an ovarian cyst on its pedicle. Spontaneous rupture of an ectopic tubal pregnancy resulting in rapid fatal hemorrhage into the peritoneal cavity is perhaps the most commonly encountered disease of the reproductive system to cause sudden death (Fig. 6-29).

Sudden death during pregnancy can occur from a massive pulmonary embolism from unsuspected static thrombosis of the pelvic veins. The same fatal complication can also happen in women suffering from large fibromyomas of the uterus. Eclamptic toxemia may develop rapidly and without warning in the latter months of pregnancy and cause sudden death during convulsions. In one such case the deceased had a negative physical examination a few days before the fatal convulsive seizure so that the possibility of a convulsant poison was considered. Since the chemical examination of the organs was negative, poison was eliminated as a factor in the case. Conversely several cases of fatal homicidal strychnine poisoning in women in the latter months of pregnancy were mistaken clinically for eclamptic toxemia with convulsions.

Severe anemia induced by prolonged severe hemorrhage from the uterus with submucous fibromyomas has caused unexpected death. Untreated carcinoma of the vulva has extended into the groin to erode the femoral vein and cause a fatal external hemorrhage.

Fatal hemorrhage from the spontaneous rupture of an ulcerated varicose vein of the vagina has been observed as a cause of unexpected death in the middle third of pregnancy in two cases.

MISCELLANEOUS AND UNCLASSIFIED DISEASES

In this category are included various conditions such as Addison's disease, constitutional diseases, blood dyscrasias, spinal deformities and hemorrhage from varicose leg ulcers, any of which may cause unexpected death. *Addison's disease,* most often resulting from the destruction of the adrenal glands by fibrocaseous tuberculosis, may escape clinical recognition and cause death unexpectedly with symptoms and under circumstances that arouse a suspicion of food or chemical poisoning. In one such case, the deceased was an adult white woman who became ill with diarrhea after eating clams; in another case, the deceased was a middle-aged white man whose gastrointestinal symptoms had led to an accusation of homicidal poisoning against his wife by other members of his family. In both cases the cause of death was bilateral tuberculosis of the adrenal; chemical examination of the viscera failed to show the presence of poison.

Metabolic disorders and deficiency diseases may cause unexpected death without producing any prior striking symptoms. Thus, occasionally, an unrecognized case of diabetes mellitus dies in coma as the result of acidosis. A case of hyperinsulinism resulting from a tumor of the islets of Langerhans may also die in coma distinguished by convulsive manifestations. In rare instances, hemochromatosis may be the underlying cause of sudden death; the authors have seen this condition in a 40 year old man whose myocardium was loaded with brown hemosiderin pigment. This had given rise to a severe myocardial fibrosis and eventually to a fatal myocardial insufficiency.

A rapidly fatal case of hyperadrenalism was encountered by the authors in a well developed white man of 32 years who suddenly collapsed with severe abdominal pain and died one hour later. The deceased had not complained previously of any symptoms. Death resulted from the massive discharge of adrenalin from a pheo-chromocytoma of the right adrenal gland (Fig. 6-32); the tumor weighed 30 gm. and when assayed contained 300 mg. of adrenalin. A similar case has been reported by Dolgin.

Rickets and *scurvy* may cause unexpected death in infants. Such cases of rickets develop fatal convulsions associated with tetany. Scurvy is characterized by extensive subperiosteal hemorrhages. The authors autopsied a case of scurvy in an infant in which death had resulted from extensive extradural hemorrhage in the spinal canal; the more usual subperiosteal hematomas were also present and one of these, located at the upper end of the humerus, had led to the mistaken clinical diagnosis of septic arthritis.

Blood dyscrasias such as *leukemias* and *anemias* may develop insidiously and cause unexpected death from some rapidly developing complication. In some leukemias, multiple brain hemorrhages may be the fatal lesion. In other cases the huge number of white blood cells and the associated anemia are sufficient to embarrass a myocardium already impaired because of coronary arteriosclerosis, and a sudden cessation of function may result. Pulmonary edema associated with fatty degeneration of the heart muscle in pernicious anemia and chronic leukemia may cause rapid death. A case of *sickle cell anemia,* with cardiac hypertrophy and sudden death from acute cardiac failure, has been observed by the authors. Vance and Fisher have reported a case of sickle cell disease in which unexpected death resulted from pulmonary fat embolism evidently caused by extensive hemorrhages and cellular necrosis in the bone marrow. *Hemophiliacs* may die as a result of a fatal hemorrhage following a slight traumatic injury.

Status Lymphaticus. Status lymphaticus is a condition which has been a center of controversy in medical circles for the past 60 years. Older and extremely competent authorities, impressed with the striking anatomic findings and association of this entity with certain rare sudden and entirely unexpected deaths of children and young adults for which no satisfactory cause or explanation could be demonstrated at autopsy, were of the opinion that status lymphaticus was a valid pathologic entity and played a role in the causation of such deaths.

Other authorities regard status lymphaticus as a normal morphologic variation without pathologic significance and maintain that it is not a cause of death and therefore not entitled to a place in vital statistics. They prefer to search intensively for some other pathologic process which can more authentically explain the death or, if a complete study has not revealed a satisfactory cause, to admit frankly that the cause of death is not demonstrable. For a more complete discussion of this viewpoint questioning the validity of the role of status lymphaticus as a cause of death, the reader is referred to the textbook, *Pediatrics,* by Holt and McIntosh.

We are in sympathy with those who consider status lymphaticus to be an inadequate explanation of a sudden death and who prefer to consider the cause of such a death as undetermined. However, we are critical of the viewpoint of those who reject status lymphaticus under all circumstances, but who are entirely willing to substitute for it another cause or category such as fulminating infection, usually in the form of an interstitial pneumonia, on extremely dubious histologic evidence. The designation of fulminating infection as a cause of the unexpected deaths in question is a far more unsatisfactory and misleading explanation than status lymphaticus, for it implies a final solution which it does not provide and is an oversimplification of an extremely complex and subtle problem of pathologic physiology, the anatomic basis of which is not evident. At least the designation of status lymphaticus, and we assume that a complete study has been made before such an explanation is offered, does not imply a mechanism by which death is brought about; indeed it is another way of saying that the mechanism of death was not revealed. The term fulminating infection does convey the impression of a specific causative process and mechanism of death and should not be used unless indubitable evidence of such infection is demonstrable. In our opinion the evidence revealed by a study of the circumstances of the death and by the essentially negative gross anatomic, histologic, toxicologic and bacteriologic findings at autopsy in many of the cases of sudden and unexpected deaths of infants and adolescents does not warrant the conclusion that such deaths have resulted from infection any more than from status lymphaticus.

The anatomic characteristics of status lymphaticus are familiar to pathologists who have performed many autopsies in cases of sudden suspicious and violent death. It has been observed in cases of sudden death of young persons that have occurred without warning after a slight degree of shock, after a blow of mild grade on the chest, after a heated argument or after being startled by a sudden loud noise. In other cases, sudden death has taken place at the very onset of inhalation anesthesia or during the injection of a local anesthetic or an antitoxin. Not all anesthesic or injection deaths reveal manifestations of status lymphaticus and lack a satisfactory explanation for their occurrence. But in some instances the death has occurred at the very start of the procedure before any appreciable amount of drug was administered and status lymphaticus was the only finding at autopsy. In such cases it is not unreasonable to consider it as a possible factor in causing the death.

Symmers on the basis of a large series of autopsied cases has pointed out that status lymphaticus has an incidence of 6.2 per cent, but that the sudden deaths associated with this condition are very rare, forming an infinitesimal proportion of the total number of cases.

The characteristic habitus of status lymphaticus reveals a well developed individual with a gracefully proportioned body, slender thorax, rounded muscular limbs, clear smooth-textured skin, scant facial and axillary hair and pubic hair in the male having a feminine distribution. The condition is less frequently encountered in women and more difficult to recognize on external examination; it is also difficult to diagnose in infants and in children before puberty. Internally there is enlargement and hyperplasia of the thymus at an age when involution is expected and hyperplasia of the lymphoid tissue in the spleen, gastrointestinal tract, tonsils, tongue and lymph nodes of the mesentery. There is hypoplasia of the cardiovascular system; the heart may be smaller than normal, the aorta delicate and narrow in caliber, and the systemic arteries, especially those in the brain, thin-walled and narrow. The adrenal glands are thin and hypoplastic; the genitalia may be underdeveloped. In some individuals of 30 years or over the recessive type of status lymphaticus may be found in which the external features of the condition are not so well marked. The lymphoid tissue has undergone different degrees of atrophy, but involution and hypoplasia of the cardiovascular system and adrenal glands still persist. In this older group sudden death with evidence of status lymphaticus is not common. In infancy this condition is difficult to recognize since hyperplasia of lymphoid tissue and a relatively large thymus are normal. Status lymphaticus is most easily diagnosed at autopsy in older children and adolescents.

The mechanism of sudden death in status lymphaticus is not clear. Symmers believed that it is the result of an anaphylactic reaction, the sensitization being expressed structurally by the necrotic germinal centers in the hyperplastic follicles and chemically by the release of nucleoproteins; the reaction is capable of taking place at certain times and not at others. Thus it may occur spontaneously or be precipitated by some external factor such as the injection of an antitoxin, the shock of a needle prick, sudden immersion in cold water or some other event. Whatever the explanation may be, sudden deaths do occur in a small percentage of individuals who show the physical characteristics of status lymphaticus under circumstances which do not cause deaths in individuals who are not so constituted; this association cannot be dismissed, even though the mechanism by which death occurs and the reason for it are not apparent in the present state of our knowledge.

Sudden deaths of infants with status lymphaticus have been attributed by Carr to pressure of the enlarged thymus upon the trachea, but such a mechanism for death by tracheal compression and asphyxia is difficult to demonstrate satisfactorily in most cases, even when the thymus is large. Pediatricians are concerned with this possibility and have resorted to radiation of the thymus to hasten its involution and forestall the possibility of death from thymic pressure.

The authors have recently encountered a death with evidence of status lymphaticus in a five month old Chinese female infant in whom there was no prior history of illness. The infant had been placed in the crib on its left side by its mother at one o'clock in the afternoon. Two hours later she discovered the infant dead in the same position in which she had placed it. The face was not covered or pressed into the bed clothes. Autopsy revealed a large thick fleshy thymus weighing 77 gm. extending from the neck to the diaphragm and laterally to obscure completely the pericardial sac (Fig. 6-34). There were petechial hemorrhages of the asphyxial type in the capsule and substance of the thymus and beneath the pleura and epicardium. The subpleural hemorrhages were more numerous on the left lung. The adrenals were small and thin, together weighing 2.82 gm. The trachea revealed slight but distinct flattening in its anteroposterior dimension. A complete autopsy did not reveal any other findings except lymphoid hyperplasia in the spleen; death was attributed to asphyxia resulting from pressure of the large thymus on the mediastinum. Why the death occurred when it did from this cause was not evident.

Sudden death in status lymphaticus may result from the rupture of a hypoplastic cerebral artery with the occurrence of a subarachnoid or more rarely a cerebral hemorrhage. Such deaths have medicolegal significance in that they may follow a sudden increase in intracranial pressure associated with physical or emotional strain during verbal or physical altercation. It is important not to confuse such hemorrhages with traumatic injury because of the suspicious circumstances. Status lymphaticus is met with in young pugilists. The authors have observed sudden deaths of such persons from subarachnoid hemorrhage which occurred during a boxing match.

Other Miscellaneous Diseases. Severe spinal deformities such as an extreme kyphoscoliosis may, by distorting and limiting the movements of the chest, cause embarrassment of the heart and respiration and sudden death. In such cases there is usually a pulmonary emphysema which has brought about the development of a right ventricle hypertrophy of the heart (cor pulmonale).

Occasionally, in a *varicose ulcer of the leg,* the large veins in the ulcer may become eroded and bleed sufficiently to cause death.

In a few cases the cause of death cannot be determined by complete autopsy even though it is supplemented by histologic, bacteriologic and chemical examinations. This is perhaps more often so in the case of infant deaths in which the autopsy findings are entirely negative; for example, *infantile convulsions* may cause death and leave no anatomic lesions. Similarly, epilepsy in children and adults is characterized by negative autopsy findings and cannot be diagnosed in the absence of a history.

DISEASES OF CHILDREN

Sudden and unexpected deaths in infants and young children may result from congenital anomalies, various infectious diseases and deficiency diseases.

Congenital heart disease causes death more frequently than any of the other developmental anomalies. Congenital malformations of other organs such as diaphragmatic hernia, urethral malformations with obstructive hydronephrosis or malformations of the intestinal tract are also encountered.

Neoplasms, chiefly of the brain, occur in children and may cause unexpected death.

Deficiency diseases such as rickets and scurvy have already been mentioned in the previous subdivision.

Obviously demonstrable infectious diseases such as diphtheria, rheumatic fever, respiratory tract infections with otitis media, mastoiditis, pharyngitis, laryngitis, tracheobronchitis and lobar, lobular and interstitial pneumonia are easy to evaluate. Meningitis, appendicitis with peritonitis, lymphadenitis and tuberculosis are readily recognizable. Fulminating meningococcic sepsis has already been described in the subgroup on the brain and meninges. The exanthemas such as measles, whooping cough and scarlet fever should be detected by the appearance of the organs and tissues and by the clinical history. Polioencephalitis can be diagnosed if the tissues of the central nervous system are examined microscopically.

The performance of the autopsy and the supplementary bacteriologic and histologic examinations in the case of older children will usually disclose the cause of death satisfactorily. The lesions encountered in this age group are as definable as those described in autopsies on adults.

Sudden deaths of infants in the first year of life are much more difficult to evaluate from the standpoint of determining the cause of death. At times the immediate cause of death is revealed but the primary disturbance escapes detection, even after the most exhaustive study.

Many apparently healthy infants are found dead in cribs or in carriages under circumstances that bring up the possibility of an asphyxial death by smothering. In some instances this is the case: the infant dangerously entangles itself in the bed clothes and is then unable to extricate itself. In many other instances the circumstances make it unlikely that the infant was mechanically smothered; it may be found dead lying face upward or to the side so that the air passages were not obstructed; occasionally the infant dies suddenly while in the arms of the nurse or mother. These crib deaths are most difficult to evaluate. Complete and careful autopsies in many of these cases have revealed no lesions that satisfactorily explain the death. In many the air passages are free of regurgitated food, the aspiration of which is often blamed for the death, and there has been no indication of smothering. Such infants have often had the best of care and nothing can be elicited to indicate previous illness, indisposition or unusual treatment. In a number of cases petechial hemorrhages were found in the thymus, scalp, pleura and pericardium such as one sees in asphyxia, but there was no indication of smothering; if asphyxia was the immediate cause of death, the primary condition that produced it was not revealed by the autopsy. During the onset of an infection infants may develop convulsions and asphyxiate. The possibility of a convulsive seizure cannot be ruled out in cases in which the infant is found dead, but in many cases it does not seem to have occurred.

The autopsy findings and the microscopic findings in these sudden deaths in infants are usually entirely negative or insufficient to explain why death occurred at the time it did. Werne and Garrow included microscopic and bacteriologic studies in a painstaking investigation of the cause of death in many such cases and believe that the sudden death is an expression, not of mechanical asphyxiation by smothering, but rather of a fulminating infection usually of the respiratory tract. Unquestionably some of these infants died of respiratory infection, but in our experience also based on many autopsies with microscopic studies, there was not sufficient evidence of inflammation in most of the cases to justify the conclusion that death was the result primarily of an infection. Most of these infants were well nourished and showed well-developed hyperplastic lymphatic tissue including a prominent thymus. The petechial hemorrhages in the thymus, pleura and pericardium would suggest that the immediate cause of death was asphyxia, even though the cause of the asphyxia was not apparent. Since the cause of death in these infants cannot be determined, it is just as arbitrary to put the responsibility on a fulminating infection, the anatomic evidence of which is lacking, as to ascribe it to status lymphaticus. As Farber has pointed out, it would be better to admit that the cause of death has not been determined than to attribute it to some condition which cannot be satisfactorily demonstrated.

Some infants die rapidly after diarrheal attacks. In such cases, aside from the dehydration and the weight loss, the autopsy reveals no positive findings and the intestinal cultures are negative or nonconclusive.

Since the autopsy findings are usually negative, the diagnosis of the cause of death in infants must depend on clinical and other data.

REFERENCES

Blumgart, H. L., Schlesinger, M. J., and Zoll, P. M.   Angina pectoris, coronary failure and acute myocardial infarction, J.A.M.A., 116:91, 1941.

Carr, J. L.   Status thymico-lymphaticus, Am. J. Pediat., 27:1, 1945.

Dolgin, W.   Pheochromocytoma and sudden death following injury of head, Arch. Path., 40:135, 1945.

Farber, S.   Unexpected death in early life, New England J. Med., 219:836, 1938.

Forbus, W. D.   On the origin of miliary aneurysms of superficial cerebral arteries, Bull. Johns Hopkins Hosp., 47:239, 1930.

French, A. J., and Dock, W.   Fatal coronary arteriosclerosis in young soldiers, J.A.M.A., 124:1233, 1944.

Helpern, M.   Multiple saccular aneurysms of cerebral arteries; rupture into subdural space, Proc. New York Path. Soc., May 26, 1933; Arch. Path., 16:754, 1933.

———— and Rabson, S. M.   Sudden and unexpected natural death. I. General considerations and statistics, New York State J. Med., 45:1197, 1945.

———— and Rabson, S. M.   Sudden and unexpected natural death. III. Spontaneous subarachnoid hemorrhage. In preparation.

Holt, L. E., Jr., and McIntosh, R.   Pediatrics, 12th ed., New York, Appleton-Century-Crofts, Inc., 1953, pp. 67, 703-704.

Horn, H., and Finkelstein, L. E.   Arteriosclerosis of the coronary arteries and the mechanism of their occlusion, Am. Heart J., 19:655, 1940.

Lauren, E.   Acta path. et microbiol. Scandinav., 14:40, 1937.

Leary, T.   Pathology of coronary sclerosis, Am. Heart J., 10:328, 1935.

Martland, H. S.   Spontaneous subarachnoid hemorrhage and congenital "berry" aneurysm of the circle of Willis, Am. J. Surg., 43:10, 1939.

———— Fulminating meningococcus infection with bilateral massive adrenal hemorrhage (the Waterhouse-Friderichsen syndrome), with special reference to the pathology, the medicolegal aspect and the incidence in adults, Arch. Path., 37:147, 1944.

Mosher, A. M., Dach, S., and Jaffe, H. L.   Activities associated with the onset of acute coronary artery occlusion, Am, Heart J., 18:434, 1939.

———— Jaffe, H. L., and Dach, S.   Prevalence of coronary artery occlusion, New York State J. Med., 39:1937, 1939.

O'Crowley, C. R., and Martland, H. S.   Association of polycystic disease of the kidneys with congenital aneurysms of the cerebral arteries, Am. J. Surg., 43:3, 1939.

Orth, J.   Was ist Todesursache? Berl. klin. Wchnschr., 45:485, 1908.

Paterson, J. C.   Capillary rupture with intimal hemorrhages, a causative factor in coronary thrombosis, Arch. Path., 25:474, 1938.

Rabson, S. M., and Helpern, M.   Sudden and unexpected natural death. II. Coronary arterio-sclerosis. In preparation.

Schlesinger, M. J.   An injection plus dissection study of coronary artery occlusions and anastomoses, Am. Heart J., 15:582, 1938.

Strassmann, G., and Goldstein, P.   Syphilis of aorta and coronary arteries, Arch. Path., 34:745, 1942.

———— and Konikov, W. M.   Sudden death from complete rupture of descending thoracic aorta with true fusiform aneurysm, caused by medionecrosis cystica, Am. J. Clin. Path., 15:250, 1945.

Symmers, D.   Status lymphaticus, Am. J. Surg., 26:7, 1934.

Vance, B. M., and Fisher, R. C.   Sickle cell disease, Arch. Path., 32:378, 1941.

Werne, J.   Postmortem evidence of acute infection in unexpected deaths in infancy, Am. J. Path., 18:759, 1942.

———— Sudden deaths in infancy, Bull. New York Acad. Med., 21:445, 1945.

———— and Garrow, I.   Sudden apparently unexplained death during infancy. I. Pathologic findings in infant found dead, Am. J. Path., 29:633, 1953. II. Pathologic findings in infant observed to die suddenly, Am. J. Path., 29:817, 1953.

Weyrich, G.   Erfahrungen über den plötzlichen Tod aus natürlicher Ursache bei Erwachsenen, Deutsche Ztschr. f. d. ges. gerichtl. Med., 18:221, 1931.

7

Natural Death and Trauma

Individuals suffering from severe organic disease may be victims of some form of trauma. In such cases the question arises as to which factor was the principal cause of death. This point may not be easy to determine.

The physician who is concerned with such a case may clarify the situation in his mind if he states the problem in this fashion:

1. Has the natural disease any connection with the trauma or is it a distinct process?

2. Is the natural disease sufficient to produce death by itself?

3. Is the traumatic condition sufficient to produce death by itself?

4. Is the natural disease merely a contributory factor in the death which is due mainly to trauma?

5. Is the traumatic condition merely a contributory factor to the death which is due to natural causes?

6. Is the death the result of traumatic injury and natural disease?

This analysis will usually enable the physician to form an opinion of the case. It may not be possible to answer every question satisfactorily. Since the natural disease and the trauma may affect the same organ and have a similar action on the system, their contributions to the death of the individual are not easily appraised. This question can be best considered by discussing the two categories of cases in which death is ostensibly due to a combination of both factors. In the first category the death occurs immediately after trauma; in the second, it is delayed.

DEATHS IMMEDIATELY AFTER TRAUMA

The first group is composed of individuals who, while suffering from a well-marked disease condition, received traumas of varying degrees of severity and then died either at the time of injury or shortly afterward. The conditions most often found under such circumstances are heart disease, especially coronary artery lesions, ruptures of aortic aneurysms, spontaneous cerebral and subarachnoid hemorrhages, syphilitic meningitis and arteritis.

Many persons with coronary artery sclerosis may die unexpectedly from acute circulatory collapse under circumstances which raise a number of medicolegal considerations, as, for example, when death occurs during an altercation with another person. When the not inconsiderable strain of emotional excitement, physical exertion or trauma is imposed upon a coronary circulation badly impaired by the extensive luminal narrowing of the arteries from arteriosclerosis, the victim may suffer a fatal collapse either in the midst of the imbroglio or soon after it has ended. The question to determine is whether or not any injury which the deceased might have received during the disturbance was responsible for his death. If the injury is severe and likely to be attended by much shock, as for example a fracture of the femur, death should be considered as primarily traumatic. On the other hand, if the trauma is a slight one and the coronary arteries are markedly sclerotic, the chief influence of the trauma would be to contribute to the death due primarily to the coronary artery disease.

The following case illustrates many of the questions which arise when death occurs at the time that an injury is inflicted on a person suffering from coronary arteriosclerosis. While crossing the street, a 48 year old white man was startled by an automobile horn and started to faint. As his knees bent, he was struck a glancing blow by a passing automobile and died immediately. The autopsy disclosed that the only injury was a 1 inch laceration of the scalp in the temple; severe coronary arteriosclerosis which in itself could have caused death was also present. The question here is whether the deceased fainted because he was actually dying of a sudden heart attack or whether his faint was merely a temporary one from which he might have recovered if he had not been struck by the automobile. In the latter event the shock of the injury might have contributed to his death, though the severe coronary artery disease must be considered as the factor principally responsible. The rapidity of the death would indicate that it was caused by the coronary arteriosclerosis and not by the trivial injury. It is also possible that the injury was not a factor per se but that the fright associated with the occurrence was the precipitating factor in the death.

It must be remembered that coronary arteriosclerosis and other lesions of the coronary circulation may be of such gradual and insidious development that the patient may not complain of such usual alarming symptoms of coronary insufficiency as pain in the chest, arms or epigastrium, dyspnea or fainting spells. However, during severe physical exertion, emotion, sexual excitement, alcoholic indulgence, disturbed sleep or while at complete rest, the individual may suddenly die because his heart with its insufficient coronary circulation cannot provide for the extra strain put upon it or continue at a minimal level of activity. In cases heard before the State Labor Commission, if the deceased died of coronary artery disease while at work, the question usually arises whether or not the exertion entailed by his labor at the time of death was sufficient to precipitate the cardiac collapse. According to the rulings of the Commission, if any unusual exertion arising out of the work is a factor that hastens the death of the workman, even though death is from natural causes, the claim would be judged compensable. On the other hand, a serious heart lesion is not always the cause of death. Many individuals with marked luminal narrowing of the coronary arteries due to advanced sclerosis have died not of that condition but of cerebral compression of traumatic origin complicating a fracture of the skull and a laceration of the brain. Evidently some hearts with severe coronary artery disease are able to function satisfactorily under rather adverse circumstances. Care must be taken to evaluate the findings at autopsy in connection with the other factors in the case in deciding the relative importance of the cardiac disease and of any injury which may be present.

Unexpected death associated with different types of trauma may occur in cases in which there is narrowing of the coronary mouths due to syphilitic aortitis, chronic valvular disease or marked hypertrophy of the left ventricle associated with arterial hypertension. The implications are the same as with a severe grade of coronary arteriosclerosis.

Aneurysm of the aorta most often ruptures spontaneously, but in rare instances the rupture may occur at the time that the victim has received an injury. In one case the deceased was struck a glancing blow by a car and falling to the ground, died in a few minutes. The autopsy disclosed a fracture of the left orbital plate but no corresponding lesion of the brain; his death was due to a hemorrhage into the pericardial sac from the rupture of an aneurysm of the ascending aorta. The trauma in this case may have caused a rise in blood pressure sufficient to burst open the wall of the aneurysm. Here the blood vessel lesion was responsible for the death, and the injury to the head merely contributed to the aneurysmal rupture and fatal hemorrhage.

Similarly, profuse subarachnoid hemorrhage may occur at the base of the brain because of the spontaneous rupture of a cerebral artery, usually in the circle of Willis, the wall of which has been weakened by a congenital defect of the muscular coat, by an aneurysm or by a syphilitic arteritis. Occasionally when a person with blood vessels of this type receives an unexpected blow against the side of the head, the vessel ruptures just at that moment because the impact caused a sudden rise of blood pressure which the weakened vessel wall could not sustain. The trauma varies; it may be slight or it may be severe enough to fracture the skull. In some cases of fatal subarachnoid hemorrhage the victim falls and the question then arises whether or not the hemorrhage preceded and occasioned the fall, or whether it occurred immediately after the head of the deceased struck the ground. This question cannot be solved by the autopsy findings alone. All the circumstances of the case must be given due consideration. In most cases of subarachnoid hemorrhage the circumstances are such as to indicate definitely that trauma played no part in the causation.

Spontaneous hemorrhages in the brain substance usually involving the basal nuclei, cerebellum or pons may also be associated with trauma; the same considerations apply to them as to the hemorrhages from cerebral arteries in the circle of Willis at the base of the brain.

Cerebral conditions such as brain tumors, pachymeningitis interna hemorrhagica or syphilitic arteritis of the vessels of the brain may develop slowly, producing indefinite symptoms of headache, vertigo and irritability without much outward change until the intracranial lesion has progressed to a degree dangerous to life. Some of these individuals may fall to the ground and die suddenly either with or without convulsions. Occasionally they may collapse during an altercation and die either with or without injury. Such deaths are likely to occur in cases of syphilitic arteritis of the brain associated with leptomeningitis. This lesion seems to increase the irritability of the individual and draw him into quarrels.

Sudden deaths during slight trauma are occasionally associated with status lymphaticus and have already been discussed on page 148.

It is important to remember that the distinctly depressing effect on the central nervous system of a severe grade of acute alcoholism may so enhance the deleterious effects of a natural disease condition as to produce unexpected death. Cardiac or cerebral lesions of moderate severity, if associated with an excess of alcohol in the system, may cause death; in the absence of alcohol a much more severe lesion of the same type would be necessary to produce a fatal result. In some instances a natural disease, pronounced acute alcoholism and a severe injury are present in the same individual; all three conditions may contribute to the death in varying proportions. Each case must be considered on its own merits in attempting to evaluate the responsibility of disease, traumatic injury or other external factors such as alcohol in causing death.

A second group includes cases of individuals who, dying from natural disease, have sustained a trauma of greater or lesser severity many days or weeks prior to death. Such cases form a large proportion of industrial death claims and the chief problem is the proper appraisal of the trauma in relation to the fatal natural disease condition. On the basis of this consideration two main categories may be differentiated: (1) in one the connection between the trauma and the fatal lesion is slight or nonexistent; (2) in the other there is a possibility that the trauma contributed to some extent in the development of the condition which caused death.

(1) When the relation between the injury and the cause of death is doubtful, the trauma is either too slight to have had any lasting effect or else it occurred so long before the final illness of the deceased that its evil consequences had long ceased to operate. An example of an insignificant injury would be a painful bruise of the shin inflicted a few weeks prior to the development of a malignant sarcoma in that same tibia. At present it is generally conceded by reliable authorities that a single trauma of this sort does not produce a malignant neoplasm. In the cases in which such a relationship has been alleged, Stewart and others have pointed out that the evidence for it cannot withstand critical analysis. The chief effect of the shin injury was to focus the attention of the victim on the affected part. He was then inclined to consider that the bruise caused the sarcoma, when in reality the succession of events was a matter of coincidence. Other examples are minor injuries to the back with the subsequent recognition of metastases in the spine and elsewhere from silent carcinomas of the bronchi or hypernephromas of the kidney.

As an example of a severe trauma which occurred so long before that all trace of it had disappeared by the time the victim died is the case of a white man of 50 years who was shocked so severely by an electric current that he was unconscious for 10 minutes. Later he returned to work and was active until his sudden death two months later from an advanced grade of coronary arteriosclerosis and myocardial fibrosis. Here the effect of the electric shock was entirely evanescent and had no influence on the course of the disease. There was no lesion in the heart, such as a recently healed infarct, which could have been interpreted as having occurred or developed just after the accident.

(2) The injury in some cases may play a distinct role in producing a condition in the body which accelerates the deleterious action of the disease processes. As examples of this type the following cases may be mentioned:

A 58 year old man who was suffering from an advanced grade of mitral stenosis sustained a fracture of the right femur in an automobile accident. He survived the injury seven days and died with all the signs of cardiac decompensation, such as dyspnea, passive congestion of the organs and general anasarca. It is obvious that the fracture of the femur, though severe, was mainly instrumental in precipitating the fatal attack of cardiac decompensation.

A 68 year old white woman who fell down a flight of stairs complained of pain in the back. In the hospital she developed a paralysis of the right side of the body and finally died nine days after the accident. The autopsy disclosed a crushing fracture of the first lumbar vertebral body but no injury of the cord, a slightly enlarged heart with slight coronary arteriosclerosis, a marked grade of cerebral arteriosclerosis with luminal narrowing of the arteries on the left side and a softening of most of the left cerebral cortex. The cerebral vessels did not contain any thrombi. The course of events here seemed to be that the deceased, fracturing her lumbar spine when she fell, was so prostrated that her cerebral circulation, already hampered by the arteriosclerosis, was further impaired. A fatal infarct of the brain resulted.

Other natural disease conditions which sometimes have an intimate connection with trauma are thrombosis and embolism of various blood vessels and septic infections of all sorts. Some of these conditions will be discussed at greater length under the headings of the various forms of trauma, as they occur fairly consistently with certain forms of injury. In other cases the connection between the trauma and the disease condition is more remote. For example, coronary artery thrombosis sometimes develops after an injury of moderate severity not directly affecting the vessel wall but producing in the victim a moderately severe degree of shock. The symptoms begin a few hours post trauma and continue until death ensues from 7 to 16 hours later. At autopsy the thrombotic process is found to have developed on the basis of an arteriosclerosis of the vessel wall which had already produced a considerable narrowing of the lumen; the only possible connection between the thrombosis and the injury is that the latter induces enough shock to cause slowing of the circulation which favors the development of the thrombus. Cerebral artery thrombosis similarly develops after trauma on the basis of an arteriosclerotic narrowing of the vessel wall and is attended by a widespread infarction of the brain and signs of hemiplegia; death may occur from 12 to 48 hours after the injury.

The following case illustrates the problems which arise when a wound dangerous to life is inflicted upon an individual with severe coronary arteriosclerosis and a fatal complication develops as a result of the arterial disease. A colored man, 48 years of age, while going up the stairs was shot in the right chest. The bullet entered from the front, passed downward and backward through the right lung, the diaphragm and the liver, and finally lodged in the right lumbar region. On admission the patient was in shock; his blood pressure remained low until he died about 40 hours later. Before his death he developed abdominal distention and an elevated temperature. There was not much evidence of blood loss.

The autopsy disclosed that the bullet had not produced an internal hemorrhage of any importance, or caused a septic infection, or traumatized the heart or pericardium in any way. There was a severe coronary arteriosclerosis with marked luminal narrowing, evidently of long standing, and a fresh infarction in the posterior wall of the left ventricle, the age of which was consistent with the survival period. The infarction was evidently precipitated by the shock and moderate hemothorax produced by the injury. These conditions further diminished the blood flow through the already narrowed coronary arteries with resultant myocardial ischemia and infarction. Death resulted from the combination of the old coronary arteriosclerosis and fresh myocardial infarction and the bullet wound of the chest, lung and liver. The injury may have precipitated the infarction but would not have done so in the absence of severe coronary arteriosclerosis. Because death resulted partly from pre-existing disease and from injury the assailant was indicted for criminal assault and not for homicide.

REFERENCE

Stewart, F. W.   Occupational and post traumatic cancer, Bull. New York Acad. Med., 23:145, 1947.

8

Types and Complications of Trauma

TYPES OF TRAUMA

Trauma may be defined as injury to the body inflicted by some form of outside force. It is divided into four categories:

1. Physical trauma, caused by physical violence
2. Thermal trauma, caused by heat or cold
3. Electric trauma, caused by electric energy
4. Chemical trauma, caused by poisons

These will be discussed in this and subsequent chapters.

1. Physical Trauma
   A. Percutaneous injuries are those which result from the penetration of the body by a force; they include:
      (1) Bullet and other missile wounds
      (2) Stab wounds and cutting wounds
   B. Subcutaneous injuries are those injuries, not necessarily penetrating, which are produced by the violence of a force exerted against the body; they include:
      (1) Blunt force injuries
         (a) Localized
         (b) Generalized
      (2) Force producing asphyxia

The lesions produced by these different types of violence are more or less characteristic.

DISTINCTION BETWEEN ANTEMORTEM AND POSTMORTEM WOUNDS

In a case of death by physical violence two points must be determined by the pathologist: (1) Is the injury ante mortem or post mortem? (2) If it is ante mortem, is it the cause of death?

1. Ordinarily it is not difficult to distinguish between antemortem and postmortem wounds. The former tend to bleed more profusely, either externally or into a body cavity, and to form pronounced hemorrhagic extravasations in the subcutaneous or interstitial tissues than do the latter. In judging different lesions by this criterion, however, it must be remembered that portions of the body may be engorged with blood post mortem, either from intense suggillations or from rapid bacterial decomposition which, increasing the pressure inside the blood vessels, forces the blood toward the periphery. Postmortem bleeding or extravasation may be pronounced under such conditions and may be confused with an antemortem process.

The most difficult injuries to differentiate are those which are inflicted upon the body just prior to death or just after death. If the lesion is a slight one like a contusion, abrasion or laceration, it may be impossible to decide this point. With

157

more severe injuries definite intravital signs are usually demonstrable: Thus, (1) a large wound of the skin may give rise to a profuse external hemorrhage with signs of loss of blood; or a severe injury of an internal organ or blood vessel may be associated with a hemorrhage of considerable size in a body cavity or in loose con-

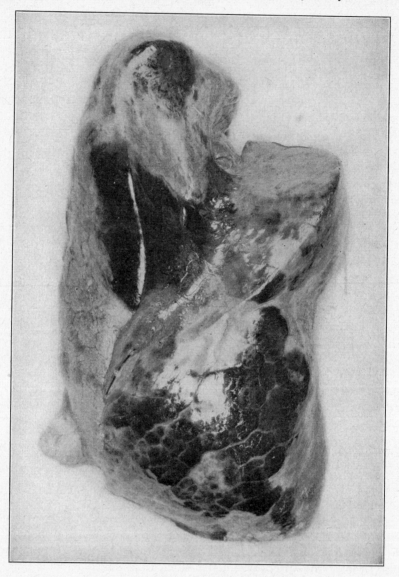

Fig. 8-1. Aspirated Blood in a Pale Lung.

The deceased died from a hematemesis which was due to a ruptured esophageal varix complicating a cirrhosis of the liver. A similar picture may result after injury in which there has been bleeding into the respiratory tract.

nective tissues. (2) If the hemorrhage communicates with the air passages, inhaled blood will appear in the bronchi and lungs (Fig. 8-1). (3) An antemortem fracture of a long bone will result in a discharge of many fat emboli from the site of injury into the lungs.

If the injury was incurred several hours prior to death, microscopic examination will show definite signs of tissue reaction, thus indicating its intravital nature. The character of the reaction may serve to suggest the age of the lesion: the appearance of polymorphonuclear leukocytes, fibrin and nuclear degeneration in a wound generally indicates an early stage, while the presence of granulation tissue, lympho-cytes, plasma cells and eosinophils is a sign that the injury was of longer duration.

2. In order to judge whether or not an injury was responsible for death, it is necessary to determine if it is of such a nature that it could result fatally, a point to be ascertained only by an acquaintance with the causation and effects of the different complications of trauma.

Some destructive injuries are obviously incompatible with survival and do not require any consideration of a complicating mechanism of death. Examples are fragmentation of the body in explosions, decapitation, transections and mangling of the body, crushing injuries of the head that demolish the brain and of the chest that tear loose the heart and lungs. A matter of concern in such cases, however, is the determination of whether the victim was alive and well, or suffering from illness or injury, or dead and from what cause, before the destruction of the body occurred. In victims already dead all evidence of the real cause of death may be destroyed or obscured by the subsequent complete or partial demolition of the body.

COMPLICATIONS OF TRAUMA

The most serious of these are shock, hemorrhage and septic infection; in addi-tion, less frequent complications such as fat embolism, air embolism, asphyxia, vascular alterations and thrombosis and embolism sometimes result from trauma and cause death.

Shock. Traumatic shock is the depressed state of the vital functions that results from severe traumatic injury. It occurs when a large portion of the body has been mangled or when an injury has been inflicted on a part liberally supplied with nerves. Shock is of two kinds: immediate or primary shock, and delayed or secondary shock.

Immediate or primary shock is caused by the overwhelming of the vital centers in the medulla by nerve impulses originating in the injured area and conveyed to the central nervous system. Death occurs in a few minutes from vasomotor collapse. Shock is a serious condition for people who are not robust; young children, elderly individuals, the severely ill and the deeply intoxicated are apt to succumb readily to this complication. If the reaction is not so intense, the patient may live for a short time; but since his low vitality is often unable to overcome the ill effects of the shock, he may die eventually of a terminal hypostatic pneumonia or some similar infection. Occasionally he may combat the noxious influences successfully and recover.

Intrinsically, immediate shock is similar to the ordinary fainting spell or attack of syncope which occurs spontaneously from such causes as poor cerebral circula-tion, weak heart action or severe emotional distress. Noxious neurogenic influences, effecting the medulla in both immediate shock and syncope, result in a vasodilatation of the splanchnic arteriolar blood vessels which in turn brings about a sudden collapse with unconsciousness and low blood pressure but without hemoconcentra-tion. The patient after the attack of syncope usually recovers quickly from his collapse and in a few minutes returns to normal, while the victim of immediate shock reacts as has already been described, depending on the severity of the trauma. At autopsy in cases either of immediate shock or syncope, lesions which are pathognomonic of these conditions are not found; in cases of immediate shock from trauma there are signs of severe bodily injury which are lacking in cases of syncope.

Delayed or secondary shock, associated especially with crushing injuries of the lower extremities, does not occur immediately after the trauma but develops a few hours later. The patient evinces signs of a general collapse with low blood pressure, subnormal temperature, cold clammy skin, perspiration, muscular weakness and incoordination, thirst, weak rapid pulse, rapid shallow respirations and suppression of urine; in the end stage he develops a short agonal rise of temperature and a period of unconsciousness just prior to death. In some cases in which the effects of immediate shock have lasted longer than usual, the symptoms of delayed shock may be added to them and confuse the clinical picture.

The basic pathology of delayed shock is a loss of tone in the smaller veins and capillary vessels of the splanchnic area. These become distended and abnormally permeable to blood plasma so that some of it is drained off into the surrounding tissues. If this condition is sufficiently widespread there is decrease of blood volume, marked hemoconcentration, deficient oxygenation of the red blood cells, lowering of the alkaline reserve and draining of the blood out of the main circulation into the dilated splanchnic capillary bed. This results in a low blood pressure and a general stagnation of the blood flow. The reduced volume of the blood combined with the expanded capacity of the capillary network is the factor which produces the damaging effects of delayed shock on the circulation.

Moon claims that the pathologic lesions described in cases of delayed shock are characteristic and are due principally to capillary atony and permeability. He enumerates among them congestion of the capillaries and venules of the trunk; edema of the lungs, of the submucous layer of different organs and of other loose tissues; and petechial hemorrhages in the serous membranes, mucous layers and parenchymatous organs. The authors have not seen any lesion which could be described as pathognomonic of delayed shock and have found at autopsy only a generalized visceral congestion, edema of the lungs of moderate grade and dark red fluid blood in the circulation. Any other lesions which were encountered could generally be attributed to other causes. The only way to establish the diagnosis of either delayed or immediate traumatic shock at autopsy is to demonstrate an injury of the body severe enough to produce death by this mechanism.

The hypotheses which have been advanced to explain delayed shock are: (1) the absorption of toxins generated in the areas of injury and (2) the neurogenic impulses which emanate from the area of injury to the brain. Both of these are supposed to produce dilatation of the splanchnic capillaries and hemoconcentration. The blood volume may be further depleted by hemorrhage, by exudation of fluid into certain areas as in the case of extensive burns, or by dehydration of blood plasma due to lack of water. At the present time the tendency is to consider delayed shock as a complicated syndrome due to a combination of neurogenic, hemorrhagic and toxemic factors associated in varying proportions in each individual case.

Surgical shock, shock in corrosive poisoning and shock associated with natural disease conditions resemble the forms just described in symptomatology and in the complexity of their component factors.

Hemorrhage. Hemorrhage in traumatic cases may be described as loss of blood from the circulation due to wounds of the heart or of the larger blood vessels, or to a severe laceration of an organ or structure which is especially vascular. The bleeding may occur at the moment of injury, in which case it is known as a primary hemorrhage, or it may take place days after the injury from a rupture of a vessel in the damaged area, in which case it is known as a secondary hemorrhage.

The result of a severe hemorrhage is a decrease in the number of blood cells in the circulation and a lessening of the volume of fluid in the blood vessels; as a consequence the circulatory flow is impaired and less oxygen is carried to the various tissues. Its chief clinical manifestations are a gradually increasing pallor, progressively lowered blood pressure, rapid feeble pulse, rapid sighing respirations, cold clammy skin, weakness, unconsciousness and finally death. In many cases hemorrhage may be associated with traumatic shock, and both complications in conjunction may exert their deleterious effects on the organism.

If the loss of blood is rapid, either externally or into a big cavity like the abdomen, chest or gastrointestinal tract, death will occur rapidly in a few minutes; in such instances the actual amount of the hemorrhage will be considerably less than in cases which have bled slowly over a long period of time. In the first type the bleeding is so rapid that the circulation, unable to adjust itself to the crisis, collapses under the strain. In the second instance it has a chance to recuperate from the drain on its resources so that death may be postponed for a few days.

A fatal hemoglobinuric nephrosis may develop after a large traumatic extravasation of blood into subcutaneous, subserous and areolar tissues and will be discussed on page 203.

Certain types of hemorrhage, such as the intracranial and intrapericardial hemorrhages, will be discussed under the injuries which cause them. The effects of such hemorrhage are dependent more on their peculiar location than on the volume of blood lost.

The pathologic findings in death by hemorrhage include, first, an injury or other lesion capable of causing hemorrhage and second, signs pointing to a fatal loss of blood. The most important signs are a pallor of the skin and mucous membranes, anemia of all viscera and a scant amount of blood in the circulation. In the typical case the heart is contracted and shows streaky minute subendocardial hemorrhages on the left side of the interventricular septum. These signs are not invariably present, however, as the heart may be distended, especially if the patient has been infused with normal salt solution, and the subendocardial hemorrhages may be absent. The autopsy lesions may be modified considerably by blood transfusions, operative procedures and the administration of general anesthesia, especially if the patient survives the injury for several days. In such instances the blood is usually dark and dehydrated; and a hypostatic bronchopneumonia or other septic infection may be present as a consequence of his weakened condition.

Infection. A fatal infection by pyogenic bacteria may follow an injury if the victim survives the immediate complication of shock and hemorrhage. In general the process takes about 12 to 48 hours to develop or, in some instances, even weeks and months.

TYPES OF INFECTION RESULTING FROM TRAUMA. Infections are caused by trauma in three ways:

(1) As the direct result of an injury which allows the entrance of bacteria into the body. Thus an injury of the abdomen and a perforation of the gastrointestinal tract by a bullet or knife blade may, by introducing pathogenic bacteria into the peritoneal cavity, cause a fatal acute suppurative peritonitis. A blunt force injury of the abdomen may rupture the intestines and be followed by the same complication.

For fuller discussion of these and similar conditions the reader is referred to the chapters on blunt force injuries, stab wounds and bullet wounds.

(2) As the indirect result of an injury which creates a local area of lessened resistance so that pyogenic bacteria may infect the area sooner or later, causing an abscess and a fatal septicemia. Abscesses of this type may form around simple fractures of the long bones, pelvis, spine, ribs and skull, or in traumatic infarcts of the liver, kidneys and spleen. They will be discussed more fully under the proper headings. This complication often occurs in persons susceptible to infection, such as diabetics, chronic alcoholics and sufferers from other chronic diseases. If these persons sustain a severe subcutaneous bruise on the abdomen or extremities they may later develop an abscess at the site of the injury. In appraising cases of this type, it is advisable to make certain that the victim has sustained an injury because many of these infections arise spontaneously without trauma.

(3) As an indirect sequel of the trauma, especially in the aged in whom the injury so depresses the general vitality that the patient succumbs either to terminal hypostatic pneumonia, pyelonephritis, ulcerative colitis or septic decubital ulcers.

Hypostatic pneumonia, a common fatal complication of chronic disease conditions, also develops after severe injury, especially in cases of head trauma, spinal injury or fractures of the upper end of the femur in elderly individuals. The basic cause of such a pneumonia is the prostration of the individual and the weakness of the circulation. By producing atelectasis, edema or congestion of the posterior portion of the lungs, a peribronchial or lobular consolidation is favored in these areas. If the trauma is instrumental in causing the conditions which precipitate the pneumonia, then the pneumonia must be considered a real complication of the trauma.

Inhalation pneumonias are apt to follow injuries which, by causing aspiration of septic matter from the mouth and pharynx into the finer bronchi, favor the formation of foul-smelling bronchogenic abscesses. This lesion is frequently associated with compound fractures of the mandible which, by lacerating the gums, favor the inhalation of blood and anaerobic bacteria into the air passages, especially when the victim is rendered unconscious by the injury or by alcoholism or is subjected to a general anesthetic in preparation for a correction of the fracture.

Lobar pneumonia may occasionally follow a traumatic injury of the chest which, by producing a contusion of the lung, forms a *locus minoris resistentiae* favoring invasion by pneumococci. In rare instances this doubtless occurs; the authors have seen an autopsy on a man of 50 years who fell and fractured his left fifth, sixth and seventh ribs at the midaxillary line; death occurred six days later. At autopsy a well developed lobar pneumonia was found surrounding a subpleural laceration of the lung adjacent to the fractures of the ribs. In most cases, however, the injury to the chest is slight, the lung is free from traumatic lesions and the pneumonia results because of a lowered resistance to infection, usually on the basis of an acute and chronic alcoholism rather than as a direct result of physical violence.

Inflammatory processes in the lung which are undoubtedly secondary to traumatic injury are the ordinary hypostatic pneumonia; the inhalation pneumonias associated with injuries of the upper air passages and mouth, such as fractures of the jaw bones; and hematogenous septic infection carried to the lungs from traumatic lesions elsewhere, as for example a septic thrombophlebitis of the uterine veins complicating a criminal abortion. Some inflammations of the lungs such as lobar pneumonia, bronchiectasis or lung abscess owe their development to some form of traumatic injury in rare instances; but strong confirmatory evidence is necessary to substantiate such a proposition. Other pulmonary infections such as viral pneumonia, tuberculosis and actinomycosis arise spontaneously and are not directly the result of trauma, though it is conceivable that external factors may be a predisposing influence in the progression of such respiratory conditions.

Many times pneumonia develops in traumatic cases independently of the trauma. Occasionally the history and the results of the necropsy indicate that the pneumonia preceded the injuries which caused death. On page 13 is described the case of a suicide who jumped off a bridge and died immediately of multiple injuries; the autopsy disclosed a fully developed streptococcic pneumonia of about 24 hours' duration at the time of death. In other instances the infection develops so long after the trauma that any direct connection between the two is out of the question; this is often seen in chronic alcoholics who, having sustained an injury which has healed, afterward die of a hypostatic pneumonia attributable to a lowered resistance from chronic alcoholism. These same considerations likewise apply to other types of septic infection which are sometimes fatal complications of traumatic injury, such as suppurative meningitis, abscesses and similar lesions.

Pyelonephritis and septic infections of the urinary tract may develop after an injury to the spinal cord resulting in trophic disturbances of the body below the level of the cord lesion (Fig. 16-56). This infection occurs less regularly in other forms of trauma but is sometimes encountered in arteriosclerotic patients who are confined to bed for a long time on account of a moderately severe injury.

Septic decubital ulcers occur after injuries of the spinal cord (Fig. 13-1) and are found in senile individuals who become bedridden after fractures of the upper end of the femur.

Acute enterocolitis is occasionally found as the terminal infection in elderly persons who have been prostrated by an injury. In these cases it is necessary to distinguish such infections from spontaneous infections by bacilli of the dysentery or salmonella groups; the latter are primary invaders and occasionally cause epidemic outbreaks.

The clinical signs evoked by septic infections are high temperature, chills and a marked polymorphonuclear leukocytosis, all of which are referable to the action of toxins formed by the pathogenic bacteria. For a while the body combats the effects of the toxins and occasionally may overcome the bacterial invasion. In other cases the pathogenic invaders defeat the resistance of the patient and kill by the effects of their toxins on the vital organs.

PATHOGENIC BACTERIA CAUSING SEPTIC INFECTION AFTER TRAUMA. The lesions in cases of septic infection complicating trauma depend upon the part of the body affected and the identity of the pathogenic microorganism invading the system. The bacteria which commonly complicate traumatic conditions are the pyogenic cocci (the staphylococci and streptococci), the pneumococci, the colon bacillus (and other intestinal bacilli), *Clostridium welchii* and the tetanus bacillus.

Staphylococcus aureus is the most important pathogenic member of its family. In the body this organism forms markedly purulent abscesses around broken bones, in subcutaneous bruises or around penetrating wounds. The infection may develop slowly and affect the system by toxemia without the appearance of the bacteria in the blood. If the blood is invaded, two types of septicemia occur: the less common type is a bacteremia without local abscess formation; the other and common type, is a septicopyemia with multiple abscess formation. The staphylococcus may produce a septic thrombophlebitis in the systemic veins near the site of an injury; this process transmits septic emboli to the lungs, producing abscesses and septic infarcts in the lung tissue. The bacteria from the pulmonary vessels may in turn invade the systemic circulation and produce multiple abscesses in the different organs. Bacterial endocarditis develops occasionally, giving rise to septic embolic infarctions or miliary abscesses in different parts of the body.

Streptococcus hemolyticus is a frequent cause of septic infection after trauma. This organism as a rule enters the body through penetrating wounds and produces an inflammation characterized by swelling, edema and cellulitis and terminating in a phlegmonous or diffuse type of suppuration rather than in a frank circumscribed abscess. The cocci may invade the blood causing a bacteremia. Bacterial endocarditis with multiple septic infarcts, suppurative pericarditis, peritonitis, pleuritis and meningitis may occur. Multiple abscess formation is not common; it may develop in the lungs as septic embolic infarcts from a thrombophlebitis of the systemic veins or in any organ as septic embolic infarcts from an acute endocarditis of the mitral or aortic valves. Petechial hemorrhages are seen frequently in the skin and mucous membranes. There is usually marked parenchymatous degeneration of organs like the liver and kidneys. The spleen may become hyperplastic and appear soft, swollen and enlarged. An acute focal nephritis or a diffuse glomerular nephritis may develop.

One type of streptococcus infection complicating wounds of the skin is known as erysipelas. It is a massive, rapidly developing edematous swelling or cellulitis of the skin and subcutaneous tissues. These tissues become infiltrated with serum, polymorphonuclear leukocytes and streptococci. Erysipelas produces a severe toxemia but is not as a rule accompanied by a general septicemia. An example of this type of infection following a puncture wound of the forehead is shown in Figure 8-2.

While the streptococci and the staphylococci cause characteristic infections in most instances, it must be remembered that the lesions may not be typical in every case. A bacteriologic examination is necessary to determine the causative organism.

The *pneumococcus* is usually the cause of suppurative meningitis in fractures of the skull involving one of the bony sinuses like the middle ear cavity, the ethmoidal, sphenoidal or frontal sinus. The lesion is usually a collection of pus in the subarachnoid space, similar to other forms of septic meningitis.

The *intestinal flora,* such as the colon bacillus and the intestinal anaerobes, are frequent causes of suppurative peritonitis and other abdominal septic infections which complicate penetrating injuries of the intestinal tract. These inflammations are often foul smelling and accompanied by gas formation, especially if the source of the infection is the stomach or the upper small intestine.

Clostridium welchii and similar anaerobic bacilli may infect a crushing injury of the extremities or a severe laceration of the perineum, producing a virulent gangrenous inflammation of the tissues, hemolysis of the blood in the area of infection and formation of gas in the tissues. The infected area swells, is crepitant on pressure, becomes necrotic and exudes a foul-smelling pus. The area of inflammation spreads rapidly along the muscle sheaths until the patient dies of the toxemia. The bacilli sometimes invade the blood during life and cause a widespread hemolysis which gives the skin a peculiar bronze tint in the agonal stage of the infection.

The *tetanus bacillus* is another anaerobic organism which, carried into penetrating wounds, causes a fatal infection. The bacillus grows in the depths of the wound but does not spread in the tissues or invade the blood. The exotoxin of great potency which it produces acts on the peripheral nerve organs in muscle to cause muscular stiffness and on the central nervous system to produce reflex spasm, convulsions and death. The symptoms begin about 7 to 14 days after inoculation. Muscular stiffness commences usually in the neck and jaws and is followed by characteristic tetanic spasms. Death occurs from asphyxia or exhaustion induced by the severe and prolonged muscular spasms. According to the older view the toxin was thought to travel along the nerves to the central nervous system, but the work of Abel and his associates has shown that it is transported mainly by the blood and to a lesser degree by the lymphatics.

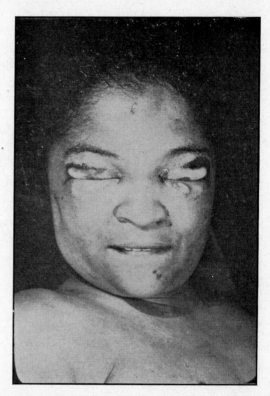

Fig. 8-2. Acute Cellulitis and Phlegmon of Forehead, Scalp and Eyelids Following Infected Superficial Puncture Wound of Midforehead Just Below Hair Line.

Other organisms causing serious but rare complicating infections in traumatic lesions will be mentioned briefly. The *anthrax bacillus* and its spores, carried by contaminated hides and shaving brushes, may cause a characteristic malignant anthrax pustule on the skin or infection of the intestines and lungs. Anthrax infections have a high mortality. *Malleomyces mallei* causes glanders which occasionally is transmitted to man from infected horses. The infection is granulomatous and may be acute or chronic; it occurs in the nose as glanders and in the skin as farcy. *Rabies* or hydrophobia is caused by a virus transmitted by the bite of dogs infected with the disease. *Tularemia,* caused by *Pasteurella tularensis,* sometimes occurs in persons who inoculate themselves while cleaning wild rabbits infected with the disease.

Fat Embolism. Fat embolism is the condition produced when liquid fat enters the circulation and is carried in the blood to block the fine arterioles and capillaries in various parts of the body. It is caused (1) by an injury to adipose tissue which forces liquid fat into the blood vessels; (2) by injecting oil into the circulation, as when oil is introduced into the uterine cavity as an abortifacient or as a medium for hysterography, or into the urinary bladder for the treatment of disease conditions; and (3) by the result in rare instances of a natural disease process without trauma, as in sickle cell anemia. In this disease the bone marrow undergoes degenerative changes and is permeated by hemorrhages. Conditions are thus produced which admit liquid fat into the blood vessels.

Cases of fat embolism occur most frequently after fractures of the long bones but have been described after injuries to subcutaneous and visceral fat and after orthopedic operations on deformed bones.

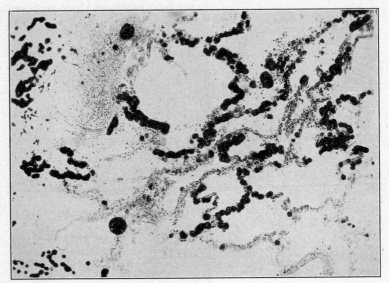

From B. M. Vance, *Proc. New York Path. Soc.*, Dec. 13, 1928

Fig. 8-3. Pulmonary Fat Embolism.

Fat droplets in the interalveolar arterioles and capillaries. Sudan III stain.

The production of fat emboli is as follows:

1. The trauma or fracture destroys fat cells, setting free a quantity of liquid oil.

2. The trauma tears some of the veins across in the vicinity of the fracture. In the bone the veins in the haversian canals, when torn, cannot collapse because of their rigid walls; the veins in the marrow space also may gape.

3. Some mechanism is present which forces the liquid oil into the veins. Pressure exerted on the liquefied fat as a result of muscular spasm and swelling of the injured soft tissues is usually responsible. Improper fixation or rough manipulation of the fracture may favor this process.

In most cases the processes of repair start early and prevent a large amount of fat from entering the circulation. In other instances, a large quantity of liquefied fat is squeezed into the circulation, is carried through the veins and the right heart into the pulmonary artery and finally blocks the arterioles and the capillaries of the lungs. When this occurs the patient will develop (1) pulmonary fat embolism, or (2) cerebral fat embolism.

PULMONARY FAT EMBOLISM. This results when the fat emboli in the capillaries impede the flow of blood through the lungs. In rare instances death may follow rapidly from an acute asphyxia if a large quantity of fat is transported in a brief interval to these organs. In one such case, a man of 54 years received fractures of the left tibia and fibula and the skull in an automobile accident. One and a half hours after the injury he developed a severe attack of dyspnea and died in a few minutes. The cause of death was pulmonary fat embolism.

Fat embolism in the lungs is not so rapidly massive in most cases and the patient's symptoms are less acute. From 8 to 20 hours after the accident the respiration and pulse begin to increase in rate. Death may occur in severe dyspnea about 30 hours after the trauma. In these cases fat globules probably are transported

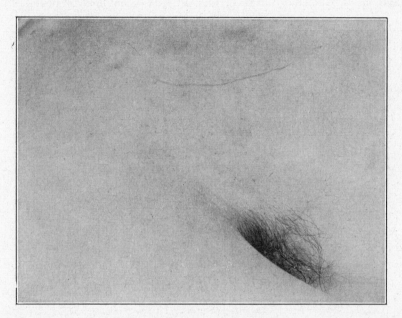

Fig. 8-4. Systemic Fat Embolism.

Clusters of petechial hemorrhages in the skin above the right axilla produced by fat emboli in the subcutaneous blood vessels.

to the lungs in moderate quantities at intermittent intervals until the circulation is obstructed. The diagnosis is established by microscopic examination of sections of the lungs stained for fat. The pulmonary vessels, arterioles and capillaries, are filled with globular fat emboli which may be sufficiently numerous to outline the alveolar capillary network (Fig. 8-3). The lung usually does not show any other characteristic lesions aside from congestion, edema and a slight hypostatic pneumonia. Other organs like the brain, heart muscle and kidneys may show a few scattered emboli because some of the fat, forced from the lungs into the systemic circulation, is carried to the organs supplied by these vessels.

CEREBRAL FAT EMBOLISM. This condition develops when the fat emboli are forced from the pulmonary capillaries into the systemic circulation in sufficient quantity to affect the brain. Some believe that the fat may be transformed through a patent foramen ovale from the right heart into the left heart but this is probably uncommon. The clinical history is fairly characteristic. About 16 to 48 hours after the injury the patient exhibits a large number of small petechial hemorrhages, grouped in small clusters, in the skin of the shoulders, neck, upper chest and in the conjunctivae (Figs. 8-4 and 8-5). At the same time he lapses into a coma which deepens steadily until his death occurs from one to five days later. At necropsy the brain is filled with small petechial hemorrhages grouped in colonies of about 3 to 10, which are confined strictly to the white matter (Fig. 8-6).

Microscopic examination of the brain discloses numerous fat emboli located in the gray matter and rarely surrounded by hemorrhages or necrosis. In the white matter most of the small hemorrhages are revealed as a ring of red blood cells around a necrotic zone of brain tissue in the center of which lies a small arteriole plugged by an embolus of fat. A few of these petechiae are undoubtedly globular extravasations or ball hemorrhages. In addition, translucent areas of necrosis, known

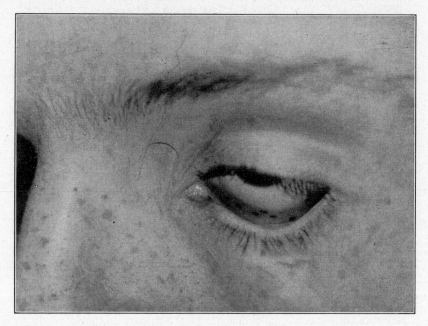

Fig. 8-5. Systemic Fat Embolism.

Petechial hemorrhages in palpebral conjunctiva produced by fat emboli in smaller blood vessels.

as areas of rarefaction, are present in the white matter; the arterioles surrounding such lesions contain fat emboli. Both the ring hemorrhages and the areas of rarefaction are infarcts of microscopic size (Figs. 8-7 and 8-8). These lesions, especially when they develop in large numbers, produce the characteristic coma previously described.

Emboli also occur in the heart muscle where they produce microscopic infarcts characterized by hemorrhage and fatty degeneration in the muscle fibers adjacent to the fat embolus. Fat emboli occur in the kidneys; they may fill the glomerular capillaries but are rarely attended by infarct formation. Although other organs may be involved, the brain lesions cause the most obvious symptoms.

Fat emboli may be found in the pulmonary arterioles after application of most generalized forms of blunt force, especially after falls from a height or highway accidents. Usually there are fractures of the long bones; in some cases, however, fractures are absent and the fat seems to be traumatized in ways not always obvious, especially when the body has been subjected to a severe jarring. The authors have seen the case of a man who fell from a height, died immediately as a result of multiple injuries and at autopsy showed numerous fat emboli in the lungs. Part of these emboli came from the fatty bone marrow of the right femur which, although not fractured, was permeated by small pinhead-sized hemorrhages. Microscopic section disclosed that the hemorrhages were caused by the impact of the fall which, by separating minute areas of the fat from their attachment to the bone, thus created

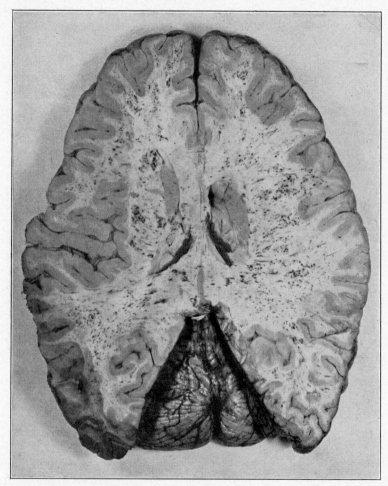

From *Am. J. Surg.*, 26:27, 1934

Fig. 8-6. Cerebral Fat Embolism.

Multiple petechial hemorrhages in cerebral white matter produced by fat emboli in the smaller blood vessels.

a condition favorable for the formation of fat emboli. This type of lesion and similar inconspicuous injuries in adipose tissue may produce a moderate grade of fat embolism in cases in which the visible injuries are not apparently severe.

The presence of a large number of fat emboli in the vessels of the lungs in a traumatic case indicates that the injury was ante mortem, provided of course that a nontraumatic cause of fat embolism is absent. If fat globules block the glomerular vessels in the kidney, the implication is even more cogent for it means that the fat in the blood was so abundant that it had been forced through the pulmonary capillaries into the arterial side of the systemic circulation and so reached the kidneys. A small number of fat emboli in the lungs may be a sign of trauma; but, as embolism of this type is sometimes seen in natural disease conditions without history or sign of injury, it cannot be accepted as a certain indication of an intravital injury unless corroborated by other findings. The explanation for scattered pulmonary fat emboli in deaths from natural disease conditions is not easy to obtain in many instances.

Fat embolism may be demonstrated in the lungs when the death of the victim occurred immediately after the injury; it may still be evident in the blood vessels

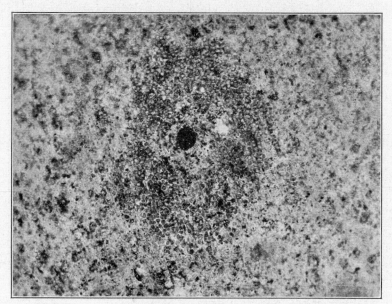

From *Am. J. Surg.*, 26:27, 1934

Fig. 8-7. Cerebral Fat Embolism.

Microscopic section of ring hemorrhage around small cerebral blood vessel plugged with a fat embolus. Osmic acid stain.

as long as 7 to 10 days post trauma. After this length of time the emboli disappear from the blood vessels. The technic used to demonstrate fat emboli is described on page 93.

Air Embolism. Air embolism results when air is introduced into the circulation during life. Its effect is to block the small blood vessels in various parts of the body with air bubbles acting as emboli. There are two varieties of air embolism: (1) pulmonary air embolism, and (2) systemic air embolism.

PULMONARY AIR EMBOLISM. This type of embolism occurs when air is introduced into the systemic veins in sufficient quantity to obstruct the circulation through the pulmonary capillaries. The air is carried in the blood stream to the right heart where it is churned into a frothy mixture which is further driven into the branches of the pulmonary artery and the lung capillaries. As a consequence of this obstruction there is a rise of blood pressure in the pulmonary arterial system and a corresponding fall in the aorta and other arteries.

There are two factors which favor pulmonary air embolism in the presence of normal atmospheric pressure: First, the fixation of the venous walls in the clavicular and pelvic regions, the upper dorsal spine and the dural membranes. When these veins are severed, they fail to collapse and hemorrhage occurs, followed by negative pressure in the vessel. Fixation of the walls may also occur in sclerosing tumors and chronic indurative inflammatory processes. Second, the suction effect of respiratory movements and heart action on such veins as the jugular, subclavian and vertebral has a tendency to create a negative pressure in the vessels during the phase of inspiration. Under these conditions air may be drawn into the veins with disastrous results.

When air is introduced under pressure into cavities or other confined spaces of

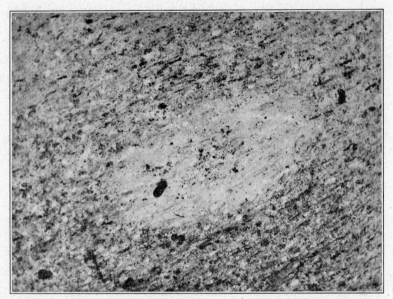

From *Am. J. Surg.*, 26:27, 1934

Fig. 8-8. Cerebral Fat Embolism.

Microscopic section of minute anemic infarct in brain showing surrounding blood vessels plugged with fat emboli. Osmic acid stain.

the body, for roentgenographic, diagnostic or therapeutic purposes, it may result in a pulmonary air embolism if it enters any of the open neighboring veins. This is apt to occur especially in the presence of ulcerative lesions or of tissues rendered friable by disease.

Pulmonary air embolism may be produced when the following circumstances and conditions exist:

1. Homicidal or suicidal knife wounds of the lower cervical or clavicular regions involving the jugular or subclavian veins, or more rarely accidental punctures by a knife during an operation. Penetration by a bullet does not usually produce air embolism.

2. Open wounds or operations such as laminectomies or chordotomies in the region of the third to the sixth dorsal vertebrae.

3. A wound of the superior longitudinal sinus inside the skull. A continued hemorrhage from this vessel while the patient is in the upright position may change the normal positive pressure to negative pressure and thus favor the entrance of air into the vein. A case of this sort was described by Doench. Similarly during an

operation for the removal of a subdural hemorrhage, the lateral sinus was accidentally entered, resulting in death from pulmonary air embolism.

4. Obstetric manipulations and gynecologic procedures on the pregnant or recently delivered uterus. Cesarian section, version or manual extraction of the placenta may introduce air into the uterus and thus into the large veins beneath the placental site. The same effect may be produced by introducing air into the recently curetted uterus with an insufflation apparatus used to distribute antiseptic powders, such as the sulfonamides, into the uterine cavity. Martland has reported two cases of fatal pulmonary air embolism following the insufflation of antiseptic powders into the vagina for the treatment of pruritus vulvae.

5. Injection of air, of fluid mixed with air, or of soap suds into the pregnant uterus for the purpose of producing abortion.

6. The injection of air under pressure into the fallopian tube to test its permeability or for the treatment of sterility. In one case seen by the authors, air was injected into the uterus following a diagnostic curettage which produced a raw bleeding surface in the uterine cavity. The air pressure was increased because of the presence of a submucous fibroid which projected from the fundus and blocked off both fallopian tubes.

7. The introduction of air under pressure into the urinary bladder in the presence of a bleeding lesion or into the accessory nasal sinuses following a therapeutic lavage.

8. Faulty technic in giving intravenous injections with the gravity or similar apparatus, such as, for example, failure to rid the delivery tube of air prior to injection, or to prevent disconnection of the tubing so that air is sucked into the open needle for several minutes.

9. The injection of air during aerography technics for visualization of retroperitoneal tumors. Such an air embolism was observed after the attempted visualization of a large hypernephroma.

Pulmonary air embolism is rarely observed following injury to peripheral veins. Kovacs has reported a delayed embolism following a scythe wound of the wrist. Generally a negative pressure from hemorrhage or other cause and a widely gaping vein are necessary for its production.

When the air enters the vein a whistling or sucking noise may be heard; immediately after there is an oppressed feeling or actual pain over the precordial area. This is followed by the rapid onset of dyspnea, cyanosis, tonic or clonic convulsions, coma and collapse. Auscultation over the precordial area may detect a churning noise caused by the movement of air and blood in the right ventricle. Fluoroscopic examination may also reveal air in the ventricle and pulmonary artery. Death may occur quickly or be delayed for minutes or hours. Recovery sometimes occurs.

The mechanism of death is a matter of controversy. Some think that the blocking of the lung capillaries is the important factor; others believe that the principal lethal effect is exerted on the heart. For further discussion of these points and of the treatment of pulmonary air embolism the reader is referred to the literature compiled at the end of this chapter.

The autopsy should be performed as soon after death as possible so as to avoid the confusion which may be created if the gases of decomposition are in the process of forming in the blood vessels. The technic of opening the heart and blood vessels under water (page 87) should be employed on all cases of pulmonary air embolism. Dyrenfurth has devised an apparatus to test for the presence of oxygen in the contents of the right heart. The theory is that this finding would indicate air embolism inasmuch as oxygen would not be demonstrable in appreciable quantity if the gases were those of decomposition.

The significant findings are a distention of the right ventricle with air under pressure and bright red frothy blood in the right side of the heart, the venae cavae, pulmonary arteries and the coronary vein; sometimes the right ventricle is tympanitic, and the air escapes visibly and audibly when it is opened under water. Occasionally the inferior vena cava as well as the right ventricle is distended with air and little or no blood is present in the vessel. The veins in the vicinity of the original point of entry usually contain air bubbles and may present a mottled semi-translucent appearance.

Systemic Air Embolism. Systemic air embolism occurs when air in sufficient quantity enters a vein of the pulmonary system and is carried through the left side of the heart to block the arterioles and capillaries in different parts of the body, most notably in the brain and heart. In most instances systemic air embolism results from penetrating wounds of the chest, treatment of pulmonary tuberculosis by artificial pneumothorax and operations on the thoracic region such as thoracoplasty, pneumonotomy or pneumonectomy. A puncture wound in a lung which is not able to collapse may penetrate a vein and a bronchiole simultaneously and allow air to enter the vein. Air embolism has also been described in cases of crushing injuries of the chest, in erosion of a pulmonary vein into a necrotizing lung cavity and in conditions which cause violent respiratory movements such as pertussis or drowning.

Occasionally a cerebral air embolism may occur as a further development of a pulmonary air embolism, the air in the right auricle passing through a patent foramen ovale into the left side of the heart; this has been given the name of paradoxical air embolism. Unlike fat, air does not readily pass through the capillaries of the lung, so that when the foramen ovale is not present, the cerebral involvement by this capillary route is rather rare. However, it has been described in a few cases of protracted pulmonary air embolism in which the action of the right ventricle had remained strong to the end.

The passage of air into the left side of the heart produces variable results. If a large quantity is distributed through the coronary arteries, the arterioles and capillaries in the myocardium are blocked and a sudden rapid death with signs of coronary occlusion occurs; this condition is known as coronary air embolism. At autopsy obvious lesions are not found in the heart muscle but air may be present in the coronary arteries.

If the arteries and capillaries of the brain are involved, the victim may die rapidly in a sudden collapse, sometimes preceded by convulsive seizures. Usually death is delayed and preceded by dizziness, faintness, visual disturbances, tonic or clonic convulsions, palsies, hyperactive reflexes and unconsciousness. Transitory blindness may occur in the early stages and is due to air emboli in the retinal arteries; the presence of such emboli may be revealed, and a diagnosis established, by ophthalmoscopic examination. Treatment of cerebral air embolism is without avail, though a few milder cases may recover spontaneously.

The autopsy should be performed under the same conditions which were observed in the cases of pulmonary air embolism. The left ventricle should be opened under water as well as the right ventricle. The air which enters the left side of the heart is dispersed rapidly and since there is little tendency to form froth, air may not be found in the arterial vascular system even in rapid deaths. When bubbles of air are found in the coronary or cerebral arteries, their presence must be interpreted with caution, as they are frequently produced as artefacts when the blood vessels are severed post mortem.

Air is never found in the cerebral blood vessels in the delayed deaths from air embolism in the brain, and the postmortem diagnosis depends largely on the correlation of the circumstances of death with the finding of petechial hemorrhages in the brain. These hemorrhages are caused by the blocking of the arterioles and capillaries in the brain tissue by air emboli so that minute areas of necrosis and ring hemorrhages are formed in the white matter. Other hemorrhages are doubtless small ball hemorrhages. The distribution is varied; the white matter may be homogeneously involved or hemorrhagic areas may be found here and there in the cortex. If the victim lives several days, microscopic areas of necrosis, as described by Spielmeyer, may be present and are to be considered as minute anemic infarcts, produced in the same way as the analogous lesions described under fat embolism. In older cases, Spielmeyer has observed reactive gliosis in these areas.

The air embolism encountered among those who work in high-air pressures, as in tunnels or in deep sea diving, will be discussed in Chapter 20.

Asphyxia. Asphyxia results whenever oxygen is prevented from reaching the red blood cells in the pulmonary capillaries and may be caused by strangulation, suffocation, pressure on the chest, pneumothorax and by other mechanisms. This subject will be discussed in Chapters 17 and 18.

Vascular Disturbances. Vascular disturbances like traumatic aneurysms and arteriovenous fistulae will be discussed in Chapters 15 and 16 under the injuries which produce them.

Noninfectious Thrombosis and Embolism. The formation of bland thrombi in the blood vessels with the occurrence of embolism is a not infrequent complication of trauma.

PULMONARY EMBOLISM FOLLOWING VENOUS THROMBOSIS. The most common sites of thrombosis are in the deep femoral, the popliteal and the posterior tibial veins of the lower extremities, the process often extending into the iliac veins. The injuries most often associated with such thrombi are traumatic lesions of the lower extremity, especially fractures of the long bones. The thrombosis usually develops in the veins of the traumatized leg but occasionally forms in the veins of both legs. For a post-traumatic period of from 10 to 24 days the victim usually suffers from the disability attendant on the local injury; then suddenly there is a severe and rapid attack of dyspnea and death may occur in a few minutes. At autopsy twisted and folded cylindric thrombi, about the diameter of the iliac and deep femoral veins from which they arise, are found blocking the main branches of the pulmonary artery (Fig. 8-9). Evidently the thrombus in whole or in part becomes detached from the iliac or femoral veins and travels through the inferior vena cava to the right ventricle and pulmonary artery, causing an overwhelming asphyxia. In some cases smaller segments of the thrombus, breaking away prior to the detachment of the main and fatal embolus, may produce small bland hemorrhagic infarcts in the lungs; clinically this lesion usually evokes a slight hemoptysis and chest pain due to the development of a fibrinous inflammation over the site of the infarct.

The emboli in the pulmonary artery may take different forms, appearing as long coherent cylindric clots with kinks and folds (Figs. 8-10 and 8-11), as shorter fragmented clots, or as thick clots with a branched form like a root. If the thrombi have developed slowly in the veins, the emboli to which they give rise are firm and mixed dark red and gray red, with well marked gray corrugations on the surface known as the lines of Zahn; microscopically they show the characteristic platelet framework with an interstitial meshwork of fibrin containing red and white blood cells. If the thrombi are formed rapidly, the emboli are soft, dark red, more homogeneous and, microscopically, composed of fibrin and red blood cells with collections of platelets here and there.

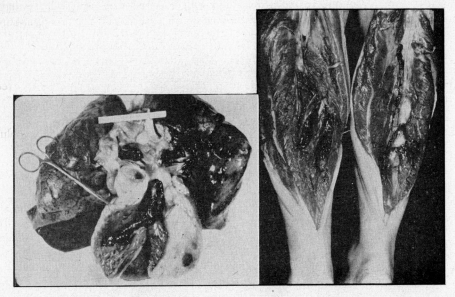

Fig. 8-9. Massive Pulmonary Embolism Following Bland Static Thrombosis of Deep Veins of Lower Extremities.

White man, 50 years old, died suddenly 14 days after sustaining fracture of skull and laceration of brain in fall from ladder while at work.

Usually the thrombotic emboli in the pulmonary arteries can be distinguished by their characteristic appearance and cylindric shape and by the haphazard way in which they are jammed into the pulmonary artery; postmortem clots have a molded appearance and form a smooth exact cast of the pulmonary conus, valve and arteries in which they arise. The extremity of an embolus may present features of diagnostic importance as it usually has the shape of a pointed or truncated cone, a feature which is lacking in postmortem clots. When the embolus is unfolded, nodal swellings are sometimes observed corresponding to the projection of the original thrombus into the venous valve cusps. A long embolus in passing through the heart may be fragmented by the churning action of that organ. In some cases of massive pulmonary embolism, Clark has described hemorrhages in the leaflets of the tricuspid valve probably as the result of trauma to the valve during the passage of the emboli. Rarely the embolus may be tied into a knot by the churning action of the right auricle and ventricle. The authors encountered one such tightly knotted embolus firmly impacted in a large branch of the pulmonary artery.

At the time of autopsy some of the larger embolic fragments may be found tangled in the right ventricle or loose in the right auricle or inferior vena cava, and they may drop out and escape detection if the heart is not opened carefully. The best autopsy technic for the demonstration of pulmonary emboli in situ is to open the pulmonary artery, right ventricle and right auricle before the heart is removed from the body. In some instances the main trunk of the pulmonary artery may contain only postmortem clots or fluid blood and the emboli are found packed in the larger branches within the lungs. These vessels should always be explored.

Dissection of the deep femoral, popliteal and posterior tibial veins in cases of pulmonary embolism usually reveals remnants of the thrombus in situ in the injured extremity, or occasionally thrombi in the veins of both extremities, or in the iliac veins. In some cases the vessel is distended with a mixed dark red and gray red thrombus, or the original site of the thrombus which gave rise to the fatal embolus

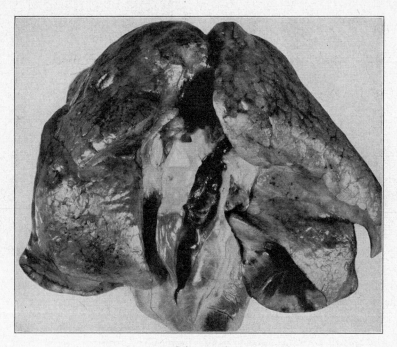

Fig. 8-10. Pulmonary Embolism.

Folded embolus obstructing the pulmonary artery which has been opened in situ. The embolus was a thrombus which formed in the right iliac vein, following an appendectomy on a four and a half months pregnant woman. Sudden death during convalescence.

is represented by a small residual fragment in one of the venous valve cusps, the vessel being otherwise empty (Fig. 8-11).

Where the process is unilateral, the wall of the thrombosed vein is often thickened in distinct contrast to the corresponding normal vessel on the opposite side. There may not, however, be any obvious difference between them. Edema of the affected extremities is comparatively uncommon. In many instances thrombi may be present in the deep veins of both lower extremities (Fig. 8-9) and exploration of the veins should be carried out on both sides. Where massive fatal pulmonary embolism has occurred, its source is obviously from the veins which are empty at the time of autopsy and not from those which are found filled with thrombi. It is noteworthy that varicosities of the superficial veins of the legs are not often observed in cases of femoral thrombosis which primarily is a lesion of the deeper veins.

Microscopic sections of thrombosed femoral or popliteal veins show typical thrombi composed of a platelet framework with interstices of fibrin containing red blood cells and leukocytes. If the thrombus is formed rapidly, the vein wall may be normal, but if the process is of longer duration, the wall may be thicker and show a round cell infiltration around the vasa vasorum in the periphery. In some cases the entire wall is infiltrated by round cells and eosinophils. Occasionally there is a definite phlebosclerosis in which the wall is thickened by a proliferation of fibrous tissue involving all layers. In a few instances some of these vessels are occluded by old canalized thrombi or sclerotic fibrous plugs.

Injuries to parts of the body other than the lower extremities or pelvis may be complicated by femoral vein thrombosis and pulmonary embolism. This process occurs even more frequently in natural disease conditions in the absence of trauma.

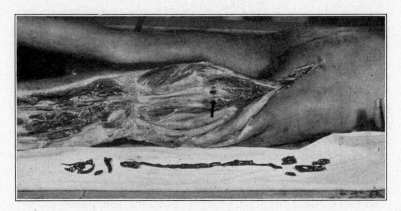

Fig. 8-11. Pulmonary Embolism.

Long fragmented pulmonary embolus removed from right ventricle and pulmonary artery. A fragment of the original thrombus visible behind the valve cusp in the right femoral vein (arrow) which has been laid open from behind to show the source of the embolus. This condition occurred in a 54 year old Negro who sustained a compound fracture of the right tibia.

Probably the correct interpretation of the thrombosis is that similar factors operate in both the traumatic and the nontraumatic cases to favor the development of the antemortem thrombus. These factors are not always easy to recognize, but stasis of the blood in the extremities, referable either to general impairment of the circulation or to some local impairment of the venous flow induced by the injury, plays an important role in producing this lesion. Alterations in the composition of the blood may favor thrombus formation or the process may start at the site of an undetected injury of the vascular intima. It is difficult to prove that these factors have been active in any particular case. In any event severe injury undoubtedly creates conditions either directly or indirectly which favor thrombus formation, and in this sense the thrombosis can be considered a complication of trauma.

The autopsy findings in each case of fatal pulmonary embolism must be correlated carefully with the history in deciding the role of traumatic injury as a factor in causing death. This is especially important at the present time when femoral vein thrombosis resulting in pulmonary embolism is considered to be invariably traumatic by many in whose estimation the diagnosis of this condition is the label of a traumatic process. This view is not justified by the facts; in many cases such thrombosis and embolism are due to natural causes, notably diseases of the circulatory system associated with sluggish peripheral circulation in which history or evidence of traumatic injury is lacking. In analyzing any particular case, a slight traumatic lesion which does not seriously inconvenience or incapacitate a person should not be regarded as a possible etiologic factor; but if the trauma is disabling, it should be given all due consideration as an influence in the production of this fatal complication.

Other veins, such as the venous sinuses of the dura mater or the subclavian and axillary veins, occasionally develop bland thrombosis after traumatic injury. Such a process in the dural veins, especially the superior longitudinal sinus, causes a retrograde hemorrhagic softening in the immediately adjacent portions of the brain. The authors have seen one case in a woman of 58 years who received a bullet wound of the right mastoid region with a comminuted skull fracture involving the right jugular foramen and traumatizing the right lateral venous sinus. She survived the injury six days and at autopsy showed a bland thrombosis of the sinus from the jugular foramen to the torcula. A retrograde hemorrhagic softening of the adjacent occipital lobe was the cause of death. The thrombus was caused by an intimal lesion in the venous sinus which in turn was the product of the skull fracture around the jugular foramen. In other cases bland thromboses of the superior longitudinal and lateral venous sinuses of the dura have resulted from a stasis of the circulation largely referable to the prostration and shock induced by injury.

A bland thrombosis does not often develop in the subclavian and axillary veins after trauma. In one case in which the deceased had been severely burned by lye thrown on his face and shoulders during a homicidal assault, such a thrombus formed in the brachial and axillary veins and gave rise to a fatal pulmonary embolism. The shock and prostration brought on by the widespread chemical burns was an important factor in producing the thrombosis.

PULMONARY THROMBOSIS. Thrombosis of the pulmonary artery occurs rarely and may arise spontaneously or develop after traumas of varying severity in different parts of the body. The thrombi are present at the bifurcation of the pulmonary artery or in the larger branches in the lung parenchyma and are either small or large enough to occlude the vessel. Most are of recent formation but a few show progressive stages of canalization and organization. They are usually found in elderly individuals whose pulmonary circulation is impaired as a result of cardiac weakness. Most if not all of these thrombi develop primarily inside the artery. Theoretically it is possible that the thrombotic process is initiated by an embolus from a thrombosed femoral vein which lodges in a branch of the pulmonary artery and grows in size centrally, until it occludes the main trunk of the vessel. This hypothesis, however, cannot be proved beyond question. The chief influence of traumatic injury on pulmonary thrombosis is to contribute to the development of the thrombus by reason of the slowing of the circulation incident to shock.

PARADOXICAL EMBOLISM. Paradoxical embolism is a phenomenon which occurs when a thrombus in a systemic vein like the femoral becomes an embolus and travels to the right auricle. From there it is forced through a patent foramen ovale into the left side of the heart and then into the systemic arterial circulation. The following case, seen by the authors, is not only a good example of this lesion but also illustrates the conditions which are necessary for its production.

A 53 year old, moderately obese, psychopathic white woman was struck on the jaw during an altercation. Three days later she was admitted to a hospital because her mental symptoms had become worse. After admission her temperature rose and remained at 106° F. On the tenth day of her stay in the hospital she displayed symptoms of shock; her blood pressure fell to a level of 70 mm. Hg systolic, 54 mm. diastolic; this improved after the injection of plasma. She died suddenly on the nineteenth day after admission.

The autopsy disclosed the following conditions: static intact thrombosis of the left iliac and deep femoral veins with early organization of the thrombus in the left common iliac, left external iliac and left femoral veins; a massive pulmonary embolism and numerous small emboli and hemorrhagic infarcts in the lungs, which arose from the right femoral, iliac and popliteal veins, the right posterior tibial vein revealing a residual thrombosis; an obliquely patent foramen ovale, ovoid in shape, 1 cm. in length and located in the anterior margin of the fossa ovalis, in which a cylindric thrombotic embolus about 1 cm. in diameter was impacted so that one end, 4 cm. long, protruded into the left auricle and a thicker larger portion projected into the right auricle (Fig. 8-12); a small embolic infarct in the brain, multiple small

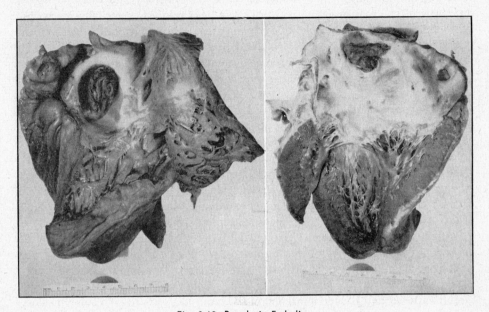

Fig. 8-12. Paradoxic Embolism.

Views of impacted thrombotic embolus protruding through both sides of patent foramen ovale. White woman, 53 years old. See text on pages 178 and 179.

embolic infarcts in the kidneys and large infarcts in a moderately enlarged spleen. The embolic lesions of the pulmonary artery and lungs and of the brain, spleen and kidneys were the cause of death.

This case is similar to those reported by French and by Taylor. French described paradoxical embolism in a woman of 36 years who died 29 days after a hysteromyomectomy with signs of pulmonary embolism. The autopsy disclosed the pulmonary arteries blocked by emboli and a cylindric thrombus projecting into the right and left auricles through a patent foramen ovale. Systemic emboli or infarcts were not found elsewhere, as the paradoxical embolism had evidently occurred just prior to death.

Taylor reported a case of paradoxical embolism in a 45 year old woman who died after a three week illness with symptoms of cyanosis, tachycardia and delirium. The autopsy revealed a massive pulmonary embolism and a long twisted embolus stuck in an open foramen ovale with infarcts in the lungs, kidneys and spleen.

The reports of these cases indicate that paradoxical embolism is rare and is produced by a combination of unusual factors: (1) A preliminary massive pulmonary embolism must occur to block the pulmonary artery enough to produce a dilatation and back pressure in the right heart and yet not cause immediate death. (2) A persistent foramen ovale, the opening not necessarily very large, must be present. As a result of the obstruction in the pulmonary artery and the back pressure created by it in the right ventricle and auricle, a sizeable cylindric thrombotic embolus is twisted and forced part way through the open foramen. Here it remains impacted, one end protruding into the left auricle and the other into the right. In our case and in that of Taylor, systemic emboli were detached from the end of the embolus projecting into the left auricle and were carried to the spleen, kidneys and brain. In the case of French the patient died of the massive pulmonary embolism before any systemic emboli were detached.

The chief medicolegal significance of paradoxical embolism is the undue importance attached to it by many physicians as a cause of death. In cases in which there has been a real or minor injury of the lower extremity and where symptoms and signs of cerebral disease have subsequently developed, some physicians have urged that the death was traumatic, postulating that a thrombosis of the femoral vein, formed as a result of injury, was followed by the discharge of an embolus to the right auricle. This then passed through a patent foramen ovale into the systemic circulation and so to the brain to result in a cerebral embolism. This theory is usually advocated when an autopsy has not been performed and the true conditions in the body have not been ascertained. Though dialectically plausible this interpretation is not justified in the light of our present knowledge because paradoxical embolism is rare and occurs only in the presence of the unusual conditions just noted. It will not occur if these conditions are absent. It is unbelievable that a small embolus will deviate in the right auricle from its direct course to the pulmonary artery to pass into the left heart through an open foramen ovale which is normally closed by overlapping of its margins unless there is a definite obstruction of the pulmonary artery to cause back pressure and force it in that direction.

ARTERIAL THROMBOSIS AND EMBOLISM. Arterial thrombosis and embolism are occasionally noted as a result of trauma. In some cases bullet wounds and stab wounds of the carotid arteries directly injure the arterial wall or the arterial intima. A thrombosis develops on the site of the injury, followed by embolism of the middle cerebral arteries and anemic infarction of the brain (Fig. 15-10). In some instances an incised wound of the subclavian artery produced a thrombosis, giving rise to emboli in the vertebral and posterior cerebral arteries. Stab wounds of the heart, especially of the left ventricle, may be survived long enough for mural thromboses to occur at the site of the injury with complicating cerebral and systemic embolism; these thrombi develop rapidly and may embolize quickly. In acute carbon monoxide poisoning, anoxic necrosis of the myocardium may occur with the development of mural thrombi in the left ventricle (Fig. 19-10). These in turn may give rise to emboli at a time when the patient is seemingly recovered from the acute dangerous effects of the asphyxiation. Thromboses of the brachial and femoral arteries have resulted from crushing injuries of the extremities and have caused gangrene of distal portions of the limbs. These lesions will be discussed fully in the chapter on blunt force. A bullet passing laterally through the body of a dorsal vertebra may force fragments of bone forward to contuse the aorta and cause the formation of a large mural thrombus over the site of injury in that vessel (Fig. 16-54).

Primary arterial thrombosis in the coronary or cerebral arteries has been discussed in connection with trauma on page 156. In these cases the artery has not been directly injured but the shock of the trauma, combined with the sclerosis in the vessel wall, may favor the development of the thrombus by slowing up the circulation of blood through the diseased vessels. In some instances the traumatic injury and shock may be so slight as to have little or no influence on the development of a thrombotic lesion in these arteries.

MULTIPLE THROMBOSES AND EMBOLISM. A few cases of multiple primary thromboses in the heart cavities, the large arteries and the large veins occur in middle-aged or elderly individuals who die a few days or weeks after a traumatic injury of greater or lesser severity. The principal findings at autopsy are chronic disease processes of moderate severity such as general arteriosclerosis, chronic alcoholism, and numerous autochthonous bland thrombi in the heart, arteries and veins, occasionally accompanied by embolic manifestations in the lungs and other organs. In these cases death is the result of thrombus formation in the heart and blood vessels, either directly or indirectly. The signs of traumatic injury may or may not be present. If it has any effect at all the traumatic injury furthers the formation of the thrombi mainly by the slowing of the blood in the vessels as a result of shock, and less often as a result of a specific injury of the vascular wall or endothelium or of any change in the composition of the blood due to trauma. The individual who is affected by this type of thrombosis is one whose circulatory system has no reserve power, even though it may operate satisfactorily under normal conditions; under a stress of any sort, whether traumatic or nontraumatic, slowing of the blood stream may occur and conditions favorable to thrombus formation may be produced. The following cases are good examples of this condition.

One case was that of a 48 year old man, a chronic alcoholic, who was removed to a hospital following a fall down some steps. He died two days after admission, showing signs of generalized weakness and gradually sinking into coma just prior to death. The autopsy disclosed none of the lesions of traumatic injury and only a minor loss of nutrition due to chronic alcoholism; there was a moderate grade of coronary and general arteriosclerosis but no serious cardiac condition. Old and recent autochthonous thrombi were present as follows: an old canalized thrombus in the left femoral vein partly blocking the lumen and a recent thrombus in the left femoral artery; recent thromboses in the right femoral artery and vein, the branches of the pulmonary artery in the lungs, the gastric artery and the left subclavian artery near its origin; an infarct of the inner surface of the left occipital lobe and a cerebral embolism of the left posterior cerebral artery, the source of the embolus probably being the left subclavian artery thrombosis. Death occurred as a result of a terminal bronchopneumonia. Microscopic examination failed to demonstrate any other lesion of importance. The formation of multiple thromboses in this case was attributed in large part to the poor physical condition of the patient and his sluggish circulation; but in the absence of a definite traumatic injury it was difficult to evaluate the influence of the fall on the course of the disease.

A 50 year old woman, struck by an auto truck, sustained fractures of the ribs on the left side. On admission to the hospital shortly after the injury, she was dyspneic and in shock and had subcutaneous emphysema of the chest wall. Several days later the left popliteal artery was obstructed; gangrene of the leg requiring amputation ensued. She died 37 days post trauma. The autopsy disclosed a woman of average stature and nutrition, with the left leg amputated in the midthigh region. Partly healed fractures of the three upper ribs on the left side were present. The heart was normal, aside from a chronic adhesive pericarditis, and was not hypertrophied; edema of the lungs was present, and there were moderate arteriosclerotic changes in the abdominal aorta and the kidneys. There was a rather extensive pseudomembranous enteritis and colitis, probably a terminal infection. There were recent thrombi in the popliteal artery and vein of the left leg, in a large branch of the pulmonary artery supplying the lower lobe of the left lung and in a large branch of the left renal artery with an infarct of the adjacent portion of the left kidney. These thrombi were probably autochthonous. In this case death was referable to the thrombotic processes combined with the intestinal inflammation. The injuries probably precipitated the fatal chain of events, but the development of the complication which caused death was largely due to the natural disease conditions already present in the body.

A 57 year old woman was admitted to a hospital with a history of having been struck by an automobile four weeks previously. Since that time she had been unable to walk. In the hospital a paralysis of the right leg, edema of both ankles and signs of arteriosclerotic heart disease were found. She died after 11 hours in the hospital. The autopsy disclosed a slightly built woman whose heart was moderately enlarged and whose coronary arteries were moderately sclerotic; there was a recent thrombus which occluded the right circumflex branch but no infarct of the heart wall; there were mural thrombi in the auricular appendages of the right and left auricles, 5 to 10 mm. in diameter, and numerous infarcts in the lungs, spleen and kidneys which probably developed as a result of embolism from the mural thrombi. There was an area of softening in the left basal ganglion due to sclerosis of the cerebral vessels and not to embolism. The thrombosis and the embolism were undoubtedly the cause of death. In the absence of any definite traumatic injury, however, the influence of the automobile accident on the course of the fatal complication must be considered as dubious.

Unusual types of pulmonary embolism are produced occasionally by trauma. Actual fragments of bone marrow have been found as emboli in smaller branches of the pulmonary artery, usually following fractures of bones containing red bone marrow. These emboli are small and are forced into the larger venous tributaries torn near the site of fracture, and from thence are transported to the lungs. Bone marrow embolism is rarely of clinical importance, but it may be accompanied by a fat embolism of greater or less severity.

After a blunt force injury of the liver, fragments of liver parenchyma may enter torn hepatic veins and be carried as emboli to the smaller branches of the pulmonary artery. In a case reported by Strauss, there was a subcapsular rupture of the right lobe of the liver with tearing of the hepatic veins and fragmentation of the liver; liver emboli of 50 μ to 2 mm. in diameter were found in the small pulmonary arteries. Lippincott and Breck reported a crushing injury of the liver with a laceration of the inferior vena cava through which a fragment of liver tissue was forced sufficient in size to block the main branch of the pulmonary artery and cause death.

Krakower described a fracture of the skull in a boy of 23 months, which was accompanied by a surface laceration of the brain and a complete tear of the superior longitudinal sinus. Small fragments of lacerated brain apparently entered the venous sinus and were found as small emboli of cerebral tissue in the lungs.

Foreign bodies may enter veins or arteries and be transported as emboli. Strauss has reported pulmonary embolism due to a lead bullet which passed into the abdomen, penetrated the inferior vena cava near the right iliac vein and at autopsy three days after the shooting was found in the left pulmonary artery covered by a red clot. The patient had been in the shock position with his head lowered and it was believed that the bullet had traveled for the most part by gravity along the vena cava to its resting place in the left lung.

Maternal pulmonary embolism from amniotic fluid has been described as an unexpected cause of death during labor. The mechanism of this sudden calamity has not been explained satisfactorily, but during delivery at the period when the placenta starts to separate and the membranes have ruptured, the mother is overcome by shock and dyspnea and dies suddenly. Histologic examination of the uterine wall and of the lungs show mucous, squamae and lanugo hairs in the uterine sinuses near the placental site, and also as emboli in the smaller pulmonary arteries in the lung tissue.

The appraisal of vascular and cardiac thromboses which develop after traumatic injury is difficult at the time of autopsy, for from the very nature of the investigation the examiner cannot obtain information which would allow him to evaluate the different factors which might produce the thrombosis. Of these the most important are: (1) Injury of the vascular endothelium or of the vessel wall. The injury of the vessel wall may be obvious, as, for example, a stab wound of the carotid artery, and may be a direct cause of the thrombus. On the other hand a lesion of the endothelium of the blood vessel is often inconspicuous and its connection with trauma less obvious, especially since this lesion is frequently the result of other factors and occurs in nontraumatic as well as in traumatic cases.

(2) Alterations in the content of the blood which predispose to antemortem thrombus formation. It is not possible at autopsy to determine with any degree of certainty whether or not such changes in the blood have or have not taken place, but they may be suspected in the presence of a chronic septic process or certain blood dyscrasias which are often attended by the production of prothrombin and other component factors concerned in blood clotting and the development of thrombi. Traumatic injury may release considerable prothrombin in some cases, but it is difficult to appraise what influence this fact may exert in antemortem thrombus formation in any particular case. (3) Slowing of the flow of blood through the blood vessels. The existence of circulatory stasis in a blood vessel, as a result either of cardiac weakness or of local obstruction to the flow of blood, is an important factor in the production of bland thrombosis. The influence of traumatic injury in producing such stasis has already been discussed.

INFLUENCE OF ALCOHOL ON TRAUMA

Alcohol is of great significance in traumatic cases. Its influence may manifest itself in three ways:

(1) The drug in excess, by increasing the irritability and decreasing the sense of responsibilty, may cause the victim to become involved in quarrels while in an unprotected state or to blunder into accidents inadvertently.

(2) If a person is intoxicated, the anesthetic action of the alcohol may obscure the pain and the other symptoms of injury so that a serious traumatic condition may be overlooked, especially if there are no external signs of its presence. Blunt force injuries of the spine, head and abdomen have been missed under these conditions.

(3) Alcohol is a severe depressant of the central nervous system; an intoxicated individual is rendered more susceptible to the effects of traumatic shock or hemorrhage.

The recognition of acute alcoholism clinically is important in a traumatic case, especially if the question of legal responsibility for the injury should arise. In New York City if a person is in such a state of alcoholic stupor that medical attention is advisable, he will be taken by ambulance to a hospital where he can be examined and given the proper treatment as a patient. Under such conditions it is legitimate for the physician to examine him for injuries and if possible to diagnose alcoholism from the behavior of the patient and from the odor of alcohol on his breath. If the clinical signs justify such procedure, the stomach contents or specimens of the blood or spinal fluid may be saved for toxicologic examination for alcohol.

If the injured person is not intoxicated to the extent that he is in need of medical attention, a medical man may be called in by the police to determine the degree of alcoholism and the extent of any injuries on the victim. Under such conditions the doctor must be careful of his legal status before conducting the examination. If he is called upon to examine the individual as a patient who is in need of treatment, he can proceed with all the freedom granted by the rules of his profession, provided that the patient does not object to the examination. If the patient objects, the physician should make a note that medical attention was refused and should not examine the patient. This question is discussed at length on page 184. If the doctor is allowed to make the examination he must be careful not to overlook the possibility that the victim may have a dangerous injury of the head or abdomen which is not easy to detect. There have been cases in which alcoholic individuals have been placed in jail and found dead the next morning, death having resulted from an unrecognized fracture of the skull or intra-abdominal injury which the police authorities or the examining doctor failed to take into consideration as a possibility when the deceased was taken into custody.

If a physician is called in simply to determine whether or not a person is alcoholic, he cannot proceed with the examination unless he obtains the consent of the individual to be examined. Both should understand that the usual relation of physician and patient does not exist under these circumstances. In rare instances the examining doctor may be authorized by a Judge of a Court of Record, in which case he can overrule the objections of the prisoner. If this type of examination is made without proper consent or authorization, the medical man will infringe upon the rights of the individual and will expose himself to a charge of assault, as discussed on page 555. For this reason the determination of alcoholism in persons who are arrested for reckless driving or criminal violence cannot always be carried out satisfactorily by the police in every locality.

Even when the prisoner gives his consent for an examination to determine alcoholism, the difficulties are not fully overcome because a chemical test on the blood, urine or exhaled breath of the prisoner is performed to supplement the clinical observations of the physicians. The problem not only predicates a chemical criterion by which degrees of intoxication can be diagnosed but also a convenient technic which would enable the toxicologist to make an accurate analysis on a small amount of organic material. Many methods have been suggested; in the United States none have been used with any consistency until recently, when a few states enacted legislation recognizing the validity of such tests including the alcohol determination on the exhaled breath. In Germany and other European countries, the process employed by Widmark (a quantitative determination of alcohol in a few drops of the person's blood) has been employed widely. Gettler and Freireich maintain that the alcohol content of the spinal fluid more closely approximates that of the brain than does the amount in the blood. For fuller details of this and other methods for the determination of alcohol in body fluids and tissues, see Chapter 46.

It is advisable in deaths from trauma in which the victim survived the injury less than 24 hours for the medical examiner to preserve the brain or liver for chemical examination in order to determine whether or not alcohol is present. In cases which live for a longer time after trauma, this procedure is useless, as all the alcohol in the system has been oxidized or eliminated long before death occurs. This question will be discussed in greater detail on page 785. The result of such an examination is a matter of importance in many legal actions. For example, if alcohol in a quantity indicating intoxication is discovered in the brain of the deceased, that fact might mitigate the responsibility of the defendant in a case of technical homicide or a civil suit for damages. In the Office of the Chief Medical Examiner in the City of New York the medical examiner, after autopsy, routinely sends parts of the liver or brain to the toxicologist for analysis of alcoholic content in all cases of trauma indicating such an examination.

The influence of trauma upon cases of chronic alcoholism is worthy of note because injuries inflicted on such persons are likely to precipitate possibly fatal attacks of delirium tremens. The traumatic lesions vary in severity from a severe bruise to a fracture of the long bone and may act as a contributing factor in causing death even though the basic process primarily responsible is chronic alcoholism.

The following case is an example of an injury which, inflicted with homicidal intent on a chronic alcoholic, was followed by a fatal attack of delirium tremens post-trauma. The deceased, a 53 year old white man, was the victim of a hold-up during which he received a bullet wound in the left side of his neck. The bullet passed downward and backward and finally lodged in the body of the sixth cervical vertebra on the left. The spinal canal was not entered but the impact of the missile caused an area of hemorrhagic softening, 1 mm. in diameter, in the adjacent left anterior horn of the cervical spinal cord. While the immediate symptoms were not alarming, a few days later the patient developed delirium tremens from which he died. In this case the assailant could not be prosecuted successfully for homicide, inasmuch as death did not result solely from the bullet wound. He could, however, be charged with the crimes of assault and robbery.

REFERENCES

Amreich, I.　Zur Ätiologie der von den Uterusvenen ausgehenden Luftembolie, Zentralbl. f. Gynäk., 9:521, 1924.

Carr, J. L., and Johnson, C.　Embolism following instrumentation and injection of oil into the urinary bladder, J.A.M.A., 104:1973, 1935.

Ceelen, W.　Luftembolie, Henke und Lubarsch Handbuch der Speziellen Pathologischen Anatomie und Histologie, Berlin, Julius Springer, 3:119, 1929.

Chase, W. H.　Air embolism (cerebral), Surg., Gynec. & Obst., 59:569, 1934.

Clark, E., and Berger, A. R.　Hemorrhagic extravasations into the leaflets of the atrioventricular valves, Arch. Path., 22:524, 1936.

Current Comment, Chemical Tests for Intoxication, J.A.M.A., 127:30, 1945.

Doench, H. O.　Luftembolie bei Verletzung des Sinus Longitudinalis, Zentralbl. f. Chir., 60:486, 1933.

Dyrenfurth, F.　Über die Anwendbarkeit des NO zur Festellung der Luftembolie und zur Atmungsnachweis beim Neugeborenen, Deutsche Ztschr. f. d. ges. gerichtl. Med., 20:391, 1933.

Editorials, J.A.M.A.　Traumatic shock, 105:1353, 1935. Confusion concerning shock, 124:1060, 1944. Toxic factors in shock, 123:485, 1943. Nervous factors in traumatic shock, 125:211, 1944.

Engelmann, F.　Über die Gefahren der sogenannten Operationslosen Schwangerschaftsunterbrechung, Deutsche Med. Wchnschr., 58:166, 1932.

Federoff, S. P., and Wischenswsky, A. S.　Luftembolie der Art. Pulmonalis bei Eröffnung des Wirbelsaulenkanals, Zentralbl. f. Chir., 57:2098, 1930.

French, L. R.　Paradoxical embolism, Arch. Path., 11:383, 1931.

Frey, S.　Experimenteller Beitrag zur venosen Luftembolie, Arch. f. klin. Chir., 148:536, 1927.

Gajzago, E.　Ein in Ausschluss Hysterographie durch Ölembolie verursachter Todesfall, Zentralbl. f. Gynäk., 55:166, 1931.

Gettler, A. O., Freireich, A. W., and Schwartz, H.　Blood alcohol and intoxication: its value in border line cases, Am. J. Clin. Path., 14:365, 1944.

――――and Freireich, A. W.　Determination of alcoholic intoxication during life by spinal fluid analysis, J. Biol. Chem., 92:199, 1931.

Gonzales, T. A., and Gettler, A. O.　Alcohol and the pedestrian in traffic accidents, J.A.M.A., 117:1523, 1941.

Ilyin, F.　Zur Frage der Luftembolie, Ber. Sitzg. Path. Gesell. St. Petersburg, 1913, Ref. Zentral. Path., 25:284, 1914.

Jehn, W., and Naegeli, Th.　Experimentelle Untersuchungen über Luftembolie, Ztschr. f. d. ges. exper. Med., 6:64, 1918.

Jockish, G.　Luftfüllung der Blase und Tötliche Embolie, Zentralbl. f. Chir., 57:1795, 1930.

Jungmichel, G.　Alcoholbestimmung im Blut, Berlin, Carl Heymann's, 1933.

Kleinschmidt, O.　Experimentelle Untersuchungen über Luftembolie, Arch. f. klin. Chir., 106:782, 1915.

Kovacs, H. J.　Über ein Fall von Luftembolie nach einer Verletzung der Hand, Zentralbl. f. Chir., 65:180, 1938.

Martland, H. S.　Fatal air embolism due to powder insufflation used in gynecological treatment, Am. J. Surg., 48:164, 1945.

Martland, H. S.   Static or spontaneous thrombosis of veins of lower extremity and pelvis, and fatal pulmonary embolism following trauma and surgical operations, S. Clin. North America, 21:383, 1941.

Moon, V. H.   Circulatory failure of capillary origin, J.A.M.A., 114:1312, 1940.

———— and Kennedy, P. L.   Pathology of shock, Arch. Path., 14:360, 1932.

Park, W. H., and Williams, A. W.   Pathogenic Microorganisms, 11th ed., Philadelphia, Lea & Febiger, 1939.

Patterson, E. A.   The danger of dilating urethral strictures with oil, J.A.M.A., 97:1147, 1931.

Puppe, G.   Atlas unf Grundriss der gerichtlichen Medizin, München, J. F. Lehmann, 1908.

Reuter, K.   Über gefährliche Methoden der Schwangerschaftsunterbrechung, Med. Klin., 28:1339, 1932.

Rukstinat, G. J.   Experimental study of traumatic shock, Arch. Path., 14:378, 1932.

Schmidt, O.   Luftbefunde im Kreislauf bei stumpfer Gewalt gegen den Brustkorb (Ein Beitrag zur Luftembolie), Deutsche Ztschr. f.d. ges. gerichtl. Med., 15:174, 1930.

Spielmeyer, W.   Über die anatomische Folge de Luftembolie im Gehirn, Verhandl. d. deutsche. Kong. f. inn. Med., 30th Kongress, Wiesbaden, 30:359, 1913.

Taylor, J.   Paradoxical embolism, Path. Soc. of Philadelphia, Nov. 9, 1933, Arch. Path., 16:901, 1933.

Vance, B. M.   Intrauterine injection of Lysol as an abortifacient, Arch. Path., 40:395, 1945.

———— Thrombosis of the veins of the lower extremity and pulmonary embolism as a complication of trauma, Am. J. Surg., 26:19, 1934.

———— The clinical diagnosis of fat embolism, Am. J. Surg., 26:27, 1934.

———— The significance of fat embolism, Arch. Surg., 23:426, 1931.

———— and Fisher, R. C.   Sickle cell disease, Arch. Path., 32:378, 1941.

Walcher, K.   Über vitale Reaktionen, Deutsche Ztschr. f.d. ges. gerichtl. Med., 15:16, 1930.

———— Über die Luftembolie, Mitt. a. d. Grenzgeb. d. Med. u. Chir., 39:314, 1926.

———— Über die gerichtlich, medizinische Beurteilung der Luftembolie in kleinen und grossen Kreislauf mit besonderer Berücksichtigung der cerebralen Luftembolie, Deutsche Ztschr. f.d. ges. gerichtl. Med., 5:561, 1925.

Wever, E.   Cerebrale Luftembolie, Beitr. z. Klin. d. Tuberk., 31:159, 1914.

Wolf, L. P.   Experimentelle Studien über Luftembolie, Virchows Arch. f. path. Anat., 174:454, 1903.

Unusual Forms of Traumatic Pulmonary Embolism

Berkheiser, S. W., and Giffen, H. K.   Bone marrow and fat embolism following multiple fractures, J.A.M.A., 147:564, 1951.

Fisher, J. H.   Bone marrow embolism, Arch. Path., 52:1315, 1951.

Jennings, E. R., and Stofer, B. E.   Pulmonary emboli composed of contents of amniotic fluid, Arch. Path., 45:616, 1948.

Krakower, C.   Pulmonary embolus containing cerebral tissue, Arch. Path., 22:119, 1936.

Lippincott, S. W., and Breck, M. R.   Embolism from liver tissue in pulmonary artery, Arch. Path., 36:423, 1943.

Rappaport, H., and others.   Bone marrow embolism, Am. J. Path., 27:407, 1951.

Strauss, R.   Pulmonary embolism caused by liver tissue, Arch. Path., 33:69, 1942.

———— Pulmonary embolism caused by a lead bullet following a gun shot wound of the abdomen, Arch. Path., 33:63, 1942.

Wyatt, J. P., and Goldenberg, H.   Amniotic fluid embolism, Arch. Path., 45:366, 1948.

9

Blunt Force Injuries of the
Skin and Subcutaneous Tissues

Blunt force produces physical trauma by the violence of its action, damaging the body without necessarily inflicting a penetrating wound. For this reason the lesions produced by blunt force are known as subcutaneous injuries in contradistinction to the penetrating wounds or percutaneous injuries caused by bullets and sharp pointed instruments. Two categories of blunt force are recognized:

1. *Generalized* blunt force, in which the violence affects the whole body or a large segment of it. Examples of this type are encountered in highway accidents, falls from a height, crushing by falling earth and similar casualties.

2. *Localized* blunt force, in which an object with a limited area of impact comes in contact with the body; for example, a blow from a fist, a blow from a weapon or a kick with the foot.

In some instances of physical trauma the blunt force causing the injuries falls not into one but into both of these categories.

1. *Generalized* blunt force acts on the body in three ways to produce injury: (a) by sudden and severe jarring; (b) by crushing; (c) by tearing.

a. Injuries due to Severe Jarring. Such injuries occur in falls, in automobile accidents in which the body is tossed into the air or knocked down and in severe impacts from moving, falling or swinging objects. These forms of trauma are sustained in two ways: by *direct* violence, in which the greatest damage is inflicted at the point of impact, as when a brick falls and shatters a person's head; by *indirect* violence, in which the injury occurs at a point distant from the area of impact. For example, a person in falling lands upon his head and shoulders and suffers a forceful distortion of the spinal column, resulting in a fracture of one of the vertebral segments.

b. Injuries due to a crushing force. Injuries of this type occur when the body is compressed by an elevator, crushed in a collision of automobiles or buried under falling masonry in the collapse of a building. The trauma is produced for the most part by direct violence.

c. Injuries due to a tearing force. A tearing force is exerted on the body when the violence is applied in a tangential direction. This occurs frequently during highway accidents in which the wheel of an automobile grinds the victim against the roadway, or during the impact of any object which is impelled against the body in a glancing fashion. External tears of the skin and severe internal tears of the viscera are produced by such violence.

2. *Localized* blunt force is a frequent cause of injury. This mechanism is encountered when an object strikes the body with forcible impact over a relatively small area. Such a force may be applied quickly, like the impact produced by the blow of a weapon. It may crush the organs, as when one man tramples on another's body. Finally, the localized blunt force may impinge on the body in a tangential

187

fashion and tear the internal structures. Examples of localized blunt force producing injury are encountered in the following ways.

a. Human Assaults. The injuries are caused by blows struck with fists or with blunt weapons such as clubs, gun butts or blackjacks, thrusts with sticks, kicks, trampling, or thrown missiles.

b. Animal Assaults. The trauma results from blows with paws, thrusts with horns, kicks and trampling.

c. Falls or Collisions. The injuries result from impact of a part of the body against a flat or projecting fixed object.

The violence in these cases is direct and confined to the part of the body which is struck. The resulting injuries are often characteristic of the object causing them.

Homicidal, Suicidal and Accidental Deaths. Homicidal deaths due to blunt force injuries fall into the following two groups.

1. The first includes those cases in which the force is applied with intent to kill. Death is produced for the most part by localized violence such as kicks, blows with the fists or blows with blunt instruments like clubs, iron pipes, gun butts, blackjacks or heavy files. In some homicides the victim is thrown or otherwise forced to fall from a height. Other types of blunt force are used rarely for homicidal purposes. The reports of the Office of the Chief Medical Examiner in New York City disclose an average of 359 homicides a year for the 33 year period from 1918 to 1951, or 2.3 per cent of the total yearly average of all deaths investigated during that period. Of the homicides a yearly average of 60, or less than one sixth, resulted from fisticuff altercations or from assaults with blunt weapons; in about one or two homicidal cases each year the victim was thrown from a building or a high place, or more rarely from or under a moving automobile, train or other vehicle, or hurled down a flight of stairs.

2. The second group includes many technical homicides or deaths in which the fatal injury was inflicted not with intent to kill but as a result of negligence, careless behavior or intoxication on the part of the perpetrator. Such deaths result from highway accidents, elevator accidents or building cave-ins. Although classified as accidental in the records of the Chief Medical Examiner, they are nevertheless referred to the Office of the District Attorney because of the possibility of criminal negligence having been a factor in their production.

Suicidal deaths from blunt force injuries occur when persons cast themselves from high places such as buildings or bridges, or throw themselves in front of moving vehicles such as trains or automobiles. Other methods in which blunt force causes death are not frequently employed for suicidal purposes. In the records of the Medical Examiner of New York City the yearly average of all suicidal deaths from 1918 to 1951 was 1030, or 0.7 per cent of all medical examiner's cases. A yearly average of 161 suicides, or less than one sixth, died by blunt force: 139 of these deaths were caused by jumping from buildings; a few by jumping from bridges, elevated railway structures or viaducts; and still fewer by the victims casting themselves down elevator shafts, dumbwaiter shafts, stairwells and chutes, or off of cliffs, poles, trees, walls or other elevations. A yearly average of 20 persons died by throwing themselves under moving trains and a smaller number under moving automobiles or street cars. In a few cases prisoners have committed suicide in jail by charging into a hard wall with the head down like a battering ram or by diving head first onto a hard floor. In one case an individual killed himself by starting a slowly moving freight elevator and allowing it to descend upon him as he squatted in the elevator pit. In another case the deceased had occupied a prison cell in which the bunks, when not in use, were swung back on a hinge and fastened against the wall like the upper berth of a sleeping car. He had seated himself beneath the folded bunk and released it suddenly causing it to drop heavily on the top of his head and to kill him by crushing the base of the skull around the foramen magnum.

Accidental injuries from blunt force are common and occur in highway accidents, falls and miscellaneous casualties. The majority of these result from generalized violence and comparatively few from localized force. The yearly average of fatal highway accidents, including the technical homicides, was 1052 cases, or about 7 per cent of all medical examiner's cases. The yearly averages for the different kinds of vehicles involved were as follows: automobiles, 518; auto trucks, 151; motorcycles, 6; subway and elevated trains, 63; street cars, 62; railway trains, 35; horse drawn vehicles, 20; run-over autobus cases were not frequent. Fatal collisions between vehicles, mainly automobiles, averaged 70 cases a year; and of automobiles or other vehicles with stationary objects like trees, pillars, walls and similar structures about 38 cases. In addition, occasional deaths occurred as the result of automobiles having overturned while being driven, of crushing of a victim between automobiles or between an automobile and a platform, or of a similar casualty.

The incidence of alcoholism among the victims of fatal highway accidents has been analyzed and incorporated in the annual reports of the Office of the Chief Medical Examiner of the City of New York since 1940. In that year, of 553 cases tested out of a total of 1,041, alcohol was found in the brain and liver in 232, or 42 per cent. This figure represents 22 per cent of the total 1,041 cases. Those not tested were victims that survived beyond the period of 24 hours during which alcohol disappears from the body so that its presence in the victim at the time of the accident could not be established by toxicologic examination after autopsy. Also, in cases in which the victim was a child, tests for alcohol were deemed unnecessary.

The yearly average incidence of deaths from falls of various types was 1393 cases or 8.5 per cent of the total. They occurred as follows: from a standing position to sidewalk or floor, 524; down stairs, 228; from a window or other part of a building, 204. A considerable number of fatal falls occurred from vehicles, elevated railway structures, bridges, scaffolds, trees, porches, chairs, beds, horses and from like elevations or down the hold of ships, into excavations and other pits. The average yearly incidence of fatal elevator accidents included 28 falls down a shaft, 15 crushings by an elevator and 2 deaths of victims in falling elevators. One or two persons were killed in a shaft by falling elevator weights. Among the great variety of fatal miscellaneous casualties, 89 were caused by missiles; others occurred in connection with the operation of machinery, during sport, from burial after the cave-in of earth or of a building, from animal assaults and from many other accidents. Fatal miscellaneous casualties had an average yearly incidence of 316 cases or 2 per cent of the total of all medical examiner's cases.

Unfortunately it is not possible in every case to establish that death from blunt force injury is homicidal, suicidal or accidental. For example, in a death after a fall from a height, there may not be any criterion in the autopsy which will enable the pathologist to distinguish the death in this regard; the only way the status of the case can be established is by a thorough investigation of the circumstances. When a violent death cannot be classified as an accident, suicide or homicide, it is listed as having occurred under undetermined circumstances; this undetermined group is included with the accidental deaths, which means that the latter category contains a number of unresolved suicides and homicides.

BLUNT FORCE INJURIES OF THE SKIN AND SUBCUTANEOUS TISSUES

The injuries produced upon the skin and subcutaneous tissues by generalized and localized blunt force are of three types: contusions, abrasions and lacerations.

Contusions. A blunt force in producing a contusion or bruise ruptures the subcutaneous blood vessels, and an extravasation of blood occurs from these into the surrounding tissues. The surface of the skin, however, is not necessarily damaged. The contused tissue exhibits a variable amount of swelling depending upon the amount of blood extravasted. Parts of the body such as the face, with abundant fatty tissue and a thin dermis, bruise easily, while regions covered by a thick dermis like the abdomen or back contuse with more difficulty. For the same reason women and children bruise more easily than men, the latter usually possessing a tougher dermis and less abundant fatty tissue.

It is unusual for blunt force to produce a characteristic contusion; it may do so if the violence is localized and the object which strikes the skin, small and hard. In one case a woman was found dead with numerous circular and crescentic bruises on the body, all evidently produced by the impact of an object of a certain size and shape; later it was discovered that the distinctive injuries had been produced by prodding with the lower end of a crutch. In some instances the distribution and location of the contusions may suggest the means by which they were inflicted. Thus if a man is found with multiple ecchymoses involving the eyelids and bridge of the nose and contusions of his cheeks and lips, the general pattern of such injuries, though not pathognomic, strongly suggests that they resulted from fisticuffs during an altercation. This subject will receive more consideration on page 261.

Some chronic disease processes are associated with changes in the composition of the blood which so hinder its clotting that the subcutaneous hemorrhages following contusions are more profuse in persons so afflicted than in normal individuals. In hemophilia the blood platelets are abnormally stable and do not disintegrate when blood is shed; an insufficient amount of thrombokinase is released and the blood does not clot readily. Dr. Jacob Werne performed an autopsy on the body of a hemophiliac who had developed massive subcutaneous hemorrhages all over the body after receiving severe blows from the fist during an altercation. Chronic alcoholics suffering from fatty infiltration of the liver with or without cirrhosis may develop a vitamin K and prothrombin deficiency and may also bruise easily after slight trauma. Extensive ecchymoses occur from minor injuries resulting when such individuals stagger, fall and strike themselves while inebriated. Occasionally such lesions have been attributed erroneously to an assault. It is also important not to confuse the extensive confluent purpuric eruptions which may occur in fulminating meningococcemia with traumatic ecchymoses; they have been mistaken for contusions and the error in such cases has resulted in unjust suspicion and accusation of maltreatment directed against the parents or guardian of the victim.

One of the most important questions concerning contusions is whether or not they were produced during life. In the early postmortem stages they may be confused with suggillation; but a distinction is possible because the latter may be blanched by continuously applied pressure which forces the blood out of the surface vessels. The antemortem bruise, on the contrary, cannot be blanched by this test as the blood is already extravasted out of the vessels into the subcutaneous tissues.

On incision of a contusion, the blood which is in the tissues cannot be washed away. On the incision of a fresh livid area the blood, which is in the vessels and not in the tissues, can be washed out of the vessels to leave the tissues clean. During gaseous decomposition the internal pressure in the circulatory system is increased and postmortem ruptures of many small vessels and hemolysis of blood take place. The resulting subcutaneous extravasation and diffusion of hemolyzed blood will first tend to enlarge the size of a pre-existing contusion. Later the putrefactive changes in the tissues make it impossible to differentiate the antemortem bruise from the postmortem decomposition.

A contusion heals after a time by destruction and removal of the extravasated blood. The duration of this process varies with the severity of the lesion, the health of the individual and the vascularity of the subcutaneous tissues affected. The more vascular the area, the smaller the contusion, and the healthier the individual, the more rapid will be the rate of healing. The first change is a subsidence of the swelling in the traumatized area and a color transformation from the bluish and reddish purple of the fresh lesion to a dark bluish-black color occurring about one to three days post trauma; after this initial darkening, the color fades, changing gradually into a greenish-blue, brown and tan and finally disappearing in about one to four weeks. If the bruise is small the extravasated red blood cells are probably removed by the phagocytic action of the histiocytes. If the contusion is larger the erythrocytes disintegrate by hemolysis and the hemoglobin is converted into hemosiderin, a brown iron-containing pigment, and hematoidin, an iron-free pigment. Toward the end stage of the healing process large histiocytes containing coarse granules of brown hemosiderin pigment can be seen microscopically in sections of the contused area. Polymorphonuclear leukocytes are not numerous in a contusion unless there has been penetration of the wound from the outside, considerable destruction of subcutaneous tissues or a complicating infection. The pathologist must be cautious in interpreting the age of contusions either from the gross color changes or from the microscopic appearance. It is possible to distinguish between a fresh or recent injury and an older one, but it is difficult if not impossible to estimate the exact age of a bruise with any degree of certainty.

In the simplest form of contusion there is extravasation of blood into the septa which carry the blood vessels from the deeper structures to the dermis through the subcutaneous fat. In most cases such a lesion heals without leaving a scar. If the trauma is more severe, blood may be extravasated in between the fat cells and some of these may be ruptured, with the formation of a localized hematoma composed of a mixture of blood and liquid fat. During the healing of the more severe injuries a scar or an area of traumatic fat necrosis may develop in the subcutaneous fat. The more extensive contusions which are accompanied by abrasions and lacerations will be discussed under those headings.

A minor traumatic lesion of the subcutaneous fat in the breast is designated as fat necrosis. It may develop after a slight injury in which free fat is liberated from the ruptured cells. The oil causes a chronic irritation and inflammation resulting finally in the formation of a hard white chalky localized mass firmly attached to the skin. Microscopically this lesion is a chronic inflammatory reaction and contains large foamy phagocytes full of lipid, foreign body giant cells, fatty acid formations with calcification, lymphocytic infiltrations and vessels showing obliterating endarteritis. It has more surgical importance than forensic significance. It has been mistaken grossly for carcinoma because of its induration and attachment to the skin.

Abrasions. An abrasion is an injury of the superficial layers of the epidermis produced by forcible contact with an object having a rough surface. In its simplest form the epidermis is compressed and its thickness decreased; the epidermal cells are flattened and their nuclei are elongated. If sufficient friction is applied, partial or complete removal of the epithelium may occur and the superficial layer of the dermis damaged. The raw surface remaining is covered by an exudation of blood and lymph which soon dries and produces a protective covering known as a crust

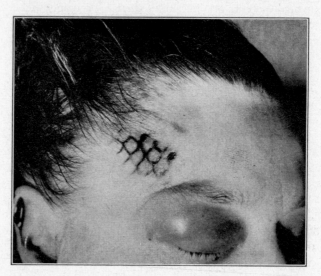

Fig. 9-1. Blunt Force: Automobile Injury.

Imprint of automobile radiator on forehead. Note hematoma of right upper eyelid from fracture of frontal bone. Vehicle homicide.

or scab. The scab consists of dried exudate and sometimes of traumatized squamous epithelium. Where the dermis is exposed, polymorphonuclear leukocytes collect adjacent to the raw area. The abraded portion heals under the scab; during the process epithelial cells extend across from the edges of the lesion and from the

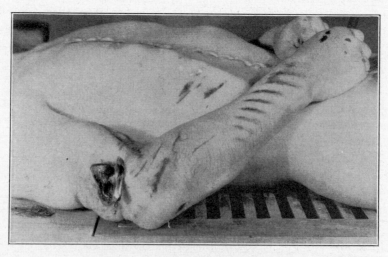

Fig. 9-2. Blunt Force: Automobile Injury.

Patterned imprint of automobile radiator on right forearm and wrist. Note broken off piece of metal radiator cap ornament embedded in arm above elbow. Vehicle homicide.

surface of the hair sheaths; the new epithelial layer undermines the scab and finally thrusts it off. The new epithelium at first consists of a single layer of cells which changes gradually into normal stratified squamous epithelium. By the time the scab is separated, the new epidermis is completely formed and ready to function. Usually no scar results from this injury.

If the skin is adjacent to bone, as it is on the scalp and face and over the inner surface of the tibia, a crushing injury such as might be inflicted by an automobile may abrade the epidermis and in addition crush the dermis and subcutaneous tissues.

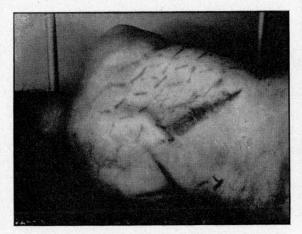

Fig. 9-3. Patterned Injury. Imprint of Tire Tread Across Back. Run Over by Auto-truck.

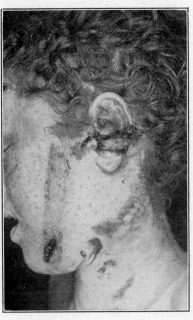

Fig. 9-4. Blunt Force: Patterned Impression of Flat Surface of Blacksmith's File on Cheek.

A similar wound was present on the other side of the face. Homicidal assault.

The dermis is decreased in thickness, infiltrated in varying degrees by blood and permeated by liquid fat expressed out of the subcutaneous tissues. The abraded area then appears translucent, dark red and parchment-like. The subcutaneous fat may be contused and even torn. When this wound heals, the traumatized area is reacted to as a foreign body and cast off with the formation of granulation tissue; a distinctly flattened scar results.

Abrasions may occur ante mortem or post mortem. As a rule antemortem abrasions display a reddish brown appearance due to a slight exudation of blood, while the postmortem variety is yellowish in hue and translucent in appearance. Postmortem abrasions generally occur over bony prominences such as the elbows, and are attributable to the rough handling of the cadaver. During advanced postmortem decomposition, patches of the entire epidermis become detached, exposing the raw surface of the dermis which then dries to form a reddish brown dark area similar in appearance to an antemortem abrasion. Microscopically this postmortem lesion shows no intravital reaction and is characterized by a separation of the epidermis from the dermis with complete loss of the former, whereas an ante-mortem abrasion usually displays signs of intravital reaction and may show the remains of damaged epithelium. In many instances, especially if the lesions are superficial or the postmortem decomposition is advanced, it is difficult or impossible to distinguish antemortem from postmortem abrasions.

The exact age of an abrasion cannot be determined with any certainty by either external or microscopic examination. From the first to the third day after the trauma the lesion is bright reddish brown, gradually changing in about two to

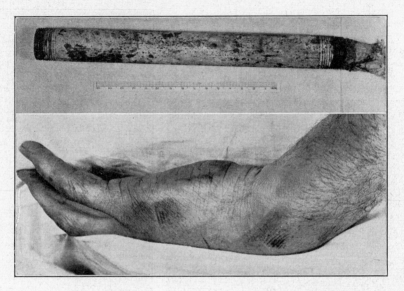

Fig. 9-5. Blunt Force: Patterned Injury Produced by Threads on Lead-Filled Metal Pipe.

Top. Grouped parallel abrasions on hand and wrist corresponding to pattern of metal threads on ends of pipe; injuries received in attempt to ward off blows which were directed toward the victim's head. Homicidal assault.

Bottom. Photograph of the weapon used showing threaded ends.

three days to a darker and duller reddish brown. The formation of the new epidermis usually starts about 7 to 14 days or sooner after the trauma, depending on the size of the lesion. Complete healing may take place in several weeks. If the area of injury has become infected the process will be delayed. Extensive postmortem decomposition and mummification in a dead body may obscure the presence of an abrasion and make any estimation of its age difficult or impossible.

Only a limited amount of information concerning the type of violence can be gained by the study of abrasions. A careful determination of the size, number, loca-tion and pattern of the lesions may furnish some clue as to its character. For example, if a rough surface scrapes the skin tangentially, linear scratch marks are produced which may taper to a fine point; the direction of the tapering corresponds to that of the abrading surface at the time of injury. Occasionally an abrasion im-printed on the skin is characteristic of the particular object or surface which pro-duced it. In highway accidents the pattern of the radiator grid or of the tire tread may be impressed in the form of an abrasion on the victim (Figs. 9-1, 9-2 and 9-3) and establish that a vehicle of a particular type was the instrument that produced the injuries. In one case a young woman was killed by blows from a large rough

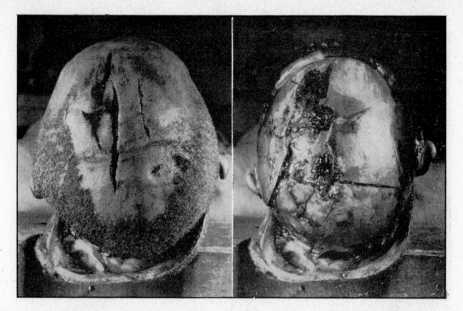

Fig. 9-6. Localized Blunt Force Injury. Lacerations of Scalp with Comminuted Depressed Fracture of Vault of Skull.

Homicidal assault with iron bar.

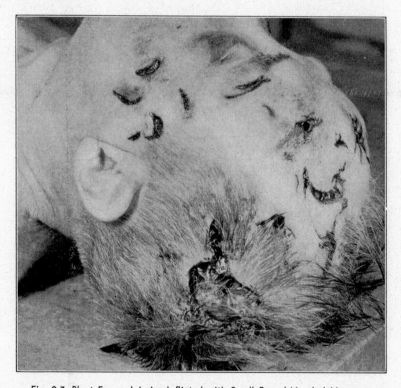

Fig. 9-7. Blunt Force: Injuries Inflicted with Small Round-Headed Hammer.

Multiple crescentic lacerations of similar pattern inflicted by blows with small round-headed hammer. Homicidal assault.

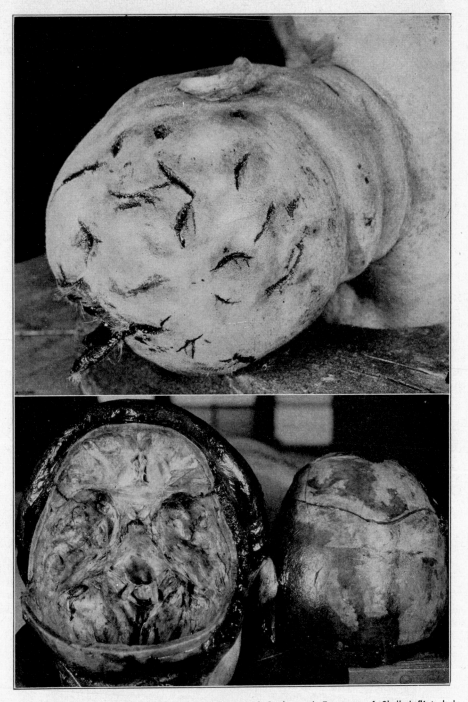

Fig. 9-8. Blunt Force: Multiple Curved Lacerations of Scalp and Fracture of Skull Inflicted by Pistol Butt.

Top. Multiple curved lacerations of similar pattern.

Bottom. Extensive fracture of vault and base of skull. Note small curved linear fracture on left parietal bone which was beneath one of the scalp lacerations. Homicidal assault.

file which produced a characteristic pattern on her face (Fig. 9-4). In another case the victim was struck with the end of a metal pipe which left the pattern of its threads on his hand (Fig. 9-5). All wounds should be carefully examined; those with the most distinctive pattern are not necessarily the fatal ones.

Lacerations. Lacerated wounds of the skin are a variety of injury caused by blunt force; in this form of trauma the epidermis is torn and the tear penetrates into the dermis and subcutaneous tissues. Lacerations are produced in various ways:

(1) By direct impact of a hard object like a bottle or club against skin stretched

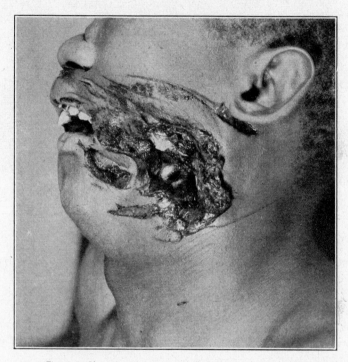

Fig. 9-9. Blunt Force: Injuries Inflicted with a Flat Iron.

Lacerations of face and compound comminuted fractures of upper and lower jaws produced by blows with a flat iron. Note the upper linear curved abrasion on the side of the cheek corresponding to the side-edge of the iron. Homicidal assault.

over an underlying layer of bone. The subcutaneous layers are contused and pulpified; the dermis and epithelial layers are split by the blow, producing stellate or angular lacerations with pointed extremities and well defined edges, often without abrasions (Figs. 9-6 and 9-7). Some of these injuries are patterned; a hammer or gun butt applied to the scalp produces lacerations which in many instances conform to the shape of the striking part of the weapon; the edges around these lacerations are usually abraded and slightly crushed and the surrounding tissues are contused (Figs. 9-8 and 9-9).

(2) By tangential impact of a rough object which tears up a flap of the skin. This type of injury is most often encountered about the head, face and extremities, parts of the body which are most often exposed to violence and less protected than the trunk. The resulting laceration is irregular and ragged and a flap of skin is usually formed at the point of impact. The edges of such wounds are often abraded and ecchymosis is present in the surrounding tissues. An injury of this type, caused

by the edge and point of a flat iron striking the left cheek, is shown in Figure 9-9;
another, inflicted on the right arm by the metal radiator cap ornament of an automobile, in Figure 9-2. A portion of this ornament was broken off in the wound,

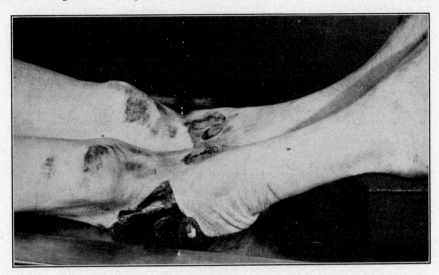

Fig. 9-10. Blunt Force: Impact of Automobile Bumper.

Symmetric compound fractures of both legs with extensive lacerations of the soft tissues
posteriorly.

which included a fracture of the humerus; it was removed at autopsy and saved as
part of the corpus delicti.

(3) By a tearing force produced by an automobile wheel. This will be described
later.

(4) By a broken bone tearing the overlying skin. Such lacerations are ragged
tears of various dimensions, most often seen on the scalp and the lower extremities.

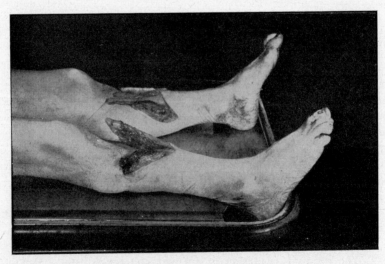

Fig. 9-11. Blunt Force: Impact of Automobile Bumper.

Symmetric compound fractures of both legs with extensive lacerations of the soft tissues
anteriorly.

Their size depends on the degree of displacement of the broken fragments of bone. For example, an oblique fracture of the shaft of the tibia may cause a small puncture wound on the anterior surface of the shin if the movement of the fragments is slight; but if the lower fragment of the broken bone is twisted by a wheel during a traffic accident, a transverse ovoid tear of the skin may result. The bumper fractures depicted in Figures 9-10 and 9-11 produced lacerations of this type. Considerable damage may be inflicted on the soft parts in the vicinity of such injuries.

The points already mentioned under contusions and abrasions apply to lacerations. An antemortem laceration generally shows an effusion of blood around its edges in contradistinction to postmortem lacerations, but the differentiation between the two may be difficult or impossible if decomposition and mummification are present or if the wound has been macerated by long contact with water. Even a large external hemorrhage is not always a reliable criterion of the antemortem origin of a lacerated wound, for postmortem lacerations inflicted soon after death in a vascular area or in a dependent part of the body may leak a large quantity of blood.

After a laceration has been inflicted blood oozes into the open wound, coagulates and then dries on the surface. Because of the damage to the tissues, polymorphonuclear leukocytes wander to the edge of the wound and are microscopically noticeable within a few hours after injury. If the wound is not infected, granulation tissue begins to form promptly and organization of the clot follows. Finally a fibrous scar is formed and is covered by epidermis in a variable period, from a week to two months, depending on the size of the injury, the vitality of the patient and the vascularity of the part. Such scars generally lack such specialized skin structures as hair follicles, sweat glands and sebaceous glands. If the wound is infected the process may take longer. Any estimation of the age of a laceration must be made with caution and all factors should be given due consideration.

REFERENCE

Reports of the Office of the Chief Medical Examiner in the City of New York from 1918 to 1951.

10

Blunt Force Injuries
of the Extremities

The injuries produced on the extremities by blunt force can be divided for the sake of convenience into those which involve (1) the soft parts alone, such as the skin, muscles, vessels and nerves, and (2) the bones and joints as well as the soft parts.

SOFT PARTS

Injuries of the soft parts are commonly produced by all types of blunt force. Most of them result from direct violence but some are caused by an indirect force. The different varieties of contusions, lacerations and abrasions of the skin and subcutaneous tissues have been described in the previous chapter.

The group of severe injuries produced by the tearing force of the automobile wheel, already mentioned in the discussion of lacerations, deserves special consideration. These wounds are avulsions resulting from the grinding action of the wheel. They occur commonly in highway accidents in which the tire on the rotating

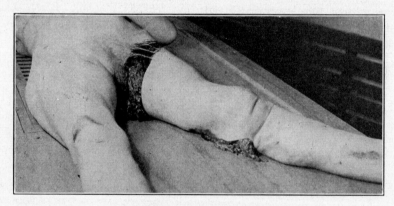

Fig. 10-1. Blunt Force: Automobile Injury.

Stocking-like downward avulsion of skin and subcutaneous tissue from left thigh. The skin of the thigh forms a loose stocking attached by a few strands of tissue at the upper end. The injury was due to the grinding action of an automobile wheel. Vehicle homicide.

automobile wheel presses the victim's limb while passing over it and exerts at the same time a tangential traction on the skin. The mildest effect of the violence is to separate the skin and subcutaneous fatty layer from the underlying muscles. This action forms a closed subcutaneous pocket of variable size containing blood and liquid fat. A more severe injury is a separation which extends completely around the circumference of the limb and results in a sleeve or stocking-like avulsion of the skin and subcutaneous fat (Fig. 10-1). If the skin is protected by clothing, the epidermis may remain intact; but in many cases the surface is abraded and the dermis and subcutaneous fat are crushed and contused; ecchymoses and brownish discoloration of the skin, due to impregnation with crushed liquid fat, are evident. The separation of the tissues in the deeper layers of the subcutaneous fat near the fascia results in the tearing of nerve fibers and small blood vessels. A person so injured suffers considerable shock. The muscles, bones and other structures may or may not be involved. In a severe avulsion, the skin is also torn through so that a communication of the subcutaneous pocket with the outside is formed. Large flaps of skin and subcutaneous tissue may be lifted up (Fig. 10-2).

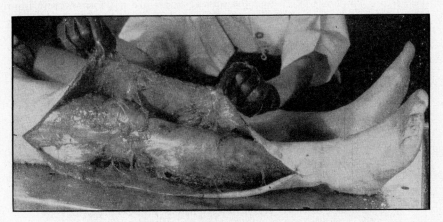

Fig. 10-2. Automobile Wheel Injury.

Extensive annular avulsion of skin and subcutaneous tissues from knee and leg.

A mild traction injury may take the form of short, irregular, incomplete or interrupted cracks or tears in the skin, usually near the junction of the thigh and abdomen. Close inspection reveals that the skin edges are split or pulled slightly apart. These lesions, also evident near the torn skin margin of a severe avulsion, are important chiefly because they suggest injury by a vehicle rather than by some other agency (Fig. 10-3). This point may have considerable medicolegal importance in a case in which death has been caused by blunt force and the manner of injury is not too obvious. The skin may show similar splitting effects as the result of sudden stretching associated with impacts and fractures of underlying bones sustained when the body falls from a height.

Occasionally the skin and subcutaneous tissues are torn and avulsed and the muscles exposed by the intense traction of the wheel (Figs. 10-2 and 10-3). While most often occurring at right angles to the direction of the tearing force, the tear is sometimes parallel to it. Sometimes one leg is involved in the injury; occasionally both are affected at about the same level. The parts first struck by the wheel may suffer the most trauma. Death usually results from shock or in some cases from external hemorrhage or septic infection. Since most severe avulsions are rapidly fatal, instances in which such injuries have undergone repair are not often encountered.

The authors have observed the autopsy findings in the case of a man who died from coronary arteriosclerosis about four months after he had sustained traumatic injury in an automobile accident. On the left thigh near Scarpa's triangle there was a closed subcutaneous pocket about four inches square, lined by a thin layer of tan-colored, fibrous tissue and containing a small amount of tan-colored fluid. This lesion was interpreted as a partly healed traumatic subcutaneous separation which had been sustained at the time of accident; during the reparative process, the blood and liquid fat had been absorbed from the closed cavity. Complications such as necrosis and infection in the injured area which usually follow such a wound were apparently prevented by the efficient collateral circulation to the overlying skin layers.

A blunt force sufficient to injure the nerve trunks and muscles usually produces severe lesions in the skin and bones. In passing over an extremity an automobile wheel may sever the muscles and nerves or separate and contuse them individually. After two to three days polymorphonuclear leukocytes in large numbers exude into the injured area and some of the muscle fibers undergo necrosis. If the trauma is slight and the muscle fibers are not too severely injured,

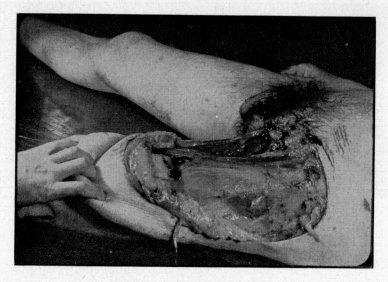

Fig. 10-3. Automobile Wheel Injury.

Avulsion in which flap of skin is separated from left thigh. Small parallel superficial epidermal tears near groin indicating traction type of injury.

the nuclei of the sarcolemma proliferate, multinucleated giant cells form around the damaged fibers and regeneration of new muscle fibers takes place without widespread changes. If the injury results in necrosis of muscle, the necrotic portions are removed by mononuclear and giant cell phagocytes and the parts are knit together by fibrous tissue repair. If neurons in a nerve trunk are severed and the torn ends are not separated by too much of a gap, the neurilemma sheaths will proliferate and bridge the defect and the neurons will establish their former continuity. If the gap cannot be bridged, a nodule or amputation neuroma composed of fibrous and nervous tissue develops at the injured end of the nerve, and axons in the distal disconnected portion of the nerve undergo wallerian degeneration.

The larger blood vessels are rarely injured by blunt force and then only in association with severe trauma to the surrounding structures. Vessels may be lacerated by broken bones. Hemorrhage is the chief complication of this injury. Traumatic aneurysm will be described in the chapter on bullet and stab wounds; it is rarely produced by blunt force.

Occasionally the intima of an artery may be injured by blunt force, and a noninfectious or bland thrombosis may develop at the site of the injury with fatal results. In one such case a 50 year old white man was run over by an automobile in a highway accident. The vehicle passed over and severely bruised the skin and muscles of both thighs. A few days later a bland thrombosis developed in the moderately sclerotic right and left femoral arteries at the level of the injury, occluding both vessels and producing moist gangrene of the feet and legs. The process eventually caused death.

Femoral vein thrombosis resulting in pulmonary embolism is an occasional complication of injuries of the lower extremity. This condition has been discussed in Chapter 8.

A severe crushing and grinding force applied to the extremities may cause an extensive extravasation of blood into the subcutaneous and intermuscular tissues, followed after a few days by hemolysis of the effused blood, a hemoglobinemia and a fatal hemoglobinuric nephrosis. As an example of this complication, a 33 year old elevator operator was crushed between elevator and floor and was taken to the hospital in severe shock. He died nine days after the injury. At autopsy extensive subcutaneous hemorrhages were present in left arm and leg, and there was a widespread separation of the skin from the muscles of the left thigh, buttock, back and flank, forming a big closed undermined cavity which contained over a pint of brownish disintegrated blood. The deceased was slightly jaundiced as a result of blood destruction. Histologic examination of the kidneys disclosed numerous blood pigment casts in the tubules of the pyramids and the cortex.

The crush or compression syndrome occurring among air raid casualties in England during the war was recognized and described by Bywaters. It is a complication of blunt force injury usually involving the muscles of the extremities. In most cases the limbs of the victim were pinned under fallen masonry and compressed for several hours. Following rescue and the release of the limbs from the crushing force, the injured extremities then became edematous, lost their power of motion and manifested hyperesthesia, anesthesia and paresthesia. Within a few hours the hemoglobin concentration of the blood increased, the blood pressure fell and the victim exhibited signs of delayed shock. Oliguria developed and many dark brown granular casts appeared in the urine. The involvement of the kidneys progressed even when the injured limb was amputated. Death occurred in about a week from renal failure. Autopsy revealed a pallid necrosis of the affected muscles and degeneration of the epithelium of the renal tubules. These contained casts full of blood pigment. The appearance of the kidneys was not unlike that encountered in deaths following transfusion with incompatible blood.

Although the kidney lesion has been a constant finding in cases of crush injury, its occurrence in a case in which a blood transfusion had not been given eliminates incompatible blood as a necessary factor in its production. Some have attributed the renal failure to the production of toxic substances in the traumatized muscle and the release from the muscle of myoglobin. Deposited in the kidney tubules in the form of casts, it causes tubular obstruction and oliguria. Others regard the drainage of blood into the liberated limb, after the pressure on it has been removed, and the consequent dangerous depletion of blood volume in the general circulation resulting in an especially severe state of delayed shock, as the noxious factor.

BONES AND JOINTS

The bones and joints of the extremities are traumatized by: (1) direct violence, (2) indirect violence, and (3) muscular action.

(1) Direct violence by its action can dislocate the joints, fracture the bones and cause considerable damage to the surrounding tissues. In elevated train or subway

accidents, joints like the knee or elbow are apt to be luxated whenever the limb is fixed at its distal end in an extended position. If the force acting on such a joint produces hyperextension, it will tear the ligaments and avulse the bone from its articulation. The bones of the extremities are frequently fractured by direct violence. The tibia and fibula may be broken across at right angles to the shaft as a result of direct impact by an automobile bumper (Figs. 9-10 and 9-11) or crushed and extensively comminuted by a wheel. A direct blow with a heavy blunt instrument may shatter the shaft of a bone like the humerus or ulna at the site of impact.

Severe and extensive fractures, crushing and mangling of the soft parts and even amputation of the extremities are produced by the metal wheels of a railway car. Other parts of the body are usually involved and there may be mangling and transection of the trunk or decapitation.

(2) Indirect violence, capable of producing injury at a distance from the point of application of a blunt force, results when the force is applied in such a way as to transmit the greatest stress to some other part of the extremity. A joint like the knee or hip can be luxated by indirect violence if one of its component bones is twisted or levered to put a strain on the joint capsule. When the violence is moderate, the synovial membrane may be contused or lacerated; bleeding may occur into the joint cavity, causing a low-grade traumatic hemorrhagic arthritis. If the violence is severe, the bone may be dislocated and the ligaments and capsule of the joint torn. In one such case, the thigh of an elderly man was pinned between a street car and the rail of a bridge. The forward motion of the car imparted a twisting motion to the shaft of the femur which dislocated the femoral head from the acetabulum. The shafts of the bones may be broken by indirect violence if they are in some way twisted or bent by a force applied to the distal end. Such injuries occur in various types of falls and in highway accidents; the fractures are either oblique or spiral, with displacement of fragments but with little tendency to comminution. The bones usually injured in this manner are the tibia, fibula, femur, clavicle, humerus, ulna and radius.

Fractures of the bones of the extremities are not usually characteristic of the type of blunt force which produced them. In some falls from a height, if the victim lands on its feet, the bones of each leg and thigh may be broken at different levels with more or less correspondence between the sides. If the wheel passes over the leg in run-over cases, a severe compound comminuted fracture of the leg bones with crushing of the tissues may be produced. In cases of assault with a heavy weapon like an iron bar, in which the victim attempted to ward off the blows, there may be transverse or comminuted fractures of one or both bones of the forearm; if one bone is fractured it is usually the ulna. Other injuries, however, may be less characteristic. The medical examiner must then describe the fractures and correlate them with the circumstances of the case as well as he can. This subject will be discussed more fully on page 324.

(3) Muscular action rarely produces serious injuries of the bones and joints and is not an important factor in their causation. (See pages 259 and 319 for types of fractures which are due to muscular action.)

FATAL COMPLICATIONS

These include shock, hemorrhage, infection, thrombosis and embolism, and the effect of such injuries on pre-existing natural disease.

Shock. Shock is a common complication of severe injuries of the lower extremities, especially when there is extensive destruction of tissue. The shock may be primary and set in almost immediately after the trauma. In such cases it is the result of the injury to the nerves and the consequent overwhelming depression of the central nervous system. Death may occur shortly after the injury. Sometimes shock is delayed or secondary and comes on a few hours after the injury. The victim undergoes a general circulatory collapse, as described in Chapter 8 under complications of trauma. Injuries producing shock are severe fractures, especially of the femur, extensive crushing of the tissues, extensive skin lacerations and avulsions such as might be caused by an automobile.

Hemorrhage. When a large blood vessel is crushed or torn or when many blood vessels are torn, a profuse escape of blood takes place externally. Extensive lacerations and traumatic amputations are often complicated by such fatal bleeding. In a compound fracture of the lower end of the femur, the sharp lower fragment, usually displaced backward, may, by tearing the femoral vessels cause a fatal hemorrhage. In performing an autopsy on cases of fatal traumatic injury in which death apparently resulted from external hemorrhage, it is important that the medical examiner confirm the diagnosis by examining the heart and other viscera for the signs denoting loss of blood described in Chapter 8.

Infection. Infection, a common complication of injuries of the lower extremities, is usually the result of the carrying of pathogenic bacteria through skin lacerations into the deeper, often traumatized, tissues. Compound fractures are apt to become infected, with the formation of abscesses around the broken ends of the bones and the development of osteomyelitis. The most common infecting organisms are the pyogenic cocci, *Staphylococcus aureus* and *Streptococcus hemolyticus*. The staphylococci may give rise to abscesses in the soft parts or to a septic thrombosis of the neighboring veins with resultant embolic abscesses in the lungs. The hemolytic streptococci after invasion produce a variety of infections which may take the form of a suppurative cellulitis, a wound erysipelas or a general septicemia.

The anaerobe, *Clostridium welchii,* may infect crushing and tearing injuries of the lower extremities, especially when necrotic traumatized tissue and numerous aerobic bacteria are present; such a combination of conditions is favorable for its growth and invasive powers. Infection with this organism causes a gangrenous necrosis of voluntary muscle and interstitial tissues with gas formation in the tissues and hemolysis of the blood. As a result the wound becomes swollen, discolored, foul-smelling and crepitant. Unless the infection is held in check by the resistance of the patient, by prompt surgical intervention or by the administration of antitoxin, it will spread rapidly and cause death by toxemia. After death the gas bacillus invades the blood vessels and is responsible for early bacterial decomposition. *Clostridium welchii* may enter the blood even during life and produce enough hemolysis to impart a slightly bronze tinge to the skin.

Some injuries, especially those which are contaminated with soil, are infected with the tetanus bacillus or its spores. The characteristic symptoms and signs of fatal tetanus may develop after several days of incubation. At autopsy, such infected wounds are deep or undermined and contain foreign material and a small amount of purulent exudate; the surrounding tissues may or may not be necrotic. Since tetanus bacilli are usually present in the wound, some of the suspected infected tissue or exudant should be removed for bacteriologic examination, as noted on page 94. The internal viscera do not reveal any characteristic lesions in tetanus. The bacillus produces its lethal effect through a potent exotoxin which does not cause any demonstrable structural changes in the tissues.

Since bruised tissue in a contusion has a lessened resistance to infection, pyogenic bacteria may gain access either through the skin or blood stream; cellulitis or an abscess may develop in such an injury and then give rise to a fatal septicemia. It should be remembered that chronic alcoholism, diabetes mellitus or some other condition may diminish the victim's resistance to infection. Similarly a closed injury of a joint or a bone complicated by a suppurative arthritis or osteomyelitis may progress to a fatal outcome.

Another type of infection which follows injury is hypostatic bronchopneumonia. This complication develops in injured patients whose vitality is low or has been lowered by the trauma. It is encountered frequently as a terminal event in feeble senile individuals compelled to lie in bed after having sustained a fracture of the neck of the femur as the result of a fall.

In evaluating the relationship of an infection to trauma it is necessary to ascertain the time of its onset. In some cases the infection is already present at the time of the injury and therefore cannot have been caused by it. In other instances it develops so long after the trauma that causal relationship is out of the question.

Thrombosis and Embolism. Some degree of pulmonary fat embolism occurs after every fracture and severe injury of the lower extremities. Fatal fat embolism, however, is a relatively rare complication of such injuries. Femoral vein thrombosis and pulmonary embolism also complicate injuries of the lower extremities. These subjects have been discussed in Chapter 8.

Effect of Injury on Pre-existing Natural Disease. Injuries of the extremities may precipitate a fatal exacerbation of a pre-existing natural disease. These disease conditions include delirium tremens, uremia, cardiac decompensation, coronary artery disease, cerebral artery disease, tuberculosis and others. In many of these cases it is difficult to say how much of the responsibility for death should be ascribed to the trauma and how much to the disease. For further discussion of this subject the reader is referred to Chapters 7 and 8.

MEDICOLEGAL CONSIDERATIONS

A physician or surgeon who treats an injured person either in the home or in a hospital is responsible not only for the professional care of the patient but also, in some instances, to the police and other law enforcement agencies. If he has reason to to believe that the circumstances are suspicious of foul play, he should report the case to the police for investigation. If during a surgical operation he recovers any foreign object such as a fragment of glass, wood or metal, for example, like the radiator ornament depicted in Figure 9-3, he should make a record of his finding, mark the object for identification and turn it over to the police as part of the corpus delicti. In such cases he may later be subpoenaed to court to identify the foreign body he removed from the wounded member.

Since a doctor may be called upon to testify in the criminal or civil courts concerning his professional attendance on an injury case, it is clearly his duty to keep an accurate record of the clinical observations which he has made. All injuries should be described as accurately and promptly as possible. The location, type and extent of the wounds may have important medicolegal significance. Questions may arise as to the manner in which an injury was produced and its duration, in addition to its nature.

Autopsies on the bodies of individuals who have sustained serious blunt force injuries present a number of problems which require solution. Among these are the cause of death; the manner in which the injury was inflicted, whether by a human assault or by the action of a mechanical agent like an automobile, or by some other form of violence; and the age of the traumatic lesion. As a rule the cause of death is determined by the autopsy findings; the other problems cannot always be answered as readily. Such answers are important in cases in which the time and circumstances of the injury are not definitely known and different possibilities are being considered by the police. The medical examiner should be cautious in giving his opinion and should obtain all information available in the case before committing himself to a definite statement. A careless, incomplete and inaccurate autopsy investigation and an ill considered opinion on the manner and duration of the injuries might mislead the police and bring an innocent person unjustly under suspicion; whereas if the police were properly guided by the medical findings, their investigation might result in the apprehension of the actual perpetrator or establish that the injuries were the result of noncriminal violence.

In traumatic amputations or in those performed surgically because of severe traumatic injury, the amputated extremity should not be destroyed. If the victim should die, the limb should be submitted to the medical examiner for his examination in connection with the autopsy on the body, especially in cases in which the amputated extremity is the only part of the body traumatized. In New York City a limb removed from a patient who survives his injuries may be disposed of by burial, arranged for either privately by the patient or by the City. A special burial certificate has to be filled out by the surgeon. In traumatic cases, the extremity should always be examined and described and the findings included in the hospital record before it is released for burial. The owner of the limb or his guardian may give permission to the hospital to dissect and dispose of it without burial. The extremity is usually buried with the body of the victim if death occurs during the hospitalization following the amputation. In such cases a separate burial certificate is not necessary.

The question sometimes arises in medicolegal cases whether or not the person could have walked after having received certain injuries of the extremities. The answer to the question must depend upon the nature, location and extent of the injuries as well as upon other circumstances of the case. The more severe traumas, such as fractures of the femur or extensive avulsions, may be accompanied by such shock and pain that the patient is not able to move. Less severe injuries, however, need not affect the individual's power of locomotion to the point of complete disability. For example, an individual can move after receiving a fracture of the tibia by using a wall or other object as a support, thus keeping his weight off the injured leg.

REFERENCES

Beall, D., Bywaters, E. G. L., Belsey, R. H. R., and Miles, J. A. R.   A case of crush injury and renal failure, Brit. M. J., 1:432, 1941.

Bing, R. J.   The etiology of renal failure following crushing injuries, M. Bull. of the New York Univ. College of Medicine, 8:107, 1943.

Boyd, W.   A Text Book of Pathology, Philadelphia, Lea & Febiger, 1938.

Bywaters, E. G. L.   Limb compression in the tube shelter disaster, Lancet, 2:273, 1943.

———— and Beall, D.   Crush injuries with impairment of renal function, Brit. M. J., 1:427, 1941.

Editorial.   Renal failure in crush injuries, J.A.M.A., 117:1019, 1941.

Editorial.   Confusion concerning shock, J.A.M.A., 124:1060, 1944.

Mayon-White, R., and Solandt, O. M.   A case of limb compression ending fatally in uremia, Brit. M. J., 1:434, 1941.

Moritz, A. R.   The Pathology of Trauma, Philadelphia, Lea & Febiger, 1942.

Patey, D. H., and Robertson, J. D.   Compression treatment of crush injuries of the limbs, Lancet, 1:780, 1941.

Puppe, G.   Atlas und Grundriss der Gerichtlichen Medizin, München, J. F. Lehmann, 1908.

11

Blunt Force Injuries of the Chest and Abdomen

The chest and abdomen together form the trunk or torso of the body. Blunt force injuries of these regions, by damaging the vital organs contained therein, are apt to have serious consequences. In addition, the skin, subcutaneous tissues, bones

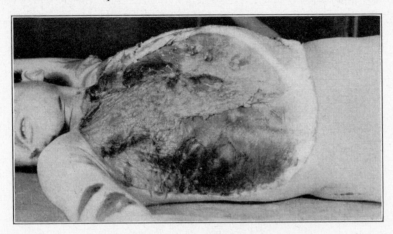

Fig. 11-1. Tearing Injury by Wheel of Motor Truck.

Avulsion of skin and subcutaneous tissues from chest wall. Fracture of spine and multiple visceral injuries. Ten year old boy run over after falling from truck on which he was hitching.

and muscles may be traumatized; the wounds produced are similar to those already described in Chapters 9 and 10 which contain illustrations of patterned injuries, severe avulsions and lacerations. Eviscerations and transections of the trunk produced by blunt force are illustrated in Figures 11-1, 11-2 and 11-3.

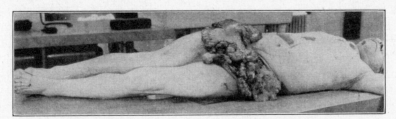

Fig. 11-2. Tearing and Crushing Injuries of Trunk Caused by Blunt Force.

Laceration of abdominal wall with evisceration, crushed chest and pelvis. Middle aged white man run over by motor truck.

CHEST INJURIES

The anatomic peculiarities of the chest must be considered before the injuries of its internal organs can be discussed. The chest is a cage supported by the spine posteriorly and the sternum anteriorly; these are joined by the ribs on each side. The heart and lungs, which it contains, are suspended from above by the great vessels and the trachea. Below, a broad arched sheet of muscle, the diaphragm, separates the chest from the abdomen. Thus its contents are protected and a blunt force, either localized or generalized, must be severe in order to injure the viscera. The ribs and sternum, however, may be fractured by a less severe grade of violence without associated injury.

SKELETAL

Ribs. The ribs are broken easily in certain places, especially on the sides of the chest just under the nipples. The third to the sixth ribs are usually involved; serious complications are rare.

Rib fractures, aside from the spontaneous or pathologic variety which occurs in such diseases as fragilitas ossium and primary or metastatic neoplasms, are of two kinds.

1. *Transverse* fractures are most common and are caused by the direct impact of a strong force or heavy object against the chest. A few or many ribs may be

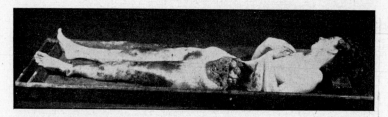

Fig. 11-3. Subway Train Injury. Transection of Body By Wheels. Suicide.

broken and any portion of the bone involved. The force may strike anteriorly and fracture the costal cartilages or the bone between the cartilages and the anterior axillary line. Violence applied to the back of the chest may fracture the ribs anywhere between the posterior axillary line and the spinal articulation. Rarely in such cases do the broken ends of the bones lacerate the parietal and visceral pleura or contuse or lacerate the lung.

2. In *oblique* fractures, caused by a crushing, bending and grinding force such as might occur in a highway accident or in a fall from height, the bones are broken by indirect violence. Generally the side of the chest first struck by the force is most severely injured. The oblique fractures are most often located on the curved lateral portion of the ribs and the fragments are sharp-pointed; the plane of the fracture may be directed either medially or laterally. When many ribs are broken, the fractures may form a vertical or oblique line with considerable abnormal mobility and deformity of the chest wall. With a severe crushing force, many consecutive ribs may be broken in two places several inches apart, the fractures forming a double row; the intervening short fragment of each rib may be pinched off, displaced inward and overlapped by approximation of the main fragments, the chest wall being pleated by this process (Fig. 11-4). Fractures of the upper ribs are not rare and not infrequently the first rib is broken without involvement of the corresponding clavicle. In oblique fractures of the ribs the sharp-pointed fragments usually lacerate the pleura and frequently injure the viscera.

Occasionally the violence is severe enough to force the lower part of the chest forward, tearing the pleura and intercostal muscles of the interspace immediately above the uppermost rib affected by the force. The tear has the shape of an elongated ellipsoid with pointed ends and varies in depth from a superficial involvement of the parietal pleura to a complete splitting of both layers of the intercostal muscles. It is parallel to the ribs and variable in length, sometimes extending from the front part of the chest to the back. The interspaces most often affected range from the third to the ninth. There may be associated fractures of the ribs and lacerations of the lungs.

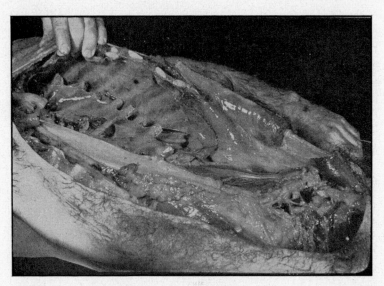

Fig. 11-4. Double Row of Rib Fractures with Inward Displacement of Short Fragments and Approximation of Ends of Long Fragments.

Other skeletal and internal injuries. Suicidal jump from sixth story to sidewalk.

Complications of rib fractures, apart from injuries of the viscera, sometimes cause death. If the force is severe and the fractures are numerous, death may result rapidly from immediate shock. Broken ribs may perforate the parietal pleura and tear the intercostal vessels to produce a fatal hemorrhage into the chest cavity. Although the rapidity of such bleeding depends on the extent of the injury, the process is usually a slow one. If the chest wall is perforated and there is free external communication, air will enter the pleural cavity and cause a pneumothorax which, by preventing the lung from expanding, may result in a fatal asphyxia. The rib fractures may be so extensive as to flatten and deform the chest, inhibiting expansion of the lung and causing atelectasis and secondary pneumonia to develop. The ecchymoses around the broken ends of the ribs may become infected by pyogenic bacteria with the development of osteomyelitis and abscesses in the chest wall, a process which may give rise to a fatal sepsis.

Sternum. Although any part of the sternum may be fractured by direct violence, the most frequent site of injury is the junction between the manubrium and gladiolus. The fractures are usually transverse and the broken fragments are angulated backward. They result from a violent impact against, or compression of, the anterior part of the chest in falls from a height, highway accidents or automobile collisions in which the breast bone strikes the steering wheel or the neck is overflexed and the chin driven against the sternum. This form of violence also fractures the cervical vertebrae. In other cases the sternum is broken transversely about the level of the second to the fourth costal cartilages by indirect violence, a severe impact forcing the lower half of the bone upward and backward and causing the gladiolus to knuckle forward and snap from the distortion. This type of injury,

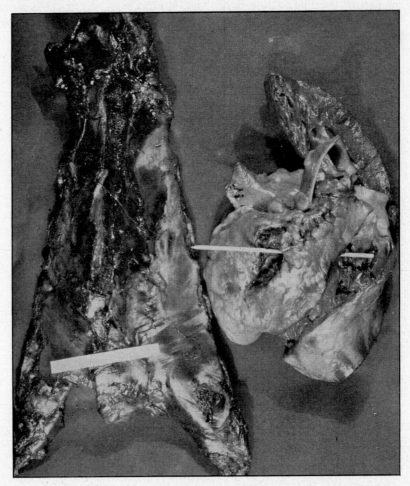

Fig. 11-5. Vertical Fracture of Sternum with Laceration of Right Ventricle Beneath Fracture without Laceration of Pericardium.

Fatal intrapericardial hemorrhage. Adult male accidentally struck by flying object.

which occurs in falls from a height, is often accompanied by symmetric bilateral fractures of the lower ribs and costal cartilages. When the violence is exceptionally severe, it produces multiple fractures of the sternum with overriding of the fragments. The vertical fractures which also occur result from the impact of a hard spinning object striking the sternum in a vertical direction. Fractures of the sternum are often associated with fractures of ribs and costal cartilages and sometimes with injuries of the cervical or thoracic vertebrae. They may or may not be accompanied by lacerations of the pericardium and heart. In some cases the heart is lacerated while the pericardium remains intact, resulting in a rapidly accumulating intrapericardial hemorrhage and cardiac tamponade (Fig. 11-5). In fatal cases, in which the sternum has been fractured, death results from the associated injuries or other causes.

Scapulas. Fractures of the scapula are comparatively rare; they are produced by direct violence in highway accidents and by falls from a height or by a severe localized blunt force. The injuries occur as cracks in the flat part of the bone or as transverse fractures of the acromion process and neck. If death occurs, it is mainly the result of associated injuries.

Clavicles. Fractures of the clavicles are common; they occur as a result of direct or indirect violence. The bone may be fractured almost anywhere along its length by direct violence like that produced by the severe impact of a blow with a heavy weapon; the fracture can be either transverse or comminuted. With indirect violence, such as may result from a fall against the shoulder, the clavicle may fracture obliquely, usually in the middle third of the shaft. In other cases there may be a dislocation of the sternal or acromial articulations. The clavicular injuries are principally important as indications of the type of violence which has been applied to the body and not as a cause of death. When death occurs, it is usually due to associated injuries or to other conditions.

THORACIC VISCERA

The thoracic organs are injured in the following ways: they may be (1) torn from their attachments, (2) contused or crushed, (3) torn, (4) burst open or (5) lacerated by broken ribs.

Wounds of the skin are sometimes absent in persons who have received severe trauma to the chest wall and fatal visceral injury, possibly because the chest is protected by clothing. In adults severe thoracic visceral injuries are usually accompanied by severe fractures of the ribs and sternum. In children and adolescents, in whom the bones are more elastic, fatal internal thoracic injuries may occur in the absence of fractures of the ribs or other bones.

Pericardium. The pericardium is sometimes torn by extreme violence to the chest such as occurs in highway accidents or in falls from a height. Such injury may be produced by the sharp-pointed ends of fractured bones, either ribs or sternum, which cause ragged lacerations of the pericardium either in front or laterally. Compression of either side of the chest produces other tears, fractures the ribs, displaces the heart in the opposite direction, forcing it against the pericardium and tearing that membrane laterally. The tears on the left side of the pericardium are ovoid in shape and vary in length from 4 to 15 cm. and in breadth from 2 to 7 cm. On the right side they are similar but as a rule smaller. Since the pericardial injuries are usually associated with bursting ruptures of the heart itself, death occurs rapidly from bleeding into the pericardial sac and through the tear in that membrane into the corresponding pleural cavity. In some cases both sides of the chest are extensively shattered with the production of ovoid tears on both the right and left sides of the pericardium.

The authors recently encountered two cases of severe pericardial and cardiac injuries in which death, occurring after an interval of several days, was not caused entirely by these injuries.

1. A 53 year old white man fell 75 feet from a scaffold. He was admitted to a hospital in shock, sweating, with rapid pulse and respirations and a blood pressure of 80 mm. Hg systolic and 40 mm. diastolic. There were tenderness and subcutaneous emphysema over the left anterior surface of the chest, an obvious fracture of the upper third of the left femur, a fracture dislocation of the left foot through the first metatarsal-phalangeal joint and a con-

tusion of the right forearm. The victim remained in shock, dying 2 days and 17 hours after the injury.

At autopsy, in addition to the above-mentioned injuries, there were fractures of the ribs on the left side and fractures of the right costal cartilages. On the right side of the pericardium there was a vertical laceration five and a half inches long extending from the upper end of the pericardial sac down to the diaphragm, through which the right auricle and part of the right ventricle projected into the pleural cavity (Fig. 11-6). There were in addition the following

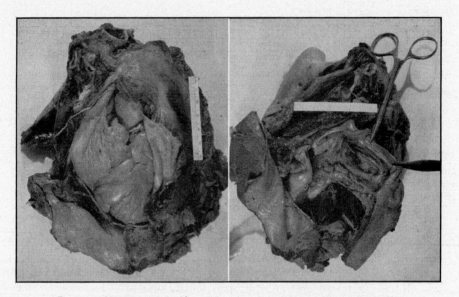

Fig. 11-6. Nonpenetrating Blunt Force Injuries of Pericardium and Heart.

Accidental fall 75 feet off scaffold. Death 65 hours after injury. See text, page 214.

Left. Vertical laceration of pericardium; protrusion of right auricle and ventricle.

Right. Right auricle opened to show contusion and laceration of endocardium and mural thrombus on injured right auricular appendage.

injuries: a superficial tear of the anterior border of the inferior vena cava in the pericardial sac which did not penetrate the wall; a dark red contusion on the inferior and medial wall of the right auricle lateral to the sulcus; a one inch tear involving the endocardium and sub-endocardial tissues and covered with a friable gray red thrombus just above the tricuspid ring on the anterior wall of the right auricle; and a mural thrombus in the right auricular appendage. There were no other pathologic changes in the heart aside from slight sclerosis of the coronary arteries and an excessive amount of subepicardial fat. The pleural cavities contained no blood and were free of adhesions. The lungs revealed considerable traumatic emphysema, the left one a small laceration at the root. Death resulted from shock produced by the injuries.

2. A 66 year old white man while seated behind the steering wheel of his automobile was injured in a collision. He was conscious after the accident but in shock and remained so until he died suddenly nine days post trauma. The autopsy disclosed lacerations of the tongue and face, a contusion of the anterior chest wall, a fracture of the sternum and multiple fractures of the ribs on the right. There was a long vertical laceration of the anterior surface of the peri-cardial sac with herniation of the heart into the left pleural cavity and compression of the left lung (Fig. 11-7). There were contusions of the anterior wall of the right auricle and right ventricle; a bulging aneurysm containing a globular mural thrombus had formed on the anterior wall of the right ventricle at the site of injury, just to the right of the interventricular sulcus. The heart was considerably hypertrophied, weighing 650 gm., and also revealed severe coronary arteriosclerosis as well as lipomatosis of the epicardium. There was chronic passive congestion of the liver. Death resulted from multiple large pulmonary emboli and multiple pulmonary infarctions, the embolism arising from a static thrombosis of the iliac and femoral veins and not from the mural thrombus beneath the contused right ventricle.

The pericardial tear by itself can be the principal cause of death. The authors have seen such a case in which a four year old boy died immediately after being run over by an auto-mobile. The necropsy disclosed fractures of the fourth to the eleventh ribs on the left side and

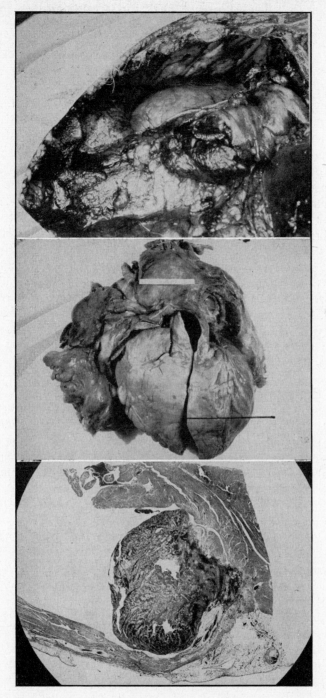

Fig. 11-7. Nonpenetrating Blunt Force Injuries of Pericardium and Heart.

Automobile collision. Victim in driver's seat. White man, 66 years old. Death nine days after trauma. See text, page 214.

Top. Vertical bursting laceration of pericardial sac with herniation of heart into left pleural cavity, photographed through autopsy incision after sternum was removed.

Middle. Contused right auricle and ventricle containing mural thrombus at level indicated by black line. Hypertrophied 650 gm. heart with severe coronary arteriosclerosis.

Bottom. Low power photomicrograph of contused right ventricle showing large post-traumatic mural thrombus. Level of section indicated by black line in middle photograph.

an ovoid tear on the left side of the pericardial sac about 3 cm. in diameter, through which the heart had been forced for a distance about half that between the apex and the auriculoventric-ular furrow. There the organ was snared and constricted as though it had been tied tightly with a piece of string. No other injuries were found, and death was attributed to the interference with heart action and to shock produced by this lesion. Crynes and Hunter have reported similar pericardial injuries.

Heart. Before discussing the various types of cardiac injury caused by non-penetrating blunt force it is worth while to emphasize certain anatomic and topo-graphic features of the heart which help to clarify the mechanism of these injuries. The heart is protected in front by the sternum and ribs. The ventricles are suspended free in the pericardial sac. The anterior surface of the heart is made up chiefly of the right ventricle. The posterior surface of the heart is composed of the fixed pos-terior surface of the auricles. Most of the left and some of the right ventricle rests on the diaphragm. The base of the heart, made up of the auricles, is more or less anchored in the pericardial sac by the pulmonary veins and the superior and inferior vena cava. Superiorly the heart is suspended by the aorta and pulmonary artery and also by the superior vena cava.

The heart and pericardium are injured only when a severe violence is applied to the chest. In the majority of chest injuries the heart escapes trauma. A slight force by itself is unlikely to produce cardiac injury. Traumatic lesions of the heart caused by indirect violence have not been encountered. The idea that the heart can be injured by a so-called contre-coup mechanism is not borne out by observation and can be dismissed from serious consideration. Indirect injury to the heart with rupture and laceration of the chambers resulting from pressure applied to the lower half of the body has not been observed in our experience. The case described by Kellert in 1917, in which extensive lacerations of the heart were found and attributed to burial of the victim in a sandpit up to his waist, is not acceptable proof of this mechanism. Prior to the autopsy the body had been embalmed and the cardiac lacerations above-mentioned are more logically explained by the postmortem action of an embalming trocar than by any other factor. The injuries were too numerous and severe to have been caused by a pressure on the lower half of the body and the question of artefact was not considered.

1. *Tearing of Heart from Attachments.* The heart is separated from its attach-ments by a violence which compresses the chest and forces the organs downward and away from the neck. The traction put on the great vessels causes them to tear transversely. Since the aorta is the main point of suspension and easily reached by severe violence applied to the front part of the chest, it suffers the most damage; its ascending portion may be torn partially or completely. The superior vena cava is not torn as frequently because, located farther back in the chest, it is less exposed than the aorta. Since the pulmonary vessels connect the heart with the lungs and do not undergo the same degree of traction, they are rarely injured. A heart torn almost completely from its attachments is illustrated in Figure 11-8.

An unusual example of extensive tearing of the cardiac attachments was noted in the case of a 55 year old man whose upper chest was run over by an automobile. The upper part of the sternum and ribs were fractured. At autopsy the heart was found free in the abdominal cavity, torn completely across through the aorta, pulmonary artery and both auricles. There were dense fibrous adhesions between the lungs and the chest wall and pericardial sac, and there was a big rent through the pericardial portion of the diaphragm. The compression was unable to drive the heart to the right or left because of the adhesions and so it forced it downward through the diaphragm into the abdomen. In other instances the heart is completely detached and found loose in the chest.

2. *Crushing and Contusion of the Heart.* The heart suffers crushing injuries infrequently inasmuch as the organ is a compact, spindle-shaped mass of constantly moving muscles lying on a soft yielding bed and well protected by the bones of the thoracic cage. Conditions are such that the heart cannot receive this type of injury unless the violence is severe enough to smash in the chest wall and crush the heart directly between the sternum and the spine. At autopsy the ventricles show varying degrees of fragmentation and a large volume of blood drained into the chest from the severed vessels.

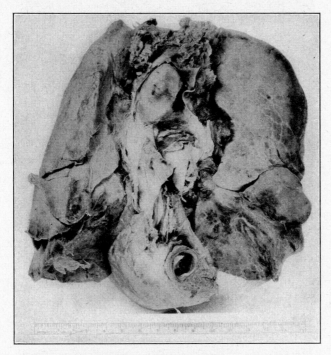

Fig. 11-8. Tearing of Heart from Attachments Caused by Blunt Force.

Complete transverse tears of ascending aorta and other vessels at base of heart with exception of a strip of the superior vena cava. The chest wall was intact except for a few fractured ribs. White boy, 4 years old, run over by a motor truck.

Cardiac contusions occur in the subepicardial fat, in the myocardium and more rarely in the valves. There is injury to the smaller blood vessels and, in the myocardium, to some of the muscles fibers, with localized hemorrhage into the tissue but without any gross loss of tissue continuity. These injuries are produced by a severe grade of violence but less intense than that which causes a crushing injury. Death is most often the result of shock and hemorrhage from other extensive, associated injuries either in the heart or in other organs.

At autopsy the cardiac contusion usually appears as a dark red, hemorrhagic area 1 to 4 cm. in diameter, either in the right or left ventricle. In the right ventricle, the muscle may be contused behind a depressed fracture of the sternum, with or without a tear of the pericardium. The traumatizing force is usually a localized direct violence applied to the sternum. Contusions in the wall of the left ventricle are more rare and, as observed by the authors, occur near the anterior interventricular sulcus, probably the result of a sudden compression of the heart between the sternum and the bodies of the thoracic vertebrae. Microscopically these injuries show extravasations of red blood cells between the muscle fibers and in the loose subepicardial tissues. The authors have not encountered any chronic fibrotic process in the heart which could be interpreted as a sequel of a myocardial contusion.

The rare instances of localized cardiac contusion observed by the authors in the absence of severe injury elsewhere were found in the anterior wall of the right

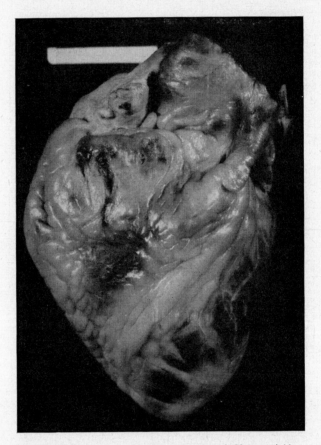

Fig. 11-9. Nonpenetrating Blunt Force Injury of Chest and Heart.

Contusion of anterior wall of right ventricle; delayed rupture and intrapericardial hemorrhage 36 hours after injury. Victim was struck on right side of chest near sternum by flying block of wood hurled by rotary saw.

ventricle a short distance below the auriculoventricular sulcus (Fig. 11-9). They resulted from a severe localized impact against the anterior chest wall usually to the right of the sternum, produced by a flying blunt object such as a block of wood hurled by a rotary saw, or by a driven golf ball. The impact may fracture several of the costal cartilages and without tearing the pericardium contuse or lacerate the right ventricle. Rupture may be immediate or may be delayed seconds, minutes or several hours. Death results from intrapericardial hemorrhage. The wall of the ventricle in this location is composed of subepicardial fat and a thin layer of myocardium, especially between the columnae carneae. This structure is easily contused and may be the seat of either immediate or delayed rupture. The right ventricular contusions and traumatic ruptures are easily recognized and evaluated; spontaneous rupture of the heart does not occur on the right side. It is this right ventricular injury which represents the only valid unequivocal example of a delayed traumatic rupture of the heart after a contusion produced by localized blunt force. The authors recently observed a case of localized contusion of the right ventricle in which a fatal rupture 2 mm. in diameter with intrapericardial hemorrhage was delayed until 36 hours after the injury. Another example of a contusion of the right ventricle complicated by aneurysm formation and mural thrombosis occurred in connection with a pericardial injury and was described on page 214 (Fig. 11-7).

Contusions or other direct traumatic injuries of the heart in human beings are not produced by comparatively mild blunt force applied to the chest. They require a degree of violence sufficient to fracture the bones and cartilages of the chest wall and to cause severe traumatic injuries of the thoracic viscera. These injuries are usually rapidly fatal. Because of the rapidity of death following the trauma, a contusion of the heart muscle inflicted along with other injuries does not have an opportunity to form myocardial scars. Any fibrosis of the heart muscle found at autopsy in the body of an individual reputed to have suffered from an injury to the chest can usually be explained more adequately on the basis of an occlusive coronary arteriosclerosis or an old myocardial inflammation like rheumatic fever than on the basis of an isolated cardiac contusion. In autopsies on a number of pugilists dying of various causes, instances of myocardial fibrosis were not encountered even though these individuals were known to have received severe bodily punishment during their various bouts. This observation does not favor the contention that myocardial contusion is easily produced and likely to form scars in the heart muscle. There is insufficient proof to warrant considering contusion of the heart as anything more than an injury sometimes found in connection with other chest or cardiac trauma. The latter is usually sufficiently severe to be immediately or rapidly fatal. Isolated contusions of the right ventricle are easily recognized and evaluated.

Some investigators in recent years have contended that cardiac contusion may occur as a result of relatively mild nonpenetrating blunt force injury to the chest wall and may produce cardiac disability of one type or another persisting for varying periods of time or even not appearing until some time after the trauma was sustained. Beck has claimed, for example, that many cases of cardiac contusion occur in automobile collisions when the anterior chest wall of the victim comes in violent contact with the steering wheel, even in cases in which the chest wall itself is not injured. According to this investigator the contused area in the heart muscle may be transformed after an interval into a myocardial scar and this lesion may be responsible for subsequent cardiac disability. The authors of this book contend that while it is possible for a cardiac injury to occur as a result of an impact of the chest against the steering wheel, such injury does not occur alone and the associated trauma must be sufficiently severe to cause rapid death. In their autopsy experience they have observed neither an isolated myocardial contusion nor a lesion of traumatic origin large enough to heal with the development of a large myocardial scar.

Bright and Beck base their claims of cardiac contusions on an analysis of 168 cases of which 157 were fatal. Of these, 152 or 96.8 per cent were found to have ruptured hearts, while 5 cases or 3.2 per cent died of myocardial failure. Some in this latter group were subjected to severe trauma and showed various injuries to which death could be attributed. Other cases lived for more than a year after the injury, dying of angina pectoris or cardiac aneurysm. Considering that these cardiac conditions are typical sequelae of occlusive coronary artery disease and are not the results of myocardial injury, it is difficult to see what direct connection there was between the trauma and the fatal lesion in this particular category.

Moritz and Atkins produced cardiac contusions experimentally in dogs by traumatizing the exposed heart and observed the different stages of healing from early extravasation of the blood in the cardiac muscle to the final stage of scare tissue formation. Of the 57 animals used in the experiments, 44 survived the infliction of the injury and remained well until they were sacrificed. None of them was subjected to tests to determine whether or not the heart was functionally impaired.

At the conclusion of their paper Moritz and Atkins stated that the "pathologic characteristics of the scars of myocardial contusion and infarction are frequently identical and the presumptive nature of their origin has to be determined by historic data rather than by postmortem examination." They stated also that the presence or absence of remote coronary occlusion did not serve to identify a myocardial scar as having resulted from infarction or contusion inasmuch as a heart, the seat of occlusive coronary artery disease, could have a superimposed traumatic lesion and a heart with a large healed infarct could have no demonstrable coronary occlusion.

The following case observed by the authors of this book makes clear the danger of interpreting the origin of a myocardial scar by historic data. A 62 year old white man who was injured by an auto truck survived 10 days in the hospital. Necropsy revealed a fracture of the left humerus and a transverse fracture of the sternum between the manubrium and the body. The immediate cause of death was an extensive hypostatic bronchopneumonia. The heart was most interesting, for in the posterior wall of the left ventricle there was a large fibrous scar in the myocardium which obviously had antedated his recent injury by many months. Although the organ was moderately enlarged and the coronary arteries were sclerotic, nowhere could an occlusion be made out. There was no prior history of heart disease. Suppose that this patient had not developed a fatal bronchopneumonia but, having survived the immediate effects of his injuries, had subsequently developed symptoms of coronary insufficiency with death occurring months after the trauma. It is fairly certain that most of the proponents of cardiac contusion as a cause of delayed disability would unhesitatingly relate the myocardial scar and the cardiac disability to the original injury and would probably argue that the fractured sternum was corroborative of a direct trauma to the heart; that the coronary arteriosclerosis, since it was not occlusive, was insufficient to explain the myocardial scar. Moreover, they would also point out that the man had had no serious heart disease before the accident because he had never complained of his heart. In other words, in retrospect they would consider the case a proved example of cardiac contusion going on to fibrosis with resultant cardiac disability and death. They would point convincingly to the history of accident and to the autopsy findings. If this person had survived a year instead of 10 days after the injury, the autopsy findings would have been much more convincing of a healed contusion than any other case described in the literature. Fortunately for the point of this discussion, namely, the danger and fallacy of interpreting a pathologic lesion on historic data, the deceased survived only 10 days, too short a time to permit any confusion as to the interpretation of the cardiac findings.

3. *Traumatic Thrombosis of Coronary Arteries.* Injuries of the coronary arteries due to nonpenetrating blunt force are exceedingly rare and do not occur in an isolated form. In the rare cases in which the coronary arteries have been directly traumatized by nonpenetrating violence there were always significantly substantial and easily demonstrable injuries to the chest wall and contents and to other parts of the heart and great vessels. When such a rare injury does occur, the very proximal segment of the right coronary artery, because of its more anterior position, is involved. In one case the authors encountered a subepicardial laceration of the proximal portion of the right coronary artery along with other severe cardiac and chest injuries resulting in rapid death from hemorrhage and shock. Among many thousands of autopsies, the authors have only once seen a traumatic, nonpenetrating, blunt force injury of the right coronary artery complicated by a very rapidly developing and propagating thrombosis of the lumen. The unusual findings are described in the following case report and illustrated in Figure 11-10.

A 52 year old white man who was driving his car alone collided with a concrete abutment. The car was severely damaged and he was immediately removed in a state of shock to the hospital where he died one hour later. Autopsy disclosed multiple rib fractures, a fracture of the sternum, an incomplete laceration of the left upper pulmonary vein, and several incomplete tears of the intima of the lower thoracic aorta in the vicinity of some atheromatous plaques. There was a small localized contusion in the subepicardial fat over the proximal segment of the right coronary artery. The artery beneath revealed an incomplete tear of the wall and a very fresh thrombus filling the distorted lumen and propagating in a retrograde direction through the ostium of the artery from which it protruded for a distance of several millimeters. At first glance the projecting thrombus appeared to be an embolus but histologic

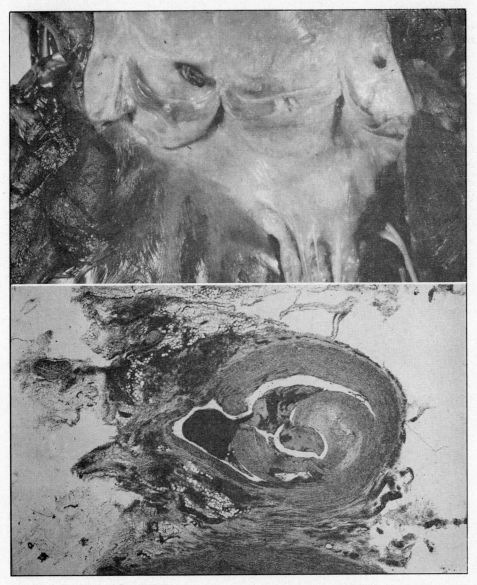

Fig. 11-10. Nonpenetrating Blunt Force Injuries of Chest, Heart and Right Coronary Artery; Very Rare Traumatic Coronary Thrombosis.

Multiple rib fractures, contusion and incomplete laceration of proximal segment of right coronary artery with rapidly developing coronary thrombosis. The victim who was in the driver's seat of an automobile which collided with an abutment was a 52 year old man who lived one hour after injury. See text, page 220.

Top. View of aortic valve and aorta to show segment of rapidly propagated thrombus protruding through mouth of injured right coronary artery.

Bottom. Low power photomicrograph of section torn right coronary artery to show injury of wall and fresh thrombus in lumen.

sections of the injured segment of the right coronary artery indicated that it had developed with amazing rapidity in the lumen of that vessel. The upper photograph in Figure 11-10 reveals the thrombus protruding through the ostium of the right coronary artery; the lower one is a low power magnification of the histologic section of the injured vessel showing the tear in the wall and the fresh thrombus in the lumen.

4. *Tearing of the Heart.* Lacerations of the cardiac muscle, especially of the ventricles, are rare. They are not encountered unless a severe grade of violence is applied to the chest, for instance, when the body is extensively mangled or crushed by being struck or run over by a heavy vehicle. The auricles are most frequently lacerated by blunt force, especially when the violence is not sufficient to separate the heart from its attachments. Although the auricular tears may be complete, they are more apt to be incomplete and to involve the endocardium and subjacent myocardium of one or both auricles. The lacerations vary in length and depth and are usually transverse, parallel to and located just above the tricuspid and mitral valves (Fig. 11-11). The interauricular septum may be torn just below the fossa

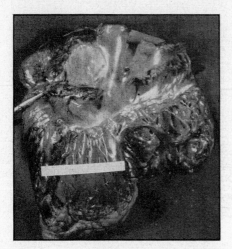

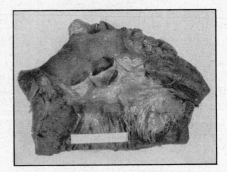

Fig. 11-11. Nonpenetrating Blunt Force Injuries of Chest and Heart.

Incomplete transverse tear of right auricle and interauricular septum below fossa ovalis with mural thrombosis. Fractured ribs. Middle aged woman struck by automobile.

Fig. 11-12. Tear of Posterior Cusp of Aortic Valve. Sinus of Valsalva Visualized by Black Paper.

Other injuries included a fracture of the dorsal spine and laceration of aorta. Struck by automobile.

ovalis. In one case observed by the authors in which the trauma was survived for two days, a bland thrombus developed on the surface of the endocardial tear in the auricle (Fig. 11-6). Rarely a papillary muscle in the left ventricle is torn across; when this occurs it is usually due to a severe distortion of the heart. The valves are sometimes torn but such injuries are rare. An aortic valve cusp may be torn as the result of a sudden increase in pressure on the aortic side produced by a sudden severe compression of the chest (Fig. 11-12). Tears of the auricular endocardium, valves, papillary muscles or cardiac muscle are usually associated with other severe injuries of the heart and thorax and require a severe grade of blunt force for their production. They do not occur as isolated injuries.

5. *Bursting Ruptures of the Heart.* The bursting rupture of the heart is comparatively common and may occur through any part of the surface of the organ.

The auricle or ventricle of either side may be the site of rupture; occasionally both ventricles are ruptured, with or without associated tears or ruptures of the inter-auricular or interventricular septum. The bursting rupture usually is a ragged circular, oval or stellate opening about 1 to 3 cm. in diameter with slight ecchymosis about the edges (Figs. 11-13 and 11-14).

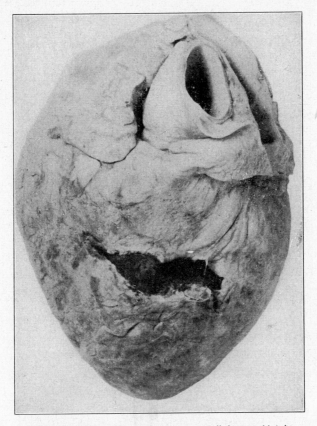

Fig. 11-13. Bursting Rupture of Heart. Fall from a Height.

Traumatic transverse rupture of heart through right ventricle. Death from intrapericardial hemorrhage.

The types of casualty which cause bursting ruptures of the heart are those which result in severe impacts, as when the body falls from a height, or in which there is a severe grinding or crushing of the chest such as might be caused by the wheel of an automobile. The violence distorts the chest, usually fractures the ribs and sternum and compresses the heart to produce a rise in pressure within the cardiac cavity. This causes the heart to rupture or burst where the strain is greatest. If the pericardium remains intact after the trauma, as it sometimes does, especially in falls from a height, it will retain the effused blood. In this case death ensues rapidly from acute asphyxia caused by compression of the heart. In run-over cases the grinding of the chest may tear the pericardium at the same time that the heart is ruptured, with rapidly fatal loss of blood into one or both pleural cavities.

A bursting rupture of the heart may occur as the result of a localized impact against the front of the chest. Such an impact may be produced by a flying blunt object such as a block of wood broken off and thrown by a rapidly revolving circular saw. If such an object strikes the chest at close range over the sternum or the right costal cartilages, it may fracture these structures from the impact of its flight and, without tearing the pericardium, may produce a small bursting rupture of the

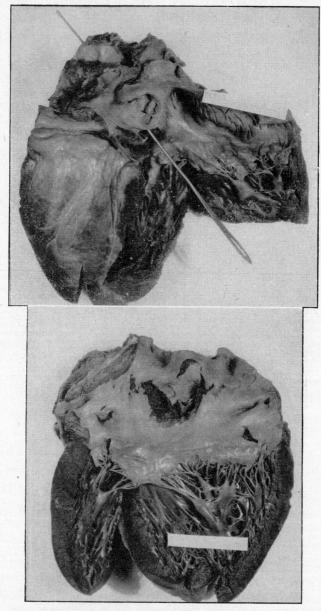

Fig. 11-14. Nonpenetrating Blunt Force Injury of Chest.
Complete interauricular septal tear and other cardiac injuries. Fall from height.

anterior wall of the right ventricle. This lesion usually occurs near the auriculo-ventricular sulcus where the muscle is thin and trabeculated and the wall composed mainly of relatively friable subepicardial fat. Fatal intrapericardial hemorrhage and cardiac tamponade result. In other cases, with the same type of localized impact, a bursting rupture does not occur immediately but the ventricular wall is contused or incompletely lacerated. Subsequent rupture may be delayed for a variable length of time as described previously in connection with cardiac contusion.

6. *Lacerations of the Heart by Fractured Bones.* The heart and pericardium occasionally are lacerated and punctured by sharp fragments of ribs during grinding and crushing injuries of the chest. At autopsy extensive hemorrhage is found in the

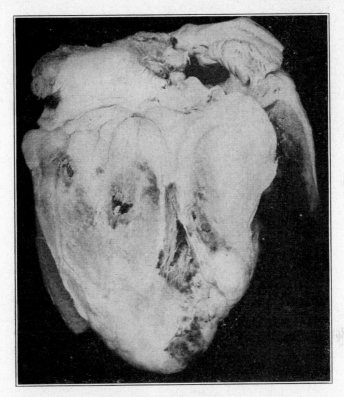

Fig. 11-15. Multiple Lacerated Puncture Wounds of the Heart.

Puncture wounds on the posterior surface of the heart produced by the sharp fragments of fractured ribs. Deceased was a white boy run over by an automobile truck. Death occurred at the scene of the accident from internal hemorrhage.

pleural cavities from these lacerated wounds (Fig. 11-15). This type of injury is described in connection with injuries of the lungs.

The sternum may be bent inward and fractured as the result of severe violence applied to the front of the chest; and it may consequently lacerate the pericardium and the heart, causing a fatal hemorrhage into the chest cavity (Fig. 11-16).

Inferior Vena Cava. The inferior vena cava is torn occasionally by a violence which forces the liver downward. The tear is transverse and partial at the point where the vessel enters the pericardium. Death results from hemorrhage into the pericardium or into the abdominal cavity.

Aorta. The aorta is ruptured traumatically inside the pericardial sac by a bursting force similar to that described in connection with blunt force injuries of the heart. The lesion is usually a transverse rent of the aortic wall located about 1 cm. above the aortic valve cusps and involving only a portion of the vessel's circumference. Death occurs from intrapericardial hemorrhage. Lacerations and

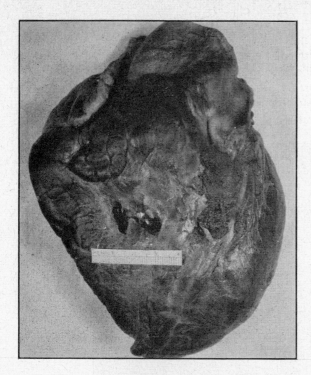

Fig. 11-16. Localized Blunt Force
Injury of Chest.

Fracture of sternum, laceration
of pericardium and right ventricle.
Intrathoracic hemorrhage. Victim
was a 76 year old man struck by
an automobile.

Fig. 11-17. Laceration of
Aorta. Fall from a
Height.

Complete transverse
laceration of descend-
ing aorta just below
isthmus (arrow). Hem-
orrhage into left chest.
White man, 37 years
of age.

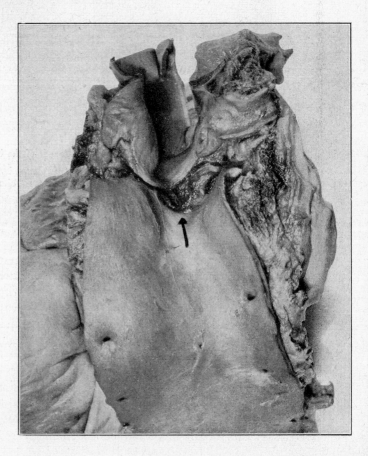

traumatic ruptures may involve other parts of the ascending portion and arch of the aorta and may be associated with fractures of the manubrium sterni and upper ribs. Forceful compression of the structures in the superior mediastinum may result in such aortic injury. A common site for a traumatic laceration of the aorta is in the descending portion just below the origin of the left subclavian artery. This is just below the isthmus where the vessel is relatively fixed and where a strong downward pull on the descending thoracic aorta may cause it to tear completely or partially. Most tears involve all the coats of the aorta and rapid fatal intrathoracic hemorrhage usually results (Fig. 11-17). The lacerations vary in shape; most are transverse but occasionally the tears are T- or Y-shaped. In some instances the aortic adventitia and the reflections of the surrounding pleura remain intact so that the hemorrhage dissects the posterior mediastinum up into the neck and down as far as the diaphragm before the mass finally ruptures and bleeds into the pleural cavity. In some cases the hemorrhage does not enter the pleural cavity.

The authors have seen the case of a young woman who was struck on the left side of the chest and abdomen by a rolling wheel which had become detached from the axle of a fast moving automobile. One week after the accident she suddenly developed signs of dyspnea, swelling of the neck, mediastinal pressure and asphyxia so that a tracheotomy was done. Death occurred two days later. Necropsy revealed a laceration of the descending thoracic aorta which almost completely encircled the vessel. There was hemorrhage in the posterior, superior and anterior mediastinum extending into the neck and causing traumatic asphyxia. Adjacent to the aortic rupture the esophagus was necrotic and suggested impending perforation and aortic esophageal fistula. The hemorrhage from the aorta had not broken through into the pleural cavities. The only other injuries consisted of contusions of the psoas and recti muscles.

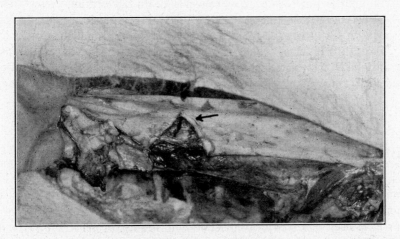

Fig. 11-18. Laceration of Aorta by Blunt Force.

Incomplete transverse laceration of descending aorta (arrow) associated with fracture of dorsal spine. Death from hemorrhage into left chest. Lesion seen through autopsy incision. White man, 56 years, struck by automobile.

Tears of the descending thoracic aorta are frequently associated with fractures and luxations of the thoracic spine caused by severe direct violence applied to the back of the chest. The laceration of the aorta and of the overlying parietal pleura is transverse and is either partial or complete; it usually occurs at the level of the fracture (Fig. 11-18). Occasionally the aorta may be lacerated between two widely separated fractures of the dorsal spine. In most cases of traumatic laceration of the descending thoracic aorta, death results rapidly from profuse intrathoracic hemorrhage.

The root of the innominate artery may be torn by a severe and rapid compression of the upper part of the chest similar to that which sometimes lacerates the arch of the aorta. In a case observed by the authors a man was knocked down and pinned under an auto truck. He survived an hour in the hospital. Necropsy revealed extensive hemorrhage in the base of the neck more abundant on the right side with extension into the superior and anterior mediastinum. The upper right four ribs were fractured and the innominate artery was completely torn across just beyond its origin.

Injuries of the aorta due to blunt force are usually recognized readily at autopsy, but the variable location of these lesions should be kept in mind. Thus traumatic ruptures may occur in the ascending aorta, a location which is also frequently the site for a spontaneous aortic rupture on the basis of medial degeneration. Superficially the traumatic and spontaneous ruptures in this segment of the vessel may resemble each other but with a careful examination it is possible to distinguish one from the other. The gross and microscopic characteristics of the lesion, the presence or absence of other associated injuries or disease, and a careful evaluation of the circumstances should enable the observer to differentiate the traumatic from the nontraumatic ruptures. In the descending aorta, excluding all perforations which arise from aneurysms, the ruptures are apt to be traumatic especially in the absence of underlying disease of the vessel wall.

Blunt force injuries of the heart and great vessels cause death by hemorrhage for the most part, and it is rare that the fatal complication is an infection. Where the cardiac injuries are severe and extensive, death necessarily ensues from the mechanical derangement of the circulatory apparatus, aside from loss of blood or severe shock. In such cases the complication causing death is not significant, for the bodily injuries in themselves are of such magnitude as to make survival impossible.

The histologic changes which take place in the repair of cardiac injuries are best studied in connection with penetrating wounds which, not being immediately fatal, undergo considerable healing. In most blunt force injuries of the heart death is too rapid for reparative changes to occur. In the early stage of a cardiac contusion, there is effusion of red blood cells in the subepicardial layer and in between the adjacent muscle fibers. If the endocardium is torn and the muscle fibers are split, fibrin is deposited on the raw surfaces, some of the muscle fibers undergo necrosis, and polymorphonuclear leukocytes infiltrate the area in the first two days post trauma. In the rare cases which survive longer, mural thrombosis beneath the contusion and aneurysmal dilatation may develop (Fig. 11-7). The later stages of repair have been observed in connection with healing of penetrating wounds of the heart. Granulation tissue develops and bridges the gap in the heart wall and later is transformed into scar tissue. Healing in heart injuries takes place as a result of the activity of the interstitial tissue, and the muscle bundles do not regenerate or proliferate to repair the damage in the heart wall.

Traumatic Intrapericardial Hemorrhage. Hemorrhage into the pericardial sac is a possible complication in all types of cardiac injuries. If the bleeding is rapid and the blood cannot escape from the sac, the heart, compressed by the effusion, will be unable to expand. The supply of blood to the lungs is curtailed and a fatal asphyxia develops rapidly. The compression of the heart by the blood in the distended pericardial sac is a condition known as cardiac tamponade. The findings at autopsy are fairly characteristic. There is usually a marked cyanosis of the head, neck and upper chest. When the body is opened the pericardial sac is distended and appears dark blue because of the effused blood within it. If the bleeding has been rapid, the contained blood is fluid or in the form of a soft homogeneous clot; if it has been slow, the blood appears as a firmer coherent clot of uneven consistency. About 200 to 500 gm. of blood may be present in the pericardial sac. The heart is contracted and firm in consistency.

If the pericardium is torn open so that blood from a cardiac injury can escape into the pleural cavity, tamponade of the heart will not occur, but death usually follows from loss of blood. As a rule this type of death is less rapid than in the case of intrapericardial hemorrhage.

If the amount of hemorrhage in the pericardial sac is insufficient to be immediately lethal, the effused blood will undergo further changes. This outcome is rare with blunt force injuries but is more apt to occur with penetrating wounds of the heart. The effused blood is hemolyzed with a change in color to brownish red; its presence in the pericardial cavity causes a reactive inflammation and brown red fibrin is deposited on the pericardial surface. Death may be caused by the increasing amount of noninfectious exudate which produces a gradual compression of the heart, or the pericardial cavity may be invaded through the wounds by microorganisms of the pathogenic type and a fatal septic infection of the cavity may follow. For further discussion of this subject see Chapters 15 and 16.

Lungs. The lungs lie in each side of the chest adjacent to the ribs and are exposed to severe violence applied to the chest wall. They are elastic spongy organs which normally contain air and have a copious blood supply.

1. *Tearing of Attachments.* The bronchi attach the lungs to the trachea and lower neck, so that when severe traction is exerted on the hilus of the lung, the bronchi are torn across. The pulmonary vessels are not torn as frequently as the bronchi for the vessels are more elastic and attached to the heart, which is not as rigidly anchored as is the trachea. The violence, usually of a crushing and grinding type which forces the lung laterally, occurs most often in highway accidents. The authors have seen one case in which one end of a falling telegraph pole penetrated the chest of the victim and tore the bronchi and pulmonary vessels directly, separating the lung from its attachments. In all these cases, death is the result of severe shock or rapid hemorrhage.

2. *Crushing and Contusion.* Crushing injuries occur when an exceptionally severe crushing or grinding force is applied to the chest wall so that the ribs are extensively fractured and the lung tissue mangled. The injury is not common and is usually associated with severe injuries to other organs. Death occurs from severe shock and hemorrhage.

Contusion of the lung may occur in connection with a laceration or as an isolated injury beneath localized fractures of the ribs when these are bent inward to impinge on the pleural surface. The pulmonary injury appears as a bluish red subpleural hemorrhagic area, roughly circular or ovoid in shape and about the diameter of the area covered by the rib fractures. Microscopically the alveoli are filled with blood. In most cases a small contusion of the lung is not sufficient to cause death; its chief medicolegal importance is that it serves to indicate the direct character of the violence which fractured the overlying ribs. At the present time many hold the opinion that a contusion of lung tissue establishes a local area of lessened resistance which, by opening the way for an invasion by the pneumococcus, produces a lobar pneumonia. Many consider that this pulmonary infection can be a direct result of the trauma. This event doubtless occurs but is quite rare. The authors have seen one case in which a lobar pneumonia developed after fractures of three left ribs and a subpleural laceration of the left lung, the pneumonia forming around the laceration as described on page 162. It is likely, in the absence of severe chest injuries, that many cases of lobar pneumonia hitherto ascribed to pulmonary contusions were nontraumatic and not infrequently preceded by alcoholism.

3. *Tearing of Lung.* Tears of the lung substance occur when a severe grinding force is applied to the chest wall, bending it in to exert compression and traction on the lung tissue. Such injuries occur when an automobile runs over the chest. If the victim is an adult, the ribs will be extensively fractured; in the case of a child or a young person, the bones are bent in and the lungs lacerated but the ribs may be soft and elastic and thus resist fracture. The tears in the lung substance may take any form, depending upon the way in which the force is applied to the chest. If the grinding occurs at right angles to the longitudinal axis of the lung, the posterior portion of the lung may be split longitudinally. This same type of violence may exert its energy on the inner parenchyma of the lung, producing an elongated longitudinal subpleural pocket filled with blood and pulpified parenchyma, which may or may not connect with the pleural cavity by a surface laceration. In other highway accidents the grinding force on the chest may be exerted parallel to the longitudinal axis of the lung and the lung tissue is torn transversely. Sometimes a flap-like tear is produced in the posterior part of the interlobar fissure between the upper and lower lobes. In some instances the lung tissue may be extensively mangled.

Transverse tears of the lung are occasionally associated with tearing of the parietal pleura and intercostal muscles in any of the interspaces from the sixth to the ninth. In these cases the lower ribs are forced forward by severe violence applied to the back of the chest. This inflicts a long elliptic tear on the parietal pleura and muscles of the affected interspace parallel with the ribs and at the same time lacerates the lung transversely.

Death in most cases is due to hemorrhage into the corresponding pleural cavity. In other cases, if a large bronchus is torn, pneumothorax occurs. Sometimes if the patient lives long enough, septic pleuritis or other infection develops.

4. *Bursting Ruptures.* Bursting ruptures of the lungs are encountered occasionally and usually are produced in falls from a height or in sudden compression of the chest by an automobile. The intrabronchial pressure in the lungs is increased, forcing the air outward toward the periphery and causing distention of the aveoli under the pleura. Subpleural air blisters about 1 to 4 cm. in diameter are formed and occasionally one of these ruptures into the chest cavity, producing pneumothorax and death by asphyxia. In some cases the ruptures are inconspicuous and cannot be demonstrated at necropsy. In rare instances there may be a bilateral pneumothorax.

5. *Lacerations by Rib Fractures.* The lungs are occasionally lacerated by rib fractures; these may occur in a number of different ways. In one type the ribs are broken by indirect violence and separate sharp-pointed fragments are forced forward or backward into the lung to produce stellate lacerations on its lateral surface. These lesions are 2 to 5 cm. in diameter, about 1 to 5 cm. in depth, and may be arranged in a row, spaced about equally. The rib fractures may be caused by direct violence. They may be bent in such a way as to lacerate the parietal pleura and the surface of the lung; the lacerations occur as ragged perforations or small flap-like tears of the lung parenchyma. Sometimes the visceral pleura is not torn, but the bone

fragments cause a contusion on the surface in the midst of which is a small ragged spherical or discus-shaped subpleural cavity filled with blood.

The complications of lacerations of the lungs caused by fractured ribs are hemorrhage into the chest, pneumothorax or septic infection.

COMPLICATIONS OF LUNG INJURIES. The hemorrhage into the chest cavity following lacerations of the lung may be fatal, in which case about 1,500 gm. of blood or blood clot can be recovered from the chest. Death in these cases is due to exsanguination and at autopsy the organs show definite signs of blood loss. The lung on the side of the hemorrhage is slightly compressed and is usually lighter in weight than the lung on the opposite side.

If the hemorrhage into the chest is not sufficient to cause rapid death, the blood gradually disintegrates and turns brownish red and brown in color in the course of a few days and a brownish fibrin is deposited on both the visceral and parietal pleura. This deposit may be considerable in amount and together with the turbid brown fluid in the pleural cavity may compress the lung. In some cases death occurs as the result of a secondary bronchopneumonia. The blood in the chest and the lung laceration may serve as a nidus for bacteria and a fatal septic pleuritis may develop, with yellowish purulent fibrin covering the pleural cavity.

A fatal pneumothorax may be produced by a laceration of the lung which communicates with a bronchus of any size. This is likely to occur if the laceration is produced by the sharp end of a fractured rib which penetrates the lung tissue obliquely in such a way that air escapes into the pleural cavity during inspiration and is trapped and prevented by the valve action of the lacerated edges from passing out of the chest through the bronchus during expiration. At autopsy air under pressure is found in the pleural cavity, sometimes unmixed, sometimes mixed, with blood. The diaphragm on the side of the lesion is pressed downward and the heart and mediastinum are displaced toward the opposite side. The lung is small and compressed by the air, and portions of it are completely airless. The interference with respiration causes a possibly fatal asphyxia. The pneumothorax which occurs from bursting ruptures of the lungs has been described on page 230.

A laceration of the lung in which there is a ruptured vein in close proximity to a ruptured bronchus may be the origin of a cerebral air embolism, as described on page 173.

Hemoptysis is another complication which occasionally results when a lacerated lung bleeds profusely in the presence of a torn bronchus. The authors have seen this complication in a man whose left chest was crushed in an automobile accident. The patient died six hours post trauma with symptoms of shock, rapid breathing and the coughing-up of much foamy blood. The autopsy disclosed, among other injuries, fractures of the seventh, eighth and ninth ribs at the posterior axillary line and near the fractures a ragged subpleural laceration of the upper lobe of the left lung 2.5 cm. in diameter. This communicated with a bronchus, evidently the origin of the hemoptysis. A similar case was described by Lester.

If the parietal pleura is torn in the presence of a lung laceration, air is forced into the tissues of the chest wall to produce the crepitant distention of the subcutaneous tissues known as subcutaneous emphysema. This condition is usually of moderate grade and in itself is not necessarily dangerous, though it does indicate that the chest has received a severe injury. In one case, a 30 year old man jumped from a high bridge into the East River, receiving simple fractures of the third, fourth and fifth costal cartilages in the front part of the left chest and a laceration of the inner surface of the left lung extending into the hilus. He died two hours after the trauma from a profuse hemorrhage in the left chest. In addition there was a massive subcutaneous emphysema in the mediastinum, face and neck from the entrance of air into the loose connective tissues by way of the laceration in the hilus. The face, neck and upper chest were ballooned out so that the features were unrecognizable until the air was massaged from the tissues post mortem. Massive subcutaneous emphysema extending from the head to the knees which followed a crushing injury to the chest in which the hilus of the lung was torn is illustrated in Figure 11-19.

The blast injuries of the lungs will be discussed in Chapter 16 in connection with bomb injuries.

Microscopically there is an extravasation of red blood cells in the alveolar spaces adjacent to a laceration of the lung; blood clot is attached to the raw surface of

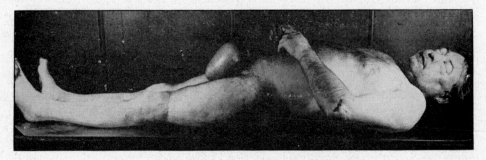

Fig. 11-19. Traumatic Generalized Subcutaneous Emphysema.
Crushing of chest by elevator.

the injury. If the lesion is small the extravasated blood is resorbed and the wound is closed by granulation tissue and fibrosis. If the blood in the parenchyma is too large in amount to be so dealt with, the injured portion may become firm like a hemorrhagic infarct until it is separated from the rest of the lung by the process of repair which stems from the alveolar walls. In the early stage polymorphonuclear leukocytes collect in the alveolar septa and the vessels are congested. Later large mononuclear cells appear in the alveolar walls. The walls become thicker, the air spaces contract and the red blood cells become formless. Organization of the area occurs and a fibrous scar is formed.

Diaphragm. The diaphragm (Fig. 11-20) is ruptured occasionally by severe violence which distorts the lower end of the chest. The left side is injured most often and the right side only rarely, as the liver protects this portion of the muscle to a certain extent. Most of the lesions are due to stretching and twisting of the membrane as a result of the distortion of the chest wall, while others are produced by forcible pressure of the viscera from the side of the abdomen. Ruptures occur occasionally near the posterior and anterior attachments of the diaphragm to the chest wall. More often the area near the central tendon on the left side is involved and the rupture is a big circular opening about 10 to 20 cm. in diameter. It is often associated with hernia of part of the stomach, small intestines, spleen and omentum into the left pleural cavity. Death may occur shortly after the injury from shock and hemorrhage into the left pleural cavity. In other cases the victim survives the injury from one to five days and dies of gastrointestinal obstruction due to con-

striction of the stomach and intestines, or of asphyxia and pneumonia induced by
compression of the left lung by the herniated abdominal viscera. In appraising the
ruptures of the diaphragm it is necessary to distinguish the traumatic rupture from
the rare congenital defect of this muscular membrane which occurs in about the
same location. The traumatic rupture shows a ragged edge with a slight ecchymosis
adjacent to the lesion while the congenital defect has a smooth fibrous edge without
ecchymosis.

Esophagus. Rupture of the esophagus from blunt force is rare and usually the
result of a severe generalized violence acting on the chest. Most cases are associ-

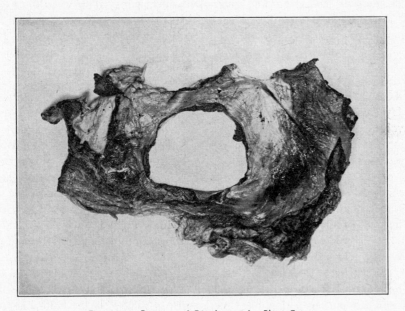

Fig. 11-20. Rupture of Diaphragm by Blunt Force.

Rupture of the left vault of the diaphragm. Death in a few minutes from shock. Adult
white man, struck by automobile.

ated with injuries of other organs and death is due to shock and hemorrhage. The
authors have seen a case in which the upper part of the chest of a workman was
compressed violently by a falling steam shovel which, striking him over the manubrium sterni, fractured the upper three ribs on both sides. The victim died two
days later of a suppurative mediastinitis, referable to two longitudinal slitlike perforations of the esophagus, each about one and a quarter inches in length situated
at the level of the manubrium and opposite each other on the anterior and posterior
esophageal walls. The violence had caused these lesions by compressing the esophagus between the sternum and the vertebral column. Fischer has described a case
of rupture of the lower end of the esophagus produced when the deceased placed a
compressed air hose in his mouth and loosed the air down his throat.

Spontaneous ruptures of the esophagus, while rare, have been described as the
result of severe vomiting. They occur as longitudinal slits which perforate the wall
of the esophagus near the cardia and allow infected material to pass into the
mediastinum, thus producing a fatal septic mediastinitis. Partial longitudinal ruptures
due to vomiting are more rare and may cause death from a profuse gastrointestinal
hemorrhage.

Postmortem digestion of the esophagus and of the cardiac end of the stomach is often associated with a marked increase in intracranial pressure either from a natural disease condition like a spontaneous cerebral hemorrhage or a brain tumor or as a result of an intracranial injury. The digestion may cause a reactionless ovoid or circular perforation or perforations of these viscera with leakage of gastric juice or food contents into the chest cavities where digestion of the pleural surface of the lungs and parietal pleura may occur. These lesions due to postmortem digestion should not be confused with antemortem injury or lesions due to disease. The chief medicolegal significance of the postmortem digestion and perforation of the esophagus or stomach, aside from any suggestion which it may offer as to the existence of an unsuspected intracranial lesion, is that it should not be mistaken for an antemortem process.

ABDOMINAL INJURIES

The abdomen is that part of the body placed just below the diaphragm and supported below by the pelvic skeleton. Its posterior portion is protected by a strongly built layer of bone and muscle so that violence applied to this region is not likely to involve any of the abdominal viscera with the exception of the kidneys. The anterior and lateral walls are a tough but compressible layer of skin and muscle and are often exposed to trauma; most injuries of the abdomen are caused by force acting on these surfaces. In many cases there are no external lesions on the skin, even when severe damage is inflicted on the internal organs, because of the nature of the abdominal wall and the fact that the trunk is usually protected by clothing.

The abdominal viscera are injured by the same types of violence which injure the viscera in the chest, that is, by (1) contusion or crushing, (2) tearing of the parenchyma, (3) rupture by a bursting force due to a rise of pressure inside the organ, (4) tearing of attachments and (5) laceration of the organ by broken bones.

The blunt force injuries of the abdominal organs are divided into (1) injuries of the parenchymatous abdominal viscera and (2) injuries of the hollow abdominal viscera and their attachments.

THE PARENCHYMATOUS VISCERA

The most important organs in this group are the liver, spleen, kidneys and pancreas. Since ordinarily their consistency is firm, they are not easily ruptured by blunt force. They are also protected by bones like the ribs or are located deep in the abdomen so that they are not easily reached except by severe violence. The principal complication which causes death in injuries of the parenchymatous organs is hemorrhage into the abdominal cavity.

The Liver. The liver is a large and firm parenchymatous organ situated in the right hypochondrium just under the lower ribs. The left lobe and a small portion of the right are located in the epigastrium and are not protected by the ribs. Because of its location and consistency, most of the injuries of the liver are associated with a severe grade of violence and are due to crushing and tearing. Lesions produced by tearing of the attachments, rupture by a bursting force and lacerations by broken bones are rare.

Contusing or crushing injuries of the liver occur when it is compressed between the anterior and posterior abdominal walls. Such injuries are produced in collisions like those in which the epigastric region of the victim is caught between the rear end of an auto-truck and a loading platform. The violence forces the liver against the anterior portion of the vertebral column, causing a partial or complete sagittal rupture between the right and left lobes (Fig. 11-21). The same type of rupture has been produced during a homicidal assault in which the epigastrium was trampled upon by the assailant. A strong localized violence applied near the edge of the liver may separate a segment of the parenchyma from the rest of the organ. In other cases it may cause a crateriform laceration at the point of application. The authors have seen a case in which a 3 year old child was violently kicked in the epigastrium by a man who wore a pointed shoe; the autopsy disclosed a stellate laceration of the right lobe of the liver 3 inches in diameter. The impact impinged on the superior

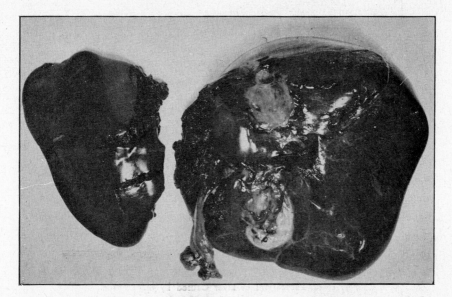

Fig. 11-21. Complete Sagittal Laceration of Liver at Junction of Right and Left Lobes.
Abdomen crushed between rear end of truck and wall.

surface of the lobe and penetrated downward as far as the inferior surface of the liver. Most of the lesions due to crushing or contusion are the result of direct impact from such mechanisms as collisions, falls from a height or severe localized violence which has come in contact with the epigastrium.

Tearing of the liver is produced in most cases by a violent grinding force, like that of an automobile wheel passing over the abdomen. The grinding force may cross the body in a transverse direction or it may pass over the trunk longitudinally or obliquely in an upward or downward direction. Several types of lesions occur. If the grinding force is applied to the right side, the result may be a huge crateriform tear of the right lobe associated with fragmentation of liver parenchyma and accompanied by numerous rib fractures in the lower right chest (Fig. 11-22). A second variety is a deep crack in the liver substance caused by forcible bending of the organ in either the longitudinal or the transverse plane. The crack occurs at right angles to the line of force and on the side of the liver rendered convex by the violence. The force may bend the left lobe of the liver upward, which results in a sagittal rupture of the hilum, occasionally associated with tearing of the left hepatic duct. Forcible bending of the right lobe may produce parallel jagged splits in the parenchyma of the surface rendered convex. In some instances ruptures arranged in a gridiron pattern occur. A third kind of injury, the subcapsular injury, is comparatively rare. In one type the force separates the capsule from the parenchyma, causing a big subcapsular hematoma (Fig. 11-23); in another type the force lacerates the liver in the depths of the parenchyma, causing a hematoma in the interior of the liver substance which does not connect with the surface (Fig. 11-24). In general the liver injuries due to blunt force are often associated with traumatic

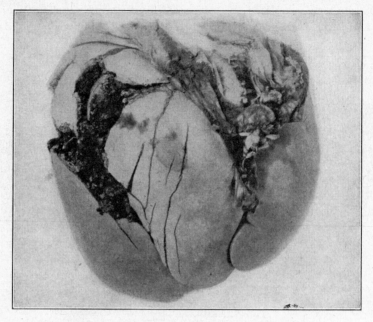

Fig. 11-22. Lacerations of Liver Caused by Blunt Force.

Crateriform laceration of the right lobe of the liver due to a crushing injury. This lesion was associated with a few fractured ribs on the right side and a sagittal tear of the lower lobe of the right lung. Death from internal hemorrhage. White boy, seven years of age, struck by automobile.

lesions of other viscera, most notably ruptures of the right lung and the right kidney.

The complications produced by ruptures of the liver are:

1. Shock. The traumatic injury to the liver sometimes produces a marked degree of immediate shock in which the patient is unconscious or in a state of severe prostration. Death may occur shortly after the trauma as a result of this complication, especially if the victim is alcoholic. In other cases the degree of shock is much less and the victim was able to walk several hundred yards from the place where he was injured, even with a severe injury of the liver.

2. Hemorrhage into the abdominal cavity. This is the most common complication and it may cause death immediately after the injury or within a few hours. Many of these patients exhibit signs of dyspnea, pallor, cold clammy skin and restlessness. Rigidity and pain in the region of the right hypochrondrium are present unless obscured by severe immediate shock. Sometimes the victim complains of pain in his right shoulder. The pain is especially severe in cases showing separation of the capsule from the parenchyma. In some instances the victim may survive the injury several days and death may occur as the result of a peritoneal infection or a secondary hypostatic bronchopneumonia. If many bile ducts are torn during

the laceration of the liver, bile may be extravasated with the blood into the abdominal cavity. After a few days this bile may be absorbed from the peritoneal cavity so that the patient develops a noticeable degree of jaundice. In rare instances a laceration of the liver near its posterior edge, where it is in contact with the posterior abdominal wall, may favor the extravasation of blood into the retroperitoneal area with the formation of a hematoma; such hematomas may become infected and a retroperitoneal abscess may form.

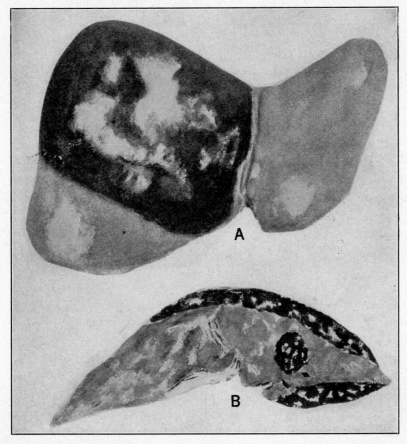

Fig. 11-23. Traumatic Subcapsular Hemorrhage of Liver.

A. Front view of liver showing large hemorrhage shining through and lifting up capsule of right lobe.

B. Cross section showing laceration in substance of liver and thickness of subcapsular hemorrhage on anterior and posterior surfaces of right lobe. Automobile injury.

3. Intra-abdominal infections. If death is delayed, the region of the liver laceration begins to show changes. The blood supply of the liver parenchyma near the lesion is impaired by the trauma and necrotic yellowish white infarcted areas develop (Fig. 11-25). These traumatic infarcts usually remain bland, but sometimes they serve as a nidus for a septic infection, so that an abscess or a septic peritonitis develops with characteristic signs of abdominal rigidity, pain, and toxemia.

Microscopically the lacerations of the liver in the early stages show blood clot and blood-stained fibrin attached to the bed and edges of the traumatized area. In about 24 to 48 hours after the injury some of the liver parenchyma at the edge of the lesion, whose blood supply has been shut off as a result of the injury, becomes anemic and yellowish white from necrosis. Histologically the typical liver structure is lost and a formless necrosis typical of anemic infarcts makes its appearance. Polymorphonuclear leukocytes gather in the periphery of such a lesion and later granulation tissue forms there. Most of the necrotic tissue is removed by phagocytes, and the laceration is finally healed by a scar. The glandular structures destroyed by the trauma are replaced not by other parenchymatous elements but by connective tissue. Lacerations in the kidneys and spleen heal in similar fashion.

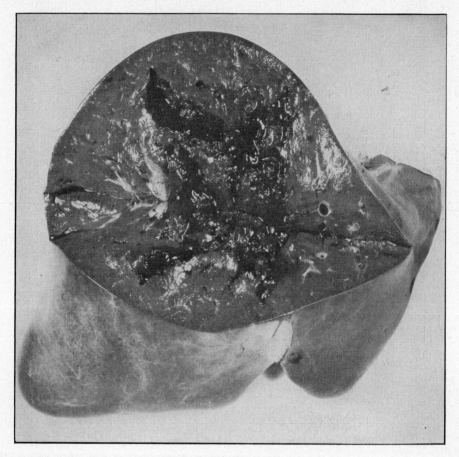

Fig. 11-24. Intraparenchymal Tears of Right Lobe of Liver.

Other associated injuries. Crushed by automobile.

The blood in the abdominal cavity undergoes the same transformation which has been described in connection with the blood in the pericardium or in the pleural cavities. In cases associated with a small hemorrhage in the abdominal cavity the blood is usually absorbed, but black deposits in the mesentery and omentum are sometimes noted at autopsy on such cases months after the injury. These are referable to the deposition of a hemoglobin-derived pigment in these tissues.

4. The extravasation of bile into the abdominal cavity. This occurs when the gallbladder or a large bile duct is torn and bile is extravasated into the peritoneal cavity. Two cases were seen by the authors in which a small sagittal rupture on the

under surface of the liver near the hilum was accompanied by tearing of the left hepatic duct. A large quantity of bile was found in the abdomen. The injury was attributed to a violence which bent the left lobe of the liver upward and to the right, so that the parenchyma on the under surface was torn and the hepatic duct was snapped across as a result of the distortion. One of the cases, not operated upon, showed clinical signs and pathologic lesions characteristic of the continued effusion of bile into the peritoneal cavity at the estimated rate of about 1,500 ml. a day. The victim was a 20 year old man who crashed into an excavation with his automobile and was taken to a hospital suffering from shock and pain in his right

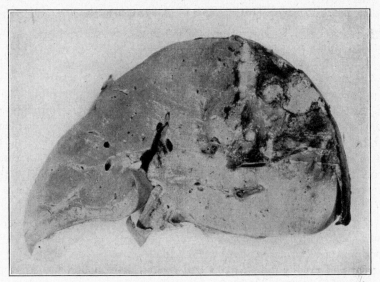

From *Arch. Surg.*, 16:631, 1928

Fig. 11-25. Transverse Section of Liver Showing Traumatic Infarcts Around the Edges of a Crateriform Laceration.

Automobile injury, 27 year old woman who lived two days after accident.

hypochrondrium. On the fourth day after the trauma, the patient became jaundiced and bile pigment was found in the urine. On the eighth day after the trauma the jaundice disappeared and the urine became free of bile, but bile-containing fluid in large quantities began to distend the abdomen. Several liters of this fluid were removed by paracentesis. Death occurred 15 days after the injury. The autopsy disclosed the following: a small sagittal laceration in the hilum of the liver and a complete transverse tear of the left hepatic duct; in the peritoneal cavity, 8 liters of bile-containing fluid which compressed the abdominal viscera; a thick fibrinous bile-stained membrane which lined the entire peritoneum including the diaphragm. The course of events in this case was, first, effusion of bile into the abdominal cavity through the ruptured duct; second, the absorption of bile into the lymphatic system and blood, producing jaundice and choluria; third, the formation of an inflammatory membrane on the peritoneal surface due to the irritant action of the effused bile which prevented further absorption of bile; fourth, the disappearance of the cholemia and the choluria and the continued collection of bile in the abdominal cavity to produce a massive biliary ascites, which finally caused death. In rare instances a retroperitoneal extravasation of bile may occur following a laceration which tears a bile duct in such a way that it communicates with the retroperitoneal tissues near the posterior edge of the liver.

Similar extravasations of bile into the abdomen are caused in rare instances by rupture of the common bile duct or the gallbladder. The common bile duct may be torn by a violence which forces the liver upward toward the diaphragm and tears the duct across near the pancreas. The ruptures of the gallbladder are due to compression of that organ when it is distended with bile and are usually stellate perforations near the fundus. In one instance a traumatic rupture of the gallbladder occurred during an automobile collision and numerous gallstones were spilled into the peritoneal cavity.

Spontaneous rupture of the liver is rare and is not likely to present a problem in diagnosis at autopsy, since it results from a pathologic process such as a malignant neoplasm or a cavernoma. A profuse hemorrhage may occur from such a rupture.

The therapeutic procedure employed in a traumatic injury of the liver will depend upon the condition of the patient at the time of examination. If a severe grade of immediate shock dominates the clinical picture, the surgeon may be reluctant to operate for fear that the performance of the operation may precipitate death. On the other hand if the degree of shock is not dangerous and the signs indicate an intra-abdominal hemorrhage, he may perform a laparotomy in the hope that he can control the hemorrhage by tamponade of the laceration, suture of the wound, or even excision of the injured area. A torn vessel or bile duct of large size is ligated if the circumstances permit. The mortality of operations on traumatic injuries of the liver is high and has been estimated at about 60 to 80 per cent.

Spleen. The spleen is an organ of varying size which is located in the left hypochondrium, well protected by the ribs and cushioned by air-containing viscera. It is vascular and usually quite fragile, and because it is mobile and well protected it frequently escapes injury.

Traumatic splenic ruptures can result from impacts produced by falls or blows over the left hypochondrium, and from the crushing and grinding action of an auto wheel passing over the left upper abdomen in highway accidents. If the violence is severe enough to involve the entire organ, the spleen may be crushed and completely fragmented. If the force is intense but localized over a part of the spleen, a crateriform laceration may occur. A tangential force may exert traction on the splenic pedicle, and separate the whole organ or a part of it from its attachments. Forcible distortion of the spleen from bending, either longitudinally or transversely, can produce tears in the capsule and parenchyma at right angles to the line of force. Transverse ruptures across the hilum are the most common injuries, and transverse ruptures on the convex surface occur next in frequency. Longitudinal tears are not common (Fig. 11-26). The splenic rupture in many cases is apt to assume a letter-like shape, such as that of a Y, H or L.

If the spleen is large and fragile from congestion, a sudden impact in the left hypochondrium may compress the organ and produce a rise of internal pressure resulting in a bursting rupture. Such injuries appear usually as cracks in the capsule and parenchyma. In diseases like typhoid fever and malaria, the spleen is swollen and may be exceptionally fragile so that a bursting rupture may occur either spontaneously or as the result of an insignificant trauma (page 144). In appraising a bursting rupture, the examiner must determine whether or not the spleen is the seat of a disease process which has rendered it abnormally vulnerable to blunt force.

The most common complication of splenic laceration is hemorrhage into the abdominal cavity, often profuse enough to cause rapid death. In such cases the abdomen usually contains a quart or more of fluid blood. If the hemorrhage takes place slowly, the blood may coagulate around the spleen, forming a clot adherent to the capsule. When the injured person survives several days, the blood in the abdomen becomes changed as has already been described in connection with injuries of the lung and liver. Traumatic infarcts develop occasionally around the edge of a lacera-

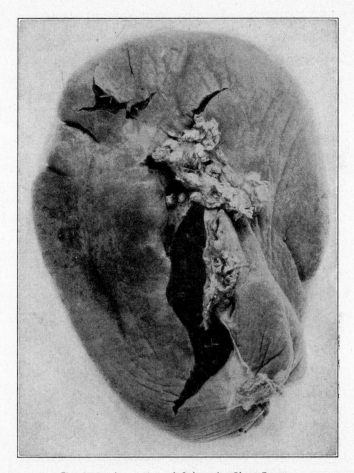

Fig. 11-26. Laceration of Spleen by Blunt Force.
Longitudinal tear of spleen with hemorrhage into the abdominal cavity. Automobile injury.

tion but rarely give rise to a septic infection. Some individuals succumb to a hypostatic pneumonia. Subcapsular injuries of the spleen are infrequent but occur and may result in delayed fatal hemorrhage into the abdominal cavity (Fig. 11-27). Retroperitoneal hemorrhages due to splenic laceration are rare.

Intra-abdominal hemorrhages from splenic lacerations are rarely as rapid as those from liver lacerations, nor as often accompanied by as much immediate shock. In some instances the victim with a rupture of the spleen is able to walk a considerable distance from the place where the injury was inflicted. Clinically patients with a splenic injury complain of pain and tenderness in the left hypochondrium, thirst, pain in the left shoulder, and exhibit pallor, abdominal rigidity, rapid pulse and dyspnea. Occasionally the abdominal hemorrhage is abundant enough to produce signs of shifting dullness in both flanks. When splenic rupture is caused by generalized violence, there may be associated injuries of other organs, especially the left lung and left kidney.

The usual treatment for a laceration of the spleen is laparotomy and removal of the spleen. The mortality with this procedure has been estimated at about 35 per

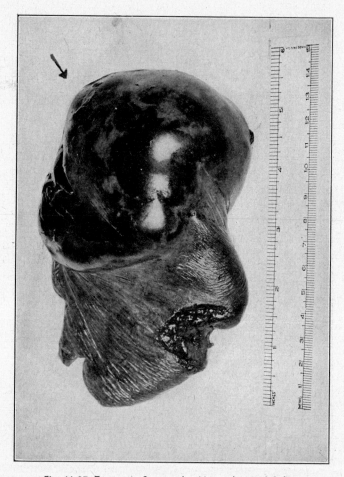

Fig. 11-27. Traumatic Suscapsular Hemorrhage of Spleen.

The capsule covering upper pole and half of the diaphragmatic surface of spleen is lifted up and distended by a large hematoma beneath (arrow). This subsequently ruptured and bled into abdominal cavity. Death 30 hours after injury. On section of organ, a laceration of pulp communicating with subcapsular hemorrhage was found (tear on lower right margin is an artifact). White man, 50 years old, struck by automobile.

cent. The prognosis is better than with operations on the injured liver, provided that other organs are not seriously traumatized. Some splenic injuries of minor grade heal spontaneously. In some instances the surgeon during a laparotomy observed that the splenic laceration was slight and had ceased bleeding, whereupon he left the spleen untouched and closed the abdomen. Full recovery of the patient has followed this conservative treatment.

Kidneys. The kidneys are a pair of parenchymatous organs, cushioned in a variable amount of fat, which lie behind the peritoneum, one in each lumbar fossa immediately in front of the twelfth rib. A moderately severe violence applied to the lumbar region may force the twelfth rib against the posterior surface of the kidney and lacerate the parenchyma transversely. These injuries may involve only the kidney substance and may produce a retroperitoneal hemorrhage. In some instances in which the victim survives a few days, the perirenal hemorrhage extends down the spermatic vessels as far as the groin. Occasionally the laceration also includes the cavity of the kidney pelvis, in which case the perirenal hematoma may consist of a

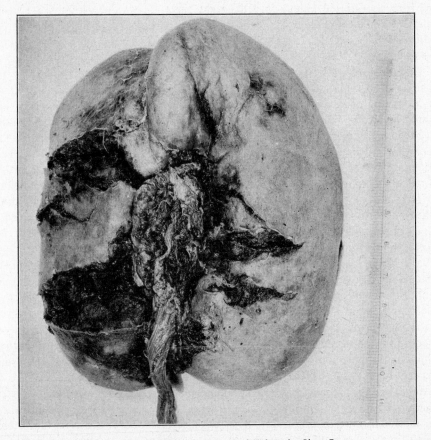

Fig. 11-28. Transverse Lacerations of Kidney by Blunt Force.

Transverse lacerations of kidney. Retroperitoneal hemorrhage. Multiple injuries and fractures, 47 year old white man, struck by automobile.

mixture of blood and urine, while blood may enter the urinary tract and appear in the urine. The type of violence which produces these injuries is an impact in the lumbar region from a blow, or from a fall from a height or from a fast moving automobile in a highway accident. The kidney may be the only structure injured, or in addition the twelfth rib or other bones may be fractured, and other organs may be lacerated.

Severe violence applied to the front of the abdomen, as for example, that resulting from a fall from a height or the grinding action of an auto wheel in a highway accident, may injure the kidney, causing small transverse lacerations which enter the hilum (Fig. 11-28), or more complete tears sometimes with extensive fragmentation of the organ. The most common complication is a perirenal hematoma composed either of pure blood or of a mixture of blood and urine. In some cases, especially in children whose perirenal fatty capsules are poorly developed, the violence lacerates the peritoneal layer and inflicts a longitudinal or stellate tear on the anterior surface of the kidney, causing death by a profuse intra-abdominal hemorrhage. In a rare case observed by the authors, the trauma produced multiple transverse ruptures of the right kidney, a perforation of the diaphragm on that side and a retroperitoneal channel between the two, permitting a fatal hemorrhage to flow from the injured kidney into the right chest. The kidney lesions are usually unilateral and occur either alone or combined with other visceral injuries. Both kidneys are rarely traumatized unless the violence is unusual in nature or exceptionally severe.

Other lesions in the kidney resulting from traumatic injury are rare. The fatty capsule may be separated from the fibrous renal capsule without actual laceration of the kidney parenchyma with the formation of a perirenal hematoma which heals spontaneously. Injuries of the renal blood vessels and ureters are rare. The authors have seen a case which occurred as the result of a highway accident in which there was an intimal injury of the left renal artery with thrombus formation in the vessel and infarction of the kidney parenchyma. For a further description of the rare complications of renal trauma, the reader is referred to the work of Vance (1928).

The symptoms and signs of traumatic injury of the kidney are pain and tenderness over the renal region and blood in the urine if the laceration has involved the kidney pelvis. Such injuries are not often attended by severe shock unless other viscera are also traumatized, and aside from rare cases of intra-abdominal or intra-thoracic hemorrhage, the bleeding from a renal laceration is retroperitoneal and not immediately dangerous. The complication which is especially feared is the development of traumatic infarct around the edges of a severe laceration of the parenchyma which can serve as a nidus for infecting organisms with the formation of an abscess and a fatal sepsis. If the kidney pelvis is lacerated, the retroperitoneal effusion of blood and urine may become infected and give rise to an extensive retroperitoneal cellulitis and phlegmon which may prove fatal. These septic complications usually require a few days to develop. A slight laceration of the kidney parenchyma is not necessarily dangerous and may heal spontaneously. The surgeon is inclined to refrain from immediate operation and to keep the patient under observation if he believes that the renal injury is not severe. The presence of blood in the urine and unmistakeable signs of a badly lacerated kidney may prompt him to remove the damaged organ in order to avoid the development of a possibly fatal septic infection.

Pancreas. The pancreas is a flat, acinose gland of tough consistency which lies across the spine behind the peritoneum. It is injured most often by the violent impact of a hard object striking the epigastrium. The force crushes the pancreas against the spinal column and ruptures it vertically (Fig. 11-29). This lesion may occur along with other visceral injuries in automobile accidents or it may be produced as an isolated injury by severe localized violence such as a kick or the thrust of a stick against the upper abdomen. Death is the result of shock and hemorrhage and usually occurs shortly after the trauma. In rare instances the pancreas may show a localized hemorrhagic contusion at the point of impact with or without laceration. If the patient lives for a few days, an extensive fat necrosis may develop, referable to the leakage of pancreatic secretion into the peritoneal cavity. The cause of death in such cases may be an acute suppurative peritonitis or a hypostatic pneumonia.

Traumatic pancreatic cysts may form in a hematoma in the substance of the gland produced by a force which does not tear the capsule or peritoneal covering. The contused tissue is soon destroyed by digestion and a cyst forms with a fibrous brownish tan colored wall devoid of an epithelial lining. In rare instances the pancreatic secretion enters the cyst and it increases in size, the walls thickening as

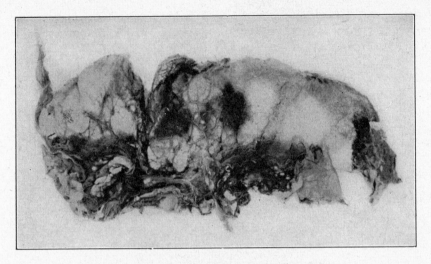

Fig. 11-29. Laceration of Pancreas by Blunt Force.

Vertical laceration of pancreas by impact against vertebral column. Death from hemorrhage and shock. White girl, 10 years of age. Struck by automobile.

a result of reactive inflammation. The fluid in the cyst may contain all three pancreatic ferments. The patient generally succumbs to shock or to septic infection after rupture of the cyst.

Adrenals. The adrenals can be contused, crushed or torn by severe violence, but the injury is usually subordinate to more serious visceral injuries elsewhere. The most common traumatic lesion is a contusion in the form of a small internal hemorrhage 2 to 3 cm. in diameter resulting from the rupture of small blood vessels near the junction between the cortex and medulla. The right adrenal is more frequently injured than the left because it is located in a vulnerable position just posterior to the right lobe of the liver where it can be crushed if the liver is violently moved.

THE HOLLOW ABDOMINAL VISCERA

The hollow abdominal viscera, including the gastrointestinal tract, the urinary bladder and the pregnant uterus, are injured by the same types of blunt force as are the parenchymatous abdominal viscera, but the traumatic lesions which are produced and the complications which ensue are characteristic and dependent on their anatomic structure and exposed position in the abdomen. The stomach, duodenum and contracted urinary bladder are fairly well shielded by the skeleton or by their position in relation to other structures, but the intestines and the distended urinary bladder are protected only by the anterior abdominal wall and are therefore vulnerable to violence applied to the lower abdomen. The structure of the hollow viscera is much more fragile than that of the parenchymatous organs and serious injury may be inflicted on them by a comparatively slight degree of violence. In spite of these facts the traumatic injuries of the solid abdominal organs outnumber the injuries of the hollow organs in a ratio of 10 to 1. The hollow viscera are more mobile and may elude the traumatizing force more easily than the solid viscera which are

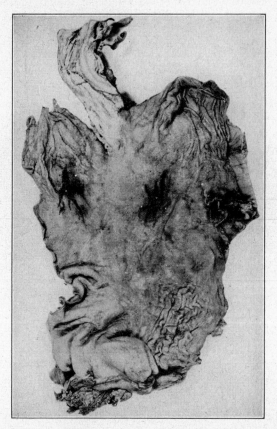

Fig. 11-30. Contusions of Stomach from Kick in Abdomen.

Contusions of anterior and posterior walls of stomach, with symmetric injuries of mucous membrane on opposite surfaces. Stomach is opened along greater curvature. White woman, 70 years of age. Lesions of this type may perforate if the patient lives long enough. Death in this case occurred shortly after the trauma from the shock and internal hemorrhage produced by associated injuries of other viscera.

anchored and less able to escape the effects of violence, a consideration which may explain the difference in the incidence of blunt force injuries of the two different types of abdominal organs.

Stomach. The greater part of the stomach is protected by the left lower ribs but a portion of the pylorus is exposed in the epigastrium. A severe thrust, especially a localized violence in the region of the epigastrium of left hypochondrium, may produce contusion, tearing and bursting rupture of the stomach wall. Laceration by broken bones is rare and tears of the stomach ligaments or omentum are not common and are not lesions of great importance. The types of blunt force which produce traumatic injuries of the stomach are encountered in run-over highway accidents, falls from a height, or the severe localized impacts applied to the epigastrium such as might be caused by kicks or trampling.

Contusion of the stomach is caused when an object with a limited area of impact strikes the epigastrium and violently compresses the stomach between the anterior and posterior abdominal walls. This type of injury may be associated with lacerations of the liver and contusions of the pancreas. In one such case the abdomen of a 70 year old woman was trodden upon during a homicidal assault and death occurred a few minutes later. The autopsy disclosed a sagittal laceration of the liver near the suspensory ligament which was the source of the fatal intra-abdominal hemorrhage. In addition there were two separate stellate lacerations of the same size and type on the mucous membrane of opposite walls of the stomach, contusions of the adjacent muscular coats, but no injury of the serous surface (Fig. 11-30). The stomach injuries played a minor role in causing death, but are important as characteristic examples of gastric contusions and as an indication of the type of violence which was applied against the abdomen. In cases in which the victim lives long enough the stomach may undergo perforation by action of the gastric juice which digests and erodes the contused areas in which the vitality of the tissues has been impaired by the trauma. In such cases death results from a rapid septic peritonitis.

Tearing of the stomach is more common and may be produced by the grinding action of an automobile wheel or any other severe tangential force which exerts a traction from right to left on the pylorus in the longitudinal axis of the stomach. Partial transverse tears of the anterior wall or complete transverse tears of the pylorus may result. Traction in rare instances may be applied from left to right to the cardiac end of the stomach and this may be torn across.

Bursting ruptures are caused by a violent force impinging upon the epigastrium while the stomach is full of contents, in such a way that the viscus is compressed and the internal pressure is increased. The stomach wall ruptures at the most dependent portion of the greater curvature (Fig. 11-31), or near the cardiac end of the greater curvature, producing a circular perforation. The edges of the rupture are ecchymotic and the lesion is to be distinguished from the reactionless postmortem digestion which may cause a perforation of the stomach wall in the cardiac area. The traumatic rupture can be readily differentiated from perforations due to an ulcerative disease process like peptic ulcer or gastric carcinoma.

The complications which cause death in traumatic gastric perforations are either shock or hemorrhage resulting from lesions of other viscera or from severe peritonitis caused by escape of gastric contents and virulent bacteria into the abdominal cavity.

Duodenum. The duodenum is a curved piece of intestine, the lower end of which crosses the vertebral column at the level of the second lumbar vertebra; practically all traumatic lesions due to blunt force are located at this point. A severe localized violence may compress the duodenum against the vertebral column and cause a contusion or perforation of its anterior and posterior walls, just as it does in the case of the stomach (Fig. 11-32). The digestive fluid, in addition, may erode the traumatized area and convert a contusion into a fatal perforation.

Partial and complete transverse tears of the duodenum also occur at this point, and are due to a severe localized violence acting on the abdomen in a tangential fashion so that the dependent portion of the loop is subjected to traction either to the right or left. Bursting ruptures occur whenever the duodenum is compressed by violence applied to the epigastrium while its lumen is distended with fluid; the pressure inside the viscus is increased so that it bursts at its most dependent portion producing a circular perforation 5 to 10 mm. in diameter.

The perforations of the duodenum allow gas-forming bacteria to enter the retroperitoneal tissues, and a gaseous gangrenous cellulitis of the right lumbar fossa results, which causes death by sepsis. Occasionally pancreatic secretion escapes through the rupture and produces multiple areas of fat necrosis.

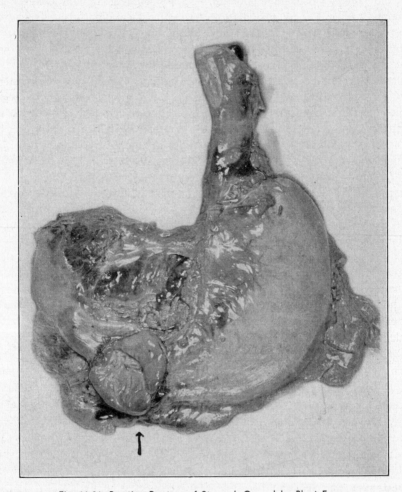

Fig. 11-31. Bursting Rupture of Stomach Caused by Blunt Force.

Bursting rupture of pyloric end of stomach with extravasation of food into abdominal cavity. Death by peritonitis. Adult Negro. Circumstances of injury undetermined.

The clinical indications of duodenal rupture are pain and rigidity in the upper part of the abdomen and other well marked signs of a septic peritoneal inflammation. An exploratory laparotomy is sometimes performed on these cases and the surgeon is not always able to find the injury because of the posterior retroperitoneal location of the duodenum in the abdomen which makes investigation of it difficult at operation. The only treatment for these injuries is early operations and suture of the rupture before the retroperitoneal cellulitis has a chance to develop, for if it is established it is usually fatal.

Intestines. The small intestine lies in the abdomen below the epigastrium and in front of the promontory of the lumbar spine. It is easily affected by violence applied to the abdominal wall in the region of the navel. The large intestine or colon is also located in the anterior part of the abdomen, but is effectively cushioned posteriorly except in such places as where the transverse colon crosses the spinal column or where the cecum and the descending colon are in juxtaposition to the

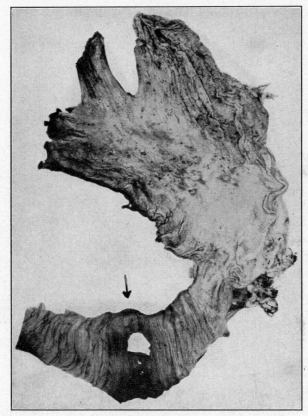

From *Arch. Surg.*, 7:197, 1923

Fig. 11-32. Contusion and Perforation of Duodenum from Pressure on Abdomen by Restraining Strap.

Complete perforation on anterior wall of duodenum and partial perforation on posterior wall. The cause of death was a gangrenous cellulitis of the right lumbar fossa. Insane person who struggled against restraining strap.

iliac bones. The small intestine is more exposed to trauma and consequently its blunt force injuries outnumber those of the large intestine by a ratio of over 11 to 1. The intestinal injuries include contusions, tears, bursting ruptures, lacerations by broken pelvic bones, and contusions and lacerations of the mesentery and mesocolon to which the intestines are attached. The intestines and mesenteries can be injured during diagnostic and surgical procedures.

A contusion of the intestine which may result in a perforation can be produced by a severe localized violence like a kick or by impact of the abdomen against a projecting object, the affected intestinal coil being bruised between the anterior and posterior abdominal walls. This injury may occur at any level in the small intestine, but in the large intestine is most often found in the middle of the transverse colon or in the cecum or descending colon, where the bowel is in close relationship to under-lying bones. An extravasation of blood may occur in the intestinal wall which may be perforated directly by the violence. The perforation is usually single with ragged edges, about 1 to 5 cm. in diameter, and surrounded by severe ecchymosis. It may involve any portion of the circumference of the bowel and even the mesentery. It is not a common lesion. In cases in which the intestinal wall is contused near the duodenum without immediate perforation, the pancreatic secretion from the duo-denum may erode the devitalized injured area into the abdominal cavity.

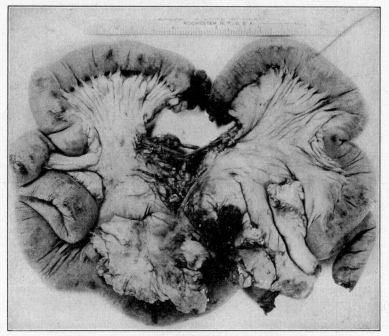

From *Arch. Surg.*, 7:197, 1923

Fig. 11-33. Tears of Mesentery and Small Intestine Caused by Blunt Force.

Complete transverse laceration of jejunum and tear of adjacent mesentery. Automobile accident. Adult white male. Deceased died as a result of associated injuries.

Tears of the intestine may be partial or complete and are caused by a tangential force acting on the abdomen and exerting traction on the intestinal wall. The com-plete tear is usually the result of a grinding action like that produced by the wheel of an automobile, and occurs most often at the upper end of the jejunum where the intestine is anchored by the ligament of Treitz. The intestine is put under tension longitudinally and torn apart somewhat distal to its upper attachment, the tear extending into the adjacent mesentery (Fig. 11-33). The circular muscle in the injured segments of bowel contracts and prevents excessive leakage, but later the muscle relaxes and the intestinal contents escape into the peritonal cavity to cause a suppurative peritonitis. The authors have seen a rare case in which the descending colon was torn across at the level of the lower pole of the left kidney by the wheel of a horse-drawn vehicle which passed over the abdomen; death occurred 42 hours later as a result of scattered peritoneal abscesses among the intestinal coils. A partial tear is the result of a severe force which crushes a portion of the intestinal wall by a tangential action and rips some of it away, leaving an ovoid opening with ragged edges about 3 to 5 cm. in diameter, usually in that portion of the intestinal circumference opposite the mesenteric attachment.

Bursting ruptures of the intestine are encountered most often in the lower ileum but can occur in any part of the bowel. The intestine is usually distended by fluid at

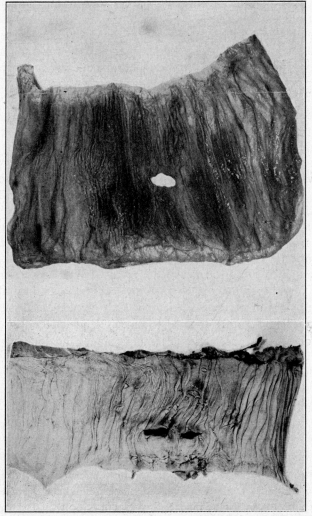

From *Arch. Surg.*, 7:197, 1923

Fig. 11-34. Bursting Ruptures of Ileum. Sudden Impact of Blunt Force Against Lower Abdomen.

Top. Single perforation, type of violence not known.
Bottom. Double perforation, struck on inguinal hernial sac by thrown brick. Death in both cases was due to an acute suppurative peritonitis.

the time of injury. The rupture is produced by an impact against the lower abdomen which increases the pressure within the intestinal lumen and causes the intestinal wall to give way at its weakest point. If the intestines are in a hernial sac, the chances of bursting are increased because the fluid and gas cannot escape from the relatively fixed intestinal loops and also because of the exposed, poorly protected position of the hernial sac. The authors have seen cases in which severe straining at stool was sufficient to rupture a coil of small intestine or a portion of the colon which was included in the contents of an inguinal hernia. When a bursting rupture of the intestine is encountered within a hernial sac, the possibility of its being caused by a slight trauma or by nontraumatic action has to be considered. Intestinal ruptures are small, single or multiple, circular or ovoid perforations about 5 to 10 mm. in diameter (Fig. 11-34), located usually in the wall of the bowel opposite the mesenteric attachment. The edges of intestinal ruptures are ecchymotic, a finding which serves to distinguish the lesions from perforations due to disease or artefact.

Sudden distention and bursting ruptures of the large intestine have resulted from the introduction of compressed air which was allowed to escape from an air jet placed near the anal orifice as a practical joke. Auster and Willard have described similar bursting ruptures of the large intestine, among other lesions, in persons floating in water, resulting from the nearby explosion of depth charges.

The appendix is rarely injured. Contusion can result from a severe localized violence which compresses the viscus against the pelvic brim. The authors have encountered only one example of contusion of the appendix and it was associated with other severe blunt force injuries within the abdomen which were rapidly fatal. An appendix in a retrocecal position is cushioned against injury by the cecum which is anterior to it.

The clinical picture when there are blunt force injuries of the intestine is variable. In some cases, there are signs of immediate shock and hemorrhage usually from associated injuries in other viscera. In others, the violence producing the rupture is not severe enough to cause shock and the victim does not experience immediate ill effects, the initial symptoms and signs often being obscured by alcoholism; but in a few hours signs of peritoneal irritation, such as pain, tenderness, abdominal rigidity and tympanites, make their appearance. If an exploratory laparotomy is performed promptly and the intestinal lesion repaired, the patient may recover; if the operation is delayed, the intestinal contents which escape into the abdominal cavity through the rupture will cause acute suppurative peritonitis which is usually fatal.

Laceration of the intestines by broken bones is rare. In one case the lower end of the sigmoid was torn by the sharp fragment of a separated sacro-iliac joint. Death was the result of a suppurative peritonitis caused by the leakage of fecal material into the abdominal cavity through this tear.

Mesentery. The mesentery is the membrane that suspends the intestines from the posterior abdominal wall. It is invested in peritoneum and contains a variable amount of fat and areolar tissue and the blood and lymph vessels which supply the bowel. Its thickness and length vary with the habitus and state of nutrition of the individual. The omentum is an apron-like appendage of the peritoneum which hangs down from the greater curvature of the stomach, anterior to the transverse colon, to which it is attached, and to the intestines. It contains blood vessels and a variable amount of fat. The structures most often affected by injury are the mesentery of the small intestine and the mesosigmoid; the other mesenteric subdivisions and the omentum are rarely involved. The injuries are classified as (1) tears, and (2) contusions (Fig. 11-35)

1. The mesentery may be torn by a grinding force like that generated by an automobile wheel, or by a severe localized violence which strikes the abdominal

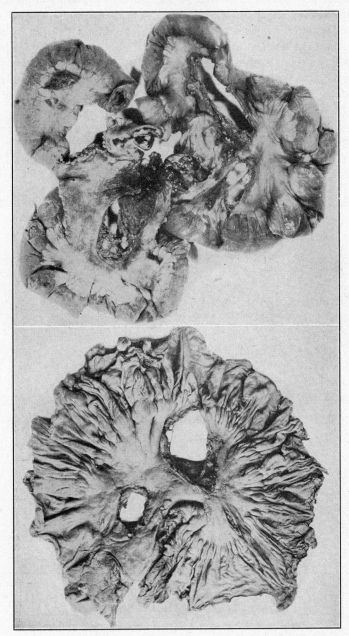

From *Arch. Surg.*, 16:631, 1928

Fig. 11-35. Injuries of Mesentery Caused by Blunt Force.

Top. Multiple tears of mesentery and small intestine. Automobile accident, 33 year old white man.

Bottom. Contusion perforation of mesentery caused by kick in the abdomen. Death in a few minutes from hemorrhage into the abdominal cavity. Homicidal assault on 50 year old white woman.

wall as a tangent. Traction is exerted on the mesentery causing circular and ovoid rents of varying size, either single or multiple.

2. The mesentery, especially one which contains much fat, may be contused and perforated by a severe local force which imprisons and crushes it between the anterior and posterior walls of the abdomen, the size of the ragged stellate or circular perforation corresponding roughly to that of the impacting surface. If several folds of the mesentery are involved, the one nearest the violence shows the

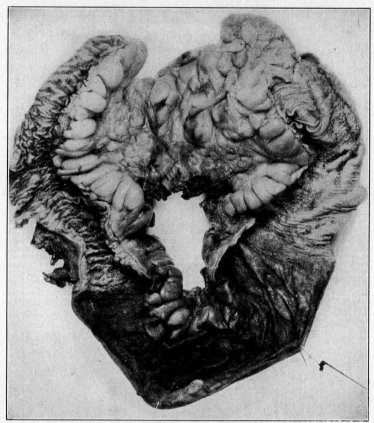

From *Arch. Surg.*, 16:631, 1928

Fig. 11-36. Perforation of Mesentery. Gangrene of Intestine.

Perforation of mesentery of small intestine with gangrene of adjacent portion of intestine. Deceased, a 36 year old white man, fell into excavation, dying of toxic ileus four days after injury.

most severe effect, the severity of the injury diminishing successively in the fold beneath. The perforations may take the form of ragged excavations near the root of the mesentery. Some of these injuries are caused by trampling or kicking the abdomen and are homicidal. In one such case the relaxed abdomen of the victim was probably repeatedly trampled on, with the production of two large ragged tears about 12 and 18 inches in diameter in the iliac portion of the mesentery.

The most common complication of a mesenteric tear or perforation is severe and often fatal intra-abdominal hemorrhage from torn mesenteric vessels. In some instances the mesenteric lesion is located close to the intestine where there are end arteries and the victim survives the immediate effects of the injury only to develop a local gangrene of the segment of intestine adjacent to the lacerated mesentery as the result of the interruption of its blood supply. Death may occur from septic peritonitis or from toxic and obstructive ileus as illustrated in Figure 11-36. Other rarer complications of mesenteric injury are mentioned by Vance (1928).

The clinical signs of a lacerated mesentery are those of severe intra-abdominal hemorrhage and shock. If the patient survives a few days there may be abdominal distention, pain and rigidity due to toxic and obstructive ileus or peritonitis. The treatment for mesenteric laceration is prompt exploratory laparotomy and ligation of torn blood vessels. It may be necessary to resect a portion of the intestine, especially if the adjacent mesentery is lacerated, in order to forestall the development of gangrene in the segment of bowel deprived of its blood supply by the mesenteric injury.

The intestines and mesentery may be lacerated in cases of criminal abortion and occasionally during a therapeutic abortion by instruments which have perforated the uterus. Martland has described patterned hemorrhagic extravasations in the intestinal wall produced by manipulation of the intestines with sponge-holding forceps and Babcock tissue forceps. In one case the intestinal injury produced by the sponge-holding forceps resulted in a fatal intestinal hemorrhage. The sigmoid colon has been perforated during sigmoidoscopic examination with the development of fatal peritonitis.

URINARY BLADDER. The bladder is a distensible muscular sac which lies in the pelvis. It receives the urine from the kidneys through the ureters, and after collecting a sufficient amount discharges it through the urethra voluntarily. The bladder when empty lies in the pelvis and is protected by the surrounding bone. As it fills with urine the bladder rises above the pelvic brim and impinges against the promontory of the sacrum.

Two types of rupture of the bladder are produced by blunt force (1) the extra-peritoneal, and (2) the intraperitoneal (Fig. 11-37).

1. Extraperitoneal ruptures. The extraperitoneal ruptures of the bladder are caused by fractures of the pelvis, especially of the pubic rami and the sacro-iliac joints. The bone fragments project inward, lacerating the bladder wall and occasionally tearing the membranous urethra across below the prostate (Fig. 11-38). As a result urine is extravasated in tissues around the bladder, and may infiltrate the subcutaneous tissues of the scrotum, abdomen or thighs. Death may occur from shock because of the pelvic fractures, or from sepsis referable to the gangrenous phlegmon and abscesses which develop in the areas where the urine is extravasated.

Occasionally an extraperitoneal rupture occurs in the absence of a pelvic fracture; the violence may act on a partly filled bladder from above, forcing it toward the pelvic floor, increasing the internal pressure and causing a rupture near the trigonum which communicates with the perivesical connective tissues.

2. Intraperitoneal ruptures. The intraperitoneal rupture is not necessarily associated with fractures of the pelvis. The bladder is easily injured when it is distended by urine and rises above the brim of the pelvis until it rests against the promontory of the sacrum. In this state, especially in a relaxed alcoholic person, a slight force against the lower abdomen may cause the bladder to rupture, because of the sudden increase in intravesical pressure. The rupture is a bursting one and is located at the fundus, appearing as an ovoid opening with slightly ecchymotic edges. Urine usually escapes into the peritoneal cavity and may give rise to a fatal

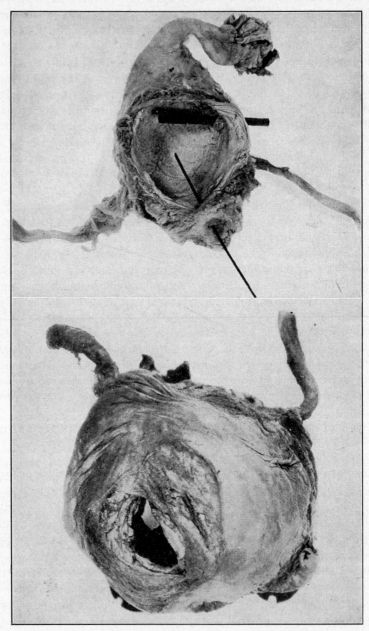

From *Arch. Surg.*, 16:631, 1928

Fig. 11-37. Ruptures of Bladder Caused by Blunt Force.

Top. Extraperitoneal ruptures of bladder caused by extensive fractures of the pelvis. There is a huge tear of anterior bladder wall, a transverse tear of membranous urethra and a small tear of left posterior bladder wall. Thick sound is in posterior rupture, and thin sound in urethra. White boy, six years old, struck by automobile, died in a few minutes of shock.

Bottom. Intraperitoneal rupture of fundus of urinary bladder. Symphysis pubis separated, seven year old white girl. Struck by automobile. Died in a few hours of shock.

peritonitis or toxemia from absorption of toxic products into the circulation. A distended bladder may also rupture spontaneously or after slight trauma especially in cases of urinary obstruction from stricture, enlarged prostrate and neoplasm.

The symptoms and signs of an intraperitoneal rupture of the bladder may be indefinite immediately after the trauma, and the victim may not realize that he has

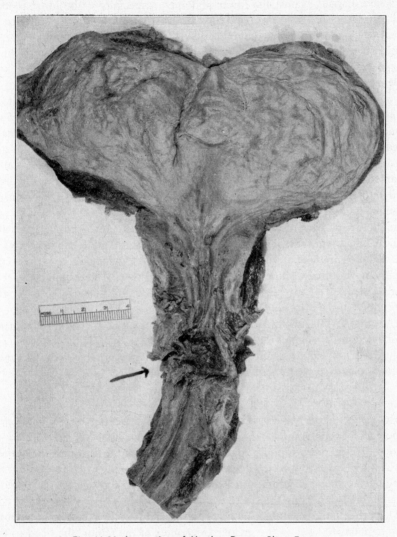

Fig. 11-38. Laceration of Urethra Due to Blunt Force.

Transverse laceration of membranous urethra associated with fractures of the pubic bones. White man struck by automobile.

been dangerously injured, especially if he is intoxicated at the time. Within a few hours peritonitis sets in and the patient if conscious complains of pain and tenderness in the lower abdomen, rigidity, tympanites and vomiting. The treatment is prompt exploratory laparotomy and repair of the rupture. With early operation there is a good chance of recovery, but if this procedure is delayed or not carried out, death will occur from peritonitis.

Ruptures of the gastrointestinal tract and urinary bladder will heal only if the edges of the wound are approximated by suture. The healing takes place by the usual stages of fibrinous exudation, leukocytic infiltration, granulation tissue formation and scar tissue replacement. The muscles which are ruptured heal by fibrous tissue growth without any proliferation of the muscle fibers.

Abdominal Aorta. The abdominal aorta and iliac vessels are injured sometimes by a severe impact against the lower abdomen, especially if the force is localized. The arterial tears are transverse and involve usually a portion of the anterior surface of the vessel. The principal complication is retroperitoneal hemorrhage. In one instance such a rupture of the abdominal aorta was caused by plaster falling upon the exposed abdominal wall of a person lying in bed in the supine position.

Uterus. Blunt force injuries of the pregnant uterus are rare. In one case a 39 year old white woman, five months pregnant, was run over by an automobile, sustaining fractures of both pubic rami on the left side, a partial separation of the left sacro-iliac joint, a fracture of the left humerus and small lacerations of the mesentery. The violence had exerted pressure on the lower portion of the pregnant uterus, rupturing the fundus and amniotic sac by an opening three and a half inches in diameter through which the fetus still attached to the placental site had been forced into the abdominal cavity. Death occurred as a result of a profuse intra-abdominal hemorrhage.

In another case a pregnant woman committed suicide by jumping from a height. She was killed outright. There were multiple injuries including fractures of the pelvis and the ribs. The uterus was enlarged with a pregnancy but appeared collapsed though not ruptured. There was a traumatic rupture of the amniotic sac and a partial separation of the placenta. A fetus of three and one half months gestation was found in the uterine cavity.

The uterine injuries and their complications caused by induced abortion will be discussed in the chapter devoted to that subject.

Injuries of the nonpregnant uterus due to blunt force are extremely rare unless the violence is exceptionally severe.

PELVIS

The pelvic girdle which surrounds the bladder, rectum and genital organs is composed of two innominate bones which are joined together in front by a cartilaginous disk at the symphysis pubis, and in back by articulation with the sacral bone at the sacro-iliac joints. The pelvis is a bowl-shaped structure of great strength absorbing the shock of the upward thrusts of the thigh bones on each side and at the same time supporting the entire trunk above the hips.

The pelvis may be broken by a severe impact as in a fall from a height. If the victim happens to land on the greater trochanter of the femur, the head of the bone is forced violently into the socket of the hip joint, splitting the pelvis transversely through the acetabulum, or producing a Y-shaped fracture in that fossa; these fractures gape widely and the head of the femur can usually be palpated through the fracture from the inside of the pelvis. If the impact acts on the pubis external to the obturator foramen, oblique fractures of the pubic rami may occur adjacent to the foramen. A severe frontal impact over the symphysis pubis may cause transverse fractures across the pubic rami. The sacrum is occasionally broken transversely by the application of direct violence.

A severe crushing or grinding force, such as might be produced by the wheels of an automobile may cause extensive luxations of the sacro-iliac joints, a wide separation at the symphysis pubis, fractures of the pubic rami and of the sacrum. In some cases there is extensive tearing of the perineum, scrotum, urethra, vagina and anus. Death usually results from immediate shock, but if the victim lives for a few hours, the hemorrhage which follows such injuries may be a factor in producing delayed shock. In a few instances the victim survives the immediate effects of the trauma, and later develops a suppurative or gaseous gangrenous inflammation in the region of the lacerations (page 255). In some cases bladder injuries produced by the fractures are responsible for the fatal complications.

Other pelvic fractures are occasionally encountered but are less important, as for example, horizontal fractures of the iliac crest, fractures of the rim of the acetabulum, or fractures of the os coccyx.

The following case, seen by the authors, is rather remarkable as an example of pelvic fractures resulting from muscular action. A 66 year old, heavily built, well nourished white man received electric shock treatment for a mental disorder. The shocks produced severe clonic convulsions. During this treatment the patient's bones were heard to crack. Death occurred several days later with signs of traumatic shock and roentgenographic evidence of pelvic fractures. The autopsy disclosed extensive fractures of the pelvis, involving both acetabula and the pubic rami. The apparent mechanism of the injury was the strong, rapidly intermittent contractions of the muscles of the hip regions which hammered the heads of the femurs against and through the acetabula, the pelvis cracking on both sides under this violence. The bones of the deceased exhibited an appreciable amount of senile osteoporosis and were probably more fragile than normal.

MEDICOLEGAL CONSIDERATIONS

The forensic importance of chest injuries due to blunt force have been discussed thoroughly in the text and will not be repeated in detail. It has been shown how extensive visceral injuries can be present without any external evidence of trauma to the skin and sometimes without fractures of the ribs. The ability of a person to move himself from the place where he was injured depends upon the severity of the thoracic injury and how much shock and hemorrhage are present. Fractures of the ribs and lacerations of the lungs if not too extensive may not interfere with a person's power of locomotion, but a serious visceral injury usually causes so much prostration that movement is impossible. Only a limited percentage of nonpenetrating injuries of the chest is brought under the clinical observation of the surgeon, and few of these cases are ever treated on the operating table. It is important that the medical attendant keep a careful clinical record of the case for reasons which have already been discussed.

The abdominal injuries deserve more detailed consideration as many of these lesions are not immediately fatal and present difficult clinical problems for the surgeon to solve. The characteristics of this type of trauma have already been discussed to the effect that visible lesions on the skin of the abdomen and elsewhere on the body may be absent, even though the abdominal viscera have been fatally traumatized. The diagnosis may be rendered more difficult by the shock displayed by the victim or by his alcoholic condition which may obscure the signs of peritoneal irritation, or by the ill-advised administration of morphine which in creating insensibility to pain may mislead the diagnostician. For these reasons the clinician occasionally fails to recognize the serious nature of the trauma, especially in the early stages, and a necessary operation is delayed. The operations for the injuries of the different abdominal viscera have already been discussed and the disastrous consequences which may follow when the performance of the operation is delayed too long have been indicated under the separate organs. Mention has also been made of the ability of the victim in some cases to walk surprising distances after receiving a severe laceration or rupture of an abdominal organ as a result of trauma.

When a laparotomy is performed, the surgeon should keep a careful record of the injuries which he observes at operation for many of these are due to criminal violence and are forensically important. The sagittal lacerations of the liver (Fig. 11-22), the perforations of the mesentery (Fig. 11-33), and injuries of the intestine, stomach and bladder are not infrequently due to blows and kicks against the anterior abdominal wall. Any case of suspicious nature should be reported to the police.

REFERENCES

Auster, L. S., and Williard, J. H.   Hydraulic abdominal concussion, J.A.M.A., 121:995, 1943.

Bacon, L. H., and LeCount, E. R.   Automobile injuries, Arch. Surg., 18:769, 1929.

Beck, C. S.   Contusions of the heart, J.A.M.A., 104:109, 1935.

Bright, E. F., and Beck, C. S.   Nonpenetrating wounds of the heart, Am. Heart J., 10:293, 1935.

Crynes, S. F., and Hunter, W. C.   Traumatic rupture of the pericardium, Arch. Int. Med., 64:719, 1939.

Editorial.   Blast injuries, J.A.M.A., 118:898, 1942.

Fischer, W.   Speiseröhre, Henke und Lubarsch, Berlin, Julius Springer, 1926, Vol. 4, part 1, page 94.

Kellert, E.   Traumatic rupture of the heart, J. Lab. & Clin. Med., 2:726, 1917.

Lester, C. W.   Compression injuries of the chest in childhood, Am. J. Surg., 66:275, 1944.

Martland, H. S.   Instrumental intestinal trauma during laparotomy, Am. J. Surg., 60:424, 1943.

Moritz, A. R.   The pathology of Trauma, Philadelphia, Lea & Febiger, 1942.

———— and Atkins, J. P.   Cardiac contusion, Arch. Path., 25:445, 1938.

Strassmann, G. S.   Relation of acute mucosal hemorrhages and ulcers of gastro-intestinal tract to intracranial lesions, Arch. Neurol. & Psychiat., 57:145, 1947.

———— Traumatic rupture of the aorta, Am. Heart J., 33:508, 1947.

Vance, B. M.   Subcutaneous injuries of the abdominal viscera, Arch. Surg., 16:631, 1928.

———— Traumatic Lesions of Intestines caused by Nonpenetrating Blunt Force, Arch. Surg., 7:197, 1923.

Warburg, E.   Subacute and Chronic Pericarditis and Myocardial Lesions due to Nonpenetrating Traumatic Injury, Copenhagen, 1938.

12

Blunt Force Injuries of the Head

Injuries of the head are the cause of death in about one fifth of the cases which are referred to the Office of the Chief Medical Examiner in New York City. They can be divided into: (1) injuries of the scalp and face; (2) fractures of the skull with intracranial injuries; (3) intracranial injuries without fracture of the skull; (4) fractures of the bones of the face.

INJURIES OF THE SCALP AND FACE

From Direct Violence. The skin of the head is comparatively delicate and covers an underlying hard base of bone. As a consequence, contusions, abrasions and lacerations (Fig. 12-1) are readily produced anywhere on the scalp and face, and often serve as valuable indications of fractures involving the bones of the cranium or face. In some cases the head does not show any sign of external injury even though the skull is fractured and the brain lacerated. This is apt to occur if the impact against the scalp is partly cushioned by a thick growth of hair or by a hat. Superficial contusions are most prominent on the lips, eyelids or ears and occur as by-products of an altercation, a highway accident or similar trauma. Hematomas can be produced in the deeper layers of the scalp and in the temporal muscles by application of a force that does not fracture the skull or lacerate the scalp, as for example, a blow with a blackjack. Abrasions of the head are not usually characteristic but may be patterned when produced by a distinctive part of an automobile or by a blunt instrument (Figs. 9-4 and 9-1). Lacerations of the head may be inflicted in any of the ways described on page 197 but the most important are those produced by blunt instruments (Figs. 9-7 and 9-8), or the grinding action of an automobile wheel. When the wheel passes over the side of the head, it may tear the scalp and ears, produce abrasions of the face and temporal regions, and cause compression fractures of the skull.

Skin injuries may be associated with severe fatal lesions inside the cranium. In such cases, the principal medicolegal significance of the external laceration or abrasion is to indicate the point where the violence was applied to the head and in the event that the wound is patterned, to suggest the type of weapon used to inflict it. Occasionally a laceration of the scalp or face gives rise to a suppurative inflammation such as erysipelas or purulent cellulitis and causes death by sepsis. The inflammatory exudate may appear as a turbid edematous infiltration of the subcutaneous fat or as a frankly purulent yellowish green exudate which causes a marked swelling and puffiness of the scalp and face. The danger of scalp lacerations which expose a fracture of the skull will be discussed later.

Injuries Secondary to Skull Fractures. An extensive hematoma in the deeper tissues of the scalp is produced by some fractures of the skull, the broken edges of the bone lacerating the pericranium and causing a massive effusion of blood to accumulate in the galea. The scalp presents a boggy swelling in the region of the hemorrhage which may be detected by palpation. The temporal muscle may

261

be involved. Hematomas with ecchymotic discoloration are produced in the eyelids (Fig. 9-1) in the same way by fractures of the orbital plates and also in the mastoid region by fractures which involve this portion of the temporal bone. The boggy palpable postauricular scalp hematoma is known as Battle's sign and is sometimes overlooked because the ecchymosis which it usually produces in the overlying skin may be either delayed in its appearance or entirely absent.

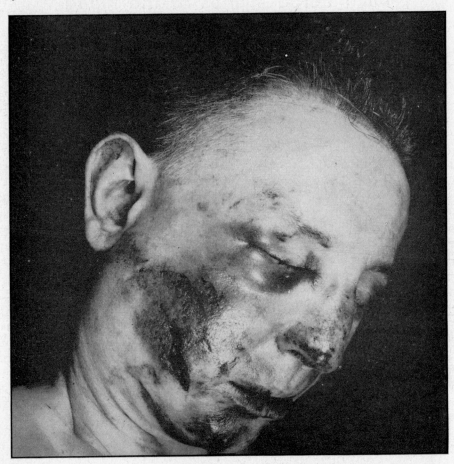

Fig. 12-1. Contusions, Abrasions and Lacerations of Face.
Homicidal assault by punching and kicking.

Bleeding from the external ear canal is caused by fractures of the middle fossa which lacerate the lining membrane of the canal or rupture the ear drum. Hemorrhages from the nose and into the throat result from fractures which involve the sphenoidal sinus or the cribriform plate, and some of the extravasated blood may be inhaled or swallowed. A fracture of the frontal bone over a hollow bony sinus may give rise to a subcutaneous emphysema of the face. Such an accumulation of air in the subcutaneous tissues may also occur after fracture of a lachrymal bone.

FRACTURES OF SKULL WITH INTRACRANIAL INJURIES

The most important injuries of the head are fractures of the cranium, the portion of the skull which encloses the brain, and the various associated intracranial injuries and complications which result from them. Before discussing these lesions it is necessary to consider the anatomic peculiarities of the skull, because they determine to a great extent the effects of trauma.

The cranium is divided into two parts, a vault and a base, which are joined and continuous. The vault, a curved dome of fairly even thickness, is architecturally strong. Its only places of weakness are the coronal, lambdoid and other sutures, and the thin squamous plates in both temporal regions. The base is an irregularly flattened plate which is formed of thick masses connected by thin fragile plates of bone. It is perforated at many points by foramina for vessels and nerves. As a consequence, the base is quite vulnerable to violence.

The masses of bone and the thin fragile plates comprising the base of the cranium have a definite arrangement and form a pattern like the hub of a wheel with six spokes. The crista galli, the right and left external angular frontal processes, the right and left petrous processes, and the basilar process of the occipital bone, are heavy osseous masses and represent the spokes; they radiate inward toward the hub, the sella turcica, and divide the base of the skull into six fossae, an anterior, a middle and a posterior fossa on each side. The floor of each fossa consists of a thin easily broken plate of bone.

The violence which produces the fracture in most cases is applied to the vault of the cranium. The force causes the skull to flatten at the point of impact, and, if the distortion is severe enough, a fracture will occur at this site.

The simplest form of fracture is a crack in the bone. It is known as a linear or fissure fracture and can result from a comparatively slight degree of violence. The fracture starts at the point of impact and travels away from it, marking the direction of the violence graphically on the contour of the skull. Its course is determined by the lines of least resistance, which are the thinnest plates of bone, the areas of gradual curvature, and the natural suture lines. The architecture of the cranium is such that the line of fracture descends from the vault into the base in between the boundaries of the fossae, and extends toward the center of the skull or one of the numerous foramina near the center. The fracture may run along the vault away from the base, but this course is not as frequent as that in which the direction is downward.

If the impact is severe, several fractures appear and radiate from the point of application to form diverse patterns on the skull, some Y-shaped or branched like a tree. In other instances, the violence may be great enough to flatten the skull and to shatter the area of impact into several fragments, producing a comminuted fracture. The term "composite fracture" is used to designate all fractures more complicated than the simple linear variety and includes those which have multiple fissures or are severely comminuted.

When an implement with a limited area of impact is applied to the skull, a depressed fracture may result and give a reasonably accurate impression of the weapon. Thus the impinging surface of a hammer produces a circular or semilunar mark on the vault of the cranium, and the point of a flatiron leaves a triangular depression. When the violence is slight, the area of impact will be suggested rather than outlined on the vault of the skull by curved cracks in the bone. A more severe blow will cause an indentation in the skull and produce a characteristic depressed fracture which depicts the area of impact with considerable accuracy. In these fractures, the inner table of the cranium will show more extensive comminution than the outer table. Figures 12-2 and 12-3 illustrate examples of depressed fractures of the skull caused by localized blunt force.

Fractures of the skull in the newborn infant are discussed in Chapter 23. The parietal bones, which are the most exposed, are the ones most frequently injured. The fractures are usually linear, angular or stellate; in the latter two types, the parietal boss is usually in the center of the fracture (Fig. 23-6).

CLASSIFICATION OF FRACTURES OF THE SKULL. Fractures of the skull are classified according to the type of violence which produces the injury, the location of the lesion, and the form and extent of the fracture.

I. *Fractures due to Impact.*

These occur when the head is violently thrown against or struck by a hard surface or object.

  A. Fractures of the vault.

    1. Variable location of impact.

      (a) Linear fractures, or simple cracks in the bone extending away from the point of impact. They are produced by a moderate grade of violence.

      (b) Composite fractures, which vary in form from a number of cracks in the bone radiating away from a point of impact to a marked comminution of the skull. They are produced by a severe violence.

      (c) Depressed fractures (Figs. 12-2, 12-3 and 12-24), or depressed sharply marked areas on the vault caused by forcible contact of an object with the limited area of impact against the head. Blunt instruments cause depressed fractures and leave characteristic lesions.

The complications of vault fractures are direct and contrecoup lacerations of the brain, with or without subdural hemorrhage; epidural hemorrhage; septic leptomeningitis. Incidence of vault fractures, 7 per cent.

  B. Fractures of the vault and base.

    1. Lateral fractures.

      (a) Linear fractures (Fig. 12-4).

      (b) Composite fractures (Fig. 12-4).

The complications of lateral fractures are similar to those enumerated under Fractures of the Vault. Incidence of lateral fractures, 40 per cent.

    2. Occipital fractures.

      (a) Linear fractures (Fig. 12-5).

      (b) Composite fractures (Fig. 12-6).

The complications are direct lacerations of the cerebellum (Figs. 12-6 and 12-7), contrecoup lacerations of the under surface of the frontal and temporal lobes (Figs. 12-5 and 12-7), with or without subdural hemorrhage; epidural hemorrhage (Figs. 12-26 and 12-27) and septic leptomeningitis are not common. Incidence of occipital fractures, 35 per cent.

    3. Frontal fractures.

      (a) Linear fractures.

      (b) Composite fractures.

The complications are direct lacerations of the under surfaces of frontal lobes with or without subdural hemorrhage; septic leptomeningitis; small hemorrhages in brain substance. Other lesions are rare. Incidence of frontal fractures, 11 per cent.

  C. Symmetrical composite fractures around the foramen magnum.

These are caused by severe impact on the top of the head, which forces the spinal column through the base of the skull (Fig. 12-8). Most of them are due to falls. Death is usually the result of shock and other complications are rare. Incidence of foramen fractures, 0.4 per cent.

II. *Fractures due to Compression of the Head.*

These fractures occur when the wheel of an automobile grinds the head of the victim into the roadway. The pressure is applied in a lateral direction and the line of fracture usually runs across the base of the skull. Death occurs in most cases from shock, but occasionally from septic meningitis. Lacerations of the brain and intracranial hemorrhages occur rarely (Fig. 12-9). Incidence of compression fractures, 6.6 per cent.

The above classification is not meant to convey the impression that fractures of the skull can always be separated into rigid categories, for occasionally individual fractures are encountered which are difficult to classify, as, for example, a depressed fracture of the vault combined with a linear fracture running into the base. The principal value of the classification is that it presents a logical schematic arrangement of this important group of injuries in the light of which they can be adequately discussed.

The authors have seen a rare fracture of the skull inflicted on a passenger during an automobile collision, probably as a result of a severe impact against the

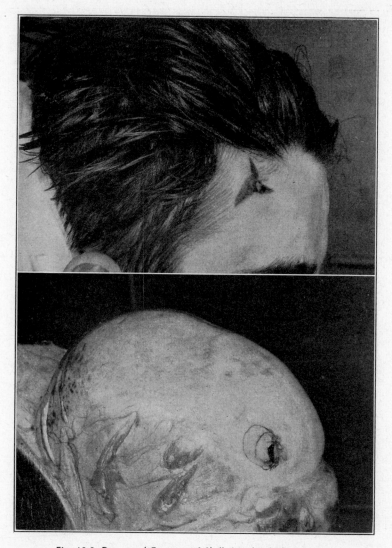

Fig. 12-2. Depressed Fracture of Skull. Localized Blunt Force.

Top. Triangular laceration of forehead.

Bottom. Underlying localized depressed fracture of right frontal bone. Brain showed direct and contrecoup contusions. Deceased thrown from motorcycle in collision.

under surface of the lower jaw which forced both mandibular condyles upward against the corresponding fossae. On the right side the articular head partly projected through a small elevated fracture in the thin floor of the fossa (Fig. 12-10); on the left side the condyle was located directly beneath a small linear transverse fracture of the middle fossa about 3 cm. in length. There were areas of contusion in the corpus callosum. Death in this case was due to other injuries.

The term contrecoup fracture is sometimes used to designate the small isolated fractures of the orbital roofs, often associated with severe fractures of the parietal and occipital regions but usually not joined to them. These isolated orbital fractures are probably produced by a pronounced change in the shape of the skull at

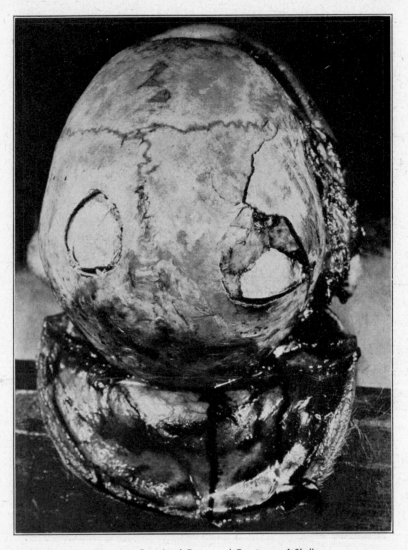

Fig. 12-3. Patterned Depressed Fractures of Skull.

Depressed punched-in fractures of the vault of the skull produced by blows with a circular hammer. Homicidal assault during robbery.

the moment of impact, and the orbital roof cracks because it is fragile and not able to stand the distortion.

INTRACRANIAL INJURIES ASSOCIATED WITH FRACTURES OF THE SKULL

Anatomic Considerations. Normally the brain covered by the meninges fills the cranial cavity and is symmetrically placed therein. Moreover it is cushioned in such a way that there is no undue pressure applied to its surface or causing any

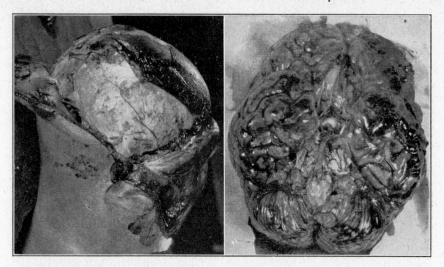

Left. Linear fracture, right side of skull in parietal and temporal regions.
   Right. Under surface of brain showing extensive contrecoup lacerations of left frontal and temporal lobes.

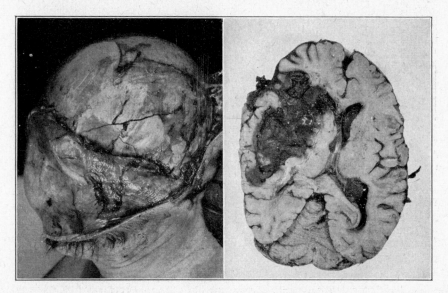

Left. Composite fracture involving left parietal, temporal and frontal bones.
   Right. Extensive direct laceration of the brain with traumatic cerebral hemorrhage rupturing into the ventricles. Contrecoup lacerations on under surface of right cerebral hemisphere not visible.

Fig. 12-4. Linear and Composite Skull Fractures. Brain Lacerations. Victims Knocked Down by Automobile.

displacement of its structure. The cerebral convolutions and sulci on its surface are well defined. The medulla and pons rest on the basilar portions of the sphenoid and occipital bones and are not compressed normally by the cerebrum or cerebellum. The brain invested by the pia-arachnoid is separated by the narrow subdural space from the inner surface of the dura which lines the cranial cavity. On the under surface of the frontal, temporal and occipital lobes, the brain is in close contact with the dura and the subdural space is only potential. The falx cerebri and the tentorium are extensions of the dura into the cavity of the skull. The tentorium separates the cerebellum from the cerebral hemispheres and the inner edges of the membrane support and surround the cerebral peduncles. The falx cerebri is a sickle-shaped membrane which separates and supports the cerebral hemispheres, and its sharp free edge rests just above the corpus callosum. The large venous sinuses which drain the brain are contained in the dura. At the foramen magnum the dura is firmly attached and is continuous with the spinal dura; the latter membrane is loosely attached to the spinal canal and differs from the cranial portion which closely invests the bone.

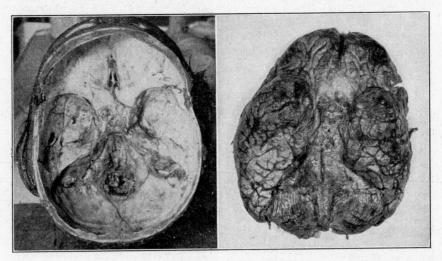

Fig. 12-5. Fracture of Skull. Brain Injury. Meningitis. Deceased Fell, Striking Back of Head on Pavement.

    A. Linear fracture in posterior fossa of the skull running down into foramen magnum and then continuing through the right petrous bone.
    B. Brain showing contrecoup contusions of temporal and frontal lobes. There was also an acute suppurative leptomeningitis which originated from pneumococcic pus in the right middle ear.

    The pia-arachnoid membranes or the leptomeninges invest the brain in two layers. The delicate pia is the innermost layer, being closely applied to the brain, even following the curves of the sulci, and extending down over the spinal cord. The arachnoid, located between the pia and the dura, is separated from the inside of the dura by the subdural space, and continues into the spinal canal where it is closely applied to the inside of the dura. On each side of the superior longitudinal venous sinus, the arachnoid is closely attached to the dura and helps to suspend the brain in the cranial cavity. At the base of the brain the arachnoid is fused into the sheaths of the vessels and nerves. As a result the subdural spaces on both sides are practically closed cavities and hemorrhages from one space do not enter the opposite side unless conditions are exceptional.

    The subarachnoid space around the brain and spinal cord presents the following peculiarities. In the spinal canal it is comparatively voluminous and forms a cistern in the lumbar region from which spinal fluid can be removed by paracentesis. In the cranial cavity the subarachnoid space invests the medulla, forming a large cistern at its junction with the cerebellum and at this point communicating

by means of the fourth ventricle with the ventricular system of the brain. The subarachnoid space on the under surface of the medulla is continued upward as a
rather roomy channel investing the pons, cerebral peduncles, the structures in
between the cerebral hemispheres and communicating through the sylvian fissures
with the subarachnoid space on the convexity of the cerebral hemispheres, which
is moderately roomy. On the under surface of the frontal, temporal and occipital
lobes, except in the sylvian fissure, the arachnoid is closely applied to the pia and
the sulci are shallow and thin so that the subarachnoid space is shallow. This is
also true of the inner surface of the cerebral hemispheres adjacent to the falx and
to the cerebellum except at the cisterna magna. Cerebrospinal fluid, blood and
inflammatory exudates accumulate in negligible amounts in such areas in contrast

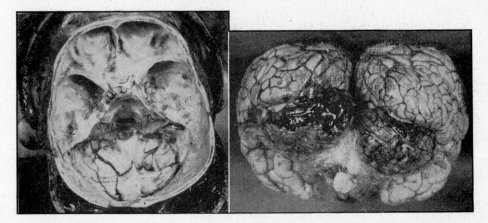

Fig. 12-6. Compound Comminuted Depressed Fracture of Posterior Fossae; Direct Lacerations of
Cerebellum.

Homicidal assault with five pound hammer. Death a few hours after injury.

to the profuse extravasions which usually occur in the more roomy subarachnoid
space over the convexity of the cerebral hemispheres, around the circle of Willis,
in the cisterna magna and in the spinal canal.

Pial venous tributaries pass through the pia-arachnoid space into the superior
longitudinal venous sinus, usually at right angles to that vessel. Similiar pial veins
on the outer surface of the temporal and parietal lobes emerge through the outer
arachnoid layer, across the subdural space and empty into venous tributaries of
the lateral sinus in the dura. These veins are sometimes ruptured by violence and
may give rise to a fatal subdural hemorrhage.

Contusions and Lacerations of the Brain. Injuries of varying severity are
produced on the surface of the brain whenever the cranium receives an impact
which brings the brain in forcible collision with the skull or the inside of the dura.
The mildest type of lesion is the rupture of minute blood vessels in the pia without
further structural damage, and the formation of a localized pia- and subarachnoid
hemorrhage on the external aspect of the cerebral hemispheres. If the impact is
more forcible, a contusion or bruise of the brain surface results, sometimes without
tearing of the overlying arachnoid membrane. The essential lesions in the contusion are small hemorrhages in the cortex and adjacent white matter due to the
rupture of small blood vessels which occur from the forcible distortion of the
surface brain tissue. The blood flows from the torn vessels into the Virchow-Robin

spaces and minute circular, ovoid or elongated hemorrhages of uneven size and irregular distribution appear in the traumatized area. The contusions are dark bluish-red in color, of varying size, intensity and depth, and they are located in the same areas of the brain where lacerations are found. There is often a small hemorrhage in the pia- and subarachnoid space adjacent to a contusion.

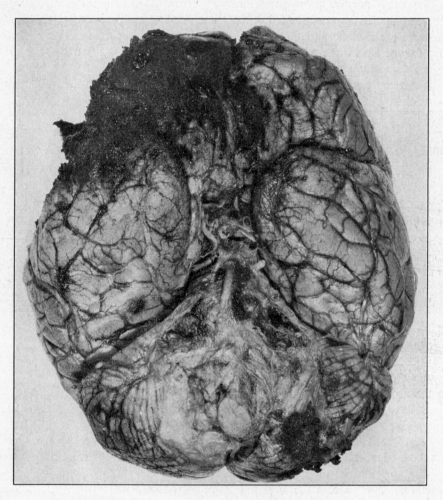

Fig. 12-7. Direct and Contrecoup Lacerations of Brain.

Under surface of brain showing direct laceration of left cerebellar hemisphere and contrecoup laceration of right frontal and temporal lobes. There was a linear fracture of the right posterior fossa of the skull. Deceased fell, striking back of head on pavement.

Cerebral laceration is the most important brain injury and is produced by a severe grade of violence which tears the pia-arachnoid and causes disruption of the brain cortex, the injury usually involving both gray and white matter. These lesions vary in size and depth depending upon the mechanism which produces them. Bleeding occurs from the surface of the lacerations, most often into the subdural space where it may be sufficient in amount to cause a fatal subdural hemorrhage. If the lacerated area communicates with the convex surface of the cerebral hemisphere a subarachnoid hemorrhage of considerable size may be the result.

The surface lacerations of the brain are classified as *direct lacerations* and as *contrecoup lacerations* (Figs. 12-4 through 12-7).

1. *Direct Lacerations*. Direct lacerations are produced during fractures of the skull in which the edges of the fractured bone injure the arachnoid and underlying brain tissue, sometimes but not always tearing the dura. Such lacerations may occur

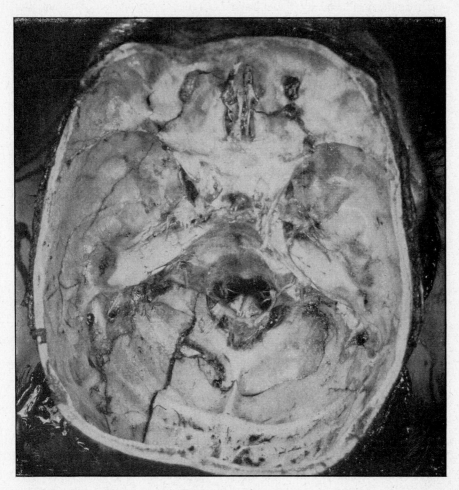

Fig. 12-8. Circumferential Fractures in Posterior Fossae Around Foramen Magnum with Involvement of Anterior and Middle Fossae.

Heavy impact on top of head.

anywhere on the brain surface and conform with the line of fracture in location, direction and general outline if not in extent. They occur most frequently on the outer surface of the parietal and temporal lobes from lateral fractures which start in the parietal bone and descend into the middle fossa on that side, because the curve of the cranium is broad in that region and more easily bent in by violence than regions of the skull with a sharper cranial curvature. Here a linear fracture may produce a shallow ribbon-like laceration 1.5 to 3.0 cm. in breadth with a superficial surface tear to which fragments of blood clot are attached; or a deep furrow may be cut into the brain tissue with blood clot filling the defect. A comminuted fracture in the parietal and temporal regions may cause an ovoid or irregular laceration of the adjacent brain surface which varies in extent, shape and depth depending upon the individual fracture. With lateral fractures the dura is most often torn in the squamous temporal region. Contrecoup lacerations of the external surfaces of the opposite frontal and temporal lobes are often associated with the direct injury of the brain. Fatal unilateral or bilateral subdural hemorrhages may be produced by these brain lacerations; the incidence of unilateral subdural hemorrhage from contrecoup laceration is 48 per cent; of unilateral hemorrhage from direct laceration, 28 per cent; and of bilateral hemorrhages from direct and contrecoup lacerations, 24 per cent.

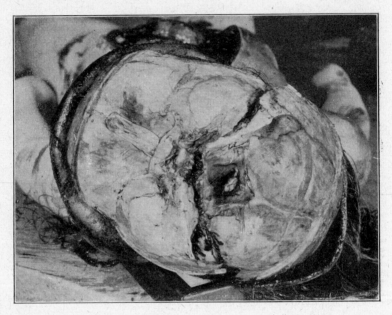

Fig. 12-9. Compression Fracture of Skull.

Compression fracture running transversely across the base of the skull. This was produced by an automobile wheel passing over the side of the child's head.

Fractures of the frontal region may lacerate the under surface of the frontal lobes, the shape and depth of the brain lesion depending upon the type of the fracture. In rare instances a fatal unilateral or bilateral subdural hemorrhage occurs from the brain injury. Contrecoup lacerations are not often produced in frontal fractures but may occur at the tip of the occipital lobe or on the cerebellum. Most rare is the occurrence of a unilateral or bilateral epidural hemorrhage (Figs. 12-26 and 12-27).

Occipital fractures may lacerate the under and posterior surfaces of the cerebellum (Figs. 12-6, 12-7 and 12-27) producing lesions of varying extent, depth and shape. In the production of this lesion the dura of the posterior fossa is often torn. In the majority of instances the direct laceration of the cerebellum is of minor importance and the most serious injuries associated with the occipital fractures are the contrecoup lacerations of the under surfaces of the frontal and temporal lobes, which produce a fatal unilateral subdural hemorrhage in about 60 per cent of the cases and a bilateral subdural hemorrhage in 35 per cent of the cases. In 5 per cent of lacerations associated with occipital fractures the cerebellar laceration is the cause of death by producing a hemorrhage below the tentorium and causing a compression of the medulla; in one instance the laceration communicated with the fourth ventricle.

2. *Contrecoup Lacerations.* Contrecoup lacerations occur on the opposite side of the brain, usually directly across from the area of impact and fracture. The force causes the brain to oscillate and strike against the opposite side of the skull, tearing the pia-arachnoid and producing lacerations of variable form and extent,

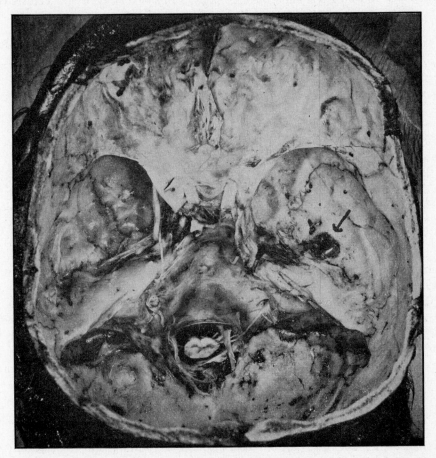

Fig. 12-10. Right Condyle of Mandible Forced Up into Middle Fossa of Skull, Impacted in Fracture Defect.

Automobile collision. Victim crushed in driver's seat.

some superficial, some deep. The contrecoup injury only occurs if the head is in motion or free to move at the moment of impact and fracture; if the skull is held immovable, oscillation of the brain cannot occur and the contrecoup mechanism cannot operate. The contrecoup injury may or may not be associated with a direct injury on the side of the fracture.

If the impact is in the occipital region the contrecoup lacerations appear on the under surfaces and apices of the frontal and temporal lobes. If the impact is directed against the lateral parietal region the external surfaces of the frontal and temporal lobes of the opposite side show the contrecoup lesions. These parts are especially vulnerable to this type of violence because the attachments of the brain are such that the organ has a greater range of oscillation in a forward or lateral direction than in any other. Moreover, the brain is in closer contact with the skull in the frontal and temporal regions than elsewhere and is likely to be lacerated by the contrecoup mechanism. In a few instances a severe force may strike the parietal or occipital region of the head without causing a fracture at the point of impact, but may produce an oscillation of the brain so as to cause severe and dangerous lacerations of the brain on the opposite side of the skull and occasionally a fatal subdural hemorrhage. Impacts in the frontal region are not so likely to produce contrecoup lacerations in the back part of the brain, as the reflections of the dura and the attachments of the brain tend to limit its oscillation in this direction.

Anatomically the lacerations are superficial broad areas, ovoid, square or rectangular in shape, with considerable blood clot attached to the surface of the traumatized cortex. On the under surface of the frontal lobe the entire surface may be lacerated (Fig. 12-7) but occasionally the laceration may be confined to the medial portion and involve the olfactory bulb and the adjacent convolutions. The temporal lobe usually shows a number of separate lacerations at the apex and on the under surface. The apex of the frontal lobe and the outer surfaces of the temporal lobes are occasionally involved. These lacerations may give rise to a fatal subdural hemorrhage. If there has been much distortion of brain tissue a large vessel may be torn and a large hollowed-out cavernous laceration filled with blood clot is produced, extending from the surface of the brain at the apex into the white matter of the frontal and temporal lobes and sometimes opening into the lateral ventricle. In a few cases, large subcortical hemorrhages are found in the form of blood cysts which do not connect with the surface though the surface of the brain may show a surface contusion. Bursting lacerations with cracking of the surface of the brain have been described as a result of contrecoup violence but are rare.

A laceration of the brain if severe enough can cause cerebral compression without the development of any appreciable subdural hemorrhage (Fig. 12-4). Such lesions as a rule are either broad superficial lacerations of the under surfaces of the frontal and temporal lobes to which considerable blood clot is attached, or big cavernous lacerations involving the cortex and white matter of the frontal and temporal lobes, which are filled with blood clot and communicate with the surface of the brain on the inferior portions of the frontal and temporal lobes; or even a large subcortical hemorrhage. In all these cases cerebral compression results from the accumulation of blood in the damaged area and from a localized edematous brain swelling in and around the traumatized tissue. The surface lacerations occur at the time of the injury. On the other hand the subcortical hemorrhages beneath the lacerations may be the result of a delayed rupture of a weakened vessel and may take several hours or more to develop. An original subcortical hemorrhage may continue to bleed until the hemorrhage is sufficiently large to cause cerebral compression. The cerebral compression is usually manifested by flattening of the cerebral convolutions especially on the vertex due to pressure against the inner lining of the dura. The flattening is either unilateral or bilateral depending upon the location and type of the cerebral laceration.

The subdural hemorrhages resulting from superficial lacerations of the brain are discussed on page 277. Discrete pontile hemorrhages may complicate cerebral lacerations (page 278); hypostatic pneumonia may also be a sequel of such injuries.

Severe impact against different parts of the head may produce multiple surface contusions and lacerations in the motor area of the parietal regions with the result that unilateral paralyses and convulsions occur as well as a certain amount of cerebral compression. In one case a man was struck with an iron bar in the right parietal region, causing a wide but shallow depression of the skull and scattered contusions without laceration in the right motor nuclei. The injury gave rise to severe jacksonian epileptiform convulsions which caused death by exhaustion. In another case the mandible of the deceased was struck and fractured on the left side in such a way that contusions were produced in the motor area of the left parietal region; unilateral convulsions and paralyses resulted as well as a certain amount of cerebral compression. The force of the blow in this case was transmitted to the articulation of the jaw on the right, causing the brain to oscillate to the left and upward against the left parietal vault.

The authors have seen another case in which the victim, a 51 year old man, was struck by a falling plank on the right lateral occipital region, and was unconscious for 20 minutes. After a brief hospitalization he was discharged but he complained for the next four months of intermittent attacks of headache and dizziness, and finally died of a suppurative leptomeningitis. The autopsy disclosed, in addition to the meningeal infection, a superficial tan-colored plaque about 1 inch in diameter on the outer surface of the right cerebellar hemisphere which was diagnosed as a healed laceration or contusion at this site, but there was no evidence that the skull had been fractured.

The healing of brain injuries consists in removal of the effused blood and traumatized brain tissue, and the final conversion of the laceration into a brown and then yellow pigmented scar. In the early stages the effused blood clots in the neighborhood of the injury, some of the fragmented brain tissue becomes necrotic, the tissue adjacent to the lesion becomes congested and leukocytes and histiocytes appear in the immediate vicinity. Strassmann observed histiocytes derived from endothelial, adventitial and microglial cells and containing hemosiderin on the sixth day after injury. During the second and third weeks the histiocytes gather in large numbers and aid in the removal of necrotic fatty myelin debris. These phagocytic cells are circular in outline and foamy in appearance from the contained fatty debris; others are large and ovoid, containing brown or yellow hemosiderin and hematoidin pigment, derived from the hemoglobin. There is an outpouring of fluid from the congested vessels, and the lacerated area and the tissue immediately adjacent may show a distinct gelatinous, yellowish-red edema. The fluid permeates the interstitial tissue and fills the perivascular and perineural spaces. During all these changes the laceration is gradually transformed in color from a red to a dark red, then to a brownish red, and finally to a brown, ending in a permanent light tan color. This last stage occurs when the debris in the lacerated area is cleared away, and granulation tissue and fibrosis have changed the area into a flat scar, termed a plaque jaune, which contains cells full of yellowish pigment. Sometimes the granulation tissue will attach the area of the old laceration by fibrosis to the adjacent dura and a brain adhesion results, which may be quite vascular. The reaction of the dura to the effused blood will be discussed later.

Cerebral Edema. Cerebral edema, whether localized or generalized, may produce a fatal cerebral compression. The localized variety, as it occurs in the vicinity of deep brain lacerations, has already been described. When the brain is sectioned in the fresh condition, the edematous area has a soft, swollen, gelatinous, yellowish-red appearance, but after the brain is fixed in formalin the color and other characteristics of the edematous area are obscured. The same type of edema is found around cerebral neoplasms and abscesses.

Generalized cerebral edema has been encountered at autopsy in association with a history of severe trauma to the head. This condition can be diagnosed pathologically on the basis of a swollen appearance of the brain, with flattening and broadening of the cerebral convolutions, diminution in the size of the ventricles, and with such signs of intracranial pressure as indentation of the lower end of the cerebellum by the foramen magnum or the protrusion of a small portion of the temporal lobe near the brain stem through an opening in the tentorium. In this generalized form the entire brain substance is affected as a whole, its weight is increased, and microscopically there is an intracellular, pericellular and perivascular accumulation of fluid. In addition to its occasional association with head trauma, cerebral edema may develop in natural disease processes. It has been encountered where death has occurred after prolonged convulsive seizures. It has been seen in a case of sudden death following the injection of tetanus antitoxin and in cases of encephalitis. It has also been observed in cases of excessive hydration resulting from the infusion into the body of inordinate amounts of fluid as a therapeutic measure.

Investigation of cerebral edema has not been successful in determining its pathogenesis, though many explanatory theories have been advanced. Some believe that the swelling of the brain is due to an increased amount of blood in the blood vessel, or to an increase of cerebrospinal fluid in the ventricles causing an expansion of the brain. Friedman has described a temporary and moderate dilatation of the ventricles of the brain soon after trauma through high roentgen-ray photographs on clinical cases. Wortis has described the same effect in his experimental work. Permanent dilatation of the ventricles from obstruction at some point to the flow of spinal fluid is rare, but has been described by Ford and Moritz and Wortman. Greenfield believes that the cerebral edema is a true interstitial edema in which the myelinated fibrils of white matter are separated by fluid. Some believe that the different glial and vascular cells in the brain may imbibe fluid, thus contributing to the swelling of the cerebral tissue. Others think that the collection of fluid in the Virchow-Robin space may also increase the size of the brain. None of these hypotheses completely explains the phenomenon of cerebral edema, and for the present the matter must be left sub judice.

Many physicians have a tendency to confuse edema of the brain with pial edema, though the two conditions are not similar and are not related. Edema of the brain is an acute increase of the fluid content of the cerebral tissue usually with compression and obliteration of the subarachnoid space and the ventricular system as the result of the swelling of the brain tissue. The brain is heavy and soggy but does not drip fluid. Pial edema, on the other hand, is a chronic accumulation of an excessive amount of cerebrospinal fluid beneath the pia-arachnoid and in the ventricles, associated with cerebral atrophy, small convolutions with widened sulci and large roomy ventricles due principally to the atrophy of the brain. The fluid is outside of the brain tissue which it seems to replace. This condition is a sequel of long-continued chronic alcoholism, general arteriosclerosis and other chronic diseases of the central nervous system. It is also known as *wet brain* because of the large amount of fluid in the pia-arachnoid which drips from the surface of the brain when it is removed from the cranial cavity.

The authors have seen a number of cases of generalized cerebral edema which displayed the following clinical picture. Symptoms of concussion were lacking, but there was a definite history of injury to the head, and after a brief interval the victim became stuporous, displayed indefinite neurologic signs, and finally died in coma. At autopsy on three of these cases, the brain was swollen and the convolutions flattened. There were no gross surface lacerations or contusions, and no hemorrhages, petechial or otherwise in the brain. In one instance, that of a prize fighter, a small thrombosed pial vein was found and the leptomeninges showed mild but definite evidence of inflammation. In another case, that of a wrestler who became ill after a bout, death also occurred with signs of cerebral compression. The brain was heavy and swollen, no contusions were present, but the leptomeninges over the cerebellum revealed mild inflammatory cell infiltration and proliferative changes. A somewhat similar case was observed in which a young woman developed signs of cerebral compression and became unconscious after a period of strenuous exercise. The brain was also swollen with evidence of pressure in those areas abutting against the tentorium and the falx. The relationship of the brain swelling and the cerebral compression is difficult to evaluate in these cases. The usual manifestations of traumatic injury were absent.

Subdural Hemorrhage. The most common cause of cerebral compression complicating fracture of the skull is hemorrhage from intracranial injuries into the subdural space. The injuries which give rise to subdural hemorrhage are: (1) laceration of the brain and pia-arachnoid; (2) rupture of blood vessels on surface of

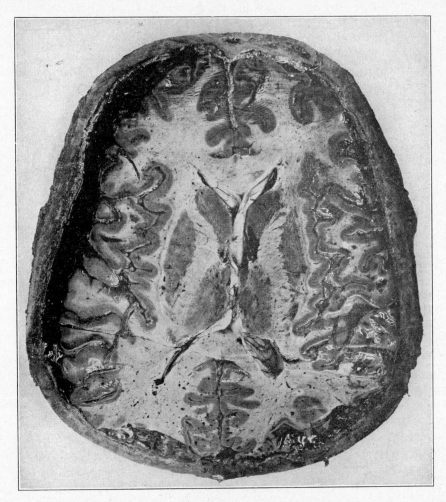

Fig. 12-11. Traumatic Subdural Hemorrhage without Skull Fracture.

Under surface of calvarium containing upper half of brain. Fresh right-sided subdural hemorrhage with molding of convolutions on side of hemorrhage and flattening of convolutions of opposite cerebral hemisphere against smooth inner surface of the dura. A contrecoup laceration of the brain was present on under surface of right frontal lobe, but the skull was not fractured. Accidental fall on street.

cerebral hemispheres; (3) re-injury of old adhesion between the brain and the dura; (4) laceration of the dura and the middle meningeal artery so that the vessel bleeds into the subdural instead of the epidural space.

1. *Laceration of the Brain and Leptomeninges.* Both direct and contrecoup lacerations of the brain bleed from their raw surfaces into the subdural space. Usually the hemorrhage is unilateral and collects as a broad and thick layer of fluid and soft clotted blood between the dura and the arachnoid, covering the cerebral hemisphere from the frontal to the occipital region and from the falx cerebri

at the vertex to the outer periphery of the fossae at the base. The blood is not found in any quantity on the under surface of the brain unless the laceration is located in this region, and it does not extend over to the subdural space on the opposite side because of the anatomic attachments of the arachnoid. The subdural hemorrhage presses the brain against the opposite side of the skull so that the convolutions of the vertex, and, to a lesser extent, of the base, are flattened against the smooth inner surface of the dura. On the side of the hemorrhage the convolutions beneath the effusion of blood and blood clot are molded and stand out prominently. If the pressure is great, the medial surface of the temporal lobe may project slightly through the tentorial opening and bruise itself, or the cerebral cortex near the lower edge of the falx may be pushed against it and also be contused or infarcted. In some cases there is an asymmetric displacement and distortion of the hemispheres with distortion and displacement of the basal ganglia, a condition readily demonstrated by a horizontal section of the brain before its removal from the skull (Fig. 12-11). Other unilateral lesions, both intra- and extracerebral will cause similar displacement and signs of cerebral compression.

Bilateral subdural hemorrhages, when present in approximately equal amounts, press the brain down in a convergent direction toward the base. The pons may be flattened against the basilar process of the occiput, the lower extremity of the cerebellum may be indented by the foramen magnum and its convolutions flattened, and the medulla may be compressed. The convolutions of both cerebral hemispheres are molded and stand out prominently. Small discrete hemorrhages may occur in the pons as a complication of a unilateral subdural hemorrhage and less frequently as a complication of bilateral subdural hemorrhages. Hypostatic pneumonia is a fairly common sequel of subdural hemorrhages if the victim survives the injury over 24 hours.

A large subdural hemorrhage is a bright crimson red when fresh, but in the course of a few days, as the blood hemolyzes, the color becomes a darker red, then brownish red and finally a yellowish brown in color. At the same time the pia-arachnoid is stained brown, and the overlying dura is similarly stained and rendered translucent. After a varying period of time, a layer of granulation tissue develops on the inner surface of the dura and organization and attachment of the partly hemolyzed and disintegrated clot begins. The inner surface of the hematoma rests directly on the arachnoid which is stained brown by diffusion of hemolyzed disintegrated blood (Fig. 12-12). During this stage the spinal fluid is xanthochromic. It is only after several weeks that the broken-down hemolyzed hematoma becomes enclosed in and separated from the arachnoid by a thin inner limiting membrane which at first is composed of a friable sheet of fibrin and later of fibrous tissue. After this inner membrane has formed, the underlying brain and its leptomeninges lose their xanthochromia and the spinal fluid again becomes colorless. The inner membrane is impervious to hemolyzed blood pigment which can no longer diffuse through it to cause xanthochromia of the brain and spinal fluid. Thus with old subdural hemorrhages, enclosed in well organized limiting membranes, the underlying brain and its leptomeninges appear clean and unstained and this is reflected in the clear colorless spinal fluid. The inner membrane, in the absence of an underlying brain laceration, does not become adherent to the arachnoid (Figs. 12-13 and 12-20).

Subdural hemorrhages arising from brain lacerations may undergo the same changes and produce the same reactions in the dura as subdural hemorrhages re-

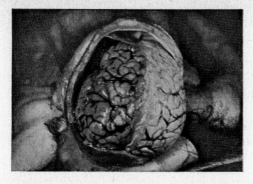

Fig. 12-12. Left sided subdural hemorrhage 10 days old. Photographed after removal of blood to show brown staining of underlying pia-arachnoid, molding of left and flattening of right cerebral hemisphere convolutions.

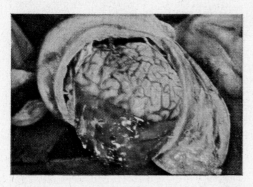

Fig. 12-13. Organizing subdural hemorrhage to show brown color and formation of inner limiting membrane separating hematoma from surface of brain. Dura with hematoma lifted up to show clear appearance of most of subjacent pia-arachnoid. Compare with Figure 12-12. Process three months old.

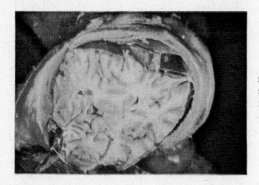

Fig. 12-14. Organizing subdural hemorrhage about two months old. Horizontal section to show brown color, adhesion of inner membrane to pia-arachnoid, and molding and compression of brain.

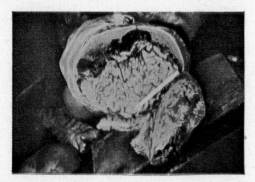

Fig 12-15. Very old organizing subdural hematoma with calcification of limiting membranes. Note large clam-shaped hematoma lifted back to show clear unstained appearance of molded subjacent brain. Death from a fresh subdural hemorrhage.

sulting from a torn pial vein or as the spontaneous subdural hemorrhages which occur in pachymeningitis interna hemorrhagica. Most small subdural hemorrhages are absorbed, leaving a slight granular tan colored pigmentation on the inside of the dura. The reactions of the dura with larger hemorrhages will be discussed on page 284.

2. *Rupture of Blood Vessels on Surface of Cerebral Hemispheres.* Violence which jars the head may cause a rupture of a blood vessel in the subarachnoid space on the lateral aspect of a cerebral hemisphere with bleeding into the sub-

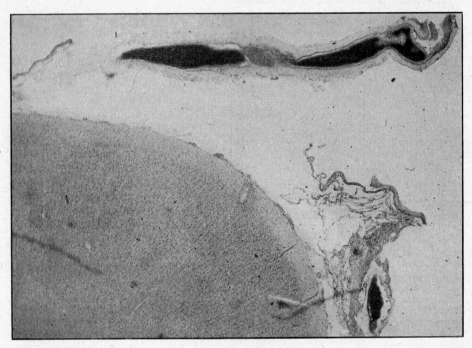

Fig. 12-16. Tear of Communicating Vein Bridging Lateral Surface of Frontal Lobe and Superior Longitudinal Sinus.

Low power photomicrograph showing platelet thrombi in torn vein. Middle aged woman punched in head. Death in two hours from rapid subdural hemorrhage.

dural space. The bleeding may be primary and continuous, or temporary closure of the vessel by thrombosis may occur, followed a few days later by expulsion of the thrombus and secondary hemorrhage. There may be a long latent interval between the time of the trauma and the onset of symptoms produced by cerebral compression, or the bleeding may be more rapidly fatal. Usually the resulting hemorrhage is unilateral but in some cases it is bilateral. Some large subdural hemorrhages of this type are accompanied by fractures of the skull and other intracranial injuries, but most of them are not.

One important variety of traumatic vascular rupture involves small bridging blood vessels (arteries, veins or a combination of the two) which cross the subdural space and connect blood vessels in the subarachnoid area with those in the dura mater. Such vessels may be torn by force applied to the front or back of the head, causing oscillation of the brain in the anteroposterior plane, and sometimes by a lateral impact which causes the brain to oscillate from side to side. Many types of physical violence produce such lesions and the causative force need be only moderately severe, as for example a fist blow struck during an altercation or a fall from the standing position with the head striking the floor.

Tears may occur in the thin-walled veins which are tributaries of the superior longitudinal sinus and bridge the subdural space near the vertex of the brain. One of these vessels may be torn across and bleed into the subdural space; at autopsy

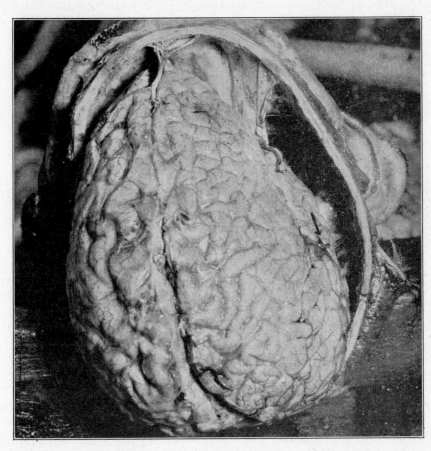

Fig. 12-17. Traumatic Subdural Hemorrhage without Skull Fracture.

Torn communicating vein on right temporal lobe (arrow) exposed at necropsy after removing large traumatic subdural hemorrhage. Skull not fractured and brain not contused. Death occurred from cerebral compression.

The tearing of these veins, which connect the pial vessels with tributaries of the dural venous sinuses, occurs occasionally when a jarring force is applied to the head as in a boxing match, a football game or a fall of an inebriated person.

it may be found closed by a cigar-shaped or a puffball-shaped bland thrombus. If the vein is torn near the superior longitudinal venous sinus, the hemorrhage may be rapid enough to cause a fatal cerebral compression in one to two hours (Fig. 12-16). Other bridging veins apt to be torn are located on the outer surface of the parietal and temporal lobes and less frequently over the frontal and occipital lobes; at autopsy such torn vessels distended by a thrombus appear as small teat-like projections (Fig. 12-17) in the center of a small subarachnoid hemorrhage, sometimes with slight contusion of the surrounding cerebral cortex.

Small arteries may also bridge the subdural space, usually on the lateral surface of the parietal and temporal lobes, and one of these may sustain an oblique ragged tear (Fig. 12-18) with resultant subdural bleeding. The arachnoid may be denuded in a small zone around the ruptured vessel and a small subarachnoid hemorrhage and cortical contusion may be present. Sometimes the bridging vessels in these areas consist of both arteries and veins included in a thick stalk, and if the violence is severe, the vessels may be torn from the arachnoid like a plant unearthed with its roots leaving only a small laceration on the brain surface. In such instances it is usually not possible to demonstrate a clear cut rupture in a sizeable blood vessel.

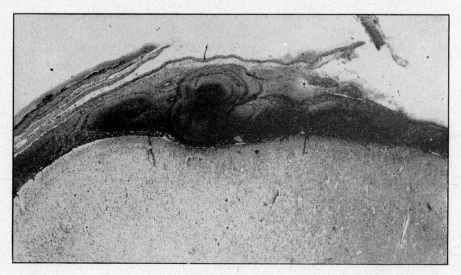

Fig. 12-18. Subdural Hemorrhage from Torn Artery on Lateral Surface of Frontal Lobe.
Low power photomicrograph. White man, 60 years old, survived 18 hours in hospital. Probable fall.

Another type of injury which occurs in the subarachnoid arteries on the lateral surfaces of the parietal and temporal lobes is the fire hose rupture. This produces a small circular hole involving the lateral aspect of the artery and extending through the adjacent arachnoid into the subdural space. This lesion is dependent upon the existence of small aberrant arterial twigs which are given off the external surface of the artery and run out toward the outer layer of the arachnoid. Such aberrant vessels are points of weakness, and may be ruptured if the brain is distorted against the inside of the skull by violence, the blow out resulting from a rise in pressure in the vessel (Fig. 12-19). These small ruptures although inconspicuous can cause a fatal subdural hemorrhage. They appear at autopsy as small pinhead to pinpoint sized dots on the outer surface of the arachnoid occasionally plugged by a fibrinous clot in varying stages of organization.

3. *Re-injury of Old Laceration.* The re-injury of an old cerebral laceration is seen occasionally. When healing occurs in such a lesion, the extravasated red blood cells are destroyed and the hemoglobin is transformed into one of the hemoglobin derivatives so that the color of the injured area changes from dark red to a yellowish brown. Vascular granulation tissue is formed in the laceration and grows so that the brain may become adherent to the dura at the site of the injury. The authors have seen cases in which such individuals have sustained a subsequent

head trauma with or without a cranial fracture, and the result was the tearing of the adhesion and its blood vessels, followed by a fatal subdural hemorrhage.

4. *Laceration of the Dura.* A fracture of the skull in the parietal or temporal regions may tear the dura and lacerate a branch of the middle meningeal artery on the outside of that membrane. In one such case seen by the authors, the torn vessel projected and bled into the subdural space. A large subdural hemorrhage in the form of a large coherent clot and weighing 220 gm. was extravasated on the upper outer portion of the cerebral cortex, pressing the brain downward.

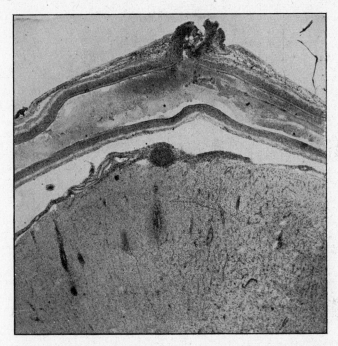

Fig. 12-19. Fire Hose Rupture of Artery on Lateral Surface of Temporal Lobe. Subdural Hemorrhage.

Low power photomicrograph. White man, 68 years old, survived 10 days in hospital. No history of injury; possible fall.

The relative frequency of the different causes of fatal subdural hemorrhages is indicated in the article by Vance (1950). In 507 cases of skull fracture, 132 cases died as a result of subdural hemorrhages of which 90 were unilateral and 42 were bilateral. Of the unilateral hemorrhages: contrecoup lacerations, 67; direct lacerations, 19; direct and contrecoup lacerations combined, 1; tearing of dura and middle meningeal artery, 1; injury of old adhesion of brain to dura, 1; rupture of communicating dural vein, 1. Of the bilateral hemorrhages: contrecoup lacerations, 18; direct lacerations of brain, 2; combined direct and contrecoup lacerations, 20; torn dural veins, 2. The average weight of the subdural hemorrhage was about 60 gm. (Vance, 1927).

The majority of recent subdural hemorrhages occur as the result of a traumatic injury, but a few have their origin in a natural disease process. The subdural hemorrhages following the spontaneous rupture of an aneurysm of the circle of Willis have been described on page 137. In addition the disease process known as pachymeningitis interna hemorrhagica may produce a sudden subdural hemorrhage of critical size, as noted on page 284. The authors have also encountered cases in which there was good reason to believe that an acute fatal subdural effusion of blood occurred as the result of a spontaneous rupture of a communicating vein between the pia and dura.

In one such case an elderly man, who had been troubled about a month prior to his death with severe paroxysms of coughing, bumped his head slightly while getting into his car but sustained no inconvenience at the time. His coughing continued. About three days after the bumping incident he became comatose and died in coma nine hours later. The autopsy disclosed a recent subdural hemorrhage on the right and a fatal cerebral compression, but not the slightest sign of an injury to the head or any other part of the body. The theory that the severe coughing had raised the cerebral venous pressure and had ruptured one of the communicating dural veins spontaneously was considered a distinct possibility, but was difficult to prove or disprove under the circumstances.

Chronic subdural hematoma is in most cases one of the many anatomic varieties of a natural process, pachymeningitis interna hemorrhagica. This condition arises spontaneously in such chronic diseases as senility, alcoholism, insanity and cerebrospinal syphilis, and is fundamentally a disturbance of the blood vessels in the inner layer of the dura which can undergo an extraordinary proliferation under the influence of circulatory or toxic factors. The vessels increase in size and ramify toward the inner surface of the dura, accompanied by a proliferation of large spindle cells; occasionally they are surrounded by an infiltration of round cells. In the early stages they appear on the inner lining as a small medusa-like tangle of vessels over the vertex accompanied by a thin hemorrhagic membrane due to capillary rupture or diapedesis. The process is usually bilateral, though one side may show a more advanced stage of the process than the other. Later when vessels of larger size are formed, these may rupture spontaneously either into the dural membrane, or into the subdural space where hemorrhages of various size appear, some large enough to cause cerebral compression. The usual course of the disease is slow, as it proceeds by a succession of hemorrhages which become organized by the formation of two limiting membranes, an outer one which becomes firmly fused to the inner surface of the dura from which it arises, and an inner one in apposition with but not adherent to the arachnoid. The inner surfaces of these membranes are lined by vascular granulation tissue which tends to organize the subdural hemorrhage between them, but under certain unfavorable conditions continues to bleed and thus increases the bulk of the hematoma by repeated fresh additions of blood. A continuation of the process of organization and recurrent hemorrhage between the limiting membranes may result in chronic cerebral compression. When the process is bilateral, the brain hemispheres are compressed downward and medially and exhibit a concave deformity so that the top of the brain has the appearance of an old-fashioned satchel (Fig. 6-22).

Chronic subdural hemorrhage may assume a great variety of anatomic forms depending on whether it is unilateral or bilateral, its age and other factors. In some cases it appears as a thick organized brown hematoma, 1 or 2 cm. thick, adherent to the dura and usually separated from the arachnoid by a smooth inner membrane on which an impression of the underlying cerebral convolutions is visible (Fig. 12-20). In rare cases the inner membrane becomes adherent to the pia-arachnoid and cerebral cortex which may exhibit extensive chronic inflammatory changes (Fig. 12-14). In other instances, there are encysted hematomas or organized hemorrhages with encysted collections of yellow fluid. Rarely the limiting membranes of the hematoma become calcified and enclose the organizing hemorrhage like the shells of a clam (Fig. 12-15).

Whether or not chronic subdural hematoma or pachymeningitis interna hemorrhagica has any connection with trauma is a point of considerable interest inasmuch as many of the reported cases in the literature stress its connection with a previous injury, generally of slight grade and sometimes occurring months or years prior to the first premonitions of intracranial pressure. It is certain that this condition develops in certain chronic diseases, as mentioned above, without any history or

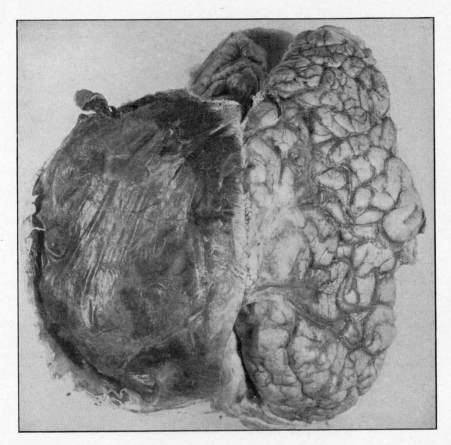

Fig. 12-20. Organizing Subdural Hemorrhage.

Dura turned back to show inner limiting membrane, disappearance of xanthochromia from pia arachnoid and intaglio impression of convolutions of underlying molded cerebral hemisphere.

anatomic signs of trauma. At the same time, the effusion of a small amount of blood from a brain laceration into the subdural space in some cases may stimulate a progressive reaction in the dura similar to that of a pachymeningitis and initiate the formation of an active chronic self-perpetuating subdural hematoma. It is possible in such cases that the traumatic hemorrhage merely accelerates the development of the hemorrhagic dural membrane which was due to form in any event or was already under way at the time of the injury. Not every case which has been inflicted with a small hemorrhage in the subdural space following a brain injury develops a pachymeningitis hemorrhagica interna. In a large number of cases in which death from nontraumatic causes occurred many months after the injury, autopsy disclosed healed brain lacerations and the old subdural hemorrhage transformed into a healed inert pachymeningitis pigmentosa. Each case of pachymeningitis must be judged with all due caution and careful consideration of the clinical history and anatomic findings in determining its possible connection with a traumatic injury.

Epidural Hemorrhage. An epidural hemorrhage is caused by a fracture of the skull which lacerates a vessel on the outside of the dura. In most cases the fracture tears the middle meningeal artery, and less often the lateral sinus, the

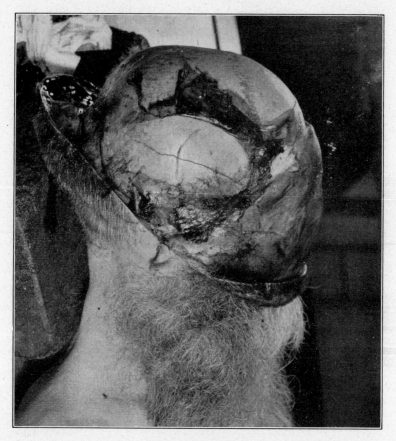

Fig. 12-21. Fracture of Skull. Tear of Middle Meningeal Artery.

Linear fracture of right parietal bone tearing right middle meningeal artery with formation of large epidural hemorrhage shown in Fig. 12-22.

Deceased, a 50 year old man, knocked down by automobile and temporarily stunned. He regained consciousness and returned home. Death occurred 10 days later.

anterior meningeal artery near the cribriform plate, or the posterior meningeal artery near the foramen magnum.

The middle meningeal artery starts from the foramen spinosum in each middle fossa and wanders out over the external surface of the dura in the parietal, temporal and lateral frontal regions, forming a dendritic pattern; grooves for the artery are present on the inside of the calvaria. Any line of fracture which crosses the arterial grooves may tear the artery and cause an epidural hemorrhage, but in the series studied by Vance, out of 268 fractures involving the lateral region of the skull, 102 showed epidural hemorrhages from a branch of the middle meningeal artery and of these only 56 were clinically important. These hemorrhages occur at any age but are most frequent in adults from 20 to 40 years especially in individuals who have a thin skull and whose dura is easily separated from the skull (Figs. 12-21 through 12-25). At the time of the fracture, the distortion inflicted on the skull separates it from the dura so that an epidural space is created into which the blood from the torn middle meningeal artery may flow. If the dura

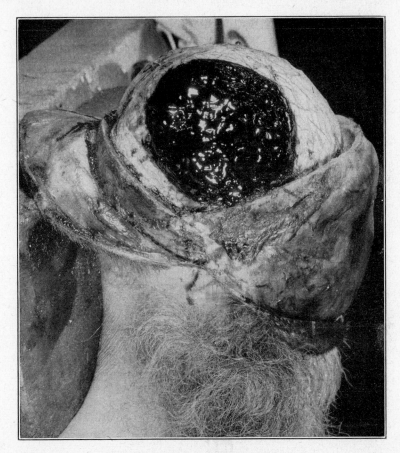

Fig. 12-22. Epidural Hemorrhage.
Same case as in Fig. 12-21. Calvarium removed to show large epidural hemorrhage.

is so adherent to the cranium that it cannot be separated or if the fracture fails to lacerate the artery, a hemorrhage will not occur.

Epidural hemorrhages produced by fractures in the lateral regions of the vault are discus-shaped clots on the outside of the dura, which press that membrane inward and cause a localized concavity on the external surface of the brain. Cerebral compression is produced and causes death. The dimensions of the clot vary. It is either ovoid or circular in outline, about 10 to 20 cm. in diameter, 2 to 6 cm. in thickness, and its average weight is about 125 gm. It may be located at almost any point under the vault and its variation in shape may be considerable, the hemorrhage taking the form of a large flat disk or of a short rather plump clot. Sometimes when the artery is lacerated near the middle fossa there may be a thin tongue of blood clot extending from that site to the main body of the hemorrhage under the vault. Occasionally the main stem of the middle meningeal artery is lacerated in the middle fossa, in which case the clot is usually globular in shape and presses up against the under surface of the temporal lobe. These globular clots are about 10 to 15 cm. in diameter and less voluminous than the discus-shaped hemorrhages. Rarely fractures which cross the vault of the skull in the parietal or frontal regions lacerate branches of the middle meningeal artery on both sides of

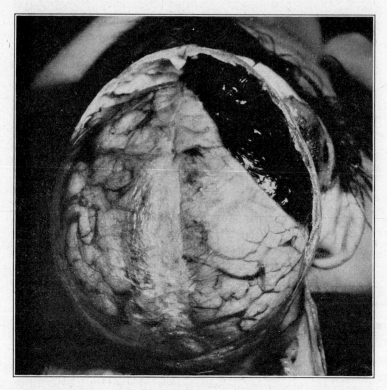

Fig. 12-23. Epidural Hemorrhage: Cerebral Compression.

Epidural hemorrhage resulted from a linear fracture of right temporal bone, and tear of anterior branch of right middle meningeal artery. Ten year old child struck on head by swing on playground. Note unusual transparency of dura which has been left intact.

the skull and produce a bilateral epidural hemorrhage with compression of both cerebral hemispheres.

The character of the epidural hemorrhage encountered at autopsy depends upon the duration of the clinical course and the rapidity of its formation. In those cases which survive only a few hours, the effused blood is like currant jelly, friable, and easily separated from the dura. In such instances it may be possible to demonstrate the tear in the middle meningeal artery which is usually lacerated transversely either partially or completely. Rarely does the hemorrhage show separation of the effused blood into a chicken-fat clot and a currant jelly clot, similar to the post-mortem clotting in the heart, and in such cases the epidural hemorrhage has probably formed immediately after the injury and has been accompanied by rapid sedimentation of the erythrocytes. If the patient has survived the injury a few days, the effused blood is firmly attached to the dura, is coherent and dark red with brownish tinge as the result of hemolysis. Occasionally small epidural hemorrhages occur as a result of fracture, or in the absence of fracture as a result of a slight separation of the skull from the dura and the tearing of many minute blood vessels extradurally. The remains of these hemorrhages can be found at autopsy, long after the injury, in various stages of healing. The old hemorrhages appear as flattened extradural tan-colored plaques due to fibrotic thickening, and on the inside of the skull as whitish, roughened, eburnated incrustations of the bone produced by the irritant action of effused blood. Microscopic examination of such lesions shows fibrous organization and the presence of yellow and brown granules of blood pigment.

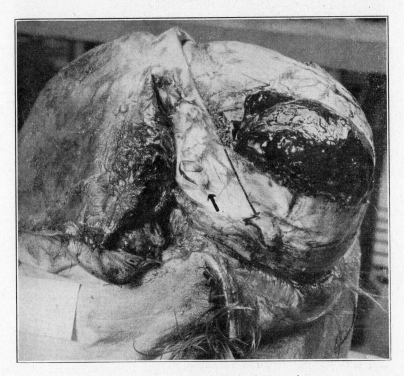

Fig. 12-24. Fracture of Skull. Epidural Hemorrhage.

Injured during altercation. Small localized depressed fracture (arrow) of especially thin squamous portion of left temporal bone. Laceration of dura and posterior branch of middle meningeal artery. Large epidural hemorrhage. Same case as Fig. 12-25.

Rarely epidural hemorrhages occur from fractures in the frontal region which lacerate the anterior meningeal artery, a branch of the ophthalmic artery which enters the cranial cavity through a small foramen near the cribriform plate. These hemorrhages are globular in shape and press in the tip of the frontal lobe. A massive frontal epidural hemorrhage pushing back both frontal lobes of the brain resulting from a linear fracture of the lateral portion of the frontal bone is illustrated in Figure 12-26. It resulted from a simple fall. Similarly a branch of the vertebral artery called the posterior meningeal artery may be lacerated by a fracture of the occipital bone and form a globular clot which presses into the cerebellum and occipital lobe. These rare epidural hemorrhages are sometimes large enough to cause fatal cerebral compression (Fig. 12-27).

Some epidural hemorrhages arise from a laceration of the posterior wall of the lateral venous sinus by the sharp edges of an occipital fracture. Globular blood extravasations are formed, about 7 to 12 cm. in diameter, which compress the vital centers in the pons and medulla, causing rapid onset of coma and death.

The superior longitudinal venous sinus is lacerated by fractures which cross the vault. The resulting epidural hemorrhage is usually not large but in rare instances may be massive (Fig. 12-28). If an ill-advised craniotomy is attempted on

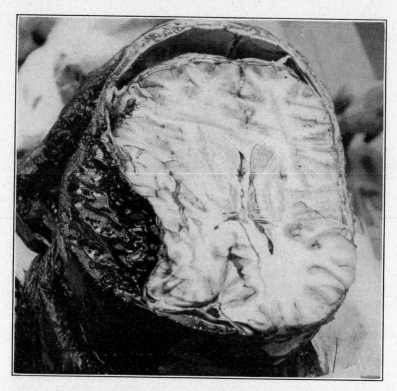

Fig. 12-25. Epidural Hemorrhage: Cerebral Compression.

Same case as in Fig. 12-24. Horizontal section of epidural hemorrhage and brain in situ to show thickness of clot and pressure on underlying dura and brain.

some of these fractures and fragments of bone are removed above the venous sinus, the lacerated vessel may bleed profusely, causing death by hemorrhage.

Traumatic Cerebral Hemorrhages. Several types of intracranial hemorrhage, ordinarily occurring spontaneously without any association with traumatic injury, occasionally follow violence to the head which may or may not fracture the cranium. Such lesions are hemorrhages in the subarachnoid space at the base of the brain, or large massive hemorrhages in the basal nuclei, cerebellum or pons, which cause death as a result of cerebral compression. Anatomically these hemorrhages are indistinguishable from the purely spontaneous type and on investigation degenerative or inflammatory changes in the cerebral arteries may be found as a basis for the rupture of the blood vessel. The head injury is responsible only in so far as it may occasion a rise in blood pressure, and thus promote the rupture of a diseased blood vessel at the time of injury. In some cases the blood vessel ruptured spontaneously while the deceased was standing, causing him to collapse suddenly and fracture his skull incident to falling. Unless a witness was present at the time of the fall it may be difficult to determine how much of a role traumatic injury played in the case.

Multiple petechial hemorrhages or hemorrhages of larger size are sometimes produced in different parts of the brain after a severe impact against the head, which may or may not cause a fracture of the skull. The hemorrhages which result

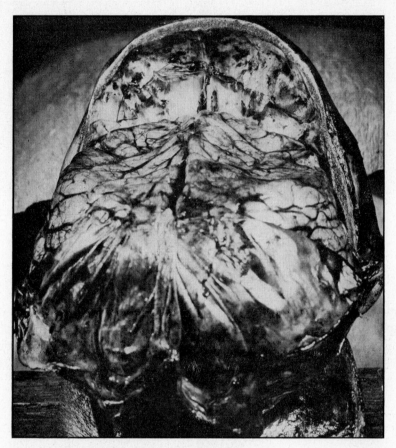

Fig. 12-26. Rare Massive Confluent Bilateral Epidural Hemorrhage in Anterior Fossae Compressing Both Frontal Lobes.

Clot, weighing 185 gm., was removed prior to photography. No brain laceration. Linear fracture of right frontal bone crossing anterior fossae. No external sign of injury. White man, 35 years old, fell down stairs. No unconsciousness; went to sleep; found dead in bed.

may be numerous or large enough to give rise to cerebral compression on account of circulatory disturbances induced in the brain. The violence causing the hemorrhages is severe enough to produce cerebral concussion and the unconsciousness that ensues favors the development of a hypostatic pneumonia. The impact causes the brain to oscillate and strike against the skull or the different reflections of the dura such as the tentorium or the falx cerebri, producing the forcible distortion of the cerebral substance which ruptures the small vessels.

Oscillation of the brain in many instances causes contusions on the outer surface of the parietal lobe and damages the motor area. This condition has been discussed under lacerations on page 275. As a result of oscillation after impact there may be enough distortion of the brain tissue near the cortex to tear a large vessel just under the surface and give rise to a subcortical hemorrhage varying in size from about 2 to 7 cm. in diameter. These lesions are most apt to occur at the usual sites of contrecoup cerebral injuries, that is on the under and outer surfaces of the frontal and temporal lobes, or on the convex surfaces of the cerebral hemi-

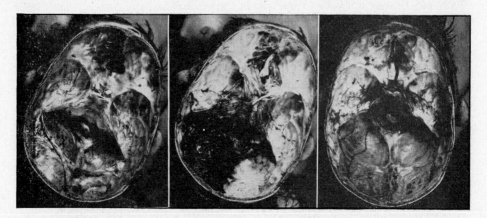

Fig. 12-27. Epidural Hemorrhage in Left Posterior Fossa Resulting from Linear Skull Fracture.

A 10 year old boy on bicycle collided with pole; survived 30 hours in coma with diagnosis of concussion.
Left. Epidural hemorrhage covered by dura.
Middle. Appearance of hemorrhage after stripping dura. Clot weighed 70 gm.
Right. Angular linear fracture in left posterior fossa.

spheres in the parietal and temporal regions. The hemorrhage is usually a blood cyst, spherical in shape, which does not communicate with the brain surface; surface contusions of the brain tissue are usually present immediately adjacent to the cyst. The hemorrhage develops at the time of the injury or soon after, or the violence may cause a slight contusion of the brain tissue, the initial injury being followed

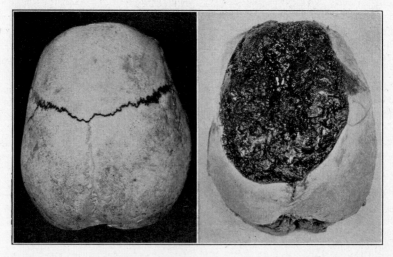

Fig. 12-28. Epidural Hemorrhage from Torn Longitudinal Dural Sinus.

Large epidural hemorrhage from longitudinal dural venous sinus lacerated by fracture of the vault of the skull which passed through the coronal suture. Impact against top of head. Automobile injury. Middle-aged white woman.

several days later by a large secondary subcortical hemorrhage. In some cases it is not easy to determine with certainty whether the hemorrhage was spontaneous or was referable to the trauma. The finding of cerebral vascular lesions and hypertensive heart disease would suggest the possibility of a spontaneous hemorrhage,

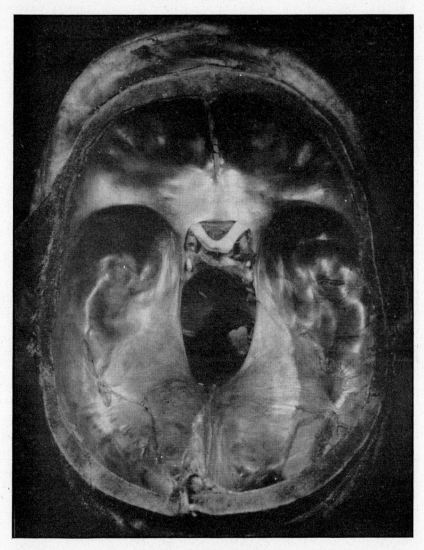

Fig. 12-29. Interior of Skull of Embalmed Body after Removal of Brain to Show Sharp Edge of Tentorium Cerebelli.

especially if signs of trauma were not present. On the other hand if injuries of the skull and brain were found, the appearance of which is consistent with the interval between the alleged injury and death of the victim, the evidence would favor the traumatic origin of the delayed secondary hemorrhage.

For example, an individual was injured about the head in an automobile accident which occurred three months prior to death. He recovered partially but not completely from the trauma. A few days before he died, he suddenly became comatose and remained in that state until death supervened. At autopsy there was no evidence of a skull fracture, but there were healed contrecoup lacerations of the frontal lobe of about three months duration and a large fresh subcortical hemorrhage in the frontal lobe. The presence of two lesions of different ages in the same area of the brain suggested that the injury may have laid the foundation for the second hemorrhage which occurred three months later.

The pons and the cerebral peduncles are often injured by an impact over the lateral parietal region, which drives the brain stem laterally, causing incomplete or almost complete laceration of a peduncle against the sharp edge of the ten-

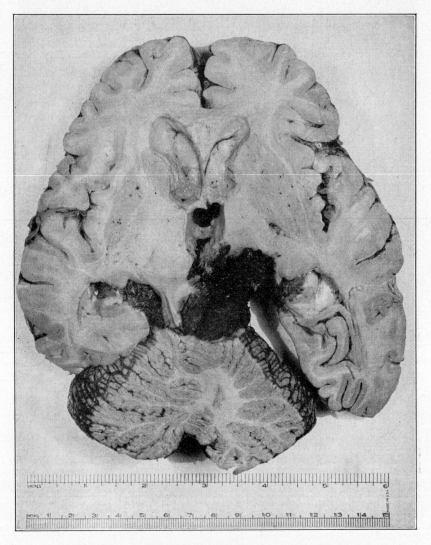

Fig. 12-30. Laceration of Right Cerebral Peduncle without Skull Fracture.

Complete laceration of peduncle caused by its impact against the edge of the tentorium cerebelli. Lateral jarring of head. Automobile injury.

torium (Figs. 12-29 and 12-30). In other cases the impact forces the brain downward so that the pons is driven against the basilar plate of the occiput, and small discrete hemorrhages, petechial in size or up to 5 mm. in diameter may occur either in the body of the pons or near the floor of the fourth ventricle where a few may rupture into that cavity. Similar lesions occur in traumatic cases in which a unilateral subdural or epidural hemorrhage presses the brain downward, and also in natural disease conditions like brain tumors which exert the same type of pressure. Under such circumstances the hemorrhages probably result from a rise in the pressure of the blood in the pontile blood vessels and from compression and distortion of the pons by the unilateral cerebral lesion. The pontile hemorrhages

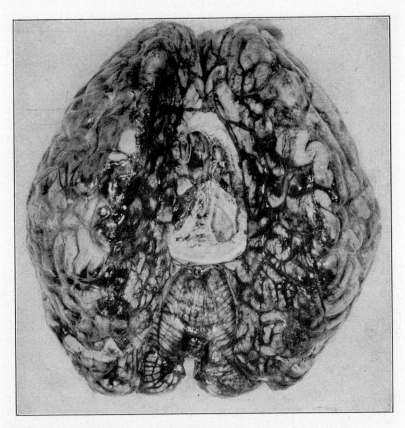

Fig. 12-31. Laceration of Corpus Callosum without Skull Fracture.

Complete laceration of the corpus callosum by impact against sharp edge of falx cerebri. Automobile injury.

of this type are usually discrete and multiple and different from the spontaneous hemorrhages of the pons which are large and massive.

The corpus callosum may be injured by impacts over the frontal or occipital regions which cause that structure to strike against the sharp edge of the falx cerebri. This may result in a complete severance of the corpus callosum (Fig. 12-31), or in widespread or localized contusions in its substance. Occasionally the ependymal surface is lacerated, and a moderate degree of hemorrhage into the lateral ventricles occurs.

Multiple small traumatic hemorrhages can occur in the white matter of the brain and in the basal nuclei as the result of an impact against the lateral frontal region. Such hemorrhages are usually petechial but may vary from 1 to 10 mm. in size. They may be spherical or elongated and are arranged in irregular groups. Some of the hemorrhages are found in the cortex as minute contusions (Fig.

12-32), and occasionally under the ependyma where they may break into the lateral ventricles to produce slight blood staining of the spinal fluid. The irregular distribution of the small traumatic hemorrhages differs from the even colony-like distribution of the punctate hemorrhages in cerebral fat embolism which are found only in the white matter and never in the cerebral cortex (Fig. 8-6). In doubtful

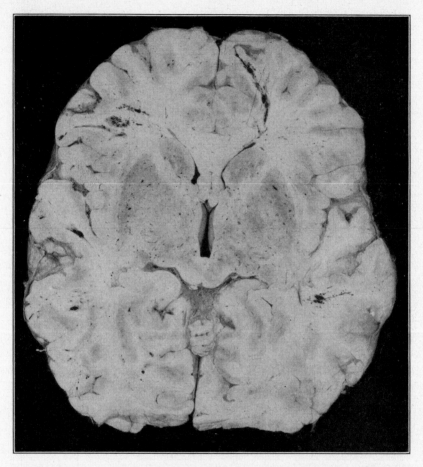

Fig. 12-32. Traumatic Concussion Hemorrhages of Brain without Skull Fracture.

Clusters of tiny hemorrhages in white matter of brain, and only a few in the cortex. They are of unequal size and uneven distribution. Deceased struck by automobile.
In such cases a fat stain should be made to rule out fat embolism.

cases microscopic sections should be made and stained appropriately to differentiate the traumatic hemorrhages from those caused by fat embolism or other conditions.

Multiple traumatic petechial hemorrhages in the brain have been suggested by Martland as the underlying condition eventually producing the punch drunk syndromes in prize fighters who have sustained severe and numerous beatings in the ring. Unfortunately the lesions in punch drunk fighters have not been described at autopsy and it is not certain whether the syndrome is entirely due to trauma. More observations are needed before this question can be decided satisfactorily. The brains of boxers who died after injuries received in the ring and were autopsied in the Office of the Chief Medical Examiner in New York City did not show small petechial hemorrhages or evidences of old petechial hemorrhages; most of them died as the result of a subdural hemorrhage from a tear of one of the veins connecting the pial vessels with the dural sinuses.

Moritz mentions lesions in cases of head injury which are of rare occurrence: among them are small reactionless hemorrhagic microscopic foci in the cortex, which are said to develop about 24 hours after trauma to the head. According to Ricker these lesions are the result of a local anoxemia produced in the smaller arteries by a reflex vasomotor disturbance due to the injury. He claims that microscopic sections of the brain have demonstrated areas of degeneration in the cerebral cortex, the optic thalamus, Ammon's horn and the Purkinje layer of the cerebellum, sometimes with loss of ganglion cells. Rarely there are capillary thromboses in the brain tissue surrounding the areas but in most cases the surrounding blood vessels do not show any obvious lesions. Helfand has also described minute foci of red softening in the brain which are believed to be due to derangement of the vasomotor mechanism.

The theory has also been advanced that the widespread, minute, traumatic hemorrhages in the brain may heal and cause minute scars in the brain tissue, a condition which has been given the name of traumatic encephalitis. Such scars are said to contract slowly, and to produce a number of progressive cerebral conditions, as for example the Parkinsonian syndrome. However, as Moritz has pointed out, the diagnosis of traumatic encephalitis should not be made in the individual case unless unmistakable signs of injury can be demonstrated elsewhere in the brain. At the same time the investigator should consider seriously the possibility that the lesions which have been attributed to traumatic encephalitis might be due to other causes.

Complications of Skull Fractures and Intracranial Injuries. SHOCK, CONCUSSION. Severe head injuries may produce typical traumatic shock (see Chapter 8). In addition, when the brain is severely jarred, deep unconsciousness or cerebral concussion results, a clinical phenomenon that can result from many different kinds of brain injury. Attempts have been made to attribute cerebral concussion exclusively to small petechial hemorrhages in the brain substance, which occasionally follow a severe impact to the head, but concussion occurs even more frequently with surface contusions and lacerations of the brain and is found with most types of traumatic cerebral lesions. Fatal concussion of the brain can be diagnosed at autopsy only by inference, that is by demonstrating severe scalp, skull and brain injuries consistent with the development of the complication.

In most cases of severe cerebral concussion, the unconsciousness occurs immediately after the injury and the individual will be incapable of locomotion. If the brain injury is a severe one, death may ensue rapidly, that is, within a few minutes or after a few hours. Needless to say a person suffering from this complication is a poor surgical risk. Death from concussion is not immediate unless the brain injury is very severe or the brain stem has been damaged. Even when the head injury is severe, as in the case of the depressed skull fractures inflicted with a hammer (Fig. 12-3), the stunned victim may retain consciousness and some orientation for a few minutes before relapsing into the coma of concussion. When consciousness is not lost immediately, the individual is usually confused and incoherent although he may be able to stagger around before collapsing.

Mild cases of concussion do occur in which the individual is stunned and rendered unconscious for only a short interval, and at the end of this period, his senses are recovered rapidly. Restoration of consciousness, however, is attended by a varying period of confusion and headache. Such mild cases are encountered in boxers who are knocked out in the ring and in individuals who receive minor blows to the head during falls or after impacts from missiles or blunt weapons. The concussion in such instances may occur in the absence of demonstrable brain injury and is not fatal. In practically all severe or fatal cases, the autopsy will reveal traumatic lesions of the scalp, skull or brain to explain why the concussion existed.

If the patient with concussion survives after 24 hours, he may succumb to hypostatic pneumonia or other complications. Some patients of strong vitality recover. Occasionally the victim may still be prostrated by concussion when cerebral compression due to intercranial hemorrhage develops and the symptoms of the former may merge with the latter.

There are several important considerations in the diagnosis of concussion. In some instances claims have been made that individuals suffering from severe coronary artery sclerosis, who suddenly dropped dead from a standing position and sustained minor scalp injuries as a consequence, died from cerebral concussion and not from their heart disease. Many unwarrantable legal actions have been filed for the purpose of collecting damages or accident insurance on the basis of such claims. The medical experts for the plaintiff usually contend that death occurred from cerebral concussion because of the insignificant scalp lacerations, even when the autopsy discloses the presence of a fatal degree of coronary artery disease and the absence of intracranial injury. There is complete disregard for the fact that death does not result rapidly or at all from mild concussion which is transitory and followed rapidly by recovery, but only occurs after severe concussion which is practically always accompanied by an easily demonstrable severe head injury and a definite period of post-traumatic unconsciousness. Without the post-traumatic unconsciousness, a diagnosis of cerebral concussion is not warranted. In some nonfatal cases it has been alleged that a postconcussion syndrome supervened, even though a period of unconsciousness did not follow the trauma. Such a diagnosis is illogical under the circumstances because proof of concussion is lacking.

Since mild cases of concussion may follow injury to the head without demonstrable injury to the brain, it is indispensable to ascertain the circumstances of the trauma and the symptoms which followed it in order to determine whether or not concussion of the brain was an actual factor in the case. Where death has occurred after trauma to the head in the absence of severe intracranial injuries, cerebral concussion can be excluded as the sole cause of death. In cases of this type, however, if there is a well authenticated period of unconsciousness after trauma, some degree of concussion may have contributed to the death. Thus an intoxicated person exhibits an increased susceptibility to this complication, because the brain is already under the influence of a depressant and even a slight brain injury may enhance the depression. In such instances death may result after a degree of violence which ordinarily would not be dangerous to life. In ascribing the cause of death in these cases the injury would only be part of it and the alcoholism or some other debilitating condition like heart disease or cerebral arteriosclerosis would also be partly responsible.

The question as to whether an injury is the sole or only a partial cause of death is important in deciding whether accident insurance death claims are to be paid and the subject of cerebral concussion is often considered in this connection. Accident insurance contracts stipulate that the accidental injury has to be the sole and exclusive cause of death independent of other disease conditions, and it is necessary to appraise the role of cerebral concussion in all cases in which that condition is suspected of being the final complication.

CEREBRAL COMPRESSION. Cerebral compression is an abnormal condition which results when any intracranial lesion arising from traumatic or natural disease processes exerts pressure on the brain. Although enclosed in a rigid cranial cavity, the brain is not subjected to any appreciable degree of compression under normal conditions. A dangerous degree of pressure may be produced by an intracranial process external to the brain, which causes a significant diminution of the volume of the skull cavity and encroaches on space normally occupied by brain tissue, as, for example, an accumulation of blood or inflammatory exudate, or an expanding meningeal neoplasm, or a depressed bone fragment. In other instances compression may be the result of a process in the brain substance, causing an undue increase in brain volume, which cannot adjust itself to the size of the cranial cavity, as, for example, cerebral hemorrhage, neoplasm, brain abscess, or obstruction to the outflow of cerebrospinal fluid out of the brain ventricles.

If the changes take place abruptly, the symptoms and signs of cerebral compression develop rapidly and terminate fatally in a short time. In such cases a localized or generalized cerebral edema may suddenly arise or a secondary cerebral hemorrhage occur, and the rapid increase in intracranial tension may precipitate sudden and violent symptoms. The same phenomena are sometimes noted in brain abscesses in which the infection erodes into the ventricles, or reaches the meninges and spreads out onto the surface of the brain. On the other hand if the changes develop gradually, as with a slowly expanding neoplasm, abscess or intracranial hemorrhage, the symptoms and signs may be insidious in their onset. It is not uncommon for a slowly growing brain tumor to compress the brain so gradually that the individual adapts himself to the changing conditions and may show no striking clinical manifestations for a considerable length of time.

Cerebral compression is produced in rare instances by some types of infection which are complications of skull fracture, such as large collections of pus in the subdural space, or by an abscess in the substance of the brain. Air inside the skull also causes death by compression of the brain (page 301).

INFECTION. The most common infectious lesion which complicates fractures of the skull is acute suppurative leptomeningitis in which a purulent exudate collects between the arachnoid and pia. In the series of 507 cases described by Vance, 48 died as the result of this complication. In some cases this infection is produced by the invasion of streptococci or other pyogenic micro-organisms into the skull cavity through a compound fracture of the vault, either at the time of injury or later by invasion of the open wound. In other cases a fracture which involves the roof of a cavity like the middle ear, the mastoid, or the sphenoidal, frontal or nasal sinuses may afford sufficient entrance to pneumococci or other infective agents, especially if the cavity contains pus, so that the subarachnoid space may be invaded and a fatal inflammation may be produced (Figs. 12-5 and 12-33). A suppurative leptomeningitis due to the meningococcus has been described by Clark and collaborators as a complication of skull fracture.

The suppurative infection may be confined to the leptomeninges in most cases, but occasionally an organism like the hemolytic streptococcus may spread throughout the body, causing a general septicemia with an acute vegetative endocarditis and septic emboli in different organs.

The *Staphylococcus aureus* or the *Streptococcus hemolyticus* may attack the dura and cause acute inflammations. In rare instances there may be a collection of pus between the outside of the dura and the inside of the skull near the site of the fracture. In other cases the inside of the dura may be lined by a purulent pseudomembrane or there may be enough pus present in the subdural space to cause definite cerebral compression. Both types of lesion are sometimes associated with signs of a general septicemia. Occasionally pyogenic cocci may invade the veins of the dura and cause a septic thrombosis in the lateral sinus or elsewhere which in turn may result in septic emboli and abscesses in the lung parenchyma.

Another infectious lesion caused by trauma is the brain abscess which develops as a result of an infection of a brain laceration by pyogenic bacteria. Such a laceration may occur immediately adjacent to a compound fracture of the vault of the skull or may be produced in the neighborhood of a fracture involving the roof of an infected bony sinus. If the laceration is a superficial one, the infective agent may cause a polymorphonuclear leukocytic infiltration and localized edema in the traumatized area, followed by swelling of the tissues and signs of cerebral compression. If a craniotomy opening is made near the abscess, the inflamed cerebral tissue may project through the opening and form a true hernia cerebri. If the laceration happens to be a deep one, pus may collect in the depths of the laceration and become walled off. The abscess may increase and burrow into the brain tissue until it invades the subarachnoid space or enters one of the ventricles of the brain, causing a fatal suppurative leptomeningitis or death by cerebral compression.

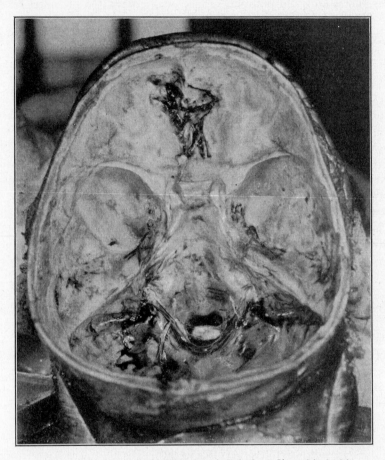

Fig. 12-33. Fracture of Nasal Bones and Cribriform Plate. Meningitis.

Fracture of nasal bones and cribriform plate with slight contusion of overlying frontal lobes of the brain. Death was caused by a complicating acute suppurative leptomeningitis, the infection entering from the nasal cavity through the fracture.

After they have become established, suppurative leptomeningitis or other infections of the brain are usually fatal. The first symptoms of intracranial infections do not develop as a rule for two or more days after the trauma, and, as many of the skull fractures which give rise to this complication are not attended by a disabling degree of cerebral concussion or cerebral compression from hemorrhage, it is not uncommon for the victim to be free of symptoms in the interval between the trauma and the onset of the fatal infection.

It must also be remembered that the intracranial infection in some cases may not be due to the fracture of the skull, for some of them, especially suppurative leptomeningitis, occur spontaneously or as a complication of natural disease processes, such as a pneumococcemia connected with a lobar pneumonia. As a general rule leptomeningitis and the other septic infections following head injury develop in about two days to two weeks, and if they appear after a much longer interval, their title as a complication of the trauma is subject to suspicion. In other cases there has been reason to believe that the meningitis found at autopsy was incurred prior to the fracture, and that the two lesions were not connected. The relation of the intracranial infection to the skull fracture must be appraised in the light of all the known facts in the case under discussion.

Persons who have sustained fractures of the skull may die after several days as a result of hypostatic pneumonia which is usually referable to the after-effects of cerebral concussion or compression of the brain produced by an intracranial injury. In such cases the concussion or the compression of the brain depresses the vital resistance of the victim so that hypostatic congestion of the lungs occurs and the hypostatic pneumonia develops in from two days to several weeks. In this connection it is necessary to consider that the victim may have been suffering from acute or chronic alcoholism or some other chronic disease condition at the time of the injury and that this process contributed to the formation of the pneumonia.

AIR INSIDE SKULL. A rare complication of fracture of the skull is the admission of air into the subdural space by a fracture which crosses the sphenoidal cavity and also lacerates the dura. Air thus enters through the opening and compresses the brain. The diagnosis of this condition during life is made by roentgenography.

Air may also enter the ventricles of the brain causing distention and death from cerebral compression. This complication occurs under rather rare conditions which allow air to enter the skull cavity and gain access to the ventricles, as in a combination of a fracture of the frontal bony sinus, a tear of the adjacent dura and a crateriform laceration of the frontal lobe which extends from the external surface into the lateral ventricle. The diagnosis has been made during life by roentgenograms which revealed the air in the ventricles of the brain. At autopsy, the brain should be removed from the skull under water so that any escape of air bubbles can be noticed.

EPILEPTIFORM CONVULSIONS. A late complication of skull fractures results from adhesions between the dura and the brain at the site of old brain lacerations. Adhesions may occur at any point on the surface of the brain but are most likely to be encountered on the under and outer surfaces of the frontal and temporal lobes where contrecoup lacerations were inflicted. The convulsions usually set in from several months to one or two years after the injuries have healed, and continue at intervals. They are either of the jacksonian or the generalized epileptiform type. Death sometimes ensues from asphyxia in the midst of a convulsion or from exhaustion due to status epilepticus.

CLINICAL CONSIDERATIONS. Many cases of skull fracture suffer at the outset such a severe grade of cerebral concussion that the victim remains unconscious or stuporous until a definite cerebral compression from an intracranial injury develops. The patient is practically unconscious and incapable of locomotion during his entire clinical course up to the time of his death.

Some fractures of the skull are inflicted with a less severe grade of concussion and remain in coma for a length of time varying from several minutes to a few hours. When consciousness returns, the victim complains of severe headache, and displays evidence of irritability, mental confusion and psychotic manifestations; he is apt to refuse medical attention. Later he becomes drowsy, aphasic and sinks back into coma, gradually or abruptly. Epileptiform or jacksonian convulsions may occur at this stage. The blood pressure and the intraspinal pressure may rise. The pupils may become unequal, and as a rule the dilated pupil occurs on the side where the cerebral compression is developing. Other neurologic signs may be present such as inequality in the reflexes or different paralyses, which show a unilateral distribution.

Other individuals sustain a fracture and a serious intracranial injury but the degree of cerebral concussion may be slight or even absent. This is especially apt to be the case if the skull is thin and the force producing the fracture not severe. In such instances the middle meningeal artery may be torn or the brain lacerated without an excessive degree of violence. The patient recovers consciousness quickly in many cases and is able to walk, but after a lucid interval of varying length during which he can wander far from the scene of the accident, he becomes unconscious a second time from cerebral compression due to intracranial injury. Epidural hemorrhages may allow a lucid interval of several minutes to a few hours; subdural hemorrhages allow an interval of a few hours to several days. In rare instances a victim with a thin skull may sustain a small depressed fracture of the temporal bone during fisticuffs without losing consciousness, but after a few hours may sink into coma as a result of a lacerated middle meningeal artery and an epidural hemorrhage.

The cases of head injury which develop cerebral compression a few hours after the trauma sometimes offer a difficult problem in diagnosis, especially if the victim is intoxicated at the time of examination. When head injury and alcoholism are combined, it is occasionally difficult to elicit signs and symptoms characteristic of the former. An inexperienced surgeon may dismiss such a case as an example of simple alcoholic intoxication, especially if there are no injuries on the surface of the body and head to suggest the possibility of serious intracranial traumatic complications. In the statistics of Vance, cases of cerebral compression due to intracranial hemorrhages or cerebral lacerations die usually in the first 24 hours after the trauma, but a substantial minority succumb after two days to a week or longer.

The diagnosis of cerebral compression is suggested by a rise in blood pressure and intraspinal pressure, and by unilateral distribution of the neurologic signs. In the early stages the pressure affects the brain on the side of the hemorrhage and the neurologic signs are contralateral. In the later stages, however, as the cerebral compression becomes generalized, the neurologic signs may change and become homolateral or bilateral, thus adding to the difficulties of the diagnosis. The spinal fluid usually contains blood if the brain is lacerated, except in rare instances in which the laceration is small. If a subdural hemorrhage from a ruptured communicating vein is present, and not accompanied by subarachnoid hemorrhage, the spinal fluid may be clear for a few days after the trauma, but later may become xanthochromic. If the injury is an uncomplicated epidural hemorrhage, the spinal fluid is usually clear.

Decompression operations on the skull, or craniotomies, are performed in cases of cerebral compression, and are frequently successful in epidural hemorrhages. The objective of the craniotomy is to remove the clot and ligate the bleeding artery. In many cases of subdural hemorrhage, the dura is opened, the hemorrhage evacuated, and recovery takes place. Craniotomies are also performed on compound fractures and depressed fractures in which loose fragments of bone are removed to lessen the danger of infection and relieve pressure.

The decision of whether or not to perform a craniotomy in the presence of doubtful signs of unilateral cerebral compression is difficult. In many cases the surgeon is guided by the history of a lucid interval between periods of unconsciousness, misinterprets the clinical picture as one resulting from head trauma, and is led to operate. Rarely cases of cerebral fat embolism from a fractured long bone of the leg, associated with superficial injuries about the head, have been subjected to a useless craniotomy because the interval between the trauma and the coma was mistaken for the lucid period of an intracranial injury and suggested an erroneous diagnosis. In elderly individuals with a head injury, a craniotomy has been performed erroneously, because the patient lapsed into coma after a lucid interval with a few ambiguous neurologic signs, which misled the surgeon into diagnosing the presence of an intracranial hemorrhage when in reality the patient was dying of a combination of traumatic shock and advanced cerebral arteriosclerosis. On the other hand an epidural hemorrhage may be located at a distance from the motor area of the cortex so that typical unilateral signs of cerebral compression may be obscured, and this may influence the surgeon not to operate when the operation would be indicated. The best results are obtained when the intracranial hemorrhages are evacuated early after the trauma, for then the brain has the best chance of recovering its normal condition and volume. If the operation is delayed for several days, the effused blood may be removed successfully at craniotomy, but the distortion of the brain may persist after operation until death occurs a few days later. In some of these cases in which operation was not attempted, a secondary pontile hemorrhage had developed as a complication.

The practice of some surgeons of puncturing the brain with a trocar during craniotomy, presumably in an attempt to discover subcortical hematomas, has produced fatal penetrating wounds of the brain (page 351). This procedure should be used with caution and is not to be recommended as a routine method of exploration during a craniotomy.

Correlation of Skull Fractures and Their Complications. Cerebral concussion accompanies most skull fractures and need not be reconsidered. The other complications vary considerably with the location of the injury.

IMPACT FRACTURES OF THE VAULT AND BASE. *Lateral Fractures.* The linear fracture starts on the vault, near or in front of the parietal boss, and descends forward and downward into the middle fossa or the anterior fossa; most of them are directed toward the central point of the skull. A few fractures may descend slightly backward into the posterior fossa. A small number may run over the vault toward the opposite side of the skull, and if the force has been intense enough the fracture may be circumferential and divide the skull into anterior and posterior parts (Fig. 9-8). Composite fractures vary from the angular and dendritic forms to those exhibiting marked comminution of the side of the skull (Fig. 12-4).

The complications are direct lacerations of the cerebral hemisphere on the side of the fracture, and contrecoup lacerations of the outer surfaces of the frontal and temporal lobes on the opposite cerebral hemisphere. Subdural hemorrhages occur from direct laceration, from contrecoup laceration, or from both together. Epidural hemorrhages are produced by this type more than by any other and usually occur in the parietal and temporal regions. Suppurative meningitis and other septic infections are common complications, because the middle ear and mastoid often communicate with a crack in the bone.

Bleeding from the ear is usually the result of a lateral fracture and is caused by direct injury of the external ear canal or by tearing of the tympanic membrane. Occasionally a small subcutaneous hemorrhage may be found in the mastoid region (Battle's sign) on the side of the fracture (page 262).

Occipital Fractures. The linear fractures start in the occipital bone or the posterior portion of the parietal bone and run down into the posterior fossae, toward the foramen magnum or the jugular foramina. Some may be directed into the middle fossae, and some involve the middle ear (Figs. 12-4, 12-5 and 12-27).

Composite fractures in the occipital region are angular and dendritic or are markedly comminuted (Fig. 12-6). Another type is the fracture which starts in the midline and diverges along the lambdoid sutures into the right and left middle fossae, meeting in the region of the sella turcica. A circular piece of bone at the base is thus separated from the rest of the skull.

Another type starts as a linear crack which passes over the vault as well as into the base, practically splitting the skull in the sagittal plane.

The complications are, first, contrecoup lacerations on the under surface and tips of the frontal and temporal lobes, which may give rise to unilateral or bilateral subdural hemorrhages, the most common lesions produced by these fractures. The lacerations are sometimes extensive and are either of the broad shallow type (Figs. 12-5 and 12-7), or of the cavernous crateriform type which extend deeply into the subcortical white matter.

Direct lacerations are encountered on the cerebellum or on the occipital lobes and are usually minor injuries. In a few cases, however, the cerebellum may be lacerated (Fig. 12-6) and bleed freely into the space below the tentorium, causing death by cerebral compression. Epidural hemorrhages (Figs. 12-26 and 12-27) are rare and occur mostly from a torn lateral sinus. Septic infections are not common with this injury.

Frontal Fractures. Linear fractures run either backward across the anterior fossa from the midline or start in the lateral frontal region, and are directed transversely toward the opposite side. Composite fractures generally show comminution of the orbital plates and extension backward into the middle fossae. Fractures of the orbital plates are accompanied by hematomas of the eyelids.

Lacerations of the brain are mainly the result of comminution of the orbital plates, and are direct lacerations of the under surface of the frontal lobes. Fatal subdural hemorrhages are produced occasionally by this lesion. Many patients with such brain injuries develop a hypostatic pneumonia which is the cause of death. Contrecoup lacerations of the occipital lobes occur sometimes but are rarely serious. Often a lateral impact in the frontal region causes small traumatic hemorrhages of petechial size in the brain substance. Epidural hemorrhages are rare and occur from a tear of the anterior meningeal artery as it enters the anterior fossa.

Suppurative meningitis and other intracranial infections are common as a complication of frontal fractures with other fractures, because the nasal cavity or accessory bony sinuses are usually involved (Fig. 12-33).

Fractures of the Vault. The linear, composite and depressed fractures may develop complications not unlike lateral fractures of vault and base. Most of the linear and composite types are located in the parietal regions.

Depressed fractures give rise to brain lacerations which are mostly direct and less often contrecoup. Epidural hemorrhages are relatively common with vault fractures. One interesting variety is a small depressed fracture which is encountered in the squamous portion of the temporal bone. This fracture can be produced by a slight degree of violence, such as a blow with the fist, and it occasionally lacerates the middle meningeal artery giving rise to a fatal epidural hemorrhage (Figs. 12-24 and 12-25).

The characteristics of symmetric fractures around the foramen magnum and of compression fractures of the skull have already been discussed (Figs. 12-8 and 12-9).

INTRACRANIAL INJURIES WITHOUT FRACTURE OF THE SKULL

Force applied to the head may cause a number of intracranial injuries without fracture of the skull.

First, a violence applied to the posterior part of the skull in some instances may cause the brain to oscillate against the frontal region of the cranium and produce contrecoup lacerations of the frontal or temporal lobes. From such lacerations a fatal hemorrhage may occur in the subdural space. A direct laceration of the brain posteriorly is not likely to occur in a trauma of this sort.

Second, numerous traumatic hemorrhages of varying size may be produced in various parts of the brain, such as the pons, basal nuclei, corpus callosum, white matter and to a lesser extent the cortex. These lesions and the manner of their production have already been described on pages 294 and 295 (Fig. 12-32). Similarly the corpus callosum can be lacerated by the sharp edge of the falx cerebri (Fig. 12-31) and the pons and cerebral peduncles torn by impact against the tentorium (Figs. 12-29 and 12-30).

Third, a force applied to the skull will tear or rupture veins, which bleed into the subdural space. The communicating veins which run from the pia to the superior longitudinal sinus may be torn by blows against the side of the head in boxing matches. Tears of communicating veins between the temporal lobe of the brain and the dura occasionally occur (Fig. 12-15). Ruptures of surface veins of the arachnoid have been described by Leary and also encountered by the authors. Sometimes a trauma will rupture blood vessels in old adhesions of the brain to the dura and cause a subdural hemorrhage. The authors have encountered a traumatic hemorrhage in the left subdural space as a result of a lateral impact in the right temporal region, which tore a communicating vein on the surface of the left parietal lobe, at the same time causing a pinpoint rupture of the adjacent cortical artery and the overlying arachnoid membrane (Fig. 12-34).

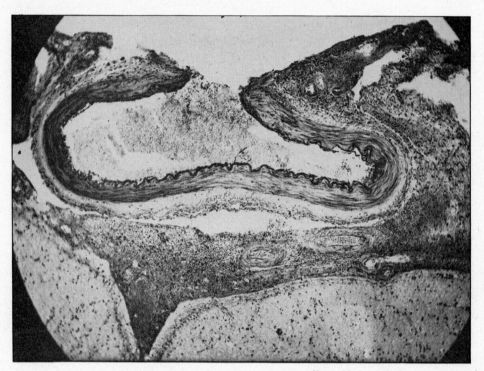

Vance, M. B., *Arch. Surg.*, 61:992, 1950

Fig. 12-34. Tear of Branch of Surface Artery on Left Temporal Lobe Resulting in Fatal Subdural Hemorrhage.

A 43 year old Negro woman, struck by chair during assault, survived 40 hours.

The subject of acute and chronic subdural hemorrhage has been discussed on pages 277 and 285 under Subdural Hemorrhage (Figs. 12-11 to 12-20).

FRACTURES OF FACIAL BONES

The malar bone is fractured by direct violence applied to the cheek by a blow from a blunt instrument or from the fist, or by a severe impact in a highway accident, or during a fall. The fractures are transverse to the long axis of the bone and are either single or multiple. Most of them are present in the posterior third of the bone, the slender portion in front of the ear canal, but may occur anywhere along its length. If the violence is severe, the malar bone may be broken off from the outer edge of the orbit. The cheek is often flattened and the bony fragments are bent inward. A marked hematoma may occur in the surrounding tissues of the cheek, which may obscure the fractures. The examiner should expose the malar bone in order not to overlook these injuries. The most serious complications of this type of fracture are traumatic lesions of the brain, especially the multiple small hemorrhages of the cerebral hemispheres, described on page 296, due to the forceful lateral impact against the cheek. After a few days a septic inflammation of the adjacent parotid gland may develop in the form of small abscesses in the parenchyma, probably referable to interference with drainage of the parotid ducts as a result of pressure from the hemorrhage in the tissues of the cheek. Many fractures of the malar bones heal without complications.

The nasal bones are fractured as a result of severe impact from direct violence. The fracture may occur at the junction of the nasal bones with the frontal or the bones may be extensively comminuted with depression and deformity of the nose. Occasionally the cartilaginous nasal septum is separated from its posterior attachment. The principal complication is a hemorrhage of greater or lesser severity from ruptured blood vessels in the nares which may be external, or aspirated into the air passages, or swallowed into the stomach. The deeper structures in the nasal cavity may be injured and fractures of the cribriform plate may be produced (Fig. 12-32), which in turn may give rise to a suppurative meningitis. Occasionally a minor fracture of the nasal bones occurs in an individual who falls from a standing position during a fatal coronary artery attack and strikes his nose against the ground. Such injuries must be correlated with the findings at autopsy in order to ascertain their significance. This subject has been discussed on pages 124 to 125.

The superior maxilla may be broken by generalized violence such as occurs in falls from a height or in highway accidents, or by severe localized violence such as repeated blows with a club. The face may show numerous abrasions, contusions and lacerations, and fractures of other bones may result with considerable deformity. The fractures usually encountered produce a separation of the superior maxilla from its posterior attachments, and in some cases from the orbits. Occasionally a midline sagittal fracture extends from the nasal opening to the posterior part of the palate and frequently the alveolar processes are broken inward or bent upward. The victims may die from shock or hemorrhage. Those who survive the immediate effects may develop some form of septic infection, such as an abscess of the antrum which may extend to the meninges and cause an acute suppurative meningitis. Most fractures of the superior maxilla are followed by inhalation of blood and infective material from the mouth; an aspiration suppurative pneumonia may result. If anaerobic organisms are inhaled, they may give rise to a putrid type of suppurative bronchopneumonia or lung abscess.

Fractures of the mandible are caused by localized impacts such as blows with a fist or blunt weapon like a club or stick or metal bar or pipe, or they may result from a generalized violence. The fractures are usually vertical, either single or multiple and may occur anywhere on the jaw bone. The most commonly encountered fracture is located in the body between the canine and the first bicuspid teeth and may be caused by a blow or punch. The authors have observed fractures through the symphysis of the body of the jaw, at the angle, through the ramus, and across the neck of the articular process. If the force and the injuries are severe enough death may result from shock. The gums are frequently torn and the teeth loosened or avulsed. Infective material may be aspirated during a period of unconsciousness or subsequently during a general anesthesia and a fatal gangrenous bronchopneumonia may develop; occasionally an avulsed tooth is found aspirated in a bronchus. Infection of the wounds may occur subsequently and an osteomyelitis of the fractured mandible ensue. Localized or spreading septic infection may complicate the process. The tongue may be contused or lacerated, sometimes resulting in severe hemorrhage or in a septic infection. In many cases, in which the mandible is fractured, there are associated intracranial injuries and cerebral concussion.

MEDICOLEGAL CONSIDERATIONS

The surgeon who attends a head injury should keep an accurate clinical record of the case, particularly noting the character and extent of any external injuries. If a craniotomy is performed, the conditions found at operation should be described. If a depressed fracture is present, the shape and size of the fragments and of the depression should be determined, especially in cases where bone is removed at operation. Such injuries may be the result of a blow with a blunt instrument and may have a characteristic pattern. Unless the surgeon enters all his observations on the patient's chart, important clues and evidence useful to the law enforcement agencies may be lost. In all cases in which criminal violence is suspected, the surgeon must make it his business to see that the police are duly informed about the injury. Any foreign fragments extracted during operation should be given to the responsible police officer without delay.

Head injuries offer many vexing diagnostic problems which occasionally have medicolegal implications. Many fractures of the skull are caused by violence which does not leave any visible mark on the head, and they occur frequently when the victim is intoxicated by alcohol. While in deep coma the injured person may come under the observation of the surgeon, and the combination of alcoholism and the absence of any external evidence of traumatic injury may mislead the doctor so that he ascribes all the clinical manifestations to alcohol alone. The situation is even more dangerous when the injured person is intoxicated and conscious, for then the tendency of the inexperienced doctor is to dismiss the case as not serious. This is sometimes followed by the death of the victim later on from cerebral compression due to intracranial injury—either in a prison cell or in some other place where medical attention is not available. The surgeon who treats head injuries must keep in mind that he may be examining the victim during the lucid interval which precedes the onset of the coma due to cerebral compression brought about by the development of a fatal traumatic intracranial hemorrhage, and should not dismiss the patient without having considered the possibility of serious intracranial injury and of the necessity for surgical intervention.

At autopsy the examiner should measure and decribe all external wounds carefully and all injuries of the skull and brain. Drawings and photographs of the important lesions are especially valuable for preserving a record of the case. Occasionally a depressed fracture of the vault may be of such a nature that it can be removed and retained as part of the corpus delicti. Any portion of a blunt instrument found in the skull should be handed over to the responsible detectives. In addition blood must be preserved in suspicious cases for determination of the groups, and hair from the scalp should be retained, for comparison with blood or fibers which may be found on blunt instruments or automobiles.

REFERENCES

Baker, A. B. Subdural hematoma, Arch. Path., 26:535, 1938.
Cassasa, C. S. B. Multiple traumatic cerebral hemorrhages, Proc. New York Path. Soc. 24:101, 1924.

Clark, E., Redish, J., and Jolliffe, N. Meningococcic meningitis complicating fracture of the skull, Arch. Surg., 35:486, 1937.

Dandy, W. E. Pneumocephalus, Arch. Surg., 12:949, 1926.

Ford, F. R. Cerebral birth injuries and their results, Medicine, 5:121, 1926.

Friedman, E. D. Head injuries: effects and their appraisal; encephalic observations, Arch. Neurol. & Psychiat., 27:791, 1932.

Greenfield, J. G. Histology of cerebral edema associated with intracranial tumors, Brain, 62:129, 1939.

Hart, C., and Mayer, E. Henke und Lubarsch: III. 1. Atmungswege und Lungen, Berlin, Julius Springer, 1928, p. 419.

Helfand, M. Cerebral lesions due to vasomotor disturbances following brain trauma, J. Nerv. & Ment. Dis., 90:157, 1939.

Leary, T. Traumatic intracranial hemorrhages, Am. J. Surg., 26:133, 1934.

——— Subdural hemorrhages, J.A.M.A., 103:897, 1934.

Martland, H. S. Punch Drunk, J.A.M.A., 91:1103, 1928.

Moritz, A. R. The Pathology of Trauma. Philadelphia, Lea & Febiger, 1942.

——— and Wortman, W. B. Post-traumatic internal hydrocephalus, A. J. M. Sc., 195:65, 1938.

Penfield, W. Mechanism of cicatricial contraction in the brain, Brain, 50:499, 1927.

Putnam, T. J. Chronic subdural hematoma, Arch. Surg., 11:329, 1925.

Rand, C. W., and Courville, C. Histologic changes in the brain in cases of fatal injury to the head. Reaction of classic neuroglia, Arch. Neurol. & Psychiat., 27:1342, 1932. III. Reaction of microglia and oligodendroglia, Arch. Neurol. & Psychiat., 27:605, 1932. V. Changes in the nerve fibers, Arch. Neurol. & Psychiat., 31:527, 1934.

Ricker, G. Die Entstehung der pathologisch-anatomischen Befunde nach Hirnschütterung in Abhändigkeit von Gefassnerven System des Hirns, Virchows Arch. f. path. Anat., 226:180, 1919.

Shapiro, P., and Jackson, H. Swelling of the brain in cases of injury to the head, Arch. Surg., 25:529, 1932.

Spielmeyer, W. Histopathologie des Nervensystems, Berlin, Julius Springer, 1922.

Strassmann, G. Formation of hemosiderin and hematoidin after traumatic and spontaneous cerebral hemorrhages, Arch. Path., 47:205, 1949.

Vance, B. M. Ruptures of surface blood vessels on cerebral hemispheres as a cause of subdural hemorrhage, Arch. Surg., 61:992, 1950.

——— Fractures of the skull, Arch. Surg., 14:1023, 1927.

Wilson, G., and Winkelman, N. Gross pontile bleeding in traumatic and nontraumatic cerebral lesions, Arch. Neurol. & Psychiat., 15:455, 1926.

Wortis, S. B. Head injuries: effects and their appraisal; experimental studies of induced convulsions and ventricular distortion in cat, Arch. Neurol. & Psychiat., 27:776, 1932.

——— and McCulloch, W. S. Head injuries: experimental study, Arch. Surg., 25:529, 1932.

13

Blunt Force Injuries
of the Neck and Spine

INJURIES OF THE NECK

The structures within the neck, aside from the spinal column, are not injured frequently by ordinary blunt force. The traumas which consistently cause strangulation and asphyxia are not included in this discussion, but, because of their highly specialized character, are considered in detail in Chapter 17. The neck organs are affected directly by blunt force, either localized like a blow or kick against the larynx, or generalized as in a fall from a height in which the neck strikes against a projection like a clothes line or other obstruction, or in a highway accident in which the neck is crushed by an automobile wheel passing over it.

A localized blunt force may not produce any external wound on the skin, or it may produce contusions, abrasions and lacerations on the head and neck not characteristic of any particular type of trauma, but always an indication that the neck organs should be carefully dissected. Thus the authors have investigated a fatal case of rape in which there were swelling and bruising of the left side of the head and neck as if from repeated blows. On dissecting the neck, hemorrhages in the cervical muscles and laryngeal mucous membrane and a fracture of the left superior horn of the thyroid cartilage were found. In some cases of blunt force injury of the neck death occurs rapidly as a result of severe shock, or laryngeal spasm, or cardiac inhibition induced by the carotid sinus reflex described by Hering. In such cases there may not be any fractures of the larynx or hyoid bone, and hemorrhage in the laryngeal mucous membrane and neck muscles may be the only sign of violence. Pressure alone on the carotid sinus may elicit the Hering reflex and cause sudden cardiac stoppage and death. In other instances the trauma also produces fractures of the hyoid bone and laryngeal cartilages and dislocations of the cartilages. Death either results from shock or may occur later from asphyxia induced gradually by hemorrhage, edema or emphysema developing in the submucous layer of the glottis and occluding its aperture. Tears of the mucous membrane of the trachea or larynx may cause submucosal emphysema extending into the neck and mediastinum and result in fatal asphyxia. In a few cases the laryngeal injury heals and the scar tissue which forms may cause obstruction of the lumen several months later necessitating operative interference.

The injuries produced by generalized blunt force on the neck are similar to those already described for the extremities. The structures in the neck, like the larynx, trachea, esophagus, muscles, nerves and blood vessels, may be contused or torn. In fatal cases death usually results from shock and localized hemorrhage and occasionally from a secondary infection; it may also occur from obstructive asphyxia induced by edema, emphysema or hematoma formation in the mucous membrane of the throat or larynx. Injuries to the recurrent laryngeal nerves may cause paralysis of the vocal cords.

INJURIES OF THE SPINE

ANATOMY. It is necessary to describe the anatomic features of the vertebral column and spinal cord before considering the injuries of these structures. The spinal cord is a strip of the central nervous system, which is suspended from the lower end of the medulla at the foramen magnum, and extends down inside the spinal canal to the level of the first lumbar segment from whence it is continued as a fine thread, the filum terminale. Nerves in pairs are given off from each side of the cord for its entire length, and at its lower end they occur in such numbers as to form a structure like a horse's tail, known as the cauda equina. Some of the nerve tracts in the white matter of the cord transmit efferent impulses from the brain to the cord, and others convey afferent impulses from the periphery to the brain. Neurons in the anterior and posterior horns of the gray matter of the cord play their part in systematizing these different impulses, the cells in the anterior horn governing the efferent impulses, while those in the posterior horn receive the afferent impulses.

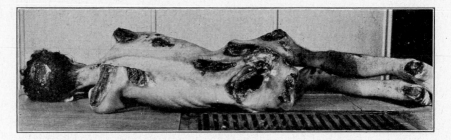

Fig. 13-1. Gangrenous Decubital Ulcerations Resulting from Spinal Cord Injury.

These have occurred over the areas of pressure on the back of the body. They involve scalp, scapular regions, length of the spine, buttocks, hips, knees and heels. The bony prominences have been laid bare. These trophic lesions and a suppurative cystitis and pyelonephritis were caused by a bullet wound of the cervical portion of the spinal cord. Death occurred four months after the shooting.

The integrity of the spinal cord is necessary if the health of the body is to be maintained. Sensory impulses, motor impulses and trophic impulses are conducted up and down the cord, and if the spinal cord is divided completely by an injury, the conduction system is deranged and disturbances occur. The muscles below the level of the cord lesion are paralyzed, visceral control is gone, sensation is lost, paralysis of the bladder occurs and trophic phenomena in the form of decubital ulcers result (Fig. 13-1).

The spinal column is the bony protection for the spinal cord and it is this function which gives it so much importance in the consideration of the different forms of trauma. Structurally the spine is composed of 7 cervical vertebrae, 12 dorsal vertebrae, 5 lumbar vertebrae, the wedge-shaped sacrum composed of 5 fused vertebrae, and the os coccyx, a small bone attached to the lower end of the sacrum. The sacrum is supported on both sides at the sacro-iliac joints by the pelvic girdle, and it in turn supports the rest of the spinal column composed of lumbar, dorsal and cervical regions. The uppermost cervical vertebra supports the skull and facial bones, while the dorsal spinal column is the mainstay of the thorax and the pectoral girdle.

The anterior portion of the spinal column is composed of segments of bone, the bodies of the vertebrae, held together by elastic disks of fibrocartilage. These disks are said to form about one quarter of the entire spinal length. From the posterior surfaces of the bodies, processes of bones extend out on each side uniting posteriorly to form an arch which surrounds the spinal cord and its membranes. Each arch is composed of a right and left anterior lamina and a right and left posterior lamina. At the junction of the posterior and anterior laminae are the right and left transverse processes. At the junction of the posterior laminae in the mid line are the spinous processes. In addition the vertebral segments have on each side of the spinal arch an articular process for the segment above and one for the segment below. The entire column is supported by ligaments of considerable strength. It can be considered as a hollow tube, well buttressed on all sides but especially in front where the vertebral bodies are articulated.

The uppermost segment of the spine consisting of the seven cervical vertebrae is the most flexible and delicate division of the column, because of the anterior curve and the oblique articulation of the bodies with the intervertebral disks which allow free play anteroposteriorly and laterally. The first cervical vertebra is peculiar in shape as it possesses cup-formed articular surfaces for the articular processes of the occipital bone. Its body is a curved piece of bone on the posterior surface of which rests the odontoid process (dens) of the second cervical vertebra or axis (epistropheus). The odontoid process projects upward from the upper surface of the body of the axis and forms a pivot around which the atlas rotates. The two bones are not joined by lateral articular processes. The other cervical segments conform to the usual vertebral types.

The dorsal or thoracic spinal segment is a comparatively rigid and solidly built structure which articulates with the ribs on each side of the body so that it forms the posterior buttress for the thoracic cage. The thoracic vertebrae have relatively slight play of movement on one another as contrasted with the mobility of the cervical segments.

The lumbar segments support the chest and all parts above it. The bodies of these vertebrae are large and composed of cancellous bone and their articular surfaces are horizontal. These vertebrae are pressed upon by the solid thoracic segments above and rest upon the rigid dense sacral bone below.

A significant anatomic feature of the spinal column is that two comparatively vulnerable divisions, the cervical and lumbar regions, are in juxtaposition to more solidly constructed segments, the thoracic and the sacral. This factor has a distinct influence upon the mechanism and location of many of the fractures and injuries which affect the spine.

TYPES OF TRAUMA. In considering the types of trauma sustained by the spinal column, the pathologist is at the disadvantage of being unable to reconstruct the accident except from information furnished him by others. Consequently, in many instances, he will not be able to tell definitely just how the deceased was injured by the violence, unless the pathologic lesions themselves furnish him with a clue.

The spinal column may be fractured by direct or indirect violence.

Direct Violence. Fractures and luxations of the spine by direct violence are produced when any force is applied directly to the back and breaks the bone at that point. Direct violence can act on any portion of the vertebral column, but the thoracic segment is involved most frequently. The injuries vary from isolated fractures of the spinous processes and laminae to complete transverse fractures and luxations through the vertebral body with crushing of the cord. The types of trauma which produce such direct injuries are encountered in automobile accidents (usually by the car running over the back), falls from a height onto a projecting object, or severe impacts of falling objects (Figs. 13-2 and 13-3).

Death may result from the shock of the trauma or from septic complications of the cord injury. A fatal hemorrhage into the chest cavities sometimes is produced when the twisting action of an automobile wheel luxates the thoracic vertebrae, usually in the region of the fourth to the ninth segments, tearing the pleura on each side of the spinal column and causing partial or complete transverse rupture of the descending aorta (Fig. 11-18). In one case a luxation of the fourth thoracic segment on the fifth was attended by a tear of the parietal pleura and rupture of the vena azygos major, followed by bleeding into the right chest. In another case, by a similar mechanism, the thoracic duct was torn by a dislocation of the tenth dorsal vertebra on the eleventh, with extravasation of a pint and a half of chyle into the right chest. Death in this instance was due to other injuries.

Indirect Violence. Indirect violence may bend or twist the spinal column in an exaggerated fashion, causing fractures or dislocations from overdistortion. This is most likely to occur when an individual falls from a height landing on his buttocks or shoulders (Fig. 13-2), dives into shallow water, is crushed under a mass of earth, or is forcibly doubled up in an automobile collision.

Fractures of the Spine. THE CERVICAL SPINAL SEGMENTS. Most of the indirect fractures involving the cervical vertebrae are caused by falls on the head or the back of the neck. An extreme overflexion is produced in this portion of the spinal column, a variety of serious injuries result, and the cervical spinal cord may be damaged.

The lesions produced by overflexion or excessive bending are:

1. Forward dislocation of the skull on the atlas, with tearing of occipito-atlantal ligaments. The caliber of the spinal canal below the foramen magnum is narrowed or obliterated and the upper portion of the spinal cord is either contused, crushed or severed by the violently displaced skull. Death usually occurs rapidly or immediately after such an injury as a result of the traumatization of the cord so near the vital medullary centers.

2. Backward luxation of the odontoid process of the axis in the cervical canal, due to the tearing of the ligaments which hold this bone in place. The luxation may be partial or complete, and the injury of the spinal cord varies from a central contusion to a complete crushing. If the odontoid is also fractured transversely through its base (Fig. 13-4), the same type of injury of the cord may result usually with rapid death. In some of these cases the fracture of the odontoid permits that segment of bone to be carried forward with the luxated atlas and spinal cord thereby may escape injury. This has been emphasized by Watson-Jones.

The upper spinal injuries are demonstrated best by removing the skull cap and brain and exposing the foramen magnum. Normally the canal through the foramen magnum into the spine is ovoid or cordiform in shape, but when a dislocation of the atlas or odontoid process is present, anteroposterior dimension of the opening is narrowed to a transverse or crescent slit. In extreme cases the cord is severed and the foramen magnum may open into the nasopharynx. In forward dislocations of the skull on the spine, fractures of the occipital condyles may occur.

Overflexion of the spine may cause a forward luxation or subluxation of the cervical segments, varying from loosening of the intervertebral cartilages to a

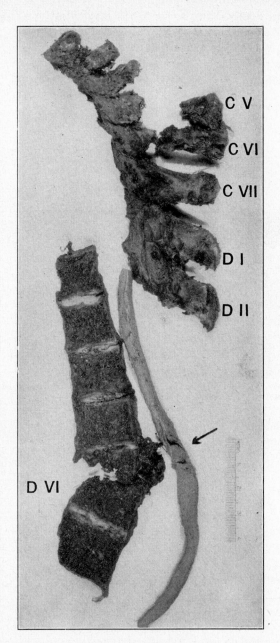

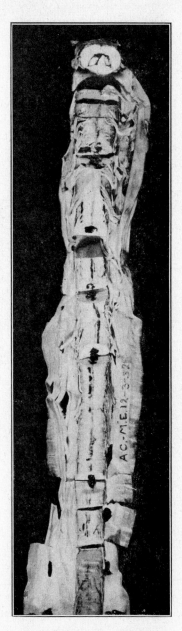

Fig. 13-2. Direct and Indirect Fractures of the Spine.

Direct fracture of spinous processes of fifth and sixth cervical vertebrae, and indirect fracture of body of sixth dorsal vertebra, with knuckling backward and crushing of the spinal cord at that level (arrow). Negro male, 39 years old, lived six hours after falling backward and head down from second story window, landing on neck and shoulders.

Fig. 13-3. Traumatic Hemorrhage in Spinal Cord: Direct Fracture Dislocation of Spine.

Hemorrhage in lower cervical and upper dorsal levels of cord; fracture dislocation of lower cervical spine; caused by sack of flour falling on back of neck.

complete dislocation of the vertebral bodies, with tearing of all attachments, ligaments and articular connections. The vertebrae dislocated in many cases are the third on the fourth, the sixth on the seventh and the seventh on the first dorsal. The spinous processes may be fractured by the ligamentary tension and muscular pull inflicted upon them during the luxation of the vertebral bodies. Occasionally the intervertebral disk is crushed with herniation of fragmented fibrocartilage posteriorly

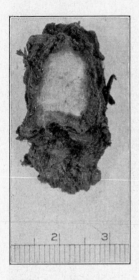

Fig. 13-4. Fracture Dislocation of Odontoid Process of Axis.

Transverse fracture and dislocation through the base of the odontoid with crushing of spinal cord. Anterior articular surface of broken-off odontoid surrounded by torn ligaments is shown. White man, 63 years old. Fall downstairs.

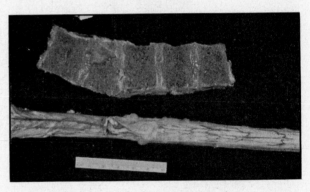

Fig. 13-5. A Healing Fracture of the Dorsal Spine with Posterior Angulation.

Thickening of pia over softened injured segment of spinal cord. Sagittal section of bodies of upper dorsal vertebrae. Accidental fall. Survived three months.

through the torn spinal ligaments into the spinal canal in sufficient bulk to compress the cord.

Overflexion may cause fractures of the sixth and seventh cervical vertebral bodies which are peculiarly vulnerable, since they are adjacent to the rigid thoracic segments. The bodies of the third, fourth and fifth cervical vertebrae are not broken as frequently. The lesion varies from a slightly oblique or transverse crack through the segment to crushing of the bone. A posterior angulation of the spine is produced and a bony projection presses backward against the cord. In addition, bilateral or unilateral dislocations of the articular processes occur. Several vertebral bodies may be fractured or luxated in the same case. The sternum and anterior portions of the upper ribs may show a few fractures in some cases of severe hyperflexion from the violent compression of the head against the upper chest.

The lesion of the spinal cord varies according to the severity of the bone injury. If the luxation is merely partial, or the fracture not marked, a small central contusion may appear in the gray matter at the level of the fracture. If the spine is markedly angulated the substance of the cord may show an extensive bruising for a few centimeters above and below the site of the lesion, due to the fact that it is violently pulled by the overflexion over the angulation so as to damage a considerable portion of its substance. With more extreme dislocation or fracture, the cord may be crushed and torn across at the level of the spinal injury. Occasionally the cord escapes injury.

The complications produced by fractures of the cervical spine depend entirely on the shock sustained and the section of the cord damaged. If the shock is severe the patient may die immediately, even without cord injury. Lesions in the upper cervical vertebrae cause rapid death because of the damage to the spinal cord and the medulla, and occasionally to the center governing the phrenic nerves. Lesions in the lower cervical spine and spinal cord cause a paralysis of the body below the neck with all the usual sensory and trophic disturbances. The patients may die in a few hours or a few days of a hypostatic bronchopneumonia, or in a week or more of severe infections of the bladder and kidneys with acute suppurative cystitis, pyelitis and pyelonephritis (Fig. 16-56), or of severe sepsis from massive decubital gangrene (Fig. 13-1). In one case a comminuted fracture of the body of the third cervical vertebra was complicated by a suppurative osteomyelitis, which caused a retropharyngeal abscess and a suppurative meningomyelitis by direct extension. In recent years complicating infections have been controlled with resulting prolonged survival by the use of antibiotic and chemotherapeutic agents.

Some of the injuries of the cervical spine caused by a twisting motion imparted to the vertebral bodies from indirect violence are unilateral, with unilateral fractures of the laminae and transverse processes and unilateral luxation of the articular processes. In fracture dislocations of the cervical spine, removal and dissection of the adjacent involved vertebrae will usually demonstrate, in addition to the injury of the intervertebral disk and vertebral bodies, either a fracture of a transverse process or of the upper part of one or both superior articular facets in the lower of the two involved vertebrae.

Other rare types of injury of the cervical spine are produced by hyperextension of the spinal column. Several cases of this type have been encountered by the authors. In two of these the individual had fallen down an embankment, lacerating his forehead. Dissection of the cervical segment of the spine revealed a bilateral fracture of the posterior arch of the atlas, a forward dislocation of the atlas still attached to the rest of the spine on the base of the occiput, and complete crushing of the cord at the foramen magnum causing immediate death. The head evidently was held stationary at the moment of impact so that the hyperextension of the spine tore the occipito-atlantal ligaments and forced the spine forward. In another case a woman seated in the rear seat of an antomobile was thrown forward during a frontal collision and lacerated her forehead against the back of the front seat. The resulting hyperextension of the cervical spinal column fractured the odontoid process at its junction with the atlas causing enough deformity of the spine at this point to contuse the cord and kill the victim outright. Other injuries due to hyperextension probably occur, but it is not easy in every instance to determine when this mechanism operates. Instances of partial luxation of the lower cervical vertebrae through the intervertebral disk without spinal cord injury are probably the result of hyperextension.

Individuals who sustain a fracture or partial luxation of the cervical vertebrae with or without damage to the cord may live for several months or years afterwards and the spinal injury usually undergoes partial or complete healing (Fig. 13-5).

A case of old subluxation between the fifth and sixth cervical vertebrae was encountered in an autopsy on an elderly white male who died of arteriosclerotic heart disease. He had sustained a fall down the stairs 11 months previously and had only complained of stiffness in the neck without any evidence of spinal cord involvement.

In another case a 45 year old white woman fell head-first down a coal chute but showed no more serious results of the accident than local pain and tenderness in the neck. After recovering from the immediate effects of the trauma she became ambulatory, complaining of pain in the neck but never displaying any signs of paralysis or trophic disturbances characteristic of a cord lesion. She died two years and four months after the fall, of acute and chronic alcoholism. Autopsy disclosed an angular deformity of the cervical spine due to an anterior flattening of

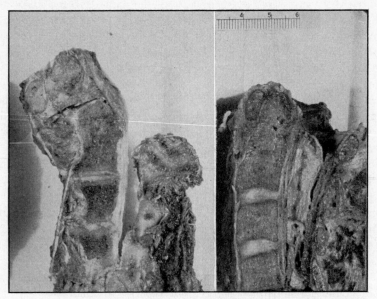

Fig. 13-6. Nine Year Old Fracture of Odontoid Process of Axis.

Fall down stairs. Progressive symptoms of spinal cord pressure associated with narrowing of spinal canal. Death from respiratory paralysis following laminectomy. Man, 52 years old.

Left. Sagittal section of thickened odontoid with pseudoarthrosis between fragments and osteoarthritis narrowing spinal canal.

Right. Similar section of normal spine to show relationship between intact odontoid and canal.

the sixth cervical vertebra, which had evidently suffered a compression fracture from overflexion during the fall and had finally healed in the shape of a wedge. The cord revealed no gross evidence of injury but microscopically a partial degeneration of the tract of Goll for a short distance above the site of the spinal injury. This lesion and the neck pain were considered to have been the probable result of injuries to the sensory nerves in this region at the time of the fracture.

In some instances an excessive amount of bony repair in a cervical spine fracture may encroach on the spinal canal and gradually cause a compression of the spinal cord.

In one such case a 52 year old white man struck his head against an iron door and sustained an injury diagnosed as a fracture dislocation of the atlas. He was hospitalized for five weeks during which time his head was kept in traction. After about a year he was able to resume work but never fully regained his strength. He remained fairly well for about four years and then gradually developed progressive weakness and stiffness first in the right lower extremity, then in the other lower and later in the upper extremities. The symptoms progressed and after a period of two more years he was unable to walk without assistance. His condition grew worse during the next two years. Roentgenography revealed a bony thickening of the upper two cervical vertebrae and a forward luxation of the atlas with anteroposterior narrowing of the spinal canal. A laminectomy with removal of the posterior arch of the atlas was performed under anesthesia to relieve the compression of the spinal cord. After the completion of the operation the patient was turned over and suddenly stopped breathing. Artificial respiration was immediately applied and he was then placed in a respirator where he regained consciousness but died 12 hours later. Death occurred eight years and eleven months after the original injury.

Autopsy disclosed an old forward dislocation of the atlas on the axis and an ununited fracture and forward dislocation of the odontoid process (13-6). The reparative bone sclerosis and hyperostosis around the pseudoarthrosis of the body and odontoid process of the axis had increased the deformity of the original injury and had further narrowed the spinal canal to compress the spinal cord which had originally escaped injury. Examination of the cord revealed atrophy of the white tracts and also fresh small hemorrhages in the gray matter of the

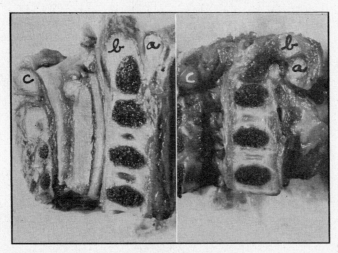

Fig. 13-7. Forward Dislocation and Downward Rotation of Atlas with Bending of Odontoid Process of Axis and Narrowing of Spinal Canal.

Birth injury during breech extraction. Lived two months. Hospitalized for swelling of posterior pharyngeal wall. Sudden death from fresh hemorrhage in compressed segment of spinal cord.

Right. Sagittal section showing forward and downward displacement of anterior tubercle of atlas (a), bending of odontoid process and displacement of its cartilaginous tip (b), narrowing of spinal canal by forward displacement of posterior arch and tubercle (c) of axis.

Left. Correspondingly labeled section of spine of normal two months old infant.

segment at the level of the laminectomy. These hemorrhages evidently occurred when the patient was turned over after the completion of the operation, and accounted for the sudden respiratory paralysis.

A somewhat similar case involved a full term newborn infant delivered by a difficult breech extraction. At birth the infant did not react vigorously and thereafter appeared listless and was difficult to feed. At the age of two months a swelling of the posterior pharyngeal wall was noted and the infant was hospitalized. Shortly thereafter it died suddenly while being fed. Autopsy revealed a remarkable spinal injury that had evidently occurred at the time of birth (Fig. 13-7). The atlas had been dislocated forward and rotated downward and the odontoid process of the axis was bent forward and its cartilaginous tip pulled downward into a position adjacent to the dislocated anterior tubercle of the atlas. These displaced structures had produced the swelling of the posterior pharyngeal wall. The spinal canal below the foramen magnum was markedly narrowed in its anteroposterior dimension and the upper cervical segment of the spinal cord revealed small old hemorrhages which had evidently occurred at birth and fresh small hemorrhages which resulted from compression of the cord at the time of death.

Fractures of the cervical spine are easily overlooked at autopsy, as external signs of violence are often absent. For this reason the neck should be examined carefully for spinal injuries to obviate such a possibility. Hemorrhage into the cervical prevertebral fascia is usually but not always encountered with these fractures. Sometimes when the head is opened a small amount of blood-stained spinal fluid is found in the cisterna magna or in the subarachnoid space around the pons and cannot be explained on the basis of any intracranial lesion. Under these conditions its presence should suggest the possibility of a fracture of the cervical spine. In many cases the brain and meninges reveal nothing abnormal.

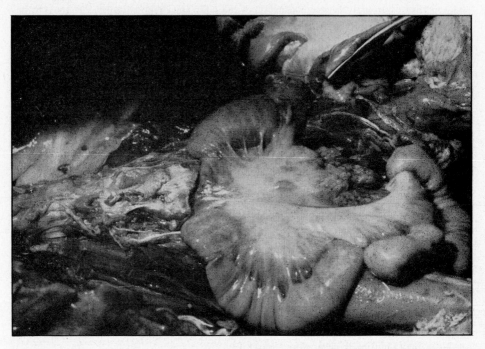

Fig. 13-8. Fracture of Lumbar Spine from Hyperextension with Separation of Second and Third Lumbar Vertebrae.

Violence resulting from a fall from third story window also caused herniation and incarceration of loop of intestine in space between momentarily separated vertebrae. Death three days after injury with signs of shock, intestinal obstruction and acute nephrosis. White woman, 42 years old.

DORSAL SPINE. Fractures of the dorsal vertebrae (Fig. 13-2) occasionally occur from indirect violence, mostly from hyperflexion. Those segments near the upper and lower ends of this region are most apt to be involved. The solidity of the vertebral bodies and the structure of the thorax protect this part of the spine against distortion. The contusion of the cord is localized fairly consistently at the level of the injury, inasmuch as there is only slight motion in the segments. The principal complications are the cord injury and intercurrent infections of the urinary tract.

LUMBAR SPINE. The lumbar vertebrae at the upper and lower ends of the segment are vulnerable to indirect violence usually in the form of hyperflexion. The body of the vertebrae is crushed from above down anteriorly and a portion is forced backward into the spinal canal to contuse the cord and the cauda equinae. This compression fracture generally results in a wedge-shaped flattening of the affected vertebral body and a slight kyphosis of the lumbar spine. Less often there is a partial or complete luxation between two vertebrae either with or without a fracture. The cord may or may not be contused. If it is injured the patient may die of a slowly developing infection of the urinary tract or a septic infection from a decubital ulcer, lasting several weeks or months. Cases without cord injury may recover after a long convalescence. These injuries are often produced by falls from a height when the victim lands on his shoulders or his buttocks, in such a way as to produce overflexion of the lumbar region. They have occurred in individuals who have been forcibly doubled up in a car during an automobile collision, and dislocations of the lumbar spine and crushing of the cord have resulted from the crash landing of an aeroplane. In some instances the injury results from a blow on the back by a falling object of heavy weight like a sack of flour. Lumbar spinal fractures have also followed the violent convulsions produced by injections of metrazol and by electric stimulation in the shock therapy of certain psychopathic disorders. Isolated fractures of the transverse processes of the lumbar vertebrae occasionally occur, but are not fatal unless combined with more serious conditions.

Forcible hyperextension of the spine may result in a fracture dislocation of the lumbar spine. The vertebrae may momentarily separate and snap back into alignment.

The rapidity with which this separation and realignment can occur is demonstrated by the rare case described by O'Sullivan and others in which the same force that produced this fracture tore the posterior parietal peritoneum and whipped a loop of intestine between the momentarily separated lumbar vertebral bodies where it became firmly trapped when the vertebrae snapped back into alignment with resultant intestinal obstruction.

The victim was a 42 year old woman who fell from a third story window and sustained an evident compound comminuted fracture of the lower third of the right femur, a comminuted fracture of the left acetabulum, bilateral fractures of the pubic and ischial rami, and fractures of the right eleventh and twelfth and left tenth, eleventh and twelfth ribs posteriorly. Death occurred three days after injury from shock, intestinal obstruction and a lower nephron nephrosis. Autopsy revealed an undiagnosed fracture between the bodies of the second and third lumbar vertebrae, multiple lacerations of the posterior parietal peritoneum, and a loop of jejunum, 35 cm. from the ligament of Treitz, firmly pinched between the bodies of the separated vertebrae (Fig. 13-8). There was complete intestinal obstruction and the bowel proximal of the compressed trapped loop was markedly distended.

SACRUM. Fractures of the sacrum are transverse and due to direct violence applied to the sacral region. They are attended by considerable shock and are similar in their effect to the other fractures of the pelvic bones (see page 258).

Os COCCYX. Fractures of the os coccyx are due to direct violence but are not dangerous to life as a rule. They are important mostly as a surgical condition.

Injuries of the Spinal Cord without Spinal Fracture. Under certain conditions the cord may be injured traumatically even though the spine is not fractured. Several such cases have been observed by the authors. In one the victim was injured during an automobile collision. At autopsy the spine was found intact but the cervical segment of the cord revealed a small contusion in the form of a hemorrhage within the gray matter. The probable explanation of this injury lies in the elasticity of the intervertebral ligaments which permits the violence to distort the spinal column momentarily, sufficient to bruise the cord without resulting in a vertebral fracture. In two of these cases the circumstances of the accident and of the death prompted the examination of the spine and the detection of the cord contusion. One case presented clinical signs of a quadriplegia; in the other the deceased died rapidly after the trauma; in neither was there any hemorrhage in the prevertebral fascia to indicate any involvement of the spine or cord.

Repair of Spinal Injuries. The repair of the bone lesions is similar to the healing of fractures elsewhere in the body. In human tissues this process can be studied to best advantage in the rib, inasmuch as the comparatively small size of the bone and the nonlethal nature of the injury allow the pathologist to observe satisfactorily all the stages of healing. The first change after the fracture is a hemorrhage around the broken ends of the bones, followed by clotting of the blood and by necrosis of the tissues at the fracture site. In about 48 hours granulation tissue invades the blood clot, removes the necrotic debris, and in about two weeks is transformed into a fibrous scar tissue which establishes fibrous union around and between the broken ends of the bone. The process after this is dependent upon the amount of motion allowed at the fracture site. If the bone is well splinted, soft osteoid tissue develops from the periosteum by the proliferation of osteoblasts, gradually extending towards the center. This holds the fracture in a bony union until permanent calcified bone trabeculae gradually replace the osteoid tissue, a process which takes several months. If there is undue motion at the site of the fracture, the osteoid tissue becomes exuberant and hyaline cartilage is laid down around the ends of the broken bone. This is then transformed into osteoid tissue and later into dense bone. The process of healing apparently occurs with greater rapidity in bones containing red bone marrow than it does in bones with fatty marrow, probably because of the increased vascularity. During healing the red blood-forming bone marrow near the site of the fracture undergoes fibrosis; later when the repair is complete the hematopoietic tissue is restored.

The repair of skull fractures occurs almost similarly, though the process varies in detail. Callus formation is usually minimal and never cartilaginous. The preservation of the periosteum at the site of injury determines how completely the fracture will heal. Some fractures do not completely heal and are visible as clefts in the bone with rounded edges; in other cases the bone is firmly knit throughout and evidence of the fracture site may completely disappear. Linear fractures without deformity may heal without a trace.

Healed or healing spinal fractures are occasionally encountered at autopsy. The most common injury is a compression fracture of the body of a cervical or lumbar vertebra which has been crushed by overflexion so that the anterior end of the vertebral body is decreased in height. There is a fragmentation of the cancellous bone trabeculae with hemorrhage and following this, granulation tissue proliferation, removal of necrotic bone, and formation of new bone occur. The injured bone, after its repair, may become sclerotic and remain deformed. Where there has been an old partial luxation between two vertebrae with traumatization of the intervening fibrocartilaginous disk, a cleavage may persist in the interior of the disk, and thickening of the bone trabeculae and fibrosis of the marrow in the adjacent portions of the vertebral bodies above and below the injured cartilage may be found.

The changes in the spinal cord are quite variable. The cord when first injured becomes edematous and soft, with hemorrhage in the interstices, chiefly in the gray matter. Depending on the severity of injury, there is more or less disruption of cord tissue, a process which may progress rapidly to liquefaction necrosis. There is usually extradural hemorrhage but almost never subarachnoid or pial hemorrhage. During repair the edema is resorbed, the effused blood is transformed into a brown pigment, degeneration of the nerve cells and axis cylinders takes place in the region of injury, and microglial cells proliferate and are transformed into the phagocytic gitter cells which remove the necrotic debris. The injured segment of cord then shrinks and is replaced by a firm fibroglial cicatrix. The nerve tracts above and below the lesion undergo degeneration with a varying amount of destruction of axones and myelin sheaths in the columns of the white matter. These degenerative lesions are best demonstrated in specially stained histologic sections. In some traumatic cases the injury may produce complete crushing or severance of the cord at a certain level and the degeneration of the afferent and efferent tracts will be maximal for that level of injury. But in other cases both the traumatic lesions at a given level and the resulting tract degenerations are incomplete. In old cases it is common to find adhesions of the injured segment of the cord to the adjacent meninges. In addition to the actual damage to the cord, the spinal nerves in the region of the fracture may also be torn and contribute to the posterior tract degeneration.

Unusual Sequelae of Spinal Injuries. The symptom complex known as railway spine was so designated because it was likely to develop after railway or other accidents in which the vertebral column has been subjected to more or less severe jarring. The individual develops a variety of neurologic phenomena, some of which are paralytic in nature, others suggestive of hysteria or neurosis. A large number of these cases appear to be functional without any demonstrable anatomic basis. The symptoms are probably dependent on many factors such as the emotional make-up of the individual, the degree of physical and psychic shock at the time of the accident, and the question of payment of damages. These cases have been known to recover completely after a satisfactory settlement. This does not imply that the patient is necessarily malingering, though it does not exclude that possibility.

Trauma is claimed by some to be an underlying factor in the production of Kummel's disease (atrophy of spinal vertebra), tuberculosis of the spine, neoplasms of the spine, and other spinal disorders. At the present time the preponderance of evidence is against any causal relation between such diseases as tuberculosis and neoplasms of the spine, and injury to that structure. Kummel's disease, on the other hand, has been regarded as the sequel of injury to the body of the vertebra in some instances an undetected fracture; in others an injury without fracture, resulting in an avascular necrosis of bone and subsequent atrophy. This question, however, has not been settled conclusively.

Other lesions of the spine, occasionally mentioned in connection with trauma, will be discussed briefly. One such condition is spondylolisthesis which affects mostly the lower lumbar spine. Two types have been described: in the first type a single vertebral body slips forward independently of the segments above and below it, and this has been ascribed to a congenital defect in the neural arches on both sides; in the second type the spine as a unity is luxated forward on one of the lower lumbar vertebral cartilages which may show extensive degeneration, usually after a slight trauma like a fall on the buttocks or after a strain like lifting a heavy weight. Such an insignificant degree of strain would be inadequate per se to produce spondylolisthesis in a normal spinal column, and the underlying etiologic factor is the degenerative or disease process in the vertebra or intervertebral cartilages.

A similar condition due to the degeneration of the fibrocartilaginous plate or the annulus fibrosus of the intervertebral disk is a herniation of the nucleus pulposus, sometimes precipitated by trauma or strain. These extrusions may extend into the bony tissue of the adjacent vertebral bodies or herniate into the spinal canal and compress the cauda equina.

MEDICOLEGAL CONSIDERATIONS

The medicolegal considerations of spinal injuries have been discussed already in sufficient detail except for a few minor points. The victim is usually not able to move after the injury, if the spinal cord is traumatized, and even if this lesion is not present the mere shock of the violence may have the same effect. Exceptions, however, do occur and the case described on page 15 indicates that a person with a fracture of the lumbar spine below the lower limit of the cord may have surprising powers of locomotion. In a few cases spinal fractures and spinal cord injuries are not suspected and diagnosed clinically. There may be no suggestive external sign of violence and the patient may be in such profound shock or so deeply alcoholic that the usual sensory and motor signs of transverse cord injury are difficult or impossible to elicit.

REFERENCES

De Costa, J. C., and Jones, F. X.   Railway Injuries, in Peterson, Haines and Webster, Legal Medicine and Toxicology, Vol. 1, Philadelphia and London, W. B. Saunders Co., 1923.

Feaster, O. O.   Delayed deformity in vertebral body fractures, J.A.M.A., 102:598, 1934.

Moritz, A. R.   The Pathology of Trauma, Philadelphia, Lea and Febiger, 1942.

O'Sullivan, W. D., Helpern, M., Correll, and Lord, S. W., Jr.   Intestinal obstruction due to compression of jejunum between bodies of fractured lumbar spine. To be published.

Polatin, P., Friedman, M. M., Harris, M. M., and Horowitz, W. A.   Vertebral fractures produced by metrazol-induced convulsions, J.A.M.A., 112:1684, 1939.

Schmorl, G.   Zur pathologischen Anatomie der Wirbelsäule, Klin. Wchnschr., 8:1243, 1929.

Sigl, A.   Ueber stumpfe Gewalteinwirkung auf Wirbelsäule und Ruckenmark und ihren Folgen, Med. Klin., 22:224, 1926.

Tillman, H.   A Text Book of Surgery, Vol. 2, New York, D. Appleton & Co., 1897.

Watson-Jones, R.   Fractures and Joint Injuries, Vol. I, Baltimore, Williams and Wilkins, 1943.

14

Correlation of the Type of Blunt
Force with the Injuries

It is not possible in every case of blunt force trauma to correlate the injuries with the type of violence. However, a brief consideration of the combination of injuries which are produced by different types of blunt force may be a helpful guide to the pathologist for determining the nature of special cases which come to his attention.

GENERALIZED BLUNT FORCE

Highway Accidents. An automobile injures the body in several different ways. The radiator or bumper may strike the victim and knock him down or toss him into the air. At the site of impact there may be definite abrasions, contusions and lacerations, arranged in a characteristic pattern (Figs. 9-1, 9-2 and 9-3) similar to that of the radiator and tire tread, or other part of the vehicle which comes in contact with the skin. The impact of the car may also fracture the skull, ribs, sternum, spine, pelvis or bones of the leg at points of contact. The bumper striking the legs frequently causes bilateral compound fractures of the tibia and fibula at the same level, the so-called bumper fracture (Fig. 9-10). Injuries of the abdominal and thoracic viscera, such as ruptures and tears of the intestines, mesentery, bladder, heart, aorta, lungs, spleen, liver, kidneys and pancreas are produced. In some instances parts of the car (Fig. 9-2) such as the door handle or radiator ornament may be driven into the body of the deceased and remain as a mute indication of the source of the injury. In one such case the door handle of the car sideswiped the deceased, entering his mouth and lacerating his throat so that the carotid artery was torn, causing death by hemorrhage. The broken handle was found in the wound at the time of autopsy and kept as part of the essential evidence in the case.

If the deceased is knocked down he may receive, characteristically enough, a fracture of the skull from impact against the roadway and suffer all the complications which attend this type of fracture. If he is tossed into the air the impact may fracture the skull and ribs by direct violence or cause fractures and luxations of the spine, bones of the pelvis and extremities both by direct and indirect violence.

Numerous automobile accidents are caused by collisions between vehicles with a telegraph pole or a steel pillar, or by the car rolling over an embankment. The bodies of the passengers are apt to be doubled up into a position of extreme anteflexion, and spinal injuries and fractures of the long bones by indirect violence are prone to occur under such conditions. In a few instances the passenger may be thrown forward from a rear seat striking his chest on the back of the seat in front so that his head snaps forward, causing a compression fracture of a cervical vertebra and a crushing injury of the cord. A few cervical spine and cord injuries may be produced by hyperextension, as described on page 315. Fractures of the ribs, sternum, skull and pelvis also occur from direct violence. In some cases, the ribs,

323

sternum and larynx are fractured when the driver of the car is the victim, if the collision has thrown him heavily against the steering wheel.

An automobile may crush an individual between itself and some other structure producing such injuries as compression of the sternum and anterior portions of the chest, sagittal liver ruptures between the right and left lobes (Fig. 11-21) or fractures of the pelvis. One case occurred in which a man was caught between a moving truck and the back of a bakery wagon in such a way that the severe impact between the truck and the step in the rear of his wagon amputated his legs completely just above the ankles (Fig. 14-1). If the crushing force imparts a twisting action to the body, luxations may occur at the hip or shoulder joints and tearing lesions of the abdominal and chest viscera may occur.

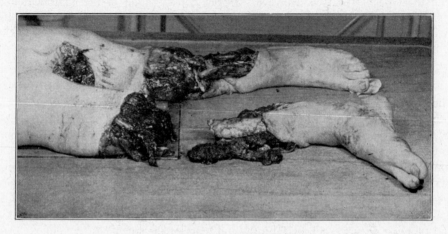

Fig. 14-1. Blunt Force: Correlation of Injury and Type of Violence.

Traumatic amputation of both legs when deceased was crushed between oncoming truck and low back step of bakery wagon which he was unloading.

The most severe and characteristic injuries are produced when an automobile runs over the body (Figs. 10-1, 10-2, 10-3, 11-1). The grinding action of the wheel causes subcutaneous separation of the skin from the muscles, or huge lacerations with stripping of the skin from the part and tearing of vessels, muscles and nerves. If the wheel passes over the legs, the lesions on both legs may be located at the level of the violence with the production of a direct transverse fracture or a comminuted fracture at that site. These injuries are not always at the same level, depending upon the way in which the wheel passes over the extremities. Occasionally the grinding action of the wheel imparts a twisting force to the legs just above the ankles causing an oblique fracture of the tibia proximal to the point where the violence was applied, which makes a ragged tear in the skin. The violence is sometimes so severe that the legs are partially or completely amputated.

The wheel may pass over the trunk, neck or head, injuring or tearing the skin, and sometimes mangling the body or head extensively. In some cases the wheel's tearing action amputates the neck partially (Fig. 14-2) or completely. Other characteristic lesions caused by this force are the compression fractures of the skull across the base (Fig. 12-9), the twisting injuries of the spine due to direct violence, grinding fractures of the ribs and pelvis, and tearing and crushing injuries of the thoracic and abdominal organs (Fig. 11-2). In some cases the marks of one wheel may appear on the legs and marks of the other wheel on the trunk or head. The treads of the tire on occasion may be imprinted on the skin (Fig. 9-3). In one case the wheel of a truck passed obliquely across the trunk tearing open the abdominal wall and squeezing out the entire contents of the chest and abdomen (Fig. 14-3).

Other types of fatal traumatic injury can result from the operation of automobiles and are discussed in other sections. These include deaths from burns when

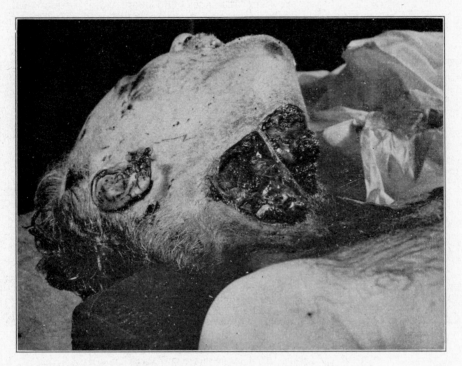

Fig. 14-2. Partial Amputation of Neck by Wheel of Automobile.

Fracture dislocation of upper cervical spine with exposure of spinal canal. Complete transverse severance of trachea, esophagus, both carotid arteries and jugular veins, with laceration of front of neck. White man, 49 years old, run over by an automobile.

the car has been set on fire from a collision, from drowning when the automobile is driven into the water either purposely or by mishap, from broken glass injuries during a collision, and from carbon monoxide poisoning when that gas is generated in the engine and carried by the exhaust to the victim.

Injuries caused by railway, subway and elevated trains are similar to automobile injuries, except that they are as a rule more extensive and more mutilating. Amputations of the head, extremities and segments of the trunk; evisceration of the cranial cavity, abdomen or chest; and extensive crushing of different parts are frequent. In subway train accidents grease from the wheels may be ground into wounds or smeared over the skin. Injuries also occur when a person gets caught in a door and is dragged along the platform, or is imprisoned between the train and the platform as the result of a misstep and ground by the forward motion of the train. Some individuals have been injured by sticking their heads out of a train in motion and shattering them against a projection.

Falls. The injuries produced by falls are the result of impact and are occasionally characteristic. In some cases the violence is a moderate one as when a person falls on the street or falls out of bed. The most common injury is an abrasion or laceration of the scalp and a fracture of the skull with intracranial complications. Many of these accidents occur when the victim is alcoholic. Often there is only slight initial concussion and recovery from the immediate effects of the trauma may be prompt, but after an interval the victim shows the effects of cerebral compression due to traumatic intracranial hemorrhage, sometimes not until he has wandered away from the scene of the fall. Old people who fall may sustain an intertrochanteric or a cervical fracture of the upper end of the femur. Less often fractures of the ribs, clavicle, bones of the extremities and internal injuries occur.

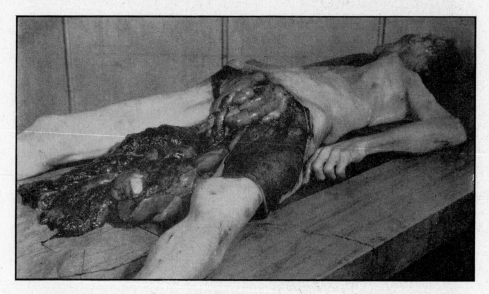

Fig. 14-3. Traumatic Mass Evisceration of Entire Contents of Chest and Abdomen.

The wheel of a truck passed over the body obliquely from right to left squeezing out all organs from the trachea on down through bursting opening in lower abdomen above the pelvis.

In many cases of simple falls of elderly people autopsy reveals injuries of greater or lesser magnitude, but the fatal lesion may be a spontaneous cerebral hemorrhage, cerebral infarction, a heart lesion, or some other natural disease condition. In many such cases death is the result of independent disease and traumatic injury. The medical examiner must appraise the significance of the traumatic lesion and of the natural disease condition in determining the cause of death (as discussed in Chapters 5, 6 and 7).

Falls downstairs or into an areaway cause more severe injuries though mostly of the same general type as just mentioned. In addition the spine may be overflexed or overextended and sustain the fractures described under that heading. The pelvis may also be fractured by a severe impact.

Many falls occur from a great height, as from the top of a tall building or high bridge, down an elevator shaft, or the hold of a ship. The violence after a drop from a great height is severe and the injuries are extensive. The bones of the extremities may be broken by direct or indirect violence and those which strike the ground first suffer the most. If the victim lands on his feet a number of fractures occur in the bones of the legs at corresponding levels; if on all fours the arms and legs both will show fractures of this type; and if he lands in a diving position the bones of the arms will be fractured at corresponding levels and the bones of the cranium and face may be comminuted. In some instances the brain may be enucleated. The spine may be shattered in different degrees by direct or indirect violence. The ribs and pelvis are injured mostly on the side which strikes the earth. Visceral ruptures due to impact are often seen. The heart may show a bursting rupture with or without a pericardial tear and the lungs often show sub-pleural air blisters. In these cases of falls from a great height the question may arise as to whether the victim died as the result of the fall or was dead before the fall occurred. Accordingly the examiner should note all signs which would indicate that the injuries due to the fall were intravital, such as fat embolism, hemorrhages around injuries, and inhaled blood, and should carefully appraise all points which might suggest that death occurred from other reasons besides the fall. The injuries which are produced by falls from a high bridge into deep water have been discussed on page 231.

Blow from a Falling Object. If an object like a brick falls from a great height and strikes the head of a person it will practically demolish the cranium, and if it strikes the trunk it will inflict severe damage there. A body of greater weight striking the back will usually fracture the spine.

Burial in Excavations or Building Cave-ins. The injuries inflicted by this type of violence are due to a crushing force or one that causes a severe distortion of the trunk. The victim may also be asphyxiated by being pinned under masonry which compresses his chest or by being buried in finely divided plaster dust which may be inhaled into his air passages (page 275). The syndrome following compression of the extremities has already been discussed on page 203.

Elevator Accidents. The injuries in elevator accidents are caused by falls down an elevator shaft either in or out of the car, by being struck by falling elevator weights or other objects or by being compressed between the elevator and the wall or landing. When the trunk is squeezed in this way a severe cyanosis of the head, neck and upper chest is produced with small venous hemorrhages in the skin and conjunctivae and peculiar changes in the eyegrounds. The condition will be discussed later under Asphyxia. The same type of injuries can occur in dumb-waiter accidents, though the most common is a severe fracture of the skull caused by a falling waiter or a compression of the head, neck and upper chest produced by its slower descent upon an individual who stuck his head into the opening of the shaft.

LOCALIZED BLUNT FORCE

The effects of localized blunt force on the body have already been considered in detail in the preceding chapters. Most of them are caused by human assaults with a blunt weapon, or by blows with the fist, or by kicking or trampling. Persons injured in an altercation may show contusions of the face from fist blows and may be knocked down during the scuffle, receiving a fracture of the skull and fatal intracranial injuries. Blows with a club or hammer on the head may produce characteristic lacerations of the scalp and characteristic depressed fractures of the skull (Figs. 9-7, 9-8, 12-2). The scalp may be lacerated by a sharp blow with a blunt weapon like a pistol butt, which produces also a localized fracture of the underlying skull. Hair from the scalp may be driven in to become tightly pinched between the edges of the fracture during their momentary separation at the time of the impact (Fig. 14-4). The patterned abrasions produced by a file or the threads of a pipe have already been described (Figs. 9-4 and 9-5). A weapon like a whip or a chain will also cause a patterned abrasion or a laceration with marked edema in the adjacent tissues of the skin so that a welt will appear on the part of the body struck. Repeated heavy blows with a blunt weapon may leave characteristic wounds on various parts of the body and cause multiple fractures of the bones of the cranium and the face. Kicks, blows or thrusts against the abdomen may give rise to localized lacerations of the parenchymatous viscera, especially the liver, pancreas and kidneys, and produce perforations of the mesentery, stomach, duo-

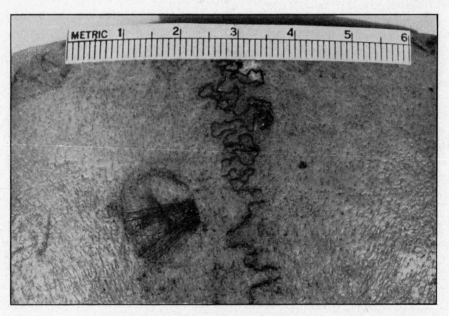

Fig. 14-4. Tuft of Hair from Scalp Driven into Skull and Held Tight Between Edges of Small Depressed Fracture.

The victim was struck on the head with a gun butt. Photograph shows the top of the skull.

denum, intestines and bladder; the abdominal wall in these cases may not show any external signs of injury. (See Chapter 11 for illustrations.)

In attacks by large animals, injuries may result from kicks, blows with the paw or hoof, thrusts with the horns or by trampling. The injuries may be similar to those produced by human assaults but are likely to be more severe. The wounds may be patterned; a person struck in the face by a horse's hoof might bear the mark of the shoe on his skin, or if struck by the paw of a leopard or bear, might show parallel scratch marks on the skin produced by the claws of the animal.

Occasionally, as the result of an impact, hairs, pieces of tissue, blood stains and fragments of cloth are deposited on blunt instruments or automobiles, and microscopic, serologic and chemical tests may be necessary in order to establish the nature and significance of such items of evidence (Chapters 38, 39 and 40).

When a physician attends an individual suffering from injuries due to blunt force which have been received under suspicious circumstances, he should report the matter to the police without delay.

Fatal injuries sustained during competitive sport are relatively uncommon and usually result from some form of impact, either bodily or by thrown or batted missiles. Injuries from bodily impact are apt to occur in football, boxing, wrestling and basketball. Injuries from the impacts of missiles are encountered most frequently in baseball, occasionally in golf and cricket. Fatalities sometimes result from falls and other mishaps during horse racing and jumping, polo, handball, basketball, and track and field sports. Drownings during swimming races, water polo matches and diving exhibitions are rare and have not been encountered by the authors. In a number of instances sudden and unexpected natural death has occurred during sport and possibly was precipitated by excitement, overexertion or exhaustion.

Such natural causes of death include spontaneous cerebral and subarachnoid hemorrhage, usually from the rupture of a cerebral artery aneurysm, occlusive coronary artery disease, syphilitic aortitis with stenosis of the coronary ostia, pulmonary infection, chronic leptomeningitis, and other natural conditions. The unusual death of a 17-year-old boy after the completion of an under-water swimming race, in which the autopsy revealed only a dilated heart and congested organs, has already been described in the chapter on sudden and unexpected natural death (page 116). Death was attributed to the unusual exertion, anoxia and cardiac strain, accentuated by breath holding while swimming under water.

In former years, before the advent of the antibiotic and chemotherapeutic agents for the treatment of infection, there were a fair number of deaths from septic infection complicating contusions and lacerations and from acute and chronic osteomyelitis complicating skeletal injuries. An occasional death resulted from tetanus. Most of these fatal septic infections followed relatively minor football and basketball injuries of the extremities. Deaths from septic infection complicating injury in sport are now rare.

Intracranial injuries, with or without skull fracture, continue to account for most sports fatalities. Subdural hemorrhage is encountered most often in boxing; fracture of the skull and intracranial injury in baseball. Intra-abdominal injuries, such as rupture of the spleen, tears of the mesentery with hemorrhage, and of the intestines with resultant peritonitis, and spinal injuries are responsible for most of the remaining deaths and occur most often in football. Intrathoracic injuries are less common. A bursting rupture of the heart and pericardial sac resulted from compression of the chest after the fall of a horse and rider during a jumping contest, the rider having fallen under the horse.

In New York City, during the 32 year period between 1918 and 1950, out of a total of approximately 190,000 accidental violent deaths, there were only 108 fatalities from injuries received during competitive sports. The distribution of these deaths is shown in the following table, which does not include deaths from recreational swimming, boating and fishing accidents, horseback riding and other forms of physical exercise. Gonzales has reported 104 of these cases (Table 14-1).

Table 14-1. Fatalities in Sports in New York City, 1918 to 1950

Baseball	43	Soccer	2
Boxing	23	Polo	1
Football	22	Cricket	1
Handball	3	Golf	1
Wrestling	3	Relay Race	1
Basketball	7	Jumping on Horseback	1
Total			108

With additions, from Gonzales, T. A., *J.A.M.A.*, 146:1506-1511, 1951.

Baseball. More than half of the 43 deaths resulted from head injury due to impact of a thrown or batted baseball. Most of the injured were amateur or semiprofessional players. Only one major league player was fatally injured when he was struck on the head by a pitched ball. There were 25 deaths from skull fracture with intracranial injuries. In 14 of these, epidural hemorrhage with only slight brain injury was found. In the other 11, brain contusions and laceration, subdural hemorrhage, small traumatic hemorrhages, and tentorial tear were the various lesions observed. Two deaths resulted from a subdural hemorrhage without skull fracture.

There were six deaths from acute and chronic osteomyelitis; in five of these the bones of the lower extremities had been injured; in the sixth case the infection involved the thoracic spine and followed an injury by a thrown bat. Three deaths resulted from septic peritonitis complicating a rupture of the intestine; one of these players was kicked, another struck by a bat and the third hit with a ball in the abdomen. In the last case the rupture of the bowel was preceded by a contusion and occurred five days after the injury. Two deaths from streptococcal and staphylococcal sepsis followed infected finger injuries. A fracture of the femur was complicated by a femoral thrombophlebitis and fatal pulmonary embolism. A death from traumatic rupture of the heart and hemopericardium was caused by a blow on the chest by a batted ball. In one case an infected laceration of the scalp caused a fatal sepsis. A collision between two players caused one to sustain a fatal contusion of the head of the pancreas with hemorrhage and fat necrosis. A player who was struck on the side of the head by a bat which flew from the hands of another player sustained a fracture of the mandible and a subarachnoid hemorrhage.

A blow on the abdomen with a batted cricket ball caused a rupture of the small intestine and death from peritonitis. A golf caddy was struck on the head by a golf ball and sustained a fatal fracture of the skull and intracranial injury.

Boxing. Injuries in this sport are usually the result of blows on the head or of impact of the head against the floor of the ring after a knockdown punch. Fifteen of the 23 deaths observed resulted from subdural hemorrhage and cerebral compression; 13 of these were due to the traumatic rupture of bridging veins between the pia-arachnoid and the dural venous sinuses, and of surface blood vessels on the cerebral hemispheres. Thirteen of these hemorrhages were unilateral; eight were on the left, five on the right and two were bilateral. Ten persons died within 40 hours of receipt of the injury, the period varying from one half hour to 38 hours; one with bilateral hemorrhage survived one half hour, the other five and one half hours. The remaining cases survived varying periods from two days to two weeks. In one case that survived eight hours after collapsing in the seventh round, necropsy disclosed only a slight amount of subdural hemorrhage in the form of a thin film of blood without evidence of brain compression; there was also a severe hemorrhagic pneumonia and laryngo-tracheo-bronchitis to which death was mainly attributed.

In addition to the conspicuously large subdural hemorrhages several cases revealed other brain lesions. Scattered small traumatic hemorrhages were found in the white matter of the parietal lobe in one case, petechial hemorrhages in the cerebral peduncles in another, small hemorrhages in the lenticular nucleus in another. These small hemorrhages were of the type which Martland was the first to consider as the basis for the later development of the punch drunk syndrome. In several cases there were streak-like hemorrhages in the pons probably secondary to the obliquely downward pressure on that structure by the subdural hemorrhage. In some cases, hypostatic bronchopneumonia was found as a complication where death was delayed. In one boxer a remarkable old cyst of the subdural space was found in association with a large fresh subdural hemorrhage.

Other lesions more difficult of interpretation are encountered after injuries during a boxing match. In one such case a heavyweight boxer collapsed suddenly in the ring during one of the late rounds of a bout. He survived three days in coma. Necropsy revealed cerebral edema, pinhead sized hemorrhages in the white matter of the basal ganglia, thrombosis of a segment of a small-calibered pial vein between the temporal and occipital lobes, and a small wedge-shaped hemorrhagic area interpreted as an infarct beneath the thrombosed vein. Microscopic examination also revealed a chronic meningo-encephalitis considered to be of several weeks duration. In another case a boxer was knocked down and struck his head against the floor. He survived four hours. Necropsy revealed hemorrhages in the thalamus, cerebellum and floor of the fourth ventricle.

Other cases difficult to assay include that of a boxer who collapsed and died in the ring, and another death which occurred after a few minutes of unconsciousness. Necropsy in these cases did not reveal any injuries and death was attributed to cardiac dilatation and hypertrophy in one case and to cerebral concussion in the other. A death from epilepsy was allegedly attributed to injuries received in boxing bouts eight years prior to the onset of the disease. The relationship between the previous boxing experiences and the illness and death is doubtful.

A fighter who received a blow over the abdomen died six days later from peritonitis resulting from the delayed rupture of a devitalized contusion of the small intestine. Another died within a half hour from a small laceration of the heart and hemorrhage into the pericardial sac. Injuries of the abdominal and thoracic organs are rare in boxing.

In the autopsies on boxing fatalities the surface injuries of the face were not conspicuous and included contusions and abrasions and an occasional small laceration of the forehead, eyelids, nose, lips, cheeks, ears and chin. In some cases such injuries were not found at all. The more pronounced lacerations, such as might induce a boxing referee to terminate a bout, were not encountered.

The most recent boxing fatality investigated by the authors was that of a 25 year old pugilist who was knocked out during the eighth round of a bout by a blow to the chin which caused him to fall backward and strike the back of his head forcibly on the floor of the ring. After regaining consciousness for a brief interval he again collapsed and became comatose. He was immediately hospitalized and a craniotomy promptly performed with the evacuation of a large left sided subdural hemorrhage. He survived in coma a total of 100 hours.

At autopsy there were no external injuries. There was evidence of the recently evacuated left subdural hemorrhage which had come from a torn communicating vein between the pia-arachnoid and the longitudinal sinus on the superior surface of the left frontal lobe. The entire brain was markedly edematous, swollen and compressed; there was some herniation of the left temporal lobe through the trephine opening in the skull. Some small hemorrhages in the cortex of the left temporal lobe and slight infarction of its medial surface were attributed to pressure resulting from the cerebral edema. A striking and most unusual lesion was an asymmetric bilateral ischemic necrosis of the globus pallidus (Fig. 14-5) more extensive on the left, and patchy ischemic necrosis in the pons and medulla, also attributed to the cerebral edema and compression. An early thrombosis of the dural venous sinuses was also found and this had given rise to small embolic pulmonary infarctions. Laryngeal edema had necessitated a tracheotomy prior to death.

The fatal outcome was attributed to the combination of the subdural hemorrhage and the cerebral edema induced by the concussion. Although the subdural hemorrhage was promptly evacuated and the pressure from that source relieved, cerebral compression was induced by the rapidly developing cerebral edema, the latter bringing about circulatory changes and the necrosis of the globus pallidus and other parts of the brain.

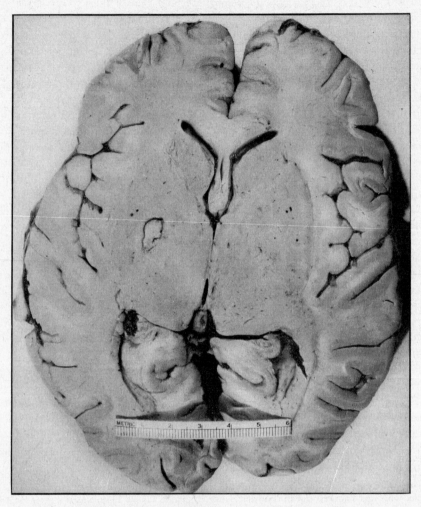

Fig. 14-5. Rare Complication of Intracranial Injury Received in a Boxing Match.

Horizontal section of brain to show ischemic necrosis of globus pallidus secondary to marked traumatic cerebral edema. A 25 year old boxer, knocked out in the eighth round by a hard left to the jaw. Prompt hospitalization and craniotomy with evacuation of a large left-sided subdural hemorrhage from torn communicating pial vein. Survived four days in coma.

Football. Ten of the 22 deaths were caused by acute or chronic septic infection following injury. There were four deaths from acute osteomyelitis; one from fulminating sepsis eight days after an injury to the iliac crest; another from septicopyemia 29 days after an injury of the ankle; the third from staphylococcal sepsis complicating an acute infection of the right tibia; the fourth from septic embolic infarction of the lungs 25 days after an injury to the os calcis complicated by osteomyelitis and thrombophlebitis of the veins of the lower extremity. There were four deaths from chronic osteomyelitis; in two of these the femur was involved, in the third the iliac crest and in the fourth the sacro-iliac joint. These cases survived from 1 to 10 years.

Intra-abdominal injury caused four deaths; three of these were from hemorrhage into the peritoneal cavity; one from a ruptured spleen with a six hour survival; another from a mesenteric laceration with slow bleeding and an 11 day survival; the third from a rupture of the jejunum with hemorrhage and shock and a 24 hour survival. The fourth death occurred one month after a laceration of the small intestine which was repaired but later caused a subacute suppurative peritonitis and bronchopneumonia.

Injuries of the head and spine caused seven deaths. There were two fatalities from acute subdural hemorrhage from the tearing of a bridging vein between the dura and pia-arachnoid, with five and seven day survival periods, and a death from chronic subdural hemorrhage of two months duration. Another death from skull fracture, epidural hemorrhage and cerebral compression occurred 48 hours after injury. Spinal injuries comprised two fractured dislocations of the cervical segment, one involving the fourth, the other the fifth vertebra with crushing of the cord in each. The survival periods were two and a half and four and a half days. A third case survived one year after a fracture of the spine and crushing and degeneration of the spinal cord. A death from tetanus occurred three weeks after a compound fracture of a finger.

Basketball. Seven deaths were encountered from injuries sustained in this sport. Most of these were from infection complicating relatively minor injuries. Thus a fatal staphylococcic sepsis developed after a contusion of the thigh; in another case fatal sepsis followed an osteomyelitis of the femur; in another it followed an abscess which developed in an injured hip; it also occurred after an osteomyelitic complication of an injury to the tibia. A death resulted from persistent hemorrhage, infection and ulceration of the nasal mucosa with severe secondary anemia following a blow to the face. A fatality resulted from subdural hemorrhage and another was attributed to post-traumatic epilepsy from a head injury sustained one year before.

Handball. This sport resulted in three deaths. In two there was a fracture of the skull and an epidural hemorrhage resulting from a fall. A third death resulted from a laceration of the brain complicated by an acute leptomeningitis, the player allegedly having been struck on the head by a handball.

Wrestling. Three deaths from activity in this sport have been encountered. In one death occurred two and a half days after rupture of the spleen with delayed abdominal hemorrhage; in another from acute lobar pneumonia 11 days after a fracture of the dorsal spine. In the third case the contestant was thrown out of the ring and rendered unconscious. He died about 24 hours later. Necropsy disclosed a marked cerebral edema and compression, and softening of one of the cerebellar hemispheres beneath an area of chronic leptomeningitis. There were no contusions or lacerations of the brain, and there was no intermeningeal bleeding.

Soccer. Two deaths occurred in connection with this sport, in each case shortly after the player had collapsed on the field. One death resulted from a fracture of the skull and an epidural hemorrhage. In the other case the victim was said to have received a blow on the abdomen. Necropsy did not reveal any evidence of injury and death was attributed to a luetic aortitis and stenosis of the left coronary ostium.

Miscellaneous. A polo player who fell from his horse sustained a fatal fracture of the cervical spine. A relay runner died from an acute suppurative peritonitis due to a rupture of the large bowel sustained by running into a railing alongside the track.

MEDICOLEGAL CONSIDERATIONS

The purely accidental character of injuries sustained in most athletic sports is generally recognized and such occurrences usually present few medicolegal difficulties. Deaths during competitive sports from natural causes or from violence may lead to inquiry as to the adequacy of medical supervision and training of contestants, the utilization of safeguards, and proper observance of the rules and regulations of the game.

Boxing differs from other sports in that the object is to knock out or win a decision over one's adversary by the delivery of stunning or weakening punches to the head and body. Because of the combative nature and great popularity of the sport, fatalities connected with it always arouse great interest and concern and usually lead to official inquiry. In such cases there may exist suspicion of an attempt or desire on the part of one participant to wrongfully injure his opponent, of tampering with a contestant before a bout, or of negligence in permitting a physically unqualified or unevently matched boxer to participate. A careful and complete necropsy including a toxicologic examination is indicated in all sports fatalities to facilitate any legal investigation which may be warranted by the circumstances.

Injuries in sport as a rule do not have any late sequelae. Most of the infections formerly seen are now effectively controlled or prevented by the use of antibiotics and chemotherapeutic agents. A post-traumatic encephalopathy with neurologic and mental disturbances develops in some poorly trained and inexpert professional boxers who have repeatedly received severe beatings about the head during bouts. Boxers who acquire this disability are spoken of by their associates as being punch drunk. Martland has attributed the development of the punch drunk syndrome to multiple small traumatic hemorrhages of the brain caused by repeated jarring blows to the head.

REFERENCES

Gonzales, T. A.   Fatal Injuries in Competitive Sports, J.A.M.A., 146:1506-1511, 1951.
Martland, H. S.   Punch drunk, J.A.M.A., 91:1103-1107, 1928.

15

Stab Wounds: Incised Wounds: Chop Wounds: Wounds Produced by Foreign Bodies: Biting, Scratching and Gouging

A penetrating wound is produced by an object which pierces the skin, enters the body and lacerates the internal structures. It is essentially a percutaneous injury and differs radically from the subcutaneous injuries caused by blunt force in which the body is damaged by the violence of the trauma and penetration of the skin is incidental and need not occur. The skin lesions of penetrating wounds are frequently characteristic of the objects responsible for the injury and therefore have considerable medicolegal importance.

An important group of penetrating injuries is caused by piercing and cutting instruments and may be subdivided as follows:

1. Stab wounds, or wounds produced by the penetration of a sharp-pointed weapon such as a knife, a dagger or an ice pick.

2. Incised wounds, or cuts made by the sharp edge of a weapon like a knife or a razor.

3. Chop wounds, or wounds inflicted by a blow with a heavy, sharp-edged instrument, as a sword, an ax, a hatchet or a cleaver.

STAB WOUNDS

Stab wounds may be inflicted with weapons such as knives, scissors, three-cornered files, or ice picks with a circular shaft, all possessing a sharp point but having blades of different shapes. Comparatively slight force is required to penetrate the body with such instruments, and as a consequence little ecchymosis is produced in the skin and deeper structures around the edges of the wounds. The depth of the stab wound is limited to a certain extent by the length of the weapon. Occasionally such injuries are produced by sharp-pointed jagged pieces of broken glass or other weapons of unusual type.

Skin Lesions. The opening in the skin generally has clean-cut edges which are rarely associated with ecchymosis in the neighboring tissues or with a thin marginal abrasion of the adjacent epidermis. If a knife is driven in at right angles to the surface the edges of the wound are sharply cut and perpendicular. If the blade enters the skin obliquely, one edge will be beveled and the opposite edge will overhang the wound. With a sharp-edged weapon like a knife the form of the skin opening is determined not only by the shape of the blade but also by the direction in which the elastic fibers in the dermis of the wounded area happen to be directed. If a flat blade enters in a direction parallel with the fibers a slit-like or elliptic wound with sharp edges and pointed ends is produced. On the other hand, if the elastic fibers are severed transversely, the wound usually gapes because of the contraction of this tissue. If the fibers are severed obliquely, the opening in the skin may gape unevenly and assume an asymmetric oval shape. If the knife blade is drawn out in a slightly different direction from that in which it entered, other fibers are cut and the wound may show a notch (Fig. 15-1). An instrument with three-cornered edges, like a triangular file, produces a three-cornered wound (Fig. 15-17). An implement with a thin circular shaft like an ice pick inflicts a round hole or slit on the skin. If the shaft is comparatively thick and roughened there

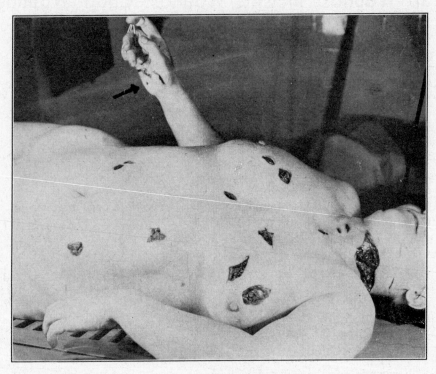

Fig. 15-1. Multiple Stab Wounds of Chest and Abdomen and Incised Wound of Neck. Defense Cuts on Right Hand.

Wounds inflicted with a knife. Note slit-like wounds on front of neck and right side of abdomen, gaping wounds and asymmetric notched wounds of chest and abdomen. Homicide.

may be a marginal abrasion around the opening (Figs. 15-2, 15-13 and 15-14). Other weapons produce their own characteristic skin lesions.

Wounds in the internal viscera also correspond to the type of the penetrating weapon, but their shape is modified in many instances by the muscular and elastic fibers in the capsule and framework of the organ.

A thin plate of bone like the vault or side of the skull may retain an accurate impression of a penetrating blade. If the penetration is at right angles to the bony surface, the wound is usually a faithful cross section of that part of the weapon passing through the bone. For example a knife blade causes a thin triangular slit, a three-cornered file produces a triangular opening, and an icepick leaves a circular hole in the bone (Figs. 15-11 and 15-12). Under some conditions a forcible withdrawal of the blade may increase the size of the perforation. Occasionally when the weapon is driven into the skull at an acute angle, the opening in the bony plate is usually an oblique section of the blade; one edge of the wound may show distinct bevelling, while the opposite edge may be slightly raised and overhang the track. There may be a slight comminution of the inner table at the point of entrance or small linear cracks may occur at the corners of the perforation, but extensive fractures are rarely produced by stab wounds of the skull.

Necropsy. The stab wounds should be described carefully in the external description of the body, and the number of wounds, their location, the dimensions and the form of the perforations in the skin noted. The most convenient method of indicating the position of the wound on the body is to give its relation to the nearest anatomic point, as, for example, a wound of the upper chest may be mentioned as two inches below and three inches to the left of the suprasternal notch.

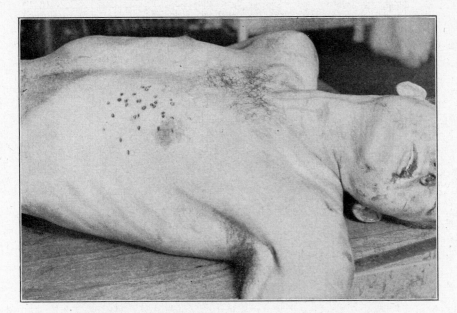

Fig. 15-2. Thirty-one Small Puncture Stab Wounds of Left Side of Chest.

The surface wounds are small slits but the tracts are deep and penetrate heart and lungs. Homicide. Such wounds are inflicted with an ice pick, skewer or similar long pointed weapon. The body was found submerged in a bathtub.

The opening on the skin is described as to the form, condition of the edges, and the size carefully determined. If the wound is elliptic its long axis and cross axis should be measured and the relation of its long axis to the planes of the body noted. Thus a slit-like wound on the chest may be described with its long axis vertical, or horizontal as the case may be, or if it is oblique, the distance of the lower end to the right or left of the upper end is noted, according to the location of the wound.

The direction and the depth of penetration must be determined as accurately as possible. The direction is usually designated (taking, as an example, a penetration of the anterior chest) as backward, downward and to the right, the principal direction being noted first and the others next, as the case may be. The depth of the wound is measured. The organs and principal tissues penetrated are described in order and the location, size, form and arrangement of the injury in each organ are noted. Each wound should be examined and described. It is important also to look for cuts and stab wounds on the hands and arms, especially the ulnar border of the forearm, as lesions of this sort suggest that a struggle had taken place, and that the victim had attempted to ward off the knife thrust with his hands (Fig. 15-1).

Sometimes it is not possible to determine the depth of penetration of a stab wound with any degree of accuracy, inasmuch as effusion of blood into the tissues, changes in the position of the viscera, or numerous other circumstances may alter the conditions existing at the time when the wound was inflicted. Consequently the depth of the track at autopsy may be different from the actual penetration of the instrument at the time of the stabbing. Moreover it is not always possible to correlate the depth of the wound with the blade of the stabbing instrument. For ex-

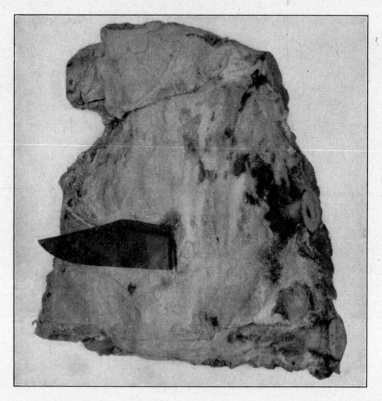

Fig. 15-3. Broken-off Blade of Pocket Knife Projecting from Inner Surface of Sternum.
The blade pierced the heart. Homicide.

ample, a short blade of two inches can penetrate four inches into a soft area like the thigh or through the anterior abdominal wall, because the force of the thrust may dent the tissues appreciably and thus deepen the wound. Conversely, a long blade may not be thrust in to its full length, and the wound may be shorter than the blade. For these reasons attempts to correlate the depth of the track and the length of the weapon should be made with caution.

If a broken-off blade is found in the wound it must be preserved as evidence for it can be fitted to the corresponding break on the original weapon and thus establish it as the instrument used. Blades are apt to break off when a knife or other weapon is driven into such bones as the sternum, spine or skull, and whenever possible it is advisable to remove a block of the bone containing the embedded blade by sawing or chiselling and to preserve the specimen as an exhibit which can be offered in evidence to show the broken weapon and its origin as well as the

extent of its penetration (Figs. 15-3, 15-4 and 15-5). Similarly a wound through
the skull without a broken blade can be removed in its entirety and preserved as
part of the corpus delicti (Fig. 15-13).

If a knife or other stabbing instrument is found at the scene of a homicide it
must be examined for finger prints, tested for human blood and scrutinized for hair
and other material. The investigation at the scene of stabbings has been discussed
on page 12.

It is also important to note whether there are any cuts on the clothing and to
determine whether or not they correspond to the stab wounds on the body. If the

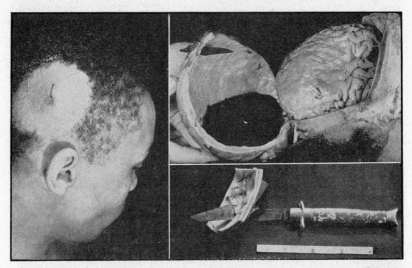

From Helpern, M., *Ann. Int. Med.*, 24:666, 1946

Fig. 15-4. Left. Homicidal Stab Wound in Right Parietal Portion of Scalp.

Upper right. Top of skull removed and laid back to show broken-off knife blade which
penetrated skull and brain. Note stab wound in dura; large subdural hemorrhage was collected
in hollow of skull at autopsy.

Lower right. Broken-off blade embedded in block of bone removed at autopsy and offered
as evidence at trial. Handle of knife with broken blade stump found on perpetrator, included
to show matching broken ends of blade. After being stabbed, victim chased his assailant for
distance of a block.

wounds have bled externally, the amount of blood which has soaked into the cloth
may give some clue to the profuseness of the hemorrhage.

The effects produced by stab wounds depend upon their location on the body.
The wounds may involve the chest, abdomen, spine, neck, head and extremities.

THE CHEST

Stab wounds may penetrate the chest from any direction. Death occurs as a
result of penetration of the heart, lungs, aorta, pulmonary arteries, venae cavae,
subclavian vessels, internal mammary vessels, intercostal vessels, diaphragm and
pleural cavities. The chief complication of these injuries is internal hemorrhage
and its effects depend upon the extent of the injury and the organs and structures
involved. Profuse external hemorrhage is not as commonly encountered, even when
there is fatal internal bleeding from penetrating injuries of the thoracic viscera.
Traumatic shock is not pronounced, as stab wounds are usually inflicted with only

a moderate degree of violence. Secondary infection and other complications are comparatively rare.

The Heart. The anatomic characteristics of cardiac stab wounds are the same as the corresponding stab wounds of the skin and depend upon the form and length of the weapon. Most of them are knife wounds and consequently the penetrating lesion on the surface of the heart is a slit or an elliptic opening with sharp edges and slight peripheral ecchymosis. The right ventricle is involved most often as it forms

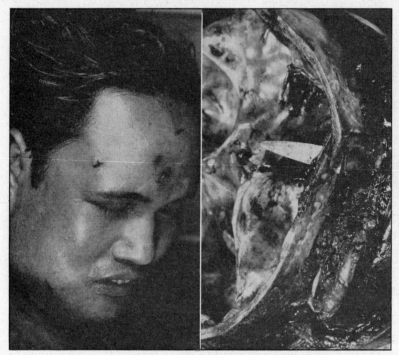

From Helpern, M., *Ann. Int. Med.*, 24:666, 1946

Fig. 15-5. Left. Small Homicidal Stab Wound in Forehead.

Right. Calvarium and brain removed showing broken-off closed scissors blades stuck in right frontal bone projecting into cranial cavity. The blades pierced the frontal lobe of the brain resulting in a delayed fatal intracerebral hemorrhage. The victim, after being stabbed, walked into accident room of hospital. The seriousness of the injury was not recognized until the onset of coma. Lived two days.

most of the anterior surface of the heart, and the left ventricle, aorta, pulmonary artery, auricles and vena cavae are next in frequency in about that order. Most of the skin wounds in cases of cardiac penetration occur on the front part of the chest and a few on the sides and back. They comprise about 25 per cent of fatal stab wounds.

In a stab wound of the heart, the perforation in the pericardial sac may not communicate with the pleural cavities or the opening may be too small to allow easy escape of blood from the pericardial into the pleural cavities. Under such conditions the effused blood compresses the heart, causing a tamponade and rapid death from asphyxia. The amount of blood in such cases varies from about 200 to 450 gm. On the other hand, if the penetrating weapon has produced a sizeable wound in the pericardial sac which communicates with a pleural cavity, the blood may readily drain out of the former into the latter. Death results from loss of blood after an interval varying from several minutes to a few hours, an interval sometimes long enough to permit surgical intervention and repair in favorable cases. The fatal hemorrhages in the chest cavities vary from about 1 to 3 liters.

The most rapidly fatal stab wounds of the heart are those which penetrate the auricles, pulmonary artery, aorta or coronary arteries, as hemorrhage from such injuries is usually profuse and rapid. Wounds of the ventricles may not bleed so freely because the contraction of the thick ventricular muscle produces a certain amount of hemostasis. Some of the penetrating lesions are amenable to cardiorrhaphy, and recovery has followed the operation. A few stab wounds of the heart undergo spontaneous healing. In some of these cases the wound is temporarily closed by the processes of repair, but after a few days the edges may break apart and death result from an intrapericardial hemorrhage. In such cases an initial fall in blood pressure may favor spontaneous closure of the wound. With restoration of blood pressure and increased heart action, reopening of the wound is apt to occur.

The blade of the penetrating instrument may be broken off and remain embedded in the heart for a long period of time without causing any serious complications. Brouardel has mentioned a rare case in which a strip of iron was driven into the myocardium where it remained for over a year until the victim's death from a cause unrelated to the injury. Two similar cases have been encountered among the routine necropsies in the Office of the Chief Medical Examiner.

One case was that of a Negro man who died of acute alcoholism. The autopsy disclosed an aneurysm of the thoracic aorta and an exuberant obliterative fibrous pericarditis. A knife blade about one and a half inches long was discovered embedded in the left ventricle, discolored black from a long sojourn in the tissues, evidently a mute relic of an old assault. The pericardial adhesions probably were the end result of an acute pericarditis which developed after the stabbing.

A more remarkable example was encountered in a 23-year-old Negro who was stabbed near the midline of the back in the region of the sixth dorsal vertebra, 7 months and 24 days prior to his death. He was treated in a hospital at the time of the stabbing but after two days was discharged on his own insistence, apparently not in serious condition. Although ambulatory, he complained of weakness and shortness of breath. About six months later, he was prevailed upon to enter the hospital because of severe pain in the left costovertebral region, radiating down to his left thigh, with evident dysuria and pyuria. A roentgenogram, fluoroscopy and angiocardiogram revealed the blade of an ice pick at the level of the midthoracic region of the spine, pointing forward and displacing the esophagus to the right. An exploratory thoracotomy through the left pleural cavity was performed, and the blade of the weapon was found embedded in the spinal column, projecting forward into the heart; its removal was considered inadvisable. The patient died during the operation.

The autopsy disclosed an ice pick blade three and one-quarter inches long, broken off, and firmly embedded in the left side of the body of the sixth thoracic vertebra. It projected forward through the posterior mediastinum lateral to the aorta and esophagus. The posterior wall of the left auricle was firmly adherent to the posterior structures and was penetrated almost in its center, the pointed slender weapon transfixing the auricle and the anterior leaflet of the mitral valve which was perforated in two places, the point of the blade reaching the upper part of the cavity of the left ventricle. The segment of blade which penetrated the heart was one and one-half inches long. The perforations in the auricle and mitral valve were 4 to 5 mm. in diameter. There was a subacute reactive inflammation with many small bland thrombotic vegetations on the valve leaflet surrounding the two perforations (Fig. 15-6). Numerous embolic, nonseptic infarctions were present in the spleen and kidneys. The weapon was discolored a bluish black as a result of its stay in the body. The blade of the instrument undoubtedly prevented a fatal hemorrhage at the time of the stabbing by plugging up the cardiac perforation.

The immediate effects of a stab wound of the heart are variable. If the wound is large, the victim dies in a few seconds. But it is possible for an individual to travel a considerable distance from the place where he was stabbed, if the wound does not bleed too rapidly and if cardiac tamponade does not occur. In one case the victim was stabbed in the heart while on the street and then ran across the roadway, up two flights of stairs into his apartment where he locked himself in the bathroom and then died. When found by the police and medical examiner, the dead body was seated on the toilet (Fig. 2-1).

Another complication of stab wounds of the heart in those cases that survive the initial and usually fatal hemorrhage is infection of the pericardial cavity and the development of a septic pericarditis or mediastinitis. The infection is caused by pyogenic bacteria carried in by the blade of the weapon. This complication ensues

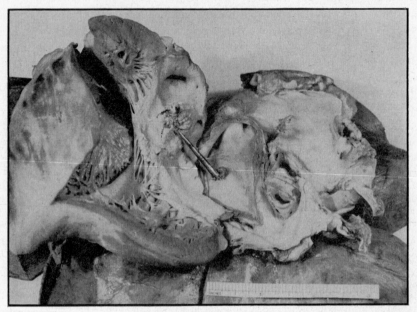

From Lowen, Fink and Helpern, *Circulation*, 2:426, 1950

Fig. 15-6. Homicidal Ice Pick Stab Wound of Back with Transfixion of Heart for Eight Months.

Victim was ambulatory for six months. Broken-off blade of weapon was embedded in the spine and impaled the heart. Its presence was not suspected until revealed by routine fluoroscopy during hospitalization about 40 days before death. Photograph of heart opened to show ice pick blade projecting into left auricle and inflamed perforations of transfixed mitral valve.

about 24 hours after the stabbing and death occurs from 1 to 10 days later. At necropsy the lining of the pericardial sac and the epicardial surface are covered with a fibrinopurulent exudate, sometimes tinged with blood. There may be sufficient purulent and bloody fluid in the pericardial sac to compress the heart. When the mediastinum is involved, there is a suppurative inflammation in the form of a phlegmon in the anterior mediastinal fat extending up on the anterior surface of the pericardium.

A rarer complication of stab wounds of the heart, observed by the authors in several instances, is massive cerebral embolism from a mural thrombosis of the left ventricle developing on the site of the penetrating wound. Such thrombosis and embolism may develop within 24 hours after the injury and death may result from massive cerebral infarction. In one such case a young woman was stabbed with a pen knife. The wound penetrated the left ventricle but there was no significant hemorrhage. Embolism into the left middle cerebral artery was produced by a portion of a mural thrombus that formed rapidly on the inner surface of the left ventricle at the site of penetration and caused death in a few days from massive infarction of the left cerebral hemisphere. Similar instances of mural thrombosis of the left ventricle and cerebral embolism and infarction are encountered in cases where the stab wound has been repaired during prompt surgical intervention.

Mural thrombosis of the right ventricle at the site of a stab wound may also occur but if embolism results, the relatively small size of the emboli is not apt to result in serious pulmonary infarction, since the lungs can absorb without difficulty many small emboli of the size that might cause a fatal cerebral embolism.

A case was encountered by the authors in which a stab wound of the right ventricle sealed itself off without any significant hemorrhage and without infection of the pericardium. The victim had also been stabbed in the chest and lung, but the lung did not collapse and the possibility of a fistulous communication between a bronchus and tributary of the pulmonary vein could not be ruled out. Before death which occurred three days after the stabbing, there was marked cyanosis of the face and venous engorgement of the neck. At necropsy a small thrombosed stab wound of the right ventricle was found and marked dilatation of the superior vena

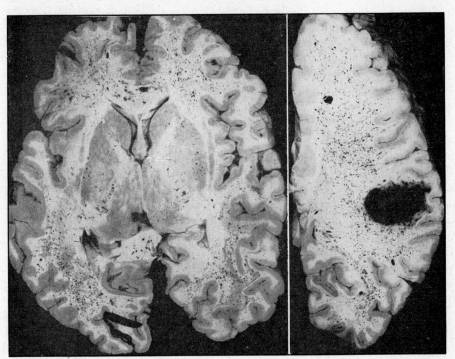

Fig. 15-7. Multiple Cerebral Hemorrhages Complicating Two Spontaneously Sealed Off Stab Wounds of the Chest, One in the Right Ventricle, the Other in the Lung.

The victim survived three days with marked cyanosis of head and venous engorgement of neck. Hemorrhages in brain attributed to venous stasis and possible air embolism. See text.

cava, the internal jugular veins and the dural venous sinuses was present without thrombosis of these vessels. There were large and small variable-sized areas of hemorrhage throughout the cerebral white matter (Fig. 15-7). The autopsy findings were explained on the basis of venous stasis secondary to the injury of the right ventricle, and possibly as the result of systemic air embolism from the lung injury, or possibly by a combination of both factors.

The authors have also observed a rare complication of a stab wound of the heart which cut the midportion of the anterior descending branch of the left coronary artery. The surgical operation was performed promptly and the severed vessels ligated. Death resulted about 50 hours after the stabbing. At autopsy there was a massive anemic infarction of the left ventricular myocardium which resulted from the interference with the coronary arterial circulation.

The Lungs. Stab wounds of the lungs comprise about 10 per cent of homicidal stab wounds, and may occur on any part of these organs, penetrating the front, sides and back of the chest, or the supraclavicular space above or the diaphragm below. Occasionally the heart, or the big vessels of the upper chest and lower neck, or the liver and other upper abdominal viscera may be pierced by the same thrust. The type of wound in the lung depends upon the shape and length of the penetrating blade. If it is inflicted by a knife, the penetration will be slit-like or elliptic with sharp edges. If an ice pick is used the resulting lesion is a circular hole. Because of the marked vascularity of the lung tissue, there is usually appreciable ecchymosis in the immediate vicinity of the wound, but it is not as marked as in cases of blunt force injury.

Death usually results from hemorrhage into the corresponding chest cavity, and this may be slow or rapid depending upon the size of the pulmonary vessels penetrated by the weapon. As a rule peripheral stab wounds do not bleed profusely, and if by any chance air enters the chest, the lung may collapse and hemostasis may result. A deeper injury involving a large blood vessel may cause a rapid hemorrhage and death in a short time. In some stab wounds of the chest wall and the lung air may escape into the subcutaneous tissues, causing a subcutaneous emphysema. If a large bronchus is entered by the weapon, blood may be aspirated into the air passages, a frothy hemoptysis may occur and areas of inhaled blood may appear in other parts of the lung. In one case seen by the authors, an ice pick was driven into the right lung, establishing a channel between a large bronchus and a large branch of the pulmonary artery and giving rise to a fatal hemoptysis.

Hemopneumothorax is a complication which occurs when air and blood enter the chest either through a wound in the chest wall or in the lung. The air passes through the penetration in the chest wall only if the stab wound is large enough to admit sufficient air to overcome the negative intrathoracic pressure. More commonly the hemopneumothorax occurs when a stab wound penetrates the lung parenchyma obliquely and severs a bronchus of appreciable size. In such cases air escapes from the lung into the chest with each inspiration and accumulates there because of a valve action at the site of the lung wound. This hemopneumothorax is gradually increased until the lung is completely compressed and the other chest organs and the diaphragm are displaced as described on page 231.

Acute suppurative pleuritis, a delayed complication of a stab wound of the chest, which may cause death by sepsis, results from infection of the pleural cavity by pyogenic bacteria. The infective microorganisms are either carried into the chest directly by the blade of the penetrating instrument, or the pleural cavity may be secondarily infected if the wound in the lung tissue attracts bacteria as a locus minoris resistentiae. In the early stages of the infection the pleural surfaces are covered by a fibrinous exudate which may be hemorrhagic. Later the exudate may increase in amount and become partly hemorrhagic and purulent in character, and the fibrin on the pleural surfaces may become exuberant and undergo partial organization. In some instances a true empyema develops and partly compresses the lung.

Cerebral air embolism results from the forcing of air from a severed bronchus into one of the pulmonary veins. The air is then carried into the systemic circulation and into the brain (page 231).

The immediate effects of pulmonary stab wounds are variable. If a large vessel is injured, the bleeding may be profuse and the victim may collapse quickly. Other wounds may bleed more slowly and the injured man may be able to move a considerable distance after the stabbing. Some of these penetrating lesions heal spontaneously by processes of repair analogous to those described on page 232, and a fibrous scar is formed in the lung parenchyma.

The Blood Vessels of the Chest. The branches of the aorta and superior vena cava may be penetrated by a weapon which is driven against the upper chest in front or directed downward through the supraclavicular space into the pleural cavity.

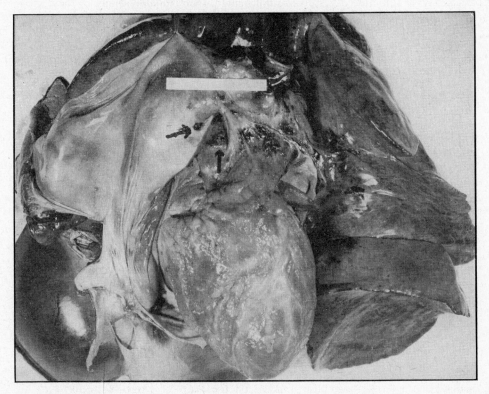

Fig. 15-8. Ice Pick Stab Wound of Pericardium and Aorta with Spontaneous Closure of Both Wounds.

Sudden death 10 days after injury from delayed secondary rupture of aortic perforation with massive hemopericardium. Oblique arrow points to healed pericardial wound; vertical arrow to wound in the aorta.

The form of the wound corresponds with that of the blade of the penetrating instrument which may pierce the blood vessel, or transfix it, or, if the blade has an edge, may sever it, partially or completely. These injuries bleed profusely, so that death is usually rapid. If the ascending aorta or superior vena cava are penetrated inside the pericardium, the fatal hemorrhage is intrapericardial or into the chest cavity as described under The Heart on page 340. Wounds of the innominate and subclavian arteries and veins generally bleed into the pleural cavity and cause death by loss of blood. In rare instances if the victim survives the hemorrhage a thrombus may form at the site of the vascular penetration and emboli may be disseminated to vessels of the brain, upper extremities or other organs. The authors have seen a case of a stab wound of the ascending aorta in which a thrombus closed the 15 mm. aortic wound and the patient lived two days after the injury. In another case, a 25 year old man was stabbed through the right side of the chest and rapidly recovered from the shock of his wound. On the tenth day he collapsed and died while seated on the toilet. Autopsy revealed small stab wounds of the right lung, pericardium and ascending aorta. There was a delayed secondary rupture of the aortic wound (Fig. 15-8) resulting in a massive fatal 600 ml. hemopericardium. There was 600 ml. of blood in the right pleural cavity. The perforation in the pericardial sac was healed.

Sometimes the internal mammary vessels or the intercostal vessels are the only ones severed, and the hemorrhage into the chest cavity is slow. Death occurs after a few days if the injured vessels are not ligated. Unfortunately many of these cases die because they are not diagnosed during life and an operation is not performed.

The authors have seen a rare complication which occurred as a result of a stab wound of the chest. A communicating opening was produced between the left innominate vein and the arch of the aorta, and an arteriovenous aneurysm resulted which dissected the anterior mediastinum. The hemorrhage caused by this process leaked slowly into the left pleural cavity and death occurred 13 days later. At necropsy, more than four liters of blood were found in the left chest, the diaphragm on that side being pushed down into the abdominal cavity.

Penetration of the diaphragm may occur in stab wounds of the lower part of the chest or upper abdomen. If the left side of this muscle is involved, in addition to the usual complications of hemorrhage and infection, a herniation of the abdominal viscera into the chest cavity may take place and shock and intestinal obstruction result from strangulation of any portion of the gastrointestinal tract which has slipped through such an opening. Among the cases of Dr. Charles Norris was a fatal strangulated hernia of this type in the left vault of the diaphragm, which suddenly developed through an old unhealed stab wound received several years before and never repaired by operation.

THE ABDOMEN

Pointed instruments may penetrate the abdomen from all directions producing wounds which correspond to the type of weapon used. These cases comprise more than 33 per cent of all stab wounds. Most of them penetrate the anterior abdominal wall, but occasionally the flanks, the lower chest, and sometimes the back and buttocks are involved. The wounds in the parenchymatous organs have the same general characteristics as those inflicted on the heart or lungs, while those in the hollow viscera are somewhat similar to aortic stab wounds in shape and extent. If the penetration is from the front, the liver, spleen, mesentery, stomach, intestines, pancreas, kidneys and bladder may suffer. If a vascular organ like the liver or spleen is penetrated, or if a large mesenteric blood vessel is cut, death may result from a profuse hemorrhage into the abdominal cavity, varying from 1,500 to 3,000 ml. Occasionally a stab wound of the liver or spleen does not cause much bleeding, but gives rise to small traumatic infarcts because of the damage to the blood supply of the tissues adjacent to the wound. In most cases these are not dangerous but sometimes they serve as a nidus for a septic infection which causes a fatal septic peritonitis. Stab wounds of the stomach, intestines and bladder allow infective material to enter the abdominal cavity and usually give rise to an acute suppurative peritonitis, especially if an operation is not performed promptly to repair the perforations. In some cases the distal portion of the duodenum may be perforated, and the outcome of such an injury is a retroperitoneal cellulitis involving the right lumbar fossa and usually fatal in a few days. Sometimes the weapon on entering the abdominal cavity does not penetrate any of the abdominal viscera but carries pathogenic bacteria into the peritoneal cavity so as to produce a fatal peritonitis. This is especially likely to happen if the intestines and omentum have protruded externally through the wound of the skin.

The weapon in some cases is driven in from the back or from the flank, and pierces the liver and kidneys. External hemorrhage may occur, or a large retroperitoneal hemorrhage results especially if the kidney is injured. Small traumatic infarcts may develop in the stabbed kidney and give rise to an abscess and general septic infection. If the pelvis of the kidney is cut a gangrenous perirenal abscess may develop. Wounds of the renal artery may result in complete infarction of the kidney. Wounds of the aorta, inferior vena cava, or iliac vessels may occur and result in a severe retroperitoneal hemorrhage at times extending into the peritoneal cavity.

If hemorrhage into the abdomen is rapid and profuse, the victim will usually collapse quickly and be unable to walk. But if the bleeding is slight, the wounded man may be able to move without difficulty, even in cases in which the intestines are protruding through the wound in the abdominal wall. As a rule external hemorrhage from stab wounds of the abdomen is not marked.

THE SPINE AND CORD

Stab wounds of the spinal canal are not common, and the penetration is usually from the back, slightly to one side of the midline. If the spinal cord is injured, paralyses, urinary tract infections, decubital ulcers and suppurative meningitis may develop and cause death. In some instances, the cord is not completely severed and the victim may survive for several years. In the case illustrated in Figure 15-9, the blade of the knife penetrated the left side of the face below the ear, passed under the foramen magnum and severed the upper spinal cord completely. The point of the weapon protruded through the back of the neck on the right side. The blade literally guillotined the spinal cord. The authors have seen a case in which the victim lived for eight years after a stab wound of the thoracic cord near the level of the fourth dorsal segment. He was paralysed below the level of the injury and during the long clinical course had periods of improvement and exacerbation, finally dying of a terminal pneumonia. Several large excavated healed scars covered with skin were found over the sacrum, representing healed decubital ulcers.

A small stab wound in the upper part of the cervical cord may damage important centers in that region. Hyperpyrexia of 106° F. or more may develop before death. The clinical picture may be one of shock.

The ability of the victim to walk after the stabbing will depend on whether or not the important fiber tracts in the cord are severed or sufficiently damaged to cause paralysis of the lower extremities. If paralysis is produced the patient cannot walk from the place of injury unassisted. The authors have seen a case in which the knife penetrated the spinal canal and barely nicked the surface of the cord, but did not cause enough disability to interfere with the movements of the deceased. The victim died six days later of an infective suppurative meningitis carried in by the knife blade.

In not a few instances broken-off knife blades have been found embedded in the spine and this possibility should always be considered. The track of the stab wound should be explored by dissection which should include the opening of the spinal canal and removal of the cord.

THE NECK

Stab wounds of the neck occur in homicidal assaults and are produced by frontal thrusts usually involving the lower anterior portion of the neck, or by round arm swings against the sides delivered anywhere between the mastoid area and the clavicle. These injuries comprise about 12 per cent of stab wounds. Suicidal and

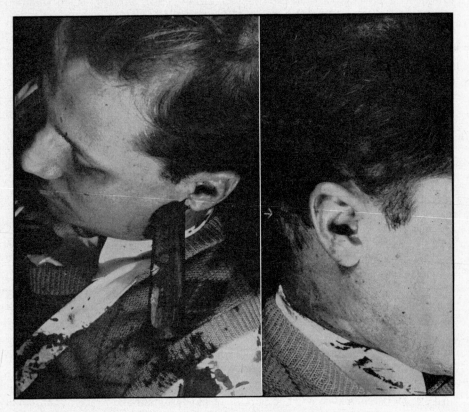

Fig. 15-9. Homicidal Stabbing.

Transfixion of neck with blade of boning knife which completely severed the spinal cord below the foramen magnum. Arrow indicates the point of the knife protruding from back of neck.

accidental stab wounds of the neck are quite rare. Death usually results from cutting of the carotid arteries or jugular veins or both, and the victim bleeds either externally or into the neck tissues. If the penetration is just below the ear or near the angle of the jaw, the jugular vein or some branch of the external carotid may be cut, and the weapon may penetrate the pharynx, larynx or trachea. In such instances blood may be aspirated into the lungs or swallowed into the stomach. The ability of the patient to move after the stabbing will depend on the rate of hemorrhage from the wound. Neck wounds may not bleed profusely but may produce a local infection such as an abscess or cellulitis of the neck, and cause death by sepsis, edema of the glottis or a secondary pneumonia.

A small stab wound of a carotid artery may become plugged by the formation of a mural thrombus which projects into the lumen of the vessel, and a portion of this thrombus may become detached and carried as an embolus to occlude one of the cerebral arteries. The result is an infarction of a portion of the brain supplied by the occluded embolized artery, the infarction causing unconsciousness and unilateral paralysis, and usually terminating fatally (Fig. 15-10).

Stab wounds of the jugular veins may be complicated by thrombosis and pulmonary embolism or by pulmonary air embolism as described on page 171. A stab wound penetrating both the internal jugular vein and the adjacent common carotid

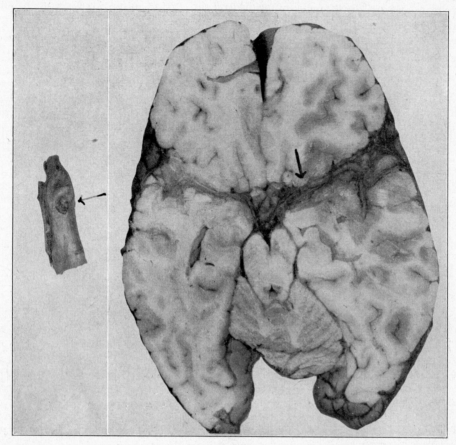

From Helpern, M., *Am. J. Surg.*, 26:60, 1934

Fig. 15-10. Stab Wound of Left Side of Neck and Left Common Carotid Artery, with Mural Thrombosis and Cerebral Embolism Occurring 36 Hours Later. Homicidal Assault with Pocket Knife.

Left. Carotid artery opened to show stab wound plugged with thrombus.
Right. Left middle cerebral artery occluded by an embolus.

artery may produce an arteriovenous fistula resulting in a serious disturbance of the circulation, or thrombosis of the injured vessels and embolization to the lungs and brain.

THE HEAD

Stab wounds in the head comprise about 5 to 6 per cent of homicidal stabbings. They are inflicted most often during an altercation in which a knife, ice pick or other instrument is thrust through the orbit into the brain, or delivered in a round arm swing against the side of the head, especially in the temporal region where the bone is thin or over the frontal or parietal regions. The force employed to penetrate the skull need only be moderately severe, for which reason concussion effects may be slight or absent. The victim may recover rapidly from the immediate effects of the injury and travel a considerable distance from the scene of the assault. Death may occur hours or days after the injury from cerebral compression produced by the traumatic cerebral or subdural hemorrhage incident to the wound in the brain, or from a septic meningitis or brain abscess caused by pyogenic microorganisms carried in on the blade of the weapon. The perforation in the skull will correspond in shape and size to the penetrating instrument and at autopsy may be removed intact with some of the surrounding bone to be preserved as part of the corpus delicti (Figs. 15-4, 15-11). Suicidal and accidental stab wounds of the skull and head are not common (page 356).

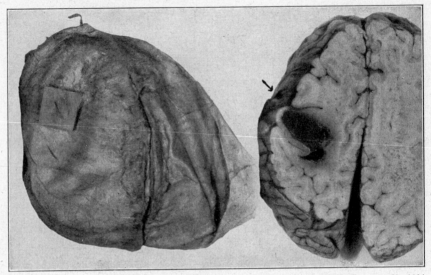

From Helpern, M., *Am. J. Surg.*, 26:59, 1934

Fig. 15-11. Thin Knife Wound Through Left Parietal Bone, Dura and Left Cerebral Hemisphere. Secondary Subcortical Hemorrhage Occurring 13 Days Later. Homicidal Assault.

Left. Square of bone containing stab wound above corresponding slit in dura.
Right. Entrance of stab wound on left cerebral hemisphere shown by arrow. Horizontal section of brain reveals large secondary subcortical hemorrhage.

Homicidal stab wounds of the head, inflicted with ice picks, knives and occasionally scissor blades have in many instances gone unrecognized during life even after hospitalization of the victim. In some of these traumatic intracranial hemorrhage was suspected and in others spontaneous cerebral hemorrhage. The true state of affairs was not discovered until autopsy, when stab wounds of the skull and brain with intracranial hemorrhage and cerebral compression were demonstrated as the cause of death (Figs. 15-12 and 15-13). The inconspicuous nature of the stab wound in the scalp where it is often concealed by hair and overlooked, or sometimes mistaken for an insignificant laceration, if observed at all, and the confusing development of intracranial complications make the antemortem diagnosis of the condition a matter of considerable difficulty. Unless the autopsy is completely performed to include the head, and the possibility of a stab wound kept in mind, the true nature of such a lesion will be unrecognized. The perforating wound in the skull may escape detection and the traumatic hemorrhage in and on the brain or under the dura may escape recognition.

In a number of these clinically unsuspected and unrecognized fatal stab wounds of the head and brain broken-off blades of ice picks, knives and scissors have been found embedded in the skull and brain.

The eye and nose area on the face, composed of soft tissue and thin plates of bone, are easily penetrated by instruments some of which, like metal rods or umbrella tips, are comparatively blunt. These instruments may be thrust into the nasal cavities or orbits, break through the thin plates of bone at the base of the skull and lacerate the brain. Death usually occurs from hemorrhage or sepsis. The authors have seen the cribriform plate perforated, and the under surface of the

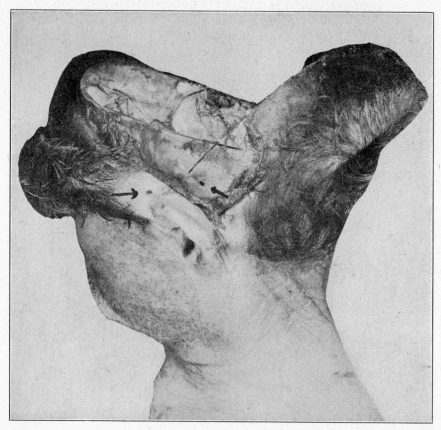

From Helpern, M., *Am. J. Surg.*, 26:55, 1934

Fig. 15-12. Small Stab Wound in Scalp above Left Ear and in Underlying Left Temporal Bone.

Scalp reflected forward and skull cap removed. The tract passed into the brain as far as the left cerebral peduncle. Lived five days. Clinically undetected. Homicidal assault inflicted with a slender pointed weapon like an ice pick.

frontal lobe lacerated by the manipulation of a nasal curet during an operation, death following a few days later from an acute suppurative meningitis. Glaister has described a penetrating wound of the orbit and brain caused by a thrust with a sharp-pointed poker. Severe damage may be done to the brain by overzealous probing with a cannula during an exploratory craniotomy, and some of the lesions are similar to those produced by an ice pick. In one such case death occurred from an intracranial hemorrhage arising from aneurysm of a cerebral artery punctured by the cannula.

Occasionally stab wounds of the brain heal, leaving a tan colored pigmented scar. In one case a knife blade was discovered years after the injury, embedded in the orbital roof and projecting into the left frontal lobe one and and a half inches where it was surrounded by tan colored cerebral scar tissue. Death was due to an entirely unrelated condition. In another bizarre case an old blackened broken-off tip of an ice pick blade was found embedded in the left petrous bone in an old

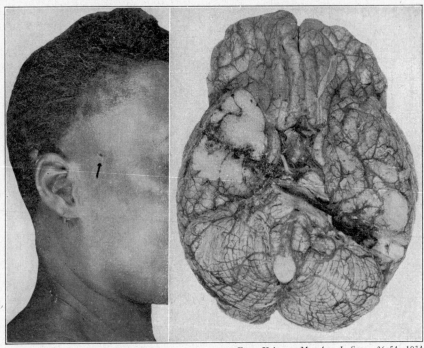

From Helpern, M., *Am. J. Surg.*, 26:54, 1934

Fig. 15-13. Penetrating Stab Wound of Right Side of Head and Brain. Homicidal Assault with Ice Pick. Lived Five Days.

Left. Small surface wound in right temple (originally concealed by hair).
Right. Diagonal slender tract of wound across brain.

scarred area of the overlying temporal lobe, the relic of an assault several years before. Death was caused by a rapidly fatal fresh stab wound inflicted with a heavy bladed knife which penetrated the left petrous bone and temporal lobe in almost the exact location as the previous wound.

THE EXTREMITIES

Multiple wounds of the arms are received most often in struggles in which the victim is trying to protect himself against a knife. If many such wounds are inflicted, the victim may die of external hemorrhage after a greater or lesser interval even though no large blood vessels are severed. In some cases the wounded person, especially if he is deeply alcoholic, may die on the operating table under the anesthetic while the surgeons are endeavoring to stop the hemorrhage. Stab wounds of the axilla and groin are apt to prove rapidly fatal, when the main arterial and venous trunks are cut, death occurring from profuse external hemorrhage shortly after the injury. Occasionally the bacteria carried into the wound produce a fatal septic infection of the extremity. In rare instances abscesses develop in the sub-cutaneous tissues and cause a fatal infection after the wounds of the skin have healed. Stab wounds of the extremities comprise about 10 per cent of homicidal stabbings.

A stab wound of an extremity involving the wall of a large artery may allow the blood to break through the arterial coats and distend the surrounding connective tissue forming a saccular swelling known as a false aneurysm. In some instances this develops a short time after the injury, but occasionally the process is delayed for days or months, the wound having weakened the arterial wall so that the disruption and swelling develop gradually after the skin wound has healed. Other penetrating wounds of the arteries, such as those produced by bullets or by the sharp end of a bone fractured by blunt force, may produce false aneurysms in much the same way as stab wounds. Occasionally both the artery and the vein are penetrated and an arteriovenous fistula is produced with all the circulatory disturbances resulting from such an abnormal channel of communication. The hazard of these lesions, especially of false aneurysms, is that they may give rise to a massive intermuscular hemorrhage in the extremity or to a fatal external hemorrhage during an open operation. Gangrene of an extremity occasionally occurs if the circulation is obstructed.

The ability of the victim to move about after receiving a stab wound of the extremities will depend upon how much blood is lost as the result of the injury. If much blood is lost rapidly, he will not be able to walk very far, but a lesser injury may not interfere with his movements. Other serious disabilities resulting from stab wounds of the extremities occur when a big nerve trunk is severed or one of the main joints necessary for locomotion is injured.

HOMICIDE, SUICIDE OR ACCIDENT

Every death from stab wounds should always be considered as possibly homicidal until proved otherwise. As a matter of fact, most deaths from stab wounds are homicidal, whether they occur on the head, neck, abdomen, chest, spine or extremities, especially if they are located in the back or in a spot where an individual could not stab himself without difficulty. Usually if the wound is so located that it could be conveniently inflicted by an assailant wielding a pointed weapon, the chances are that it was so inflicted. The wound in many cases is a single penetration at a vital spot, like the left supraclavicular region, or the groin, most apt to occur in a sudden surprise attack. If there is an altercation followed by a scuffle, there may be a number of wounds, occasionally associated with defense cuts on the hands and arms. Multiple wounds which penetrate into different parts of the body generally indicate an intent to kill (Fig. 15-1). In a few homicidal cases a number of stab wounds may be inflicted in a circumscribed area as shown by the case of two men who were found dead with multiple penetrating injuries on the front parts of their necks. Later it was discovered that the perpetrator had knocked them unconscious and had repeatedly punctured their necks with the sharp blade of a scissors. The 31 stab wounds on the chest (Fig. 15-2) at autopsy were homicidal in character in that each was discrete and of uniform depth, differing from multiple suicidal perforations which may be encountered in the same body region but generally show evidence of incomplete perforation.

The yearly Reports of the Office of the Chief Medical Examiner in New York City indicate that out of a yearly average of 378 homicides (2.6 per cent of the total number of medical examiner's cases), an average of 80 was listed as homicide by stabbing which includes four to six deaths from homicidal incised wounds and chop wounds. The number of homicidal stabbings together with incised and chop wounds has averaged over 100 yearly since 1937 and in excess of homicidal shootings. Homicidal shootings were more frequent than stabbings up until 1937.

Suicidal stab wounds occur over those areas of the body on which the deceased can inflict a stab wound easily with his own hands. The most frequent site is the chest over the heart region. Usually the person grasps the knife in his right hand and directs it upward and to the right into the cardiac region on the left side of the

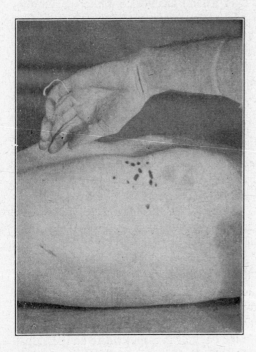

Fig. 15-14. Multiple Self-inflicted Stab Wounds of Left Chest with Penetration of the Pericardium. Suicide.

Note superficial cut on left wrist. Deceased stabbed himself with a pair of scissors.

chest. Occasionally he accomplishes his purpose in one stroke and may leave the knife sticking in the wound. In one suicidal case seen by the authors a bread knife was driven in through the left costal cartilages to the depth of 5 inches, missing the heart but penetrating the left pulmonary vein at the hilum of the lung, causing a fatal hemorrhage into the left chest. In other cases the instrument is jabbed into the chest a number of times, in a circumscribed area (Fig. 15-14). The wounds are variable in depth, some barely penetrating the chest wall, and others entering the pericardium and heart; the superficial thrusts are hesitant in character. Frequently the suicide does not withdraw the point of the weapon from the skin but may stab himself repeatedly in different directions through the same skin perforation. In several cases there have been more stab wound tracks below the surface of the skin than perforations in the skin. The suicide in stabbing himself, whether one or more times, is apt to open up his clothes and drive the blade through the uncovered skin (Figs. 15-15 and 15-16).

In many cases of suicide the attempt even with multiple stab wounds is not always successful and the individual may resort to other means which present a puzzling picture to an inexperienced investigator. Thus if a body is found which has obviously died of a fall from a height, or as a result of submersion, and on its

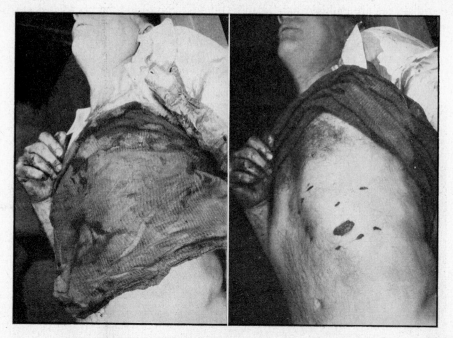

Fig. 15-15. Multiple Suicidal Stab Wounds of Left Side of Chest.

Note absence of perforations in the undershirt which had been pulled up by the victim prior to stabbing. Body found as shown in photograph on right.

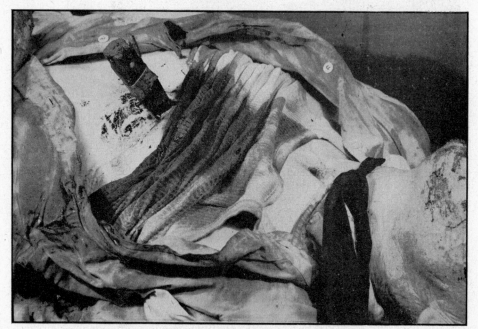

From Lowen, Fink and Helpern, *Circulation*, 2:426. 1950

Fig. 15-16. Suicidal Stabbing with Kitchen Knife.

The weapon was found in the wound. Note shirt opened and undershirt pulled up by victim prior to stabbing.

precordial area are multiple stab wounds, the first impression may be that death is homicidal, but careful autopsy and investigation may disclose its true suicidal character. Occasionally small transverse incisions may be found on the flexor surfaces of the wrists or thighs suggesting the self-inflicted nature of the injuries (page 13).

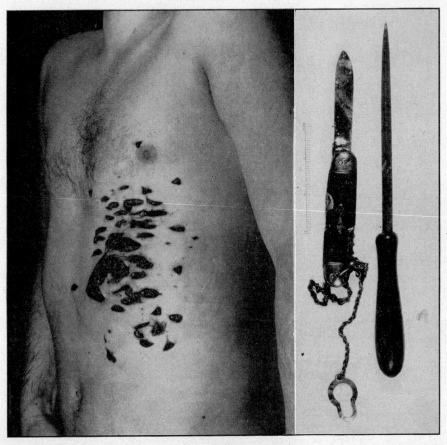

Fig. 15-17. Multiple Suicidal Stab Wounds Inflicted with a Pocket Knife and Triangular File; Total of 50 Wounds.

The heart was not penetrated and there was little bleeding from the wounds. The victim also drank mercurochrome and then jumped from a fifth story fire-escape to the sidewalk.

In one remarkable case the deceased first attempted suicide by drinking an ounce of aqueous mercurochrome. He then stabbed himself over the left side of the chest a total of about 50 times with a pocket knife and a triangular file. Despite extensive mutilation of the thoracic cage none of the wounds penetrated the heart. After the unsuccessful stabbing the deceased jumped from the fifth floor fire escape and died of the blunt force injuries associated with the fall (Fig. 15-17).

Attempted suicidal stab wounds of the head are encountered occasionally, but the entrance of the knife is blocked by the skull. Generally a large number of small puncture wounds are noted in the temporal region, where the attempts are made, but they extend only to the bone. One successful suicidal attempt by a stab wound was performed by an insane individual who drove a knife into his brain through an old healed craniotomy opening (Fig. 15-18). In the case illustrated in Figure 15-26 multiple attempts to stab through the skull were unsuccessful. Suicidal stab wounds of the spine and extremities are not common. Self-inflicted stab wounds of the abdomen and of the neck are not frequent. Among the yearly average of 1,241 cases of suicide in New York City (8.7 per cent of all medical examiner's cases),

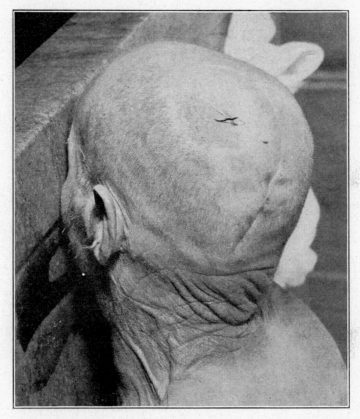

Fig. 15-18. Suicidal Stab Wound of Scalp and Brain Through an Operative Craniotomy Defect in the Skull.

The healed operative scar is plainly visible on the scalp.

an average of 42 cases resulted from incised wounds and stab wounds of which only 3 to 5 were by stabbing.

Accidental stab wound cases are rare and are caused by falling against projecting sharp objects like broken pieces of glass, in which event pieces of glass may be found in the wound. The authors have seen a fatal penetrating wound in the neck of an alcoholic individual who fell on the sharp projecting point of a broken bottle neck and died of external hemorrhage from the severed jugular vein. A remarkable accidental fatal stabbing, autopsied by Dr. Robert C. Fisher, resulted from the fall of an elderly obese woman against a dresser, in such a way as to dislodge a heavy plate glass mirror which dropped on the floor and smashed. The victim in falling was completely transfixed from back to front on a large pointed saber-shaped piece of broken glass (Fig. 15-19). Other accidental stab wounds occur when a butcher or a cook lets a knife slip as he is drawing it toward himself in carving, so that the sharp point penetrates the lower abdomen and the intestines or the groin. Penetrating wounds may be inflicted by the assault of an animal. Thus a person may be gored by the horn of a steer or the tusk of a boar, but such occurrences are rare. Penetrating wounds by sharp pointed missiles are unusual but generally are easily identified.

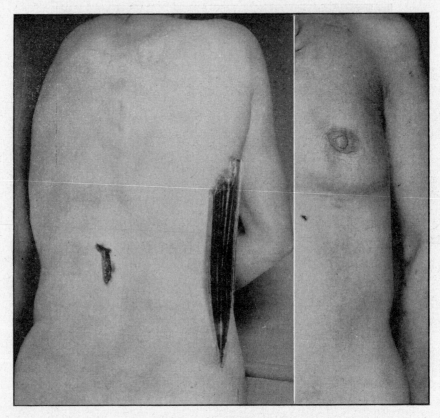

Fig. 15-19. Accidental Stabbing Resulting from a Fall on Broken Glass.

The elderly obese victim fell against a dresser, dislodged the mirror and impaled herself on a large saber-shaped fragment of glass which transfixed the body from back to front. The large posterior entrance wound and the smaller anterior exit wound are shown in the photographs, also the glass fragment removed from the body.

In one case a plank containing a projecting nail dropped on the head of the victim, the nail penetrating the skull, dura and part of the cerebral hemisphere. Death occurred after four days from a brain abscess and a suppurative pachymeningitis which developed from this injury. The authors have seen a case of accidental stabbing by a wood carver's gouge which was thrown loose from its handle when the person using it attempted to shake some wood shavings from its cutting end. The long metal shaft shot out, tumbling in the air, and the conical sharp-pointed end which had been inserted in the holder struck a nearby person on the side of the neck, penetrating the spinal canal and cord just below the foramen magnum, causing immediate death by shock.

In another remarkable case a 45-year-old longshoreman was struck on the left side of the base of the neck by the end of a wooden plank and sustained what appeared to be a one and one-quarter inch gaping laceration of the skin, for which he was treated without hospitalization for 11 days, until evidence of infection caused him to be hospitalized. He survived six more days. At autopsy a broken-off prismatic-shaped splinter of wood, 5 inches long and 1 inch in diameter, was found embedded obliquely in the posterior mediastinum, transfixing the esophagus. The tapered end of the missile penetrated the upper medial portion of the right lung. Death resulted from pulmonary suppuration, empyema, mediastinitis, and hemorrhage into the esophagus from erosion of the azygos vein (Fig. 15-20).

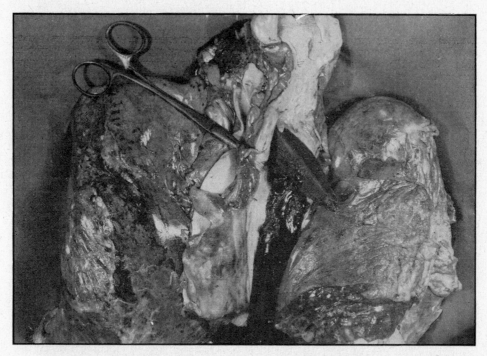

Fig. 15-20. Accidental Penetrating Wound of Neck and Chest Produced by a Large Broken-off Splinter of Wood.

The victim was struck by the end of a plank. The fragment of wood discovered at autopsy is shown in the rear view photograph. It obliquely transfixed the esophagus and posterior mediastinum, its distal end eroding the right lung and azygos vein. See text.

CUTS OR INCISED WOUNDS

Incised wounds are inflicted by an instrument with a sharp edge, like a knife, a razor or a piece of glass. In making the incision the edge is pressed against the skin and then drawn along the surface. The degree of force required to inflict this injury is relatively slight, so that traumatic shock does not occur unless precipitated by other factors such as hemorrhage. The most common fatal complications of incised wounds are hemorrhage and septic infection.

Incised wounds are noted most often on the exposed portions of the body, the neck, the head and the extremities. The abdomen and chest are not as frequently involved (Figs. 15-21, 15-22 and 15-23). The majority of fatal incised wounds are suicidal, such cases averaging about 35 to 40 a year in New York City; homicidal cases of this type average four or five a year; fatal accidental incised wounds are rare.

Suicidal incised wounds are most commonly inflicted on the throat. The individual usually holds the weapon in his right hand and starts the incision on the left side drawing the blade to the right, or he may incise the right side of the neck, drawing the blade forward and downward. A left-handed person would cut himself in the same way, usually starting the incision on the right side of the neck. The

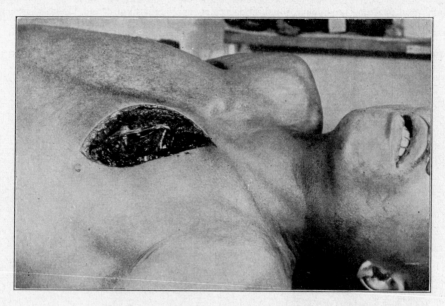

Fig. 15-21. Deep Incised Wound of Chest Wall, Ribs and Heart.
Homicide.

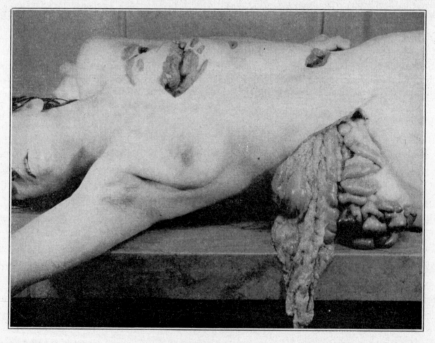

Fig. 15-22. Multiple Incised Wounds of Left Chest, Breast and Abdomen Inflicted with a Long-bladed
Knife. Evisceration Through a Large Abdominal Wound.
Homicide.

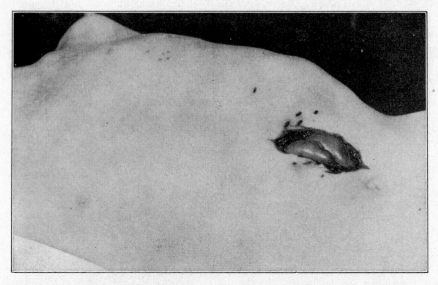

Fig. 15-23. Self-inflicted Incised Wound of Upper Abdominal Wall with Partial Evisceration.

Note small superficial hesitation cuts. Wounds made with a razor blade. Suicidal. Death occurred under anesthesia during attempted surgical repair.

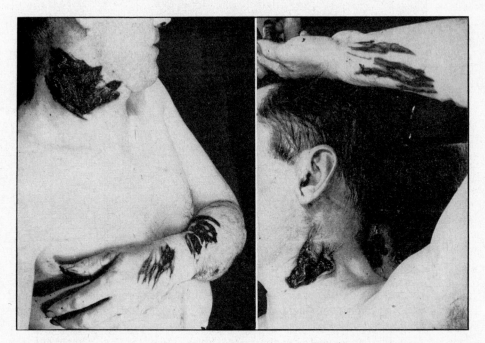

Fig. 15-24. Suicidal Incised Wounds of Both Sides of Neck with Hesitation Cuts.

Note self-inflicted incised wounds of the forearms are on the radial borders in contrast to homicidal cases in which defense cuts are frequently sustained along the ulnar border of the hand and forearm.

suicide may incise both sides of his neck and the opposite wrist and forearm (Fig. 15-24). In rare instances repeated horizontal shallow cuts are made on the back of the neck. The characteristic pattern of the suicidal wound reveals repeated hesitant attempts to slash the throat in the same line of incision; the edges are usually ragged

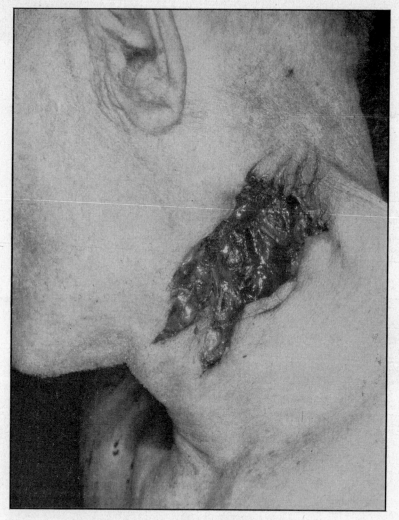

Fig. 15-25. Multiple Suicidal Overlapping Incised Wounds and Hesitation Cuts of Neck with Severance of Jugular Vein.

due to the overlapping of numerous superficial incisions more or less parallel and merged with the main component of the wound (Figs. 15-25 and 15-26). Or the attempt may start as a scratch or a shallow cut, gradually growing deeper as the incision continues and penetrates the large vessels (Fig. 15-27). The blade may penetrate the external jugular vein through a relatively short shallow incision (Fig. 15-28), or may cut deeply, severing the muscles, vessels, trachea, larynx, esophagus, and even scratching the spine (Fig. 15-29). In most cases death results from profuse external hemorrhage, occasionally attended by inhalation of effused blood if the air passages are punctured. If the jugular vein is cut, pulmonary air embolism may supervene. If the victim survives the immediate effects of the injury, fatal septic infections of the neck or lungs may develop. Some cases of cut throat recover and are marked by an unsightly depressed scar on the front of the neck. Ineffective self-inflicted incised wounds of the throat, at times accompanied by similar unsuccessful slashes on the wrists, are not infrequently found in suicidal deaths from other

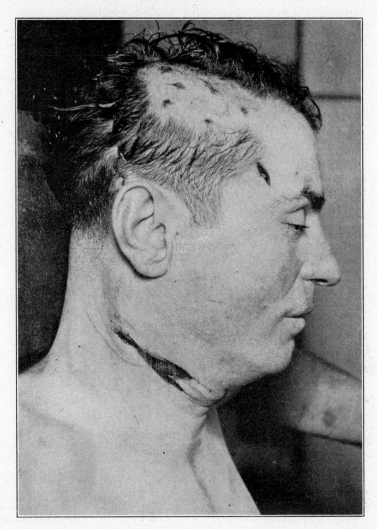

Fig. 15-26. Self-inflicted Incised Wounds on Right Side of Neck and Superficial Stab Wounds on Right Side of Scalp.

Note hesitant overlapping character of superficial repeated cuts on neck. Scalp wounds exposed by cutting away hair. Deceased also attempted to hang himself from gas pipe which broke under the weight of his body. Death finally from carbon monoxide poisoning. Same case as in Fig. 4-6.

forms of violence and help to establish the suicidal character of the death (Fig. 18-12).

A rare complication of an incised wound of the neck is illustrated in the following case. During an altercation, a 37 year old Negro man received a gaping incised wound of the left shoulder and neck, eight and one-half inches in length and one and one-quarter inches in depth, with complete severance of the left common carotid artery and internal jugular vein, the wound extending through the left lobe of the thyroid and anterior portion of the trachea. After admission to the hospital shortly after the injury, the bleeding vessels were all ligated and the hemorrhage stopped. The victim lived about 14 hours, apparently dying of loss of blood. Autopsy disclosed that the distal ligated segment of the severed carotid artery had become plugged with a soft intact thrombus. Although there were no emboli in the cerebral arteries, the left cerebral hemisphere with the exception of the frontal and occipital poles revealed early infarction. There was evidence also of considerable blood loss. Death was attributed in part to hemorrhage and in part to the cerebral infarction.

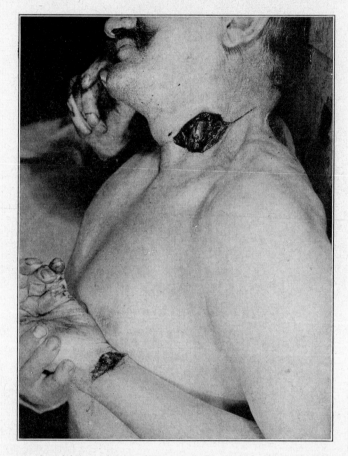

Fig. 15-27. Suicidal Incised Wound on Left Side of Neck, Cutting Jugular Vein.

Note hesitant superficial commencement of cut at its posterior end. The left wrist has also been slashed.

The homicidal incised wounds of the neck and throat usually have sharp clean-cut edges, penetrate deeply and do not show any hesitation marks (Fig. 15-30). Such wounds may be multiple, cross each other at a deep level, and involve the head and other parts, as well as the neck. The homicidal incision may take the form of a single deep slash on the side of the face or neck as shown in Figure 15-31. During an assault the victim may attempt to ward off the thrusts and sustain wounds on the fingers, palms, forearms and wrists that are readily identified as defense cuts. In the natural blocking position with the forearm bent and raised such wounds are apt to be received along the ulnar border and are easily distinguished from the self-inflicted incisions on the flexor surfaces of the wrists and forearms in suicidal cases, which will be described later. They are not to be confused with the less common self-inflicted incised wounds along the radial border of the forearm (Fig. 15-24).

Homicidal cuts in some instances resemble the suicidal, for it is not only possible for an assailant to stun the victim and then cut his throat with ease in such a way as to simulate a self-inflicted wound, but also in rare instances the resemblance is produced fortuitously as illustrated in Figure 15-32. In this case, before several fatal deep slashes of the throat, each penetrating to the spine, were inflicted by the

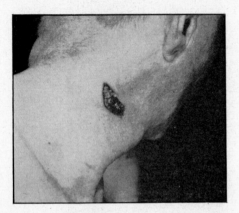

Fig. 15-28. Superficial Suicidal Incised Wound of Neck with Severance of External Jugular Vein and Fatal Hemorrhage.

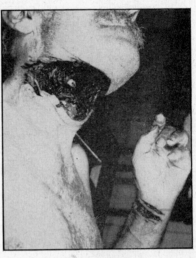

Fig. 15-29. Suicidal Incised Wound of Throat with Severance of All Structures to the Spine. Hesitation Cuts on Neck and Multiple Parallel Cuts on Left Wrist.

assailant, the victim by dodging the weapon had received several superficial cuts on the right side of the neck, resembling the hesitation cuts of a suicide.

In homicides occurring during a gang vendetta, the face of the victim may be mutilated by multiple slashes having a crude symbolic pattern. Thus the long slash on the cheek crossed by two shorter ones (Fig. 15-33) would seem to denote that the victim had double-crossed his assailants and was paying the gang penalty for his indiscretion. Other bizarre patterns of mutilation by cutting are encountered in gang murders and in assaults arising out of heterosexual or homosexual infidelity or jealousy (Fig. 15-34).

Homicidal incised wounds of the extremities may result in fatal hemorrhage especially if the axillary, brachial or femoral vessels are cut. The incised wounds of lesser severity received during an assault and designated as defense cuts are usually associated with other more serious or fatal injuries. They may, however, give rise to septic infection.

Suicidal incised wounds of the extremities are usually inflicted with a knife or razor, most often on the flexor surface of the wrists and elbows, and in some cases on the groins, thighs, ankles or knees. They are sometimes found on the radial border and exterior surface of the forearm. The cuts are usually multiple, parallel, more or less transverse, and located in circumscribed areas. They are variable in length and depth, and often show evidence of hesitation (Figs. 15-14, 15-24, 15-27, 15-29 and 18-12). Several regions of the body may be incised. Such wounds are usually not fatal but occasionally death results from slow hemorrhage from the incised vessels, or from septic infection of the extremity. In rare instances the severance of a vein may be followed by a fatal air embolism. Self-inflicted wounds of the extremities, although usually not fatal, are an important indication of the suicidal character of a violent death otherwise not recognizable as such.

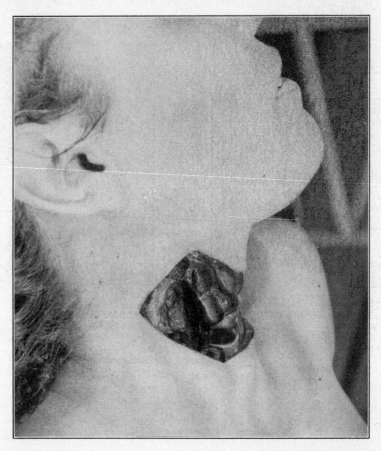

Fig. 15-30. Homicidal Deep Incised Wound of Throat with Severance of Trachea, Carotids and Jugular Vein.

Another cut was present on the left side of face and neck. Note absence of hesitation marks and clean-cut edges of wound. Compare with Figs. 15-26 and 15-27.

Homicidal incised wounds of the chest and abdomen are illustrated in Figs. 15-21 and 15-22. A suicidal incised wound of the abdominal wall is shown in Figure 15-23 and is characterized by hesitation cuts. The Japanese method of suicide is to make a large angular incision of the lower abdomen with a sword while in a sitting posture. Death is caused by sudden evisceration, release of the intra-abdominal pressure and cardiac collapse. In this country the method is rare. In a recent case the perpetrator, following the commission of a homicide by cutting, incised his own abdomen and cut off a loop of eviscerated small intestine, which he left behind on the floor at the scene of the killing. He then walked down several flights of steps to the street and when found, it was at first thought that he had been assaulted. He was taken to a hospital where he notified the authorities of what he had done. A laparotomy was performed, the severed bowel was successfully repaired and recovery ensued.

The ability of an individual to walk after having received incised wounds will depend upon the severity of the injury and the rapidity of the hemorrhage from the severed vessels. With rapid loss of blood locomotion is usually limited; with less profuse bleeding, movement is possible and usually will be marked by a trail of

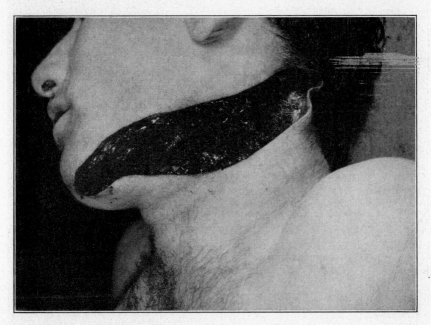

Fig. 15-31. Homicidal Incised Wound on Left Side of Neck with Severance of Internal and External Carotid Arteries and Jugular Vein.

Note absence of hesitation marks and clean-cut edges of wound. Compare with Figs. 15-26 and 15-27.

blood. In cases of profuse bleeding, the clothing of the victim may be soaked with blood, and blood may be gathered in a pool on the floor around the body. Study of the blood distribution at the scene may furnish important information to the examiner. If the bleeding is from a small artery like the radial, the blood will be spurted and the appearance of the drops of blood when they strike a surface is characteristic. If they strike at right angles they flatten out into crenated circular spots; if a drop strikes obliquely its base will be held by the impinging surface and its convexity projected forward by the momentum, forming a characteristic pattern of bowling pin shape, the narrow end indicating the direction of the spurt (Fig. 26-1). A larger drop may show several narrow parallel forward projections. If a large artery is cut, the hemorrhage will be rapid and profuse and the blood will not spurt as far or in as fine a stream as when a smaller artery is severed. If a vein is cut the blood will flow or gush out depending on the size of the vessel. Spurted drops of blood found on a surface do not always indicate arterial bleeding; blood that has accumulated on a part of the body or extremity may be spattered or splashed by a weapon or by the motion of the bloodied part.

Accidental incised wounds serious enough to cause death are rare. They occur when a person is cut by coming in contact with broken glass, with moving machinery, or is inadvertently injured by an implement like a scythe, a sickle or a knife. In these cases unless the history and circumstances clearly establish the nature of the occurrence, the diagnosis of accident should be made with caution.

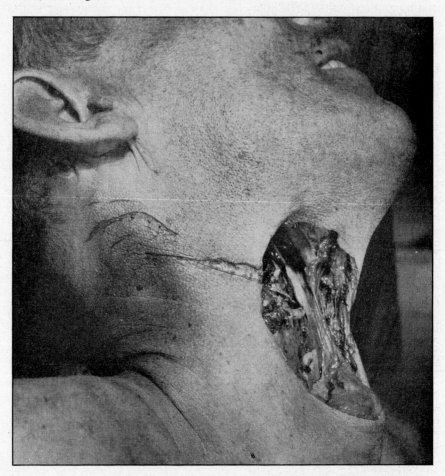

Fig. 15-32. Homicidal Cut Throat.

The single horizontal incised wound on the front of the neck severed all structures down to the spine. The superficial cuts on the right side of the neck were also inflicted by the assailant during the struggle and on casual examination they resembled suicidal hesitation cuts.

Glass cuts commonly result when a person is violently thrown against or through a sheet of plate glass, such as the windshield of an automobile (Fig. 15-35), or crashes heavily through a pane of glass after falling (Fig. 15-36). The sharp uneven edges and spicules of glass fragments may produce extensive abrasions, lacerations, puncture wounds, and incised wounds, the latter sometimes involving important blood vessels and causing severe or fatal hemorrhage. Wounds of the neck are most dangerous. In the extremities the blood vessels, nerves and tendons may be cut and fatal hemorrhage occur (Fig. 15-37). Air embolism and septic infection are occasional complications of these injuries, whether inflicted on head, neck or extremities. Cuts produced by glass have a distinctive form at times. The part of the skin first injured is cut deeply, the wound may taper off into a scratch mark and the edges may be sinuous, giving the gash a saber or comma shape. At times glass cuts resemble a knife wound and are only to be distinguished by finding glass fragments in the cut. When multiple cuts are inflicted at the same time from a single impact against a pane of glass (Fig. 15-35) they may be parallel or slightly divergent.

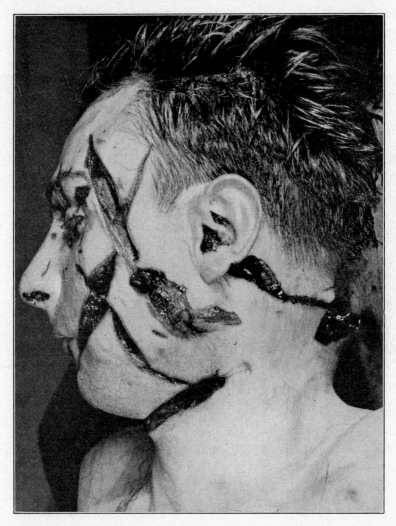

Fig. 15-33. Vendetta Murder. Multiple Wounds of Face and Neck with Pattern of "Double Cross" on Cheek.

There were numerous stab wounds on the chest and abdomen.

CHOP WOUNDS

Chop wounds are wounds caused by a blow with the sharp splitting edge of a fairly heavy instrument like a hatchet, an ax, a saber or a cleaver (Fig. 15-38). The vast majority of these injuries are homicidal; a few are accidental and usually caused by power fans, band saws, circular saws or ship propellers which may lacerate the soft tissues extensively or amputate parts of the body. Suicidal injuries are rare; an example is the case described by Glaister of an insane person who struck herself on the head with a hatchet.

The homicidal chop wounds are usually inflicted on the exposed portions of the body like the head, face, neck, shoulders and extremities. The chest and abdomen are also attacked but not as frequently. Death is most often due to shock or hemorrhage, especially with multiple injuries. In these cases the deceased usually has been killed instantly and so has been unable to move by his own volition.

The wounds left on the skin by a chopping instrument have about the same dimensions as the cross section of the penetrating blade and sharp edges though

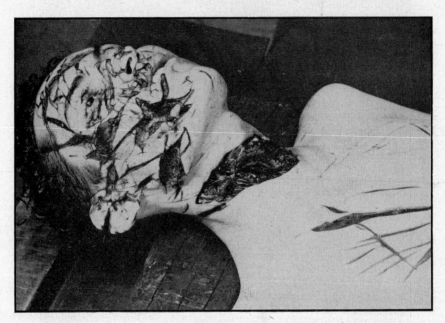

Fig. 15-34. Mutilating Homicidal Incised Wounds of Face, Neck and Chest Inflicted with a Straight-edged Razor.

the margins may show a slight abrasion. The cranium may be depressed in the region of such a laceration and display a wound which is almost an exact reproduction of the cross section of the blade. If the blow against the head is a glancing one, a piece of the skull may be removed in much the same way that a chip is chopped off a piece of wood. The facial bones may be penetrated and the lower jaw cut across. The neck may be almost completely severed by the blows. In such cases it is important to examine the air passages and the lungs for signs of aspirated blood. If the upper extremities are attacked there may be complete or incomplete amputations of the fingers or other bones of the hand and joints like the wrists or elbows may be severed or disarticulated.

EXAMINATION OF WEAPONS

Knives and other weapons found at the scene of a crime are collected and preserved as evidence by a police officer or other responsible person and also examined for clues. The presence of finger prints on the weapon are determined whenever possible, and the presence or absence of foreign material on the blade or handle recorded. Hair, pieces of cloth, blood and sometimes tissue are the most important substances encountered in this investigation. The hairs, pieces of cloth and tissue fragments must be examined microscopically, according to the procedure described in Chapter 28. When found on the blade of a knife or an ax, the immediate problem is to determine if the hair on the weapon is human, and if it resembles that of the deceased, for this discovery may help to identify the weapon used in the homicide. For further discussion on this subject, the reader is referred

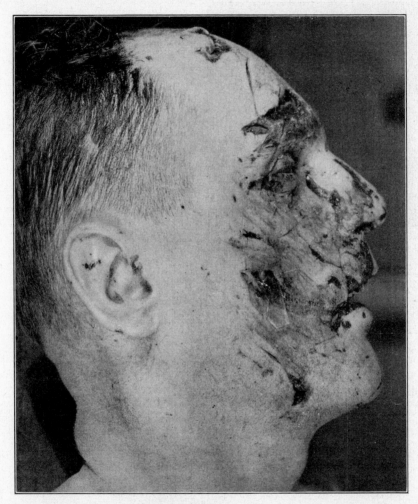

Fig. 15-35. Wounds Produced by Impact with Breaking Glass. Automobile Accident. Head Thrown Through Windshield.

to Chapter 28. The same implications also exist in regard to blood stains, for the examiner must determine whether or not the blood is human and, if possible, the group to which it belongs. The blood of the deceased should be similarly examined to determine its group for comparison with that of the blood stains on the weapon. This subject is fully discussed in Chapters 26 and 27.

HEALING OF WOUNDS

The same pattern of healing occurs in connection with stab or incised wounds as has already been described under lacerations of the skin and injuries of the internal organs. There is primarily a hemorrhage into the wound, followed within several hours by an infiltration of polymorphonuclear leukocytes into the surrounding tissues. Granulation tissue is then formed and the clot is invaded and organized. The process results in closure of the wound by scar tissue formation. The scar that forms on the skin is pale and elliptic or long and tape-like with pointed ends, depend-

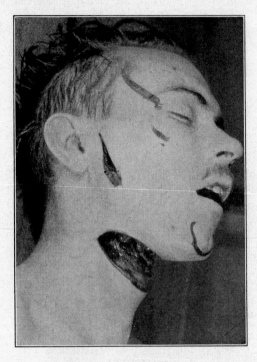

Fig. 15-36. Multiple Incised Wounds of Face and Neck Produced by Broken Glass.

Glass fragments were found in fatal wound of neck which otherwise resembled a knife wound. Deceased, while intoxicated, accidentally fell down a flight of stairs crashing through a heavy plate glass door at the bottom.

ing on the nature of the original wound. These healed lesions are covered by stratified squamous epithelium, but the skin adnexae such as hair follicles, sebaceous glands and sweat glands are lacking.

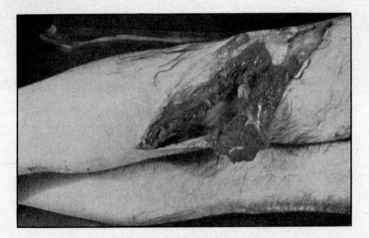

Fig. 15-37. Fatal Incised Wound of Left Leg with Severance of Popliteal Vessels Produced by Heavy Fragment of Plate Glass Window Which Broke When Victim Was Thrown Against It. The Severed Ends of the Vessels Are Seen in the Center of the Oblique Wound.

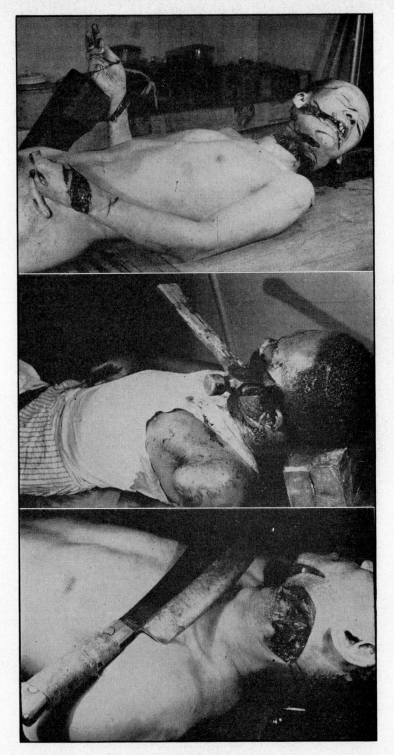

Fig. 15-38. Homicidal Chop Wounds.

Top. Multiple chop wounds inflicted with a cleaver.
Middle. Hatchet wound with weapon embedded in head.
Bottom. Multiple cleaver wounds of neck. Weapon placed on body for photograph.

MEDICOLEGAL CONSIDERATIONS

The surgeon who is called upon to treat stab wounds and incised wounds must always consider the possibility that they were inflicted with felonious or homicidal intent. If there is the slightest suspicion of this he should report the matter to the police. As most of these cases are criminal in nature, the surgeon should be especially meticulous in the compilation of the clinical record and in his description of the wounds on the body of the victim. If he operates so as to repair or obliterate injuries on the head, chest, abdomen or elsewhere, he should make careful notes of

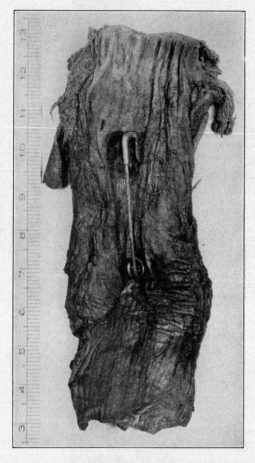

Fig. 15-39. Injury by Swallowed Foreign Body.

Perforation of esophagus by open safety pin, secretly swallowed by insane person. Point of pin penetrated into pericardium causing suppurative pericarditis. The pin was revealed at autopsy.

his findings, for he may be the only medical person to see these wounds in their original state. He will be almost certainly called in to testify if the case is tried in court. Any fragment of a weapon found in the body should be delivered to the police detectives as part of the corpus delicti.

Other considerations have been discussed in the previous paragraphs, and it only remains to emphasize a few clinical points which are sometimes overlooked by surgeons. Usually the lesions on the skin are obvious enough and indicate to the clinician what his treatment should be. However, as has been noted, stab wounds of the head are sometimes inconspicuous, difficult to find and not infrequently missed. In operations on the abdomen, when the stomach and intestines are involved, the surgeon must be careful that he has closed all perforations in these viscera, before sewing up the anterior abdominal wall. In a few cases the authors have seen the stab wound in the anterior surface of the stomach carefully sutured but the perforation in the posterior wall untreated. Wounds in the duodenum also are easily overlooked because of their location deep in the abdominal cavity.

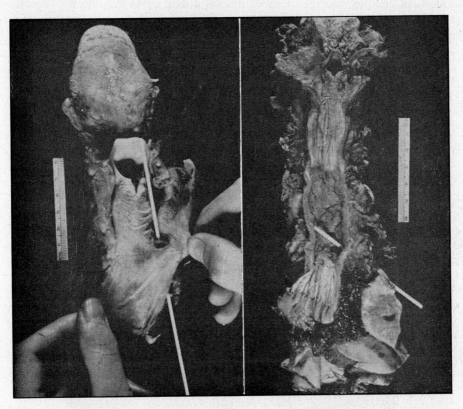

Fig. 15-40. Perforation of Esophagus During Diagnostic Esophagoscopy.

The instrument pierced the upper end of the esophagus, penetrated the mediastinum and pericardial sac and exposed the auricular appendage which was mistaken for a cauliflower-like neoplasm. Death resulted from phlegmonous mediastinitis. A probe is inserted in the perforation.

Fig. 15-41. Perforation of Lower End of Esophagus by Esophagoscope Through Site of Lye Stricture. Fatal Suppurative Mediastinitis.

FOREIGN BODIES

Foreign bodies, such a nails, needles, pins, toothpicks, fish bones, and numerous other objects are introduced into the body in various ways and sometimes cause death. Some of these objects may penetrate the skin, embed themselves in the tissues and give rise to a fatal septic infection. In one case a 10 year old boy drove a splinter of wood 2 inches long into the sole of his right foot and died two weeks later of tetanus. The splinter had evidently not been detected by clinical examination and it was recovered from the right foot at autopsy.

Pins and needles have been jabbed into the cardiac region for suicidal purposes, and after penetrating the myocardium, have been pulled into the pericardial sac by the movements of the heart. The authors have encountered two cases of this type. In one a sewing needle was found in the heart muscle at autopsy and the epicardium was scratched several times indicating a number of attempts to drive the needle in before the heart muscle snatched it away. Death in this case was due to multiple fractures received when the patient committed suicide by jumping from a third story window. In another case the deceased pushed a darning needle into his precordial area and died 14 days later of an acute suppurative pericarditis, the autopsy revealing a 4 inch needle embedded in the interventricular septum.

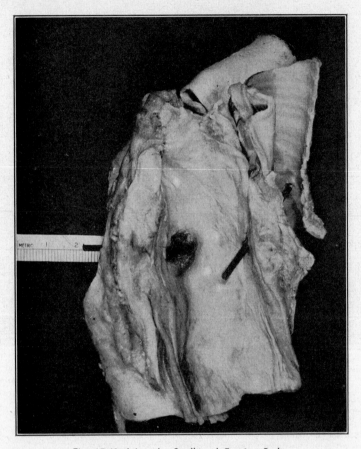

Fig. 15-42. Injury by Swallowed Foreign Body.

Same case as Fig. 15-43. Multiple perforations of esophagus by swallowed chicken bone, causing traumatic fistulae between esophagus (center) and trachea (reader's right) and between esophagus and aorta (reader's left) as shown by probes. Death from hemorrhage into esophagus and stomach from aortic puncture.

Children and insane individuals sometimes place small objects in the nose, mouth, ears, urethra or bladder, but the results are rarely serious, except when an occasional septic infection is produced. Sometimes children place small objects in the mouth and aspirate them into the air passages, causing death by asphyxia; in one case a sunflower seed was inhaled and blocked the bronchus of the right lung, and in another case a small lima bean obstructed the trachea. Other foreign material has been inhaled into the lungs and has given rise to abscesses.

Various foreign bodies have been placed in the vagina or rectum but rarely cause serious complications unless they are inserted to induce abortion or for perverted sexual purposes. A fatal septic infection may occur in some cases. These subjects are discussed in greater detail in Chapters 22 and 24.

Most foreign bodies gain entrance to the system by being swallowed either accidentally or intentionally. A sharp, thin and smooth object like a needle or a fish bone may penetrate any portion of the gastrointestinal tract and cause death by septic infection. If the pharyngeal wall is penetrated, a suppurative cellulitis of

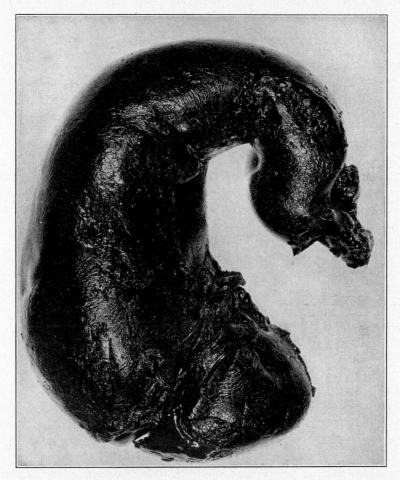

Fig. 15-43. Massive Cast of Clotted Blood Found in Stomach at Autopsy as a Result of Hemorrhage from Aortic Wound into Esophagus.

Same case as in Fig. 15-42.

the mouth and neck result. If the esophagus is perforated, a suppurative mediastinitis or pericarditis is often produced (Figs. 15-39, 15-40 and 15-41). If the stomach or intestine is pierced, septic peritonitis or abdominal inflammation is caused. In a case seen by the authors a piece of wire one and one-half inches in length perforated the wall of the upper jejunum and was recovered by laparotomy free in the abdominal cavity, death occurring 12 days later from abdominal sepsis. The complications following the accidental swallowing of a tube of radium are discussed on page 758. If the duodenum is perforated a retroperitoneal phlegmon may develop. In a rare case, a fragment of chicken bone lacerated the esophageal wall and eroded into the aorta, causing a fatal hemorrhage into the esophagus and stomach (Figs. 15-42 and 15-43). In a case described by Bailey, a swallowed toothpick passed through the duodenum into the inferior vena cava and was transported by the blood to the right ventricle of the heart.

Many foreign bodies which are not sharp may be swallowed and accumulate in the stomach in large numbers. This condition is discovered not infrequently among the inmates of insane asylums. Hair and other fibers may collect and form large tangled masses known as phytobezoars.

BITING, SCRATCHING, GOUGING

Bites are injuries inflicted by the teeth of animals and the bills of birds. Among the animals whose bites are most important are mammals, reptiles and fish. In this group the mammals most worthy of mention are the carnivora like dogs, cats, foxes and wolves; rodents like rats and mice; and the horse. The group of reptiles contains several animals whose bites are poisonous (e.g., serpents and lizards) which will be discussed in Chapter 32, and others whose bites are mutilating (e.g., large turtles or alligators. The most serious fish bites are caused by tropical varieties ranging from the injuries inflicted by sharks which can mangle a human body to those produced by smaller fish which nip and tear the flesh from the exposed parts like the face and hands. The bites of fish may be inflicted both ante mortem and post mortem.

Injuries inflicted by the bills of birds are rare antemortem lesions. In civilized life they are caused mostly by pet birds, such as parrots which may nip the finger of an incautious person. Such wounds are complicated by septic infection of the wound or in rare instances by an attack of psittacosis. Birds also may devour a dead body which is lying in the open; buzzards tear and rend the flesh; crows perforate the body with their sharp bills, leaving characteristic puncture wounds.

The bite made by a dog depends upon the action of canine teeth and the cutting molar teeth, along with the tendency of the animal to tear and worry his prey. Dead bodies which have been partially eaten by dogs show tearing and fraying of exposed parts and crushing of bones. In the case described on page 71 the body was decapitated, the head was stripped of flesh and the neck was eaten away so that the dogs could get at the parenchymatous viscera (Figs. 4-21 and 4-22). The intravital bite is a lacerated wound which is fatal in some instances and may be inflicted on the neck, face, arms and legs. On the neck the jugular vein may be torn. Death may occur from external hemorrhage, rarely from air embolism, or the trachea may be compressed and death result from asphyxia. In other cases the crushing of the shaft of a long bone may give rise to fat embolism. The most frequent method of transmitting rabies to man is by the bite of an infected dog. The most common complication of a dog bite is a septic infection of the wound caused by pyogenic bacteria.

The cat possesses sharp premolar teeth and bites into flesh without worrying it, so that the injury is clean-cut as though caused by a pair of shears. Cats, unless they are the larger members of the family like lions and tigers, rarely attack dead bodies and rarely bite the living.

Rats bite mainly with their incisor teeth producing a gnawed surface. Their attacks on the dead body have been described (Figs. 4-19 and 4-20). Rats bite live persons who are helpless, such as a small infant or a moribund sick person.

The principal complications of rat bite are septic infection, infectious jaundice and rat bite fever.

Horses occasionally nip stable attendants and others with their front teeth, leaving an ovoid tearing wound. The head and the arms are the parts most often attacked. Death may take place as a result of septic infection of the wound.

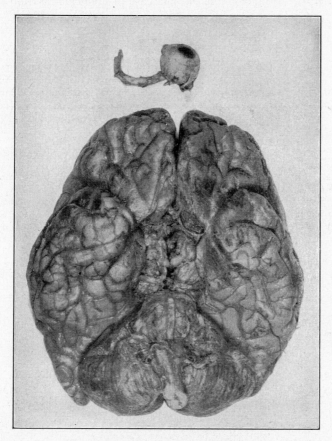

Fig. 15-44. Manual Enucleation of Eyeballs.

Both eyeballs were gouged out by fingers of assailant. The optic nerve and tract are attached to eyeball shown in illustration. Victim, an attendant in a mental hospital, assaulted by insane patient. Death from subarachnoid and subdural hemorrhage.

Human bites are inflicted on the face and hands during assaults, and on the breast, neck and face during sexual excitement. Many of the bites are contusions and abrasions of the skin of an indefinite ovoid shape with a pattern corresponding to the teeth in the dental arch (Fig. 24-2). Sometimes actual lacerations are caused on the nose and fingers. Septic infections, tuberculosis and syphilis may be transmitted by human bites. Human dentition furnishes a means of identification inasmuch as the teeth may be as individual in different people as finger prints. The marks of teeth on such articles as apples, tobacco plugs or chewing gum may be the means of detecting the identity of the biter.

Injuries by scratching may occur with the cat family either with the front paws or with the hind paws. The typical wound consists of long parallel furrows which are dug into the skin and flesh by the four claws. In the case of the larger carnivora there may be considerable blunt force applied to the body and fractures, lacerations and internal injuries may be produced. Septic infection of a lacerated wound also occurs.

Injuries due to gouging and scratching are observed in cases of death by criminal violence but usually do not present any diagnostic difficulties. Most of them are of secondary importance though in one case of homicidal assault both eyeballs were pulled from their sockets by the fingers of the assailant (Fig. 15-44).

REFERENCES

Bailey, C. H.   A case of foreign body in the heart, Arch. Int. Med., 11:440, 1913.

Brouardel, P.   Les Blessures et les Accidents du Travail, Paris, J-B. Ballière et Fils, 1906.

Glaister, J.   Medical Jurisprudence and Toxicology, 7th ed., Baltimore, Williams & Wilkins Co., 1942.

Helpern, M.   The postmortem examination in cases of suspected homicide, Ann. Int. Med., 24:666-700, 1946.

———— Unusual stab wounds of head and neck, Am. J. Surg., 26:53, 1934.

Henke and Lubarsch.   Handbuch, Berlin, Julius Springer, 1926, Verdauungsschlauch IV, 1, 21:598; Herz und Gefasse II, 599-919.

Houtrouw, T.   Uber die gerichtlich-medizinische Wurdigung von Bissverletzungen durch Mensch und Tier, Deutsche Ztschr. f. d. ges. gerichtl. Med., 16:89, 1930.

Lowen, H. S., Fink, S. A., and Helpern, M.   Transfixion of the heart by embedded ice pick blade with eight months survival, Circulation, 2:426-433, 1950.

Martland, H. S.   Medical Examiner's Findings in Deaths from Shooting, Stabbing, Cutting and Asphyxia, Symposium on the Medicolegal Necropsy, Baltimore, Williams & Wilkins Co., 1934, pp. 50-66.

Moritz, A. R.   The Pathology of Trauma, Philadelphia, Lea & Febiger, 1942.

Puppe, G.   Atlas und Gundriss der Gerichtlichen Medizin, München, J. F. Lehmann's Verlag, 1908.

Reports of the Office of the Chief Medical Examiner in the City of New York from 1918 to 1951.

Vance, B. M.   Bullet wounds of the heart, Am. J. M. Sc., 169:872, 1925.

16

Bullet and Other Missile Wounds

Many penetrating wounds are produced by various types of metallic missiles propelled at high velocity. The most common missile encountered in civil life is the bullet, usually fired from a pistol and propelled by the force of expanding gases produced from the explosive charge of gunpowder in the cartridge shell. Bullets are also fired from weapons such as the rifle and machine gun and occasionally from crudely improvised firearms made of wood or metal with a cylindric barrel fashioned to hold a cartridge and to direct the passage of a projectile. Blank cartridge pistols when fired at very close range can also produce penetrating wounds.

Other missiles are metallic pellets and slugs fired from shotguns, and miscellaneous slugs and fragments of metal discharged during the explosion of crudely fabricated bombs and infernal machines. Metal shell-casing fragments from exploding military bombs and shells are infrequently encountered among civilian populations except in wartime. The deliberate bombing of cities and civilian populations in World War II with weapons such as aerial bombs, rocket bombs fired from great distances and bombs powered with the terrific force of atomic energy have increased the variety of missile injuries with which the physician in civil life should be familiar.

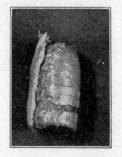

Fig. 16-1. A .38-Caliber Lead Bullet with Attached Splinter of Rib.

This bullet had passed through the chest of the deceased and was found on the floor at the scene of the homicide.

Wounds Caused by Pistol Bullets. TYPES OF WEAPONS AND AMMUNITION. The two types of pistols commonly used are the *revolver* and the *automatic*. In a revolver, the cartridges are loaded into the chambers, usually six in number, of a revolving cylinder. Each chamber in succession is aligned with the barrel of the pistol by the rotation of the cylinder. In the single action revolver, after a cartridge is fired by pulling the trigger, the hammer is hand cocked, the cocking action rotating the next chamber into firing alignment. In the double action weapon, the rotation of the cylinder, the cocking of the hammer and the dropping of the hammer are accomplished by completing a single pull on the trigger; most double action pistols can also be hand cocked. To unload and reload the revolver, the cylinder is exposed either by releasing it and swinging it out sideways or by bending down the barrel; empty shells and undischarged cartridges are extracted from the chamber and new cartridges inserted.

Most revolver ammunition in the past was loaded with black powder; the newer cartridges contain so-called smokeless or semismokeless types of powder. The bullet is made of lead or lead hardened by alloying it with small amounts of antimony or tin. The segment of a bullet within the cartridge case is cylindric and the projecting portion is ogival and rounded at the tip or dome. Illustrations of lead bullets recovered in fatal shooting cases are shown in Figures 16-1 and 16-2. Such missiles are readily deformed and fragmented by passing through hard bony structures.

During its passage through the pistol barrel, the cylindric surface of the bullet is indented with a set of parallel slanting grooves, 4 to 7 in number, corresponding in number, with, direction and pitch to the lands inside the barrel. The lands are elevated surfaces between the spiral grooves or riflings cut into the inner surface of the barrel for the purpose of imparting a spin to a bullet squeezing through it. The grooves and lands on the bullets corresponding to the lands and grooves in the pistol barrel are important for the identification of the weapon used. Certain variations and imperfections in these rifling marks on the bullet are produced by corresponding imperfections in the bore of the pistol barrel and may serve by comparison with identical markings on test bullets fired from a suspected weapon to establish it as the one from which the bullet in question was fired. The grooves produced by most pistols, including the Smith and Wesson and the Webley, slant or twist to

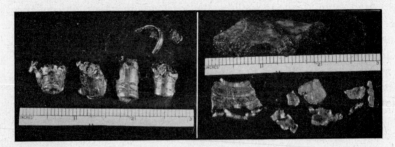

Fig. 16-2. Deformed and Fragmented .38-Caliber Revolver Bullets Recovered at Autopsy.

Left. Four bullets found in victim's head.
Right. Eight fragments of a single bullet flattened and deformed by impact against shaft of femur. Loose bone fragment above ruler.

the right. Those produced by the Colt pistol riflings slant toward the left. The directions indicated are from the base to the dome of the bullet.

Revolver cartridges have a cylindric brass shell with a small projecting rim around the edge of the base. The primer is located on the inside of the shell just under the center of the base. When the trigger is pulled and the hammer is dropped, the impact of the firing pin detonates the primer and this explosion ignites the propelling charge of powder in the cartridge case with the rapid production of a large amount of gas which forces the bullet through the barrel and on its course. In older ammunition, the primer contained a mixture of mercury fulminate, stibnite (antimony sulfide), potassium chlorate and powdered glass. In recent years, the composition of this mixture has been changed; the mercury has in large part been replaced by lead compounds such as the azide and styphnate, and the potassium chlorate by barium nitrate.

The caliber of bullets and of pistols is expressed in hundredths of an inch in Great Britain and the United States; in Europe and in Asia it is expressed in millimeters. The calibers of revolver bullets and of revolvers most commonly encountered in the United States are .32, .38 and .45. The .32 and .38 caliber bullets are made in two sizes, long and short.

An *automatic pistol* is one which when fired ejects the empty cartridge shell and delivers another cartridge from a magazine clip in the handle into the chamber for the next shot. The process is repeated each time the gun is fired. Most automatic pistols work on the blowback principle. The recoil of the gases forces the breech mechanism to slide back ejecting the empty shell and permitting another cartridge to slide into the chamber from the magazine as the slide moves forward again; both slide and magazine are activated by strong springs. The magazines vary in capacity from 5 to 10 cartridges. The shell of the cartridge is rimless with a deep circumferential groove just above the base, which distinguishes it from a revolver cartridge. The shell contains smokeless powder, and the mechanism of firing it is similar to that described for revolver cartridges. The bullet fired from the automatic pistol is ogive-shaped like a revolver bullet, and its cylindric surface is indented with grooves as the result of passing through the rifled pistol barrel. It has a central core of lead covered with a casing or jacket of hard metal, such as copper, cupro-nickel, cupro-zinc or steel (Fig. 16-3). Although more resistant to deformity than a lead bullet, a hard jacketed bullet may become fragmented on

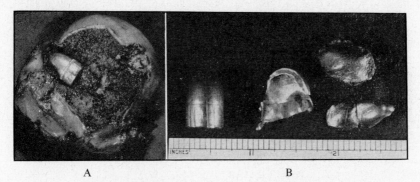

A   B

Fig. 16-3. Hard Metal-Jacketed Automatic Pistol Bullets Recovered at Autopsy.

A. Undeformed .32-caliber bullet embedded in head of humerus.
B. Two .45-caliber bullets, the one on the left undeformed, the one on the right deformed and broken into three fragments of separated core and jacket by striking bone.

striking heavy bone. Revolver ammunition can be fired from an automatic pistol of similar caliber if the rim is filed away. Automatic pistol ammunition can be fired from a revolver with the aid of an adapter.

The calibers of automatic pistols used in the United States are mostly .25, .32, .38 and .45 inch. The weapons of Colt manufacture and some foreign makes have riflings with a left twist; those with a right twist are all of foreign manufacture and have calibers of 7.65 mm. and 9 mm.

The characteristics of weapons in common are shown in Table 16-1.

POWDERS. The *black powder* in revolver ammunition is composed of 60 to 75 per cent potassium nitrate, 10 to 20 per cent sulfur and 2 to 8 per cent of charcoal. One grain of powder forms 200 to 300 ml. of gas composed of 50 per cent carbon dioxide, 10 per cent carbon monoxide, 35 per cent nitrogen, 3 per cent hydrogen sulfide and 2 per cent hydrogen with traces of methane and oxygen. After the cartridge is fired, a residue remains composed of 56 per cent potassium carbonate, 25 per cent sulfides, 16 per cent sulfates, 0.5 per cent thiocyanate and traces of nitrate, thiosulfate, ammonium carbonate, sulfur and carbon.

The black powders burn with the production of much heat, flame and smoke, and many of the powder grains are only partly burned or remain unburned. After detonation of the explosive charge in the cartridge, the bullet is propelled through the barrel of the gun by the after-coming column of expanding compressed gases, smoke and flame intermingled with burned and unburned powder grains, all travel-ing at approximately the same velocity. Some of the gas, flame, smoke and powder

Table 16-1. Weapons in Common Use

REVOLVERS	NUMBER OF GROOVES	DIRECTION OF RIFLINGS
Webley, .455, .38, .32	7	right
Webley, Fosbery, .450	7	right
Colt, all calibers	6	left
Smith and Wesson, .45, .32	5	right
J. T. & Co., S. & W. model	4	right

AUTOMATIC PISTOLS		
F. D. Leige	7	right
Webley, .455, .32, .25	6	right
Browning	6	right
F. N.	6	right
Savage	6	right
Infallible	6	right
Harrington & Richardson	6	right
Express	6	right
Mauser, .25	6	right
Helfricht	6	right
Steyr (Pieper's Patent)	6	right
Surete, M. F. (St. Etienne)	6	right
Le Francais (St. Etienne)	6	right
Ortgie's Patent (Deutsche Werke)	6	right
V. Bernedo	6	right
Colt, .45, .38, .32, .25	6	left
Delta	6	left
Errasti	6	left
Victoria (Spanish make)	6	left
Stosel	6	left
Eibar	6	left
Bayard (Pieper)	6	left
Unique	6	left
Libia	6	left
Reims	6	left
Mauser, .311	4	right
Dreyse	4	right
R. F. M.	4	right
Haenel Suhl	4	right
Frömmer (Budapest)	4	right
Luger P-08, 9 mm., German	6	right
Walther P-38, 9 mm., German	6	right
Walther PP & PPK, 7.65 mm., German	6	right
Sauer & Sohn, 7.65 mm., German	4	right
Fabrique National, 9 mm., Belgian	6	right
Fabrique National, 7.65 mm., Belgian	6	right
Ceska Zbrojovoka, 9 mm., short Czech	6	right
S. A. C. M., 7.65 mm., long French	4	right
Beretta, 9 mm., short Italian	6	right
Beretta, 7.65 mm., Italian	6	right
Glisenti, 9 mm., Italian	6	right
Nambu, 8 mm., Japanese	6	right
Radom, 9 mm., Polish	6	right
Tokarev, 7.62 mm., Russian	4	right

From Smith and Glaister, *Recent Advances in Forensic Medicine,* modified by H. L. Butts.

grains leak past the bullet and emerge in front of it. The bulk of the gas and its products escape immediately after the bullet, however, and on passing the muzzle expands and diverges into the shape of an elongated cone. The powder grains may travel 18 to 24 inches or more, depending on the length of barrel, caliber and type of weapon, and the type of ammunition. The flame and the smoke do not travel as far as the powder grains, both having a shorter range and more restricted dispersion dependent on the character of the weapon and the ammunition. The flame travels ahead of some of the powder grains but is preceded by others at the time of discharge. Whenever the gun is fired close to a target, characteristic marks are left on its surface, varying with the distance and angle between the muzzle and the target.

If the muzzle is held in contact with the target, the perforation will usually be large from the explosive force of the gases, the products of discharge will be blown

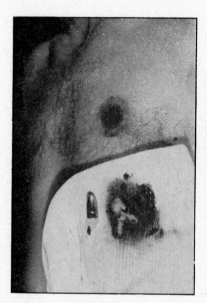

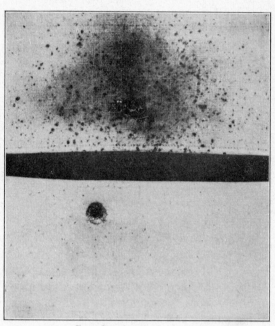

From Gonzales, T. A., *Am. J. Surg.*, 26:43, 1934

Fig. 16-4. Suicidal Contact Bullet Wound of Precordium from A .45-Caliber Automatic Pistol.

Bullet shown was found in back. Characteristic cross tear and burning of fabric of undershirt through which shot was fired. Note circular burn and smoke halo around entrance hole in skin.

Fig. 16-5. Comparative Effects of Black and Smokeless Powder on a White Target. The Gun Was Fired at a Distance of Six Inches.

Top. Black powder. Bottom. Smokeless powder.

into the bullet track and this will be blackened by powder and smoke and seared by flame for a varying distance below the surface. The edges of the bullet hole may be blackened and seared by flame and the skin surrounding it blackened by a ring or halo of smoke, especially if the shot is fired through clothing, in which case the cloth will show a large cruciate perforation with burning of the edges of the fabric (Fig. 16-4). In contact wounds, the skin surrounding the perforation will not be tattooed with embedded powder grains as in a close-up shot, although occasionally some unburned powder grains may be deposited loosely on the skin in and around the margin of the perforation. Small calibered pistols such as .22 and .25 produce correspondingly small and regular contact wounds in contrast to those of larger caliber. Contact wounds of the skin will be described later in more detail.

If the gun is held at a slight distance from the target within range of the powder blast, the products of discharge will produce marks around the bullet hole. If the target is within range of the flame discharge, the area around the perforation will be singed or branded by the flame and smudged by smoke in varying degree, and in and surrounding the area of the flame burn there will be a compact zone of densely packed powder grains driven into the target in an unburned, partly burned or still burning state, producing the peppered stippled pattern or tattoo. If the weapon is fired beyond the range of the flame, the flame burn and smoke stain will be absent and the powder grains may be sprinkled in a wide circle around the bullet perforation. The closer the muzzle of the revolver is to the target, the more concentrated and intense the areas of flame burn or brand, and the areas of tattooing with powder grains.

In close-up revolver shots the marks of the products of discharge on the target in relation to the bullet perforation are modified by the kick of the gun. As the bullet and the gases pass through the barrel and out of the muzzle the recoil tilts the barrel upward; the bullet strikes the target as directed in the original line of fire, but the flame and powder grains are directed to the target along the line produced by the recoil; as a consequence the bullet perforation is slightly below the center of the flame burn and even more below the center of the area encompassed by the embedded powder grains. This eccentricity is evident in the upper photograph in Figure 16-5, and in the close-up revolver bullet and black powder wounds illustrated in Figures 16-23 and 16-24. Both victims were shot at close range while lying on the floor after having been shot through the back of the head. With the automatic pistol the pattern of the close-up shot is usually concentric as there is little tendency for the muzzle to tilt when the gun is fired. The characteristic action of black powder fired on a surface at close range is the production of severe flame marks, conspicuous smoke stains and coarse black stippling or tattooing by partly burned or unburned powder grains (Fig. 16-5).

If the gun is discharged at a distance from the target beyond the range of flame, smoke and powder grains, only the bullet perforation is produced. The bullet may soil or foul the edges of the perforation with substances deposited on its surface during its passage through a fouled gun barrel and, if the target is abrasive, some of the metal from the bullet surface may also be rubbed off. The fouling effect is likely to be conspicuous around holes in light colored cloth produced by lead bullets. The margin of the perforation may also be stained with oil from the gun barrel, deposited on the surface of the bullet. It is important not to confuse the fouling stain around a bullet perforation with the marks of a close-up or contact shot.

Occasionally when a lead bullet is fired from a defective barrel with a roughened bore, small particles of lead are scraped from its surface and propelled forward as molten droplets for a considerable distance before striking the target. These are usually small but their metallic character is easily recognized. Such lead particles may be found embedded in the victim's skin or on the clothing near the site of the bullet perforation, or as the only missiles to strike a given area. They should not be confused with powder grains (Fig. 16-6). If the cylinder of a revolver is not properly aligned with the barrel, when the gun is fired particles of lead from the bullet and components of the exploding powder may be deflected and discharged in a radial direction at right angles to the barrel through the space between the cylinder and the barrel. This effect is known as cylinder flare and in some cases the pattern and its location in relation to a contact entrance hole may serve to indicate the length of the revolver barrel.

The powder loaded into automatic pistol cartridges is known as *smokeless* and is composed of nitrocellulose (single base powder), or nitrocellulose and nitroglycerine combined (double base powder). The explosion of one grain of these substances forms about 800 to 900 ml. of gases, about three times the volume as the same amount of black powder. The gases produced consist of carbon dioxide, carbon monoxide, nitrogen, hydrogen and traces of methane. In the solid residue nitrates and nitrites are present, with traces of other substances such as barium nitrate, potassium bichromate, potassium oxalate, potassium bicarbonate, diphenylamine, nitrobenzene, camphor, Vaseline, graphite and sawdust.

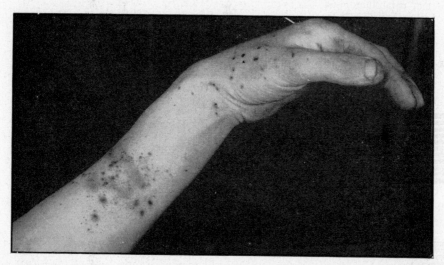

Fig. 16-6. Irregular Sprayed Pattern of Lead Spicules in Skin of Forearm and Hand.

These particles were scraped from the surface of a .38-caliber bullet during its passage through the barrel and traveled eight feet to the target. They should not be confused with powder grain tattooing.

The smokeless powder for pistol cartridges is gelatinized, to retard the rapidity of the explosion thus tending to keep up an even regular pressure on the bullet. The explosion of smokeless powder usually is attended by much less flame and smoke and is more completely combusted than black powder. As noted in Table 16-2 only about one-third the weight of smokeless as compared with black powder is sufficient to impart the same muzzle velocity to a projectile of given weight and caliber. Most revolver cartridges are now loaded with smokeless or semismokeless varieties of powder and the effects of black powder cartridges are now only occasionally encountered. Semismokeless powder consists of a mixture of 80 per cent of the black and 20 per cent of the smokeless types.

In recent years there has been considerable improvement in handguns in relation to velocity and kinetic energy. The modification of the frontier model .44 caliber weapon into the Smith and Wesson .44 Special and the development of the .357 caliber Magnum are examples. The .44 caliber Special shoots a 235 grain lead bullet, usually of the gascheck variety, with a muzzle velocity of 1,200 feet per second and energy at the muzzle of 751 foot pounds, and at 100 yards of 522 foot pounds. The muzzle velocity of the Magnum firing the 158 grain bullet is 1,510 feet per second with the hand loaded cartridge and 1,450 with the factory loaded type.

Table 16-2. Commonly Used Cartridges *

DESCRIPTION	POWDER GRAINS	BULLET GRAINS	MUZZLE VELOCITY FEET PER SECOND
5—4 Velo dog revolver	1¼ S	45 M C	650
.297/.230 Morris short	3½ B	37 L	870
	1¾ S	37 L	870
6.35 mm. (.25 inch) automatic pistol	2 S	50 M C	625
7.5 mm. Nagant revolver (Swedish)	10 B	105 L	725
7.5 mm. Nagant revolver (Swiss)	5 S	105 M C	725
.300 inch Mauser pistol	7 S	85 M C	1400
7.65 mm. (.32 inch) automatic pistol	3½ S	72 M C	875
7.65 mm. parabellum pistol	5½ S	92 M C	1200
8 mm. Lebel revolver	11 B	120 M C	625
	4 S	120 L	725
.32 inch Smith and Wesson	4½ B	85 L	550
	2 S	85 L	550
.32 inch Colt new police revolver	11 B	100 L	725
	4 S	100 L	725
9 mm. automatic pistol	5½ S	110 M C	1000
.360 inch revolver	16 B	125 L	1050
.38 inch Smith and Wesson revolver	10 B	145 L	625
	2½ S	145 L	650
.38 inch Smith and Wesson special	18 B	158 L	875
	6 S	158 L	875
.38 inch Colt police positive revolver	10 B	150 L	660
	2¾ S	150 L	660
.38 inch revolver	10 B	124 L	625
	3 S	124 L	625
.38 inch automatic pistol	6 S	130 M C	1050
.45 inch Colt automatic U.S.A.	7 S	200 M C	870
.455 inch Webley automatic pistol	7 S	224 M C	710
.450 inch revolver	13 B	225 L	660
	6 S	225 L	710
.455 inch revolver	18 B	265 L	710
	7 S	265 L	600

From Smith and Glaister, *Recent Advances in Forensic Medicine.*

* S = smokeless powder, B = black powder, L = lead, M C = coated.

The energy of this load at the muzzle and at 100 yards is 754 and 566 foot pounds respectively. Hollow pointed bullets fired from these guns mushroom on striking flesh and cause considerable tissue destruction.

The marks produced by smokeless powders vary greatly from those produced by the black variety. In contact shots the explosive force of the gas is pronounced, but searing and power smudging are slight. In shots fired a few inches from the target surface flame effects are not as conspicuous and tattooing by powder grains is not as marked. The comparison of black and smokeless powder effects in close-up shots on the same white target at the same distance and with the same weapon are shown in Figure 16-5. The tattoo marks vary with the shape of the powder grains; some of the round flat smokeless grains produce circular abrasions, but when they strike on edge they produce fine short linear cuts in the skin; other smokeless grains with a tubular or square flake form leave longitudinal cuts on the surface when they strike on edge (Fig. 16-25). Some of the unburned grains may be discovered with characteristic forms such as squares, circles or triangles, either solid or with punched-out centers.

Powder marks on clothing, skin or other surfaces should be sought for by a careful naked eye examination and with the use of a hand lens; in most cases this type of investigation will yield sufficient information. The examination of powder marks around a skin wound should be entrusted to a medical man; to the attending physician if the patient is still alive, and to the pathologist if the body is up for autopsy. Photographs of the powder mark pattern should also be taken. In doubtful cases additional microscopic and chemical examinations should be made of powder deposits and residues to determine the type of powder.

Black powder grains have no characteristic shape when magnified and are usually amorphous, having a black or brown appearance. They can be distinguished from granules of smokeless powder but are difficult to differentiate from other black powders. At present black powder is used mainly in blank cartridges, fired to produce a noisy and flashy effect.

Smokeless powders, which have largely supplanted black powders for the loading of pistols as well as other types of ammunition, contain granules of a great variety of shapes and colors. Different lots prepared by the same manufacturers vary from time to time, the colors ranging from bright orange to bluish black and the shapes taking the form of minute globules, cylinders and flakes of different sorts. The amount of residue from smokeless powder is usually small and a complete chemical analysis is not always practicable. It is possible to demonstrate the presence of nitroglycerine or nitrocellulose and, in addition, other substances added to the powder to moderate the explosive force and render it more stable.

Nitrocellulose is insoluble in water, alcohol and ether but is soluble in acetone. If the powder residue is extracted with acetone, the nitrocellulose will be dissolved with related substances and can be tested with an aqueous solution of potassium hydroxide or a dilute solution of alcoholic ammonia. Color reactions of light yellow, intense red violet, orange and blue result, depending on the nitro bodies present.

Nitroglycerine is a viscous substance which may be extracted from the powder residue with ether. It is obtained by letting the solvent evaporate and heating the residue on a water bath with an 80 per cent methyl alcohol solution. The nitroglycerine will dissolve; a piece of filter paper saturated with this solution and ignited, will burn with a green flame.

After the ether extraction the powder residue can be treated with water, and such materials as barium and potassium nitrates, chlorides, starch, gum and gelatin may be separated and identified. To test for nitrates, brucine and sulfuric acid are added to the solution which turns a bright orange-red color if the test is positive. The residue left after the water extraction consists of such insoluble substances as charcoal, graphite, wool meal, lime and magnesium carbonate, which may be tested for microscopically and chemically. Camphor used in some powders may be recognized by its characteristic odor. Diphenylamine, or diethyl diphenyl urea, or diphenyl urea are occasionally present and may be recognized by the intense blue color given with sulfuric acid containing a trace of nitrite.

Guareschi has shown that the mercury fulminate in the primer of a cartridge contributes its decomposition products to the powder residue during its discharge and has demonstrated mercury by appropriate tests around the entrance wound of a close-up shot. The mercury in the primer in recent years has been replaced by lead compounds. Spectrography and roentgenography have also been used to identify metallic elements in bullet tracks in order to differentiate entrance and exit wounds and to determine direction of the missile. When spectrography is used for this purpose, more metal will usually be found around the entrance hole than in the vicinity of the exit perforation, provided that the bullet has only traversed soft tissue. Walker and others have pointed out that the metallic residues in the edges of a bullet entrance perforation may have been carried there as fouling on the surface of the bullet derived from the gun barrel without inclusion of any metal from the bullet surface. If bone has been struck or perforated, considerably more metal will be found in the tissues of the track beyond the bone, than if the track had only involved soft tissue. If, in a skeletonized body, two perforations are found through the skull, suspected of being entrance and exit bullet wounds, spectrographic proof of the presence of lead in specimens removed from the edges of the perforations strengthens the evidence in favor of a gunshot wound. If the bone happens to have been struck near the end of the track, the exit perforation may contain more metal than the entrance wound. In all doubtful cases the track should be accurately determined, and any involvement of bone should be noted. The practical value of such methods of investigation in the study of bullet wounds and other missiles cannot be appraised completely at the present time and much careful correlated work has yet to be done in order to avoid mistakes in interpretation which may have far reaching consequences. Fortunately in almost every case of a gunshot wound, it is possible by unassisted painstaking observation of the details of the entire track, to determine the character of a bullet wound with sufficient accuracy and to differentiate entrance from exit wounds, thus establishing the direction of the bullet track.

A method of detecting gun powder residue on the hands of a suspect in a homicidal shooting or of a victim in a suicidal shooting has come into vogue in localities where little attention is given to the autopsy or to a careful study of the bullet track. This method is commonly known as the paraffin test and depends on the fact that when a poorly constructed revolver is fired some of the invisible powder residue may escape from the breech to contaminate the hand that holds the weapon. If the hand is examined soon enough these substances may be detected. A paraffin impression is made of the surface of the hand which is then tested for nitrites with diphenylamine. The test is fallible inasmuch as the hand may have been contaminated with nitrogenous compounds, a common source of which is urine. In such a case a positive test would be of doubtful significance; a negative result is not conclusive, for a well-constructed revolver will not discharge any residue on the hand. The most serious objection to the test is the delay in its use during which time the substances tested for may have been washed away or other substances, giving a similar reaction and positive test, may have been added either deliberately or by chance to the skin surface in question. A competent chemist is needed to perform the analysis on powder or its residues, and the foregoing description is intended only to indicate the problems that must be faced in the analysis.

Tests for Powder Residues. The late Joseph T. Walker devised a method for demonstrating the pattern of powder residues on fabrics by printing it onto gelatinized paper treated with either "C" acid (2-naphthylamine-4, 8-disulfonic acid), or "H" acid (1-amino-8-naphthol-3, 6-disulfonic acid), or with alpha-naphthylamine and sulfanilic acid. The procedure is carried out as follows: Glossy photographic paper is fixed thoroughly in hypo solution to remove all the silver salts and then washed and dried. It is either placed in a warm 5 per cent solution of the "C" or "H" acid for 10 minutes and dried, or soaked in a 0.5 per cent solution of sulfanilic acid for 10 minutes, dried and then swabbed with a 0.5 per cent solution of alpha naphthalamine in methyl alcohol and again dried. A sheet of the prepared paper of sufficient size is placed face up on a towel or pad of cotton cloth and the material to be tested is placed face down on the paper. The preparation is then covered with a thin dry cloth or towel slightly moistened with a 20 per cent solution of acetic acid, and then by another layer of dry cloth. The entire pack is pressed with a warm iron for several minutes. If unburned powder grains are present, the nitrites they contain will result in the production of dark red or orange-brown spots on the prepared paper.

EXAMINATION OF WEAPON, CARTRIDGE SHELLS AND BULLETS. In all cases of shooting, whether the wounding is fatal or nonfatal, the suspected weapon and the exploding cartridge shells, and any bullets recovered from the scene of the shooting or from the body of the victim are examined by the ballistics experts of the police department. The procedures include an examination of the weapon for fingerprints, and of the barrel and empty shells chemically and microscopically for powder residues, and also similar examinations of such materials as blood stains or hair fibers which may be on the weapon.

The cartridge case is examined for any distinctive marks that the firing pin, the breech block, the ejector or the barrel may produce on it; comparisons are then made between test cartridge shells fired from the gun and shells under investigation. The shells usually recovered at the scene of a shooting are those mechanically ejected from an automatic pistol when the gun is fired. They should always be saved as evidence for comparison with test shells fired from the suspected weapon.

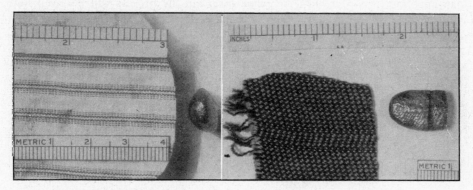

Fig. 16-7. Separate Imprints of Two Cloth Fabrics on the Same Lead Bullet.

Left. Finely woven pattern of cotton shirt on nose of bullet.
Right. Coarser pattern of weave of overcoat on side of flattened bullet.
The victim was shot while standing with his back against a tiled wall. The bullet turned and flattened against the wall and dropped out inside the overcoat.

Other pistols besides automatics and revolvers are encountered and have been used in fatal and nonfatal shootings. One type is the single shot target pistol that fires a .22 caliber lead bullet. Another is the old fashioned single action .44 caliber revolver. Derringers, four barreled pistols, homemade weapons and other freak guns are sometimes used for homicidal and suicidal purposes. Many automatic pistols of foreign make have been brought back as souvenirs by returning members of the armed forces. A considerable number of such weapons find their way into the possession of persons who use them for criminal purposes. Ballistics bureaus of most police departments have acquired or should acquire samples of such weapons and of the ammunition used in them for purposes of recognition and testing.

The examination of bullets found at autopsy or surgical operation is an important part of the procedure in any suspected criminal case. First, the nature of the projectile is determined, whether lead or hard-metal coated, and then its caliber, the riflings, length and weight. The presence of any substances found on the bullet such as lubricants or paints is noted; for example, some lead bullets are painted with a copper colored paint known as lubaloy, a lubricant intended to minimize fouling of the barrel during the passage of the lead bullet. Marks on bullets are described in detail. A cruciform incision may be found on the dome of a lead projectile for the purpose of causing it to spread like a dum-dum bullet when it comes in contact with its target, a device which is rarely successful with pistol ammunition. Other deformities are caused by the impact of the bullet against other surfaces. Thus a lead bullet in penetrating cloth may obtain an impression of the weave of the fabric on the tip or side. Figure 16-7 illustrates such a bullet with the imprint of the fine weave of the shirt fabric on the nose and the coarser weave of the overcoat on the side, the bullet having turned a right angle to strike the inside of the coat before dropping out of the track. The victim was shot while standing against a tiled wall. In another case, a lead bullet struck against an inscription on a metal plate, and letters on the plate were imprinted on the surface of the lead. Many deformities of the bullet are due to its passage through bony structures in the body (Fig. 16-2).

The examination of the markings upon bullets for the purpose of identification is an important procedure in a homicide case, but the process will be given here only in outline as it is properly a part of the science of ballistics. The suspected gun is fired into a cotton or sand bank so as to obtain a test bullet which will show

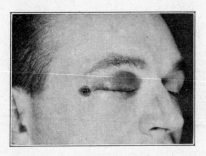

Fig. 16-8. Distant Bullet Wound of Entrance on Face.

Punched-in circular perforation surrounded by a concentric abrasion collar produced by bullet entering at right angles to skin. Note absence of brand and tattooing. Homicide.

characteristic riflings on its base, impressed there by the lands and grooves of the gun barrel. This test bullet is then compared with bullets recovered at the scene or from the body of the victim, to see if the riflings correspond in any way. The apparatus for the examination consists of two microscopes, each of which contains a stage with a turning arrangement designed so that a bullet can be held under each objective and rotated at will. The objectives are low-powered lenses. The two microscopes are joined at their oculars by a comparison eye piece. The test bullet is adjusted to the stage of one microscope and a bullet recovered from the body of the victim or the scene of the crime is adjusted to the stage of the other. By looking through the comparison eyepiece, the riflings from both projectiles will appear in the same ocular field and can be compared. If necessary the bullets can be photographed from all points. Rolled impressions of riflings on a bullet can be made upon a plasticene plate which has the advantage of giving a plane surface for comparison. Test firing of the gun may also reveal individual peculiarities in the weapon which may help in the identification of missiles. If the bullet is broken, the fragments may be collected and weighed, as the caliber of the projectile can sometimes be estimated from its weight, even if it is shattered and deformed. See Table of Weights, page 388.

VELOCITY AND WOUNDING POWER OF BULLETS. Pistol bullets are propelled at a relatively low velocity, usually not exceeding 1,000 feet per second at the muzzle. In most revolvers the muzzle velocity of the bullet is between 550 and 850 feet per second, but in some automatic pistols, such as the .30 caliber Mauser, the 85 grain bullet is fired at a muzzle velocity of 1,400 feet per second. High velocity missiles, such as projectiles from military rifles, or machine guns, or shell fragments from high explosive cannon, mortar shells or aerial bombs may travel at speeds in excess of 2,500 feet per second. The amount of damage inflicted on a

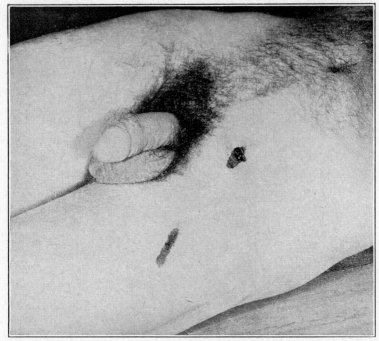

From Gonzales, T. A., *Am. J. Surg.*, 26:46, 1934

Fig. 16-9. Tangential Bullet-slap Abrasion on Left Thigh with Oblique Re-entrance Wound in Groin.

The abrasion on the thigh is in line with the beveled lower border of the re-entrance wound and indicates that the bullet track is directed upward and to the right. Homicide.

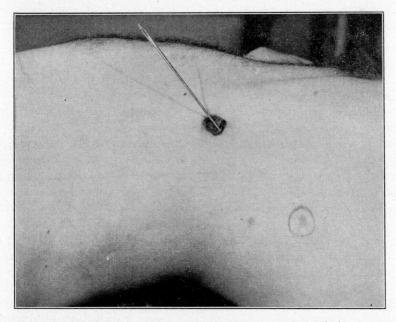

Fig. 16-10. Tangential Bullet Wound of Entrance in Right Flank.

A probe inserted into wound indicates direction of track; the bullet is located beneath faintly contused skin in inked circle. Note beveling of upper and undermining of lower borders of wound. Homicide.

target depends on the striking energy of the missile which is the product of its mass or weight multiplied by the square of its velocity, or MV^2.

The efficiency or wounding power of the missile is dependent upon its ability to expend its striking energy on the tissues. Thus to have wounding power it is required that the missile have a sufficient amount of kinetic energy to reach and penetrate the target, after which the effects will be determined by its size, shape, spin, orientation, resistance to deformity and fragmentation, and by the character and resistance of the tissues traversed. In the case of pistol bullets and shotgun pellets which have a relatively low velocity, the initial striking energy is limited and

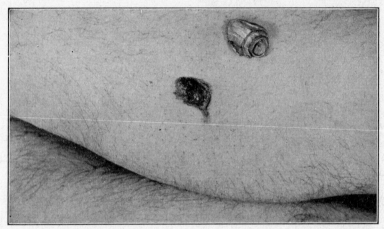

From Gonzales, T. A., *Am. J. Surg.*, 26:44, 1934

Fig. 16-11. Ricocheted Bullet and Its Entrance Wound on the Calf.

The bullet was flattened when it struck the floor before passing upward into the soft tissues of the leg.

the resistance of the tissues may be sufficient to cause the missile to expend all its energy and to stop in its track. A limited and insufficient amount of damage may result from failure to penetrate deeply enough into a vital region. With low velocity pistol bullets, optimum destructive effect is obtained only at relatively close range at which the striking energy is most efficient.

Bone, over all other tissues, offers the greatest resistance to the passage of a bullet because of its density, and the skin is second only to bone in this respect. For this reason bullets which have penetrated the body may have sufficient energy to traverse all tissues including bone, but are stopped just under the skin at the point where they might be expected to emerge, as they lack sufficient remaining energy to perforate the tough and unyielding dermis. Such spent bullets may frequently be palpated at the end of their track just under the skin (Fig. 16-29) from which they may be removed for examination by a small incision. In other cases pistol bullets have just enough residual energy to make their exit through the skin only to drop into the clothing, a fact important to remember when clothing is removed from the body in a homicide case, in order to avoid losing the bullet during this procedure. Occasionally a spent bullet is found with its nose protruding from an exit wound (Fig. 16-31). In most cases, even when the bullet passes through body and clothes there is usually not enough residual energy to carry it far and it may be found in the vicinity of the shooting.

Fig. 16-12. Multiple Contact and Close-Up Bullet Wounds of Entrance. Black Powder and Lead Bullets from a .38-Caliber Revolver.

Homicide. Three large lacerated contact wounds on left side caused by subcutaneous explosion of gases with tissues deeply burned and blackened by flame, smoke and powder.

On right side of cheek a close-up wound with flame burn, smoke smudge and tattooing from embedded powder grains.

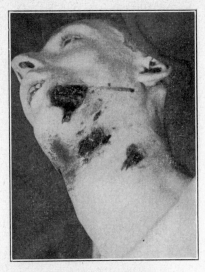

Fig. 16-13. Contact Bullet Wound of Entrance.

Left. Large gaping entrance wound of right temple caused by subcutaneous explosion of gases.

Right. Smaller lacerated wound of exit of bullet in front of left ear. Suicide.

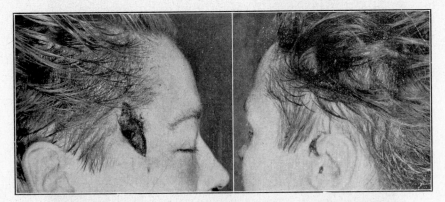

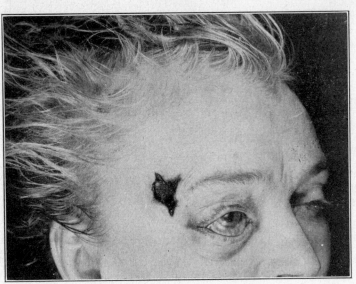

Fig. 16-14. Contact Bullet Wound of Right Temple.

Subcutaneous tissue in wound blackened by flame and powder. Traumatic exophthalmos of right eye caused by explosion of gases deep in track. Homicide.

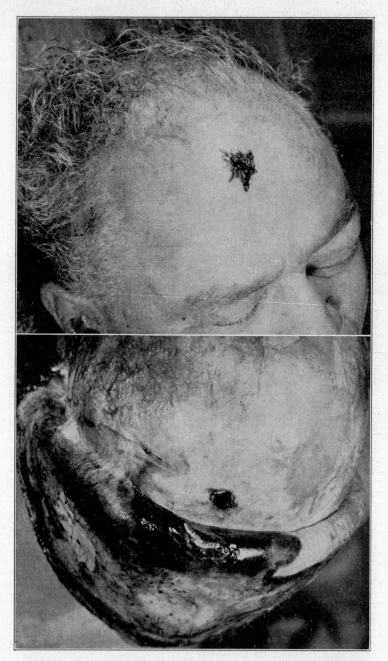

Fig. 16-15. Contact Bullet Wound of Forehead.

Top. Stellate lacerated wound of entrance. No burn or powder grains on surrounding skin.
Bottom. Bullet hole in skull shown by reflection of scalp, with the edge blackened by powder and rimmed by lead. Fragment of lead has been shaved from bullet by its passage through the skull and is embedded in the scalp. Suicide.

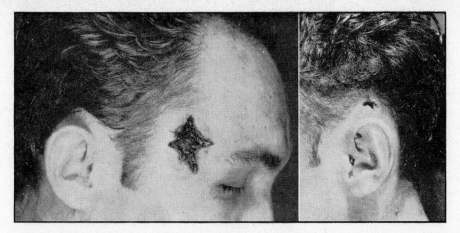

Fig. 16-16. Suicidal Bullet Wound from a .38-Caliber Automatic Pistol.

Large cruciform contact entrance wound of right temple. Smaller exit wound above left ear.

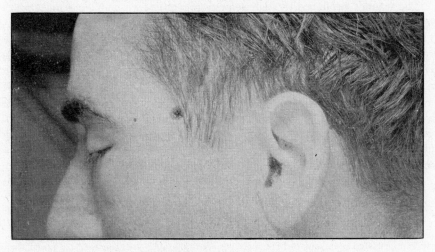

Fig. 16-17. Small Contact Bullet Wound Inflicted with .22-Caliber Pistol.

Note superficial resemblance to a distant shot. Powder effects were found in deeper tissues. Suicide.

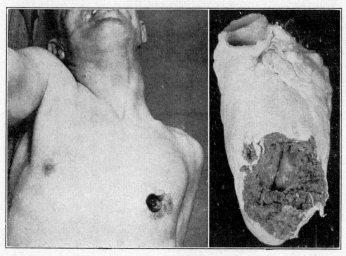

Fig. 16-18. Contact wound, lead .38 bullet, black powder. Suicide. Left. Circular powder burn and smudge around wound of left chest. Right. Extensive laceration of heart due to explosion of powder gases deep in bullet track. Black powder embedded in heart muscle.

The wounding effects of pistol bullets for the most part are confined to those tissues which are perforated by the missile and the damage is limited to the bullet track. Exceptions occur when bullets strike bone and fragments of the latter are driven into surrounding structures. Thus a passage of a missile through the spine may displace bone fragments into the spinal canal to contuse or lacerate the spinal cord or forward to lacerate the aorta; similarly a tangential bullet wound of the skull may drive bone fragments into the brain, and in long bones, fragmentation by a bullet may result in injury to adjacent blood vessels and nerves. In contact pistol wounds with the larger caliber bullets, additional damage is caused by the explosive effect of the powder charge which is blown into the track along with the missile. Such a wound in the head may result in extensive bursting fractures of the skull from the force of the exploding gases added to the energy of the missile. Separation of the sutures is not uncommon and traumatic exophthalmos may also occur. These effects are taken up in detail in the descriptions of bullet wounds in different parts of the body.

The wounds produced by high velocity projectiles which have a muzzle velocity greater than 2,500 feet per second may be very extensive and out of all proportion to the size of the missile, in distinct contrast to the wounds produced by low velocity pistol ammunition and shotgun pellets, which cause considerably less damage to the tissues unless the weapon is fired at contact range and additional injury is received from the explosive effects of the powder. When a high velocity projectile passes through the tissues, the injury produced usually extends for a considerable distance radial to the path of the missile and its pattern depending on the tissue involved may be radically different from the wounds produced by low velocity bullets. Friable organs like the kidney, spleen or liver usually manifest injuries much greater in extent and with a conspicuously larger cross sectional diameter than the caliber of the bullet would suggest, even when the missile is of relatively low velocity.

The mechanism of extensive wound production by high velocity missiles has been studied by Callender, Zuckerman, Harvey and their associates. With the use of special fragment guns capable of firing small steel spheres at velocities between 3,000 and 4,000 feet per second, they have demonstrated by means of high speed photography and synchronized high speed roentgen-ray equipment that such a missile in passing through a gelatin block or through the hind legs of an animal forms a large momentary cavity in its wake. There is violent swelling and deformity of the gelatin or tissue and the cavity that develops does not attain its greatest size until after the missile has passed through. The cavity results because the material in the path of the missile is displaced, not only in the direction of its forward progression but also in lateral directions, and, as a consequence the diameter of the cavity is many times the diameter of the missile. The motions set up create stresses which disrupt the tissue, and for this reason a small high velocity projectile can produce a relatively enormous wound. The momentary cavity soon subsides leaving a smaller zone of residual permanent disruption as an indication of the track taken by the missile.

Harvey and his associates have demonstrated by their studies that the volume of the temporary cavity produced by a high velocity projectile and the size of the residual permanent wound depend upon the quantity of kinetic energy which the missile loses in passing through the tissue. At any particular point in the track of the missile, the size of both the temporary cavity and of the permanent wound will depend upon the rate at which the kinetic energy is being expended per unit distance traveled at that point. For a given type of tissue, the over-all size or volume of the wound depends upon the total kinetic energy expended by the projectile in passing through that tissue and the general shape of the wound depends upon the amount of kinetic energy expended at successive depths of penetration. The greater the quantity of energy expended per unit distance, the greater will be the diameter of the wound.

In considering wounds made in various regions of the body by missiles of different shapes, the problem becomes more complex. It is apparent that the nature of the tissues penetrated is just as important in determining the size and shape of a wound as the properties of the projectile. The relative density, cohesive strength and actual mass of different tissues involved,

Fig. 16-19. Contact Bullet Wounds of Entrance.

Contact bullet wounds of entrance caused by revolver, showing a small wedge-shaped patterned abrasion above each perforation produced by impact of rib of pistol. Homicide. Muzzle and rib of revolver shown in insert.

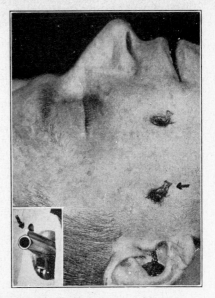

Fig. 16-20. Contact Bullet Wounds of Entrance.

Left. Skin around bullet perforation bruised and burned. Beneath perforation is a small circular abrasion produced by impact of retractor spring rod of automatic pistol.

Right. A .25 caliber pistol with slide drawn back to show retractor spring rod. Suicide.

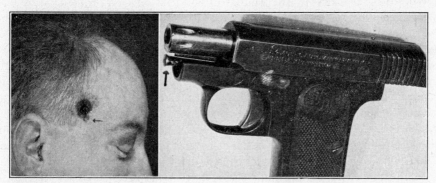

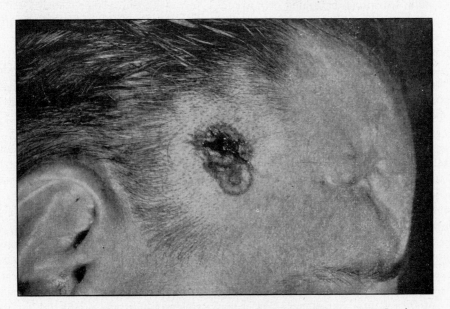

Fig. 16-21. Patterned Impression of Muzzle of .32-Caliber Colt Automatic Pistol.
Contact wound. Suicide. Compare with Figure 16-20.

especially the presence or absence of bone, all are important factors in determining the amount of resistance which will be offered to the passage of a projectile. The greater the resistance encountered by a missile in perforating a given type of tissue, the greater will be the expenditure of energy by the missile in penetrating a given distance into the tissue, and the more voluminous will be the hole made by the missile. The mass of the projectile is also important, since for a given velocity the kinetic energy and potential wounding power of a projectile are directly proportional to its mass. Other factors being constant, the greater the mass of a projectile and the longer it can continue to expend large quantities of energy in traversing the tissues, the more pronounced will be the destruction produced in its passage. Any increase in the mass of a projectile, in the size of its presenting surface and in its striking velocity will cause a corresponding increase in the resistance encountered, the kinetic energy spent and the total disruption it may produce on any given tissue.

Helpern and Hickam have shown that the pattern of wounds made by high energy military bullets or shell fragments of comparable weight and velocity assume one of three basic shapes; they are: (1) cylindric; (2) conical, with the apex of the cone directed toward the entrance side; or (3) conical with the apex directed toward the exit side. Combinations of these shapes occur and considerable irregularity in their form may result depending upon the types of tissue traversed by the projectile.

A bullet in passing through the body inflicts a wound at the point of entrance on the skin and if it emerges another wound is produced at the point of exit.

WOUND OF ENTRANCE. The wounds of entrance inflicted on the skin by pistol bullets are characteristic of a hard projectile varying in size from .25 to .45 caliber, traveling at a muzzle speed ranging from 550 to 1,400 feet per second. When the penetration occurs the skin is dented in and stretched, the bullet punching its way through epidermis and dermis and producing a roughly circular opening with slightly ragged edges, and a narrow zone or collar of reddish brown abrasion on the immediately surrounding epidermis. If the bullet strikes the skin perpendicularly, this zone may be uniform in width, but if it penetrates at an acute angle, the zone of abrasion is usually wider on the side from which the missile comes, characteristics which are sometimes helpful in determining the probable direction of the track. A faint zone of ecchymosis may surround the wound of entrance, but may be absent. In some cases, the projectile passes tangentially over the skin without penetrating it, leaving an elongated ovoid reddish furrow on the surface, called a bullet slap or graze. In other cases the missile may penetrate the skin tangentially and produce a deeper furrow in the subcutaneous tissues. Figures 16-8, 16-9 and 16-10 show these different types of entrance wounds on the skin, which are made by the bullet alone without any contribution from the products produced by the powder charge; this means that the muzzle of the gun was fired beyond the range of these products or that they were filtered out by cloth or other substance which intervened between them and the skin.

The size of the wound of entrance may correspond somewhat to the caliber of the penetrating bullet, but the correspondence is not close enough to allow the examiner to use the diameter of the skin perforation as a reliable criterion for estimating the size of the bullet. In a particular case factors may be introduced which may lead to erroneous conclusions. After the passage of the bullet, the resilient skin may return to its original condition, and by the contraction of muscular and elastic elements in the dermis the wound of entrance may be actually smaller than the caliber of the projectile. On the other hand the bullet may be deformed and flattened before striking the skin, as in a ricochet from a hard flat surface, and leave a wound of entrance larger than the original missile, usually of an irregularly ovoid or triangular shape (Fig. 16-11). The same effect is produced in a re-entrance wound. Sometimes a bullet may strike an object and tumble, hitting the body side on, in which case an elongated wound of entrance like a keyhole will

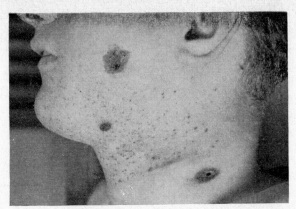

From Gonzales, T. A., *Am. J. Surg.*, 26:47, 1934

Fig. 16-22. Contact and Close-up Bullet Wounds of Entrance on Face and Neck.

Large contact wound on cheek with absence of brand and tattooing. Close-up wound on chin surrounded by wide zone of embedded powder grains, but with absence of flame burns, indicating that muzzle of gun was held beyond range of flame but within range of the powder grains. Close-up wound on neck, showing embedded powder grains and powder smudge above the collar line. Homicide.

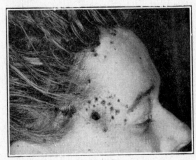

From Gonzales, T. A., *Am. J. Surg.*, 26:48, 1934

Fig. 16-24. Close-up Revolver Bullet Wound of Entrance.

Circular bullet perforation and flame burn in skin surrounded by zone of tattooing with unburned and burning powder grains. Unburned powder grains produce punctate abrasions, whereas burning powder grains are each surrounded by a small halo of reddened skin. Homicide.

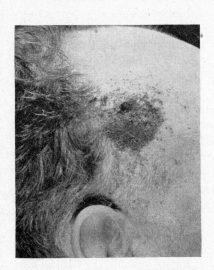

Fig. 16-23. Close-up Revolver Bullet Wound of Entrance of Right Temple.

Bullet perforation is eccentrically placed in a large area of flame burn, in which white, burned, shriveled hairs are visible. A narrow zone of embedded powder grains is shown in the skin beyond the brand.

Location of bullet hole in area of burn indicates that trigger was pointed upward in relation to position of head when pistol was fired. Homicide.

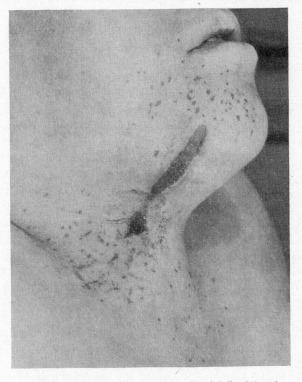

Fig. 16-25. Close-up .38-Caliber Pistol Bullet Wound. Smokeless Powder.

Note more compact tattooing by powder grains on chin and wider dispersal on neck. Bullet grazed chin and then entered neck. The small square flakes of powder produced square and linear abrasions of the skin. Homicide.

be produced. The deformities of the wound of entrance caused by the powder explosion in contact wounds will be discussed later.

If the gun is discharged with its muzzle close to the body, the products of the powder explosion will produce characteristic effects on the skin and clothing. The nature of these products and the way in which they are discharged at the time of firing have been discussed on page 386. If the muzzle is held against the skin at the moment of discharge, a contact wound will result, and the wound of entrance will be large and crateriform in type and triangular, stellate, cruciate or elliptic (Figs. 16-12, 16-13, 16-14, 16-15 and 16-16), due to the explosive effects of the powder gases; these large irregular contact wounds are usually produced by large-calibered pistols and are most commonly encountered on the scalp and face where delicate skin is in close juxtaposition to a hard underlying layer of bone. Contact wounds are not always large and irregularly lacerated, they may superficially resemble a distant shot in size and regularity (Fig. 16-17). This is especially true in the case of small-calibered pistols. With black powder the skin around the opening may be blackened by smoke or seared by flame (Fig. 16-18), and the bullet track in the subjacent tissues may be blackened to various depths. The smoke stains may be removed easily with a damp cloth and thus are easily distinguished from the other products of the powder explosion. With a smokeless powder the searing and smoke staining effects are usually less conspicuous. In some contact wounds, the imprint of the muzzle of the gun is found stamped as a patterned abrasion on the skin around the bullet perforation, an effect produced by the kick of the gun at the moment of discharge. This is seen in the homicidal shooting depicted in Figure 16-19, in which the rib of the revolver barrel produced a characteristic patterned abrasion above the wound of entrance. In a suicidal shooting the impact of the retractor spring rod of the automatic pistol inflicted a small circular abrasion on the skin below the bullet perforation (Fig. 16-20). In another the entire muzzle of an automatic pistol was imprinted on the temple (Fig. 16-21). Examples of contact bullet wounds in suicidal and homicidal cases are illustrated in Figures 16-4, and 16-12 to 16-22, inclusive.

If the gun is fired at close range, the skin around the bullet hole may be seared or branded a brownish red by the flame and peppered by the powder grains which are driven into the surface. The different powders vary in their effects and produce the types of tattooing already described. At close range black powder produces a roughly circular reddish brown flame burn with closely packed powder grains near its periphery. The seared hairs in the burned area have a beaded and shriveled appearance (Fig. 16-23). At slightly greater distances the flame marks disappear, and the powder grains are more dispersed, appearing as small black and red dots tattooed on the skin. Burning powder grains produce punctate marks with halo-like burns in the surrounding skin (Fig. 16-24), whereas unburned grains produce a punctate abrasion in which the powder grain may sometimes be found. Revolvers firing cartridges loaded with black powder discharge flame for a distance of approximately six to eight inches and powder grains in a diverging conical pattern with decreasing concentration and with dispersal up to about 18 inches. Smokeless powder with less flame and fewer unburned powder grains in the discharge produces less burn, smoke and tattooing than black powder (Fig. 16-5). The tattooing by smokeless powder grains may consist of patterned marks corresponding to the shape of the grains and the manner of impact (Fig. 16-25).

If a revolver is fired at close range and at right angles to the skin surface, the

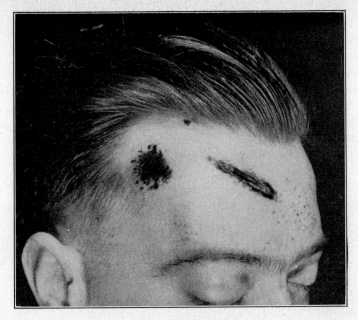

Fig. 16-26. Two Close-up Bullet Wounds of Forehead.

Wound on right temple shows bullet perforation, brand and a narrow zone of tattooing; the muzzle of the pistol was held close to the skin at right angles.

The other wound is an abraded furrow produced by tangential impact of the other bullet. The scattered powder grains on the left side of the forehead indicate that the direction of the bullet is upward and to the right. Homicide.

Fig. 16-27. Close-up Bullet Wounds of Entrance with Corresponding Exit Wounds.

Top. The bullet wounds of entrance are located on the left side of the head. They show a small abrasion collar, a small zone of flame burn and a narrow zone of tattooing. The ear lobe is lacerated by explosion of gases. These signs indicate that the shots were close-up.

Bottom. Corresponding larger stellate wounds with everted edges made by exit of bullets from right cheek. Homicide.

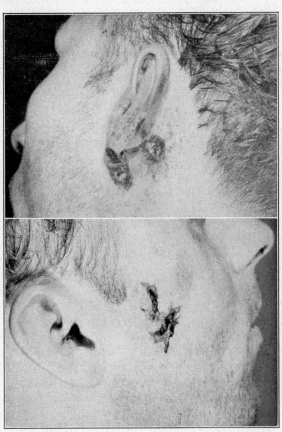

bullet perforation will be slightly below the center of a zone of flame marks and powder grains, for reasons already described (Figs. 16-23 and 16-24). If the line of fire is oblique to the skin, powder grain and flame marks will be more intense and in a narrower zone on the side which the bullet strikes first. Such marks may be absent from the distal area, or if they reach the distal zone will be more broadly diffused and scattered. The markings will indicate the direction of fire with a fair degree of accuracy (Figs. 16-25 and 16-26). Examples of close-up entrance wounds produced by black powder and smokeless powder cartridges are shown in Figures 16-22 to 16-28.

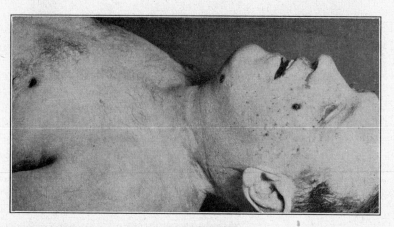

Fig. 16-28. Comparison of Close-up Bullet Wounds of Entrance on Exposed and Clothed Surfaces of the Body.

Wound on cheek shows perforation surrounded by a wide zone of embedded powder grains. Wound on left chest consists only of bullet perforation, the powder grains having been filtered out by clothing. Homicide.

Bullet wounds of entrance give some indication of the distance from which the gun was discharged, only when the contents of the cartridge have left marks on the person or clothing of the deceased. A contact bullet wound is usually identified without difficulty, but should be verified by detailed exploration of the track at autopsy. If marks of flame and powder grains are concentrated in a small circle, the indications are that the gun was discharged a few inches away from the victim. If powder grain tattooing alone is found in a wide cirle, it would indicate that the muzzle of the gun was held at a slightly greater distance, beyond the range of flame. The best method of ascertaining the approximate distance from which a close up shot was fired is by comparing the marks on the deceased or his clothing with those made by similar cartridges fired from the suspected gun at varying distances from the target. If one of the test shots produces marks similar to those found on the body or clothes, the known distance of the gun from the target during the test would best indicate the distance the weapon was held from the body at the time of the shooting.

If the bullet wound of entrance is on an unclothed part of the body and is a simple perforation without surrounding powder marks, it is not possible to estimate the range except to say that the shot was fired from a distance beyond the range of the powder discharge. If the shot is through a clothed surface, only an examination of the clothing can indicate its range and establish whether it was contact, close up or from a distance. In a contact shot, the clothing will usually reveal a cross-shaped burned perforation and the skin around the bullet hole will be surrounded by a halo of smoke. The smoke halo surrounding the bullet hole may also be found on

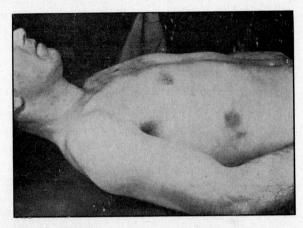

Fig. 16-29. Contusion of Skin Overlying .38-Caliber Bullet at End of Track on Right Lateral Surface of Chest. Homicidal Shooting. Multiple Tracks.

the deeper layers of the cloth. In a close-up shot, the clothing may absorb or filter out all of the products of the discharge including the flame burn, smoke deposit and powder grains, the bullet alone passing through to produce a perforation in the skin indistinguishable in appearance from a distant shot (Fig. 16-28). It is absolutely

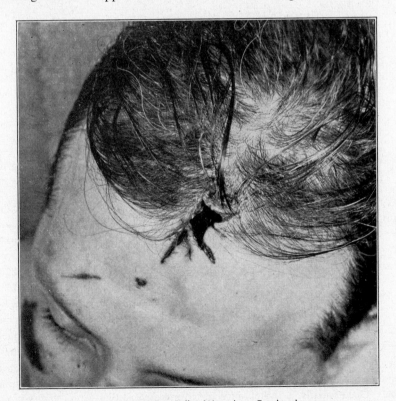

Fig. 16-30. Exit Bullet Wound on Forehead.
Large stellate lacerated wound with everted edges made by exit of bullet and fragments of bone. Entrance wound on back of head. Homicide.

essential that the clothing be examined to determine a close-up shot through the clothing. In many cases, such examination can be made with the naked eye or small hand lens or low power binocular microscope. With dark colored heavy-napped fabrics, infrared photography may prove helpful, and the surface of the cloth around the perforation can be tested chemically for dotted nitrite deposits according to the method recommended by Walker, page 390. The detection of invisible cartridge discharge residues including those of the primer on clothing and on the skin around the bullet perforation is usually not practicable. It requires the help of the expert chemist and physicist and may require the use of infrared photography, radiography with soft x-rays, low power microscopy, microchemical analysis and spectrography. Fortunately, the cases which require such technics and special equipment are rare.

WOUNDS OF EXIT. The bullet may penetrate the body to a variable depth and may stop at any point in its course. It may travel the width of the trunk and finally

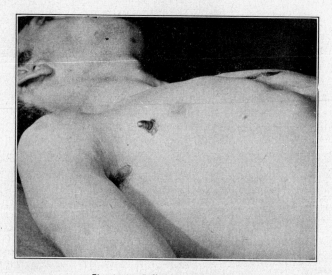

Fig. 16-31. Bullet Wound of Exit.

A .38-caliber lead bullet protrudes from the exit hole. Entrance wound not visible on side of left chest. Homicide.

come to rest just under the skin of the opposite side where it may be located by palpation; under such conditions a hematoma may form about the bullet and appear as a bluish swelling beneath the skin (Figs. 16-10 and 16-29) surmounted in a few cases by a reddish brown abrasion. In many instances the bullet passes out of the body and leaves a wound of exit which varies much in size and appearance; some are stellate in shape, usually larger than the wound of entrance and show everted edges as a result of the bullet erupting through the skin with diminished velocity. Large exit wounds are likely to occur if the bullet has been deformed or has tumbled in its passage through the body or if other hard substances like bone fragments, are carried out with it. Other wounds of exit are mere slits of the skin, especially when the bullet is undeformed and is propelled with just enough force to drive it through the tissues without causing undue disruption at the point of emergence. Occasionally a bullet may be found protruding from an exit wound. Various types of exit wounds are illustrated in Figures 16-13, 16-16, 16-27, 16-30 and 16-31.

Typical wounds of entrance can usually be distinguished from wounds of exit, but sometimes differentiation on external examination alone is difficult. If the perforations have been macerated in water, as in submerged bodies, entrances and exits may appear alike, as in the case depicted in Figure 4-26. Tangential wounds through soft tissues with entrance and exit close together, are difficult to distinguish from one another unless other evidence is available to establish the course of the bullet. In doubtful cases the perforations in the clothing must be examined and signs may be discovered which indicate the way in which the bullet entered the body, as for example, powder marks, flame marks and fouling marks of the bullet on cloth. Examination of the bullet track may help for sometimes pieces of cloth or minute fragments of lead are carried into the wound of entrance and may identify it. If the bullet has passed through bone, small bony fragments are often carried forward with it, thus disclosing the direction of the track. Entrance and exit wounds through the skull are readily distinguished as described on page 419.

Examination of the clothing in shooting cases is important not only because it enables the examiner to determine whether a wound on a covered portion of the body resulted from a close up or distant shot, but also because it may reveal the direction of the bullet track, in cases in which the bullet has passed completely through the body, producing entrance and exit wounds which are not readily differentiated. In such cases, the bullet may pass out of the skin through the exit wound but not completely through the clothing, which circumstance will indicate its direction.

In a murder trial in New Jersey presided over by the late Judge Egbert Rosecrans, the defendant admitted the fatal shooting but claimed that he acted in self-defense and there seemed to be strong corroborative evidence that this was so. The fatal bullet had passed completely through the body. The victim was operated upon and during this procedure, a bullet wound on the front of the abdomen was obliterated. At necropsy, the bullet perforation on the back was interpreted as an entrance wound by the pathologist. Because of this interpretation, the self-defense plea of the perpetrator was not believed and he was indicted and tried for murder. Upon inquiry, it was learned that the articles of clothing worn by the deceased when he was shot had not been examined. Fortunately they had been kept and were examined during the trial. The fatal bullet had perforated all the garments in front but not in the back, indicating clearly that it had entered through the front of the body, a fact consistent with the claim of self-defense. The defendant was acquitted.

Bullet wounds of entrance in some instances do not bleed externally and may be so concealed as to escape detection. Small calibered bullets may produce fatal wounds with inconspicuous perforations in the scalp, axillary, scapular and buttock regions usually in clothed regions of the body. A bullet may enter the head between the open eyelids and either perforate the eyeball or pass between the eyeball and the orbit into the cranial cavity and brain. After death, the closed eyelids may conceal the entrance of the track (Figs. 16-32 and 16-33).

REPAIR OF BULLET WOUNDS. The process of healing is somewhat similar to that described under stab wounds. There is hemorrhage into the bullet track, extravasation of blood into the tissues around the wound, infection, necrosis and polymorphonuclear leukocytic invasion of the traumatized areas. Afterwards granulation tissue is formed, the necrotic debris is removed, organization occurs, the skin wound is closed and the track is converted into a solid fibrous strand. If the bullet remains embedded in the tissues, it is surrounded by a fibrous capsule in which it becomes tarnished.

The flame burn on the skin produces a reaction similar to any third degree burn, as discussed on page 526. In close up wounds, the powder grains, driven into the

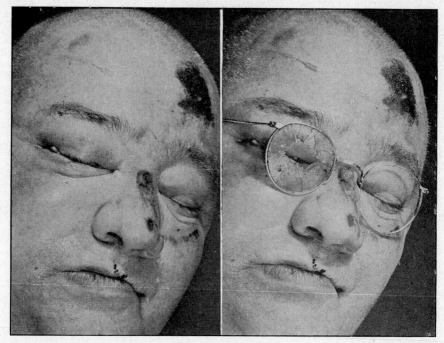

From Helpern, M., *Ann. Int. Med.*, 24:666, 1946

Fig. 16-32. Homicidal Bullet Wound of Right Eyeball Concealed by Eyelids.

When the body was found, the wound was not suspected. Victim's eyeglasses with bullet hole in right lens, shown replaced in photograph on right, were found on ground. Bullet recovered in brain.

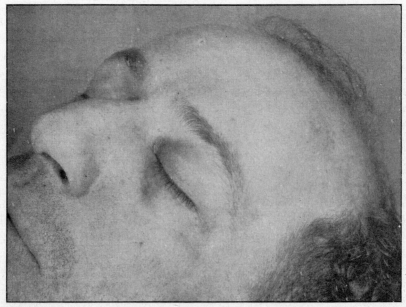

From Helpern, M., *Ann. Int. Med.*, 24:666, 1946

Fig. 16-33. Homicidal Bullet Wound Through Inner Canthus of Left Eye, Concealed by Closed Eyelids.

Bullet passed medial to eyeball and was recovered in brain.

skin with the discharge, penetrate into the epidermis and superficial layers of the dermis, and those that are burning cause a local destruction and distortion of the epithelium, followed by exudation of serum and fibrin, crusting and epidermization about the grain and a leukocytic infiltration into the adjacent portion of the dermis.

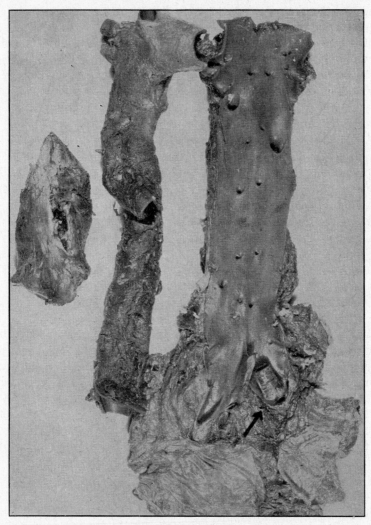

Fig. 16-34. Bullet Wound of Dorsal Spine (Left) and Thoracic Aorta (Middle). Bullet After Entering Lumen of Aorta Dropped into Left Common Iliac Artery (Right with Arrow).

The powder tattoo persists in the skin for about two to three weeks, after which it is thrust off; in some cases the tattooing may be permanent.

NECROPSY PROCEDURE. Bullet wounds at necropsy must be described with care. The character of the perforation, its shape and size should be determined, with careful measurements taken of its dimensions. The location of the wound is important and the part of the body perforated, the relation of the wound to the nearest anatomic point, its distance from the midline of the front or back, its distance above the heels and buttocks, and any other points worthy of record such as flame and powder marks should be mentioned. Photographs, diagrams and drawings are valuable to show the number, character and location of the wounds on the skin. After the body is opened, the direction and length of each of the bullet tracks must be ascertained and the organs which have been perforated must be noted. The complication which has caused death should be determined specifically; this subject will be considered further in a discussion of the bullet wounds of different regions. If the bullet track passes through the body the wound of exit must be identified and adequately described. If the bullet stops in the body, it should be located and carefully recovered without further mutilation for ballistic examination and as important evidence in establishing the corpus delicti. If it is delivered to the police officers, the medical examiner should mark it on the nose or base for future identification, and avoid damaging the riflings on the sides.

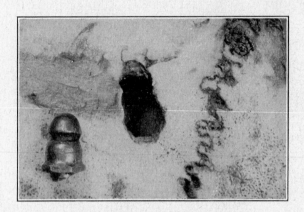

Fig. 16-35. Broken-off Metal Curtain Fastener from Automobile, Embedded in Skull.

Deceased was struck on head by automobile and the piece of metal driven into the bone. During life, this was mistaken for a bullet on x-ray examination.

At autopsy in rare cases it is difficult to locate a bullet because of postmortem wandering and a roentgenogram may be required to accomplish this end. The bullet may be loose in a large body cavity, in the gastrointestinal tract, or spinal canal or it may be fragmented inside the skull. In one case a bullet entered the right subclavian vein and, in some way, was shifted through the right auricle and both venae cavae to the right common iliac vein where it was located by a roentgenogram. In another instance, a .38 caliber lead bullet had penetrated the spine and perforated the thoracic aorta; it was found in the left common iliac artery where it had dropped or embolized (Fig. 16-34). At autopsy an old bullet with a blackened surface occasionally is found encapsulated in scar tissue at the end of an old bullet track, and may cause confusion if it happens to lie in the path of a fresh gunshot wound.

In blunt force injuries, a small metal object may perforate the skull and break off and on roentgen-ray examination simulate a bullet. In one such case, a broken-off metal button, a curtain fastener from an automobile, was found embedded in the skull (Fig. 16-35). The roentgen-ray examination during life had given the mistaken impression that it was a bullet.

HOMICIDAL, SUICIDAL AND ACCIDENTAL BULLET WOUNDS. Bullet wounds, like all other types of physical injury, from a medicolegal standpoint must be classified as homicidal, suicidal or accidental. In deciding the status of a particular case it is necessary to obtain all the available information, including the facts brought out by the autopsy, by the investigation of the scene of death and the circumstances attending the shooting. The data discovered by the medical examiner, though important and revealing, must be supplemented by police investigation before the nature of the shooting is classified. Each individual case will present its own problems, and it is difficult to formulate a set of general rules which can be applied to all cases with equal cogency.

Bullet wounds inflicted with homicidal intent are the most common, and account for about 53 per cent of all homicidal deaths. In New York City, in recent years, the average yearly number of homicides by shooting has been about 200, outnumbering the suicidal and accidental shootings by a considerable margin. A review of 274 homicidal shootings selected at random, indicates that in about 70 per cent the wounds resulted from a single bullet penetrating a vital portion of the body; 25 per cent involved the abdomen, 23 per cent the chest, 10 per cent the head, 7 per cent the spine, 3 per cent the neck and 2 per cent the extremities. In the remaining 30 per cent of the total, wounds by more than one bullet were encountered, and these multiple tracks sometimes involved one region, sometimes two or more.

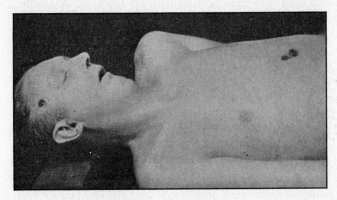

Fig. 16-36. Three Self-Inflicted, Closely Placed, Contact Bullet Wounds on Left Upper Quadrant of Abdomen; Parallel Tracks; Three Bullets Recovered in Left Posterior Chest Wall. Fatal Contact Wound of Right Temple. 32-Caliber Revolver.

Bullet wounds of the homicidal type can assume a great variety of forms, and for this reason the possibility of homicide should be considered in every death by shooting until investigation shows this interpretation to be incorrect. The most important point which the examining physician must decide is whether or not the bullet wound could possibly have been inflicted by the deceased himself, as indicated by the location and character of the wound of entrance, the direction of the track and other features typical of suicidal bullet wounds which will be discussed later. If the wound of entrance is a contact wound, there is always the possibility that it is suicidal, unless the gun has been fired into a part of the body not easily reached by the deceased such as the back of the chest or neck. A bullet wound of the non-contact type, either a close-up or a distant shot, is only very rarely self-inflicted. Multiple bullet wounds are usually homicidal, especially if they occur on the back or sides of the body, or involve different regions of the body, or are noncontact shots; most multiple contact shots are also homicidal, though a few occur in the temple, anterior abdomen or cardiac region which are undoubtedly suicidal (Fig. 16-36). In accidental shootings, the wounds are most often produced by single shots and are not distinguishable anatomically from those which are homicidal. The circumstances of every shooting should always be investigated by the police, especially those which are purported to be accidental.

Correlation of bullet wounds and tracks with the circumstances of the shooting may be possible in a particular case, if the investigation by the police has revealed the essential facts. Without investigation of all the circumstances, the postmortem findings in deaths from single bullet wounds yield only medical information subject to variable medicolegal interpretation. Though important as evidence, this information alone cannot reveal the manner in which the shooting occurred. On the other hand, the autopsy findings in some cases of multiple bullet wounds give valuable hints concerning the manner of their infliction, which must be interpreted with caution. It must always be remembered that deductions from such facts are properly clues for guidance of the police and prosecutor and not necessarily evidence which can be presented on the witness stand.

In one type of multiple bullet wound homicide the perpetrator, alarmed at a threatened attack or moved by a feeling of injury, pulls out his gun on the impulse of the moment and blazes away at the object of his animosity; or he may be a nervous hold-up man who fires because he loses his head. A scuffle may result, or the victim may turn and flee, or attack the perpetrator. A great variety of wounds can occur depending upon the circumstances: if there is a scuffle, some of the wounds may be close-up and the bullets may strike the body in various places and at different angles; if the victim flees, most of the entrance bullet wounds will probably be in the back; if the victim rushes at the assailant the bullets will usually strike and produce entrance perforations in the front of the body. In this type of case where the assailant is in a panic or under strong emotion, a number of shots may go wild or graze the skin. Some bullets after passing through the upper extremities may re-enter the body, in which case it would be necessary for the medical examiner to determine if the perforations through the arm are in alignment with those on the body or represent separate bullet tracks. Excusable homicides, which occur when police officers shoot individuals who are resisting or fleeing arrest, may reveal similar patterns of multiple bullet wounds, but in most instances death is caused by a single bullet which may strike the body at an unusual angle, as in the case in which a policeman fired upward at a burglar who was running up the fire escape; the bullet entered the left lower region of the abdomen, ranged upward through the intestines, stomach, liver and right lung, and finally emerged through the top of the right shoulder.

Premeditated, calculated homicide by shooting can occur in a variety of ways. If the deceased is killed as the result of a gang feud, he may be surprised and shot by his enemies who then may dump his body on the highway or in a building, with one or more close-up or contact wounds of entrance in the back of the neck or head. Occasionally the victim is waylaid by the killers and a number of bullets are pumped into him from different directions; in such cases bullets of different types and calibers may be found in the body, thus indicating that more than one gun was used. Another type of premeditated killing is committed by a perpetrator who is known to the victim and not suspected by him, and so accomplishes his crime in a deliberate and even leisurely fashion. In some instances the victim is lying in bed and shot a number of times at close range; in such cases, there may be several close-up wounds of entrance surrounded by flame burn and powder tattoo, grouped on one side of the head and neck with the bullet tracks parallel or deviating only slightly. In one such case the perpetrator fired six shots into the deceased at close range, then calmly reloaded the gun and fired a seventh. In a similar case four bullets were fired at close range into the right chest, right flank, right hip and right thigh of the victim, all spaced at equal intervals and all in the same straight longitudinal line. In another case the perpetrator first shot the deceased in the back of the head and then when the victim crashed to the floor, discharged one bullet into his forehead and three into his right chest; all four bullets entering the front of the body were distant shots and their tracks were practically parallel. Multiple parallel tracks produced by bullets entering the same side of the body usually indicate that the victim was a quiescent target and thus suggest a certain amount of deliberation on the part of the person firing the pistol. An example of homicidal, multiple, close-up and closely placed bullet wounds with parallel tracks is shown in Figure 16-37.

An important consideration in homicidal shooting is that an individual who has received a fatal bullet wound may not realize that he has been injured. In one case

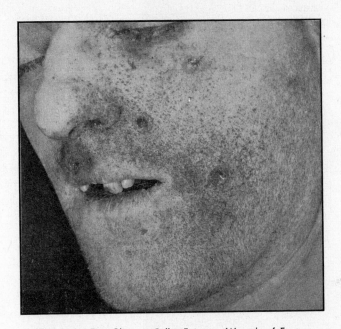

Fig. 16-37. Five Close-up Bullet Entrance Wounds of Face.

Overlapping powder tattoos. Branding of skin around three lower perforations. Lead bullets; smokeless powder; .38-caliber revolver.

a police sergeant captured a subway bandit after the prisoner had fired a gun at him point-blank; 10 minutes later he delivered the bandit to the patrol wagon and then suddenly collapsed, dying several hours afterwards of a hemorrhage from a bullet wound of the liver. A second case was that of a patrolman who suddenly collapsed, apparently without cause, while talking with a friend on the street and died a quarter of an hour later. The autopsy disclosed that the cause of death was a bullet wound of the back from a .22 caliber lead bullet which entered between the shoulder blades, perforated the aorta and trachea and caused a profuse fatal internal hemorrhage. Apparently the deceased died without realizing that he had been shot. Under some conditions an impact of the projectile is not sensed by the injured person.

Suicidal shootings in New York City average about 112 cases a year and comprise about 10 per cent of all suicides. The perpetrator usually holds the gun against his person at easily accessible points, and practically all the wounds of entrance are contact wounds. The most common point of application of the muzzle of the weapon is the right temporal region if the individual is right-handed, and the left temporal region if he is left-handed. The entrance wound may be located as far forward as the middle of the forehead or as far back as the occiput; the bullet track is directed towards the opposite side, usually slightly upward, and with a slight lateral deviation

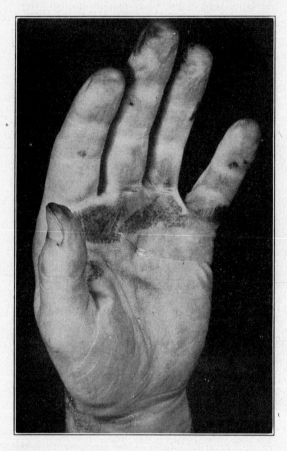

Fig. 16-38. Burn of Left Hand in Suicidal Shooting.

Burns across distal part of palm and on tips of fingers of left hand caused by hot gases of discharge. Pistol was fired with the right hand and clenched in the left hand to steady it against the temple.

to one side or the other. Sometimes the gun is put into the mouth, nose, ear, or on the face or under surface of the chin and fired upward into the brain. In one instance the deceased held the gun vertically downward on the top of his head and pulled the trigger with his thumb while he steadied the barrel with his other hand, receiving a burn on that hand from the flame which passed out of the gun muzzle. In another case, Figure 16-38, the deceased fired the pistol against the side of his head while

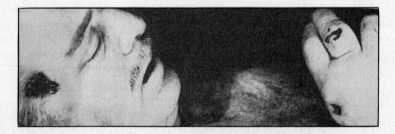

Fig. 16-39. Suicidal Contact Wound of Right Temple from .32-Caliber Automatic Pistol.

Note in-and-out bullet wound of right hand with fractures of second metacarpal and proximal phalanx of middle finger produced by prior shot.

holding the barrel in his free hand and branded the palm of that hand with the flame of the discharge. In a few cases the suicide interposes his hand between the pistol and his head, shooting himself through the palm of the hand. In one instance the deceased, using an automatic pistol, shot himself through the hand that held the weapon, presumably in testing it, fracturing the bones of his hand and middle finger; he nevertheless used the weapon to fire a contact shot through the right temple (Fig. 16-39). In another case the deceased rigged up a special complicated apparatus so arranged that the gun pointed at his occipital region; when it was properly adjusted he fired the weapon by pulling a string attached to the trigger. Suicidal bullet wounds of the head are illustrated in Figures 16-3, 16-4, 16-15 through 18, 16-20 and 21, 16-36, 16-39 and 40, 16-46 and 16-51.

Bullet wounds of the chest and abdomen inflicted with suicidal intent are less common than those of the head. On the chest the gun is fired into the cardiac region in a backward direction with a slight deviation upward or downward and either to right or left. In the case depicted in Figure 16-18, the skin revealed a large circular flame burn around the contact wound of entrance, and the explosion of the heavy charge of black powder in the track lacerated the heart and deposited black powder in the torn edges of the myocardium. Another example of a contact bullet wound of the chest is seen in Figure 16-4. The suicidal bullet wounds of the abdomen are most often inflicted in the epigastric region and produce perforations and lacerations of the upper abdominal viscera. In one case a contact shot was fired through the left breast in a direction downward, backward and to the left, followed by a second self-inflicted contact shot just over the ensiform which took a parallel direction; the second bullet pierced the diaphragm, liver, stomach and spleen and caused death by hemorrhage into the left chest from the liver and diaphragm perforation. The abdomen is more apt to be selected as the site of a suicidal shooting when a rifle or shotgun is the weapon used.

Multiple suicidal bullet wounds are occasionally encountered and may involve a single region like the temple, chest or abdomen, or a combination of two different regions such as the chest or temple, abdomen or chest, and so on (Fig. 16-36). In one case the suicide fired five shots into the anterior portion of his right temple, perforating the skull five times without touching his brain; he lived several days after the shooting, finally dying of sepsis. In another case, Figure 16-40, the deceased shot a bullet from a defective cartridge into his right temporal region and the missile stopped in the scalp, from which its base was found protruding; he then fired the fatal shot into his brain, the bullet entering the scalp just anterior to the first shot. When multiple suicidal bullet wounds are fired serially, the first bullet either does not take effect or the injuries inflicted do not incapacitate the victim immediately, enabling him to fire other bullets into his body. As a rule a bullet traversing or jarring the brain causes immediate unconsciousness, but if bone is involved without injury of the brain or a large vessel, the individual may retain his sensibility and power of motion. A bullet passing through the chest or abdominal viscera in some cases does not incapacitate the victim, and he may be able to shoot himself again. In one such case, the first bullet passed through the chest and heart but rapid exsanguination was prevented by extensive old adhesions in the chest and pericardial cavities; the second bullet was fired into the temple and brain. The authors have also seen a case in which a Chinese, in the presence of witnesses, fired two pistols simultaneously, one into his head and the other into his chest, exemplifying another method of inflicting multiple suicidal bullet wounds. A rare type of suicidal shooting was recently encountered in which a 9 mm. bullet fired from an automatic pistol propelled another bullet which was already stuck in the barrel from a shot fired previously with a defective cartridge; both bullets entered the temple in tandem through the same entrance hole and were found on the opposite side of the head just inside the calvarium in which they had produced two perforations about one half inch apart. The base of the stagnant bullet was indented by the nose of the propelling missile so that it was possible to stand the bullets up one on the other as shown in Figure 16-41; in addition the single discharged shell found at the scene revealed evidence of excessive breech pressure.

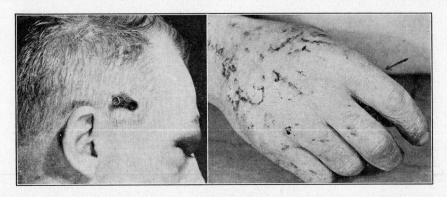

Fig. 16-40. Multiple Suicidal Bullet Wounds of Right Temple.

Left. The first bullet was fired from a defective cartridge, and did not perforate scalp. Its base is shown protruding from the wound. The entrance of the second fatal bullet wound is shown just anterior to the first.

Right. Blood is spattered on dorsum of right hand and hairs are burnt short on dorsum of first phalanx of index finger. The trigger was pulled with the thumb and the hairs were burnt by the backflash from a defective revolver.

Circumstances corroborating the suicidal character of a shooting are the presence of a note or of preparations indicating the intention of the deceased to kill himself. In cases of suicidal shooting, the gun is usually found near the corpse and in rare instances in the hand of the deceased. It is possible on the other hand for the bullet wound to be self-inflicted but for the gun to be missing, because another person removed it from the scene. Confusion may arise if the gun has been tampered with by some one after the shooting; in one such case, the owner of the revolver used by the deceased removed the empty cartridge shell and substituted a single un-exploded cartridge for it. In some instances of homicidal shooting, the scene may be dressed up to simulate suicide in order to cover up the crime. After inflicting a contact wound on the anterior surface of the body or on an area of the head accessible to the victim, the perpetrator could plant the weapon in the open hand of the deceased in such a position that a casual examination would suggest that the hand had been used to fire the weapon. The hand after death relaxes with the fingers slightly flexed allowing the index finger to be easily placed through the trigger guard and next to the trigger of a weapon placed in the palm of the hand. In such factitious cases, the thumb will usually be found under and not around the gun handle. Such cases obviously need a thorough investigation by both police and medical examiner, and where there is suspicion that the weapon has been planted in the victim's hand, the scene should not be disturbed and no object moved until photographs have been taken. A gun may discharge powder residues in the form of grains, smoke and invisible chemical substances through a defective breech onto the other hand which fires the weapon, and such residues should always be looked for and checked against the condition of the weapon. Blood may be spattered back from the entrance wound onto the trigger hand (Figs. 16-40, 16-42 and 26-1). For a discussion of the chemical tests for powder residue on the hands see page 390.

Accidental bullet wounds are comparatively rare, the number of fatal cases in New York City each year averaging about seven. In most accidental shootings the wound results from a single bullet. Usually the victim is shot unintentionally by a person who is ignorant of firearms or careless of their use. In one case a hotel

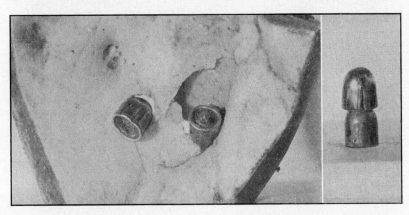

Fig. 16-41. Tandem Bullets Which Entered Through Single Contact Wound in the Right Temple.

Left. Two .32-caliber automatic pistol bullets found at end of track under left parietal bone. Right. Bullets placed in tandem. Base of first bullet dented by nose of second. See text.

employee found an old-fashioned four-barreled pistol discarded in rubbish and, without thinking, pointed it through an open doorway, pulling the trigger just as a fellow employee stepped into the opening; the gun happened to be loaded and was discharged, killing the victim instantly. Similar cases occur when boys discover a gun or pistol and fire it either accidentally or without the knowledge that the weapon is loaded. Occasionally when police are shooting it out with law violators, an innocent bystander is struck by bullets from the police guns; in one such case a stray bullet fractured the tibia of an elderly man, causing death from suppurative osteomyelitis and general streptococcic septicemia six days later. In a few instances bullet wounds, either self-inflicted or involving others, result when a gun is discharged accidentally while it is being cleaned or as the result of having been dropped on the floor. All such cases should be thoroughly investigated by the police and medical examiner in order to ascertain the true circumstances of the shooting; many bullet wounds are claimed to be accidental when in reality they are homicidal or suicidal.

BULLET WOUNDS IN DIFFERENT BODY REGIONS. The most convenient method of considering the anatomic features of bullet wounds is to discuss them as they occur in the different regions of the body as: the head and face, neck, chest, abdomen, spine and extremities.

Head and Face. About ten per cent of all homicidal bullet wounds occur on the head and face. In a group of 55 such cases studied, 18 wounds of entrance were located in the frontal region, of which 13 were found above a line drawn through the eyes and 5 below this level. Nineteen wounds of entrance were present on the sides of the head about equally divided between right and left, and 15 of these were located above a horizontal line drawn through the ear. Fifteen wounds of entrance were present on the back of the head, 12 of which were found below and 3 above a horizontal line connecting both ears.

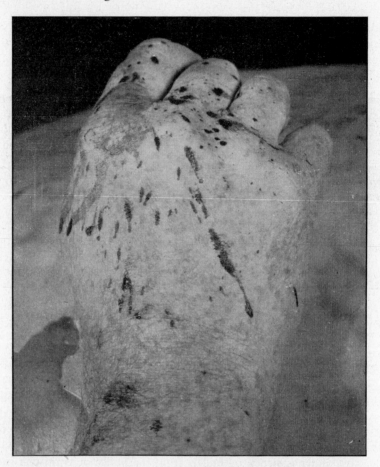

Fig. 16-42. Blood Splashed Back on the Right Hand in Which Pistol Was Held.
Suicidal shooting through right temple.

The homicidal bullet wounds of this region are especially notable in that about one-half were close-up or contact shots, showing flame burns and powder marks about the wound of entrance, while the other half were distant shots. In about one third of the cases the bullet passed in and out of the head, but in two thirds of the cases the bullets were recovered and of these almost 80 per cent were lead bullets fired from revolvers, many propelled with black powder, and about 20 per cent were smokeless powder driven, hard-metal jacketed bullets fired from automatic pistols.

Head. The direction of the bullet track in the head depends on the location of the wound of entrance, for as a rule when the skull is penetrated the projectile is directed toward the opposite side. Most of the shots range upward with a few exceptions in which the bullets are directed downward, and lateral deviations to right or left also occur. The majority of these perforations are present in the vault portion of the cranial cavity, fewer pass through the base upward to the vault and still fewer enter by the vault and pass downward into the base.

The most characteristic wounds in the skull are due to bullets which penetrate the bones of the cranium and produce holes similar to the perforation resulting from the passage of a bullet through a pane of glass. When the surface of the glass is struck, the forward motion of the bullet causes a clean-cut opening at that point, corresponding to the caliber of the projectile, but as it passes through the bullet

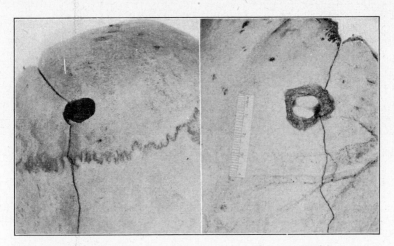

Fig. 16-43. Penetrating Bullet Wound of Entrance in Skull.

Left. Punched-in hole in outer table of bone.
Right. Larger beveled hole in inner table of bone. Linear fractures extend from margins of perforation.
A bullet on exit from the skull produces a punched-out hole on the inner table and a beveled hole of the outer table, each respectively larger than the corresponding holes made by the bullet entering the cranial cavity.

exerts a lateral expansive force on the substance of the glass in addition to the forward propulsive force; this lateral disruption chips away pieces of glass on the surface where the bullet emerges, leaving a larger hole with beveled edges which shelve in a concentric fashion towards the smaller opening of entrance. This appearance is characteristic and serves as a reliable diagnostic criterion in determining the direction of the missile through the glass pane. If the bullet strikes the pane at right angles the opening of entrance is roughly circular and is centrally placed in the zone of beveling; if the bullet strikes the pane obliquely, the opening of entrance is usually ovoid and is eccentrically placed in the zone of beveling which is wider on the side opposite to the starting point of the missile.

The same mechanism operates when a bullet passes through the skull, perforating the cranial bones. At the wound of entrance the missile leaves a punched-in hole in the outer table, while the opening on the inner table is large and shows beveling (Fig. 16-43). Pieces of bone from the wound of entrance are often driven into the cranial cavity and may aid in establishing the direction of the bullet track. At the point of exit the bullet strikes the inner table first, leaving a punched-out opening usually larger than the perforation in the skull at the point of entrance, and the increased expenditure of energy by the bullet in passing through results in a larger beveled opening on the outer table (Fig. 16-44). The bullet, especially if it is lead, may become deformed on entering the skull and this deformity and the fact that the bullet may tumble on its axis after entering the skull, may be factors in the increased size of the skull perforations at the point of exit. Occasionally the bullet does not have enough momentum to force its way out of the cranium, and may be

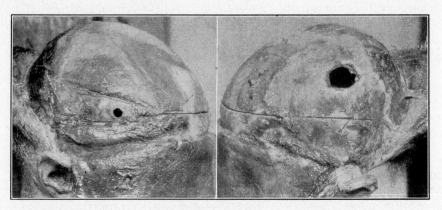

Fig. 16-44. Bullet Holes of Entrance and Exit in the Skull as Seen from the Outer Surface. Compare with Figure 16-43.

Left. Small punched-in wound of entrance in right temporal bone. A circle of bone was driven into brain.

Right. Larger beveled wound of exit in left parietal bone. A circle of bone from exit hole was found comminuted beneath intact scalp. A .32-caliber lead bullet was found beneath these bone fragments. Suicide.

found in the midst of a localized, comminuted eruptive fracture at the point of emergence, or the impact of the bullet may separate a disk-shaped button of bone by its impact against this area. This plug of bone may have the shape of a truncated cone, the base formed by the outer table.

Contact bullet wounds of the head introduce the element of exploding gunpowder and its residues which modify the appearance of the bullet track around the wound

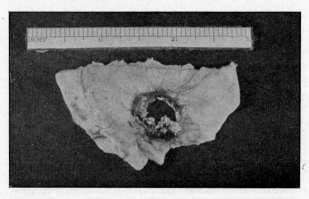

Fig. 16-45. Smoke Halo Surrounding Perforation on Outer Surface of Dura in a Contact Pistol Bullet Wound of Head.

A similar effect was found on the adjacent inner surface of the skull around the hole in the bone. Suicide. Black powder; .32-caliber lead bullet.

of entrance, the more so if the powder is black. Not only the subcutaneous tissues but also the opposing surfaces of the skull and dura (Fig. 16-45) are blackened by a ring of smoke which surrounds the perforations and serves as a valuable point of identification of a contact wound in doubtful cases. If the powder charge is exceptionally heavy, the bullet channel through the brain may be blackened and

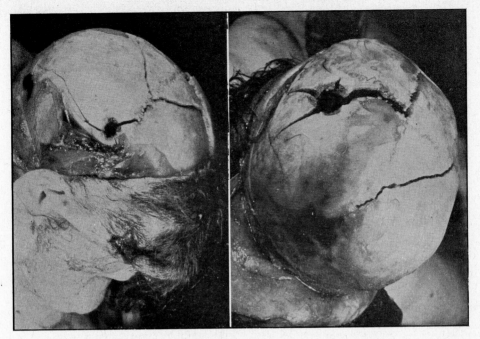

Fig. 16-46. Entrance and Exit Holes in Skull with Extensive Connecting Bursting Fractures.
Single suicidal contact shot through right side of head with .38-caliber automatic pistol.

widened and the skull extensively fractured. Smokeless powder produces less stain-ing of the tissues. In contact shots, the explosive force of the powder and the energy released by impact of the bullet may produce extensive bursting fractures of the skull (Figs. 16-46 and 16-47).

Fig. 16-47. Bursting Fracture of Skull with Separa-tion of Sagittal Suture.

Homicidal contact wound from a .38-caliber pistol bullet in the right parietal region. Note faint smoke ring on inner surface of bone around entrance hole.

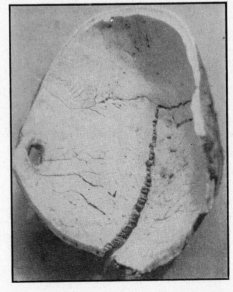

Bullets may graze the top and sides of the cranium without entering it, and in such cases in and out wounds are found on the scalp about an inch or so apart, while the skull in between shows an ovoid or elongated gutter-like depression, pro-

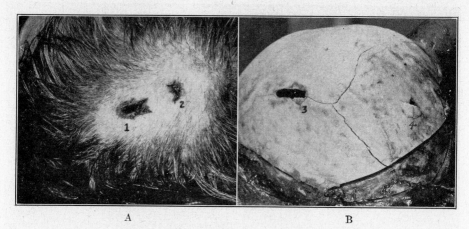

A   B

Fig. 16-48. Wounds Produced by Lead Bullet Striking Scalp and Skull Obliquely and Splitting into Two Fragments.

A. Beveled oblique entrance wound of whole lead bullet in scalp at 1. Exit wound made by fragment of split lead bullet at 2.

B. Elongated wound of entrance made by other fragment of split lead bullet in the calvarium. The bullet was cut lengthwise by the sharp distal edge of the perforation produced in the skull at the time of impact. Note beveling of outer table in posterior portion of entrance hole at 3, caused by exit of a fragment of split bullet which then passed out of scalp at 2 in A. Note comminuted elevated fracture at 4 caused by impact of bullet fragment which entered cranial cavity.

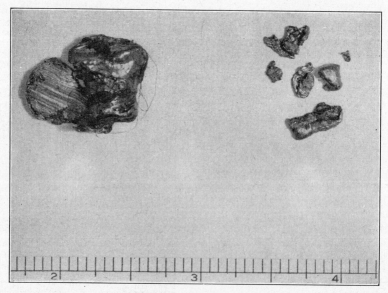

Fig. 16-49. Deformity of Lead Bullet.

Left. Badly deformed .38-caliber lead bullet found on floor at scene of homicide. Deceased was a young Negro woman with an entrance and an exit bullet wound of the head. Note single hair torn out and entwined around bullet as it left scalp. Hair similar to that on head of deceased.

Right. Fragments of lead shaved off of same bullet and found in scalp tissue under entrance wound. This occurred when the bullet entered the skull.

duced by the tangential impact of the bullet. In one such case the bullet passed on its way but the impact against the skull drove small pieces of bone through the dura into the brain. A lead bullet striking the convexity of the skull obliquely, may cut a furrow or gutter in the cranial vault, and split on the sharp distal edge of the furrow, one fragment penetrating the brain and another emerging from the scalp, Figure 16-48. Examination of the elongated perforation in the skull will usually reveal the proximal portion of the outer table to be punched in and the distal margin of the outer table to be beveled, the perforation containing component characteristics of an entrance and exit wound.

The impact of bullets, especially those made of lead, against the skull may cause them to be deformed in various ways. If the projectile fails to penetrate it may become mushroomed or indented by striking the outer table; a lead bullet may strike the outer table at an angle, slide along the surface of the skull and become flattened into a thin ovoid disk. If penetration occurs, the bullet may be deformed, indented, mushroomed, partially or completely divided by striking a sharp edge, or fragmented by striking sharp bony fragments. Not infrequently, a collar-shaped fragment of lead is shaved off around the wound of entrance and is found embedded in the surrounding scalp tissue (Fig. 16-15). In one case a deformed lead bullet in passing out of the head of a Negro girl carried away some of her kinky hair on its rough projections, and was found a few feet away from the body with the hair still attached (Fig. 16-49). Hard-metal jacketed bullets usually show little deformity except for indentations near the nose or base, but in rare cases may be fragmented, the jacket sometimes separating from the core, (Fig. 16-3).

A bullet which enters and traverses the cranial cavity may ricochet inside the skull—that is, glance or bounce off the inner table and then continue to travel in a different direction. This occurs in about 20 per cent of bullet wounds of the head. The type most commonly encountered is that in which the bullet, after passing through the brain, strikes the opposite portion of the cranial vault obliquely, and is then deflected into the brain again at an angle, like the carom of a billiard ball against the edge of the table. In a few instances the bullet follows the curve on the inside of the skull, as in a suicidal case in which the gun was fired obliquely upward into the right temple, the bullet traveling in a complete semicircle inside the dura across the vertex, ploughing a furrow on the surface of the cerebral hemispheres, perforating the superior longitudinal sinus and finally coming to rest with its base upward in the petrous portion of the left temporal bone. An unusual ricochet was encountered in another case in which a lead bullet was fired into the back of the head, traveling through the brain in a direction upward, forward and to the right, until it was indented by the outer portion of the curved rim of the lesser wing of the right sphenoid; then, traveling inward along this curve, it was deflected upward, backward, and to the left through the brain in the manner of the hai-alai ball caught in the scoop and returned to the wall by the player.

One of the secondary lesions produced by a bullet perforation of the skull is a linear fracture which may extend from the wound of entrance or exit, and occasionally connect the two. Such fractures may be extensive and two or more lines may radiate out from the bullet hole in different directions but they tend to be horizontal. Unlike those caused by blunt force, the fractures resulting from bullet wounds are more often found on the vault and occur less frequently on the base. The extent and pattern of the fractures depends on the mass and velocity of the bullet, its direction and site of impact on the skull, and in contact shots, on the added explosive force of the gases. A heavy bullet, traveling at high velocity may shatter the skull into plates of various sizes (Fig. 16-50).

In an unusual case of a suicidal contact wound of the right temple inflicted with a .32 caliber revolver, the entrance perforation in the thin right lateral portion of the frontal bone was circular and revealed a characteristic smoke ring around its margin. The exit perforation was located in the left parietal bone, but curiously, although beveled on the outer table, instead of being round, was semicircular in shape and delimited by a linear fracture, the edges of which

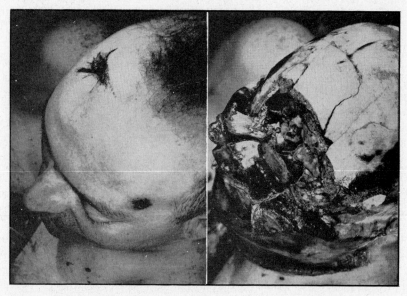

Fig. 16-50. Homicidal In-And-Out .45-Caliber Automatic Pistol Bullet Wound of Head, at Range of Eight Feet.

Entrance in left temple, exit in right frontal region. Note extensive comminuted fracture of frontal bone resulting from oblique impact and track of heavy high-velocity bullet.

were in apposition (Fig. 16-51). The fracture extended around the vault of the skull from the entrance perforation, and was evidently initiated at the time the entrance hole was produced by the bullet and exploding gases. The fracture line actually must have traveled faster than the bullet traversing the brain, for at the split second when the bullet arrived at the other side of the skull to make its exit, the fracture must have been in existence with its edges separated sufficiently for the bullet to clear the lower edge and to produce a semicircular nick in the upper one where it struck. The semicircular exit hole furnished graphic evidence of the distortion of skull and separation of the edges of a fracture at the time of its occurrence and also of the greater speed of a fracture line as compared to that of a bullet which produced it.

Bullet wounds of the brain involve the cerebral hemispheres in the majority of cases, and less often the cerebellum, pons and medulla. The most common lesion is a ragged cylindric tunnel through the brain substance, considerably larger in diameter than the caliber of the bullet, with ecchymosis in the brain tissue surrounding the track and considerable blood and clot and comminuted tissues debris in the perforation itself. Small bone fragments from the entrance perforation in the skull are usually carried into the brain for a variable distance and are found embedded in the main track or at the end of short divergent tracks which they produce in the surrounding brain tissue. The surface furrows of the cortex described under ricochets present the same features. Numerous large vessels like the venous sinuses and the arteries of the circle of Willis may be perforated or torn and give rise to considerable hemorrhage.

In the vast majority of cases, death from bullet wounds of the skull and brain is due to shock resulting from the forcible and destructive trauma caused by the missile. If the brain is penetrated, the individual is rendered instantaneously unconscious and incapable of movement. If the medulla or pons is penetrated, death occurs immediately, but if other portions are involved, the victim may die shortly thereafter or live for several hours or days before succumbing.

In some cases, the bullet penetrates the large dural venous sinuses causing rapid death from profuse external hemorrhage. Arteries of the circle of Willis may be severed by a bullet and death occur rapidly as a result of cerebral compression

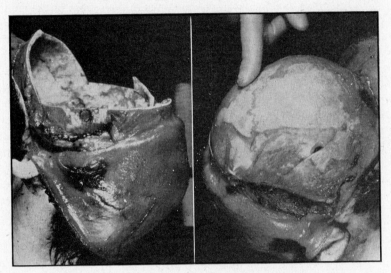

Fig. 16-51. Unusual Semicircular Exit Perforation of .32-Caliber Bullet.

Left. Circular entrance hole visible in lateral surface of right frontal bone below horizontal saw cut.

Right. Semicircular exit hole in left parietal bone above the fracture line which connected the two perforations.

Suicidal contact wound of right temple. See text.

from subarachnoid hemorrhage. Bullets passing through the brain may perforate the choroid plexus or arteries on the surface causing fatal cerebral compression from hemorrhage into the ventricles or subdural space, the victim dying in a few minutes or after a lapse of a few hours.

If the immediate effects of the injury are survived, death may take place within several days from septic infection carried in by the bullet. This usually takes the form of an acute suppurative leptomeningitis, or a localized brain abcess.

A rare complication of a bullet wound of the skull is an arteriovenous fistula between the cavernous sinus and the internal carotid artery. In one case the two vessels on the right side were perforated and a communication between them established by a single bullet fired into the right ear. The victim died 22 days later of an acute hydrocephalus induced by circulatory disturbances in the cerebral venous system as a result of the fistula.

In rare instances a bullet wound which involves the brain undergoes healing leaving a tan colored scar in the brain substance. If the brain during the healing process becomes adherent to the dura, epileptiform convulsions may develop and cause death. In other cases healing occurs without sequelae.

Bullet wounds may involve one or both eyeballs from behind and usually cause blindness. These injuries are noted most frequently in self-inflicted wounds of the temples, in which the projectile may cut across the optic nerves. A curious effect sometimes encountered in suicidal contact wounds of this type in which the bullet passes through the posterior part of both orbits, results from the explosive force of the gases blowing the eyes forward from their sockets and protruding them on the face. Such traumatic exophthalmos caused by a homicidal contact wound of the temple is shown in Figure 16-14. Bullet wounds entering the ear canal or mastoid region are uncommon; but cases of this type are described on pages 178 and 425.

Face. Bullet wounds of the face are less common than those of the cranium and many of them show close-up or contact wounds of entrance. Many projectiles entering on the side of the face pass through the facial bones and make their exit on the opposite side without causing any serious trouble, except as a potential avenue for septic infection. Some bullets enter the face and take a course upward and backward, causing the fatal injury of the skull and brain. Others pass downward and backward into the organs of the neck and the cervical spine injuring these structures and giving rise to a fatal complication. In one case the victim was shot on the right cheek, the bullet entering the back part of the throat severing the right internal carotid artery near the base of the skull; this was followed by a retropharyngeal hematoma which reached such proportions in 30 hours that the laryngeal inlet was occluded and death occurred as the result of asphyxia. The most important injuries in this region are bullet wounds of the lower jaw, causing compound fractures of that bone, and not infrequently resulting in an infection of the fracture and inhalation of septic material which may give rise to a gangrenous inhalation pneumonia with abscesses. Shock and hemorrhage are rare unless other structures are injured, and the victim may well be capable of locomotion. Many of these wounds heal.

Some suicides insert the muzzle of the gun in the nares or in the mouth. The track of the projectile is usually upward and backward and the structures involved depend upon the angle of the shot and whether it is directed vertically, horizontally or toward the right or left. In both nasal and buccal contact shots the bones are shattered, the soft tissues torn and powder residue is deposited in the area. In the midline nasal shot, the walls of the sphenoidal sinus and sella turcica are shattered, the pituitary body and optic chiasm disrupted and the anterior branches of the circle of Willis are torn. The missile continues through the cisterna basalis and the base of the brain, the third ventricle and posterior part of the corpus callosum and usually grooves the medial surfaces of the cerebral hemispheres. The bullet may ricochet on striking the inner table of the skull or penetrate the superior longitudinal sinus and be found in the vicinity; in rare instances it is found in the sinus. Not infrequently, the missile passes through the sinus and makes its exit through the vault of the skull leaving the characteristic beveled exit defect described on page 420. Shots which deviate to right or left may involve the internal carotid artery in the carotid canal and the cavernous sinus. If the direction of the bullet is more vertical, it may pass in front of the sella turcica through the ethmoid bone and injure the frontal lobes of the brain.

Similar effects are observed in wounds of the hard and soft palate. These structures and the tongue are disrupted and powder residue deposited on the parts. The tissues injured in nasal shots may be involved or a more horizontally directed projectile may pass through the naso-pharynx and the basilar process of the occipital bone injuring the pons, cerebellum and the basilar artery. At a lower level, the missile may shatter the atlas, enter the foramen magnum and pierce the medulla or comminute the axis and injure the upper part of the spinal cord. Death is usually due to hemorrhage and shock. If the medulla and upper spinal cord are injured, death occurs rapidly from disturbance of the vital centers.

Homicidal bullet wounds of the nares or buccal cavity are rare. Conspicuous powder residue deposits on the face in close up shots and their absence in distant shots will establish the diagnosis. Homicidal contact wounds in the mouth or nose, inflicted on a victim stuporous or unconscious from alcohol or drugs, may simulate suicidal wounds.

Neck. Bullet wounds of the neck comprise about 2 to 3 per cent of the total number of homicidal shootings. Some of these injuries involve the muscles and vertebral column without seriously damaging other structures and are not dangerous except as a nidus for a septic infection. In one case a bullet was embedded in the transverse process of the cervical spine where it remained quiescent several years; an operative removal was attempted but the patient died during the operation, probably as the result of the administration of a general anesthetic. On page 185, a case of a bullet wound of the neck is described in which the bullet was embedded in the spine and death occurred from delirium tremens some days subsequent to the injury.

The wounds of entrance occur mostly on the sides of the neck near the angle of the jaw, but some are encountered in the lower lateral part of the neck, in the front or in the back. Some of these shots enter the spinal column and may lacerate the cord; others in the front part of the neck range upward through the base of the skull and pierce the brain; some bullets entering the lower portion of the neck range downward and perforate the subclavian vessels or the lungs causing death by intrathoracic hemorrhage.

The structures in the neck which are most vulnerable to bullet perforations are the carotid arteries, the jugular veins and the air passages such as the pharynx, larynx and trachea. A perforation of the carotid artery or the jugular vein may be followed by a profuse rapidly fatal external hemorrhage. In some cases the bullet wound communicates with the pleural cavity and hemorrhage occurs into the chest; the air passages may be perforated and an hemoptysis may follow; or the bullet may enter the esophagus and blood may be swallowed into the stomach. Death is apt to occur in a few minutes and the victim is likely to be prostrated soon after the shooting though in some cases he may live several hours. Sometimes a bullet wound of a large artery or vein causes a hemorrhage to collect in the interstitial tissue of the neck. In one case the left jugular and innominate veins were perforated, resulting in a big cervical hematoma in addition to the external hemorrhage, the victim living six hours after the injury. In some cases the bullet grazes a carotid artery injuring the intima with the subsequent development of a mural thrombus, and from this, either with or without subsequent embolism to a cerebral artery, fatal cerebral infarction may occur. It is also possible for a similar injury of the jugular vein to result in a bland thrombosis of that vessel, with subsequent pulmonary embolism. Air embolism is a rare complication of bullet perforations of the veins of the neck.

Perforations of the air passages may occur from bullet wounds of entrance high in the neck involving the pharynx and larynx, or from entrance wounds lower down which pierce the trachea. The complications of such injuries are various: blood may enter the lumen of the air passages resulting in hemoptysis of foamy blood, or inhalation of blood into the lungs, with death a combination of hemorrhage and asphyxia; those cases which survive the immediate effects of the injury may develop a suppurative inhalation pneumonia. In some perforating bullet wounds of the trachea or larynx, an appreciable obstruction of the air passages by the inward displacement of their cartilages at the site of the perforation may occur, occasionally combined with a hematoma in the muscles of the neck or in the submucous layer of the larynx or pharynx. With such wounds a delayed submucous hematoma or a submucous emphysema may develop and increase the laryngeal or tracheal obstruction. In a few instances the victim survives the injuries for several days and then succumbs to a septic cellulitis in the submucosa of the larynx or pharynx, or to an intermuscular phlegmon in the neck.

Chest. Bullet wounds of the chest are encountered in about 23 per cent of homicidal shootings, and of these over one half of the wounds of entrance were in front, one-quarter in the back, and one-quarter in the axillary and lateral regions of the chest. Most of the entrance wounds in the front of the chest were encompassed in an area about 14 inches in diameter, covering the region between the lower end of the manubrium and the ensiform cartilage with the lateral boundaries represented by two vertical lines drawn just external to the nipples; the greatest concentration was over the precordial area. Over the sides and back of the chest the entrance wounds although less numerous were evenly distributed.

The tracks of most chest bullet wounds were toward the opposite side from the wound of entrance, the vast majority ranging downward, with deviations to right or left. Few passed upward into the neck or head. Some shots directed against the lower chest passed downward into the abdomen injuring the abdominal viscera. A few bullets entering through the anterior abdominal wall or the lower back penetrated the chest from below through the diaphragm and injured the chest organs. The bullets did not pass out of the body in about two thirds of all the cases and of these about two-thirds were black powder-driven lead bullets and one-third were smokeless powder-driven, hard-metal jacketed bullets. Probably if there had been a higher proportion of smokeless powder cartridges, fewer bullets from such ammunition would have remained in the body. Some bullets, especially those composed of lead, were deformed by striking the spine, ribs or sternum and occasionally deflected from their course. The proportion of close-up and contact shots was much less on the chest than on the head and face.

Lungs. Bullet wounds are encountered more frequently in the lung than in any other chest organ and are produced by projectiles passing through the chest in almost any direction. Their numerical ratio in comparison with bullet wounds of the heart is about two to one. In spite of this preponderance, only about a third of the fatalities from chest bullet wounds results from pulmonary injuries, the other two-thirds of the deaths resulting from the more serious bullet perforations through the heart or the large vessels of the chest. The right and left lungs are about equally involved and so are the upper and lower lobes of each lung. In a few cases, both right and left lungs are perforated by the same bullet crossing the chest from side to side.

The reaction of the victim to a bullet wound of the lung is variable and depends on whether or not a large vessel has been involved. If a sizeable branch of the pulmonary artery or vein is perforated, bleeding into the chest will probably be rapid and profuse, and death may occur in a few minutes; with a wound of this type the individual may not be capable of locomotion. In other cases, the bullet does not lacerate a large vessel so that only slight bleeding results, permitting the victim to walk a considerable distance after being shot. Where death is due to hemorrhage, the autopsy may disclose from 500 to 1,500 or more grams of blood in one thoracic cavity, and where both chest cavities are involved 1,200 to 2,500 gm. of blood may be variously distributed between them. The victim may die at the scene of the shooting, or may survive the pulmonary perforations several hours or even days. In the cases that die soon after the injury the blood in the chest is fluid or clotted and dark red in color. If the hemorrhage is profuse and confined to one side of the

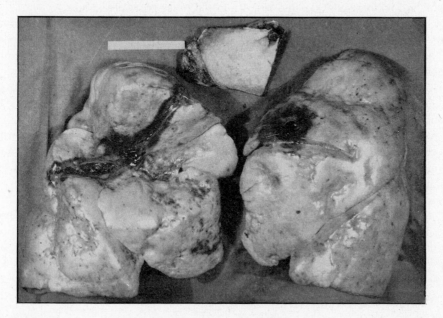

Fig. 16-52. Bullet Track Involving Both Lungs.

Missile penetrated left upper lobe, pulmonary artery, root of right lung, interlobular fissure grooving adjacent lobe surfaces (shown separated in photograph). A .32-caliber bullet was recovered in the right scapula (block of bone containing bullet included in photograph).

chest, the corresponding lung will be compressed and lighter in weight than the one on the opposite side. The victim who survives several days usually shows changes in the extravasated blood which turns brown in color and forms a rusty brown fibrinous deposit on the pleural surfaces as described on page 231, while the lung may show a marked compression atelectasis and a peribronchial hypostatic pneumonia. In some of these cases, the pleural cavity becomes infected and a septic pleuritis or an empyema of the chest may develop, and death may result from such complicating septic infection. a septic pleuritis may follow a thoracotomy performed in an attempt to stop bleeding from the bullet perforations.

Some complications of bullet wounds of the lung are dependent on whether or not a sizeable bronchus is perforated as well as a blood vessel. The most common of these is a hemopneumothorax following the type of bullet wound which causes blood and air to enter the pleural cavity where an increasing amount of air is trapped. The mixture of blood and air in the pleural cavity compresses the lung, displaces the thoracic viscera, and may cause death by a combination of asphyxia and hemorrhage. The chest wall may also be the seat of a subcutaneous emphysema as a result of such a wound. In rare instances cerebral air embolism occurs when the bullet track has established a connection between a bronchus and a pulmonary vein of moderate size; in one case seen by the authors, the victim suddenly became unconscious about an hour after receiving a bullet wound of the right lung, dying 24 hours later; the autopsy disclosed small discrete hemorrhages in the white matter of the brain and diffuse areas of patchy hemorrhage in the gray matter of the cortex which were attributed to a sudden cerebral air embolism. In other cases where the bullet has lacerated a fairly large branch of the pulmonary artery near a sizeable bronchus, an hemoptysis may ensue, the victim spitting up large quantities of frothy blood and inhaling considerable blood into the other parts of the lung.

The bullet in its passage through the lung produces a cylindric tunnel, much larger than the diameter of the projectile (Fig. 16-52). This track is surrounded by a wide zone of ecchymosis and the lining of the cavity is ragged and usually contains blood clot. If the bullet first perforates a rib, small bone fragments may be driven into the track in the lung for a short distance. In through and through wounds of the chest, such bone fragments in the lung indicate the direction of the track. The wound of exit from the lung is usually greater in diameter and shows a broader zone of ecchymosis than the wound of entrance. These injuries may heal according to the process described on page 232, and the track finally closes and is eventually transformed into a fibrinous scar. Surgical operations are performed occasionally on pulmonary bullet wounds and usually for the purpose of closing the pleural perforations in order to stop hemorrhage.

Heart. Bullet wounds involve the heart about half as frequently as the lung, but are much more dangerous to life. In most of these, the bullet enters the chest in the precordial area anteriorly, but some occur when the bullet penetrates the sides and back of the chest. The ventricles are pierced in about four fifths of the cases, the right and left chambers being about equally involved, while the two auricles are wounded in one fifth of the cases, the right about three times as frequently as the left.

The bullet wound of entrance in the heart appears as a small circular or stellate perforation through the epicardium, surrounded by a thin zone of abrasion and a slight ecchymosis in the subepicardial tissues. The wound of exit is frequently larger and is roughly circular or ovoid in shape. The bullet causes a variable amount of damage to the cardiac muscle, sometimes producing a simple circular channel and sometimes tearing a large ragged hole, the form of the lesion depending on the size of the projectile and the manner in which the myocardium is lacerated. Contact wounds in the precordial region may cause considerable shattering and blackening of the myocardium, especially if the charge in the cartridge is black powder in sufficient quantity to have a high explosive force (Fig. 16-18).

Bullet tracks may penetrate the heart in all directions, but one of the most common is a wound of the right ventricle which passes backward and downward, traversing the septum and emerging by the left ventricle posteriorly. Projectiles entering the left side of the chest may pierce the apex of the right or left ventricle, and travel through the heart, finally making their exit through the right auricle. If the bullet enters the side of the right chest, it may penetrate the right ventricle and pass out of the heart near the apex. The auricles are usually entered by frontal shots which pass backward either causing an in and out wound or cutting a furrow in the auricular wall. The same type of lesions are sometimes produced on the

ventricles by missiles which graze those cavities. Occasionally a coronary artery or
venous sinus is perforated by the track of a bullet wound through the heart.

Cases have been described in which a bullet has passed over the anterior surface
of the pericardium without entering it, but at the same time causing a rupture of the
right ventricle. The authors have seen such a case in which .32 caliber lead bullet
penetrated the lateral portion of the left chest in front, traveled horizontally to the

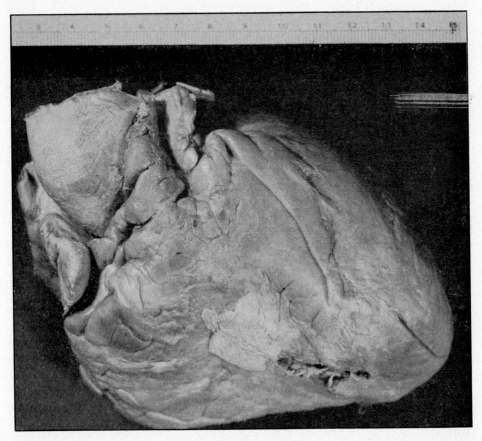

Fig. 16-53. Tangential Horizontal Furrowed Bullet Wound of Anterior Wall of Right Ventricle Without
Penetration of Pericardial Sac.

Hemopericardium and cardiac tamponade. Wound from .32-caliber bullet. See text.

right over the front of the pericardium and lodged in the right portion of the anterior
mediastinum. The pericardium was not entered, but there was an elongated ovoid
furrow of the anterior wall of the right ventricle (Fig. 16-53), 30 mm. by 5 mm.,
parallel to the bullet track and immediately adjacent to it; this caused a hemorrhage
into the pericardial sac and a fatal tamponade of the heart. An unusual feature of
this case was that the bullet passed through a box of safety maches in the left hand
coat pocket of the deceased, igniting them and carrying some of the burning match
heads to the right side of the anterior mediastinum where they scorched some of the
adipose tissue.

The principal complications of cardiac bullet wounds are hemorrhage into the
pericardial cavity, hemorrhage into one or both pleural cavities, or septic infection
of the pericardial sac. Fatal hemorrhage into the pleural cavities is fairly common,

occurring in over two thirds of the cases, and is encountered when the pericardium is perforated in such a way that blood can escape from that sac into one or both sides of the chest. The escape of blood may be so rapid that death occurs in a few minutes after the shooting as a result of acute blood loss. In other cases, the bleeding is slower and the blood escaping into the pericardial sac is constantly drained through the pericardial perforation into the pleural cavity, thus lessening the pressure around the heart; under these conditions the victim may survive a few minutes or hours and in favorable cases long enough for surgical intervention. In fatal cases the amount of blood found in the pleural cavities may vary from about 700 to 3,000 gm., and about 100 or more grams are found in the pericardial sac.

Sometimes a bullet of small caliber perforates the pericardium in such a way that blood cannot escape through the perforation into either chest but is retained in the pericardial sac, causing death in a few minutes by asphyxia from cardiac tamponade; see pages 228 and 340. At autopsy the amount of pericardial hemorrhage in this type of case may vary from 200 to 450 gm. and the heart is found markedly contracted. In rare instances the hemorrhage does not take place immediately, but occurs secondarily after several days as the result of a sudden rupture of the wound in the heart wall, followed by a fatal cardiac tamponade. In a case of his type, the blood in the pericardial sac will present all the appearances of having been rapidly shed and will not show any of the changes which ensue if it had been in the sac for several days.

In rare instances, the cardiac wound may not cause a marked effusion of blood into the pericardium so that the patient may survive the immediate effects of the injury, but after a few days the serous membrane reacts to the presence of the blood and a mechanical inflammation results. The blood becomes brownish red in color, an exuberant layer of brownish red fibrin forms on the pericardial layers with effusion of serous fluid, and the gradual compression of the heart; this in itself may be the fatal complication. A more likely result is the introduction of pathogenic bacteria into the pericardial sac and a septic inflammation of that cavity with exudation of purulent fibrin or frank pus on the serous surface, causing death by compression of the heart or by septic toxemia.

In cardiac bullet wound cases which survive the injury a few days, it is possible for a thrombus to develop on the injured endocardium, and become a source of embolization to the systemic or pulmonary circulations, depending on its location. In some instances a bullet may penetrate into one of the chambers and serve as an embolus. D. H. Collins has reported a remarkable case of bullet embolism into the right lung with the production of a massive pulmonary infarction, following a self-inflicted 9 mm. bullet wound of the chest and right ventricle, the bullet first having lodged in the interventricular septum before embolizing into the right pulmonary artery.

The question frequently arises in cases of cardiac bullet wounds, whether or not it is possible for a victim to move after a fatal shooting. All cases must be judged individually, and the answer to that question on the basis of the results of the autopsy, would depend largely on the nature of the cardiac wound, the presence or absence of a cardiac tamponade and the amount of the hemorrhage. Reports in the literature and case records in the office of the Chief Medical Examiner indicate that wounds of the heart do not prevent the victim from walking, running or climbing stairs, at least for short distances. Generally wounds of the auricles are more rapidly fatal than those of the ventricles, because the comparatively thick muscle of the latter may contract and produce hemostasis and temporary closure of the opening. Wounds of the heart sometimes undergo spontaneous healing and many remarkable cases have been reported. Vance has described a case in which a .38 caliber lead bullet was found encapsulated in the wall of a right auricle of a Negro man who had been shot some years previously, and who had died of a totally unrelated condition. Delayed rupture of a partially healed bullet perforation of the heart also occurs occasionally. In some cardiac bullet wounds cardiorrhaphy is attempted if the victim is not overwhelmed by shock and hemorrhage, but in spite of dramatic success in a few cases, the mortality is appreciable.

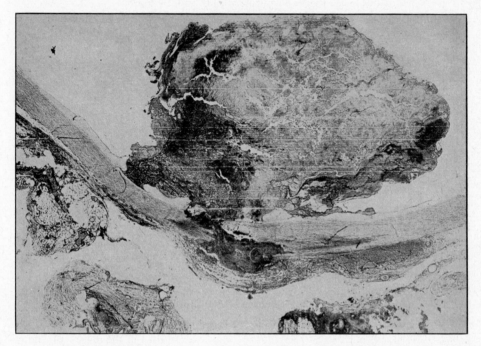

Fig. 16-54. Traumatic Mural Thrombosis of Aorta Complicating Bullet Wound of Dorsal Spine.

Bone fragments from the perforated vertebral body were displaced forward and contused the aorta with resultant thrombosis. Low power photomicrograph of histologic section of aorta showing large bland mural thrombus at site of injury.

Arteries and Veins of Chest. The ascending aorta, the arch and the descending thoracic aorta are occasionally perforated by a bullet, and death occurs rapidly as a result of an intrapericardial or intrathoracic hemorrhage. The perforations may be paired and close together, denoting entrance and exit wounds in which case they have a stellate shape or a distorted H shape somewhat larger than the projectile. The bullet may penetrate one side of the vessel leaving a ragged stellate opening at that point; or the vessel may be grazed by the missile and show merely checker-board or linear ruptures of the wall. Rarely a bullet may perforate the spine from the rear and lacerate or contuse the aorta by displacing bony fragments forward; a mural thrombosis may develop at the site of the injury (Fig. 16-54).

Perforations of the pulmonary, innominate, carotid and subclavian arteries are similar to those of the aorta but the vessels are smaller and they may be partially or completely severed by the bullet. The innominate and subclavian arteries may be perforated by shots which range downward from the lower neck into the chest, or enter the chest and range upward and back through the lower neck, death usually occurring as a result of hemorrhage into the corresponding chest through the communicating bullet wound.

The venae cavae, innominate, subclavian, jugular and pulmonary veins are sometimes perforated by bullets, showing lesions similar to the wounds of the arteries but smaller and more circular in shape. Death is usually the result of pericardial or intrathoracic hemorrhage. The innominate and subclavian veins are sometimes wounded by bullets which pass from the neck into the chest, or upward from the chest into the neck, followed by a fatal hemorrhage into the chest cavity. Air embolism is not a common complication of a bullet wound of these vessels.

The internal mammary and intercostal arteries and veins may be severed by a bullet and bleed slowly into the corresponding pleural cavity, and death may occur after several days unless these vessels are ligated. One case was observed in which the right internal mammary vessels were severed near the first costal cartilage by a .25 caliber hard-metal jacketed bullet, death occurring four days later with 1,500 ml. of blood in the right chest and 300 ml. in the left chest, the bullet having entered the left pleural cavity also where it tore the intercostal vessels in the second interspace.

Abdomen. The abdominal cavity is involved in about 25 per cent of all homicidal bullet wounds, over one half of the projectiles entering the anterior abdominal wall between the ensiform and the umbilicus, about one-sixth penetrating the lower anterior abdomen between umbilicus and symphysis, about one-sixth entering the lumbar region and the buttocks, and almost one-sixth passing into the abdomen through the flanks. A few bullet wounds of the lower chest ranged downward and involved the abdominal viscera, and others which penetrated the thighs were directed upward into the abdominal cavity.

The bullet wounds of the abdomen, unlike those of the head and chest, were operated upon in over one half of the cases, the operation usually being an exploratory laparotomy, followed by repair of stomach or intestinal perforations, resection of intestines or tamponade of lacerations of the liver or other solid viscera with gauze or fiber sponge. In slightly more than five sixths of the cases of bullets remained in the body; three fifths of these were lead bullets and two fifths hardmetal jacketed missiles. In about one sixth of the cases the bullet made its exit from the body. The high percentage of retained projectiles depended largely on the fact that many were stopped by the spine and the pelvis. Close-up and contact bullet wounds of entrance occurred but were relatively less frequent than in the category of shots directed against the head. The missiles entering the abdomen were occasionally deflected in ricochets off the lumbar vertebrae, the pelvic brim, the transverse spinal processes or the lower ribs.

The shots entering the upper anterior abdomen generally took a backward and downward course with occasional deviation to the right and left; comparatively few were directed upward and backward. The organs penetrated in order of frequency were the small intestine, liver, stomach, mesentery, duodenum, pancreas, abdominal aorta, kidneys, large intestine, inferior vena cava, portal vein and spleen. Various combinations occurred as it was rare to have only one organ or structure perforated; the commonest were liver and stomach, liver and intestines, stomach and intestines, and less frequent combinations involving the other abdominal viscera and structures. The most frequent cause of death was intra-abdominal hemorrhage in over one third of the cases, intestinal hemorrhage in less than one-sixth, suppurative peritonitis in about one-sixth, and other septic conditions in about one-sixth, such as retro-peritoneal abscesses, retroperitoneal cellulitis or hypostatic pneumonia induced partly by exploratory laparotomy and general anesthesia.

Bullets entering the lower anterior portion of the abdomen were directed back-ward, some downward and some upward, usually with lateral deviation to the right or to the left. The organs perforated were mainly the small intestine and the large intestine, less often the kidneys, and rarely the liver, duodenum, left external iliac artery and uterus. The principal fatal complication was an acute suppurative peritonitis. Intra-abdominal hemorrhage caused death in comparatively few instances.

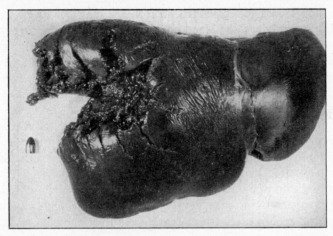

Fig. 16-55. Massive Stellate Wound of Right Lobe of Liver Produced by High-Velocity 9 mm. Bullet Fired from Luger Automatic Pistol.

Bullet included in photograph to show disproportion between its caliber and diameter of the wound.

The wounds of entrance in the back were located in the buttocks and in the lumbar region. The bullet tracks usually ranged forward, upward and with deviations to the right or left, but a few were directed in a downward direction. The organs involved were the small intestine, large intestine, urinary bladder, kidneys, abdominal aorta, left external iliac vein, liver and gallbladder. The most common cause of death was intra-abdominal hemorrhage, less often an acute suppurative peritonitis, and one case of a bile peritonitis due to perforation of the gallbladder.

Some projectiles entered by way of either the right or the left flank and ranged toward the opposite side with various deviations in an upward or downward and a forward or backward direction. The organs and structures perforated were mainly small intestine, large intestine and mesentery, but occasional wounds occurred in the liver, stomach, duodenum, kidneys and abdominal aorta. The principal cause of death was an acute suppurative peritonitis, and less often the victim died of intra-abdominal hemorrhage. In one case in the series analyzed there was a supera-tive retroperitoneal cellulitis due to a penetrating wound of the duodenum.

The vertebral column and spinal cord are frequently injured in bullet wounds of the abdomen, but they are not included in the list of lesions in as much as they did not contribute materially to cause the death of the victim in this particular series of cases. The fatal bullet wounds of the spinal cord will be considered later.

Liver and other Parenchymatous Viscera. The bullet wound of the liver appears as a stellate perforation (Fig. 16-55) on the peritoneal surface considerably larger than the caliber of the projectile, with the exit wound usually larger than the wound of entrance. The bullet produces a large ragged cylindric tunnel through the parenchyma with fragmented tissue, blood and blood clot in the lumen. Most of these tracks enter the diaphragmatic surface and pass downward out of the under surface; others range through the organ laterally; occasionally the tracks take an upward direction; in some instances the surface of the liver may be furrowed by a glancing shot. The principal complication of such injuries is a profuse intraperitoneal hemorrhage, varying from 1,500 to 3,000 ml., due to laceration of large intra-phepatic blood vessels. In most cases such hemorrhages cause death in a few minutes or in several hours; in a few cases the hemorrhage may not be excessive and the victim may live several days, the blood undergoing the various changes described on page 238. Sometimes a large bile duct is lacerated causing a mixture of blood and bile to be extravastated into the abdominal cavity. In one case the gallbladder was penetrated by the bullet and at autopsy a slight degree of icterus was noticeable and a marked bile peritonitis was present with 1,000 ml. of pure bile in the abdominal cavity, similar to the case described on page 239. In some cases the patient survives the wound a few days and changes occur around the perforation through the liver; the blood supply of the tissue immediately adjacent to the wound is impaired by the disruption of tissue, and some of it becomes yellowish white in color and necrotic, forming a lesion known as a traumatic infarct. This condition, not dangerous in itself, may be a nidus for pathogenic bacteria and an abscess followed by a suppurative peritonitis may develop. The bullet wound may heal without complication, and a fibrous cord may form in the liver substance as a remnant of the old perforation.

The other parenchymatous abdominal organs, kidneys, pancreas and spleen, like the liver, are also injured by bullets and may give rise to an intra-abdominal hemorrhage of severe grade. The wounds present morphologic features similar to the wounds of the liver, and may show similar traumatic necroses, and may undergo a similar type of healing. Sometimes a bullet passing through the kidneys may enter the pelvis and cause blood to appear in the urine. In rare instances a shot through the pancreas may sever a large secretory duct and give rise to a widespread fat necrosis in the abdominal fat, occasionally complicated by septic infection. In a few cases a bullet may cause adjacent perforations of the pancreas and duodenum, or of the right kidney and duodenum, and the injury of the parenchymatous organ may bleed profusely through the duodenal perforation into that portion of the intestine; at autopsy a large amount of blood or a massive blood cast is found in the stomach, duodenum and upper jejunum, sufficient in amount to cause death.

Blood Vessels of the Abdomen. Bullet perforations of the larger blood vessels in the abdomen such as the abdominal aorta, the inferior vena cava, the portal vein and the iliac, renal and mesenteric vessels occur, similar to the same injuries already described in the large vessels of the chest. The usual result is a severe hemorrhage into the abdominal cavity which causes death in a few minutes to a few hours. Rarely a bullet wound of the abdominal aorta, or of the inferior vena cava occurs in close proximity to a bullet perforation of the duodenum and a fatal hemorrhage takes place into the gastrointestinal tract as described above. Occasionally a wound of the renal vessels gives rise to a large retroperitoneal hematoma in the lumbar fossa and sometimes is accompanied by infarction of the kidney due to disturbance of its blood supply.

Stomach and other Hollow Viscera. Bullet wounds of the stomach and intestines occur as small stellate or circular holes through the wall of the viscus, the opening at the point of entrance being usually smaller than the opening at the point of exit. The stomach is often perforated by a bullet entering the anterior surface and the greater curvature and passing downward and backward and out through the posterior wall and lesser curvature; less frequently the stomach is transfixed by a bullet entering by the back and traveling forward. Projectiles ranging across the abdomen from right to left may pierce the stomach near the pylorus and emerge from it near the cardiac end, and those missiles passing from left to right may cross from cardia to pylorus; in some instances the same bullet may re-enter the stomach and produce three or four wounds of the stomach wall. Occasionally the gastric wall is grazed by the projectile which produces a single elongated perforating furrow. The principal complications of such gastric perforations is a marked septic peritonitis of the fibrino-purulent or necrotic type. Unless the stomach wounds are promptly sutured, they may cause death by this infection in a few days. The surgeon in operating on this type of case should be careful to close all the perforations, including those on the posterior wall.

The perforations of the small intestine are similar to those of the stomach, the chief difference being that the bullet may perforate several coils of the intestine so that there may be as many as two to six entrances and exits and furrows of the wall. The mesentery may also be wounded and many blood vessels may be severed and bleed intra-abdominally. Intestinal wounds do not heal spontaneously and if allowed to remain unrepaired usually cause death from a septic peritonitis. If the perforations are sutured, healing occasionally occurs. Wounds of the upper jejunum in addition to a septic peritonitis may cause a widespread fat necrosis due to the escape of pancreatic secretion into the abdominal cavity.

Rarely a tangential grazing shot of the anterior abdominal wall may cause such a large perforation that the small intestines slide through the opening and are exposed on the surface of the body, where they are in danger of becoming infected with pathogenic microorganisms. This injury is most likely to occur as a result of a laceration by a bomb fragment, but in several cases has been produced by pistol bullets. It is also possible for a bullet to lacerate the vault of the diaphragm and produce a diaphragmatic hernia, but this complication is rare.

Bullet wounds may occur in all parts of the large intestine. In most cases a single shot will cause a wound of entrance and a wound of exit, or a single furrow, but occasionally a projectile entering by the flank may perforate and re-enter the large intestine inflicting three or four wounds. The most common fatal complication is an acute septic peritonitis due to the invasion of bacteria from the intestine or from the outside. If the posterior wall of the cecum is perforated, a fatal retrocecal cellulitis may be produced in the right lumbar fossa. Sometimes bullet perforations of the rectum and other parts of the large intestine may give rise to a hemorrhage of appreciable size in the intestinal lumen.

The bullet perforations of the duodenum are similar to those of the stomach. Ordinarily a single bullet produces an in and out wound, but sometimes a bullet track ranging to the right and downward, may perforate the wall and reenter it, leaving three or four wounds. Wounds of the anterior wall may give rise to an acute suppurative peritonitis associated with fat necrosis in the abdominal cavity. Wounds of the posterior wall may cause a gaseous, gangrenous cellulitis of the right lumbar fossa similar to the condition described on page 248. The relation of bullet wounds of the duodenum to gastrointestinal hemorrhage has already been discussed.

Bullet wounds of the bladder, kidney pelvis or ureter may produce an extravasation of urine into the abdomen and give rise to a suppurative peritonitis, or they may cause an extravasation into the retroperitoneal tissues which finally ends in a gangrenous infection of these areas.

Another type of sepsis occurs when a bullet passes through the abdomen without seriously injuring any of the viscera, and then lodges in the spine, pelvis or posterior abdominal muscles where it acts as a foreign body which forms the nidus for a huge retroperitoneal abscess. The process is slow and the patient may waste away from septic intoxication, resulting from the size and extension of the abscess.

The behavior of an individual after a bullet wound of the abdomen is variable. In cases where a large blood vessel is severed the hemorrhage may be sudden and profuse and the victim suffers an immediate collapse. On the other hand some abdominal wounds do not cause such overwhelming prostration so that the victim may be able to travel a considerable distance from the scene of the shooting. Many bullet wounds of the abdomen are amenable to surgical operation, and many can be cured if treated promptly.

Spine and Spinal Cord. Bullet wounds of the spine and spinal cord comprise about 7 per cent of all homicidal bullet wounds, but in only about a third of these was the wound itself responsible for the death; in the remaining two-thirds, the victim died of a fatal complication originating in other organs. In the fatal spinal cord cases, the wounds of entrance occur mostly on the back near the mid-line, extending from the neck to the lower lumbar region; some occur in the lateral portions of the back, a few in the sides of the neck and trunk, and a very few in the front part of the neck and trunk. The segments of the spinal cord involved are the cervical region in a trifle less than one half of the cases, the dorsal region in slightly more than one-third and the lumbar region in a little more than one sixth of the cases. In many of these cases the wounds of entrance were contacts or close-ups. About two thirds of the cases were treated by laminectomy. A large proportion of the bullets did not pass out of the body and some were removed by the surgeon at operation.

The spinal cord is injured by bullets in one of two ways: (1) the projectile may traverse the spinal canal and sever the cord, partially or completely, producing a ragged perforation with ecchymosis in the adjacent tissue, or it may pass through and graze the cord producing a contusion in its substance adjacent to the track; (2) the bullet may strike the laminae, the spinous processes or the vertebral bodies and fracture the bone without penetrating the cord, but causing a contusion in its substance at the point of impact. Many of these cases of bullet injuries of the cord live for weeks or months after the shooting and the cord and its membranes may show different stages of the processes of repair. A contusion of the substance may be transformed into a tan colored cavity which on section shows fibrous tissue replacement, large foamy cells containing fat droplets and large cells containing brown pigment. Where death is long delayed, the cord becomes shrunken and fibrous, the dura becomes thickened, and adherent to both bone and cord. If the lesion is completely transverse, the segment below the level of the perforation will show motor tract degeneration, and above that level will show sensory tract degeneration (see page 321).

Bullet wounds of the upper cervical spinal cord may cause sudden death as a result of shock, or the victim may die in from 18 to 24 hours with a derangement of the heat regulating mechanism, a prominent sign being a persistent high temperature. The most characteristic reaction, not only for the cervical region but for all other spinal segments, is an obliteration of all sensory feeling, a removal of all trophic control and a total motor paralysis in that part of the body below the level

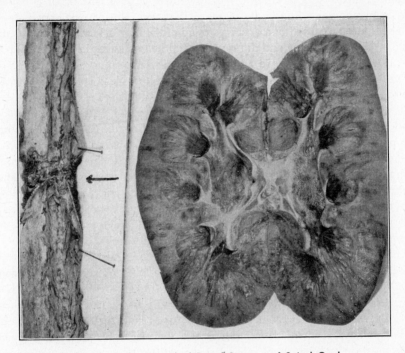

Fig. 16-56. Bullet Wound of Dorsal Segment of Spinal Cord.

The deceased lived six weeks after the shooting, suffering from paralysis of the bladder, bilateral ascending pyelonephritis, uremia and sepsis. Homicide.

of the injury and a condition rendering the victim vulnerable to all types of septic infection.

Hypostatic pneumonia is apt to occur in cervical cord perforations a few days after the shooting as the lungs are markedly congested and edematous. In injuries of the dorsal and lumbar spinal cord a pneumonia may occur as the terminal infection which supervenes at the end of a long period of illness.

Suppurative cystitis, pyelitis and pyelonephritis may develop in a few days to a few weeks after the trauma in the form of small hemorrhagic areas of inflammation or gangrenous grayish yellow pseudomembranous deposits on the lining of the bladder or kidney pelvis with thickening of the wall in some cases. The kidneys may show a subacute interstitial inflammation composed of a marked infiltration of round cells and leukocytes, but in many cases, a suppurative bilateral pyelonephritis with abscesses in the kidney parenchyma is encountered (Fig. 16-56). In one case of a perforating bullet wound of the tip end of the lumbar cord, the patient survived the injury two years and eight months, showing signs of a chronic septic condition of long duration, the spleen being the seat of a chronic enlargement of 500 gm., and the kidney pelves the seat of a chronic septic pyelonephritis with numerous renal calculi which had developed since the injury. In other cases intermuscular abscesses may develop in the thighs and peripelvic tissues as the result of a septic infection following a cord injury.

Occasionally pyogenic microorganisms may invade the spinal canal and affect the cord and its membranes, either carried in by the bullet or in some other manner. The infection usually takes the form of an acute suppurative leptomeningitis, most pronounced in the area of injury or slightly above it, or it may occur as a localized septic pachymeningitis at the site of the perforation. In one case, however, which lived about three weeks after a grazing wound of the cervical cord, there was marked edema, swelling, softening and diffuse petechial hemorrhages in the cord for a zone which extended an inch above and an inch below the injury; microscopic section showed that this lesion contained many polymorphonuclear leukocytes and was an acute septic transverse myelitis due to the bullet wound.

In cases which live for a matter of months, usually characteristic of bullet wounds of the thoracic and lumbar cord or of the cauda equina, the victim may develop huge gangrenous decubital ulcers of the back, buttocks, sacral regions, hips, heels and other points of pressure and may show extreme emaciation and muscular atrophy. (Fig. 13-1). He may succumb to the septic condition thus induced or die of a secondary bronchopneumonia. In one case of over nine months duration after a bullet wound which injured the spinal cord at the level of the seventh cervical vertebra, the victim developed a huge decubital ulcer which eroded the sacrum and the upper ends of both femurs, the autopsy disclosing amyloid infiltration of spleen and kidneys, probably the result of the chronic suppurative osteomyelitis.

A laminectomy performed on bullet wounds of the spinal canal is intended to relieve compression on the cord and to permit extraction of the bullet if it is within reach. If the cord is perforated or otherwise badly injured the operation has little if any influence on the outcome. The prognosis is bad, for whether the cases live from a few days to many months, they usually succumb to the septic infections already mentioned. Even those rare cases which live for years do not regain normal health.

An important consideration in connection with bullet wounds of the spinal cord is that the body is paralyzed below the level of the lesion, but at the same time consciousness is usually retained. A victim whose cord is injured by a bullet will not be able to walk unassisted from the place where the shooting occurred.

Extremities. Fatal bullet perforations of the lower extremities are encountered about 2 to 3 per cent of homicidal bullet wounds. A few of these injuries enter from the front or back of the thigh and range upward through the lower abdomen, perforating the small intestines, cecum, rectum or bladder and causing death by an acute suppurative peritonitis or pelvic abscess. The majority, however, injure the structures in the thigh, such as the femur, the femoral vessels, muscles, joints and nerves, and occasionally produce a fatal complication as a result of these injuries.

The wounds of entrance are about equally distributed over the front, back and outer lateral aspect of the thigh from hip to knee. The direction of the track is toward the opposite side with varying lateral, and upward and downward deviations. Most of the bullets pass in and out of the thigh and few remain to be recovered at operation and at autopsy. Most of the shots are are fired from a distance and closeup and contact shots are not common. In some cases when a wound of entrance occurs on the outer lateral aspect of one thigh the bullet may emerge on its inner lateral aspect and penetrate or transfix the opposite thigh.

The most serious injury occurs when a bullet completely or incompletely severs a femoral artery, or femoral vein, or one of the larger branches, producing an external hemorrhage which may cause death in a few minutes to several hours. Occasionally a few of these cases are saved by the prompt application of a tourniquet around the thigh above the site of the injury or by prompt ligation of the bleeding vessel. Anatomically the bullet perforations of the femoral vessels are similar to corresponding injuries of the iliac arteries described on page 435. In one case a bullet shattered the lower end of the femur in such a way that one of the sharp bone fragments lacerated the femoral artery; the immediate hemorrhage was controlled by a gauze pack, but 72 days later, the artery ruptured and the victim died of a secondary hemorrhage.

A bland thrombosis may be produced in a femoral vein or artery as the result of a bullet injury of the vessel wall, and sometimes a bland thrombus forms in a femoral vessel which is adjacent to an abscess of the thigh complicating a bullet perforation. A thrombosis of the femoral vein may follow a slowing of the venous circulation in that thigh referable to local conditions produced by the injury or to general circulatory disability following the systemic effects of the trauma; a fatal pulmonary embolism may occur as the end result of a lesion of this type (page 176).

If a bullet perforates the femoral or popliteal artery, a false aneurysm may develop quickly, or the bullet may weaken the wall of the artery without immediate effect, but with the occurrence of a rupture and false aneurysm weeks later at the injured site. If an artery or vein are joined by a bullet perforation, the two communicate, and an arteriovenous fistula results. These lesions produce circulatory disturbances and local pressure signs of greater or lesser importance, but only occasionally do they cause a fatal complication. In one case the victim had sustained a tangential, nonperforating bullet injury of his left femoral artery which after 32 days of quiescence, suddenly ruptured forming a large crural hematoma; the surgeon made an incision in an attempt to ligate the injured vessel, but the patient promptly died of a severe external hemorrhage.

Septic infection may occur from any bullet wound passing through the thigh, especially one involving muscles or bones. The bullets may carry in infected foreign material which would find a favorable nidus in extravasated blood, following the perforation. The infection may take the form of extensive intermuscular abscesses, a phlegmon of the subcutaneous tissues, or a suppurative thrombosis of the femoral vein or its tributaries, all of which may produce a general septicemia or a general septic intoxication. The bullet may strike the heavy shaft cortex of a long bone producing a comminuted fracture of a "butterfly" or "multiplication sign" type with shattering of the shaft and this may be the starting point for a purulent osteomyelitis and a fatal sepsis. Bullets are likely to perforate the spongy cortex and bone at the ends of the shaft without comminuting it. Wound tetanus and gas bacillus infection of the extremity may also occur.

Bullets may also perforate the arm or the leg, but do not cause wounds as often fatal as those in the thigh. However there is always a possibility of a fatal hemorrhage from a severed vessel and a chance that some form of septic infection may follow the perforation.

An individual with a bullet wound of the extremities may display different degrees of incapacitation. If the muscles alone are penetrated, the victim will probably be able to move a considerable distance, at least for a short time after the shooting. A fracture of the thigh bone or a severe hemorrhage from a large vessel usually prostrates the victim and prevents him from traveling any great distance without assistance. Fractures of the tibia and fibula, however, will not necessarily prevent a wounded man from limping a considerable distance with the aid of a crutch or stick.

MEDICOLEGAL CONSIDERATIONS. If a physician treats any bullet wound in his office or in a private home, he should report the case as soon as possible to the police. It is important for him to keep an adequate record of the case and to describe the nature and location of the bullet wounds, and to note the direction of their tracks as far as he can ascertain them. A photograph of the wound in its original state is invaluable. These records are especially important if an operation has to be performed which obliterates the bullet wound, for then the surgeon may be summoned to testify as to the nature of the injury, as he probably would be the only medical observer to have seen the wound in its original state. Any bullet which the surgeon removes from the body must be delivered to the police as an important part of the corpus delicti, and a receipt should be obtained from the police officer to whom the bullet is delivered. All gunshot wounds must be reported to the police by the attending physician regardless of their nature.

Blank Cartridge Wounds. A blank cartridge is a cartridge case with a percussion cap primed with fulminate of mercury and filled with powder held in place by a paper wad or similar material instead of a metal bullet. Blank cartridges are employed mostly in army rifles during practice maneuvers in the field, or in pistols fired on the stage, in Fourth of July celebrations, sporting events or in situations where the use of the loaded shell would be unnecessary and dangerous.

Blank cartridges may be dangerous when used under certain conditions. Those used in the United States Army rifle contain enough explosive to cause a severe wound at close range. Even the cartridges fired in Fourth of July pistols are capable of producing a fatal injury. On one occasion a small thin boy of 14 years, fired a pistol containing a .32 blank cartridge as a contact shot into his fifth left interspace near the sternum, blowing a hole through his skin, intercostal muscles, pericardium and right ventricle, death resulting from intrapericardial hemorrhage. Deaths from blank cartridge pistol wounds have resulted from the discharge of the weapon held in contact against the palm of the hand, usually during Fourth of July celebrations. The wounds so inflicted have been complicated by fatal tetanus infections.

Rifle Wounds. A rifle is a gun with a long barrel the bore of which is rifled like a pistol barrel. A carbine is a short-barreled rifle. Rifle cartridges contain a heavier charge of gunpowder and a heavier projectile than the pistol cartridges of the same caliber and, when fired, produce more damage upon a target. In the United States Army rifle and caliber of the bullet is .30 inch; the projectile weighs 150 grains, and is quite pointed and elongated. Its lead-tin base is covered by a hard cupronickel envelope. The initial velocity at the muzzle has been estimated to be 2,700 feet per second. The bullet has a clockwise spin in its flight, and during the first 200 yards of its course it gyrates slightly around its long axis. The wounds inflicted on the body are similar to pistol wounds when soft tissues are penetrated, but more destructive when bone is struck. The wound of exit may or may not be much larger than the wound of entrance depending on the amount of energy expended by the missile which is determined by striking velocity, resistance of the tissues and the yaw or precession of the missile. The great explosive force of the gases together with the energy of the bullet has a very destructive effect in close up wounds especially if bone is struck, and in contact shots may blast a sizeable hole in the skin; a contact rifle shot directed against the cranial cavity may shatter the head (Fig. 16-57).

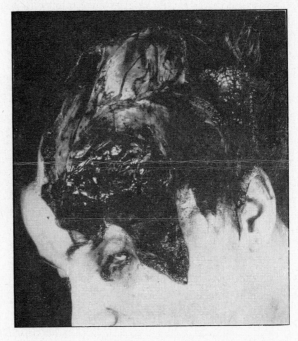

Fig. 16-57. Destructive Contact Wound of Head.

Produced by shot from 30-30 gage hunting rifle. Homicide.

Some rifle bullets, especially those used for big game, have a hollowed-out tip, which results in their becoming deformed on striking skin or bone, the larger irregular striking surface and oscillation or yaw of the missile causing more energy to be expended during its passage and a more destructive wound. This type of

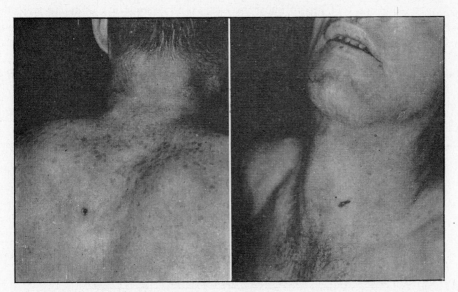

Fig. 16-58. Homicidal In-And-Out .22-Caliber Rifle Wound of Back and Neck.

Shot from a distance of several hundred yards while exercising dog on roof of tenement. Small round entrance hole on back; slit-like hole on neck anteriorly. Spent bullet found near body. Carotid artery perforated.

missile is known as a dum-dum bullet and is designed primarily to stop a large charging animal.

Most of the fatal rifle wounds encountered in New York City have been inflicted by .22 inch caliber rifles firing lead bullets from cartridges containing black powder. The surface wounds are small and inconspicuous but the missiles can penetrate deeply and produce fatal injuries similar to those produced by pistol bullets. Some

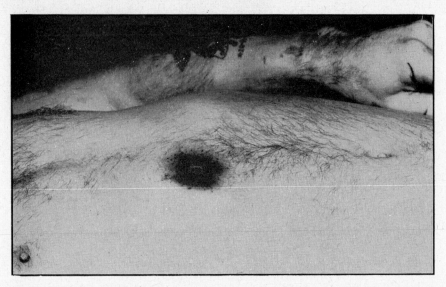

Fig. 16-59. Suicidal Contact Rifle Wound of Upper Abdomen Inflicted with 7.7 mm. Japanese Rifle.
Perforation surrounded by wide circular flame and powder burn. Exit hole in back.

cases are homicidal and occur when a person in a building snipes another on the street or from one roof top to another (Fig. 16-58). Some are unintentional and result from careless use of the weapon by irresponsible adolescents eager to try out a new gun purchased for them by a thoughtless parent. The individual may unintentionally shoot himself or some one else. The range of rifle bullets, even of .22 caliber, is great, and fatalities have resulted from partly spent stray bullets finding a human target.

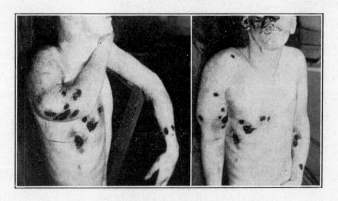

Fig. 16-60. Submachine Gun Bullet Wounds.
Large wounds of head, trunk and extremities made by .45-caliber bullets fired at close range. The right humerus is shattered. Gang murder.

In suicidal rifle wounds, the muzzle of the gun may be placed in the mouth or against the front or side of the head, or against the chest or upper abdomen (Fig. 16-59), then fired. Such contact wounds of the head are the most destructive.

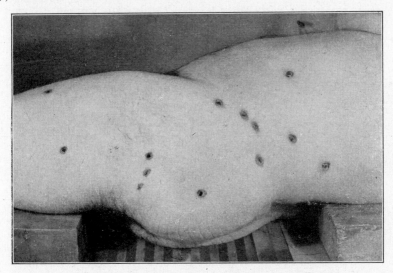

Fig. 16-61. Multiple Shotgun Wounds Produced by Buckshot (000).
Fired from double-barreled shotgun. Homicide.

Machine Gun Wounds. Machine guns are automatic rifled guns with a complicated mechanism capable of firing large numbers of bullets in succession as long as the trigger is pressed and ammunition is fed to the gun. Machine guns are used in times of war, and vary in caliber from .30 to .50 inch. The bullets are large and heavy and covered with a hard-metal jacket. They are propelled at high velocity and produce destructive shattering wounds, especially when hard bone is struck. If such bullets are made to tumble before striking the target, they produce large,

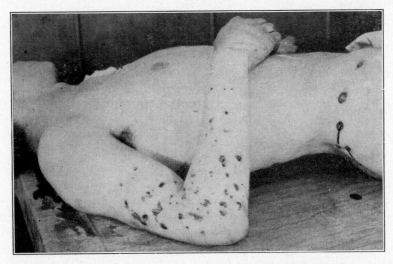

Fig. 16-62. Multiple Shotgun Wounds from Double-Barreled Weapon.
One barrel was loaded with small birdshot and the other with large buckshot. The small shot are embedded in the upper extremity and the large shot in the flank and back. Homicide.

channeled, destructive wounds in the soft tissue out of all proportion to the size and caliber of the bullet, as noted on page 444. On the other hand, a machine gun bullet of high velocity traveling through soft tissues while spinning, undeformed, on its long axis, will produce a fairly clean track with the entrance and exit wounds of regular and comparable size. Such a missile expends a minimum of energy in traversing the tissues and does relatively much less damage than a tumbled bullet or one that strikes bone in its track.

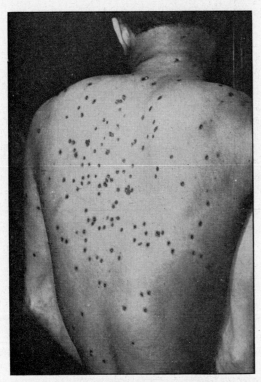

Fig. 16-63. Homicidal Shotgun Wounds of Back.

Constellation pattern of perforations produced by unevenly dispersed small shot. Twelve-gage gun fired at a range of about 10 yards.

In gang wars submachine guns, shorter but just as destructive as the military variety, have been used. The bullets are hard and metal coated and are usually .30 to .45 inch caliber (Fig. 16-60).

Shotgun Wounds. The shotgun is a firearm equipped with one or two barrels of the smooth bore type, firing metal slugs designed for shooting game or clay pigeons. This weapon has become an implement of homicide, especially when the barrels have been shortened to render it easier to handle. The riot guns used by law enforcement agencies are short-barreled shotguns.

Shotguns have barrels of different diameters or gages. At the present time, 12, 16 and 20 gage barrels are in common use; larger gage, 10 and 8, were manufactured in the past. The diameter of the 12 gage is 0.738 inches, the 16 gage, 0.671 inches, and the 20 gage, 0.623 inches. The cartridge of the gun varies in size for the different gages. It is composed of a metallic base with a projecting rim joined to a cylindric shell which is made of heavy oiled paper. The ammunition is held in the opening by a circular cap, and behind the shot is a wad of coarse felt which holds the powder charge at the base near the centrally placed percussion cap. The powder in the shell, whether black or smokeless, is quick burning, and gases form in the barrel rapidly.

The barrels of shotguns are either cylinder bore, in which the entire barrel is the same diameter from breech to muzzle, or choke bore, in which the diameter of the barrel narrows as the muzzle is approached. This degree of constriction varies, and the different degrees are spoken of in terms of full choke, half choke and

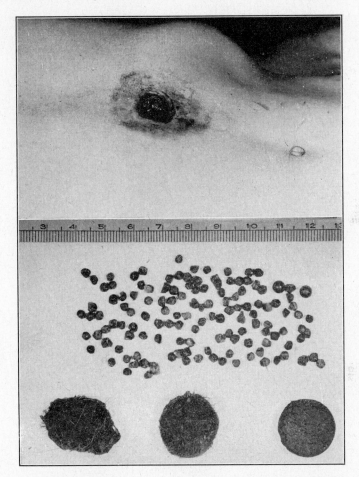

Fig. 16-64. Contact Wound of Abdomen with Single-Barreled Shotgun.

Top. Large single wound of entrance in abdominal wall with powder smudge and burn in track and on surrounding skin.

Bottom. Numerous small birdshot, felt and paper wads removed from abdomen. Suicide.

quarter choke. The practical aspect of this differentiation is that the cylinder bore tends to throw the shot in a cloud which scatters easily while the choke bore holds the shot together for a longer distance before they scatter; the full choke holds them longer than the half choke, and the half choke longer than the quarter choke (Table 16-3).

Table 16-3. Spread in Inches of Shot at Various Distances

	5 YARDS	10 YARDS	15 YARDS	20 YARDS	30 YARDS	40 YARDS
Cylinder	8	20	26	30	45	60
Half choke	5	12	16	20	32	45
Full choke	3	9	12	15	25	40

From Smith and Glaister, *Recent Advances in Forensic Medicine,* 1939.

The various bores of the barrels of shotguns used in the United States are designated as full choke, modified choke, improved cylinder and cylinder. The choke involves only the three or four inches of the distal portion of the barrel, the remainder having a cylinder bore.

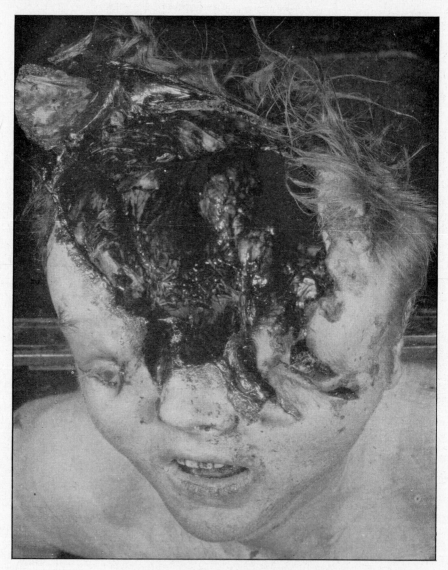

Fig. 16-65. Suicidal Contact Wound of Head from Double-Barreled Shotgun.

Muzzle placed above nose. Top of head demolished and brain blown out and found on grass in three pieces near body. Trigger finger contused.

The shotgun, up to a yard distance, produces a single wound with much burning, blackening and tattooing. From 1 to 3 yards the wound becomes larger, burning and blackening are not present, but tattooing of slight grade occurs. At greater distances the tattooing disappears and the shot disperses (Figs. 16-61, 16-62). The perforations of the shot are somewhat similar to perforations of pistol bullets, and they tend to form astronomical patterns on the skin like constellations of stars (Fig.

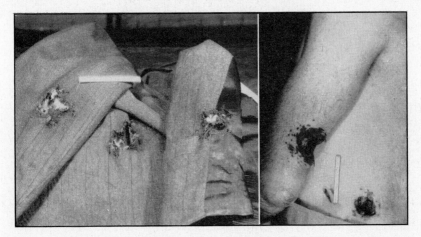

Fig. 16-66. Homicidal Shotgun Wound at Range of Eight Feet; 12-Gage Gun; Small Shot.

Full load of shot passed through border of left arm and re-entered upper left flank. Pellets and wads recovered near kidney. Note small satellite perforations of scattered pellets around large wounds produced by main load. Similar effects visible in sleeve, coat and vest.

16-63). Contact wounds made by a shotgun are destructive because of the explosive force of the gases. Sometimes the wound of entrance is cylindric, slightly larger than the size of the barrel and smoke stained. In contact and also in close up shots the cartridge wads are frequently driven into the track along with the slugs or pellets (Fig. 16-64). The authors have seen a case in which the gun was fired with the muzzle in contact with the bridge of the nose, the explosive force bursting open the base of the skull and the vault of the cranium (Fig. 16-65); by some freakish

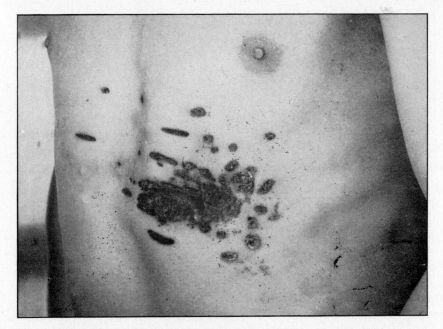

Fig. 16-67. Tangential Shotgun Wound of Anterior Surface of Chest.

Twelve-gage gun; small shot. Load grazed chest from left to right. Small groups of dispersed pellets penetrated the heart. Some pellets visible under the skin on right side.

quirk of the explosion the brain was blown outside of the head comparatively intact except at points where it was torn from its attachments. In close up shots with ammunition containing small pellets, the bulk of the pellets and the wads may penetrate for a variable distance through a single large entrance wound, and a few pellets which have scattered slightly from the main charge may produce a zone of small

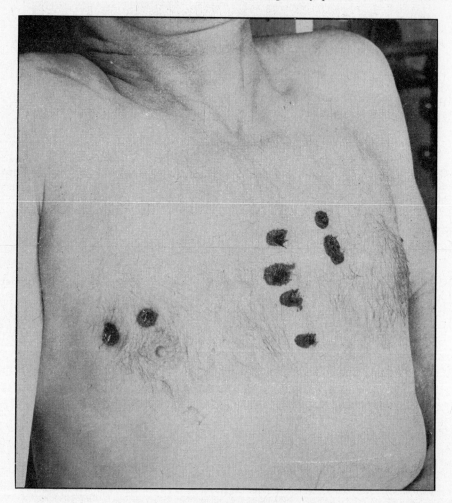

Fig. 16-68. Homicidal Shotgun Wounds of Chest.
Twelve-gage shell, (000) buckshot. All nine slugs in the load entered the chest separately.

satellite perforations around the main large entrance wound (Fig. 16-66). A tangential shot may produce a broad, composite, abraded wound on the skin and the direction may be evident from the location of single pellets under the skin on the far side of the track (Fig. 16-67).

The size of the shot varies from a single large mold shot (cast in molds) to multiple shots. The Eastern U.S. (000) have a diameter of 0.360 inch and are known as buckshot; in a 12 gage shell they are nine in number. The entrance holes on the chest produced by all nine pellets of such a shell are shown in Figure 16-68. The number and pattern of distribution of the entrance wounds will depend on the distance of the weapon from the target. Shotgun pellets range in size from buckshot to dust; with the latter there are 2,600 minute shot in a 12 gage cartridge. The smaller the shot, the larger the number in the cartridge. This is true for almost all shotgun ammunition.

English (L-G)	Eastern U.S. (000)	Western U.S. (2)
6 pellets	9 pellets	9 pellets

Homicidal, accidental and suicidal shotgun shootings occur and the large pellet wounds and tracks individually are similar to those produced by pistol bullets. The suicidal injuries are inflicted against the abdomen, chest and the head. The pellets and wads obtained from shotgun cases should be examined by the ballistics expert.

The late Detective Sergeant Harry L. Butts, Ballistics Bureau, New York City Police Department, described to the authors how the perpetrator of a homicide may alter a shotgun shell containing bird shot to produce a more destructive wound. The cartridge is prepared by making a circumferential incision at right angles to its longitudinal axis, cutting almost but not quite through the case, at a point where the missile portion of the charge impinges on the powder. When the shell is fired, the missile end becomes detached at the incision from the rest of the case, and is propelled as a single projectile, composed of cartridge case, wads and shot. After it penetrates the body and strikes forcibly against bone or a firm viscus, the impact produces a bursting of the case and violent spreading of the shot in all directions with much damage to adjacent viscera.

BOMB EXPLOSION WOUNDS

A bomb is a container filled with an explosive mixture which is fired either by a detonator or a fuse. The explosive mixture is composed of nitrocellulose, nitroglycerine combined with an absorbent, dynamite, trinitrotoluol, or gunpowder of different sorts. The container is usually made of metal and strongly built so that when the explosion occurs its devastating effect will be enhanced by the resistance which must be overcome. The fragments of the container or bomb casing act as penetrating missiles. Most deaths from explosions in civil life are the result of accidental dynamite blasts, or homicidal cases in which infernal machines, operated by clockwork, are planted in a crowded locality in order to cause as much destruction as possible. The military types of bombs are discussed on page 453. The effects of atomic explosions are discussed on page 763.

Several phenomena take place during an explosion. First, there is a disruptive effect of the expanding gases which may shatter or even obliterate a body at close range. If the bomb bursts at a slightly greater distance, the explosion may hurl the victim against a wall or toss him through the air, causing characteristic blunt force injuries. The blast may drive numerous fragments of the bomb or pieces of nearby objects, such as gravel, glass, wood particles or stone through the air into the skin of the deceased, causing ragged perforations of all sizes and shapes on that surface of the body exposed to the explosion; death may be the result of shock and hemorrhage following such perforations. At autopsy all foreign material found in the body should be preserved for chemical examination, as it may be possible to ascertain the nature of the bomb and trace the materials used in its manufacture. Burns of the body may occur as a result of the flame generated in the explosion (page 528). If the bomb explodes in a confined space enough carbon monoxide may be generated to cause asphyxiation of a trapped person. Similar fragment missile injuries are occasionally observed in boiler explosions on steamboats, or in explosions of gasoline or carbon monoxide in buildings.

Blast Injuries. The air raids in London disclosed that many individuals near an exploding bomb were not touched by flying fragments or by flame, but were struck by the blast wave, or the sudden expansion of gases formed in the explosion. The wave by its impact against the chest wall causes a number of injuries to the lungs, but in many cases these effects were averted when some screen like a wall intervened between the exposed person and the blast. Some of the individuals affected died immediately, while others lived for a few hours to a few days. The animal experiments of Hooker and of Zuckerman suggest that when death occurred soon after the explosion it was the result of a circulatory collapse due to immediate shock, such as might follow any blunt force injury.

The cases which survived the effects of the blast for a longer period, showed signs of severe prostration, shock, restlessness, respiratory difficulties and pain in the chest. The most prominent physical signs were bulging of the chest and signs of consolidation in the lungs. The findings at necropsy were massive hemorrhages in the lung tissue with a consistency of pneumonic consolidation, acute pulmonary emphysema, lobular pneumonia and hemorrhages in the mediastinum. On microscopic examination in the cases reported by Cohen and Biskind, numerous red blood cells were described as distending the alveoli, separation of the epithelium of the bronchioles from its basement membrane was noted, and a few ruptures of the elastic tissue and capillaries in the alveolar walls were mentioned. These authors believe that the high pressure blast wave on passing from a medium of greater density like the soft tissues and the solid viscera to a medium of lesser density like the air-containing viscera of the lungs and gastrointestinal tract, produces a disruptive effect at the interface of these media. Injuries of the lung and less frequently of the gastrointestinal tract are more frequent and serious than the injuries inflicted on the brain and the solid organs. Robb-Smith claimed that a fatal fat embolism was present in some of his cases but others have not found any significant degree of this condition in blast injuries.

Hydraulic Concussion. A depth bomb is a high explosive bomb which is detonated by a spring-plunger-trigger mechanism, adjusted to a suitable water pressure so that it is set off when the bomb sinks to the depth giving this pressure. The explosion causes water to shoot upward and at the same time produces lateral concussions of sufficient strength to damage the steel seams of vessels within a radius of several hundred yards. Men floating on the sea within the range of effectiveness of such a bomb may be affected by the explosion, feeling first a compression of the abdomen and then a sharp pain and a sense of fulness and later cramps, nausea, vomiting, shock and bloody diarrhea. Death may occur as a result of shock or from an acute suppurative peritonitis after an interval of several days. At autopsy, some cases show miliary submucous hemorrhages and large subserosal hemorrhages in the large intestine. In other cases there may be a longitudinal tear in the large intestine, either in the sigmoid, transverse colon or cecum, apparently similar to the ruptures of the large intestine caused by the introduction of compressed air into the anus. The mechanism is conceived as a violent compression of the abdomen, combined with a forcible impact of water which forces its way through the anus in considerable volume into the large intestine and causes an hydraulic rupture of that viscus. Lesions of other abdominal organs are rare, and injuries of the lungs in humans are rare in this type of trauma. Experimental work on animals has produced injuries in the lung by underwater explosions.

REFERENCES

BULLET WOUNDS

Black, A. M., Burns, B. D., and Zuckerman, S. Wounding Mechanism of High Velocity Missiles, in War Medicine, W. S. Pugh, ed., New York, F. Hubner and Co., 1942.

Callender, G. R. Wound ballistics; mechanism of production of wounds by small bullets and shell fragments, War Med., 3:337, 1943.

Collins, D. H. Bullet embolism: a case of pulmonary embolism following the entry of a bullet into the right ventricle of the heart, J. Path. & Bact., 60:205, 1948.

Eidlin, L. M. Röntgenographischer Nachweis des Metallringes am Einschuss, Deutsche Ztschr. f.d.ges. gerichtl. Med., 22:204, 1933.

Gerlach, W., and Werner. Spektrographische Untersuchungen alter Schussverletzungen, Deutsche Ztschr. f.d.ges. gerichtl. Med., 23:204, 1934.

Gonzales, T. A. Wounds by firearms in civil life, Am. J. Surg., 26:43, 1934.

Guareschi, G. Der Nachweis des Quecksilbers bei Schussverletzungen, Deutsche Ztschr. f.d.ges. gerichtl. Med., 23:89, 1934.

Harvey, E. N., Butler, E. G., McMillen, S. H., and Puckett, W. O. Mechanism of Wounding, War Med., 8:91, 1945.

Helpern, M., and Hickam, J. B. Wounding effect of high energy missiles, J. Aviation Med., 17:504, 1946.

Kockel, H. Kriminaltechnisches Neues zur Frage des Nahschusses, Deutsche Ztschr. f.d.ges. gerichtl. Med., 24:55, 1934.

Reports of the Office of the Chief Medical Examiner in the City of New York from 1918 to 1941.

Smith, S., and Glaister, J.   Recent Advances in Forensic Medicine, New York, Blakiston Co., 1939.

Smith, W. H. B.   Pistols and Revolvers, vol. 1., Washington, D. C., The National Rifle Association of America, vol. 1.

Vance, B. M.   Bullet wounds of the heart, Am. J. M. Sc., 168:872, 1925.

Walker, J. T.   Bullet holes and chemical residues in shooting cases, Am. J. Police Sc., in J. Crim. Law & Criminol., 31:497, 1940.

Blast Injuries and Hydraulic Concussion

Auster, L. S., and Williard, J. H.   Hydraulic abdominal concussion, J.A.M.A., 121:995, 1943.

Cohen, H., and Biskind, G. R.   Pathologic aspects of atmospheric blast injuries in man, Arch. Path., 42:12, 1946.

Fulton, J. F.   Blast and concussion in the present war, New England J. Med., 226:1, 1942.

Goligher, J. C., King, D. P., and Simmons, H. T.   Injuries produced by blast in water, Lancet, 2:119, 1943.

Greaves, F. C., and others.   Experimental study of underwater concussion, U. S. Nav. M. Bull., 41:339, 1943.

Hooker, D. R.   Physiological effects of air concussion, Am. J. Physiol., 67:219, 1924.

O'Reilly, J. N., and Gloyne, S. R.   Blast injuries of the lungs, Lancet 2:423, 1941.

Robb-Smith, A. H. T.   Pulmonary fat embolism, Lancet, 2:135, 1941.

Wilson, J. V., and Tunbridge, R. E.   Pathologic findings in a series of blast injuries, Lancet, 1:257, 1943.

Zuckerman, S.   Experimental study of blast injuries to the lung, Lancet, 2:219, 1940.

17

Traumatic Asphyxia: Strangulation

ASPHYXIA

Asphyxia is a condition which results when the respiratory interchange between the air in the lung alveoli and the blood in the pulmonary capillaries is interrupted; the red blood cells cannot replenish their oxygen supply and the carbon dioxide cannot be discharged from the blood into the lungs. Its continuation beyond a few minutes will so harm the respiratory mechanism that death results. Traumatic asphyxiations conform to this definition; in such cases air is prevented from entering the pulmonary alveoli either because of interference with the respiratory movements or of obstruction within the air passages. Fatal asphyxia may also result if the respiratory interchange in the pulmonary alveoli is interfered with by blocking the flow of blood through the lungs as in massive pulmonary embolism or tamponade of the heart by an intrapericardial hemorrhage.

The term asphyxia is also used in the broader sense of anoxia, and designates the state of tissue asphyxiation produced when the oxygen and carbon dioxide interchange between the blood in the capillaries and the tissue cells in all parts of the body is prevented. Such tissue asphyxiation may result from disturbances in circulation or from diminution in the blood of hemoglobin available for the transportation of oxygen in the absence of any disability in the mechanism of pulmonary respiration. The term asphyxia as generally employed refers to an interference with the oxygen interchange in the lungs.

Symptoms. Asphyxia is manifested in a well-defined sequence of symptoms, which Puppe has divided into four stages: dyspnea, convulsions, apnea and the final stage. This division is valuable principally because it provides a convenient way to describe the pathologic physiology of the asphyxial process. At times the sequence of events may be modified by a number of factors and not be amenable to division into four distinct stages.

STAGE OF DYSPNEA. The deficient oxygenation of the red blood cells and the accumulation of carbon dioxide in the plasma stimulates the respiratory center in the medulla, with resultant rapid and forceful respiratory movements, rapid pulse, rise in blood pressure, and cyanosis, especially noticeable in the face and in the hands.

STAGE OF CONVULSIONS. Convulsions then set in; at first they are clonic, then tonic, finally taking the form of opisthotonic spasms. The pupils become dilated and the heart rate slows. These effects are referable, probably, to increasing paralysis of the higher centers in the brain from lack of oxygen.

STAGE OF APNEA. The respiratory center becomes so deeply depressed that breathing becomes weaker and may cease. Unconsciousness sets in, and an involuntary discharge of spermatic fluid may occur, and less often, a discharge of urine and feces.

FINAL STAGE. In this stage, complete respiratory paralysis ensues. After a few automatic contractions of the accessory muscles of respiration in the neck, the breathing stops. The heart may continue to beat for a brief period after respiration has ceased.

Lesions Found at Autopsy. The general postmortem appearances in asphyxial deaths result from the presence of unoxygenated blood in the tissues. Thus the face has a dusky purplish blue or plum color (Fig. 4-2), the conjunctivae are injected, the organs cyanotic and congested, and the blood in the heart dark and fluid. Small hemorrhages may be found in the thymus, lungs, pericardium, pleura, larynx, conjunctiva, scalp and skin. In rare cases in which factors leading to rapid clotting and sedimentation of blood are present at the time of asphyxiation, postmortem currant jelly or chicken fat clots may be found in the heart cavities and larger vessels. Such a finding is not incompatible with a diagnosis of asphyxia if other evidence favors that interpretation.

The recognition of asphyxia as a cause of death at autopsy is occasionally difficult and requires considerable care, skill and understanding based on experience on the part of the autopsy surgeon. Needless to say, a complete autopsy including a careful examination, removal and dissection of the neck and throat organs is essential. From the medicolegal standpoint, the performance and interpretation of the autopsy in cases of asphyxial death are more difficult than in any other type of case. The findings are rapidly obscured by postmortem putrefaction, and for this reason the autopsy should never be delayed.

Etiology. Fatal asphyxia may result from either natural disease processes or from traumatic causes.

NATURAL CAUSES. Asphyxia may result from natural disease conditions which obstruct the upper air passages, such as laryngeal edema, Ludwig's angina, diphtheritic laryngitis, tumors of the larynx and masses in the neck. Bronchial asthma and anaphylactic reactions following injection of foreign protein or serum may give rise to a fatal asphyxia as a result of the spasmodic contraction of the bronchial musculature. A pneumothorax may produce a fatal asphyxia by restricting the respiratory movements of the lungs. Interference with the blood supply to the lungs, such as the complete blocking of the pulmonary artery in massive pulmonary embolism, or the compression of the heart by a hemorrhage into the pericardial sac from a ruptured aneurysm, are examples of asphyxial death. Marked emphysema which reduces the capillary bed of the lungs, or a pulmonary fibrosis from pneumoconiosis or chronic pneumonitis, which also constricts the pulmonary circulation, can cause considerable asphyxia.

TRAUMATIC CAUSES. A number of traumatic conditions produce complications which cause death by asphyxia. These include pulmonary embolism from femoral vein thrombosis complicating an injury of the lower extremities, pulmonary fat embolism from a fracture of a long bone, pulmonary air embolism from an incised wound of the internal jugular vein, traumatic intrapericardial hemorrhages from ruptures or penetrating wounds of the heart, and bilateral pneumothorax from injuries to the chest wall or lung. These in whole or in part cause asphyxia by hindering the circulation of blood through the pulmonary blood vessels, thus interfering with the respiratory interchange in the lungs. They have been described in Chapters 7 to 16.

The most important variety of asphyxia from the medicolegal standpoint is that which results when air is forcibly prevented from entering the air passages; it is consistently produced by the following types of violence:

1. Strangulation including hanging, strangulation by ligature and manual strangulation.
2. Suffocation including smothering and choking.
3. External pressure on the chest.
4. Drowning.
5. Inhalation of suffocating gases.

STRANGULATION

Strangulation is the closure of the air passages as a result of external pressure on the neck which prevents the ingress or egress of air during respiration.

Hanging. Hanging is a form of strangulation in which the pressure on the neck is caused by a noose, band or other external mechanism tightened by the weight of the body in such a way as to constrict the throat and close the air passages. The lumen of the upper portion of the larynx is effectually occluded by the direct pressure of the ligature which forces the base of the tongue upward and backward against the posterior pharyngeal wall, pushes the soft palate and uvula upward and depresses the epiglottis over the laryngeal opening. The compression applied to the throat from front to back and from the sides affects the superior laryngeal nerves, the carotid arteries and the jugular veins, causing shock and direct disturbances of the cerebral circulation. After the hanging starts there is a rapid loss of consciousness. The individual cannot free himself, but if cut down shortly after suspension may be revived sometimes by artificial respiration. Usually death occurs in a few minutes from the combined effects of asphyxia, cerebral circulatory disturbances and shock.

Suicidal hanging is comparatively uncommon, with a yearly average of about 177 cases or about 13 per cent of the total number of suicides. Accidental and homicidal hanging is rare. In hanging himself an individual may place the noose around his neck, and then stand on a stool and attach the free end of the ligature, usually a length of rope or other material, to a peg or similar fixture; by stepping off the stool he will suspend himself free of the floor with the weight of the body drawing the noose tight. He may also accomplish his purpose by bending his knees from a standing into a half kneeling position so that only part of his weight is exerting traction on the cord. Similarly a person can hang himself in a sitting posture, or while reclining in a prone or supine position with the cord holding his head from the floor, the only requirement being that sufficient traction is put on the constricting band to compress the neck. In hanging, consciousness is lost so rapidly after the constriction is effected that the victim is unable to free himself.

A visit to the scene of a hanging is necessary, especially if the nature of the death is under suspicion. All the circumstances must be carefully investigated and evidence sought which might indicate that the death was not suicidal but homicidal and that another person or persons attempted to create the impression of a suicide. There is always the possibility that the victim of a homicide by other means was strung up after death in order to deceive the authorities into believing that death was self-inflicted. The medical investigation must search for discrepancies which would cast doubt on the seemingly obvious interpretation. Especially the location and character of the postmortem lividity on the skin surface must be noted as its distribution may be at variance with the position of the suspended body. However, if the body was suspended immediately after death the distributions of the suggillations would be the same as in a bona fide hanging. In such cases the cause of death

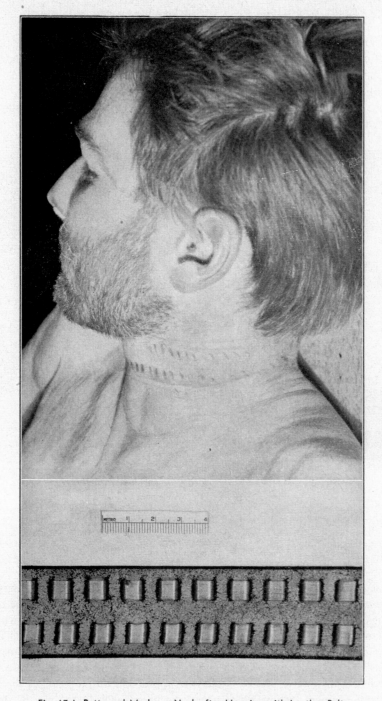

Fig. 17-1. Patterned Marks on Neck after Hanging with Leather Belt.

Top. Double row of vertical abrasions on side of neck made by pressure of woven leather belt.

Bottom. Woven leather belt used. Suicide.

must be carefully determined by a complete autopsy and a thorough laboratory investigation.

The marks on the neck must be examined closely, for the ligature leaves a distinct furrow of its own width and pattern on the skin surface. The bed of the furrow may be pale and the edges brownish red from abrasion caused by the constriction, or the entire mark may take the form of a reddish brown abrasion. The skin surface adjacent to edges of the furrow may exhibit slight engorgement of the dermal vessels and ecchymoses which some consider a sign of intravital reaction.

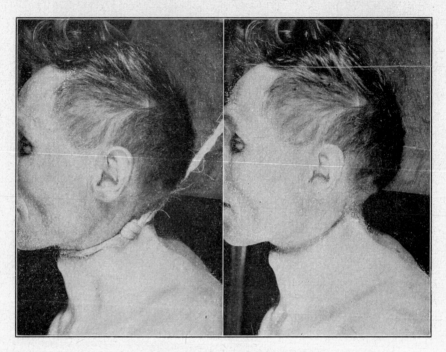

Fig. 17-2. Asphyxia by Hanging. Production of Furrow on Neck.

Left. Noose of double twist hemp rope with slip knot on left side of back of neck in original position as found on deceased who was suspended from a tree.

Right. The rope has been removed to show the abraded furrow encircling neck. Note prominent depression above thyroid cartilage, impression of knot and upward cant of furrow on side of neck characteristic of hanging. Suicide.

The thinner the ligature and the tougher the material of which it is composed, the more pronounced will be the mark on the skin of the neck; the softer the material in the ligature and the broader the constricting band, the less distinct will be its impression on the skin of the neck. The form of the furrow will depend on the type of the ligature, the number of its loops around the neck and the point of suspension. If the band has a distinctive pattern like the woven belt depicted in Figure 17-1, it may produce a distinctive and characteristic impression on the neck. If the ligature is a piece of hempen rope with fine projecting fibers, such fibers may be deposited in the mark. In the fresh state, the furrow may be indistinct, but after postmortem drying the characteristic features become more pronounced. Microscopically the ligature mark has many of the characteristics of an abrasion, showing slight desquamation and flattening of the cells of the epidermis; death usually occurs so quickly that an intravital reaction is difficult to demonstrate.

Ligatures commonly used in hanging are lengths of cord or rope, leather belts, packing wires, twisted sheets or garments (Figs. 17-1 through 17-5). The arrangement of the loops and knots in the constricting band varies considerably, the most common form being a simple noose from a single strand and less often a noose formed from a double strand of ligature. The impression made by such a ligature is symmetric or non-symmetric depending on the location of the knot at the point of suspension. If the knot is in the midline at the back of the head, or in front under the chin, the marks on the neck are usually symmetric, that is, those on the sides are horizontal at about the level of the upper border of the thyroid cartilage of the larynx, and cant upward toward the point of suspension. If the knot is placed laterally behind one ear, the marks of the ligature are asymmetric, canting upward and converging on the side where the knot is located, and horizontally placed on the opposite side. In some cases a rough ligature is used, and the noose adjusted at a low level on the neck; the weight of the body during the suspension may then displace the ligature upward to the level of the thyrohyoid ligament, leaving strand marks indicating the original and final position of the noose, and a broad abrasion to show its upward displacement. Occasionally the arrangement of the constricting band may be complex with considerable overlapping of many folds and knots.

In most hanging deaths, dissection of the throat and neck organs and tissues does not reveal any sign of traumatic injury. Fractures of the superior processes of the thyroid cartilage and hemorrhages in the neck muscles have been encountered occasionally. Ruptures of the sternomastoid muscles and of the thyrohyoid ligament, and fractures of the cornua of the hyoid bone have been described. Fractures of plates of the thyroid cartilage and of the cricoid cartilage are rare. Rarely small transverse intimal tears of the carotid arteries are caused by the ligature; intimal tears of the jugular vein are even less common. In most cases the other

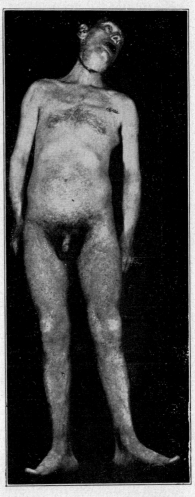

Fig. 17-3. Dependent Lividity after Hanging.

Note dried abraded furrow around neck and deep purple dependent postmortem lividity with Tardieu spots in lower extremities and hands. The body had remained suspended for several hours after death. Suicide.

organs in the body do not show characteristic findings aside from the general signs of asphyxia and the marked hypostatic congestion of some of the lower abdominal viscera.

The color of the face is variable; it may be either pale or cyanotic, depending on the circumstances. Small circular and punctate hemorrhages may be present in the galea of the scalp and in the laryngeal mucous membrane, but they are usually absent. Postmortem suggillations are noted in the most dependent portions of the body, usually in the legs, thighs, hands and penis, especially if the body is suspended; the lower extremities have a dusky bluish-purple color and the livid skin is heavily sprinkled with Tardieu spots. The upper part of the body is pale by comparison (Fig. 17-3). In some cases a postmortem greenish discoloration from early bacterial decomposition appears on the lower abdomen fairly soon after death because of

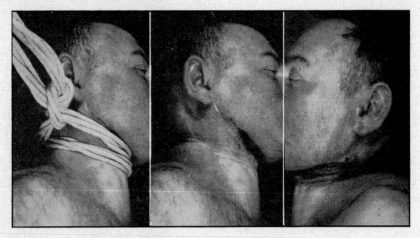

Fig. 17-4. Suicidal Hanging.

Quadruple strands of rope looped twice around the neck and then knotted with suspension point behind right ear. Photographed before and after removal of rope.

the hypostatic engorgement of the intestines (Fig. 4-3). The tongue may protrude between the teeth because of the upward compression of the ligature against its base, but this does not occur invariably. When it does, the tip of the tongue and the lips may appear dry and livid. In some hangings emission of semen occurs, and occasionally an escape of urine and feces.

Rarely a person who is released from a noose after hanging for a minute or two lives for a few hours only to succumb to the aftereffects of shock or damage to

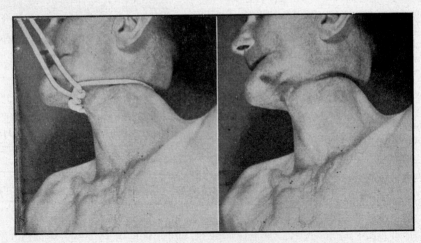

Fig. 17-5. Suicidal Hanging.

Rope looped around neck with knot and suspension point at side of chin. Note corresponding pattern of furrow and rope on neck in photographs.

the medullary centers, or to die later from hypostatic pneumonia. The autopsy in such cases may reveal little that is characteristic, or, in cases that survive more than 24 hours, may show patchy anoxic necrosis in the brain similar to that encountered after cardiac arrest during anesthesia with temporary resuscitation by cardiac massage. Even more rarely, a victim may be revived by artificial respiration and recover without sequelae.

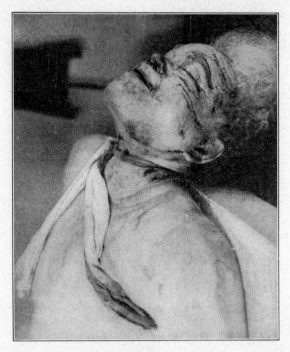

Fig. 17-6. Strangulation by Ligature.

An example of garroting by means of a stocking tied tightly around the neck. The deceased was also stabbed in the neck. Homicide. Rape.

Accidental hanging occasionally occurs; usually the victim is one of a group of children playing realistically with a lasso, or an individual who has fallen and entangled himself in a coil of rope in such a way that he is hanged or strangled by a loop around his neck. In one case a person fell while climbing a ladder, and caught his neck in between the rungs; his air passages were fatally compressed while he was thus suspended and large irregular abrasions were inflicted on the anterior surface of the neck. Homicidal hanging is rare and usually perpetrated by a mob.

Hanging as a method of legal execution is employed in some states and countries. Such judicial hangings have little similarity to the ordinary suicidal types encountered among the civilian population. The condemned person, with the noose adjusted around his neck, is made to fall six feet or more, and brought up with a jerk at the end of the rope; death occurs from a combination of shock, crushing of the spinal cord by dislocation and fracture of the upper cervical vertebrae and asphyxia. If the drop is insufficient, the cervical spine may not break and the victim dies of asphyxiation.

Strangulation by Ligature. The pressure on the neck in ligature strangulation is applied by a constricting band which is tightened by some force other than the body weight.

Most ligature strangulations in New York City are homicidal; they comprise about 1 per cent of all homicides and are encountered on an average of three to four times a year. In some instances the victim is surprised by the assailant and easily overcome, or stunned by a blow and then strangled. The implement used may

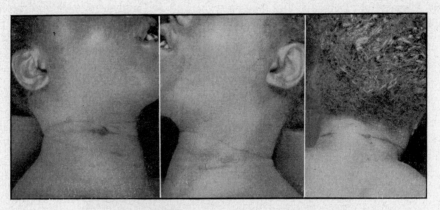

Fig. 17-7. Homicidal Ligature Strangulation.

Ligature marks produced by thin twine looped three times around the neck.

be a handkerchief or towel which is thrown around the neck and twisted tight with the hands as in the bow string strangulations formerly carried out in Turkey. A coil of rope is sometimes used, and either twisted or pulled tight in the form of a noose. In some cases a stocking is tied around the neck by the assailant. Neckties,

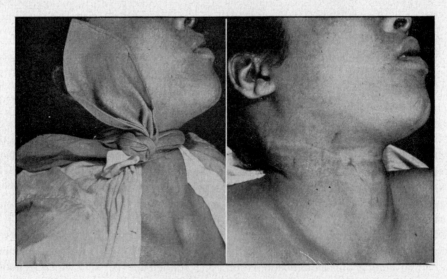

Fig. 17-8. Homicidal Ligature Strangulation.

Necktie tied with a double knot. Note corresponding shallow impression of knot on neck.

leather belts, electric cords, twine and other ligatures are also employed (Figs. 17-6 through 17-10). Ligature strangulation is sometimes used as a method of infanticide (Fig. 23-4). Another variety of strangulation is encountered in gang murders in which the victim, usually a member of a rival gang, is trussed up with coils of rope which constrict the neck, mouth, cheeks, arms and legs; the autopsy reveals death by asphyxia and marks on the bodies caused by the binding rope. In overcrowded and understaffed mental hospitals, psychopathic patients have strangled one another with strips of cloth. In a recent case the victim was helplessly restrained in a camisole at the time she was killed by strangulation. Judicial strangulation was formerly a method of execution in Spain; it was carried out with a constricting device known as a garotte which when tightened also pierced the back of the neck and spinal cord with a dagger attachment.

Strangulation with a ligature is sometimes employed as a means of suicide; a cord, rope or other ligature appropriated from the clothing such as a bath robe cord

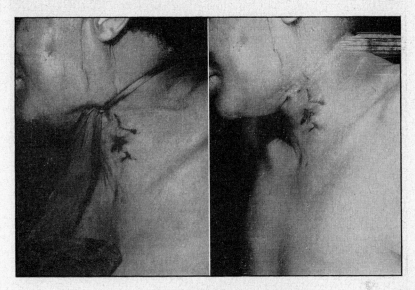

Fig. 17-9. Homicidal Ligature Strangulation.

Silk stocking knotted tightly in front of neck. Grouped abrasions on side of neck produced by fingers of assailant.

or a dress belt, can be looped and tied tightly around the neck, or can be applied and tightened as a noose by the hand of the victim himself. In several suicidal cases, a leather belt was looped one or more times around the neck, tightened and then secured by merely fastening the buckle. Puppe has described a strangulation in which the deceased placed a noose around his neck, fastened the free end of the noosed ligature to a fixed point near the floor, and then by assuming a supine position strangled himself by pushing himself away from the point of attachment with his legs; in such a case the mechanism of asphyxiation is similar to hanging. In suicidal strangulation, the ligature may be wrapped around the neck one or several times but the knot is usually a simple one such as the victim himself could tie before losing consciousness. Examples of suicidal strangulation are illustrated in Figures 17-11 through 17-14.

Accidental death by ligature strangulation is rare, but it may occur when an individual becomes entangled in a rope while at work, or is the victim of a practical joke. If he is very drunk, a comparatively slight degree of constriction of the neck may cause a fatal asphyxia; an alcoholic may strangle himself by clumsily wrapping the bedclothes around his neck or by inadvertently resting his throat against the projecting side of the bed. Occasionally infants in cribs are strangled by becoming

tangled in the clothes, or by forcing their heads under the snug ties of a restraining
garment or blanket intended to prevent them from falling out of the bed. A violent
psychopathic patient may strangle himself if left unattended in improperly applied
restraints. In a few instances, a victim has strangled himself inadvertently while
constricting his neck for the purpose of arousing erotic sensations.

In most ligature strangulations as in hanging, death occurs rapidly. Examination
of the undisturbed body at the scene of death is most important. The arrangement

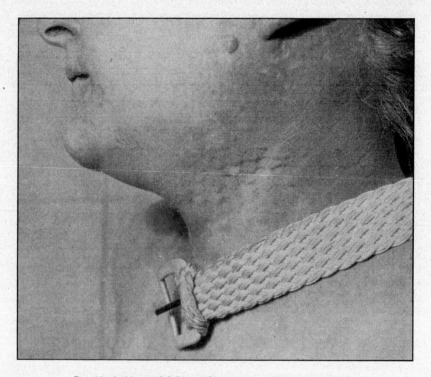

Fig. 17-10. Homicidal Strangulation with a Woven Cord Belt.

Note pattern of fabric imprinted on left side of neck. Perpetrator surrendered and confessed strangling victim manually, not mentioning use of belt until confronted with it. Belt
had been removed and was found on chair near body. Necropsy did not reveal evidence of
manual strangulation.

of the ligatures and of the knots as well as the surroundings will enable the trained
observer to distinguish the homicidal, suicidal and accidental cases. If ligatures
which were present on the body are untied or removed before the medical investigator has examined them, he may find it difficult if not impossible to determine the
nature of the strangulation. In homicidal cases, the perpetrator may remove the
ligature and the examiner will have to depend on the presence of marks produced
by it together with the asphyxial signs to diagnose the case correctly. The absence
of the ligature generally precludes a suicidal or accidental interpretation except in
suicidal cases in which there are indications that it has been removed by someone
who desired to conceal the fact that death was self-inflicted.

In an unusual homicidal ligature strangulation, encountered by the authors, the
victim in his struggle tore loose a tightly knotted heavy twine ligature which was
found in his hands at the scene of death. In another case the victim, an elderly

woman, was strangled with a stocking. This had evidently been removed at some later time for a conspicuous dry furrow was found on the neck and the rolled-up ligature, cut across with a knife or scissors but with the knots undisturbed, was found on the floor next to the bed in which the body of the deceased was discovered. It is not an overstatement to say that in all deaths from traumatic asphyxia, such as strangulation, suffocation or smothering, the preliminary examination of the body and the surroundings is fully as important as the autopsy. It should never be omitted from the investigation.

In cases where the ligature has been promptly removed before it has produced any pronounced pressure marks on the neck, the development of postmortem putre-

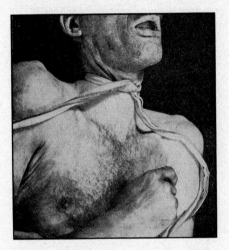

Fig. 17-11. Suicidal Ligature Strangulation.

Dressing gown belt around neck and tied in front with single knot. Body found in prone position.

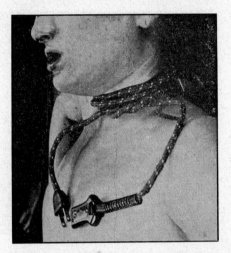

Fig. 17-12. Suicidal Ligature Strangulation.

Multiple turns of electric cord around neck. Body found in prone position on floor.

faction may completely obscure the ligature marks as well as the general signs of asphyxiation. In hot weather the examination of the dead body at the scene and the autopsy should not be delayed longer than is absolutely necessary. The same difficulty may arise with smothering asphyxiation.

Before performing the autopsy in a death from ligature strangulation, the body should be photographed with the undisturbed ligatures in place to show the looping and the arrangement of the knots. In removing the ligature, it is best to cut the strands in a region where they are not overlapped and away from the knots which should be preserved. The cut ends can be made secure with adhesive tape or tied with string to prevent their unraveling. The entire ligature with the knots intact should be preserved as an important part of the corpus delicti. After the ligature has been removed, the neck should be photographed to show the furrowed impression produced by it. In cases where the ligatures are multiple and applied in layers, the photographs should be taken serially to show the details of the application and the multiplicity of the devices employed. Figures 17-8, 17-9, 17-10 and 17-13 illustrate homicidal and suicidal ligature strangulations before and after the ligatures have been removed.

The constricting band in ligature strangulation is horizontally pressed against the larynx and produces a horizontal mark on the neck, similar to but usually at a lower level than the marks produced in hanging; in the ligature cases the element of bodily suspension is not present so that the marks do not slant upward as a rule. In a few instances the ligature may constrict the upper portion of the neck and produce a dislocation of the tongue upward and backward as already described under hanging on page 456. In most cases, however, the larynx is pressed backward against the posterior pharyngeal wall, the anteroposterior diameter is shortened and its lumen is closed; in a few cases the larynx may be compressed laterally and the air passages occluded. The great blood vessels of the neck are constricted, the veins usually more than the arteries. The compression is not as severe as in hanging so that the veins may be closed while the arteries remain patent; as a result a marked

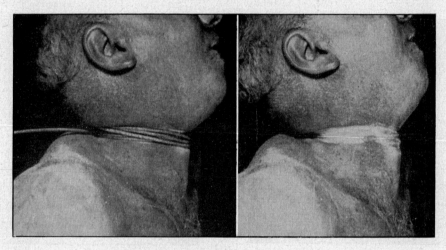

Fig. 17-13. Suicidal Ligature Strangulation.

Multiple turns of rope around neck. Body found in prone position. Note contrast between pallor of broad composite furrow and adjacent livid skin.

cyanosis of the head and neck may be produced. The compression of the jugular veins and the incomplete closure of the carotid arteries also results in the development of fine punctate and coarser hemorrhages in the skin of the face, in the conjunctiva (Fig. 17-15), and in the lining of the scalp and fascia over the temporal muscles, the latter evident when the scalp is reflected. Injury to the vagus nerve and its superior branches may cause shock and be a factor in the rapidity of death in some cases.

In deaths from ligature strangulation, the usual findings at autopsy are the ligature marks on the neck, cyanosis of the head and face, blotchy and punctate hemorrhages in the bulbar and palpebral conjunctiva, very fine or irregular punctate hemorrhages on the face, discrete and confluent hemorrhages in the galea of the scalp and over the temporal muscles, mucosal and submucosal hemorrhages in the pharynx and larynx, and general signs of asphyxia such as congestion and cyanosis of the organs, an abundance of dark red fluid blood in a dilated heart and in the large vessels, subpleural and subpericardial hemorrhages and overaeration of the marginal alveoli of the lungs. Hemorrhages in the brain have not been encountered by the authors although there is usually marked venous engorgement in that organ. The number of petechial hemorrhages beneath the visceral pleura and the epicardium may be very few. Protrusion of the tongue may or may not occur. Hemorrhages in the muscles of the neck, fractures of the laryngeal cartilages and hyoid bone, intimal tears of the cervical blood vessels and tears of the neck muscles, although described in the literature, have not been encountered by the authors in ligature strangulation.

Among the ligature strangulations investigated by the Medical Examiner's Office in New York City, there was a case in which the asphyxiation was produced gradually. The victim, profoundly alcoholic, was found dead on his back in bed, his necktie tied snugly around his neck; the face was cyanotic and there was foam oozing from his mouth. There were no furrow

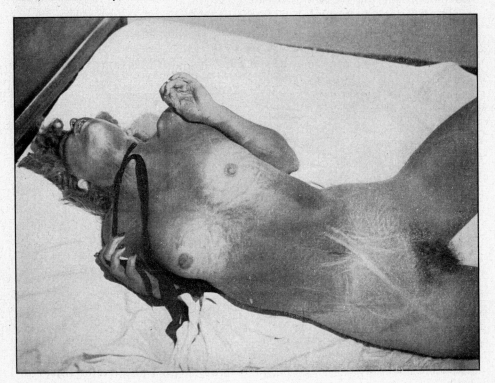

Fig. 17-14. Suicidal Ligature Strangulation.

Cloth dress belt around neck and tied tightly in front with a single knot. Body found nude in prone position on bed. Complete statute-like rigor mortis evident in photograph of turned over body.

marks around the neck, indicating that the necktie had not been exerting extraordinary compression. The lungs were very heavy and edematous. All the findings indicated that there was sufficient pressure to induce a certain amount of asphyxia without the respiratory passages being completely closed off. This effect, together with the depressing action of the alcohol, caused a slow respiratory paralysis and a gradual circulatory failure.

Occasionally after the prompt removal of the ligature in a case of strangulation, the victim can be revived by artificial respiration and by other measures. Even though he is revived, he may have been so affected by the trauma as to die from shock within a few hours, or later from a complicating bronchopneumonia.

Manual Strangulation or Throttling. Throttling is produced by pressure of the hand or forearm against the neck and air passages. Practically all of these cases are homicidal. In New York City, there are about three such cases a year, comprising about 1 per cent of the total number of homicides. Using one or both hands the assailant may grasp the neck and compress the sides of the larynx, thus closing the opening of the glottis. In other cases, the hand exerts pressure against the front of the larynx and closes the lumen by shortening its anteroposterior diameter. In some cases of throttling, the base of the tongue is forced backward and upward as described under hanging and the opening of the glottis is closed. Unfortunately it is not always possible to ascertain from the findings at autopsy how the strangling force has been applied, since the compression of the neck is temporary and the normal elasticity of the involved structures tends to return them to their customary relationships after the pressure is released.

The force may be applied in several ways. If one hand is used, either right or left, it may grasp the neck in front, the thumb exerting pressure on one side, the fingers on the other, and the palm of the hand forcing the neck organs backward at the same time. Both hands may be applied to the throat from in front, the thumbs

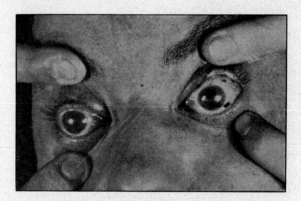

Fig. 17-15. Homicidal Ligature Strangulation.

Punctate asphyxial hemorrhages in conjunctivae. Eyelids held separated during photography.

digging in over the anterior part of the larynx and pressing the air passages back, and the fingers grasping the sides and back of the neck; or the assailant may be behind his victim, his fingers grasping the throat in front and exerting backward and lateral compression while his thumbs press against the sides and back of the neck.

Manual strangulation has been accomplished by pressing the palm of the hand on the front part of the neck without employing the fingers. This method was used by a man who strangled his two children, aged 5 and 7 years, as they lay sleeping on their backs, one at the foot and the other at the head of the bed; he pressed one palm on the throat of one child and his other palm on the throat of the other simultaneously, until they ceased to struggle. The autopsy disclosed only the signs of asphyxiation, without any marks on the skin and without injuries to the deeper structures of the neck.

In the method of strangulation known as mugging, the assailant, standing either in front or in back of the victim, applies his forearm against the front of the neck in the laryngeal region. In wrestling this type of violence is known as the strangle hold, and it is strictly barred because of its danger. In a case of homicidal assault with intent to rape, the perpetrator lay on top of the supine victim and strangled her by pressing the ulnar side of his flexed forearm against her larynx; at autopsy there were no external marks of violence on the neck but the cricoid cartilage of the larynx was found extensively fractured. In street robberies, the assailant may attack the victim from the rear, bringing the radial side of his bent forearm against the front part of the neck so as to compress the air passages. Fatal mugging usually results in extensive injuries to the deeper structures of the neck but produces few or no cutaneous lesions. In some instances a foot is pressed against the front part of the neck during a scuffle and causes severe injuries to the throat organs.

During manual strangulation, the neck receives considerable mauling, and strong pressure is applied intermittently to the region of the larynx. The air passages are blocked and the vessels of the neck are compressed, with resulting asphyxiation and disturbance of the blood supply to the brain. The nerves are also traumatized, especially the superior laryngeal branches of the glossopharyngeal and hypoglossal

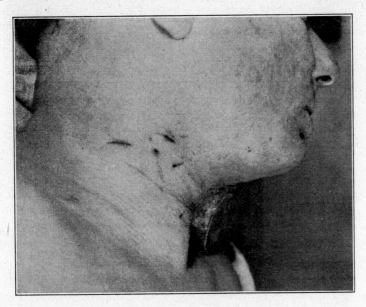

Fig. 17-16. Manual Strangulation, Throttling.

The grouped linear and curved abrasions on the side of the neck were made by the finger-nails of the assailant.

nerves, and the plexuses surrounding the bifurcation of the common carotid arteries which are formed chiefly by fibers from the vagus and sympathetic nerves. Death may supervene abruptly from shock and cardiac inhibition at any time during the manual strangulation as the result of sudden pressure on this plexus, inducing the carotid sinus or Hering reflex, even before asphyxia is far advanced. Death is apt to occur more readily from shock if the victim is under the influence of alcohol.

The findings at necropsy in manual strangulation are more variable than those encountered when the neck is compressed by a ligature. The general signs of asphyxia, such as cyanosis; suffusion of blood in the head, neck and fingers; small hemorrhages in the galea of the scalp, conjunctivae, face, eyelids, shoulders and chest; congestion of the brain, lungs and other viscera; fluid blood in the heart; distention of the right ventricle; and petechial hemorrhages over pleurae and peri-cardium are not always developed to a conspicuous degree. In a few instances, the tongue is found protruding between the teeth. Very rarely are small hemorrhages found in the brain substance and its membranes. Overdistention of the lungs and of the air vesicles and interstitial emphysema are occasionally encountered, more especially in infants.

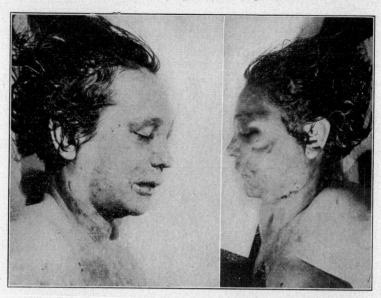

From Gonzales, T. A., *Arch. Path.*, 15:55, 1933

Fig. 17-17. Manual Strangulation. Fingernail Impressions.

Curved impression of thumbnail on right side of neck. Grouped abrasions on left side of neck probably produced by other fingers. Neck grasped from the front. Homicide and rape.

External marks of injury may be found on the neck after manual strangulation but not invariably. In some cases in which the palm of the hand or part of the forearm has been pressed against the throat, there are no external signs of violence evident on the skin even though the cartilages of the larynx are fractured. In other cases there is a profusion of indefinite abrasions and contusions on the face and

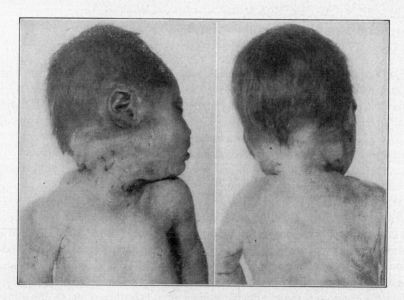

Fig. 17-18. Manual Strangulation. Fingernail Impressions.

Curved thumbnail impression on back of neck. Grouped fingernail impressions on right side of neck. The neck was grasped from behind and on the right side. Infanticide.

neck, not characteristic of any particular kind of violence. When the neck is grasped by the fingers, the fingernails may produce small semilunar abrasions of one fourth to one half inch in length and about a sixteenth of an inch or less in width. If only one hand has grasped the throat, it may be possible to recognize the thumb impression on one side of the neck and the other finger nail marks on the opposite side; in other cases the skin injuries may suggest a different application of the hands. The curved abrasions, variable in number, may be arranged discretely in groups, confined to small circumscribed areas, usually on the sides of the larynx, but they may occur on the front, sides or back of the neck. In some instances the finger nails may penetrate more deeply into the skin, especially if they are long and the victim struggles, and inflict larger grouped excoriations with a geographic pattern and also scattered irregular scratch marks. Figures 17-16 through 17-19 illustrate various

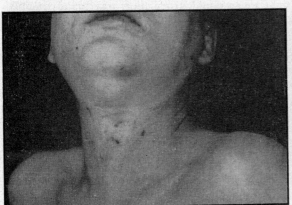

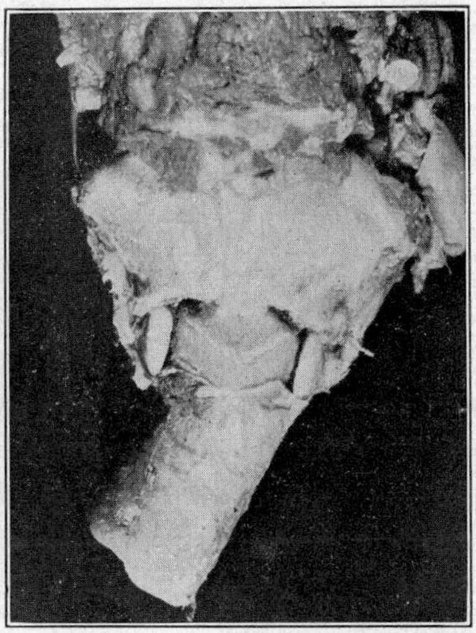

From *Arch. Path.*, 15:55, 1933

Fig. 17-19. Homicidal Manual Strangulation.

Grouped abrasions on front of neck produced by fingers of assailant. Victim also raped. Dried semen found on pubic hair, thighs and vulva. Spermatozoa found in vaginal smears.

Fig. 17-20. Manual Strangulation. Fracture of Laryngeal Cartilage.

Double symmetric fracture of cricoid cartilage. Homicide.

types of skin injuries produced during manual strangulation. Histologic examination of skin lesions reveals the characteristics of abrasions, including flattening of the squamous epithelium, with elongation of the cell nuclei, and defects in places from which the epidermis was removed. The skin marks are associated with and indicative of the more serious injuries of the deeper structures of the throat and neck. Not frequently contusions and abrasions of the skin are found elsewhere on the body and on the mucous membranes of the lips, tongue and mouth and usually but not necessarily indicate a struggle during the perpetration of the crime.

The injuries within the throat and neck produced by manual strangulation include contusion hemorrhages in and between the muscles, in the thyroid gland and salivary glands, and asphyxial petechial hemorrhages in the pharyngeal and laryngeal mucous membranes. Contusions and tears of the thyrohyoid membrane, and fractures of the cartilages of the larynx and of the hyoid bone are also produced; the thyroid and cricoid cartilages and hyoid bone are injured most frequently (Figs. 17-20 and 17-21).

In a series of 24 cases of manual strangulation described by Gonzales, 13 showed the following fractures: lateral ala of thyroid cartilage, 3; anterior arch of cricoid cartilage, 2; cricoid and thyroid combined, 3; superior cornua of thyroid cartilage, 1; hyoid bone, 4 (body, 1, right greater cornu, 1, right greater cornu and tearing of right thyrohyoid membrane, 1, left greater cornu associated with injury of cricoid cartilage, 1). Tears of the sternomastoid muscles and injuries of the arytenoid cartilages of the larynx, tracheal rings, cervical vessels and nerves were not encountered in this series but have been described by others.

The fractures of the thyroid cartilage are usually longitudinal, involving the mid portion or the ala, and rarely running in a crosswise or oblique direction. The cricoid cartilage is usually injured in front or on the sides and the fractures are vertical. The superior horns of the thyroid may be broken, while the arytenoid cartilages are rarely involved. The body and greater cornua of the hyoid bone may be fractured, usually in a vertical direction, and the thyrohyoid ligament contused or torn. In rare instances some of the upper tracheal cartilages sustain vertical fractures anteriorly. As a result of a mugging, the right thyrocricoid articulation was found forcibly luxated and its ligaments torn. Hemorrhages occurring around the fractures and in the laryngeal and adjacent structures are an important indication that the damage was inflicted during life. In this connection it must be remembered that the greater cornua of the hyoid are sometimes loosely attached to the body of the bone by fibrous union and the mobility of the process may lead the inexperienced observer to diagnose such an articulation erroneously as a fracture. Similarly the superior process of the thyroid cartilage may be loosely attached to the body by fibrous tissue and be mistaken for a fracture. However a careful dissection of the neck organs should reveal the true nature of such articulations.

Hemorrhages of varying size from petechiae to large effusions of blood are often present in the submucous layer of the larynx and pharynx. The muscles of the neck and the intermuscular tissues may also reveal hemorrhages of different size. Injuries caused by manual strangulation are similar in infants, adolescents and young adults to those produced in more mature victims, except that in younger persons fractures of the laryngeal cartilages and of the hyoid bone may not occur because of the greater resiliency and elasticity of these structures in young people. The important consideration in such cases is to establish the antemortem nature of the injuries and also indications that they were produced by violence of a type sufficient to cause a fatal compression of the throat organs.

Some victims of manual strangulation die after comparatively slight pressure on the throat, without fracture of the laryngeal cartilages or hyoid bone and with characteristic grouped abrasions on the neck present or absent. Alcoholic individuals may be asphyxiated easily by manual compression of the neck and succumb without revealing any demonstrable sign of violence at autopsy. If localized pressure is applied to the carotid plexus or sinus, death may occur suddenly without any trace of violence to the neck organs or elsewhere; even the general signs of an asphyxial death may be lacking.

The attending circumstances in all cases of manual strangulation are important. The crime is usually committed in a fit of anger or jealousy, and the victim is weaker than the perpetrator, or is temporarily helpless from alcohol, drugs or sleep. If two persons have about the same physical development, manual strangulation is not a likely method of homicide unless the perpetrator manages to catch his victim at a disadvantage. A number of throttlings occur during rape or violation, and the victim is either a woman or a child. Some infanticides are carried out by manual strangulation. Occasionally the method is used during the perpetration of a robbery if the chances are favorable. There are reports of individuals who have recovered from the effects of manual strangulation, even with laryngeal fractures, but such cases are rare.

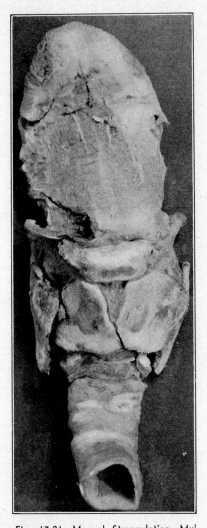

Fig. 17-21. Manual Strangulation. Multiple Fractures of Laryngeal Cartilages.

Double fractures of hyoid bone, thyroid and cricoid cartilages. Homicide.

Each case must be evaluated carefully and all the circumstances thoroughly investigated. The marks on the skin, the signs of asphyxia, the injuries within the neck and the presence of alcohol in the body, are criteria which must be considered before finally classifying the death. It is important to determine reliable criteria which will establish that the injuries of the neck are antemortem; thus if grouped abrasions are present on the skin of the neck, and hemorrhages are found in the submucosa and intrinsic muscles of the larynx, it is correct to conclude that the trauma was inflicted during life; similarly if there are fractures of the laryngeal cartilages and hyoid bone, accompanied by small hemorrhages in their immediate neighborhood, that fact would establish the intravital nature of the injury even in the absence of any skin abrasions.

The medical investigator must be cautioned that a group of abrasions on the front of the neck does not necessarily mean that death is due to manual strangulation, although such a possibility should always be considered and the death investigated with that possibility in mind. In one instance a 50 year old white man was found dead, partly dressed in a shirt with a collar button attached, his neck revealing a small group of indefinite abrasions and scratch marks over his adam's apple. The autopsy and chemical examination later disclosed that there were no significant injuries in the neck and that death was the result of alcoholism. The abrasions of the neck were evidently produced by the collar button which scratched the skin, possibly during the violent convulsive movements incident to the alcoholism.

Whether a man can strangle himself by squeezing his own throat with his hands is a disputed point. Puppe described such a case in which an insane individual had done this but doubted if the death could be considered suicide by manual strangulation alone inasmuch as the deceased was partly smothered in bed clothes at the same time. In a case recently commented upon in the Journal of the American Medical Association the death of a boy occurred while he was practicing jiu jitsu holds on his own neck. The commentator discounted the possibility that death was asphyxial but suggested that the deceased may have inadvertently exerted pressure on his carotid sinus, causing death by reflex stoppage of the heart or the Hering reflex.

Fractures of the laryngeal cartilages and hyoid bone can result from blows or kicks directed against the front part of the neck. The resulting damage may be slight, involving only the superior processes of the thyroid cartilage or the cornua of the hyoid bone, or the injury may be severe and the cartilages of the larynx extensively shattered. Death may occur immediately at the time of the injury from severe shock; occasionally it is delayed several hours, as in the case of a woman who was brought into the hospital with fractures of the cricoid cartilage and a hematoma in the submucous layer of the larynx which gradually increased in size and caused death by obstructing the air passages. Similar delayed deaths may occur from laryngeal edema or emphysema following blunt force injuries to the larynx. In some cases, a sudden blow over the larynx without fracture of the cartilages causes a fatal collapse because of the Hering reflex in which cardiac paralysis is brought about by stimulation of the carotid sinus nerve plexus; this is especially liable to occur in persons who are profoundly alcoholic or who are suffering from cardiac or cerebral disease.

REFERENCES

Current Comment. Can self-applied jiu jitsu cause death? J.A.M.A., 123:152, 1943.
Gonzales, T. A. Manual strangulation, Arch. Path., 15:55, 1933.
Puppe, G. Atlas und Grundriss der Gerichtlichen Medizin, München, J. F. Lehmann, 1908.
Reports of the Office of the Chief Medical Examiner in the City of New York from 1918 to 1951.

18

Traumatic Asphyxia: Suffocation; External Pressure on Chest; Drowning

SUFFOCATION

Suffocation may be defined as a form of traumatic asphyxia which results when an obstruction of the air passages prevents the entrance of air into the lungs. By strict interpretation, the different forms of strangulation belong to this category, but they have been considered separately because of their well-defined charactertistics which distinguish them from the other forms of traumatic asphyxiation. The varieties now to be discussed are smothering and choking in which the asphyxia is caused by substances blocking the lumen of the air passages.

Smothering. Smothering occurs whenever the external openings of the air passages, the nose and mouth, are mechanically closed off by a solid object or finely divided material. Most fatal smotherings are accidental and in New York average about 45 cases a year; homicidal and suicidal deaths from this cause are relatively uncommon. An intoxicated person may smother himself accidentally by burying his face in a pillow or covering it inadvertently with the bed clothes, especially when the depression of the central nervous system from alcoholism renders the victim easily susceptible to asphyxiation. Young infants are sometimes accidentally smothered as the result of carelessness on the part of the mother or nurse who arranges the bed clothes so that they cover the nose and mouth of the baby. If the mother is in bed with the infant she may smother it accidentally by overlying it during sleep. An individual unable to help himself may accidentally fall into a large quantity of semisolid or finely divided material like mud, plaster, ashes, feathers, grain or coal so that his mouth and nose are engulfed by the substance. If the air supply is completely cut off and at the same time the movement of the chest is hindered by the compression, death may occur rapidly from asphyxiation, but if the obstruction of the air passages is partial and the chest is free to expand, the asphyxiation is more gradual in its onset and death may not occur for several minutes or hours. The victim may struggle, inhale some of the material into his air passages and gulp some into his stomach in an intense effort to breathe. Usually the head and the upper part of the body become markedly cyanotic. Several cases have been encountered in which the victims were buried under an avalanche of pea coal after falling into a coal chute. Two of the victims were rescued alive, one dying within a short time, the other surviving for a period of two hours; the body of another was found dead. The autopsy in each case revealed a marked cyanosis of the head, inhalation of fine coal into the trachea and larger bronchi (Fig. 18-1) and a small amount of swallowed coal in the stomach. If the victim does not aspirate too much of the material and manages to survive the immediate effects of the suffocation, the substance inhaled may cause an aspiration pneumonia or a lung abscess.

Some smotherings are homicidal (Fig. 18-2). During the commission of a

475

robbery, the victim may be bound and gagged and the gag so arranged as to cover both nose and mouth. A towel may be used and wrapped around the lower part of the face, or a pad is held in place with strips of adhesive tape in such a way as to block both orifices. In some cases the nose is not occluded but the gag is crammed into the mouth so forcibly as to displace the soft palate and the tongue back against the posterior wall of the pharynx and cause a fatal occlusion of the air passages. In one such case almost an entire towel was stuffed into the mouth.

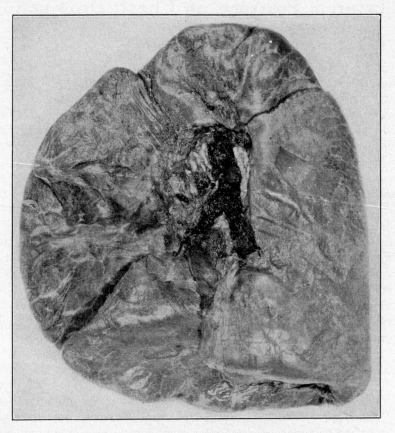

Fig. 18-1. Accidental Smothering in a Coal Pile.

Deceased was buried under a pile of falling coal. The trachea and larger bronchi of the lung have been cut open to show the inhaled coal fragments. The deceased lived two hours after his rescue.

Another method of homicidal smothering is known as burking and derives its name from the fact that it was employed by Burke and his accomplice Hare to obtain a supply of bodies which were then sold to the medical schools in Edinburgh during the early part of the nineteenth century. The victim rendered helpless by drink was thrown to the ground and held by the weight of the assailant's body on his chest; one hand was then placed over the victim's nose and mouth and the other hand pressed the lower jaw towards the upper, the combined maneuver causing rapid asphyxiation and little if any external evidence of violence. Smothering has also been accomplished by pressing a pillow over the face of the supine victim (Fig. 18-3), or by forcing the face of a victim lying prone into the pillow (Fig. 18-4).

The case illustrated in Figure 18-3 is an excellent example of the importance of the medical examiner's visit to the scene and examination of the undisturbed dead body in its surroundings. When discovered, the body of the young white woman had been dead about 24 hours and post-mortem decomposition had already begun to set in. Examination of the supine body revealed small pin-point sized asphyxial hemorrhages in the whites of the eyes, a finding especially significant in a supine body in which decomposition had not yet advanced too far. There were no other signs of traumatic injury and the only other finding in the room to suggest a violent death by smothering was a blurred lipstick impression of the mouth of the deceased on a rumpled pillowcase next to her head. A police investigation resulted in the apprehension of the victim's estranged husband with whom she had registered at the hotel. He at first denied any knowl-

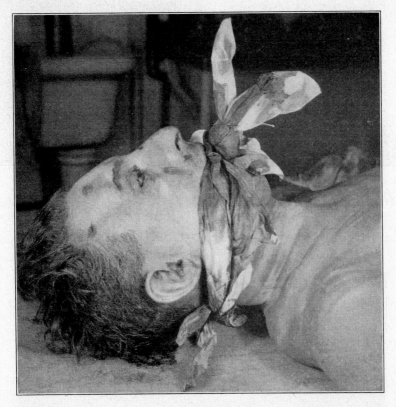

Fig. 18-2. Homicidal Smothering with Handkerchief Used as a Gag During Robbery.

edge of her death but when confronted with the red smudge on the pillowcase, confessed that he had smothered her and then arranged the body and scene to make it appear as if she had died in her sleep. By the time the body had been moved to the mortuary for autopsy the next morning, postmortem decomposition had been accelerated and was so far advanced as to destroy the significance of the asphyxial hemorrhages in the eyes had they been seen for the first time without a firsthand knowledge of the circumstances under which the body was found. The visit to the scene in a smothering case is as important as if not more important than the autopsy in determining the cause of death and character of the violence.

When such homicidal methods are used there is generally a considerable preponderance of strength of the perpetrator over that of the deceased, and such crimes are usually committed in the heat of anger or passion. Similar methods are used in committing infanticide. In rare instances, homicidal and infanticidal smothering is accomplished by throwing or causing the victim to fall into semisolid or finely divided material like coal dust, sand, ashes or similar substance.

Suicidal smotherings are comparatively rare. In one such case the deceased

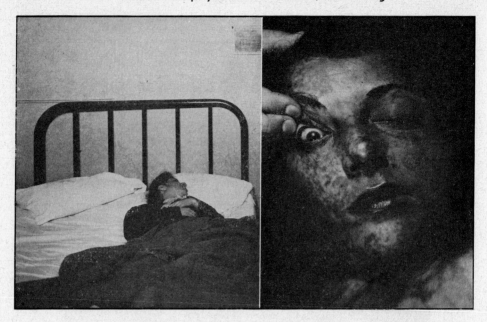

Fig. 18-3. Homicidal Smothering with a Pillow.

Left. Photograph of scene of undisturbed dead body where examination revealed no signs of violence except punctate asphyxial conjunctival hemorrhages, and smudged lipstick impressions on pillow case near head.

Right. Hemorrhages in conjunctiva photographed at autopsy. See text.

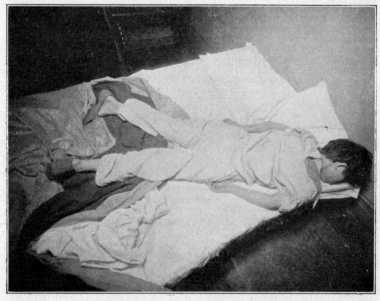

Courtesy Police Dept., City of New York

Fig. 18-4. Homicidal Smothering with Pillow.

Undisturbed position of body as discovered at scene. There were no external marks of injury. Only signs of asphyxia were found at autopsy. Perpetrator confessed that he forced face of deceased down into pillow to stifle her screams.

crammed a bath towel into her mouth, forcing the tongue back far enough to block the nasopharynx. In another the suicide tied a small pillow over her face so that it covered her nose and mouth; it was held in place with two stocking ligatures wrapped around another small pillow placed at the back of the head, so that the head

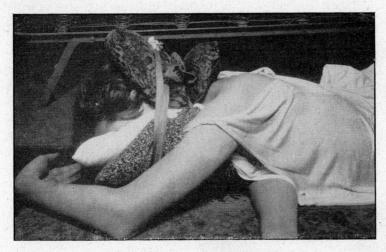

Fig. 18-5. Suicidal Smothering with a Pillow.

The pillow covering the face was tied in place with stockings. Additional pillows were placed in front and in back, over which the stockings were tied. Body found on floor in prone position next to bed.

was cushioned between them (Fig. 18-5). Another person smothered herself by placing two broad pieces of adhesive plaster across her nose and mouth (Fig. 18-6).

The anatomic findings at autopsy in cases of smothering are those of asphyxia, and in addition there may be evidence indicating the method by which the victim

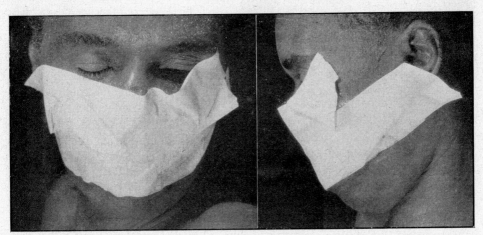

Fig. 18-6. Suicidal Smothering.

Two wide overlapping strips of adhesive plaster covered the nose and mouth.

was smothered such as the presence of a gag on the face or in the mouth, or of finely divided material in the air passages; in cases in which the hand or a pillow has been held over the face, abrasions and a faint scuffing of the skin from rubbing may be seen on the tip of the nose and around the mouth, or the features may show distortion from continuous violent compression if the object used was allowed to remain in place for any length of time. If the smothering has been rapid and sudden, the principal signs will be those of asphyxia, such as cyanosis of the face, small circular ecchymoses in the galea of the scalp, punctate hemorrhages in the conjunctivae, and dark red fluid blood in the heart. If the process of smothering is less rapid and asphyxiation takes longer, marked cyanosis, hyperaeration, and edema of the lungs may develop. The larynx and pharynx may or may not show any cyanosis or submucosal hemorrhages. If the death is homicidal, it is necessary for the medical investigator to establish the method of smothering; the diagnosis cannot be made with certainty until a complete autopsy has been performed and the scene and circumstances of death investigated. In smothering cases the prompt examination of the undisturbed dead body at the scene is of prime importance, almost as much so as the autopsy, and may be the only means of obtaining the information that will conclusively establish whether the smothering was homicidal, suicidal or accidental. Postmortem decomposition may destroy or obscure subtle evidences of asphyxial death resulting from smothering, especially in cases in which the smothering device has been removed or the body not examined at the scene.

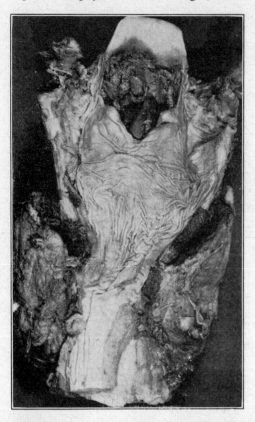

Fig. 18-7. Asphyxia by Choking on Bolus of Food.

Sudden death caused by the aspiration of a piece of frankfurter into larynx. The deceased was a 37 year old woman who was suffering from postencephalitic Parkinson's disease.

Choking. Choking occurs when solid objects or materials enter and obstruct the lumen of the air passages, preventing air from reaching the lungs. Most cases are accidental. An individual, suffering from acute alcoholism or severe cerebral arteriosclerosis to the extent that the deglutition reflex is disturbed, may attempt to swallow too large a bolus of food with the result that the bolus enters the larynx instead of the esophagus, causing sudden death by laryngeal obstruction, asphyxia and shock (Fig. 18-7). In some cases the bolus may be held in the pharynx and close the laryngeal opening. In the case of a body whose tonsils were removed under ether anesthesia, a long gauze pad was left in the throat and was aspirated into the opening of the larynx, causing a rapidly fatal asphyxia (Fig. 18-8).

Other accidental chokings have occurred in which older infants have aspirated objects such as coins, marbles, sunflower seeds, lima beans (Fig. 18-9) or similar foreign bodies into the larynx and trachea. If the object passes the narrow laryngeal aperture and reaches the trachea or bronchi, the obstruction is not always complete and death may not occur for several hours; the chief findings at autopsy are marked cyanosis, hyperaeration of lungs, over distention groups of alveoli and scattered areas of atelectasis, probably the result of excessive mucus in the bronchi.

Vomitus in many cases is regurgitated and aspirated into the lungs. This phenomenon is common in acute alcoholics or during operations under ether anesthesia, or in young infants who may regurgitate some of their food into the laryngeal open-

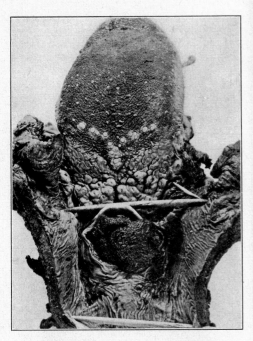

Fig. 18-8. Asphyxia by Choking on Inhaled Gauze Pad.

Aspiration of gauze pad into larynx. Gauze was left in throat after tonsillectomy under ether anesthesia.

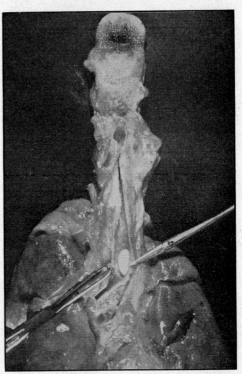

Fig. 18-9. Accidental Choking.

A lima bean was aspirated into the trachea by a young child. Trachea opened to show the bean blocking a main bronchus.

ing. Death from asphyxia may result sometimes rapidly or sometimes slowly. In the latter event, stomach contents may be carried down into the finer ramifications of the bronchial tree, and considerable cyanosis and acute pulmonary distention may be present. If the victim survives the first effects of the aspiration, a necrotic pneumonic infiltration may follow and cause death by sepsis.

Occasionally blood is inhaled into the lung because of various injuries of the head and throat, but death is usually due to some other factor. In one case, however, in which the victim was shot through the pharynx, the bullet wounds oozed blood which was swallowed and then molded into long cylindric clots by the rugae of the stomach; these clots were subsequently regurgitated and aspirated, completely filling and closing the laryngeal aperture and extending down into the trachea (Fig. 18-10). In a few of the traumatic cases, the aspirated blood undoubtedly favors the development of a subsequent bronchopneumonia or lung abscess.

Rarely choking is suicidal; in an autopsy by Dr. Henry Weinberg it was found that the deceased had stuffed his necktie into his pharynx and larynx, thus producing a fatal asphyxia. This case is discussed on page 104.

Choking as a means of infanticide may be effected by the perpetrator stuffing a wad of toilet paper or gauze into the pharynx or larynx (Fig. 18-11).

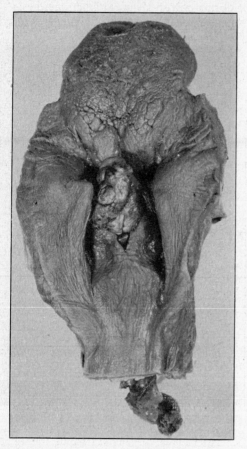

Fig. 18-10. Choking by Aspiration of Regurgitated Swallowed Blood.

The blood, which oozed from a homicidal bullet wound of the pharynx and was molded into long clots in the stomach, blocked the larynx.

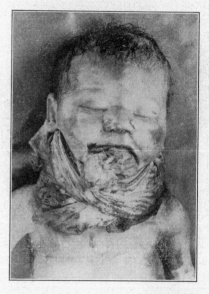

Fig. 18-11. Infanticidal Smothering with Gauze Gag Stuffed into Mouth.

Gauze ligature tied around neck. The violence is often excessive as illustrated.

ASPHYXIA BY EXTERNAL PRESSURE ON THE CHEST

Asphyxia may be produced by external pressure on the chest, which prevents air from entering or leaving the lungs by stopping the respiratory movements of the chest. In homicidal cases the assailant may kneel on the chest of the victim, or squeeze it with the arms or legs as in wrestling. The process of burking has been described. Accidental deaths are more common and are encountered when persons are crushed in a theater panic by the crowd which has become jammed in a doorway. The body of the victim exhibits a purplish black cyanosis of the face and neck; small subcutaneous petechial hemorrhages on the face, chest, shoulders and neck; congestion and petechial hemorrhages in the sclerae, conjunctivae and in the galea of the scalp, all attributable to compression of the trunk which prevents respiration and causes venous engorgement in the upper part of the body. The same effects are seen in accidents in which the body of the victim is squeezed between an elevator and one of the floors. In addition to the findings already described, there is usually a broad transverse abrasion across the front and back of the trunk due to pressure from the edges of the elevator and the floor. Similar compression of the chest may be produced when the victim is buried under a pile of sand or coal, or under rubble in a building collapse, or is crushed in a highway accident. In a recent catastrophe, a building collapsed while most of the occupants were asleep; some of the fatalities from compression asphyxia and smothering also exhibited conspicuous patterned imprints of the bedsprings on the otherwise livid back (Fig. 18-12).

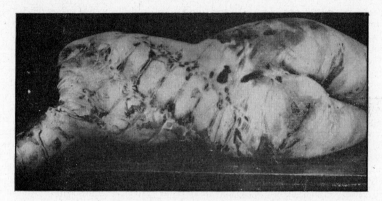

Fig. 18-12. Patterned Impression of Bedspring on Back.
The victim was crushed and smothered while in bed by the collapse of a tenement building.

DROWNING

Drowning is a form of suffocation occurring when the victim is submerged in water or other liquid which is inhaled into the air passages and pulmonary alveoli. The cause of death in 90 per cent of drownings is asphyxia resulting from the inhalation of water into the pulmonary alveoli and bronchi and the exclusion of air from the lungs. About 1 to 2 per cent of deaths occurring during submersion are the result of circulatory collapse or syncope, attributable to the shock of immersion in cold water, especially if the victim is physically weak or sick. The remaining 8 or 9 per cent of drowning deaths probably result from a combination of asphyxia and circulatory collapse. However, it would be a matter of considerable difficulty to determine just what did actually occur during a death from submersion unless an eyewitness was present. Drowning can occur if only the mouth and nose of the victim are covered by fluid without immersion of the entire body.

The symptoms displayed during drowning vary, depending upon circumstances. A few victims die of immediate shock shortly after they are plunged into cold water and cannot be revived even though rescued quickly. The asphyxial cases manifest different signs. In one type there is sudden chilling of the neck and chest, followed by an immediate inhalation of water at the moment of submersion, reflex spasm of the larynx, early unconsciousness and a rapid asphyxia. This reflex spasm is more likely to occur if the person is submerged with his face upward for then water flows readily through the nose into the laryngeal opening. In most instances, the victim after submersion, struggles to get to the surface, inhales water and becomes panicky; when he does emerge, he gulps a mixture of water and air and severe coughing and expiratory efforts follow. There is urgent need of oxygen, more water is inhaled and also swallowed, the respiratory movements become more violent, the face becomes cyanotic, the bladder and rectum may be emptied and unconsciousness sets in. During the period of unconsciousness before death, the respiratory movements of the submerged victim result in the inhalation of varying and considerable amounts of water. The process of drowning may take three to five minutes but may be prolonged to 10 minutes or more. After the respiratory movements stop, the heart may continue to beat for a short time. The relative coldness of the water in which most drownings occur usually causes a contraction of the arrectores pilorum muscles and the appearance of cutis anserina or goose flesh.

The treatment of persons rescued from submersion is the removal of water from the air passages and the manual application of artificial respiration. This is done usually by placing the victim in a prone position with the head and shoulders depressed so that water can flow from the trachea and bronchi out of the nose and mouth; the tongue may be drawn forward with gauze to facilitate drainage. In the Schafer method, rhythmic pressure is applied over the lower ribs posteriorly to expel the air and water, with alternate release of pressure to allow passive expansion of the elastic chest wall and inspiration of air; the pressure is applied about once every 5 seconds to simulate as nearly as possible the normal respiratory rate. The operator in a kneeling position straddles the lower part of the victim's prone body, resting each hand on the corresponding lower portion of the chest, and exerts pressure by leaning forward as described above. The prone pressure method of Schafer because of its simplicity and the ease with which it can be performed has enjoyed wide and successful use for many years as a means of manual artificial respiration. It replaced to a great extent the older arm lift-chest pressure method of Silvester in which the victim was worked over while in a supine position which is particularly disadvantageous in submersion cases.

The Silvester method accomplished some degree of active inspiration during the arm lifting phase of the procedure. In recent years, the advantage of providing an active inspiratory phase during manual artificial respiration has become recognized and various push-pull methods have been devised to provide an active inspiratory as well as expiratory phase. These are carried out with the victim in a prone position and have been recommended as more effective than Schafer prone pressure or Silvester arm lift-chest pressure methods. The newer methods represent a combination of prone pressure to produce active expiration and a pulling or lifting phase to actively induce inspiration which is more effective than that accomplished by the passive phase of the Schafer method. The push-pull technic of artificial respiration most recommended at the present time is the arm lift-back pressure method devised by Holgar Nielsen in Denmark in 1932. This procedure has been adopted in place of the Schafer method by the American Red Cross, the United States Armed Forces and by various police departments including that of New York City. Other modifications of the pull-push methods are the hip lift-back pressure and hip roll-back pressure methods, performed on the prone victim. The various methods of manual artificial respiration are critically surveyed in the article by Gordon, Sadove, Rayman and Ivy and are also described by Cole and Puestow in their book, First Aid, Medical and Surgical.

The procedures must be continued until the respiratory centers in the medulla begin to function and breathing is resumed, which may be a matter of minutes or hours. Artificial respiration should be persisted in until it is evident that the victim is beyond any hope of revival. Other measures such as cardiac stimulation and warmth are helpful after respiration has been restored.

The postmortem appearances after drowning are variable and none of them is absolutely pathognomonic. If the body has been removed from the water a short time after death, the clothing is wet, and the skin is wet, cold, clammy and pale because of the contraction of the surface blood vessels. The postmortem lividity is usually not deep and is light red in color after submersion in cold water, but in some cases it is dusky and cyanotic, or it may be a mixture of the two. There may be an early rigor mortis of the contracted arrectores pilorum muscles especially on the thighs, hips, arms and shoulders, resulting in a persistent cutis anserina, or goose flesh appearance, of the skin (Fig. 4-5). The face may or may not be cyanotic, the conjunctivae are usually markedly congested and a few subconjunctival ecchymoses may be present. A variable amount of fine white cohesive foam composed of small bubbles usually escapes from the nose and month (Fig. 18-13), and watery fluid generally flows from the nose and mouth when the body is turned on its side. The hands may contain various objects which they have grasped in struggling. Rigor mortis as a rule makes its appearance early in submerged bodies because of the cold temperature of the water and strenuous muscular activity of the victim during drowning.

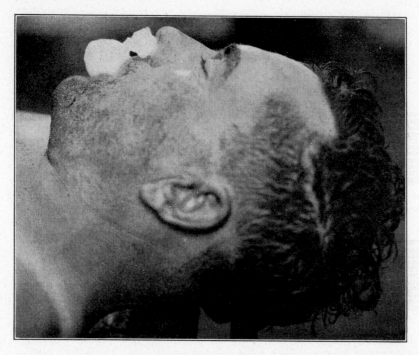

Fig. 18-13. Foam in Fresh Drowning.

Fine foam exuding from mouth and nostrils of a drowned body which has been submerged only a short time.

The air passages from nasal cavities to bronchi, when investigated at autopsy, may contain stiff foam or frothy fluid, and sometimes fragments of water-borne material such as sand, sea weed, mud, algae and other objects, but such substances may be absent. The lungs are usually large, distended, cyanotic, congested, edematous, stiff and heavy (Fig. 18-14). Areas of inhaled water mixed with air in the alveoli may be distinguished on close scrutiny, appearing as irregular, subpleural patches of gray blue to dark red color interspersed between salmon pink and yellowish gray more aerated lung tissue. The lungs in drowning have a marbled appearance, and the surface may pit on pressure. Histologically the lung reveals distention of the air vesicles and congestion of the capillaries. When drowning has occurred in fresh water ponds containing algae, the latter are sometimes found in the bronchioles or alveoli. In some cases in which the victim has struggled during submersion, considerable water may be swallowed into the stomach. The heart is distended and usually contains fluid blood, but in some instances the blood in the heart has been found clotted. Most of the other viscera show marked congestion. In fresh cases, the findings at autopsy are sufficiently characteristic of inhalation of water and death by asphyxia to allow the diagnosis of drowning to be made.

After it has been in the water a few days, the condition of the body changes. First there is bleaching, maceration, swelling and wrinkling of the cornified epithelium of the hands and feet especially the palms and soles, which become evident in from 24 to 48 hours; later as a result of bacterial decomposition the epidermis separates from the dermis. Bacterial decomposition makes its appearance in the first two days after submersion during the summer months and after a week of submersion during the winter time. The body has a tendency to float in the water head down, so that the formation of gas occurs first in the head and upper part of the trunk, and with its appearance the remains rise to the surface and become what

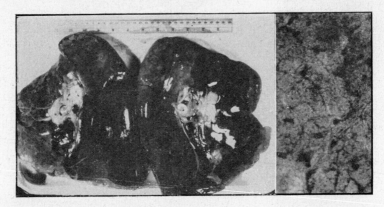

Fig. 18-14. Appearance of Lungs in Drowning.

The victim was submerged in salt water. Body recovered in fresh state. Lungs are smooth, heavy, large, stiffened and distended by inhaled water. Bronchi filled with foam. Photograph of lung surface at low magnification to show vesicles distended with air and water, shown at right.

is known as a floater. In the rivers and inlets around New York City many floaters rise to the top in May and June when the warm weather of the late spring raises the temperature of the water and speeds up the decomposition of those bodies drowned during the winter months. The postmortem changes which take place in bodies submerged in water have been discussed on page 73 and have been illustrated in Chapter 4; they must be considered by the medical investigator as they sometimes simulate antemortem injuries and in other instances tend to obscure them.

The autopsy on a body decomposed by prolonged submersion reveals changes caused by the decomposition which usually obscure and even obliterate the signs which would be suggestive or indicative of death by drowning. During decomposition the foam and water disappear from the air passages, and damage is inflicted on the alveolar structure of the lung which causes that organ to diminish in size and to assume a dirty, dark red, water-logged appearance which disguises the signs by which inhaled water can be recognized. Sometimes the pleural cavities in these cases are filled with a dirty, red, blood-stained fluid; this has been attributed by Sydney Smith to transudation of inhaled water from the lungs to the chest cavities as a result of postmortem changes. Such postmortem pleural effusions are encountered in many cases of drowning, but in some they are absent; furthermore decomposed bodies which have not drowned or have not been submerged may reveal the same type of pleural fluid but in lesser amounts. Unless corroborated by other evidence, blood stained fluid in the chest cavities of a floater cannot be considered a reliable criterion of death by submersion.

Because of the difficulty in diagnosing drowning by postmortem examination alone, numerous chemical tests have been devised to corroborate or disprove such a diagnosis in a suspected case. These tests are based on the principle of dilution and change in concentration of various substances in the blood by the diffusion of inhaled water into the blood returning from the lungs into the heart. The test which has given the most consistent results was devised by Gettler, and is based on the

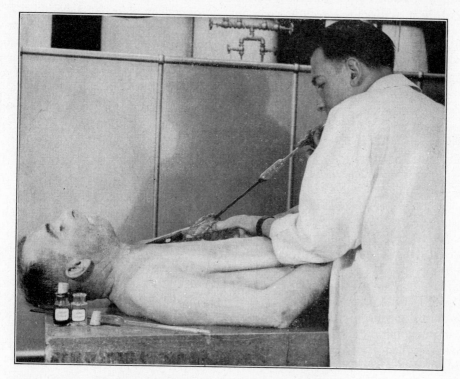

Fig. 18-15. Removing Blood from Heart for Drowning Test.

A sample drawn from the right heart is in the small bottle. Blood is being drawn into the pipet from the left side of the heart.

difference in the sodium chloride concentration of the blood on the right and left sides of the heart in most cases of drowning.

The blood is collected with separate dry pipets from the right and left sides of the heart before any of the organs are disturbed or removed. The surface of the heart is wiped dry before it is punctured with a dry knife, then samples of blood are placed in labeled clean dry flasks. About 20 ml. of blood should be withdrawn (Fig. 18-15).

Three milliliters of blood from each sample are treated separately as follows: 27 ml. of distilled water and 30 ml. of saturated picric acid solution are added and the mixture is allowed to stand for 10 minutes. The solutions are then filtered through dry filter paper. Exactly 40 ml. of each filtrate is pipeted into a dry Erlenmeyer flask and 10 ml. of M/29.25 silver nitrate solution is added to each. The preparations are allowed to stand several hours and then mixed thoroughly. Four milliliters of starch citrate mixture are added and the resulting mixtures are titrated with a standard M/117 potassium iodide solution.

The silver nitrate solution is made up of 5.812 gm. of silver nitrate, 250 ml. of concentrated nitric acid, and water to make 1 liter.

The starch-citrate mixture is prepared by dissolving 2.5 gm. of soluble starch in 500 ml. of warm distilled water, to which are added 446 gm. of sodium citrate and 20 gm. of sodium nitrite. The ingredients are dissolved by heat, the solution filtered through cotton and diluted with water to make one liter.

The potassium iodide solution is made by dissolving 1.419 gm. of potassium iodide in 1 liter of water.

The result is calculated as follows:

$$1,000 - \left(\frac{\text{ml. KI used}}{2}\right) = \text{mg. of NaCl in 100 ml. of blood.}$$

The sodium chloride content is determined for the blood from each side of the heart. In nondrowning cases, the concentration of sodium chloride in the blood is normally the same on both sides. During drowning, water is inhaled and diffuses into the pulmonary venous circulation which conveys it to the left side of the heart where the concentration of sodium chloride as well as of other substances in the blood, becomes altered; an appreciable difference in the salt contents of blood may result between right and left sides of the heart. If the body is submerged after death, inhalation of water does not occur, and the sodium chloride content of the blood would not be altered and would be equal on both sides of the heart. According to Sydney Smith, water does not enter the lungs or stomach of a body submerged post mortem if the pressure of the surrounding fluid is not very great. Whether or not it enters a body which sinks to a great depth is uncertain.

The finding of algae and other water organisms in the bronchi and alveoli of submerged bodies is considered by some to be an indication of the inhalation of water. Investigations have been made by the authors on many of the submerged bodies recovered from the waters in and around Manhattan Island. The technic consisted in opening the bronchial tree, scraping off the contents of a small bronchus with the spatula end of a small probe, mixing them with a drop of water on a microscope slide and examining the preparation under a coverslip as a wet smear. The bronchial contents in cases recently submerged usually contained much fluid or mucus and many cells of human origin such as large macrophages, bronchial epithelium and red blood cells but no algae or similar plants. In cases which were submerged longer, the bronchi had lost their excess secretions and contained a little sanguineous fluid which on microscopic examination showed a varying collection of algae such as volvox, thread-like segmented organisms and diatoms. The bronchial contents of bodies recovered from the turbulent estuaries of the North and East rivers yielded few algae, but those from bodies drowned in the sluggish Harlem River and in the Central Park lakes contained many microscopic plants.

The significance of these findings is not easy to determine, and depends upon the validity of the assumption that water does not enter the lungs or stomach of a body which is submerged post mortem. Sydney Smith holds this opinion, but Kasparek and others consider it a distinct possibility that water may seep through the air passages of a person submerged after death carrying in microscopic water plants. At present this question cannot be answered satisfactorily, and the medical examiner can only correlate his observations with the other findings in the case.

The water inhaled during drowning is absorbed by diffusion and osmosis into the blood in the pulmonary veins, and is carried to the left side of the heart. If it is sea water with a high concentration of sodium chloride, the blood in the left side of the heart will acquire a much higher salt content than the blood in the right side. If fresh water is inhaled, the blood in the left side will have a lesser sodium chloride concentration than the blood in the right side. A pronounced difference in salt concentration between the blood on both sides of the heart is a fairly reliable criterion of inhalation of water into the air passages and lungs, but a slight difference is not conclusive. Whenever possible, the sodium chloride content of the water in which the victim's body is found should be determined, especially from bathtubs and artificial swimming pools which may contain salt water, chlorinated water or a considerable amount of urine.

Unfortunately a number of factors may interfere with the validity of the test. A wide persistent foramen ovale, or any other large communicating defect between the right and left sides of the heart may permit the blood in the two sides to mix and thus equalize any difference in salt concentration. If the drowning occurs in mildly brackish water with about the same sodium chloride content as normal blood, the test might be inconclusive since inhalation of such water might not cause an appreciable change in the salt concentration of the blood. Postmortem putrefaction alters and destroys the blood and the gases formed usually force the blood out of the heart so that the test cannot be employed. Cases of submersion in which death occurred from laryngeal shock without the inhalation of water, may not show any difference in the sodium chloride concentration of the blood. The test, when positive, merely indicates the inhalation of water into the lungs, and does not prove or disprove death by drowning. The autopsy findings and the circumstances must always be considered in determining the cause of death.

The sodium chloride chemical test for drowning gives most consistent results in cases of salt water drowning in which the bodies are promptly recovered and thus have not undergone postmortem decomposition. In such cases, the postmortem appearances are also usually characteristic or very suggestive of drowning and offer little difficulty in interpretation. The test has not proved as helpful in fresh water drownings in some of which the postmortem findings are not as pronounced. It has not been helpful when it would be most useful in cases in which the usual anatomic evidences of drowning have been obscured by postmortem decomposition and where the diagnosis of drowning is difficult or impossible to establish or prove. With early postmortem decomposition, rapid changes in chloride content of the blood are apt to occur by diffusion and some have advocated magnesium determination on the blood in addition to sodium chloride content on the principle that the magnesium concentration does not become as rapidly altered after death. However, it seems to the authors that, with the onset of decomposition, the same objection would apply to that substance, magnesium, as applies to chlorides.

Inhalation of salt water also increases the salt concentration in the lungs as well as in the blood. In the laboratories of the Chief Medical Examiner, Dr. A. O. Gettler and his staff have made determinations of the sodium chloride concentration in the blood, lung tissue and pleural fluid from fresh and decomposed bodies drowned in salt water and have found concentrations much higher than determinations made on similar material taken from nondrowning cases. The results are suggestive but must be interpreted with caution in the individual case as criteria for diagnosing death by drowning, since there is no definite information available as to sodium chloride concentration in the lung tissue and pleural fluid in cases in which the body is definitely known to have been dead before submersion and decomposition.

Drownings are homicidal, suicidal, accidental or undetermined as to classification in these categories. Accidental and undetermined cases are the most common, occurring on an average of 400 a year in New York City. Many adults and children drown while swimming in pools, in lakes or at the seashore, and some of these have also sustained fractures of the skull and the spine after diving into shallow water. Other persons become ill in the water, then submerge and die even though promptly rescued. Such deaths may occur in shallow water; in such cases the autopsy usually discloses some disease process such as a severe grade of coronary arteriosclerosis either as the cause of death or of the submersion. Many people fall into the water from piers or boats while intoxicated; similar accidents occur during work. Occasionally a ship sinks or capsizes with a large number of people on board. Sometimes a drunken motorist drives his car off a pier and drowns along with other trapped occupants in the car. Children, elderly or intoxicated persons may drown accidentally in a bathtub. An individual may faint or suffer a convulsion seizure

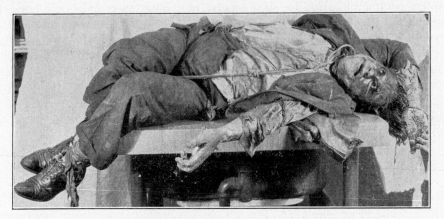

Fig. 18-16. Suicidal Drowning.

Swelling and wrinkling of epidermis of hands with beginning separation from dermis, resulting from long submersion. Deceased tied himself with rope and jumped into river. Note that arms are free.

and submerge his head in a sink full of water and drown because no one is nearby to rescue him. The undetermined category of cases will be discussed later.

Proved suicidal drownings average about 30 a year, about 3 per cent of the total number of suicides in New York City. Sometimes they are recognized as such only after an investigation of the circumstances of death and previous history of the deceased, which may reveal financial troubles, mental depression, previous attempts at suicide or definite indications of preparation for the final act. When a body is found in the water, trussed up with ropes and attached to heavy weights, the question of the possibility of the deceased having rigged up the harness or of some one else having tied the ropes has to be considered. If the victim is not firmly bound by the ropes and some freedom of movement, particularly of the arms, is possible (Fig. 18-16), the diagnosis of suicide is reasonable especially if supported by other evidence. Some suicidal cases reveal characteristic self-inflicted parallel cuts on the wrists and neck, strongly suggesting the suicidal nature of the drowning (Fig. 18-17).

Another suicidal case was encountered when an autopsy on a body recovered from the Hudson River disclosed not only evidence of death from drowning but also a moderately severe corrosion of the stomach mucosa by a solution of copper sulfate obviously swallowed just prior to the submersion. Similarly a bather at a beach attempted to simulate an accidental drowning in committing suicide. He was observed to be in acute distress, but despite an immediate rescue he could not be revived. The autopsy revealed that the death was caused by a large amount of cyanide which the deceased had ingested while swimming.

Some people commit suicide by jumping from a high bridge into the water; they usually sustain fractures of the sternum, costal cartilages or ribs in the front of the

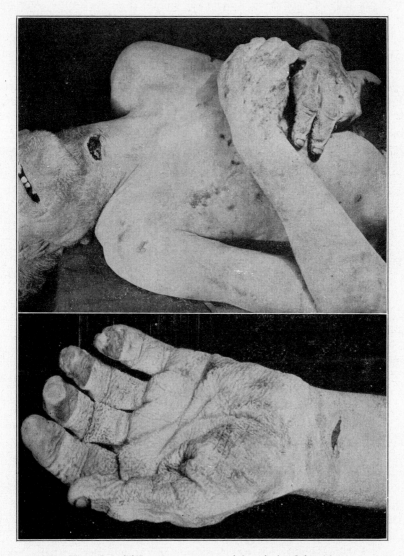

Fig. 18-17. Suicidal Drowning. Attempted Suicide by Other Means.

Note self-inflicted superficial cuts on front of neck (top) and on flexor surface of left wrist (bottom). The bleached wrinkled skin on the hands indicates moderately prolonged submersion. "Washerwoman hands."

chest, or fractures of the thoracic spine from overflexion of the trunk, and lacerations of the heart and lungs. These injuries result from the severe impact against the surface of the water and are generally fatal, even though they are less extensive than injuries which result after falls from a similar height against the ground. Others drive an automobile off a pier into the river. A number of suicidal drownings occur in bathtubs, the deceased assuming a supine or lateral position and submerging the head so that water flows readily into the air passages. Some of these suicides take a large dose of narcotics or barbiturates prior to the submersion to render the process easier or to make the result more certain.

Homicidal drownings are rare, comprising about 0.4 per cent of all homicides in New York City. In some cases they are identified as such only after the circumstances of the crime are made clear by police investigation. However, if a body is fished out of water, trussed up in such a way that it could not have been done by the deceased but must have been done by another person (Fig. 18-18), and the autopsy reveals death by drowning, suspicion of foul play would be more than justified. If wounds are present, the question arises as to whether they were inflicted with homicidal intent, and in all cases it is necessary to determine whether the injuries are ante mortem or post mortem; this may be difficult if the body is badly

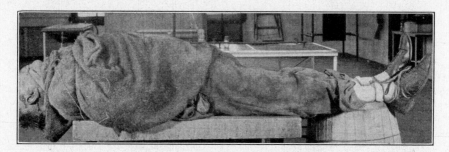

Fig. 18-18. Homicidal Drowning. Sack Murder.

The victim was gagged, tied up in a burlap sack with rope and wire and then dumped into the river.

decomposed. In some homicidal cases, obviously antemortem and not self-inflicted bullet wounds or stab wounds have been found on a submerged body which has also shown signs of inhaled water in the lungs. A correct appraisal of the cause of death would depend on the nature of the wounds, for if they are slight, death would be due to drowning, but the presence of a serious injury attended by considerable shock or hemorrhage would indicate that the injury was the cause of death.

Some homicidal drownings do not reveal any signs of injury or other evidence on the body which would cause the death to be considered suspicious. The homicides committed in England by George Joseph Smith indicate that a person can be drowned in a bathtub without much difficulty; Smith drowned three of his wives in that manner. From the information available, he would wait until the woman was supine in the tub, whereupon he would seize and elevate her feet suddenly so that her head would be submerged; water rushing in through her nostrils apparently caused a laryngeal spasm and rapid death by asphyxia. The authors have encountered a case of homicidal drowning in a bathtub, in which a man killed his seven year old stepson by forcing the child's head back under water as he lay supine in the tub. At autopsy the lungs were pale and hyperaerated and dark red patches of inhaled water were plainly visible against the paler lung tissue; the air passages were filled with stiff white foam. In another case the perpetrator, intent on robbery, confessed to stunning and then throttling his victim, after which he forced her face while she was still alive into a saucepan full of water on the kitchen floor. The body was found with the face submerged in the pan which contained blood tinged frothy fluid.

It is obviously easy for one or several people to push an individual unable to swim into deep water and cause him to drown, and the autopsy would reveal only signs of asphyxia by submersion without indicating or suggesting the way in which it occurred. In all these cases a thorough investigation by the police is necessary to determine the character of the death.

A number of drownings are presented to the examiner as bodies recovered from the bays, inlets, reservoirs, lakes or ponds in New York City in various stages of postmortem decomposition following submersion. Clues which might lead to prompt identification are sometimes lacking, and even when the corpse is finally identified, a satisfactory history may be difficult to obtain. The circumstances of death are usually not ascertainable, for the chances are that the drowning occurred in the absence of eyewitnesses. Subsequent investigation may fail to elicit evidence which would justify classifying the drowning specifically as homicidal, suicidal or accidental. These cases are designated as submersion deaths under undetermined circumstances.

REFERENCES

Cole, W. H., and Puestow, C. B.   First Aid, Surgical and Medical, New York, Appleton-Century-Crofts, Inc., 1951, pp. 236-239.

Gettler, A. O.   A method for the determination of death by drowning, J.A.M.A., 77:1650, 1921.

Gordon, A. S., Sadove, M. S., Rayman, F. and Ivy, A. C.   Critical survey of manual artificial respiration, J.A.M.A., 147:1444, 1951.

Jetter, W. W., and Moritz, A. R.   Changes in the magnesium and chloride contents of blood from drowning in fresh and salt water, Arch. Path., 36:601, 1943.

Kasparek, B.   Beitrag zur Diagnose des Ertrinkungstodes durch den Nachweis von Planktonorganismen in Lunge und Duodenum, Deutsche Zeitschr. f.d. Gesamte Gericht. Med., 27:132-142, 1936.

Puppe, G.   Atlas und Grundriss der Gerichtlichen Medizin, München, J. F. Lehmann, 1908.

Reports of the Office of the Chief Medical Examiner in the City of New York from 1918 to 1951.

Smith, S.   Forensic Medicine, London, J. & A. Churchill, Ltd., 1940.

19

Asphyxiating Gases

The atmosphere is a mixture of gases, ordinarily containing by volume about 21 per cent of oxygen, 78 per cent of nitrogen, 0.94 per cent of argon and 0.04 per cent of carbon dioxide, also traces of helium, xenon, krypton, niton and hydrogen, and varying amounts of ammonia, ozone and water vapor. This mixture at the barometric pressure encountered at and not too far above sea level is best suited for the support of animal and plant life. Its most important component is oxygen which is essential, either in an atmospheric or dissolved state, for all living matter with the exception of the anaerobic microorganisms which can obtain it from the oxygen-containing compounds. Nitrogen and argon are inert substances which dilute the atmospheric oxygen, while the amounts of the other gases are too minute to have any direct influence on the animal organism. If the amount of oxygen in the air is diminished considerably as in the rarefied atmosphere of high altitudes, the unadapted or unprotected individual may suffer seriously and even fatally from oxygen lack. If the components of the atmosphere are inhaled in stronger than normal concentration, the effect may also not be beneficial. Pure oxygen breathed in over a long period of time undiluted by nitrogen may cause a slight irritation of the air passages. Nitrogen and argon, although inert and without specific toxic action, could induce asphyxia if inhaled in the pure state because of the absence of oxygen. Gases other than those occurring in the atmosphere are produced by natural or artificial means and may when inhaled cause injury or death by asphyxia or by toxic action.

CARBON DIOXIDE

Carbon dioxide, CO_2, besides being a constituent of the atmosphere, is formed in large quantities by natural and artificial chemical processes. It is produced by the oxidation and respiration of animal and plant tissues, by the combustion of fuel, by organic decomposition and by fermentation in nature and in brewery vats; it is contained in solution in effervescent mineral spring waters, it issues from the ground in large quantities in certain localities, and it is produced by the burning of lime in the preparation of quick lime and by the action of acids upon carbonates. It is a colorless, odorless, heavy gas having a specific gravity of 1.52 in comparison with air; that is, it is one and one-half times heavier. If it is not diffused by ventilation into the atmosphere, it tends to seep down and stagnate at lower levels.

In urban surroundings carbon dioxide accumulates in manholes, cellars and beer vats; in the country districts it is found in wells, silos, caves and mines. Sometimes it is present in sufficient quantity to cause fatal asphyxiation. Concentrations of carbon dioxide from 0.1 to 0.5 per cent in air may produce symptoms of languor and headache; if 8 or 9 per cent there is danger of suffocation, while exposure to higher percentages is likely to be fatal. Naked flame has been used as an indicator of a dangerous quantity of the gas but cannot be relied upon as a danger signal, since

494

lighted candles can burn in an atmosphere containing more than 12 per cent of carbon dioxide, a concentration dangerous to life.

Typical cases of poisoning by carbon dioxide occur when individuals descend into manholes, wells or brewery vats which have not been ventilated for some time. The victims may collapse suddenly and rapidly after inhaling the poisonous atmosphere; would-be rescuers frequently are also overcome unless they are protected by an oxygen mask. In the records of the Medical Examiner's Office fatal carbon dioxide poisonings are not common, 20 cases having occurred in the 24 year period from 1918 to 1941 inclusive. Most of these fatalities were the result of workmen entering manholes and brewery vats without due precautions. In 1936, several persons in Brooklyn were fatally asphyxiated while working in the hold of a ship in which solid carbon dioxide, so-called dry ice, was used as a refrigerant; enough carbon dioxide gas had been liberated to produce a dangerous concentration in the poorly ventilated surroundings. In 1945 a pipe in the refrigerating system of a factory suddenly burst and filled a small room with carbon dioxide, asphyxiating several workmen and causing one death. More recently, Lovelace has pointed out a hazard connected with the use of carbon dioxide gas to extinguish a fire in the sealed pressurized cabin of a large commercial aircraft. The use of carbon dioxide in the sealed plane was believed to have resulted in the asphyxiation of the pilot when the heavy gas gravitated to the forward end of the plane during a rapid descent impelled by the fire. The asphyxiation of the pilot was believed to have been the cause of the plane's crashing.

Carbon dioxide induces asphyxia through the exclusion of oxygen, a process which is accelerated in the early stages by the stimulating effect of the gas on the respiratory center, resulting in deeper and more rapid respirations. The inhalation of air containing a poisonous concentration of carbon dioxide will suddenly produce giddiness, a sensation of ringing in the ears and tingling in the nose, a sense of pressure in the head, nausea, perspiration, muscular weakness and marked somnolence. After an initial rise of blood pressure accompanied by intense cyanosis, rapid respirations and increased pulse rate, the symptoms and signs of general collapse quickly ensue, with rapidly developing coma and death. If the atmosphere is almost pure carbon dioxide, the toxic action is even more startling and is marked by spasm of the glottis, convulsions, sudden coma and rapid death from respiratory paralysis.

If a victim is rescued after having been overcome by carbon dioxide, he should be promptly removed from the danger zone and given artificial respiration with oxygen inhalations. The effort toward resuscitation should be continued for a long time as surprising recoveries have occurred even after protracted insensibility.

The postmortem findings are those of death from acute asphyxia. The face may show a marked bluish cyanosis but occasionally it presents a pasty pallor. All the organs including the brain are intensely congested, the blood is dark red in color and the right side of the heart distended. Minute asphyxial hemorrhages may be present in the pericardium, pleura and galea of the scalp.

It is not possible to establish by chemical tests performed on the dead body that a lethal amount of carbon dioxide was inhaled. The only practical procedure is to demonstrate the presence of a poisonous concentration of the gas in the atmosphere of the locality where the deceased was asphyxiated. The nature of the death should suggest itself by the circumstances even before the autopsy. Samples of air should be collected immediately at the scene of the poisoning and later tested to determine the presence of a dangerous concentration of carbon dioxide. For this purpose, a bottle of 5 to 6 liters capacity is filled with water and lowered by a cord into the space where the victim was found. At the desired level the bottle is tilted by means of another cord attached to its bottom, so that the water runs out and is replaced by a sample of the poisonous atmosphere. The bottle is allowed to right itself and is pulled out with its mouth directed upward after which it is tightly corked, sealed and labeled. It is kept until the air it contains can be tested for carbon dioxide content (Chapter 42).

Fatalities have occurred among persons imprisoned in a small room, closet or safe without ventilation. In such cases, asphyxiation is due as much to the insufficient oxygen supply as to the excessive collection of carbon dioxide. It is likely that the heat, humidity and other deleterious effects produced by such confinements contribute to the fatal outcome.

CARBON MONOXIDE

Carbon monoxide, CO, is a colorless (and in pure form, odorless) gas slightly lighter than air. It is produced during any process in which there is incomplete combustion of carbon, and is generated in stoves, furnaces, gasoline engines, conflagrations, explosions, around electrodes of electric furnaces, and during combustion of natural gas, coal, charcoal and coke. Carbon monoxide is one of the inflammable components of manufactured illuminating gases, in amounts varying from 20 to 30 per cent, and imparts to such mixtures its own poisonous properties; all the gaseous fuels containing carbon monoxide produce the same effect on the human organism as the pure gas. Other constituents such as cyanogen, hydrocarbons and sulfur compounds furnish the pungent odors characteristic of these mixtures.

The monoxide is an unsaturated carbon compound which can be ignited in the presence of oxygen to form carbon dioxide. A mixture of one volume of carbon monoxide with one half its volume of oxygen, or two and a half times its volume of air, is explosive in the presence of a flame. Such explosions may occur when persons commit suicide with illuminating gas in a kitchen in which the pilot light on the stove is burning. In some cases, the explosive mixture is ignited by a spark from an electric appliance like a refrigerator or a door bell. In other cases the source of the ignition is not always evident. Illuminating gas explosions at times are very destructive (Fig. 19-1).

Carbon monoxide forms colorless liquids, known as carbonyls, with nickel and iron which decompose into their gaseous and metallic components in the presence of heat; poisoning by these substances is described on page 764. If chlorine is passed over glowing charcoal, carbon monoxide combines with chlorine to form phosgene, one of the lethal war gases (page 518).

In cases of carbon monoxide poisoning the gas is inhaled into the alveoli of the lungs where it comes in contact with the red blood cells in the pulmonary capillaries and combines with their hemoglobin to form the compound carboxyhemoglobin. The affinity of carbon monoxide for hemoglobin is 210 times greater than that of oxygen, and carboxyhemoglobin is more stable than the loosely combined oxyhemoglobin. As a result, carbon monoxide binds the hemoglobin firmly and rapidly, preventing oxygen from entering into combination with it. When a large amount of carboxyhemoglobin is formed in the blood, oxygen cannot be supplied to the vital organs in sufficient quantity and a fatal anoxemia develops. About one half of the total amount of carbon monoxide is absorbed during the early part of the exposure. The reaction is a reversible one, and as the blood becomes more and more saturated with carboxyhemoglobin, carbon monoxide is absorbed more slowly. If the intake of this poisonous gas is checked before a lethal concentration is reached in the blood and oxygen is introduced in the respired air, the hemoglobin molecule will be freed of its carboxy component, carbon monoxide will be eliminated during

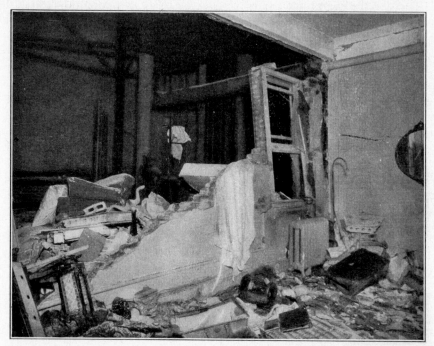

Courtesy Police Dept., City of New York.

Fig. 19-1. Wreakage Caused by Explosion of Illuminating Gas in an Apartment.

Deceased committed suicide by allowing illuminating gas to escape from four jets in kitchen stove. When the carbon monoxide concentration in the air had attained the explosive percentage, the gas was ignited, possibly by the spark from an electric refrigerator, causing a destructive centrifugal explosion. Fragments of a suicide note were found in the debris. There were no injuries on the body of the deceased but his blood revealed 60 per cent carboxyhemoglobin saturation.

expiration, oxyhemoglobin will be re-formed, and the victim may be started on the road to recovery (see treatment, page 501).

The reversible reaction may be stated as follows:

Oxyhemoglobin plus CO $\leftrightarrows$ carboxyhemoglobin plus O_2 (Henderson and Haggard). The rapidity and amount of absorption of carbon monoxide in the blood depends upon the amount of gas in the air and the amount of carboxyhemoglobin already present in the victim. With 0.1 per cent of carbon monoxide in the atmosphere, owing to the greater affinity of that gas for hemoglobin (210 times more) than the affinity of oxygen, one half of the available hemoglobin will be converted to carboxyhemoglobin and one half will remain oxyhemoglobin. At this point an equilibrium in the blood is reached which is reversible according to the law of mass action. If the percentage of carbon monoxide in the air is increased, more carboxyhemoglobin is formed; but, on the other hand, if carbon monoxide is kept from the victim, and oxygen is available, carboxyhemoglobin will slowly disappear from the blood.

Carbon monoxide does not have any known deleterious effect on the red blood cells, aside from the formation of carboxyhemoglobin; after the elimination of the carbon monoxide from the blood, the red cells are unaltered. The principal damage to the organism occurs while carboxyhemoglobin is present in the blood in sufficient amount to impair the oxygen interchange in the pulmonary and systemic capillaries, and to induce anoxemia and widespread tissue anoxia which produce characteristic symptoms and signs. The various pathologic lesions occurring in carbon monoxide poisoning are the direct result of this anoxemia.

Clinical Considerations. Acute carbon monoxide poisoning produces at first headache and languor accompanied by a rapid, forceful heart beat, a primary rise in blood pressure, and an increase in the respiratory rate. In a short time the pulse becomes small and rapid, the respiration labored and the blood pressure is lowered. In severe cases, headache, drowsiness, faintness, motor weakness, anesthesia, hyper-reflexia, ankle clonus, generalized spasticity and stupor supervene. Bright red flushes may appear on the skin. Prior to or after sinking into a deep coma there may be vomiting and involuntary evacuation of urine and feces. The temperature may become subnormal, and death occurs from a few minutes to an hour later while the victim is in coma.

The poisonous concentration of carbon monoxide in the air is estimated at 0.02 to 0.05 per cent by volume, and any atmosphere containing a higher percentage of the gas is dangerous (Table 19-1, and reference to Henderson and Haggard). Moreover, if a person breathes carbon monoxide in low concentration for a con-

Table 19-1. Physiologic Response to Various Concentrations of Carbon Monoxide

	PARTS OF CO PER MILLION PARTS OF AIR
Concentration allowable for an exposure of several hours	100
Concentration which can be inhaled for 1 hour without appreciable effect	400 to 500
Concentration causing a just appreciable effect after 1 hour exposure	600 to 700
Concentration causing unpleasant but not dangerous symptoms after 1 hour exposure	1,000 to 1,200
Dangerous concentration for exposure of 1 hour	1,500 to 2,000
Concentrations which are fatal in exposures of less than 1 hour	4,000 and above

From Henderson and Haggard, *Noxious Gases.*

siderable length of time, especially during sleep, he will be poisoned just as effectively as though he were exposed to a high concentration for a shorter period. When low concentrations of the gas are inhaled, coma does not supervene immediately but a state of complete helplessness may develop and the victim may not be able to save himself.

The blood in cases found dead in the atmosphere of the gas usually contains carboxyhemoglobin in concentrations over 50 per cent saturation, which means that the hemoglobin combining power of the blood is appropriated to that extent by the gas. Differences in susceptibility to the asphyxial power of carbon monoxide depend upon the victim's resistance, on the percentage of hemoglobin in the blood, on the depth and rapidity of his respirations and on the conditions of exposure. Usually when two or more persons are poisoned by carbon monoxide in the same room, it has been found that the percentage of carboxyhemoglobin in the blood of the different victims is approximately the same, if they are equally healthy and have been subjected to the same conditions of exposure. For example, in one case the percentage of carboxyhemoglobin in the blood of one victim was 65 per cent and for his companion was 60 per cent. In another case, the blood of one of the victims contained 70 per cent carboxyhemoglobin, but the blood of his companion, evidently less susceptible, contained 40 per cent. In still another case, one of the occupants of the premises was found dead with 55 per cent of carboxyhemoglobin in the blood, but another person in the same room, evidently not exposed in the same way, escaped with a severe headache.

In some cases of poisoning the victim is rescued while in deep coma and saved from immediate death. Some individuals revive promptly after restorative measures have been administered, showing as the most prominent symptom an intense headache which may pass off in a few hours without any other aftereffects. Other cases slowly recover consciousness but manifest distressing sequelae as the result of damage to the central nervous system and other organs from the initial anoxemia produced by the large amount of carboxyhemoglobin in the blood. Lesions resembling frost bite and scattered blebs and bullae (Fig. 19-2) may appear on the skin of

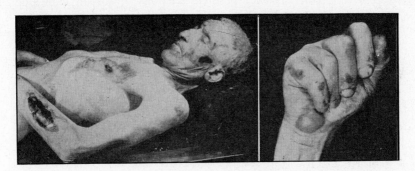

Fig. 19-2. Bullae of Skin Following Acute Carbon Monoxide Poisoning.

Unruptured bulla on right wrist; dried open bullae on face, forearms and trunk. These lesions are sometimes mistaken for burns.

the face and extremities; these are frequently mistaken for burns. Decubital ulcers may develop. Neurologic and mental symptoms and signs resembling those of ascending paralysis, chorea and imbecility may make their appearance.

The anoxemia resulting from carboxyhemoglobin in the blood, unlike the asphyxia produced by carbon dioxide, is not rapidly alleviated when the victim is removed from the poisonous atmosphere and is supplied with oxygen or an oxygen-carbon dioxide mixture. During such resuscitation, carbon monoxide is slowly dissociated from the hemoglobin of the erythrocytes and eliminated, the speed of the elimination varying with the amount of the carbon monoxide originally absorbed. If a moderate amount of carboxyhemoglobin is present, about one half of its carbon monoxide is removed during the first hour of therapy, but complete elimination is delayed for several hours. If large amounts of carboxyhemoglobin are in the blood, the removal of the gas is slower and the period of anoxemia during elimination will be prolonged. In carbon monoxide poisoning another factor which interferes with the oxygen supply available to the tissues is the abnormal type of oxygen dissociation curve encountered in the presence of large concentrations of carboxyhemoglobin. The oxygen tension of the blood is lowered, and an adequate transfer of oxygen from the blood to the tissues does not take place in a period of suddenly increased need, even though the blood contains oxygen ordinarily in excess of such requirements. In this respect carbon monoxide poisoning differs from severe anemia in which there is a corresponding or even greater reduction of the oxygen-carrying capacity of the blood because of the lack of hemoglobin. The blood in severe anemia retains the normal elastic type of oxygen dissociation curve and provides additional oxygen to the tissues needed if there is increased demand occasioned by sudden increased activity. An individual with an anemia in which the hemoglobin is reduced 50 per cent can carry out activities after a state of rest without difficulty. The victim of carbon monoxide with 50 per cent of his hemoglobin combined with carbon monoxide may retain consciousness or recover consciousness while at rest, only to collapse and become unconscious if he attempts to walk or otherwise become physically active.

The investigations of Gettler and Mattice have shown that many individuals such as traffic policemen and taxi drivers who are exposed on the street to gases from automobile exhausts, have as high as 6 to 19 per cent of carboxyhemoglobin in the blood day after day without suffering appreciable ill effects. There is reason to believe that the daily presence of small amounts of carbon monoxide in the

Table 19-2. Percentage Saturation of the Blood with Carbon Monoxide and Corresponding Physiologic Effects

PER CENT OF HEMOGLOBIN IN COMBINATION WITH CO	PHYSIOLOGIC EFFECT
10	No appreciable effect except shortness of breath on vigorous muscular exertion
20	No appreciable effect in most cases except short wind even on moderate exertion; slight heachache in some cases
30	Decided headache, irritable, easily fatigued, judgment disturbed
40 to 50	Headache, confusion, collapse and fainting on exertion
60 to 70	Unconsciousness, respiratory failure and death if exposure is long continued
80	Rapidly fatal
Over 80	Immediately fatal

From Henderson and Haggard, *Noxious Gases.*

blood is not as harmful as has previously been supposed (Table 19-2, and reference to Henderson and Haggard). On the other hand, some investigators believe that there is a chronic form of carbon monoxide poisoning, developing in individuals who are exposed day after day to an atmosphere containing a small amount of carbon monoxide. A variety of symptoms and signs have been described as characteristic of such repeated exposures; among them are included muscular weakness, a high hemoglobin percentage, a high erythrocyte count and, in more serious cases, fatty degeneration of the viscera, severe anemia, gray pallor of the skin, digestive disturbances, loss of memory, psychic manifestations and convulsions. It is highly questionable whether the repeated inhalation and excretion of small quantities of carbon monoxide insufficient to produce symptoms of poisoning at the time of exposure are a valid cause of the varied clinical manifestations and disabilities designated by some as chronic carbon monoxide poisoning. A critical analysis of such cases will usually disclose some other process (generally of disease) as a more reasonable explanation of the illness.

Carbon monoxide may be detected in the blood during life, provided that the specimen is collected within 1 to 2 hours after exposure, for after that time most of the carbon monoxide would be eliminated from the body. About 10 ml. of blood may be removed from an arm vein with needle and syringe and placed in a stoppered bottle. In a fatal case the specimen of blood may be taken at any time before decomposition sets in; the blood may be collected from the chambers of the heart or from large vascular trunks like the femoral vessels near the surface of the body. The bottle in which the blood is collected, should be dry, clean and tightly stoppered, to prevent escape of any carbon monoxide from the blood.

A small portion of the blood may be greatly diluted with distilled water and subjected to spectroscopic examination. The absorption bands of carboxyhemoglobin are similar to those of oxyhemoglobin, both compounds giving two bands between D and E in the yellow and green divisions of the spectrum. A narrow band lies near D in about the same position for both pigments, and a broader band is present near E, the carboxyhemoglobin band being slightly nearer E than the oxyhemoglobin band. The two spectra may be differentiated by adding a drop of freshly prepared ammonium sulfide solution to the blood solution; if the pigment is oxyhemoglobin the absorption bands will change to those of reduced hemoglobin but if carboxyhemoglobin is present the absorption lines will not change. The spectroscopic test is not satisfactory unless the blood contains at least 10 per cent carboxyhemoglobin, and this is also true of many other qualitative tests for this compound. For further discussion of the qualitative and quantitative tests for carbon monoxide in the blood, see Chapter 42.

Protection and Treatment. Protection against carbon monoxide in concentrations which might be encountered in a conflagration may be obtained by wearing a special gas mask with a canister, similar to the masks used as protection against poison gases in war. It possesses a face piece, an inlet tube which connects with a canister, and a separate outlet tube with a valve. The face piece fits airtight and on inhalation the incoming air passes through the canister into the mask and the outlet valve closes; on expiration the inlet valve closes and the expired air escapes by the outlet valve. The canister contains hopcalite (MnO_2, 50 per cent; CuO, 30 per cent; CO_2O_3, 15 per cent; Ag_2O, 5 per cent) which is a catalyst, oxidizing CO to CO_2. The inhaled air is dried by passing through calcium chloride, since water vapor will affect the hopcalite. This mask does not protect the wearer against atmospheres which are deficient in oxygen.

Coal mines sometimes contain carbon monoxide in dangerous quantities, frequently associated with carbon dioxide and other gases. The oxygen in such atmospheres may be insufficient, and the only protection is to wear a self-contained breathing apparatus with an oxygen tank, which will enable the worker to enter dangerous levels with a minimum of risk. In some cases, canaries and mice are used as physiologic indicators of the presence of carbon monoxide; canaries, especially, give signs of distress in the presence of dilute concentrations of the gas.

The treatment for acute carbon monoxide poisoning is to remove the victim to an uncontaminated but not too cold atmosphere, and to administer artificial respiration. The prone pressure method of Schafer or preferably the newer arm lift-back pressure method of Nielsen (page 484) may be used if necessary, but most large communities have emergency squads supplied by the gas company who carry out this duty and also administer artificial respiration with a mixture of oxygen and 5 per cent carbon dioxide through a special inhaler apparatus. The carbon dioxide component of the mixture stimulates the respiratory center, deepens the respirations and ventilates the lungs; oxygen is inhaled in large quantities and the elimination of carbon monoxide is speeded up. Many advise against the use of pulmotors or lungmotors which may injure the patient if they are used by an inexperienced operator. If the patient is brought into a hospital, he may be put into a Drinker respirator, a special apparatus for supplying artificial respiration by alternately applying positive and negative air pressures to the chest; this apparatus also should be operated only by one who is experienced. For a more complete description the reader is referred to the orginal article by Drinker and McKhann. Artificial respiration should be maintained until it is absolutely certain that resuscitation is no longer possible. Other methods such as venesection or partial exsanguination followed by transfusions have been tried but are not consistently beneficial. Caffeine may be useful as a cardiac stimulant.

Pathologic Lesions. At necropsy, acute cases of carbon monoxide poisoning dying soon after exposure show a marked cherry red color of the blood, tissues and viscera, and a pink or rose red color of the postmortem suggillations. This color is evident if there is 30 per cent or more of carboxyhemoglobin in the blood, and is easily distinguishable from the reddish purple lividity of oxyhemoglobin or the dusky violet hue of reduced hemoglobin (Figs. 4-4 and 4-6). The cherry red color of carboxyhemoglobin is not discernible under the pigmented epidermis of dark colored races and is often not typical in hue when it occurs in a slightly dark skinned individual. However, at autopsy the viscera, especially the voluntary muscles, brain, heart and lungs, are characteristically colored a bright cherry red in typical cases of carbon monoxide poisoning, regardless of the appearance of the suggillations in the skin. The cherry red color of carboxyhemoglobin persists in the dead body until advanced putrefaction occurs, and the presence of the pigment may be demonstrated by appropriate chemical tests even in cases with decomposition. In embalmed bodies, the lividity of carboxyhemoglobin remains characteristic and the compound may be demonstrated toxicologically.

The question sometimes arises in legal proceedings, whether or not a body, dead from another cause, could absorb carbon monoxide through the skin in the areas of postmortem lividity, if it is placed in an atmosphere containing this gas. Experiments conducted in the Office of the Chief Medical Examiner under the supervision of Dr. Alexander O. Gettler indicated that carboxyhemoglobin is not formed in the blood in any demonstrable amount under these conditions nor are the internal viscera colored a cherry red, though it is possible that a minute quantity might be produced in the more exposed suggillations. If a high percentage of carboxyhemoglobin is present in the blood of the heart, the presumption would be that the gas was absorbed during life.

Carbon monoxide is claimed by some to be transmitted through the placenta from the blood of the mother into the fetal circulation and sometimes to kill the fetus by anoxemia even when the mother is not harmed. Petri mentions a case reported by Maresch of delayed carbon monoxide poisoning by placental transmission of carbon monoxide from mother to fetus, in which the pregnant woman was resuscitated after exposure to illuminating gas and gave birth to an infant 13 days later. The child died nine days after birth, and the autopsy revealed degenerative changes in the brain which were attributed to carbon monoxide anoxemia.

Helpern and Strassmann point out that this case does not prove the transmission of carbon monoxide through the placenta to the fetus for the lesions in the brain of the infant might have been caused by simple anoxia from the mother's carbon monoxide poisoning; a high percentage of carboxyhemoglobin in the maternal blood merely deprives the fetus of oxygen, but none of the carbon monoxide is transmitted to the fetal blood across the placental barrier. These authors cite a case of their own concerning a pregnant woman who at full term committed suicide by inhaling carbon monoxide; her blood and tissues showed the typical bright red color at autopsy.

Chemical examination of her blood revealed a 65 per cent concentration of carboxyhemoglobin. In contrast the fetus was cyanotic, and its organs and blood were dark and free of carbon monoxide. Its death resulted from simple asphyxia due to lack of oxygen brought about by the carbon monoxide in the maternal and not in the fetal blood. Carbon monoxide does not diffuse across the placental barrier after it is bound by the hemoglobin in the mother's blood.

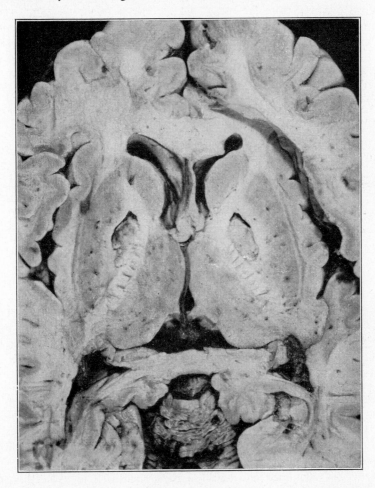

Fig. 19-3. Carbon Monoxide Poisoning: Bilateral Symmetric Softening of the Globus Pallidus.
Death in coma, two days after exposure to illuminating gas. Suicide.

In rare instances anoxic pathologic lesions are produced in brain and myocardium when the victims have died during a prolonged exposure to dilute concentrations of illuminating gas. In one case two young white women in their early twenties were found dead, poisoned during sleep by the illuminating gas from a leaking fixture, after a probable exposure of one and a half hours. The autopsy disclosed a bright red color of the blood and viscera, and chemical examination demonstrated 60 per cent of carboxyhemoglobin in the blood of both victims. Numerous petechial hemorrhages were found in the white matter of the brain and also in the heart muscle; histologic examination of both organs disclosed hyalin thrombi in the finer arterioles with numerous ring hemorrhages and minute areas of rarefaction necrosis in the white matter of the brain, and hemorrhagic areas in the myocardium, conditions all attributable to anoxemia.

Delayed fatal carbon monoxide poisoning occurs when the percentage of carboxyhemoglobin in the blood of the victim is not sufficient to cause death at the time of exposure, but is sufficient to produce a prolonged unconsciousness which later results in death. The victim may survive for 2 to 10 days after all carbon monoxide is removed from the blood, but the effects of the anoxemia persist and fatal complications supervene. The pathologic lesions encountered in autopsies on delayed carbon monoxide poisonings occur as a direct result of anoxemia and are

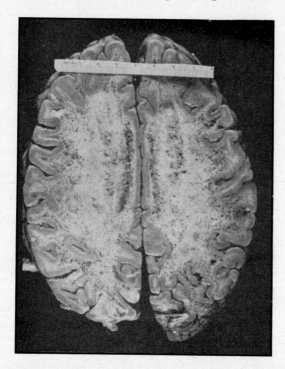

Fig. 19-4. Punctate Hemorrhages in Cerebral White Matter Following Acute Carbon Monoxide Poisoning with Prolonged Exposure Prior to Rescue.

Survived 48 hours. Brain sectioned horizontally.

characteristic of that complication. In rare instances other pathologic lesions, not specific for any particular traumatic or disease condition, develop secondarily from the anoxemic lesions themselves, and sometimes cause death.

The effect of continued anoxemia on the organism is to cause dilatation and engorgement of the smaller blood vessels, especially in the brain, as a result of vasomotor paralysis; the blood stagnates in the vessels, becomes laked, and hyaline thrombi may be formed. The victim remains in coma, his vitality is depressed, and a hypostatic pneumonia of the peribronchial or lobular type may appear about 24 to 48 hours after exposure. Aside from the pneumonia, dark dehydrated blood, vascular congestion and a postmortem lividity of dusky, bluish violet hue are encountered at autopsy, for at this stage the blood does not contain carboxyhemoglobin.

If the victim survives the exposure 48 hours or more, areas of symmetric softening may be found in the anterior portions of the right and left globus pallidus (Fig. 19-3). In the early stages these lesions are roughly spherical foci of reactionless necrosis, 10 to 15 mm. in diameter, either pale and anemic, or pink from congestion, and faintly distinguishable from the surrounding normal tissue. Later the necrotic area is sharply marked off from its surroundings, shrinks, becomes formless and shows a tendency to crumble; a reactive process, microglial in type, begins in the periphery and soon invades the necrotic area. In these foci the smaller blood vessels stand out prominently, containing red blood cells, white blood cells or hyaline thrombi; others are surrounded by microglial clumps or red or white blood cells. In some of the older lesions, globules or beaded rings of a dark blue staining material, may be present in the periphery of the arterial vessels of smaller size. Kolisko interprets the symmetric areas of softening as a delayed result of anoxemia affecting the globus pallidus, a part of the brain which requires a relatively large amount of oxygen and which is supplied by long and thin arteries with few anas-

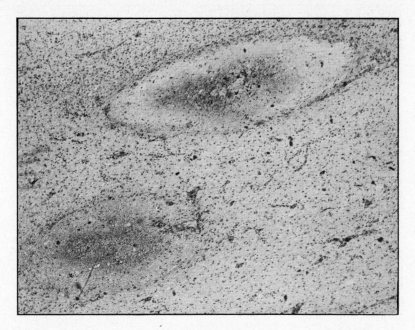

Fig. 19-5. Patchy Demyelinization of Cerebral White Matter due to Anoxia Resulting from Acute Carbon Monoxide Poisoning.

Death 6 days after exposure. Photomicrograph, 16 mm. objective.

tomoses. Under normal conditions the blood supply is adequate but in a state of anoxemia from carbon monoxide poisoning, the oxygen needs of the globus pallidus are not met and bilateral necroses occur in the anterior portions of these nuclei. The lesion is not pathognomonic for carbon monoxide poisoning, as it has been encountered in barbiturate poisoning (page 819) and in cases of marked scleroses of the vessels of the corpus striatum.

If the anoxemia is prolonged, lesions may develop in other portions of the brain. In the white matter, especially of the cerebrum where the small arteries are almost end vessels with but few anastomoses, anoxemia causes sluggishness of the circulation and dilatation of blood vessels which may be engorged with normal blood, laked blood, neutrophil leukocytes or hyaline thrombi. Shortly thereafter microscopic areas of rarefaction necrosis appear in the white matter along with ring hemorrhages which are sometimes visible as punctate red dots in the brain; these lesions are associated with the occlusion of the minute arteries by hyaline thrombi which form in the vessels and produce microscopic infarcts in the white matter (Figs. 19-4 and 19-5). The rarefaction necrosis appears as an ovoid translucent area surrounded by thrombosed vessels or as a perivascular circular zone around a single thrombosed vessel. The myelin in the necrotic tissue is destroyed and removed, leaving a mesh-like structure which contains edematous fluid, hemolyzed red blood cells or even fibrin deposits. (See reference to Petri.) The ring hemorrhages are similar to the lesions described under fat embolism (page 168), showing a central vessel obstructed by a hyaline thrombus, a circular zone of necrotic brain tissue around the vessel, and a ring hemorrhage forming the outermost zone (Fig. 19-6). In other cases a small arteriole may become necrotic as a result of anoxemia, and rupture,

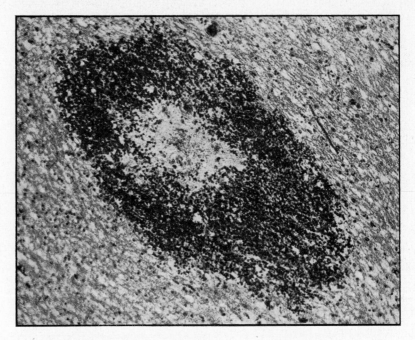

Fig. 19-6. Ring Hemorrhage in Cerebral White Matter.

Acute carbon monoxide poisoning. Survived 6 days after exposure. Same case as Figure 19-5. Photomicrograph, 16 mm. objective.

producing a small ball hemorrhage. In some carbon monoxide poisonings with a protracted clinical course, the blood vessels of the white matter may contain hyaline thrombi in large numbers and may be surrounded by microglia, leukocytes and round cells; occasionally microglia may show mitotic figures and may permeate the surrounding brain tissue which is usually edematous. In a few instances dark, blue-staining beaded deposits may be encountered, encircling the peripheral zone of the smaller blood vessels.

Necroses in the heart muscle may occur as a result of anoxemia in delayed cases of carbon monoxide poisoning which have survived the exposure 36 hours or more. The most common sites for such necroses are the papillary muscles of the left ventricle whose tips are not as well supplied with blood vessels as the rest of the myocardium. Macroscopically longitudinal incision of the papillary muscles may show patchy hemorrhages at the tips or a fan-like hemorrhagic striation branching out from the tendinous insertion into the muscle (Fig. 19-7). Histologic examination discloses vascular dilatation and congestion, intermuscular hemorrhages, necrosis, atrophy or eosinophilic staining of the muscle fibers, and a slight neutrophil, leukocytic infiltration in the periphery of the necrotic areas. In rare instances the ventricular muscle of the heart is involved, the chambers are dilated, and the myocardium is permeated with hemorrhagic infiltrations especially near the pericardium and endocardium (Fig. 19-8). Histologically there is dilatation and engorgement of blood vessels, some intermuscular extravasation of the red blood cells, hyaline thrombi in the smaller blood vessels, eosinophilic staining and swelling of muscle

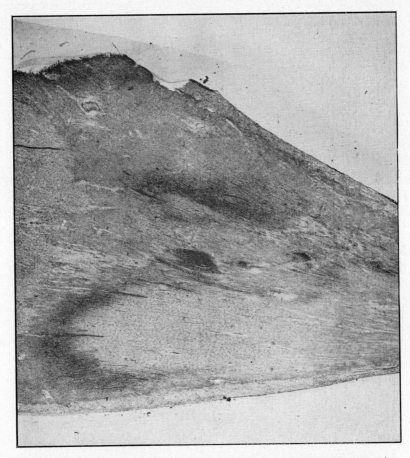

Fig. 19-7. Anoxic Necrosis of Tip of Papillary Muscle of Left Cardiac Ventricle.

Acute carbon monoxide poisoning. Death 4 days after exposure. Low power photomicrograph.

fibers and a slight leukocytic infiltration at the periphery of the necrotic areas. If the heart is extensively involved, circulatory disabilities may follow (page 123). Petri has mentioned cases of subacute myocarditis in delayed carbon monoxide poisoning, but whenever such a condition is encountered at autopsy, trichinosis, chronic infections, coronary artery disease and similar processes must be eliminated as possible etiologic factors before accepting the lesion as a possible result of carbon monoxide anoxemia.

Other complications of delayed carbon monoxide poisoning occur as areas of trophic erythema and blister formation in various places on the skin of the trunk, face and extremities, not necessarily at the points of pressure (Fig. 19-9). These lesions are few or many in number, are roughly geographic in shape, and vary in size from a few millimeters to 20 cm. or over. In the early stages the epidermis is intact, and the dermis and subcutaneous fat are markedly injected; histologic examination of the area may show a thick infiltration of neutrophilic leukocytes in the arterial walls. Collection of fluid between the epidermis and dermis may occur and the epithelial cells in the region of the blister may undergo swelling and

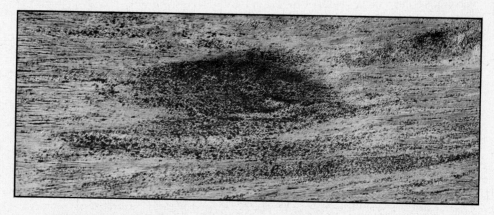

Fig. 19-8. Higher Magnification of Hemorrhagic Area in Lesion shown in Figure 19-7.

degeneration. The epidermis may break, a raw surface is exposed and an ulceration may develop. The nature of the lesion indicates a necrosis similar to a decubitus, occurring as a direct result of the initial anoxemia. In some cases typical decubital ulcers may occur at the various points of pressure. Uncommon conditions, such as localized myositis of the buttock, and pathologic lesions in other viscera may occur. For discussion of these the reader is referred to Petri.

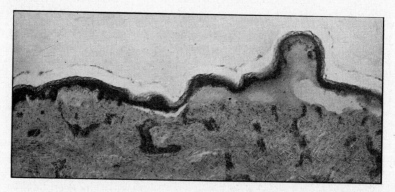

Fig. 19-9. Photomicrograph of Skin Blister from Same Case Illustrated in Figures 19-7 and 19-8. 16 mm. objective.

If the exposure to carbon monoxide results in severe anoxemia over a long period of time, the primary lesions may be the basis for other fatal complications. If considerable degenerative changes have occurred in the heart muscle, the myocardium is weakened, the circulation of the blood is slowed and conditions favorable for thrombus formation are produced. Mural thrombi sometimes form in the left ventricle (Fig. 19-10) and on occasion are detached as an embolus to one of the cerebral arteries, causing an infarct of the brain. A thrombus may form in the femoral vessels and cause gangrene of the leg. The authors have observed thrombus formation in the pulmonary artery in delayed carbon monoxide poisoning from slowing of the circulation secondary to myocardial involvement. If the victim is an elderly individual, arteriosclerotic changes and other chronic disease processes may materially abet the development of anoxemic lesions and precipitate the onset of fatal complications. In autopsies on delayed cases of carbon monoxide poisoning, it is necessary to distinguish the pathologic conditions which are due to anoxemia from the poisoning, and those which are the result of disease processes or other causes.

Types of Poisoning. ACCIDENTAL. Many types of carbon monoxide poisoning are accidental, and most of them in large urban centers are cases of illuminating gas poisoning. In many instances the deceased is an intoxicated or an arteriosclerotic individual who blunders into a dangerous situation with the gas fixtures. Some turn

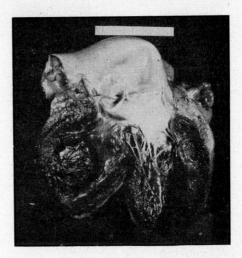

Fig. 19-10. Large Globular Thrombus in Left Ventricle at Site of Anoxic Necrosis of Endocardium and Myocardium.

Acute carbon monoxide poisoning. Death several days after exposure. Elderly white woman.

the gas on and then forget to ignite it, some allow a pot to boil over and extinguish the gas flame, others stumble over and disconnect a gas hose which extends from a stove to a wall fixture allowing gas to escape into a room; a tube joining a wall fixture with a stove may have a deficient connection which allows a dangerous leakage. In some cases the victim has gone to sleep with a gas stove burning, and during that period the main for the house was turned off, extinguishing the fire in the stove; later, while the victim was still asleep, the gas main was turned on again and the gas escaping into the room without igniting, asphyxiated him.

Carbon monoxide may be released into a room in poisonous amounts, even when illuminating gas or other fuel is burning, because the flame does not completely consume all of the carbon components of the gas. Ordinarily a blue flame on a burner burns all the carbon monoxide and hydrocarbons to carbon dioxide, but under some conditions some of the carbon monoxide escapes combustion and the hydrocarbons are partially oxidized to carbon monoxide. Henderson and Haggard assert that when a blue flame is brought in contact with a cold object, like a utensil, it is chilled and incomplete combustion occurs. If the gas is driven at a forced blast through a burner or if the edges of the burner are fouled by carbon deposit, insufficient oxygen will reach the flame and carbon monoxide will escape into the room in dangerous quantity. For these reasons, gas stoves, gas heaters and refrigerators operated by illuminating gas may be dangerous appliances to operate in a confined space (Figs. 19-11 and 19-12). Coal, coke and charcoal stoves may generate sufficient carbon monoxide to cause fatal asphyxiation. A large coal furnace in the cellar of a small building may produce carbon monoxide in sufficient quantity to permeate the house and fatally asphyxiate several occupants. The central heating furnace of a large building discharges smoke and carbon monoxide into the flues and if these crack in different places at various levels, carbon monoxide may escape into different floors of the building with resulting fatalities. The close association of carbon monoxide with fuel combustion is illustrated by the higher incidence of such asphyxiations in winter.

The exhaust gases from internal combustion engines contain on the average 7 per cent of carbon monoxide and are therefore dangerous. Accidental cases of

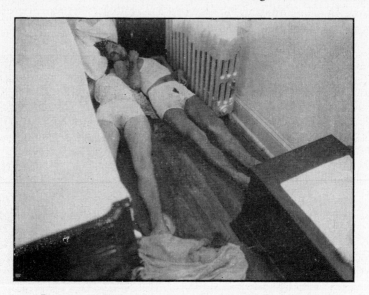

Fig. 19-11. Multiple Deaths from Carbon Monoxide Poisoning.

Prolonged inhalation of relatively low but lethal concentrations (0.05 to 0.1 per cent) of carbon monoxide generated during faulty operation of gas flame refrigerator. Note bizarre position of bodies at scene, the circumstances at first suspicious of homicide.

poisoning may occur quickly if the engine of a motor car is allowed to run in a small closed garage. In a closed traveling automobile they have also resulted from the escape of exhaust gases into the body of the car from a defective exhaust pipe which ran under the back part of the floor. In conflagrations enough carbon monoxide is generated by the combustion to be fatal for any person forced to inhale the smoke.

SUICIDAL. Suicidal deaths from carbon monoxide poisoning are common, and most of them are due to illuminating gas. In the typical case, evidence of preparation for the event is present; a note may be left indicating a suicidal intention, or the cracks of the windows and doors may be stuffed with cloth or paper to prevent the escape of gas from the room, or there may be a gas tube leading from a fixture which is attached near the mouth and nose of the deceased. Occasionally the suicide holds his head over the gas jets of a cooking stove, impressing the gratings on his face, or he may place his head inside an oven and then turn on the burners. In one instance the suicide covered his head with a blanket as he lay in bed, conducting illuminating gas through a long tube from a wall fixture to his face under the blanket. A few individuals commit suicide by running an automobile engine in a closed garage and inhaling the gases from the exhaust.

HOMICIDAL. Homicidal carbon monoxide poisoning is not as common as the other two types, but has been encountered occasionally. With gas fixtures in a room and an intoxicated victim, it would be an easy matter to set the stage for an innocent interpretation of a homicidal death. To discover the truth it would be necessary to detect some discrepancy between the story and the circumstances. The case of Malloy who was insured for an expensive life insurance policy by a group of men illustrates these points. They made several attempts to kill him by running him down with an automobile, by feeding him poison and by other means. Finally they

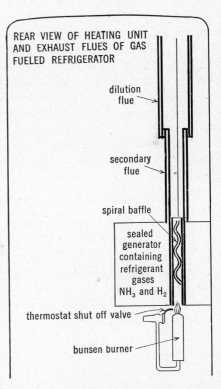

Fig. 19-12. Diagram of Gas Flame Refrigerator Showing Arrangement of Flues Which Discharge Products of Combustion into the Closed Atmosphere of the Room.

Carbon monoxide generated by incomplete combustion of fuel gas during faulty operation of the heating unit of the refrigerator may contaminate the air of a poorly ventilated room to a dangerous degree and cause serious or fatal acute poisoning, characteristically slow and manifested by progressive headache, mental confusion, nausea, vomiting, involuntary bowel action, stupor, unconsciousness and death. Poisoning by carbon monoxide in the raw gas is prevented by an automatic thermostatic shut-off valve should the flame be extinguished. Improper alignment of the bunsen burner, impingement of the flame, inadequate supply of primary air, overgassing, blockage of the flue by accumulated soot and scale are factors favoring generation of carbon monoxide.

REAR VIEW OF HEATING UNIT AND EXHAUST FLUES OF GAS FUELED REFRIGERATOR

dilution flue

secondary flue

spiral baffle

sealed generator containing refrigerant gases NH_3 and H_2

thermostat shut off valve

bunsen burner

asphyxiated him with illuminating gas while he was insensible from alcoholic intoxication. The homicide was discovered several months later, after the deceased had been buried with a cause of death certified to by a physician as lobar pneumonia. The true cause of death was apparent and easily demonstrated on the exhumed and embalmed body.

If several persons are asphyxiated in the same room, the chances are that the poisoning is accidental. On the other hand, such deaths may be homicidal, or the result of a suicidal pact, or homicidal and suicidal, and the case can be solved only after an investigation. The authors have seen a case of the last mentioned type which had some bizarre features, the perpetrator binding his wife to the bed, turning on the gas jets, and then lying down beside her while asphyxiation occurred.

The yearly average of deaths from carbon monoxide in New York City is about 842 cases, of which the great majority are cases of illuminating gas poisoning. Of these, 440 are suicides, carbon monoxide being the most common form of suicide, and of that number 435 cases are illuminating gas poisoning and 5 cases are the result of poisoning from the gases in a motor exhaust. Accidental cases number

395, with illuminating gas cases 370 and carbon monoxide poisoning by combustion of fuel 25. In many instances the circumstances were not determinable. Homicidal cases are rare, about 7, and are generally associated with the suicide of the perpetrator.

In New York City in 1950 and 1952 respectively, throughout the Boroughs of Richmond and Brooklyn, natural gas was substituted for the old illuminating gas which was manufactured from coal and contained carbon monoxide as its chief ingredient. Natural gas contains methane (CH_3), 94.1 per cent; ethane (C_2H_6), 3.6 per cent; propane (C_3H_8), 1.0 per cent; higher paraffin hydrocarbons, 0.7 per cent; and carbon dioxide (CO_2), 0.6 per cent. There is no carbon monoxide in natural gas so that if it is inhaled directly with plenty of oxygen, the victim is not seriously affected but only rendered uncomfortable. Of course if the gas were inhaled in a closed chamber without oxygen, it would cause death from asphyxia like carbon dioxide. As it is rich in hydrocarbons containing much carbon, natural gas on combustion might form considerable carbon monoxide and be a source of poisoning, especially if burned under conditions in which complete combustion did not occur.

The statistics of the Chief Medical Examiner for Richmond from 1947 to 1951 show a striking decrease in fatal cases of gas poisoning after the substitution was made:

   1947—fatal cases of gas poisoning, 13 (suicide, 8; accident, 5).
   1948—fatal cases of gas poisoning, 16 (suicide, 9; accident, 6; homicide, 1).
   1949—fatal cases of gas poisoning, 9 (suicide, 3; accident, 6).
   1950—fatal cases of gas poisoning, 0.
   1951—fatal cases of gas poisoning, 0.

Investigation of the scene of death is important in all suspected cases of carbon monoxide poisoning. If the asphyxiation is due to illuminating gas, the odor of this substance may be detected by persons discovering the dead body; on the other hand, if the carbon monoxide is formed by fuel combustion of any sort, such odor is usually lacking. It is important in every case for the examiner to determine the possible source of carbon monoxide, whether from a gas pipe, a burning stove, a leaky flue, a running motor or some other appliance like a gas refrigerator or a gas heater. In many cases in which asphyxiation is caused by unconsumed carbon monoxide escaping from a burning gas stove or heater into a small room, the temperature may be quite warm and the body of the deceased may show considerable decomposition. In cases of doubt, the body should be examined in a good light, an autopsy performed and blood and other tissues kept for chemical examination. In some instances the routine examination for ethyl alcohol may be important in determining the nature of the case. If the skin of the deceased is at all dark in color, the postmortem lividity may not show a typical cherry red color, but the blood, muscles and viscera usually do. If postmortem putrefaction is present and has reached the stage of complete blood destruction, it will not be possible to test for carboxyhemoglobin by chemical examination.

HYDROCARBONS

Methane, CH_3, is one of the hydrocarbons formed from decaying organic matter in marshes and mines, and is a constituent of natural gas. It is odorless, colorless and inflammable, burning with a blue flame. Methane diffuses easily into air and in proportions of 1 to 18 of air by volume it forms an explosive mixture which is often encountered in mines and is known as fire damp. The principal toxic action of methane is to cause asphyxia, merely because it replaces oxygen. Some claim that it has a slightly toxic effect on the central nervous system but as a lethal poison it is not of much importance. The higher homologues of the methane series such as acetylene, found in some illuminating gases, have a slight anesthetic action on the central nervous system, but are not very toxic. Other aliphatic hydrocarbons are discussed under volatile organic poisons on page 804.

SULFUR COMPOUNDS

Hydrogen Sulfide. Hydrogen sulfide, H_2S, is a colorless transparent gas which has an odor like rotten eggs. It is soluble in water, and is inflammable, burning with a blue flame; when mixed with half its volume of oxygen, it is explosive. Its specific gravity is 1.1912, slightly heavier than air.

The gas is produced by the decomposition of organic matter containing sulfur and is found in sewers, cesspools, tannery vats, glue factories, fat rendering plants and privy vaults. It is formed in the human intestine during life, and in the body after death as a result of bacterial putrefaction. Hydrogen sulfide is produced in laboratories by the action of acids on metallic sulfides, and is set free in mines by analogous reactions. Some manufacturing processes which use sulfur compounds are accompanied by the formation of considerable hydrogen sulfide. The gas is found naturally in volcanic regions and in the waters of mineral springs.

Poisoning by hydrogen sulfide is likely to occur in places where large quantities of the gas are produced, such as chemical laboratories, manufacturing plants, sewers and big cesspools. Hydrogen sulfide is one of the components of a mixture, known as sewer gas, which contains in addition, hydrocarbons, carbon dioxide, ammonia, nitrogen and air. The poisonous concentration of hydrogen sulfide in the air is 0.02 per cent, while 0.1 per cent is distinctly dangerous. The authors have encountered one case in which four workmen were descending a ladder into a cesspool pit and, overcome by the exhalations of the sewer gas, suddenly tumbled to the bottom; all were rescued but one man died as a result of smothering in the mud.

Externally hydrogen sulfide is a moderately severe local irritant, and after absorption is a virulent systemic poison. The gas irritates the conjunctivae and, on inhalation, causes a slight inflammation of the air passages combining with the alkali in the cells to form sodium sulfide. If a small portion of this compound is absorbed into the blood stream it is finally converted into innocuous sulfates and excreted in the urine. If pure hydrogen sulfide is inhaled and absorbed into the blood in large quantity, the poison paralyses the central nervous system, causing rapid death by overwhelming the respiratory center. If the concentration is less intense, giddiness, nausea, pains in the abdomen, labored breathing, irregular heart action, delirium, convulsions, coma, collapse and death may occur. In more dilute concentrations, conjunctival irritation, sleepiness, headache, dizziness and fever may follow a long exposure. Individuals in daily contact with the gas may develop a chronic poisoning which is marked by headache, gastric colic, constipation, malaise, anemia, conjunctivitis and furunculosis. A person who has recovered from one exposure to hydrogen sulfide seems to be rendered more susceptible to the poisonous effects of the gas during any future exposure.

Hydrogen sulfide acts on the blood in cases where the gas is inhaled over a long period of time to form a compound known as sulfmethemoglobin; this compound has a specific absorption spectrum of two bands, one in the red zone between

D and C, while the other is more indefinite and runs from D nearly halfway to E. Formerly it was supposed that sulfmethemoglobin was derived by the action of hydrogen sulfide on oxyhemoglobin, but now it is considered that it is not formed unless methemoglobin is present. As the formation of sulfmethemoglobin is slow, this pigment is absent in cases of rapid poisoning.

If a rapidly fatal case of hydrogen sulfide poisoning is autopsied soon after death, little will be disclosed that is characteristic. Later the body undergoes rapid bacterial decomposition with congested organs, dark blood sometimes bluish green in color, dark red muscles, and rapidly spreading, greenish discoloration of the tissues of the abdomen. If death is delayed after the poisoning, especially after a long exposure to a low concentration of the gas, edema of the lungs and a dark cyanosis are found at autopsy. The treatment and prophylaxis are practically the same as in carbon monoxide poisoning.

Sulfur Dioxide. Sulfur dioxide, SO_2, is a colorless gas, heavier than air (specific gravity, 2.25), and so pungent that it is not respirable. It is formed when sulfur is burned and is found around towns which use coal containing a large amount of this substance; in nature sulfur dioxide occurs near volcanoes. The gas is employed in industry as a disinfectant, as a bleach and as a powerful reducing agent.

Inhalation of the gas produces sneezing, coughing, irritation of the air passages and conjunctivae, followed by dyspnea, cyanosis and convulsions. If a large quantity is inhaled, spasm of the glottis occurs and death from rapid suffocation supervenes. In the later stages the blood is affected and may be brownish red from the formation of acid hematin. The cornea may be rendered opaque by inflammation. If those exposed to the gas are habituated gradually, they are often able to endure high concentrations.

Autopsy discloses cyanosis and other asphyxial signs, inflammation of the respiratory tract, and dark blood with an acid reaction and appreciable amounts of acid hematin. Prophylaxis and treatment are practically the same as for carbon monoxide poisoning.

THE OXIDES OF NITROGEN

Nitrous Oxide. Nitrous oxide, N_2O, is a colorless gas with a sweetish odor and taste, slightly heavier than air, the specific gravity being 1.53. The gas is prepared for anesthetic purposes by heating ammonium nitrate to form nitrous oxide which is stored in wrought iron cylinders after proper purification. In administering the anesthetic, nitrous oxide is mixed with 20 per cent oxygen or less in a special apparatus in order to reduce the danger of asphyxia. When inhaled, the gas produces a tingling sensation, rapid unconsciousness and anesthesia, accompanied by cyanosis and an elevated blood pressure. Under the influence of nitrous oxide patients may become hilarious or display some other emotional reaction and, because of such effects, the compound has long been known as laughing gas. Nitrous oxide is mostly employed in minor surgical and dental operations of short duration for which it is well suited, as the patient recovers consciousness rapidly and suffers few after-effects. In major surgical operations, it is used to induce anesthesia which is then maintained by other anesthetics such as ether or cyclopropane, substances safer for prolonged use. Fatal poisoning by nitrous oxide during its use as an anesthetic sometimes occurs but is not frequent.

Courville classifies nitrous oxide poisoning as: (1) Acute. This category includes cases in which death occurs suddenly and early during the anesthesia, and also those in which the victim dies after prolonged anesthesia while under the influence of the gas. (2) Delayed. In this group the victim may die after a long survival period of days or weeks, or recover with sequelae resulting from cortical or lenticular brain damage. This group of delayed poisonings also includes cases in which the patient recovers, after having shown transitory emotional and mental disturbances.

Courville has listed a number of predisposing factors which render a patient susceptible to untoward effects of nitrous oxide. (1) Congenital predispositions which include personal idiosyncrasy to nitrous oxide, robust habitus and status lymphaticus. (2) Acquired conditions such as alcoholism, pulmonary disease, blood dyscrasias and preexisting cerebral conditions, all of which may react unfavorably to the induced anoxemia associated with nitrous oxide anesthesia. (3) Disturbed reflex actions, especially from the carotid sinus, or from the lower abdomen, which may lead to unfortunate results during the course of the anesthesia. These factors may operate in either acute or delayed poisoning.

ACUTE POISONING. Acute poisoning during the use of nitrous oxide as an anesthetic may occur, because the anesthetic effect of the gas is due in part to its direct depressant action on the brain, and in part to the associated asphyxia. To obtain a loss of sensibility, the amount of oxygen in the anesthetic mixture must be diminished to a point where the patient is on the threshold of lapsing into a dangerous state of anoxemia and cerebral anoxia. In some cases sudden death may occur from paralysis of the respiratory and vasomotor centers in the medulla at any time during the administration of the anesthetic. The postmortem findings are those of asphyxia with marked cyanosis, congestion of viscera and dark red blood. In other cases in which the patient has been exposed to a long period of anesthesia death may occur from cerebral anoxia while still under the influence of the anesthetic. The treatment of the acute poisoning is artificial respiration, inhalation of oxygen and appropriate stimulation.

DELAYED POISONING. In rare cases in which nitrous oxide anesthesia has continued for a long period of time the immediate effects of the anesthetic may be survived but the patient may remain in stupor for an interval varying from 36 hours to weeks. At the end of that time he may die as a result of severe degenerative lesions in the central nervous system induced by the anesthesia, or he may recover gradually retaining permanent disabilities consequent upon anatomic lesions in the central nervous system, or his recovery may be complete after transient emotional and mental manifestations. The underlying cause of these conditions is the anoxemia and tissue anoxia produced by the prolonged administration of nitrous oxide, the effects being enhanced by the reduction in the quantity of oxygen necessary for induction and maintenance of anesthesia. As the anoxemia progresses the oxygen tension is diminished in the blood which is then unable to give up its oxygen to the tissues as readily as under normal conditions. The combined effects of the anoxemia and the direct depressant, toxic action of nitrous oxide on the medullary centers may cause the circulatory and respiratory mechanisms to fail. In delayed poisoning, the most characteristic feature is the variety of symptoms and signs referable to the central nervous system resulting from the pathologic changes in the brain produced by the tissue anoxia. In such cases, the more pronounced the degree of respiratory and circulatory failure, the more severe will be the neurologic and mental effects, the more marked the pathologic lesions in the brain and the more unfavorable the prognosis.

In the delayed fatal cases, the victim remains unconscious and may manifest muscular activity varying from twitching to gross convulsive seizures, signs which are suggestive of decerebrate rigidity; the temperature rises and death in coma occurs after a long interval. In a few cases the patient may recover consciousness and exhibit physical helplessness, apraxia and motor speech disturbances; death may then occur after a long period of debilitating illness. Albumin may be present in the urine denoting damage to the renal epithelium from the asphyxia.

Rarely a patient may regain consciousness after a lengthy period of stupor and recover after a long convalescence but is left with serious residual mental and neurologic symptoms and signs such as dementia, delirium, choreiform and athetoid movements, muscular rigidity and flexion deformities, due to structural changes in the cortex and the lenticular nucleus. A few fortunate individuals recover, displaying only temporary emotional and neurologic manifestations.

Autopsies reported by Courville on the fatal delayed nitrous oxide poisonings which have survived the administration of the anesthetic 36 hours or more, usually show pathologic conditions in the brain. The lesions may take the form of focal necroses, similar to those found in carbon monoxide poisoning, in which areas of rarefaction and ring and ball hemorrhages are found in the cerebral hemispheres, and bilateral necrosis is found in the globus pallidus and other parts of the lenticular nucleus. The cerebral cortex may exhibit varying degrees of necrosis; the process may be focal, diffuse or so extensive that most of a cerebral hemisphere is involved.

The changes which occur in the necrotic areas are mainly the result of tissue anoxia. The nerve cells undergo swelling and lipoid material accumulates in the cytoplasm, or the cells shrink and undergo a process of sclerosis. Some cells exhibit ferrugination, the cytoplasm being transformed into a dark blue staining substance. The tigroid material near the nucleus of the nerve cells degenerates and the nucleus undergoes dissolution or degeneration. The Purkinje cells in the cerebellum may contain iron deposits. The nerve fibrils undergo dissolution. The blood vessels may be surrounded by microglia which may be transformed into foamy compound granular corpuscles filled with fatty deposits; the perivascular cells may show mitotic figures; the necrotic tissue may be permeated with reacting and proliferating microglia. The vessels in the degenerated areas may proliferate to form a vascular scar; calcium deposits may occur in the blood vessel walls within the lenticular nucleus. Central necroses of the liver lobules, acute degeneration of the kidney tubules and pulmonary edema and congestion were also observed.

Nitric Oxide. Nitric oxide, NO, is a colorless, corrosive gas which is nearly insoluble in water. It is never found in the atmosphere because in the presence of oxygen it is transformed into a yellowish gas, NO_2, or a brownish gas, N_2O_4, both of which are soluble in water. These compounds are formed when nitric acid acts on metals, and may be produced in large quantities in chemical laboratories. The gases are generated also during the manufacture of explosives such as nitroglycerine and guncotton, and during the burning of nitrate celluloid photographic film. The toxicity of these oxides of nitrogen is indicated by the fact that an inhalation of 0.6 to 1.0 mg. concentration of the gas in a liter of air may cause rapid death, while lesser concentrations may be distinctly dangerous.

Death may occur soon after exposure or in 5 to 40 hours. Inhalation of a small quantity of the gas produces a spasmodic contraction of the bronchi with cough, tightness of the chest and a cramp-like pain in the abdomen. These symptoms occur immediately or are delayed a few hours, especially if the concentration of the gas is dilute. If a large quantity is inhaled there is sudden collapse, marked by dyspnea, coughing, cyanosis, tightness of the chest and death as the result of shock. At autopsy the lungs are markedly congested and edematous, the mucous membrane of the air passages is reddened, the bronchial epithelium is desquamated and the secretion in the bronchi and alveoli may have a brownish tinge. If much mucus is swallowed the stomach mucous membrane may be discolored by a yellowish brown tinge. The viscera are markedly congested and the blood in the vessels may have a black red or chocolate colored hue from the formation of methemoglobin, produced by the nitrite action of the gas on the blood; in a few cases the blood may be almost black and have an acid reaction. Death may occur as the result of a secondary pneumonia. The diagnosis of acute poisoning by nitric oxide derivatives is made on the basis of a history of exposure, of the results of the autopsy and of the chemical examination of the poisonous atmosphere.

The treatment of the acute poisoning is to remove the victim from the poisonous atmosphere as soon as possible and administer artificial respiration, preferably with inhalation of 5 per cent carbon dioxide in oxygen. Weak alkaline salt infusion may be used to combat the acidity in the blood. Venesection and intravenous injection of normal saline solution may be indicated.

Some cases show delayed symptoms with continual recurrences for several weeks. Wood has reported a case in which an obliterating bronchiolitis developed as a sequel to the acute lesions in the air passages. Carnified pneumonias and chronic pneumonitis have been described in similar cases (Petri). Small hemorrhages in the brain and degenerative changes in myocardium, liver and kidneys have been reported but are not common (Petri). A chronic poisoning has been described in workers continually exposed to nitric oxide derivatives; the victims show cachexia, pallor and yellow discoloration of skin, hair, gums and incisor teeth (Petri).

Other gases, responsible for cases of fatal poisoning, such as hydrocyanic acid, chlorine, phosphine and arsine, will be discussed in Chapters 28 and 29.

WAR GASES

The term gas, as used in the vocabulary of chemical warfare, does not designate the physical state of a substance but rather its applicability as an agent fitted to carry destruction or damage to the enemy forces. Thus the actual combat gases are either true gases, smokes, volatilized liquids or finely divided solids, but in spite of their physical differences they have many features in common, referable to their employment in warfare. These chemicals are designed to harass troops in a battle zone, and to accomplish this purpose effectively they must be used in considerable quantity over a broad segment of the terrain.

A chemical compound, to be acceptable as a war gas, must be capable of being manufactured cheaply in enormous quantities, preferably as a by-product of some industry. It must be definitely toxic in low concentration, otherwise it will not be effective against troops distributed over a wide area. The substance must be heavier than air so that it will not be easily dispersed, but it must be capable of enough volatilization to pervade the terrain which is assailed. Finally its chemical composition must be stable and not of a type to corrode the containers in which it is stored.

In World War I, toxic chemicals were directed against the enemy in three different ways. The earliest method was to transport large containers charged with such poisonous gases as chlorine and phosgene to the front lines and there open the valves, allowing a favoring breeze to carry the toxic fumes to the lines of the enemy.

Later this was superseded by more effective methods: in one, large canisters containing the gases were thrown by trench mortars in a concentrated attack on a sector of the enemy front, and automatically discharged of their contents after landing; in another method the chemicals whether gas, liquid or solid were enclosed in special artillery shells which were fired in a barrage on a definite area, the explosion of the shell setting free the noxious substance in such a way that it permeated the atmosphere near the ground. Gas shells are most effective on a damp foggy day without much wind, for under such conditions the fumes are less likely to be scattered. Four types of poison are employed as war gases, (1) lacrimators, (2) lung irritants, (3) vesicants and (4) sternutators.

1. **Lacrimators.** Lacrimators or tear gases are fired in artillery shells and are ordinarily harmless to life in the concentrations obtainable under such conditions, but they produce severe lacrimation and temporary blinding of those in the neighborhood of the explosion. One of the lacrimators is chloracetophenone, a finely divided powder with an odor like locust flowers. Brombenzyl cyanide is another lacrimator in the form of a powder with an odor like sour fruit. The regular gas mask protects against these substances. The treatment after exposure is to bathe the eyes in boric acid solution and to apply sodium bicarbonate solution to any irritation which might develop on the nose or face.

The authors have seen a case in which chloracetophenone in tear gas produced a more severe reaction. A white man in the early forties locked himself in a room and successfully resisted all attempts to eject him. The police were called and injected tear gas to drive him from his stronghold, but were not able to enter for an hour and a half; during this time the man was exposed to the chemical fumes. He was found unconscious and taken to the hospital where he died two days later. The autopsy disclosed a light purplish brown discoloration of face, neck and shoulders with a few indolent blisters here and there, and a suppurative pseudomembranous inflammation of larynx, trachea and bronchi even involving the smaller branches. The conjunctivae were congested but not noticeably inflamed. Death was due to secondary bronchopneumonia from the inflammation of the air passages. The lesions were similar to those encountered in mustard gas poisoning but not as severe. They were probably due to the protracted exposure of the deceased to the tear gas.

2. **Lung Irritants.** The group of lung irritants are lethal chemicals used to kill the enemy and, as they are soon dissipated from the terrain, they are often employed as a preparation for an infantry attack. Some, such as chlorine and phosgene, are gases and can be released from tanks, canisters and gas shells. Chloropicrin, on the other hand, is an oily liquid with an odor like fly paper and is used in gas shells. The regulation gas mask if put on in time is sufficient protection against any of the lung irritants. If they are inhaled, these chemicals cause dyspnea, tightness of the chest, coughing and varying degrees of irritation of the conjunctivae; chloropicrin causes also a severe conjunctival irritation and has the inconvenient effect of producing vomiting, sometimes in the gas mask.

PHOSGENE. Phosgene, a colorless gas with an odor like moldy hay, is one of the most lethal of the lung irritants. When it is inhaled in overwhelming amounts, death may occur in a few minutes to an hour from acute asphyxia associated with marked cyanosis, shock and suddenly falling blood pressure. At autopsy the lungs show areas of hyperaeration mingled with areas of collapse, presenting a marbled appearance, and the pulmonary blood vessels are engorged, the capillaries are distended, but the alveoli are not markedly edematous. The gas in encountering the air passages is partially decomposed into hydrochloric acid, and may produce a slight inflammation of the mucous membrane, destruction of the neighboring erythrocytes and a brownish discoloration of the surface layers from acid hematin formation.

Most of the cases of phosgene poisoning die in 24 hours, with an average duration of 12 to 14 hours. Such victims usually show a distressing asphyxia, severe coughing, marked cyanosis, rapid pulse and falling blood pressure; some of them may die in a rapid collapse, marked by a pasty pallor, weak pulse and complete circulatory failure. Autopsies on such bodies disclose markedly edematous, cyanotic lungs, voluminous and heavy, with foam in the air passages and fluid pouring from the tissues on cut section; the lungs have a marbled appearance because of the lighter areas of hyperaeration and interstitial emphysema which are mixed in with the darker areas of edema and pulmonary congestion. There may be irritation and desquamation of epithelium in the upper respiratory tract, and moderate irritation and inflammation of the conjunctivae and lids. The heart is usually distended and contains fluid blood and the viscera are congested. The treatment employed in the early cases is oxygen inhalation, cardiac stimulation or venesection as the symptoms indicate. If the eyes are inflamed they may be bathed in boric acid solution. The milder cases usually recover without sequelae.

Some patients who survive the acute stage for two days or more, may die of a terminal pneumonia, usually peribronchial in type; rarely the victim may recover from this complication but may develop chronic obliterative bronchitis, bronchiectasis or similar lung conditions as sequelae. After World War I, many of the victims of a wartime gas attack had a tendency to attribute to that episode all subsequent lung infections which they might incur, even though several years might have elapsed during the interval. Most of those claims were erroneous and the causal connection in most cases was dubious; the evidence should be unimpeachable to render a claim of this sort valid.

Other lesions in delayed cases of poisoning are small petechial hemorrhages and minute areas of rarefaction necrosis in the white matter of the brain, similar to those described in carbon monoxide poisoning. Some consider the possibility that carbon monoxide may play a role in producing these lesions as it is formed during gas shell explosions and may be inhaled (see Petri). In rare cases, thrombi are said to be formed in the heart and blood vessels as a result of cardiac weakness and may produce infarcts and other embolic phenomena in some of the other organs.

3. **Vesicants.** The vesicant war chemicals are yperite or mustard gas (dichlorethyl sulfide) and lewisite (chlorvinyldichlorarsin), both of which are volatile irritant liquids, discharged in artillery shells so as to impregnate the area of attack. The vesicants are persistent after they have been deposited on their objective, and a terrain covered with mustard gas is poisonous to human occupation for two to four days. The shells are usually fired against a segment of the battle front which an army does not wish to occupy, but from which it desires to keep the opposing army.

YPERITE. Yperite or mustard gas is a volatile liquid with a pungent but not overwhelming garlicky odor, which is irritant whether the skin is exposed directly to the liquid or to its fumes. The action of mustard gas is insidious, for the irritative effects do not occur immediately, but develop about 2 to 4 hours after exposure. The conjunctivae and eyelids are congested, swelling and edema of the submucous tissues are present, profuse lacrimation occurs, and the victim complains of local pain and photophobia. In severe cases a mucopurulent inflammation develops, sometimes resulting in scarring of the cornea and blindness. The oily portions of the skin may be inflamed, such as the face, axillae, pubes, scrotum and similar areas, starting usually as erythema and congestion and soon followed by swelling and edema of the subcutaneous tissues, a bright red color of the surface layer and the formation of blisters varying in size from a few millimeters to many centimeters in diameter. The victim complains of pain and itching in the affected areas. Yperite penetrates to the deeper layers of the epidermis where it is partly decomposed with the release of chlorine; irritation follows and blister formation may result from the exudation of fluid between the epidermal layers. The superficial layer may become necrotic and rupture, leaving a raw surface; the blister fluid apparently does not possess any irritative properties and does not cause further inflammation. The skin lesions inflicted by mustard gas are slow to heal and on recovery become brown in color like sunburn.

A severe inflammation appears in the respiratory tract about the same time as the skin burns, and is most severe on the third day after exposure. The lesion begins as a marked necrosis of the upper respiratory tract, larynx, trachea and bronchi down to the finer branches, and soon becomes pseudomembranous in character with congestion, edema and swelling of the submucous layer. The most prominent symptoms are fever, painful cough, dysphonia, difficult respirations and a variable degree of asphyxia. Many of the victims die of a terminal bronchopneumonia which develops as a direct result of the bronchial inflammation. In rare instances the stomach is inflamed as the result of swallowing the chemical. Some cases which recover may show residual lesions of the bronchial and pulmonary inflammation such as squamous epithelial metaplasia of the bronchial mucous membrane, chronic obliterative bronchitis, and other pulmonary conditions. Systemic effects due to the absorption of mustard gas have been described; leukopenia and bone marrow necrosis in human battle casualties were reported by Krumbhaar and Krumbhaar. For the results of the intravenous injection of dichlorethyl sulfide into rabbits, causing leukopenia and bone marrow necrosis, see reference to Pappenheimer and Vance.

The treatment is symptomatic. The burns are treated as soon as possible by sodium bicarbonate dressings. The regulation gas mask protects the wearer from inhaling the vapor, but does not protect the skin from burns; that is only possible by wearing clothes made of specially prepared cloth.

NITROGEN MUSTARDS. The nitrogen mustards, methyl bis (Beta chlorethyl) amine hydrochloride and tris (Beta chlorethyl) amine hydrochloride are similar chemically to dichlorethyl sulfide, the chief difference being that nitrogen replaces sulfur in the molecule. They are also similar toxicologically, for the nitrogen mustards are vesicants when applied externally and when absorbed or injected intravenously exert a destructive action on lymphatic tissue, bone marrow cells, intestinal mucosa and growing tissue with mitotic figures. The drugs have been employed in the treatment of various lymphatic and bone marrow dyscrasias, with some success in Hodgkins' disease but with indifferent results in most of the other conditions. They are given by intravenous injection on four successive days in doses of 0.1 mg per kilo of body weight; larger doses are considered dangerous. In rare instances local corrosion may occur at the injection site; a general reaction similar to the toxic effects of roentgen-ray therapy may supervene with nausea, vomiting, weakness and transient headache, and sometimes with leukopenia, normocytic anemia and thrombocytopenia. Serious complications are not common.

LEWISITE. Lewisite is a volatile colorless liquid with an odor like geraniums, which rapidly blisters the skin and inflames the mucous membranes. After absorption it causes hemolysis of the red blood cells and afterwards may produce signs of arsenic poisoning. Therapy and prophylaxis are similar to those of dichlorethyl sulfide.

4. **Sternutators.** The class of sternutators is represented by sneeze gas, diphenyl chlorarsin, a dark brown liquid with an odor of shoe polish, and adamsite, diphenylamine chlorarsin, a brown powder usually odorless. Less often employed sternutators are arsinmethyldichloride and arsinethyl dichloride. These compounds are fired in artillery shells and after the explosion permeate the air and cover the landscape. A person inhaling the air or swallowing food or water contaminated by the chemical would be stricken with coryza, nausea, malaise, headache, salivation, pain in the chest and prostration. A few cases develop symptoms of arsenic poisoning but a fatal outcome is not common. These compounds are efficient in destroying morale and are not used for their lethal action. The regulation gas mask will protect against the sternutators. The treatment is mostly symptomatic, sodium bicarbonate is useful as a mouth wash.

5. Goldman and Cullen recognize a fifth class called *nerve and blood poisons* to which belong the gases carbon monoxide and hydrocyanic acid. Carbon monoxide may be formed by the combustion of the explosive when a large shell bursts in a dugout, and poisoning has resulted if soldiers are trapped in such cavities. In spite of their toxicity both hydrocyanic acid and carbon monoxide are not suitable as war gases and have not been employed in that role to any extent. For further discussion of these gases see pages 498 and 802.

Toxic chemicals known as nerve gases were developed during World War II, but the important facts about them have been kept as military secrets. These nerve gases are practically colorless and odorless liquids which produce a poisonous vapor on evaporation. The victim may inhale the vapor, or swallow it or absorb it from his conjunctivae or skin. After absorption the chemical causes an inactivation of cholinesterase with the result that acetylcholine accumulates in the central and peripheral nervous systems, producing acetylcholine poisoning.

Absorption of a small amount of the vapor is followed in a few minutes by a contraction of the pupils to pin point size, a paroxysmal constriction of the bronchi and a running nose. A slightly larger dose produces a ciliary spasm, disturbances of vision, pain in the back of the eyeballs and photophobia. As these symptoms are highly disagreeable, the effect of much diluted nerve gas is regarded as an efficient destroyer of morale. The absorption of larger amounts of the chemical causes death with severe bronchiospasm which interferes with both inspiration and expiration of air, a low blood pressure falling to shock levels, sudden unconsciousness and bradycardia ending in cardiac arrest.

REFERENCES

Beck, H. G., Schulze, W. H., and Suter, G. M.   Carbon monoxide—a domestic hazard, J.A.M.A., 115:1, 1940.

Courville, C. B.   Untoward Effects of Nitrous Oxide Anesthesia, Mountain View, Cal., Pacific Press Publication Ass., 1939.

Doremus, C. A., and McNally, W. D.   Gaseous Poisons, from Peterson, Haines and Webster, Legal Medicine and Toxicology, Vol. II, Philadelphia, W. B. Saunders Co., 1923.

Drinker, P., and McKhann, C. F.   The use of a new apparatus for the prolonged administration of artificial respiration, J.A.M.A., 92:1658, 1929.

Freireich, A. W.   Hydrogen sulphide poisoning, Am. J. Path., 22:147, 1946.

Gettler, A. O., and Mattice, M. R. The "normal" carbon monoxide content of the blood, J.A.M.A., 100:92, 1933.

Gilman, A., and Philips, F. S. The biological actions and therapeutic applications of the beta-chloroethyl amines and sulphides, Science, 103:409, 1946.

Golden, L., and Cullen, G. E. Some medical aspects of chemical warfare agents, J.A.M.A., 114:2200, 1940.

Helpern, M., and Strassmann, G. Differentiation of fetal and adult human hemoglobin, Arch. Path., 35:776, 1943.

Henderson, Y. Dangers of carbon monoxide poisoning, J.A.M.A., 94:179, 1930.

────── Lack of evidence for chronic carbon monoxide poisoning, Correspondence, J.A.M.A., 115:796, 1940.

────── and Haggard, H. W. Noxious Gases, New York, The Chemical Catalog Co., Inc., 1927.

Kolisko, A. Die symmetrische Encephalomalacie in den Linsenkernen nach Kohlenoxydgasvergiftung, Beitrage z. Gerichtl. Medizin, Leipzig und Wien, Franz Deuticke, 1914.

Krumbhaar, E. B., and Krumbhaar, A. D. The blood and bone marrow in yellow cross gas (mustard gas) poisoning, J. Med. Research, 40:497, 1919 to 1920.

Maresch, R. Ueber einen Fall von Kohlenoxydgasschädigung des Kindes in der Gebärmutter, Wien. med. Wchnschr., 79:454, 1929.

Pappenheimer, A. M. The pathology of the poisonous gases used in the war, Proc. New York Path. Soc., 19:97, 1919.

────── and Vance, M. The effects of the intravenous injection of dichlorethylsulphide in rabbits, J. Exper. Med., 31:71, 1920.

Petri, E. Vergiftungen, in Henke und Lubarsch, Handbuch, Vol. X, Berlin, Julius Springer, 1930.

Reports of the Office of the Chief Medical Examiner in the City of New York from 1918 to 1951.

Rhoads, C. P. Nitrogen mustards in the treatment of neoplastic disease, J.A.M.A., 131:656, 1946.

Therapy, Conferences on. Carbon monoxide poisoning, New York State J. Med., 43:1-9, 1943.

Trichter, J. B., and Helpern, M. Accidental carbon monoxide poisoning due to domestic gas appliances and gas refrigerators, Am. J. Pub. Health, 42:259-267, 1952.

Webster, R. W. Legal Medicine and Toxicology, Philadelphia, W. B. Saunders Co., 1930.

Wood, F. C. Poisoning by nitric oxide fumes, Arch. Int. Med., 10:478, 1912.

Wood, J. R. Medical problems in chemical warfare, J. Roy. Army M. Corps, 96:169-173, 1951.

20

Thermic Trauma: Electricity: Roentgen Rays: Starvation: Atmospheric Pressure

THERMIC TRAUMA

Thermic trauma occurs when the body is subjected to an extreme degree of heat or cold. If the entire organism is affected so that the normal temperature of 98.4° F. is altered markedly, a general reaction is produced. On the other hand, if merely parts of the body are brought in contact with the extremes of heat or cold, the tissues are damaged at these points and local lesions make their appearance.

Cold. LOCAL REACTION. The cold temperature in winter may attack the exposed parts of the body such as the hands, feet, ears and nose. Its first action is to blanch the skin by causing contraction of the superficial vessels, but later when the vasomotor control of the part is paralyzed, the vessels become distended, a dusky flush suffuses the affected area and itching, tingling and swelling occur. In the milder cases, the exposed part returns to normal in the course of time, but in the severer cases, especially where feet are exposed to cold for days, more serious lesions are produced. In the cold winter of 1934 to 1935 cases of gangrene of the feet caused by exposure to cold were found among the indigent in New York City. Exposure of the skin to extreme cold such as might be produced in the manufacture of liquid air may give rise to a severe burn analogous to the burns produced by heat.

GENERAL REACTION. The effect of cold on the human organism as a whole is to induce pallor and chilling of the skin over the entire body accompanied by goose flesh, or cutis anserina. Later the skin vessels become paralyzed and distended, followed by congestion of the internal viscera, which drains the skin of blood and leaves it in a blotchy state of mixed pallor and cyanosis. The individual so exposed, develops an overpowering state of lethargy and finally dies in coma. In other cases a person who is exposed to cold, but who is rescued before the fatal symptoms begin, may die of internal congestion and delayed shock a few hours later. Other cases may develop a lobar pneumonia as a result of their chilling.

The postmortem appearances of death by freezing are usually not characteristic. The heart contains fluid blood of bright arterial hue, and there is marked visceral congestion. The postmortem lividity often shows a bright red appearance, occasionally mixed with patches of dusky red. If the body continues to be frozen after death, whether death was due to exposure or some other cause, ice develops in the body fluids, and the corpse acquires a board-like rigidity and a firmness of the flesh like a metallic statue. Freezing may cause expansion of the fluid contents of the skull and may crack the cranial vault, especially along the suture lines.

Most fatalities from exposure to cold are the result of misadventure, as when an intoxicated individual falls asleep outdoors in freezing weather. Exposure to cold has been used also as a means of homicide or infanticide.

Heat. GENERAL REACTION. The general effects of heat on the human organism as encountered in the temperate zone are usually seen in the hot, humid summer months and may take one of three forms: (1) heat exhaustion, (2) heat stroke (sun stroke or insolation), or (3) heat cramps.

Heat Exhaustion. Heat exhaustion may result from a combination of prolonged exposure to excessive heat and humidity and of physical exertion, and is prevalent under working conditions where such stresses prevail. The person affected may first experience a subjective sensation of heat and of headache, followed by pallor, profuse perspiration, subnormal temperature, muscular weakness, irregular pulse, circulatory collapse, and sometimes death. The basic condition is an acute circulatory failure, the greatest stress from the exposure to heat falling on the medullary centers and the cardiovascular system; many of the victims are abnormally susceptible to heat or are suffering from some chronic disease process. In some of the fatal cases the autopsy may show a moderately severe coronary arteriosclerosis or some other form of heart disease. Dark fluid blood is present in the heart and the viscera are congested, but otherwise the postmortem findings are not characteristic.

Heat Stroke. The principal action of heat in this condition is to cause a paralysis of the heat regulatory center in the medulla. After a few premonitory symptoms of headache, dizziness and subjective heat sensations, the victim suddenly becomes unconscious and falls. The surface of the body is flushed, dry and hot to the touch, the pulse is full and rapid, the respirations are stertorous, and the temperature is elevated from 107° to 110° F. In some fatal cases there is a rapid circulatory collapse, and death may occur after a few hours from shock. Other cases may survive a few days and develop a fatal bronchopneumonia. At necropsy, the principal findings may be congestion of the organs, dark red fluid blood in the heart, degenerative changes in the ganglion cells, marked cerebral congestion and cerebral edema. Postmortem decomposition sets in rapidly as a rule. Cases of heat stroke are apt to occur in hot humid weather with the temperature consistently in excess of 100° F. for several days. Chronic alcoholics, persons with chronic disease conditions, or individuals abnormally susceptible to heat are the types likely to succumb to heat stroke.

Malamud and his collaborators on the basis of a study of 125 fatal cases of heat stroke occurring in military personnel describe three types of clinical onset: (a) an acute type with persistent coma or delirium; (b) an acute type with initial coma or delirium followed by a remission of symptoms and then a final relapse; (c) an insidious onset with the late development of coma. The fatal illnesses lasted from an hour to 12 days, about 30 per cent of the cases surviving the onset 24 hours or longer. At necropsy the principal lesions were encountered in the central nervous system and less often in other viscera. They were of two classifications:

1. Lesions produced by hyperthermia. These were manifested in the central nervous system by progressive degeneration of the nerve cells in the cerebral cortex, cerebellum and basal ganglia but not in the brain stem and hypothalamus; later the degenerated cells were replaced by glia. The degree of involvement was the more intense the longer the patient survived with a high temperature. When the survival period was more than 24 hours, degenerative changes in the megacaryocytes sometimes followed by regeneration, small central necroses in the liver lobule, degenerations in the adrenal cortex, lobular pneumonia and lower nephron nephrosis were encountered (see below).

2. Lesions produced by shock. These consisted of congestion and edema of

brain tissue and small hemorrhages in the walls of the third ventricle, fourth ventricle and aqueduct, probably of terminal nature. Small hemorrhages were also found in the lung tissue, and in the heart in the epicardium, endocardium and bundle of His.

The term lower nephron nephrosis has been applied to the renal lesion described in a great variety of conditions such as transfusion with incompatible blood (page 666), certain types of poisoning such as from phenol or sulfonamides (pages 730 and 830), crushing or trauma to muscle (page 203), heat stroke (page 524), burns (page 527) and many others. The development of the kidney lesion is preceded by a state of shock, usually associated with hemolysis in the blood vessels or marked destruction of striated muscle tissue; in some cases these conditions are absent. Clinically the nephrosis sometimes produces oliguria or anuria; hemoglobin-derived pigment may appear in the urine; and azotemia, uremia and hypertension may occur. At autopsy the gross lesions in the kidneys are not pathognomonic; the cortex may be pale and swollen and offer a vivid contrast to the dark bluish red pyramids, but this does not invariably occur. Microscopically there is focal degeneration and necrosis in the lining epithelium of the thick tubules of Henle and the distal convoluted tubules. If the patient survives three or four days after the onset of symptoms, regeneration of the epithelial cells may occur, and occasionally edema and round cell infiltration in the adjacent interstitial tissue and thrombosis in the adjacent venules may be encountered. Casts of hemoglobin-derived pigment or of hyaline-like material are found in the collecting tubules and occasionally in the cortical tubules; a pink albuminous fluid is often found in Bowman's capsule. The victim may die in about 10 days after the onset of symptoms. The pathogenesis of lower nephron nephrosis is not fully understood but in many cases it is doubtless a disturbance in the renal excretion of disintegration products of hemoglobin or myohemoglobin in combination with other factors. Many investigators apply the term hemoglobinuric nephrosis to this condition because of the hemoglobin-derived casts in the renal tubules and consider it an accurate description of the actual lesion.

Patients incubated in a hot air cabinet for the treatment of an acute gonococcal infection sometimes are overcome by the heat. The body of the patient except the head is subjected for a few hours in the cabinet to a temperature of 107° F., the thermal death point of gonococci. The ordeal is a severe one; in a case observed by the authors the deceased, a girl of 19 years, was fatally prostrated with a high temperature and all the other signs of heat stroke. In his series of cases, Hartman has described edema of the brain, ganglion cell degenerations and necrotic hemorrhagic areas in brain tissue which he attributes to anoxia produced by exposure to heat.

Heat Cramps. Heat cramps are a minor condition which occurs in workmen, especially those laboring in hot surroundings and perspiring excessively; by this the body is drained of its chlorides and the sarcoplasm of the voluntary muscle is depleted. If much water is ingested without restoring the lost chlorides to the system, violent muscular cramps ensue, and the body may become rigid from tetanic muscular spasm. The condition is treated prophylactically by furnishing the workers sufficient common salt in the drinking water to replace whatever chlorides are lost during sweating. If convulsions set in, intravenous infusion of a dilute saline solution is indicated.

LOCAL REACTION. Excessive heat acting locally on the skin and more exposed mucous membranes produces characteristic injuries known as burns. The most common causes of burns are sunlight, Finsen light, hot liquids, flame and hot objects. Four degrees of burns are recognized:

1. First degree. Burns of the first degree commonly result from the action of sunlight which produces the characteristic sunburn, or from overexposure to ultraviolet light, or from the heat of a flame, hot water or hot objects which have a brief contact with the skin. In the early stages the epidermis remains intact, but the skin is reddened due to the marked injection of the blood vessels in the dermis immediately under the epithelial layer. The erythema of the skin blanches on pressure.

The subepithelial tissues may become edematous and there may be a slight infiltration of polymorphonuclear leukocytes in the involved area. This inflammation subsides in time, and during healing there may be a surface desquamation of the superficial layers of the epidermis. A scar does not ordinarily result, but after the more severe grades of sunburn have healed, the subsequent pigmentation in the skin is often uneven. Rarely xeroderma pigmentosa results from repeated excessive exposure to sunlight and may end in the development of epithelial carcinomas of the skin.

2. Second degree. Second degree burns are produced usually by a hot liquid, flame or a hot object, and rarely by overexposure to light. The typical lesion is a bleb or a blister with reddened edges which is produced by the action of heat on the superficial vessels in the dermis; these are rendered permeable and serous fluid containing a high proportion of albumen and chlorides exudes into the surrounding tissues and through the deeper layers of the epidermis, elevating the superficial layers of the epithelium to form a watery vesicle. There is usually an infiltration of polymorphonuclear leukocytes in the tissues below the blister. If the blister ruptures, the epithelial covering is removed and a raw surface remains, which dries forming a parchment-like, reddish brown or rusty area on the skin. Microscopically the bed of the ruptured blister shows patches of elongated epithelial cells with elongated nuclei, accompanied by varying degrees of epithelial desquamation. In time the dried area is covered by regenerated epithelium, similar to the process described in the healing of abrasions, and a thin flat white scar develops.

A blister does not form post mortem on the application of heat, except on rare occasions immediately after death when the molecular life of the tissues is still present in which case albumen is absent in the blister fluid and there is an absence of any inflammatory reaction. Blisters formed as a result of postmortem putrefaction differ from the antemortem burn by the absence of inflammatory reaction and by the elevation of the entire epidermis from the corium to form the covering of the blister.

3. Third degree. Third degree burns are associated with an actual loss of skin substance. They are usually produced by flame or a red hot brand and less often by hot water or by prolonged contact with an object emitting less heat, like a hot water pipe. The heat sears the skin, causing a coagulation necrosis of the surface layers which are first rusty brown in appearance and later turn dark brown and then black. There is a pronounced infiltration of polymorphonuclear leukocytes into the surrounding tissues with much inflammatory edema, and the small blood vessels in the deeper layers adjacent to the burn may show thrombi and leukocytes in their lumens. The necrotic tissue after a while is separated by granulation tissue and is shed as a slough. The gap gradually closes with the formation of a wrinkled cicatrix which is covered by squamous epithelium but does not usually contain any of the accessory skin structures such as hairs, sebaceous glands or sweat glands. The scar may present itself as a wrinkled contracture or it may develop into a large surface keloid. Postmortem desquamation of the epidermis due to putrefactive changes may dry and leave rusty brown areas which sometimes simulate burns, but such artefacts are free from any signs of inflammation.

4. Fourth degree. The fourth degree burn is similar to the third degree burn but is more destructive, as it is associated with actual charring of the tissues.

The distribution of the burns on the body of the victim depend upon the source of the heat and the manner of its application. When burns are due to light, certain parts of the body are exposed to the action of the rays, as for example the head, neck, shoulders, arms and back in the case of sunburn, and such regions show a marked erythema in contrast to the paler unburned skin. Flame produces geographic patches of reddish brown hue, so called because they have the varying sizes, shapes and arrangements of land and water areas on a map, and the skin may be stained by smoke and the hairs singed; in some cases the entire skin may be involved. If the burn is caused by an explosion, that part of the body nearest the blast will be affected the most; thus if the victim faces the burst of flame the face, hands and front part of the trunk will be burned, and the scalp hair and eyebrows will be singed. If the burn is caused by a hot object, a brand having the form and dimensions of the area of contact will be impressed on the skin.

The general effect of burns is to produce severe pain and shock because of the extensive injury to the sensory nerves in the skin, and death may occur quickly from immediate shock with vasomotor collapse. In some cases, the victim lives for a few hours and dies of delayed shock which is in part referable to the damage inflicted on the sensory nerves, in part to the absorption of toxic substances from the burned tissues, and in part to the exudation of serum into the inflamed areas in amounts sufficient to deplete the volume of the circulating blood. In general the symptoms are more severe the greater the extent of the burned areas on the skin, and the intensity of the burns is less significant than the amount of body surface involved. If the lesions are not sufficient to cause death in a few hours the victim may survive a few days and die of a hypostatic pneumonia. In some cases a fatal septic infection may develop from the local lesions which are inflamed and necrotic as the result of infection by pyogenic bacteria. When these complications supervene the temperature usually shows a sharp rise and pulse and respiration may become more rapid. In a few cases a lower nephron nephrosis appears on the second day post trauma and dominates the clinical picture with oliguria, albuminuria, hematuria, hemoglobinuria and other signs of kidney dysfunction.

If the victim dies shortly after the burning, the internal lesions found at necropsy are not characteristic; the blood may be dark, dehydrated, thick and decreased in volume, but in the event of copious intravenous infusions and transfusions, these findings may be modified. If the victim has lived a few days, there may be a hypostatic pneumonia, and degenerative changes in the parenchyma cells of the liver and kidneys. A marked parenchymatous degeneration with swelling of the epithelium may be noted in the cortical tubules of the kidneys a few hours post trauma. On the second day or thereafter a nephrosis with albuminous, granular and pigment deposits distending the tubules of the lower nephron segment may be encountered. In the liver there may be mild degenerative changes in the cells adjacent to the central venules with swelling and a deposition of yellow brown pigment in the cytoplasm; in rare instances a slight jaundice may be present.

The great difficulty in appraising the significance of the hepatic and renal lesions, is that the therapeutic procedures usually employed with burns may be possible causes of the parenchymatous degenerations. Some investigators have described necrotic changes in the livers of fatal cases of burns which were treated with applications of a solution of tannic acid and have attributed such changes to the action of the drug. Sulfonamide administration sometimes produces renal and hepatic lesions, and transfusions in rare cases of mismatched bloods may be the cause of a hemoglobinuric nephrosis. The pathologic physiology in deaths from burns is complicated and is not wholly determined by the thermic lesion alone;

therapeutic measures, secondary septic infections and even preexisting chronic disease conditions may help to shape the pathologic picture at autopsy, and all factors must be considered before deciding upon the significance of the different lesions. Many pathologic lesions, in the past attributed to burns, were probably due to other causes. Ulcerations in the duodenum mentioned in the literature in connection with extensive burns of the body have not been seen by the authors.

Most fatal cases of burns are accidental, an average of 370 cases a year occurring in New York City. Over three fifths of these are due to flame in conflagrations; from fires started in clothing or furniture by burning stoves, lighted matches, smoldering cigarettes or bonfires; or from explosions of inflammable liquids like

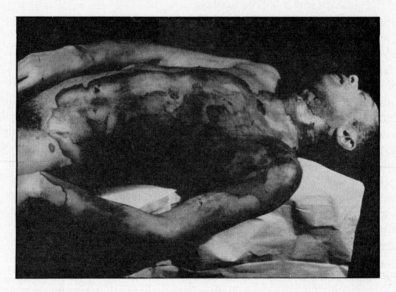

Fig. 20-1. Homicidal Third Degree Burn Produced by Flaming Gasoline.

gasoline, naphtha, benzine, kerosene and alcohol. About one fifth of the cases are scalds caused by hot liquids or steam. A small number are due to hot objects or ultraviolet light. Burns from lightning and electricity will be discussed later. Homicidal burns are rare: in one instance a woman during an altercation was thrown against a hot stove which set her dress on fire; in another case the victim was drenched with gasoline and then ignited (Fig. 20-1). Suicidal burns are rare, as in the case of a psychopathic woman who saturated her clothing with kerosene and then ignited herself.

CONFLAGRATIONS. A conflagration is the burning of a building or some other large structure, and as a result its occupants are overwhelmed by the flame or are overcome by the inhalation of smoke containing carbon monoxide which is produced by the combustion. The victims are affected in different ways by these factors, depending on the conditions which are present during the conflagration. Some who die in a fire may receive few and slight burns of the skin but show inhalation of carbon monoxide in fatal amounts. The bodies show smoke stains on the face and elsewhere, slight singeing of eyebrows and scalp, a deposit of soot in the nostrils, and the postmortem lividity has a cherry red tinge because of the presence of carboxyhemoglobin. Soot and mucus may be present in the air passages down to the finer bronchi and the bronchial mucous membrane is reddened because of the injection of vessels in the submucous layer (Fig. 20-2). The blood, muscles and internal organs are cherry red in color, and the percentage of carboxyhemoglobin varies from 30 to 60 per cent. In other cases, third degree burns of geographic form are present, especially on the exposed parts, the clothing is burned in places, the hair may be singed, and the skin colored brown by the smoke. Burns of the first and second degree may be present and are probably due to heated air and not to flame; occasionally the hot air is inhaled with the soot and causes surface necrosis of the laryngeal and tracheal epithelium and edema of the submucous layer. If the victim

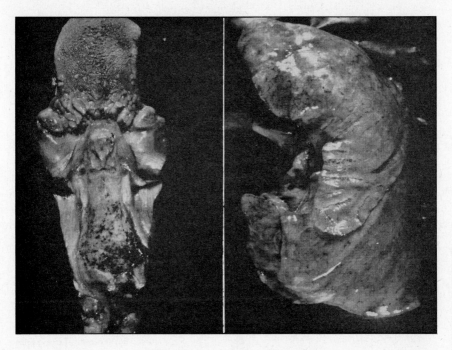

Fig. 20-2. Effects of Inhalation of Smoke.

Left: Edema of larynx, inhaled soot and inflammatory membrane lining tracheal mucosa.
Right: Obstructive interstitial emphysema in the lung which also revealed severe necrotizing aspiration bronchopneumonia. Twelve year old victim trapped in burning building, lived 12 hours after rescue.

survives for a few days after the conflagration, the carbon monoxide is eliminated from the system; a mucopurulent or pseudomembranous inflammation may develop in the air passages and terminate in a bronchopneumonia.

After the death of the victim the flame may continue its action and cook the body, causing blackening and contraction of the skin which becomes brittle so that the dermis splits in long and wide elliptic cracks. The hair is burned off, the skin is drawn tight over the face, the eyelids are sometimes closed, the cornea becomes opaque and edema of the loose tissues is present. The voluntary muscles are pale and cooked, and the internal viscera are cooked, dull and shrunken. With longer exposure to the fire, the skin is charred and removed, and the skeletal muscles are heated to a dark red-brown color and are dry and contracted. The limbs are flexed to varying degrees causing the body to assume a pugilistic attitude and the fingers to become hooked like claws (Fig. 20-3). The bones may be extensively charred, especially the extremities and face, artificial fractures are produced by the heat, and with further action by the fire, the extremities are burned away, close to the trunk. In some cases, one surface of the corpse may be exposed to the flame and may show considerable destruction while the other side may be protected and comparatively intact.

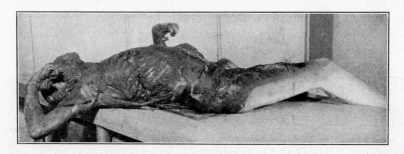

Fig. 20-3. Burns of Head and Body from Fire.

Fourth degree burns of head and body from flame which started in an upholstered chair accidentally set on fire by a cigarette. Note pugilistic attitude of upper extremities as a result of postmortem contracture of burned muscles.

In cases in which the flame is in contact with the head, resulting in extensive charring of the skull, the intense heat may cause a postmortem transudation of blood between the dura and bone, which appears as an amorphous brownish-red deposit (Figs. 20-4 and 20-5), totally unlike the discus-shaped traumatic epidural

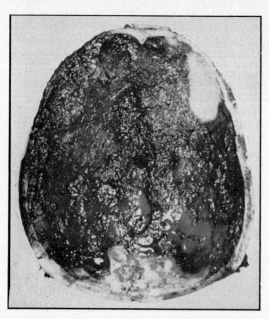

Fig. 20-4. Postmortem Extravasation of Blood in Epidural Space Resulting from Action of Flame on Skull.

View of inner surface of skull cap. Victim trapped in burning building; body and head extensively incinerated. This finding must not be mistaken for antemortem injury.

hemorrhage. This postmortem extradural hemorrhage is probably the result of a combination of factors produced by the intense heat which causes a local shrinkage of dura and brain and postmortem rupture of vessels on the outside of the dura; during the burning of the body blood is also forced from the trunk into the head and then into the extradural space through the ruptured vessels. Postmortem fractures of the vault of the skull may result in connection with the charring, and if associated with extradural hemorrhages, may be mistaken for antemortem injuries and erroneously interpreted as evidence of foul play. With extensive charring and incineration of the body, little if any fluid blood is present in the remains.

If the flame is unchecked the body will be reduced to a shapeless carbonaceous mass, and finally to a heap of gray and yellow ashes. The distal portions of the extremities and the features are usually destroyed first, and then the larger portions

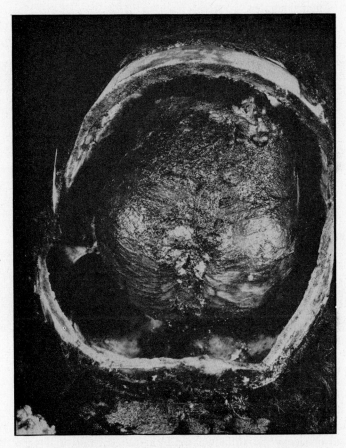

Fig. 20-5. Unusual Effect of Incineration of Heart in a Conflagration.

Shrinkage of brain and dura. Rendered brain tissue percolated through dura into extradural space. Photograph taken after removal of skull cap.

of the trunk. The bones and teeth are more resistant to the action of the flame, and may persist when the other tissues are destroyed. The teeth become charred and brittle and break off easily. The body is not usually completely consumed by the fire unless the conflagration is intense or prolonged, or unless the body is subjected to professional cremation. See page 32 for a discussion of cremation as a means of disposing of a body after homicide. An unsuccessful attempt to dispose of a body by dismemberment and incineration in a bonfire after murder is shown in Figure 3-10. A similar attempt to conceal a murder by placing the body under the bed and then setting fire to the premises is shown in Figure 20-6. The fire was extinguished before extensive burning occurred, and the ligature used to strangle the victim and a head injury were plainly evident. In each of these cases the blood did not contain any carbon monoxide.

Most conflagration deaths are accidental, and there may be several fatalities in the same fire. The question of identification of bodies burned beyond recognition in conflagrations has been discussed on page 32. If the fire can be traced to an incendiary, the deaths would be considered homicidal. If it occurs in a building in which there are violations of the fire prevention laws, the owner can be prosecuted on a charge of manslaughter.

Other types of flame burns occur when the clothing of women and children are accidentally set on fire at the kitchen stove or in some other fashion; in such cases

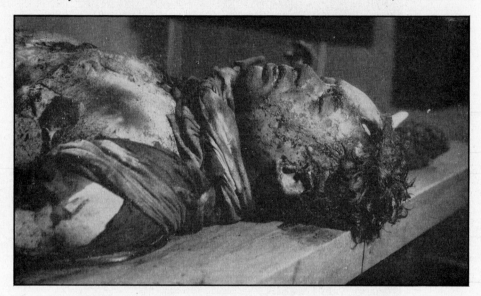

Fig. 20-6. Crude Attempt to Conceal Homicidal Strangulation by Incineration.

Body was placed under bed and room set on fire. Carbon monoxide absent from blood and soot not found in air passages, indicating that deceased was dead before fire was started.

a burn is sustained around the upper thighs and abdomen, which has been designated as the bathing suit burn because of its characteristic distribution. In other instances an intoxicated or sleepy individual seated in a stuffed chair or lying in bed has set it on fire with a lighted cigarette (Fig. 20-3). In such cases, the victim sustains the most severe burns on the back or on that part of the body in contact with the flaming material and also exhibits signs of inhalation of smoke and carbon monoxide. A person while driving or riding as a passenger in an automobile or an auto truck which collides with a tree or a steel pillar or is rammed by another car may be trapped and burned to death if the gasoline tank is smashed and ignited. Extensive incineration of the body can occur as in a building conflagration (Fig. 20-7). In cases in which a charred body is found in a burned automobile, a careful investigation is in order to determine whether the deceased was alive at the time of the fire. The characteristics of burns due to explosions have been described.

The same difficulties are encountered with burns as with other injuries, in ascertaining whether the lesion was inflicted before or after death. An antemortem burn exhibits distinct reddening of the skin and a definite intravital reaction (see pages 526 and 527 for detailed description). Under some circumstances it may be difficult to demonstrate the intravital nature of the lesion satisfactorily, especially if postmortem decomposition is present, or if the remains are badly burned. A burn inflicted just prior to death is often difficult to distinguish from a burn produced immediately after death. In conflagrations, when the body is severely charred, the

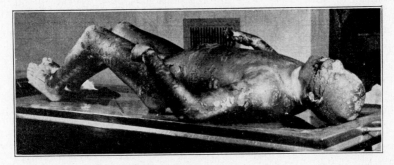

Fig. 20-7. Burns of Entire Body from Flame.

The deceased was trapped in the driver's seat of an automobile which was set on fire by explosion of gasoline tank after collision.

presence of inhaled soot in the air passages and of carboxyhemoglobin in the blood is helpful to the extent that it indicates that the deceased was alive during the conflagration; it does not prove the antemortem occurrence of the burns inasmuch as the victim may have suffocated before the flame reached him. *A routine examination of the blood for carboxyhemoglobin* should be made on all cases found dead at the scene of a conflagration.

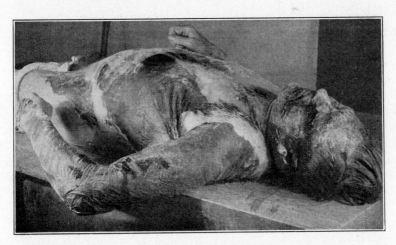

Fig. 20-8. Third Degree Steam Scalds of Face, Trunk and Upper Extremity.

The scalds were incurred accidentally when a steam pipe burst in a Turkish bath. The denuded areas of skin have been treated with tannic acid. Note geographical distribution of lesions on trunk.

SCALDS. Scalds are burns caused by hot liquids and hot vapors, in most cases by water near the boiling point or by steam which may be superheated. Such effects as singeing of the hair, charring of the skin and burning of clothing do not occur. There are three degrees of severity in scalds: the first degree characterized by erythema; the second degree by blister formation which is the most characteristic lesion; the third degree by destruction of tissue due to coagulation necrosis of the affected region.

The same distribution of the lesions may occur in cases of scalding as with flame burns; the tissue destruction is not as intense, since there is no charring or incineration. Reddish brown, patchy geographic lesions may be produced on the skin, or the entire body surface or a large part of it may be involved. Persons scalded by steam may inhale the hot vapor; at autopsy in such cases a grayish-red coagulation necrosis of the mucous membrane and edema of the submucosal tissues of the air passages may be encountered.

Most scaldings are accidental. A child may pull and spill a kettle of boiling water over himself, or a cook may upset a pot of simmering soup over herself with resulting geographic scalds on head and shoulders and other parts of the body. A

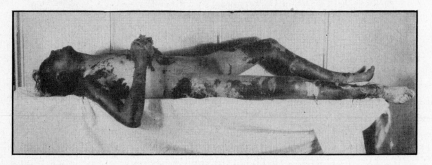

Fig. 20-9. Body Scalded and Boiled by Superheated Steam which Escaped Through Burst Valve in Engine Room of Ship.

person may fall into a bath tub filled with boiling water and sustain extensive scalding, or he may slip in the tub and inadvertently grab hold of and turn on the hot water faucet and scald himself. Severe scalds can result from the premature opening of home steam-pressure cookers and are apt to involve the face and hands. Persons are occasionally scalded in Turkish baths (Fig. 20-8), or in the engine room of a ship when a steam pipe bursts, the superheated vapor under increased pressure producing severe extensive burns. Prolonged exposure to such superheated steam results in a cooking and coagulation of the tissues (Fig. 20-9).

Rare homicidal cases occur in which the victim is doused with boiling water; angry-looking, reddish-brown, second and third degree scalds on face and trunk are produced. Suicidal scalding is very rare.

TRAUMA CAUSED BY ELECTRIC ENERGY

Electricity is a form of energy which under certain conditions can injure the body and cause death. In nature, it is produced by the storm clouds and is discharged as lightning. By human ingenuity, electric energy is generated from mechanical energy by dynamo-electric machines and distributed for use in the form of an electric current. Electricity has a potential and flows through a conducting medium eventually dissipating or grounding itself in the earth. The human body is a good conductor of electricity and if placed in the path of the charge, serious injury and death may result from paralysis of the heart or of the medullary centers. In addition to this shocking action on the body, electric energy is transformed into heat which in sufficient quantity may produce electric burns; heat production sufficient to produce enough elevation of temperature to cause a burn occurs at points of resistance, usually on the skin, where the current enters and leaves the body. The over-all resistance of the tissues within the body to the passage of the current is low, because of the large cross sectional area involved.

The ability of an electric current to effect a burn on entering or leaving the body is dependent upon the temperature to which the tissues are raised by the heat produced by the current flow. The burning temperature is determined by the intensity of the current, the duration of its action and the resistance at any given point of contact. Electric energy available for conversion into heat is expressed in watts and is the product of the electromotive force or voltage (V) multiplied by the intensity (I) of the current or amperage. The heat production, expressed in watts, is VI. According to Ohm's law, the intensity of the current or amperage is equal to the voltage divided by the resistance (R) of the conducting medium or I equals V/R so that V equals IR. Substituting IR for V in the above formula VI, heat production can be expressed as I^2R, in which I is the amperage or intensity of the current and R the resistance. Heat production is thus proportional to the square of the intensity and to the resistance; but for a current of a given voltage, if R is increased in the circuit, I is diminished in accordance with Ohm's law, and heat production I^2R falls off in greater proportion because of the lowered I^2. Since the rise in temperature is the result of I^2R, the maximum temperature will be produced where R is maximum along the path of the current, and consequently the greatest burning effect will take place in the skin where R is greatest.

Thus if the resistance of the skin is high as when it is dry, and the voltage or tension of the current is low, the intensity or amperage of the current may not be sufficient to produce a serious shock or to effect a burn. Conversely if the resistance is reduced as it would be if the skin were moist or covered with sweat, then even a current of low voltage would have sufficient amperage to produce a severe and even fatal shock without necessarily producing a skin burn, especially if the contact is only for a brief interval. If the voltage of the current is sufficiently high to overcome the resistance of the skin, a shocking intensity of current may pass through the body, and burns may be produced at the points of contact where the resistance is great; the extent and degree of the burns varies with the area over which the heat production or I^2R is distributed and also with the duration of its action. In some cases, especially with high-tension currents, the heat production is sufficient to produce a severe burn even when the skin is dry (Figs. 20-13, 14 and 15). In other instances, a current of low tension flowing through a contact for sufficient time may produce a severe and deep burn (Fig. 20-16). If the electric contact is diffuse as with a body submerged in a bath tub full of water into which a live wire has fallen, the heat production may be insufficient to produce any burns at all, despite the fatal shocking effect of the current. There are cases of fatal electric shock in which low-tension currents have entered through a moist area of skin without the production of a burn because the contact was not sufficiently long. As a rule, severe burns by low-tension currents are most apt to occur when the skin resistance is low and the electric contact of sufficient duration. Severe burns, however, can occur fairly rapidly under these conditions. The fatal shock may kill instantaneously or very quickly, so that in most cases of electrocution with low-tension currents, death has occurred before the burn has been completed, much of the burn occurring post mortem. With high-tension currents, the burns can occur almost as rapidly as the shock, and in some instances severe electric burns are produced with nonfatal shocks.

It is the shocking action of the current that is responsible for immediate death in electrocution; the burns are incidental to the passage of an adequate amount of current through the resistant skin of the victim. The heat production of most currents passing for only a brief period through the relatively nonresistant tissues of the body is not sufficient to produce an elevation of temperature that will result in any demonstrable heat effect away from the sites of contact.

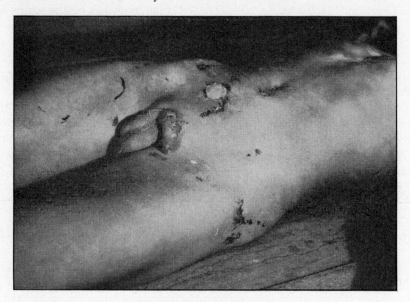

Fig. 20-10. Lightning Burns.

Victim killed by bolt of lightning after swimming. Irregularly distributed superficial burns of abdomen, hips and penis in area covered by swimming trunks.

Lightning. Bolts of lightning are discharged in the form of a giant spark similar to, but infinitely more huge, than those generated by a static electric machine. Lightning usually strikes the tallest object on the landscape, and many persons have been struck by it while prominently exposed in an open field. Some have been killed while standing near a tall tree, or while wet with rain or sea water, or wearing a metal object about their persons, circumstances which may favor the attraction of lightning bolts. In most instances, the victim who is struck dies immediately from the paralyzing effect of the charge on the nervous system.

The action of a lightning bolt is unpredictable. If it strikes in a crowd, it may kill a few people and injure others, while some persons may escape injury altogether. Under such circumstances usually more people are injured than killed. In some cases the violence of the bolt is expended on the clothing of the victim, which may be ripped and torn, the individual himself remaining unharmed.

Persons who survive after having been struck by lightning may exhibit symptoms and signs of great diversity, mostly neurogenic in type. The milder manifestations are severe mental shock, prolonged and intense nervousness which in women may be accompanied by suppression of the menses. More severe effects are unconsciousness, numbness in various parts of the body, paralyses, deafness and blindness, but these are usually transient phenomena.

The lesions in fatal cases of lightning stroke are varied and depend on how smoothly the body has served as a conductor of the charge. In some cases, the bolt passes through the body easily without producing any demonstrable injuries externally or internally. In other instances, the skin resists the entrance and the exit of the bolt, and the electric energy is transformed into heat, producing burns on the skin. These burns exhibit a great variety of forms; sometimes the lesions can be identified as the points of entrance and exit of the bolt, and occasionally they are produced by charged metallic objects in contact with the skin. In a case seen by the authors, the bolt struck a boy wearing a pair of bathing trunks, apparently entering through a metal buckle and branding the skin at that point; it then traveled through

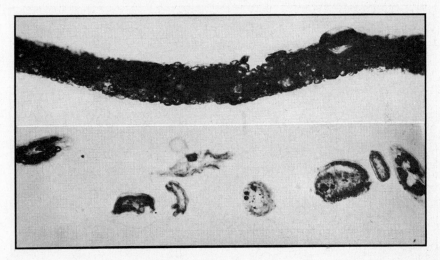

Fig. 20-11. Lightning Effect on Hair.

Victim killed outright. Burned hairs from thigh shown in whole mount and cross sections. Adjacent skin and clothing not damaged. No other injuries noted.

the wet trunks producing geographic third degree burns over the groins and hips without singeing the cloth (Fig. 20-10). Sometimes the hair is charred without other external signs; Dr. Richard Grimes investigated a case in which the hair on the thighs was burned, the adjacent skin and clothing not being affected (Fig. 20-11). In other cases, the clothing may become ignited and thus burn the skin.

Rather bizarre figures on the skin, known as lightning marks, may be produced when lightning is conducted to a nearby person after striking a tree or building. The bolt enters the skin, producing a burn, and then travels down the body, forming an irregular pattern of arborescent ecchymoses along its course which may end at the nates or the groin or extend down to the heels. The lesion results from the resistance of the smaller blood vessels in the skin which are ruptured by the violence of the charge with the production of the peculiar mossy dendritic figures. If the victim is struck while leaning against a tree, a burn may occur over the area of contact such as the shoulder or neck, and extravasation of blood and injection of blood vessels may occur, forming subcutaneous hand-like or leaf-like blotches; this lesion is also due to the resistance of the subcutaneous blood vessels to the passage of the bolt.

The injuries which are occasioned by the outgoing electric charge usually occur on the hands and feet. Minute, punctate, blackened burns are occasionally found on those sites. If the bolt emerges from the feet, the adjacent portions of the shoes may be perforated or even destroyed. In some cases the charge making its exit from the palms and soles causes violent disruption of the flesh.

The internal effects of lightning are sometimes severe and are in most cases attributable to the variable resistance of some of the tissues to the massive electric charge. Fractures of the bones, gross injuries of the brain, ruptures of blood vessels and abdominal viscera have been noted. In evaluating cases of this sort the possibility of blunt force injuries must also be considered before attributing all these effects to electric action alone, especially since the lightning bolt sometimes has a

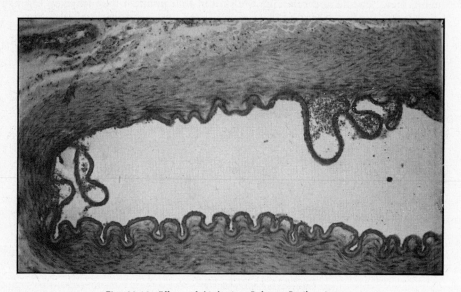

Fig. 20-12. Effect of Lightning Bolt on Basilar Artery.

Note disruption of intima and partial detachment of internal elastica. Low power photomicrograph. Same case as Figure 20-10.

disruptive action on its targets which may supply the means of blunt force injuries. In a case of lightning death autopsied in the Office of the Chief Medical Examiner, the only internal lesion produced by the bolt was a rupture of the intima and elastica of the basilar artery (Fig. 20-12).

The determination of death by lightning is corroborated in most cases by the fact that the deceased was exposed outdoors in a thunder storm, in a situation where it was possible for him to have been struck by lightning. If the variable lesions characteristic of severe electric trauma are found on the skin in a case of this type, and if there is no other cause of death demonstrable at autopsy, the diagnosis of death by lightning can be made with reasonable certainty. The Office of the Chief Medical Examiner in New York City does not encounter many deaths from lightning. The records reveal an average of three such cases every two years.

Electric Current. The electricity that is generated artificially for human use has caused serious injury and a large number of deaths. By far the greater proportion of such injuries and fatalities arise out of accidents along the transmission systems which carry electric energy to the distant points where it is used. A much smaller number of electric accidents occur in power plants where electric energy is generated, and in the homes and in industry where low-tension currents are employed.

Currents of electricity are either direct or alternating, and are transmitted through metal wire conductors. In the direct variety the current flows continuously in one direction. In the indirect, alternating or alternate type, the flow of current undergoes a rapidly alternating change in direction; the alternating current that is generated in this country has a frequency of 60 cycles per second. This is in the dangerous low range of frequency as far as shocking potentiality is concerned. The shocking effect of the alternating current is more dangerous than the direct. The high frequency currents used in diathermy, which oscillate at 1,000,000 cycles a

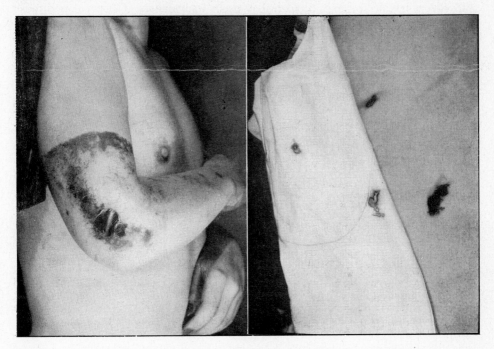

Fig. 20-13. Electrical Burns Produced by Contact with High Tension Current.

Large burn on right forearm. Two smaller deeper burns on left hip; note corresponding holes with charred edges burned in laboratory coat worn by victim when she was accidentally electrocuted while operating an x-ray machine.

second, and carry 20,000 to 40,000 volts at 1 to 2 milliamperes, are comparatively harmless in that they do not cause shock. They may, however, produce severe burns if the electrodes are applied loosely to the skin.

The tension of electric currents is measured by the voltage. Currents of low tension are utilized in the home and in industry, and are usually 110 or 220 volts, the former being employed for lighting and for most household appliances, the latter for electric motors, ovens and for other special purposes. Heavy motors such as those used on elevators and street cars obtain power from voltages of 440 or 660. Currents in excess of 1,000 volts are high tension. One hundred thousand volts are used to transmit electric power over long distances, and from 20,000 to 1,000,000 volts are used in deep roentgen ray therapy.

The intensity of the current which may act on the body is expressed in terms of amperage and depends upon the voltage and upon the resistance of the tissues, especially of the skin, which is a variable factor. If the body is well insulated and cannot conduct the current, it may not be damaged even by a high-tension voltage.

On the other hand, when the body is moist and well grounded it is an excellent conductor of electricity, and currents of low tension such as are encountered in the home and in industry may cause immediate death. Currents of 110 volts have caused death and fatal shocks have been reported with 25 volts. The fatal shocking power of low-tension currents is not generally recognized. Poorly designed and defective electric appliances and equipment have been responsible for fatal accidents with low-tension currents.

When a person receives an electric shock, the muscles of the body are thrown into violent tetanic spasm and death may occur immediately. The peculiar disposition of the individual may favor the fatal action of the electric charge; neurotics, cardiacs and some with status lymphaticus are most prone to succumb. On the

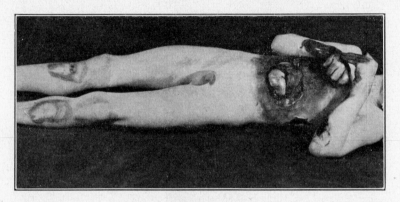

Fig. 20-14. Electrocution by Contact with High Voltage Current.

The deceased, a young boy, tripped while running across tracks of elevated railway and fell across third rail with legs grounded on steel car rail. Extensive charring of tissues of trunk and upper extremities from contact with third rail. The burns on the legs were caused by the current passing out of the body.

other hand, Jellinek believes that if the individual is braced mentally to meet an electric shock he can successfully withstand a charge which might be fatal otherwise. Sleep is supposed to make the body more refractory to the shocking effect of the electric current. In some cases, the victim is rendered unconscious by the shock of a high-tension current and may die later, or he may recover completely or suffer later from various sequelae. Electric shocks by low-tension currents either kill immediately or not at all and, when nonfatal, are usually without sequelae.

Accidental electrocutions by high-tension currents have occurred in power houses, roentgen-ray laboratories and in experimental electric laboratories (Fig. 20-13), or from contact with a third rail on electric railways (Fig. 20-14). The currents in such accidents have ranged from 1,000 to 200,000 volts. As a curious example of an electrocution by a current of high voltage, Jellinek describes the case of a boy who was killed when he urinated upon a high-tension wire, the current being conducted to the body by the urinary stream. The current from a high-tension wire that has fallen on an automobile may electrocute the occupants when they leave the vehicle and ground themselves. The rubber tires on the wheels may insulate the car sufficiently from the ground so that the occupants who do not attempt to leave remain unharmed.

The electric current diffuses through the body from the point of entrance and emerges at the point or points of exit. Burns may occur at these sites because the

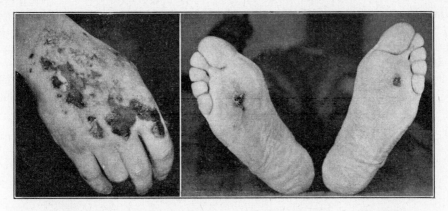

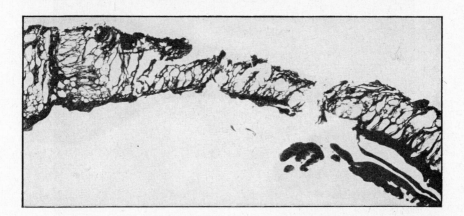

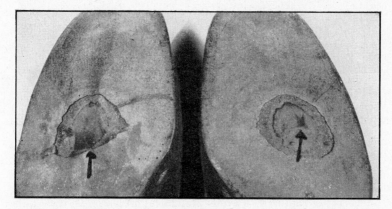

Fig. 20-15. Electrocution by Contact with High Voltage Current.

The deceased was electrocuted by the current from a high voltage condenser, which he had inadvertently touched with the back of his right hand, while both feet were grounded. Irregular broad burn on the back of the right hand where the current entered. Symmetrical deep electrical burns on ball of each foot through which the current escaped. Low power photomicrograph of histologic section of deep burn of sole of foot; note vacuolated honeycomb-like effect in horny layer of epidermis and detachment from dermis. Old shoes worn by the deceased when electrocuted; note the small perforations (arrows) in worn-out portions of the soles produced by the exit of the current. There were corresponding holes burned in the socks.

skin offers resistance to the passage of the current with the result that the electric energy is transformed into heat sufficient in intensity to raise the temperature to the burning point (page 535). The skin lesion at the point of entrance of the current is frequently located on the hand, often on the fingers (Figs. 20-16 and 20-17), but depending on circumstances may occur in other places on the body (Figs. 20-13, 14 and 15). In some instances the burn is a slightly depressed brand

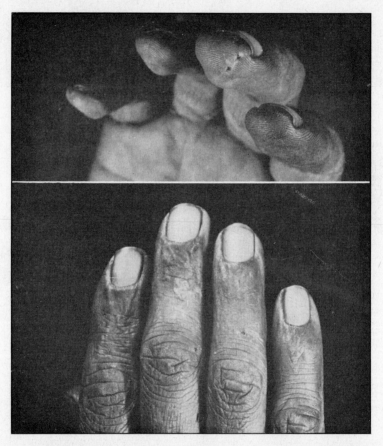

Fig. 20-16. Small Inconspicuous Burns on Tip of Middle Finger and on Back of Index and Middle Finger.

Accidental electrocution while tampering with a small radio set powered by 110 volt low tension current. See Figure 20-18.

which is gray or grayish yellow in color, and its shape may correspond with some portion of the electrically charged object which was in contact with the burned area. In other cases the heat produces a blister between the layers of the epidermis, which remains intact or is ruptured, leaving a reddish brown area with a border of wrinkled epidermis (Fig. 20-17). If the skin remains in contact with the electrode, cooking and charring of the skin and underlying tissues may occur, even with currents of low tension (Fig. 20-17). Jellinek has described other marks produced by the current on the skin near its entrance; there may be zigzag lightning-like figures in the skin; metallization or blackening of the skin surface around the entrance of the current may occur as the result of the volatilization of the metal of the electrode by the intense heat and the deposition of the metallic compounds that are formed.

A burn may be produced at the site where the current emerges, depending upon the resistance of the skin where this occurs. The skin may be ruptured as though by a minute explosion, or punctured by an emerging electric spark with the production of a small carbonized hole. Perforations may also appear in clothing and shoes which cover the points of exit. The current may emerge from an upper extremity, opposite to the one through which the current enters, or from one or both lower

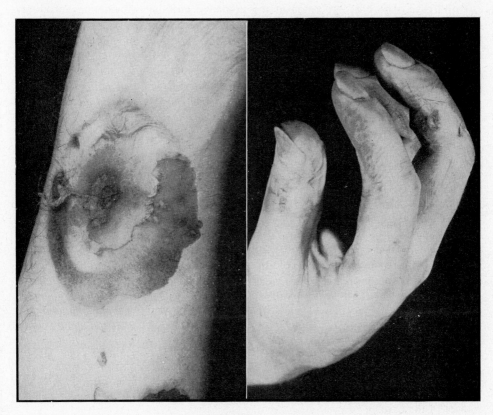

Fig. 20-17. Severe Electrical Burns from Prolonged Contact with Low Tension Current.

Extensive charring and blistering of skin of fingers and palm of right hand and deep burn on volar surface of left forearm. Deceased accidentally electrocuted while operating improperly insulated 110 volt hand drill. Duration of contact 10 to 15 minutes. Found dead in cellar, grasping drill which was still running.

extremities, or from other locations depending on the circumstances and how the body is grounded.

In high-tension electrocutions, in addition to entrance and exit burns, other electric burns may be produced at various points where the clothing is in contact with the skin and these appear usually as reddish brown geographic areas of varying size. Occasionally the clothing is set on fire and flame burns are produced. If the current enters and leaves the body over a wide area of low resistance, the amount of heat produced by the passage of the current is insufficient to raise the temperature to the burning point and neither current marks nor burns will be produced on the body. In one such case a workman stepped into a puddle of water covering a high-tension wire and was instantly killed by the electric shock without any burns or current marks having been formed on the skin. In some deaths caused by low-tension currents, burns are not produced; in 11 out of 37 cases of low-tension electrocutions the circumstances were such that neither current marks nor burns resulted. In deaths caused by high-tension currents, burns are more likely to be produced except under special circumstances.

The microscopic characteristics of the current marks, although not specific for electric injuries, are nevertheless helpful at times in establishing the diagnosis in a doubtful case. The heat generated at the points of entrance or exit may produce small circular vacuoles in the stratum corneum, a lesion that is most striking when it occurs in the thick horny layer of the skin on the fingers and palms or on the soles of the feet. The vacuoles form in the sweat ducts probably as the result of steam production and expansion in those structures. A honeycomb or Swiss cheese-like appearance is produced (Figs. 20-15 and 20-18). The epidermis in the center of the burned area may be denuded of its superficial layers. In the deeper layers of the epidermis, there is elongation and palisading of the cells and nuclei and the distortion gives the epidermal cell pattern a whorled appearance (Fig. 20-18). In some cases, the epidermis and corium are compressed, and the latter may assume a lilac color when stained with hematoxylin and eosin. The cells and nuclei of the hair follicles and sweat glands may also show a spindling distortion. Vesiculation of the epidermis and also charring of the skin and subcutaneous tissue may be found in some cases but the other changes are usually encountered in the margins of such charred and blistered areas.

Current marks can usually be distinguished from abrasions or postmortem artefacts produced by artificial respiration for the last two do not show any signs of burning. A distinction can also be made between current marks and postmortem blisters, for the electric lesion splits the layers of the epidermis (Fig. 20-18), while the bullae of decomposition separate the entire epidermis from the corium. The microscopic appearance of an electric burn does not establish that it was intravital for similar lesions can be produced by the action of electricity on a dead body, and the electric lesions are not pathognomonic inasmuch as they can be simulated by the application of a red hot object to the skin. Nevertheless, the current marks are valuable criteria of electrocution, when considered in connection with the circumstances of the case.

The mechanism of death from electricity has been a matter of much dispute. Some consider that the current traverses the heart and causes immediate death by ventricular fibrillation. Others believe that death results from the paralyzing action of the electric current on the respiratory center in the medulla. Mild cases of electric shock that are revived by artificial respiration lend support to the theory of paralysis of the medullary center, but do not disprove the cardiac theory. In some high-tension electrocutions, death results from a combination of electric shock, burns and blunt force injuries which are occasionally produced when the victim is thrown from an elevation on being shocked. In some cases, the individual survives the immediate shocking effect of the current, but dies later of burns or blunt force injuries. Electric burns tend to heal slowly because of the deep necrosis that may develop in the lesions; Jellinek has described rapidly forming edema around the burns especially on the face and limbs. Some of the cases which survive high-tension electric shock and burns develop neuropathic symptoms such as neuritis, muscular atrophy and paralysis. Low-tension currents can cause immediate death from shock but if the shock is not fatal, there are usually no sequelae.

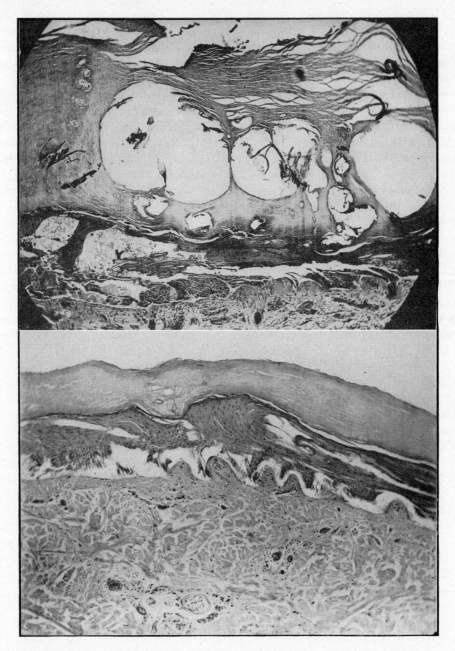

Fig. 20-18. Histologic Sections of Electrical Burns Produced by Low Tension Current Shown in Figure 20-16.

Upper: Burn of finger tip. Note honey comb effect in the horny layer resulting from disruption of sweat ducts, shrinkage and irregular splitting of the epidermis with elongation and spindling of the cells.

Lower: Burn on dorsum of finger. Note irregular shrinkage and splitting of the epidermis and spindling of the nuclei.

The pathologic findings at autopsy in cases of electrocution, aside from the current marks and burns, are not characteristic. In those seen by the authors where death had occurred immediately after the shock, there was fluid blood in the heart, congestion of viscera, slight edema of the lungs, and a few petechial hemorrhages in the conjunctiva, pleura and pericardium. A number of lesions produced by high-tension currents have been described in the literature, such as hyaline change in the muscle fibers, rupture of muscles due to spasms, hemorrhages in the floor of the fourth ventricle, microscopic changes in the ganglion cells, formation of pearl-like bodies in the bones from fusion of calcium phosphate, fractures, necrosis and ruptures of blood vessels in the extremities with hemorrhage and gangrene of the extremities in cases in which the victim had survived for a time. In judicial electrocution, the brain is heated by the current and vacuolization of the tissues around the vessels has been noted. Lesions in the heart are rare.

Helpern and Strassmann have analyzed the statistics of 144 cases of accidental electrocution; of these 101 deaths were caused by high-tension currents of 600 volts or more, and 43 deaths were due to contact with low-tension currents of 110 or 220 volts, usually of the alternating type. In the high-tension group, there were 64 immediate deaths and 37 delayed deaths; of the latter 23 persons died within 48 hours and 14 died in from 2 days to two and a half months after the accident. In the low-tension group there were 37 immediate deaths and 6 delayed deaths caused by ignition of clothing by burning insulations or short circuit sparks rather than from the effect of the electric shock.

Of the deaths due to high-tension currents, 65 occurred during work, 29 from contact with high-tension wires and third rails while trespassing, and 7 from contact with fallen high-tension wires. In the low-tension group 26 fatalities occurred during work, and 11 in the home. In both low- and high-tension groups most victims were in the third and fourth decades of life; but there were a considerable number of children in the high-tension group. One hundred and thirty-five cases were males. In 13 of the low-tension cases the victim cried out when the shock was received; in 24 the victim was found dead, the accident not having been witnessed. The accidents occurred mostly in warm weather and were most numerous during July and August. The seasonal incidence was especially striking in the low-tension group. Hot humid weather induces sweating and the moist skin has a lessened resistance to the current. Wet soil and damp shoes and feet supply excellent conditions for grounding. Many low-tension accidents occurred while the victim was washing out a boiler and standing in water, holding an electric extension lamp in one wet hand and manipulating a hose in the other, conditions ideal for the passage of a current through the grounded body. In some cases electrocution occurred when the victim touched a defective electric appliance or fixture while taking a bath. In other cases electrocution by low-tension currents resulted while the victim was installing electric apparatus in a damp cellar or elsewhere, testing bells, changing electric light bulbs, operating a defective switch board, repairing or tinkering with radio sets, operating electric machines such as a hand drill, repairing an elevator motor, and coming in contact with poorly insulated wires or a fallen wire in water or in damp soil.

Most deaths by electrocution are accidental, occurring at a yearly rate of about 24 cases. Electric deaths of a suicidal or homicidal nature are rare. Dr. Charles Hochman investigated one suicidal case in which the deceased rigged up an elaborate apparatus, using it to electrocute himself. In all electrocution cases the circumstances of death must be thoroughly investigated in order to determine the nature of the occurrence.

The legal execution of criminals by electrocution is now carried out in many states and this method has been employed in New York State since 1889. In the preparation of the condemned person the hair is shaved from the scalp and one leg, and the trouser leg is slit upward so as to give access to the electrode. After he is strapped to the chair, an electrode in the form of a metal cap is placed on his head and the other electrode is fastened around his leg. An alternating current of 1,700 volts and 7 amperes is then passed through the body for a minute; it produces a tetanic spasm and immediate loss of consciousness. The voltage of the current is then reduced and its flow through the body continued. The process is repeated a second time to make sure that life is extinct. The law provides for an immediate autopsy after the execution.

ROENTGEN RAYS

Roentgen rays which are also commonly designated as X-rays, are a form of energy having the power to penetrate some materials which are opaque to light, and because of this property they have two important uses in the practice of medicine:

1. The visualization of the internal structures of the human body by means of the roentgen ray photograph is an important aid in diagnosis. Roentgenograms may be introduced as legal evidence if they are properly identified by the roentgenologist who took them.

2. Roentgen rays are used as a therapeutic agent for the treatment of certain malignant tumors and blood dyscrasias. The rays affect the lymphatic and embryonic tissues readily and are valuable in treating and combating diseases like lymphosarcoma and the leukemias, and anaplastic neoplasms such as embryonal carcinoma of the testis or endothelial myeloma of bone (Ewing's tumor). Other tumors like melanoma, epidermoid carcinoma or osteogenic sarcoma are highly resistant to roentgen ray therapy.

The effect of roentgen rays on the cell is to destroy the nucleus primarily, and to inhibit the multiplication of proliferating cells. This is its chief therapeutic action against the blood dyscrasias. In affecting neoplasms the rays not only destroy the cells but excite an inflammatory reaction in the stroma of the tumor and in the surrounding tissues so that the affected portion undergoes necrosis and sloughs away. During this process, cellular elements are destroyed and toxic products are released, producing both local and systemic effects on the body.

Local Effects of Radiation. The roentgen rays consist of alpha rays, soft beta rays, hard beta rays and gamma rays. The alpha and soft beta rays are resisted by the skin where they are prone to cause severe burns, while the hard beta rays penetrate easily and are less liable to produce local effects. The use of an appropriate screen to filter out the harmful rays has considerably reduced the incidence of skin burns in roentgen ray therapy.

The rays when applied therapeutically in large doses without due precaution may produce an erythematous burn on the skin which is difficult to cure. The signs of injury do not appear immediately, and a latent period of about 14 days intervenes before the onset of the inflammatory changes in the skin; these are variable in degree and include erythema, epilation and blister formation. Indolent, necrotic ulceration with fibrosis of the corium and subcutaneous tissues may supervene, and the healing of these lesions is slow and incomplete. The microscopic picture resembles that found in ordinary burns except that in the lesions produced by roentgen rays, the vessels in the skin are apt to become thrombosed and telangiectases may develop with impairment of the nutrition of the affected area.

Roentgenologists and technicians who are repeatedly exposed to the action of the rays over a long period of time may develop a severe dermatitis around the finger nails which tends to spread over the entire hand. The lesions consist of patches of atrophic skin intermingled with areas of hyperkeratosis, generalized scaliness of the epidermis, a process resembling xeroderma pigmentosum, brittleness of the nails, painful fissures in the skin, and telangiectatic dilatation of the capillaries. The intimal layer of the arteries becomes thickened and the lumen of the vessels narrowed or occluded by this process or by thrombosis. If the exposure is continued for a number of years, epidermoid carcinoma may develop in the area of dermatitis.

Systemic Effects of Radiation. The systemic effects produced by the roentgen rays are referable to the destruction of cellular tissue and the liberation of toxic products. After exposure many individuals show an acute toxemia of varying severity. In mild cases the patients may complain of giddiness, headache, malaise, anorexia, nausea, vomiting, salivation, fever and chilly sensations. In severe cases, nausea and vomiting, the latter sometimes uncontrollable and bloody; offensive and bloody diarrhea; abdominal pain and distension; fever; restlessness and dyspnea may occur; the patient may die of cardiac collapse several days after the onset of symptoms. In these cases the intestinal tract may show numerous ulcerations, and the liver and bile ducts may be damaged.

Chronic systemic effects have been described, such as sterility, attributed to the action of the rays on the germinal cells. Rolleston mentions reports which indicate that the rays have a deleterious action on the fetus in utero, causing malformation and deformities. Long exposure to roentgen rays may produce changes in the bone marrow and blood, such as mononucleosis, leukopenia, aplastic anemia and rarely a leukemoid reaction. The gamma emanations of radium compounds produce effects similar to those of roentgen rays, in most cases causing aplastic anemia as discussed on pages 757 and 758.

STARVATION

Cases of starvation are occasionally encountered, but only rarely are they important from the medicolegal standpoint. Instances are met with in mentally deranged persons who starve themselves voluntarily, and among unfortunates who have been without food. In other cases the victims have been imprisoned and starved for homicidal purposes.

The length of time required for fatal starvation depends on whether or not the victim can obtain water. Without food and water, he may survive from 6 to 10 days; without food but with water, he may be able to live considerably longer, even a month or more.

The lesions that develop as the result of starvation are progressive emaciation, disappearance of fat, drying and shriveling of the skin, atrophy of the muscles and viscera, dehydration of the tissue and blood, congestion of the brain and meninges, and contraction of the gastrointestinal tract. Acidosis develops and acetone appears in the urine. Furunculosis and other secondary infections are apt to complicate the progress of starvation.

Incomplete starvation occurs when the body is deprived of a necessary component of the diet, such as protein, carbohydrate, fat, minerals, water and vitamins. The deprivation of protein reduces the amount of protein in the serum, and edema of the subcutaneous tissues and effusions into the body cavities, diarrhea, secondary anemia, leukopenia, polyuria and weakened cardiac function may develop. If the deprivation is continued, a complicating fatal secondary infection may occur. The depletion of the blood proteins resulting from dietary insufficiency can be corrected by adding an adequate amount of protein food to the diet. The deprivation of sugar, fat and minerals in a poorly balanced diet produces various disturbances of nutrition rather than a real starvation and such disorders are not forensically important.

The absence of the various vitamins from food over a long period of time can cause striking nutritional disturbances. Some of these have considerable medicolegal significance, inasmuch as they are encountered in nursing homes and insane asylums. The lack of vitamin A tends to produce hyperkeratoses of the skin, atrophy of the mucous membranes, drying up of the salivary and lachrymal glands, chronic conjunctival and corneal infections and night blindness. A deficiency of vitamin D and calcium may be followed by respiratory catarrh, anemia, osteomalacia and skeletal deformities characteristic of rachitis in children. The lack of one of the fractions of vitamin B (thiamine) may produce neuritis, sore tongue, hypertrophy of the heart and the other manifestations of beriberi. The absence of another vitamin B fraction (nicotinic acid) is responsible for the dermatitis, diarrhea and mental symptoms occurring in pellagra.

The most striking nutritional disturbance is scurvy which is due to lack of vitamin C. This is apt to occur among children in nursing homes where the inmates are not properly fed and also in adults deprived of fresh food for some time. The underlying defect is a failure in the deposition of intercellular material by the supporting tissues of the body, resulting from the absence of or an inadequate amount of vitamin C in the diet, Hemorrhages in various parts of the body are the chief clinical manifestation. In children they are found under the serous surfaces and skin, in the kidney, and under the periosteum near the junction of the epiphysis and the shaft; there is a distinct osteitis and disturbance of bone growth at this site and the lesion may present itself as a swelling near the joint. In adults a massive hemorrhage may develop in the intermuscular tissues of the thigh or leg, and the gums exhibit a hemorrhagic inflammation which in severe cases may progress to gangrene. Anemia and emaciation occur in the later stages of the disease. The condition can be alleviated if the patient is fed an antiscorbutic like orange juice, tomato juice or ascorbic acid (vitamin C).

INJURIES PRODUCED BY CHANGES IN ATMOSPHERIC PRESSURE

Barotraumas include the effects of exposure to diminution of barometric pressure at high altitude and also those which follow sudden transition from increased to normal atmospheric pressure in individuals who work at low depths.

Low Atmospheric Pressure at High Altitudes and in Aviation. Exposure to low atmospheric pressure at high altitudes, in mountainous regions or during the ascent of aircraft, produces a variety of harmful effects on the body. At altitudes above 10,000 feet, the oxygen content of the air is diminished sufficiently to produce physiologic disturbances. There is deficient oxygenation of the blood and the resultant anoxia places a strain on the circulatory, respiratory and nervous systems. Giddiness, cyanosis, dyspnea especially on exertion, nausea, headache, nosebleed, muscular weakness, lethargy and syncope may develop; memory and judgment may become impaired. If the heart is not organically sound, exposure to a rarefied atmosphere may cause it to fail. Prolonged exposure to low atmospheric pressure at high altitudes occasioned by a sojourn in a mountainous region, results in an adjustment of the body to the lowered oxygen supply. There is a compensatory increase in the number of erythrocytes and in the amount of hemoglobin in the blood.

Sudden ascents in aircraft to altitudes above 10,000 feet may produce a variety of effects on the occupants. A state of anoxia will ensue if supplementary oxygen is not available to compensate for its lack in the atmosphere; those exposed may suffer from giddiness, nausea, muscular weakness, dyspnea and tachycardia. The symptoms of oxygen want may come on insidiously and first manifest themselves by a feeling of exhiliration, impairment of judgment and memory, lack of coordination and delay in reaction time. At altitudes above 10,000 feet, respirators are provided which automatically deliver increasing amounts of oxygen as the altitude is increasing. Above 20,000 feet elevation, failure to provide supplementary oxygen will result in severe anoxia with loss of consciousness, circulatory collapse and death. Fatalities from anoxia occurred during balloon ascents to high altitudes in the days before the heavier than air aircraft were devised.

Other hazardous phenomena are encountered during high altitude flying. Thus the temperature steadily falls as the altitude increases and at 25,000 feet is 40° below zero Fahrenheit. Proper protection with electrically heated clothing is necessary to prevent frostbite and fatal freezing. The effects of the cold are obviously more rapid if the occupant of the plane is not protected from the wind. To overcome the effects of oxygen lack and severe cold in high altitude flying, aircraft have been designed equipped with sealed heated pressurized cabins.

Rapid ascent to elevations above 25,000 feet may result in the release of the nitrogen which is dissolved in the blood and tissues, in the form of bubbles producing a modified form of air embolism and tissue emphysema similar to that encountered in compressed air illness or caisson disease. Symptoms of the bends may develop and involvement of the spinal cord may produce paralysis. The breathing of pure oxygen or of a mixture of oxygen and helium prior to taking off in rapid ascents may forestall the development of symptoms of this phenomenon at altitudes where it usually occurs.

Rapid accelerated descents from high altitudes such as occur in dive bombing in which the speed of the plane may reach 500 miles per hour and sudden changes in direction at high velocity, bring into play centrifugal forces which tend to drain the blood from the brain into the lower part of the body resulting in a momentary blacking out or in longer periods of unconsciousness. In addition, repeated rapid ascents and descents, chiefly the latter, may produce harmful effects on the auditory apparatus. Otitis media may result from barotrauma where there is failure to equalize the pressure in the middle ear. Fowler has pointed out the factors that predispose and contribute to its production; these include extremely rapid descent, infection of the upper respiratory tract especially acute sinusitis, acute nasopharyngitis, catarrhal inflammation of the eustachian tube with closure, and previous otitis media, and above all deficient knowledge or carelessness about opening the eustachian tubes during descent to keep the pressures on both sides of the tympanic membrane equalized. Various degrees of deafness, transient and permanent may ensue.

Sudden Changes from High to Low Atmospheric Pressure. Caisson Disease. After exposure to high atmospheric pressure of two or three times or more above normal, such as would be encountered during the construction of deep underground tunnels or in deep sea diving, too rapid removal and decompression of the individual to normal atmospheric pressure may produce severe and sometimes fatal manifestations of a malady which has come to be known as caisson disease or the bends. It is more properly designated as compressed air worker's sickness and the manifestations are similar to but usually more serious than those encountered in aero-embolism and emphysema associated with rapid ascent to rarefied atmospheres.

Exposure to high atmospheric pressure in a compressed air chamber results in increased solution of air in the blood and tissues, especially the fatty and lipid tissues which absorb nitrogen five times as rapidly as other tissues. The oxygen is absorbed and utilized but the large excess of inert nitrogen and carbon dioxide remains dissolved. If a diver is brought to the surface gradually or if a worker in a caisson is decompressed by gradual passage through a series of decompression chambers until the pressure of the outside atmosphere is reached, the accumulated nitrogen in the tissues and blood will escape imperceptibly by diffusion, bubbling of the dissolved gases will be avoided and no serious consequences will ensue. But if the person who has been exposed to an increased atmospheric pressure is suddenly decompressed and brought into an atmosphere of normal pressure, the excess nitrogen and carbon dioxide dissolved in his tissues and blood are suddenly released from solution, appearing in the form of gas bubbles which produce an emphysema of the tissues and a modified form of air embolism in the blood vessels. In milder cases the gases trapped in the less vascularized tissues and in the joints may be liberated to produce symptoms of the disease without any bubbling taking place in the blood. A definite train of symptoms follows the sudden release of gases into the tissues and into the circulation. The victim is doubled up by the severe muscular pain and abdominal cramps, from which effect the designation of the bends has been derived. Pains in the joints, vertigo, deafness, paralysis of the extremities, cyanosis, mottling of the skin and coma may supervene. In fatal cases death usually occurs within 24 hours.

If the victim dies shortly after an attack and an autopsy is performed soon after death, the blood especially in the right heart and veins may be found foaming with nitrogen and carbon dioxide bubbles. Bubbles may also be present in the mesenteric, meningeal and coronary vessels, in the omentum, cortex of the brain and cerebrospinal fluid. Emphysema of the subcutaneous, joint and areolar tissues may be present. Minute hemorrhages may occur in the spinal cord, forming destructive lesions of varying size near the center; in cases which survive these may cause signs of myelitis. Blebs are occasionally seen in the brain substance. Myocardial degeneration, softening of the voluntary muscles and mottling of the skin have been described.

In some cases of caisson disease, the immediate attack is survived and serious complications develop later. These may be grouped into three categories:

1. Caisson myelitis. This is produced by air embolism in the thoracic region of the spinal cord, most involved because of its comparatively rich blood supply as compared with the cervical and lumbar regions. The destructive lesions involve most intensely the gray and white matter in the central portions of the dorsal cord, and give rise to a paraplegia which in turn may be complicated by septic, occasionally fatal, infections of the urinary tract. Lichtenstein and Zeitlin have described a case

of caisson myelitis in a Negro male of 63 years who died of natural causes, surviving the primary injury of the cord 25 years, during which time he remained disabled.

2. Permanent involvement of the joints and bones. The joint lesions may consist of gas in the articular cavity and bubbles in the periarticular tissues; in other cases aeropathic changes in the bones may also affect the joints. A persistent arthralgia may result. In the long bones the lesions usually take the form of an aseptic necrosis or infarct, occurring mostly in the metaphysis but sometimes in the diaphysis or articular portions. Early stages in the development of such bone infarcts have not been described in human cases of caisson disease, for they develop slowly and manifest themselves years after the primary attack; they are encountered as an area of necrosis which may be encapsulated, cystic or partly calcified. Their formation is attributed to disturbances of circulation in the osseous tissue from the

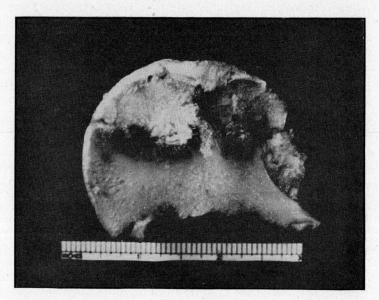

Fig. 20-19. Avascular Necrosis of Head of Femur. Complicating Caisson Disease.

Both femoral heads were involved and surgically removed. Appearance of lesion in bone 4 years after its inception during an attack of "bends." Case of Dr. F. Vom Saal, Hospital for Special Surgery, New York.

presence of air emboli in the blood vessels and in part to pressure and stress of body movement on the affected area. For further discussion see reference to Colonna and Jones.

The following nonfatal case of Dr. Frederick Vom Saal is an illustration of aeropathic necrosis in bones. A white man of 40 years, a tunnel worker, after a severe attack of the bends returned to work four days later, complaining of pain in back, hips and shoulders. His disability grew worse and after four years he could do only light work. A roentgen ray examination disclosed deformity of the femoral heads and wedgeshaped areas of rarefaction near the joint surface, ostensibly the cause of the arthralgia. After surgical resection of the affected bones, the heads of the femurs were flattened to the shape of door knobs, and yellowish gray, pyramidal-shaped infarcts, from 25 to 30 mm. in diameter, were found in the cancellous bone near the articular surface, surrounded by a thin zone of dark red congestion about 1 mm. thick (Fig. 20-19). Microscopically the joint cartilage was cracked in places and the adjacent cancellous bone was sclerotic; in the center the bone was necrotic in some areas and was absent in others showing beginning cyst formation. In the interosseous tissues there were large mononuclear cells containing fine particles of brown pigment.

3. Permanent impairment of hearing referable to damage inflicted on the auditory apparatus. This is due to sudden variations in atmospheric pressure resulting in unequal pressures on both sides of the tympanic membrane and in anatomic or functional disturbances of hearing.

Caisson disease is averted by gradually transporting workers from deep levels where the atmospheric pressure is high to the surface through a series of decompression chambers. Many persons are abnormally susceptible to atmospheric pressure changes, and great care must be exercized in restoring them to normal pressure levels. Compressed air workers, or sand hogs, wear identification tags which direct that they be sent to decompression chambers should they develop symptoms of the bends or lose consciousness as a delayed result of a too sudden return to normal atmospheric pressure. Physical activity may sometimes precipitate delayed symptoms of caisson disease in a case in which the decompression has not been complete.

REFERENCES

Armstrong, H. G. Principles and Practice of Aviation Medicine, Baltimore, Williams and Wilkins Co., 1943.

Ash, J. E., and Spitz, S. Pathology of Tropical Diseases, Philadelphia, W. B. Saunders Co., 1945.

Baker, R. D. Untoward effects of various substances recommended for burns or wounds, Arch. Surg., 48:300, 1944.

———— The internal lesions in burns with special reference to the liver and splenic nodules, Am. J. Path., 21:717, 1945.

Behnke, A. R. Concepts derived from investigations pertaining to high altitude flight, J.A.M.A., 133:450, 1947.

Boyd, W. A Text Book of Pathology, Philadelphia, Lea and Febiger, 1938.

Colonna, P. E., and Jones, E. D. Aeroembolism of bone marrow, Arch. Surg., 56:161, 1948.

Erdmann, S. Aeropathy or compressed air illness among tunnel workers, J.A.M.A., 49:1665, 1907.

———— The acute effects of caisson disease or aeropathy, Am. J. M. Sc., 145:520, 1913.

Fowler, E. P. Causes of deafness in flyers, Arch. Otolaryngol., 42:21, 1945.

Friedman, N. B., and Kritzler, R. A. The pathology of high altitude frostbite, Am. J. Path., 23:173, 1947.

Glaister, J. Medical Jurisprudence and Toxicology, 7th ed., Baltimore, Williams & Wilkins Co., 1942.

Hartman, F. W., and Major, R. C. Pathological changes resulting from accurately controlled artificial fever, Am. J. Clin. Path., 5:349, 1935.

———— Lesions of brain following fever therapy, J.A.M.A., 109:2116, 1937.

Helpern, M., and Strassman, G. Circumstances and postmortem findings, especially skin lesions, in accidental electrocution. Am. J. Path., 16:592, 1941.

Jackson, C. N. Inanition and malnutrition, Arch. Path., 7:1042, 1929; 8:81, 1929.

Jaffe, R. L. Electropathology, Arch. Path., 5:836, 1928.

Jellinek, S. Elektrische Verletzungen, Leipzig, Johann Ambrosius Barth, 1932.

Kahlstrom, S. C., Burton, C. C., and Phenister, D. B. Aseptic necrosis of bone: infarction of bone in caisson disease resulting in encapsulated and calcified areas in diaphyses and in arthritis deformans, Surg. Gynec. & Obst., 68:129, 1939.

Lichtenstein, B. W., and Zeitlin, H Caisson disease, Arch. Path., 22:86, 1936.

Lucké, B. Lower nephron nephrosis, Mil. Surgeon, 99:371, 1946.

Malamud, N., Haymaker, W., and Custer, R. P. Heat stroke, Mil. Surgeon, 99:397, 1946.

McWhorter, J. E. The etiological factor of compressed air illness, Am. J. M. Sc., 139:373, 1910.

Moyer, H. N. Medico-Legal Relations of the X Rays, Radium and Ultra-Violet Rays, in Peterson, Haines, and Webster, Legal Medicine and Toxicology, Philadelphia, W. B. Saunders Co., 1923, Vol. 2, p. 954.

Puppe, G.   Atlas und Grundriss der Gerichtlichen Medizin. München, J. F. Lehmann, 1908.

Reports of the Office of the Chief Medical Examiner in the City of New York from 1918 to 1951.

Rolleston, H.   The harmful effects of irradiation, Quart. J. Med., 24:101, 1931.

Wade, W.   Diseases due to Physical Agents, in Cecil's Text Book of Medicine, Philadelphia, W. B. Saunders Co., 1933, pp. 541-548.

Walker, J. Jr., Saltonstall, H., Rhoads, J. E., and Lee, W. E.   Toxemia syndrome after burns, Arch. Surg., 52:177, 1946.

21

Pregnancy: Puerperium: Illegitimacy

PREGNANCY

Pregnancy is that state which occurs in the female when an ovum, discharged from an ovary into the genital tract, is fertilized by a spermatozoon in the semen, introduced by the male during coitus. It can also occur after artificial insemination. Pregnancy lasts from the time of conception to the birth of the child and its usual duration is about 10 lunar months or 9 calendar months.

Pregnancy is most apt to occur between the ages of 14 and 45 years. Its possibility commences with the onset of the menses, which normally begin at about 12 to 16 years, depending on race and climate. Menstruation may be retarded until 18 or 20 years of age, but occasionally may start precociously in children of four years or even younger. Pregnancy has been described in children of 8 to 10 years, many of whom have had a precocious menstruation. As long as menstruation persists, the possibility of pregnancy exists. The menses stop in many women shortly after the forty-fifth year, and pregnancy after that age is not common, though cases have been described in older females.

The assertion is often made that a woman can become pregnant to full term without being aware of her condition. Considering the fact that this state is preceded by sexual intercourse, begins with suppression of the menses, and is marked by a progressive enlargement of the abdomen, it is difficult to see how it could pass unnoticed. There is a possibility that a woman could be impregnated in deep sleep or unconsciousness, and later attribute the menstrual and abdominal signs to some other condition. Some women do not associate pregnancy with sexual intercourse, and may not recognize their plight through ignorance.

Situations occasionally arise under the criminal or civil law when it is necessary to determine whether or not pregnancy exists in a certain case. A charge of concealing the fact that she is pregnant may be brought against a woman who has been separated from her husband or who is not married. Actions for divorce or slander may follow such accusations. In other instances a woman may claim that she is impregnated with a posthumous child, to secure for herself a greater share of her deceased husband's estate. She may feign this condition for the purposes of blackmail, to extort extra damages in an accident case, to substantiate a charge of alleged rape or seduction, to avoid a prison term or to escape a sentence of death. In any of these situations a physician may be called upon to examine a woman to solve the problem of whether or not she is pregnant.

Before starting the examination, the physician must obtain the consent of the woman in the presence of witnesses, or better still, get a signed statement from her that she agrees to the examination and understands that the usual relation of physician and patient does not exist between them. Without a definite court order the physician cannot examine the woman against her consent, and if he does he is not only liable for civil damages, but also may be subjected to criminal prosecution.

The same restrictions apply when the examining physician is a woman. The requests of other members of the family who may be in favor of the examination do not give him the authority to proceed without the woman's consent, unless she is a mental defective, in which case consent can be given by next of kin. If the medical attendant, however, is acting through a court order served upon him or is directed by a judge of a court of record in open court, he can overrule the objections of the woman (page 606). A record should be made of the time and place of the examination. In arriving at a diagnosis the physician must take into consideration all the symptoms and signs present and sift the available evidence with considerable care. A false diagnosis under such conditions is not only damaging to the woman, but may be disastrous to the reputation of the physician.

Diagnosis. The symptoms of pregnancy are subjective phenomena which the woman recounts to the physician. They are, therefore, only hearsay evidence as far as he is concerned, and of no value unless confirmed by positive objective signs which the physician discovers on physical examination or by laboratory tests.

SUBJECTIVE SIGNS. The most important subjective sign of pregnancy is the cessation of the menstrual flow. The monthly periods stop in most cases during the first month after conception and do not commence again until three months or more after delivery. Variations occur sometimes, and at best the sign is merely a suggestive item of information. One should remember also that the woman may not be telling the truth. In addition, the cessation of the periodic flow may be due to a variety of conditions, such as ovarian dysfunction from emotional disturbances, general organic disease and definite pathologic lesions in the genital tract.

A woman may attempt to simulate menstruation by sprinkling blood from some other source on her clothing or pads. Microscopic examination may be sufficient to establish the nature of such a stain; if it is menstrual blood, it should contain numerous vaginal epithelial cells. The precipitin test can be tried to determine if it is human blood or animal blood. If the stain is human blood it may also be possible to determine its group by the isoagglutination tests and to compare this result with the result obtained from the agglutination test on the woman's blood. Unless the results are consistent the stain may be considered as having come from some source other than the woman (Chapters 26 and 27).

The other subjective signs, such as nausea and quickening (that is, subjective sensations of fetal movements), are likewise unreliable as diagnostic criteria in a medicolegal case.

OBJECTIVE SIGNS. During pregnancy the uterus enlarges inside the abdominal cavity, and this enlargement is a great aid in making the diagnosis. The increase in size takes place according to a well-defined schedule.

The nonpregnant uterus is pear-shaped with a slight flattening of the antero-posterior diameter. The average dimensions are: 2½ inches to 4 inches in length, 1½ to 2 inches in breadth, and 1 inch to 1½ inches in thickness. Usually these measurements are expressed in the simple formula of 3 inches by 2 inches by 1 inch.

When the uterus becomes pregnant and enlarges, its body tends to become ovoid in shape. After the third calendar month the enlarging uterus rises above the brim of the symphysis pubis and is about 4 to 5 inches long, the corpus containing the fetus is 3 to 4 inches, and the cervix one inch in length. In the fourth month the uterus is about 5 inches long, and its fundus can be palpated midway between the symphysis and the umbilicus. In the fifth month the uterus is 6 inches long, and is definitely flask-shaped, with an ovoid globular body and a cervix which begins to shorten. In the sixth month the uterus is 7 inches long and its fundus is as high as the umbilicus. In the seventh month it is 8 inches long and its fundus is midway between the navel and the ensiform cartilage. In the eighth month it is 9½ inches long and the fundus is level with the ensiform cartilage. In the ninth month the uterus is 10 to 12 inches long and has widened. Its lower end may sink into the pelvis so that the fundus will be at the seventh month level. In most cases the diagnosis of pregnancy can be made from the enlargement of the uterus. There are, however, numerous other conditions which simulate the uterine swelling in pregnancy and make differentiation difficult; pathologic processes such as ovarian tumors, ascites, obesity and uterine fibromyomas are some of these.

The other objective signs are considered in connection with the period of pregnancy during which they generally appear. For the sake of convenience, the nine calendar months of gestation are divided into trimesters or subperiods of three months each.

A. *First Trimester*. The first three months of pregnancy are characterized by the suppression of the menses, nausea and vomiting. The base of the bladder is compressed by the enlarging uterus, and more or less vesical irritability develops.

The breasts commence to enlarge and become boggy. The areolae of the nipples increase in size and become more pigmented. Montgomery's glands grow and appear as small elevated nodules in the areola. Further changes in the breast during pregnancy are described on pages 561 and 577.

The uterus in this period has not enlarged enough to be recognizable from external examination, but a few uterine changes can be elicited. They are:

1. Goodell's sign, the softening of the cervix in the early stages of pregnancy, beginning about the third week.

2. Hegar's sign, softening and compressibility of the lower uterine segment, which can be elicited between the second and fifth month.

3. A softened and boggy uterine fundus which can be demonstrated about the third month by bimanual examination.

All these signs in conjunction cannot be considered as anything more than strong presumptive evidence of pregnancy. For this reason a positive diagnosis of pregnancy cannot be made on the physical signs alone before the second period of pregnancy.

B. *Second Trimester*. The second period of pregnancy includes the fourth, fifth and sixth months. The signs that appear in this stage are of considerable diagnostic importance. They are:

4. Jacquemin's or Chadwick's sign. This is a bluish or purplish discoloration of the vaginal outlet, due to the increasing pelvic congestion with advancing gestation. It occurs early, but is rarely well marked prior to the fourth month.

5. Braxton Hick's sign. This is the elicitation of intermittent uterine contractions of which the patient is unconscious.

6. Ballottement or the bouncing of the fetus in the uterus. This can be demonstrated from the fourth to the eighth month.

7. Active fetal movements, when elicited, are a positive proof of pregnancy. They are noted as distinct taps against the abdominal wall, probably from movements of the fetal limbs, or as undulating movements from side to side of the abdomen, from movements of the fetal trunk. They are not noted before the middle

of the sixth month and are not demonstrable in all cases. Increased abdominal fat and excess liquor amnii obscure this phenomenon.

8. If the fetal heart sounds are heard the diagnosis of pregnancy is positive. The sounds are like the ticking of a watch placed under a pillow, 120 to 160 beats per minute, about twice as fast as the maternal heart beat. They can be heard best by the stethoscope over the uterine enlargement, near the umbilicus. They cannot be heard with any degree of certainty until the fifth month, and in cases with thick abdominal walls or excess of amniotic fluid, they are hard to hear at all.

C. *Third Trimester.* In the third period of pregnancy, which includes the seventh, eighth and ninth months, the diagnosis can be made with much more certainty by physical examination. Bimanual palpation of the vagina and abdominal wall, in this stage, may enable the examiner to identify fetal parts as they present themselves at the vaginal outlet. Palpation of the abdomen alone may show the position of the fetus as it lies in the cavity of the uterus.

SUPPLEMENTARY TESTS. A number of supplementary tests have been employed in an attempt to establish a definite criterion for pregnancy.

Roentgen Ray. Roentgenography has been employed and reveals characteristic pictures in cases where the fetal ossification centers have become well developed, which includes cases from the fourth intra-uterine month onward. However, on the living patient, the method must be used with caution on account of the possible deleterious effect which the rays might exert on the ovaries or on the fetus in utero. It is valuable in cases where the woman is dead and where an autopsy is not immediately possible. The roentgenogram might demonstrate the necessity for an autopsy in a case in which the indications for it were otherwise not clear.

Aschheim-Zondek Reaction. A biologic test for pregnancy devised by Aschheim and Zondek depends upon the increased amount of gonad-stimulating hormone secreted into the blood and then excreted in the urine of pregnant women. This substance can be detected early by injecting small amounts of the woman's urine into immature virgin female mice. In these animals, hemorrhages into the immature ovarian follicles, or corpora lutea are produced about four days after the injection if the donor of the urine was pregnant. The reactions are usually visible to the naked eye.

The Aschheim-Zondek technic for the test in mice is as follows:
Five infantile female mice, about three to four weeks old and weighing about 6 to 8 gm. apiece, are selected. On the first day each one is given three doses of the suspected urine by subcutaneous injection in the amount of 0.5 ml. at a dose. On the second day three similar doses are given. Ninety-six hours after beginning the test, the animals are killed and the ovaries are examined for corpora lutea or for punctate hemorrhages into the graafian follicles. Both reactions can be seen with a small hand lens or with the naked eye and represent a positive test.
The Friedman modification of the test is based on the same principle, but employs rabbits in place of mice. The technic is as follows:
Ten cubic centimeters of suspected urine are injected into the ear vein of a mature virgin female rabbit which has been isolated for at least three weeks. The ovaries are examined 24 hours later. A positive reaction is indicated by recent hemorrhages into the follicles.

The reactions are positive in 98 to 99 per cent of the pregnancies. Aschheim, after injecting 3 ml. of urine into mice, reported positive results as early as 10 to 16 days after the fruitful coitus. The test is almost always positive three to four days after the expected date of the first missed menstrual period. The reactions continue to remain positive throughout pregnancy, as long as the placenta remains alive. The test becomes negative in about seven days after the termination of pregnancy. In cases of abortion in the early months it may remain positive for about 10 days. A negative test following an abortion may help to fix approximately the date of the abortion.

The test is valuable in confirming the diagnosis of pregnancy in cases of criminal abortion, for occasionally in this condition the anatomic indications are not clear cut. It may be helpful as a corroboration of pregnancy which has followed a case of rape. It would also detect spurious cases of gestation.

A negative Aschheim-Zondek test in a known case of pregnancy indicates death of the placenta and embryo. It is conceivable that an abortionist might allege that the reaction was negative and that the embryo was dead, as an excuse to induce abortion. The statement could be checked, however, by repeating the test and if it was positive his allegation would be discredited.

The Aschheim-Zondek test is not specific for pregnancy, but is also positive in cases of hydatid mole, ectopic gestation, chorio-epitheliomas in both sexes and certain tumors of the pituitary.

PUERPERIUM

A situation sometimes may arise which necessitates the medical examination of a woman to discover whether or not she has been recently delivered of a child. In conducting such an examination the physician will be obligated to obtain the consent of the woman, as has been discussed previously under Pregnancy. Determination of the puerperal state is important in cases in which a woman is trying to conceal a birth or feign one, and may arise in trials for abandonment, infanticide, abortion, slander, inheritance, fraud or blackmail.

Examination upon the Living. Legally the expulsion of a fetus prematurely from the uterus is termed an abortion. In obstetric practice the custom has been to call all such expulsions in the first three months, abortions; in the middle three months, miscarriages; and in the last three months, premature deliveries. These distinctions, though useful in a medical sense, do not have any application in law. In the examination of a patient for signs of a recent delivery, much will depend upon how far advanced pregnancy was at the time of expulsion, and how soon after the expulsion the patient is examined.

In an abortion between the second and third months, the uterus may expel the fetal remains without incurring laceration, and in any event, as it is only slightly enlarged it quickly returns to normal; after two or three days, there is no sign of the gravid condition which ended a short time before. It is only when the examiner obtains a part of the fetus or some uterine curettings, and identifies them microscopically as products of conception that he can form a positive judgment concerning recent pregnancy.

If the abortion occurs between the third and the fifth months, the expulsion of the fetus will distend the cervix and the vaginal canal, possibly producing a few contusions and lacerations. The cervix uteri is described as having the shape of a funnel and the vulvar tissues are congested and patulous. This condition will persist for a few days and then disappear gradually. However, if a septic infection develops in the uterus, the patulous condition will remain longer. In addition the breasts are larger, are congested and contain serous or milky fluid known as colostrum.

It is possible in this period to make a diagnosis of recent abortion upon the physical examination alone, but such examination must be made soon after the event, because the signs will disappear. The difficulty in diagnosis is to distinguish a menstrual uterus, in which there is a certain amount of relaxation and bleeding, from a uterus after a recent abortion. If fetal remains can be demonstrated microscopically, however, they will be positive evidence of the postabortal state.

If the woman has been delivered at full term the signs are much more definite and persist longer. Nevertheless, it is desirable that the doctor should make his examination as soon after delivery as possible, because the genital organs return to almost normal in about two or three weeks. An examination at the end of that period might fail to establish the delivery of a child at full term.

Changes occur in the breasts, abdomen and genital organs after delivery at full term. The breasts will be enlarged, boggy and nodulated, and will contain colostrum or milk. The areola will be dark and wide, the nipples will be prominent, and the stage will be set for lactation which commences shortly after.

The abdominal walls, immediately after delivery, are pendulous, relaxed, wrinkled, and may show numerous linear striae. The uterus can be readily palpated well above the symphysis pubis. Other conditions may give a similar picture, but the uterine enlargement and the relaxation of the abdomen and the breast changes are characteristic of a recent delivery. In the first two days post partum, the uterus contracts to a size about 7 inches long and 4 inches in width. At the end of one week post partum it is about 5 inches long; at the end of two weeks it is 4 inches long. After two months it may be normal in size.

Vaginal examination discloses smooth and relaxed genital passages. The internal os closes during the first 24 hours. The external os is patulous and shows lateral transverse tears. Other birth tears may appear in the vagina and the perineum. The labia majora and minora may be enlarged and contused. Carunculae myrtiformes, or remains of the hymen, are apt to be more obvious in primiparae. The lochia or puerperal discharge from the uterus starts in the puerperium and normally lasts one or two weeks. For the first three or four days it is bloodstained and is termed lochia rubra, for the next four days it is serous and is labeled lochia serosa, and for the last period it is a yellowish white color and is termed the lochia alba. It has a peculiar and characteristic odor; when examined microscopically it may contain placental debris.

A woman who has been delivered of a child at full term has passed through a strenuous ordeal. Ordinarily she will lie in bed and receive postnatal care during the puerperium before resuming her ordinary activities. However, it is possible for some women to be up and around immediately after the birth of a child, and they may do it for the purpose of misleading the examining physician. It is a well known fact that primitive people like certain Indian tribes on the march, allow the woman in labor to drop behind in a secluded spot, have her child and then catch up with the tribe afterward.

In the normal postpartum state practically all the diagnostic signs will disappear shortly after two weeks. Any examination subsequent to that period will not discover any criteria which will enable one to tell how long an interval has passed since childbirth, and this is especially true of multiparae. In them, signs are usually present which indicate previous pregnancies, and these tend at times to confuse the signs of recent delivery. The abdominal wall is more or less flaccid and numerous longitudinal white scars of old striae can be seen; the same phenomena, however, can follow any other abdominal enlargement. The breasts will be large and pendulous with prominent nipples, quite in contrast to the firm breasts of girls. The fourchette is absent, the hymen may be replaced by carunculae myrtiformes, the vaginal tract is open and birth scars may be present on the perineum and cervix uteri. In a certain percentage of these cases, however, these signs are not distinct, and it may be difficult to state positively whether the woman is multiparous or nulliparous. In primiparae, the effects of recent birth are more marked than in multiparae. The question may arise whether a woman can undergo labor without knowing that she is giving birth to a child. Dorland says: "It is well recognized that unconscious delivery is possible, though rare, during profound sleep, during a state of coma or syncope, in an apoplectic, eclamptic, hysteric or asphyxiated woman, and under the influence of an anesthetic, narcotic or intoxicating liquor." This condition is more apt to occur with multiparae than with primiparae.

Examination upon the Dead. This subject is treated in Chapter 22.

LEGITIMACY AND PATERNITY

Legitimacy is the status of any person who has been born in lawful wedlock. In law the general presumption is that if the person is born during the continuance of a legal marriage the birth is legitimate. If he is born within a reasonable length of time after the dissolution of a marriage by divorce or death, his birth is presumed to be legitimate.

The question of illegitimacy, however, can be raised and sustained if it can be proved that the husband could not possibly be the father of the child. This can be done if the evidence is sufficient to show that:

(1) the alleged father is under the age of puberty, (2) the alleged father is physically incapable of procreation because of illness, old age, or congenital or acquired deformities, (3) the alleged father did not have access to his wife during the time that the child was begotten.

The legitimacy is clearly impossible in cases in which both parents belong to one race and the child in question unmistakably belongs to another race; or if the blood group of the child is not consistent with that of the parents as determined by the isoagglutination tests.

In the treatment of this subject by law, the complications which may arise in any given case are many and various, and the legal practice has not been determined conclusively for many of these points. In any event, the presumption of legitimacy is strong in most jurisdictions, and proof advanced to establish illegitimacy must be absolutely convincing to override this presumption.

An unmarried woman, inspired by hopes of gain through blackmail, may claim that a certain newborn child is her own and was fathered by a certain man. In such instances considerable medical investigation must be made. There are the questions of the pregnancy of the mother, the probable date of impregnation, the date of birth of the child and the evidence on the alleged mother of the delivery of a child. In addition, there are the questions of the resemblance of the child to the alleged father and the scientific isoagglutination tests on the blood which may confirm or deny the possibility of his parentage.

It is important that a physician who is consulted in a legitimacy case should have a comprehensive knowledge of the normal duration of pregnancy, and of the degree to which it may be shortened or lengthened, compatible with the birth of a viable child. This question is complicated at the start, because it is not possible to set the date of actual conception, even when the date of the fruitful coitus can be ascertained. In some cases, the union of the ovum and spermatozoon may occur within a few hours after intercourse; in others, it may not take place for a number of days.

A further point of uncertainty is that ovulation is not synchronous with menstruation. As a consequence the onset of the pregnancy cannot be determined with exactness. The most that the examiner can attempt is to compute 280 days (10 lunar months, 9 calendar months, 40 weeks), from the date of the last menstrual period; the date obtained from this calculation is somewhere in the middle of the last two weeks of pregnancy. The calculations can be further complicated by the fact that it is possible for pregnancy to occur at a time when the menses are suppressed for some other reason, so that it is not possible in such circumstances to calculate the date at all. On the average, the gestation in the human female is 280 days, but it may last only 240 days or extend to 300 days or longer.

The size of the child is important in the consideration of protracted or shortened pregnancies and, as a rule, the longer the gestation, the larger the infant. However, this is not invariably so, for it is by no means unusual to find rather large infants occurring in short periods of gestation, and for cases of protracted pregnancy to give rise to comparatively small infants. The average weight of full term infants is 7½ pounds, but they may vary from 3 pounds to 15 pounds.

It may be important in cases of inheritance to determine whether or not the infant was born alive. This means that it must be separated from the mother and achieve respiration and an independent circulation. It is not essential in some jurisdictions that it should be capable of survival. Thus, it is sufficient for a fetus of four or five months' development in utero, to be born alive and live a short time, to fulfill the conditions of live birth. Viability, or the ability of the child to survive after birth, does not exist until the infant has had at least six months of gestation.

Superfetation. Another question which is debated occasionally is that of superfetation. This means the impregnation of a second ovum in a woman already pregnant, and the subsequent birth of twin children at the same time, one of which may be mature and the other immature. They can be born, also, at full term, the one a few weeks ahead of the other. This condition, for a long time denied by obstetricians, while theoretically possible, is difficult to prove. The pregnancy does not close the cervical or tubal orifices immediately, and so if a second ovulation occurs after the first, the ovum may be impregnated, and the second embryo take root and develop.

Superfecundation. This is a phenomenon, denoting pregnancy with two or more children, the result of separate fertilizations of two or more ova liberated at the same ovulation, by spermatozoa introduced during successive acts of coitus. Superfecundation has been offered as an explanation of those cases, a few of which have been described, where a woman was delivered of twins, one white and the other black, presumably the products of coitus with different men. The application and limitations of the isoagglutination tests in trying to prove superfecundation are discussed on page 644.

Paternity. The question of paternity arises in contests over legitimacy, posthumous births or suppositive children. It is a point difficult to decide in many instances, and hitherto has been unraveled from the point of view of resemblance or lack of resemblance, between the child and the alleged father. Such characteristics as the form of the features, color of eyes and hair, peculiarities of manner and stature, are of value only to a limited degree. For example, the color of the eyes is a mendelian trait and subject to the limitations of Mendel's law. Thus it is possible for two brown-eyed persons to produce brown-eyed offspring and sometimes blue-eyed offspring. If one of the parents is brown-eyed and the other blue-eyed, the children would occur in the proportions of three brown-eyed to one blue-eyed, but this distribution would hold only if a large number of children were produced. Two blue-eyed persons would not produce children with brown eyes, but only children with blue eyes, as blue eyes are recessive characteristics and do not carry the dominant brown-eyed genes. On the other hand, some brown-eyed persons may carry a few recessive genes along with the dominant ones, which explains the occasional appearance of blue eyes in a brown-eyed family.

The question of telegony and maternal impressions may come up in a case in which the child has not any resemblance to its alleged father. The advocates for the mother urge that she has transmitted the characteristics of a former mate to her child by the alleged father, or she has received a strong visual impression from some source, which is transmitted to the child. This question has excited much controversy and has been discarded as a possibility in maternity cases.

The question of resemblance is, at best, a tricky proposition, and each case of paternity must be decided on its own merits. Fortunately, the problem has received considerable aid from the isoagglutination tests on blood. By establishing the type of the child's blood, and the type of each of the alleged parents, it is often possible to determine whether the alleged father could have been the real father of the child or not. This is discussed in detail in Chapter 27.

REFERENCES

Aschheim, S. Pregnancy tests, J.A.M.A., 104:1324, 1935.

Dorland, W. A. Legal Aspects of Pregnancy in Peterson, Haines and Webster, Legal Medicine and Toxicology, Philadelphia, W. B. Saunders Co., 1923, Vol. 1, p. 929.

Eastman, N. J. Williams Obstetrics, 10th ed., New York, Appleton-Century-Crofts, Inc., 1950.

Herzog, Alfred W. Medical Jurisprudence, Indianapolis, The Bobbs-Merrill Co., 1931, Sections 860-907.

22

Abortion

Abortion may be defined as the premature expulsion of the fetus from the womb at any time before its term of gestation is complete. Medically the term abortion is applied to the termination of pregnancy during the first three months of intra-uterine life, while an abortion occurring during the middle period of pregnancy is designated a miscarriage, and one taking place after the seventh month is called a premature birth. Legally there is no distinction made between abortion, miscarriage or premature delivery and all are known by the name of abortion.

Abortions may be divided into three categories: spontaneous and accidental, therapeutic, criminally self-induced or induced by others.

Spontaneous and Accidental Abortions. Pregnancy may terminate at any time during the period of gestation, either as a result of natural causes without any obvious underlying disease process, or because of its association with certain diseases such as syphilis, malposition and malformation of the uterus, acute infections with high fevers (such as pneumonia and trichinosis), ovarian dysfunction or placental inflammations which favor the spontaneous separation of the fetus from the uterus. In women who are prone to abort easily, external causes of a trivial nature may precipitate the expulsion of the fetus. In such persons accidental falls, trauma to the abdomen or elsewhere, fright, electric shock, and exercises such as jumping, skipping rope, bicycle riding or horseback riding may bring about this condition. In most women, the fetus clings rather tenaciously to the uterus and even severe physical trauma or shock may not be attended by abortion. In women who are prone to abort spontaneously, either as a result of disease or external trauma, the process usually occurs before the third or fourth months of gestation, and as a result the whole ovum is expelled. In all cases the possibility that the abortion is spontaneous must be considered, but undoubtedly many of those alleged to be spontaneous in nature are the result of wilful interference for the purpose of terminating pregnancy.

If an abortion occurs in a pregnant woman who has been the victim of an accidental trauma, the person responsible for the injury is open to a civil suit for damages. The same rule applies to a physician who inadvertently administers any medicine to a pregnant woman which may cause her to abort.

Therapeutic Abortions. If a disease condition is present which will make continued gestation and delivery perilous for the woman, the physician in attendance may be compelled to terminate the pregnancy. The diseases in which an abortion of this type may be indicated are death of the fetus, toxemia of pregnancy, heart disease, kidney disease, tuberculosis, some forms of insanity, bony deformities of the pelvis and such intra-uterine conditions as hydatidiform mole. Before inducing the abortion, the medical attendant must call in another physician in consultation, and review the indications for the proceeding. In some cases it may be better and less dangerous for the woman to continue with the pregnancy than to have an abortion performed. The indication for the interruption of gestation should be evident and not merely an excuse for the induction of a criminal abortion.

CRIMINAL ABORTIONS, SELF-INDUCED

The self-induced abortion occurs when the woman attempts to end her pregnancy by the self-administration of some drug, or by such mechanical means as bicycle riding, hot baths, the insertion of slippery elm sticks into the cervix, or the introduction of darning needles into the cavity of the uterus. In some instances, the woman herself may force a sharp instrument through the vault of her vagina into the abdominal cavity and lacerate her abdominal viscera, causing death by sepsis. In investigating a case of this type at autopsy, the question must be decided whether the findings are compatible with the proposition that the woman could cause the injuries by her own efforts, or whether the manipulations of an abortionist would offer a more logical explanation for their presence. It is often necessary to supplement the medical evidence with the investigations of the police department in order to reach a decision on this point. In the United States unless there is a definite statute in the jurisdiction concerned, a woman is not criminally liable for producing an abortion on herself, though she is liable if she procures somebody else to perform the operation. A fatal self-induced abortion has a status similar to that of suicide. In New York State a pregnant woman is criminally liable for performing or attempting an abortion on herself and may be punished by imprisonment for from one to four years.*

CRIMINAL ABORTIONS INDUCED BY OTHERS

A criminal abortion is the induced destruction and expulsion of the fetus from the womb of the mother by another person unlawfully, that is, when there is no therapeutic indication for the operation. This crime is considered a felony whether or not the abortion results fatally. If the woman dies as a consequence of the procedure the abortionist and anybody else who is concerned with the crime, such as an anesthetist or nurse, can be charged with homicide. Even a relative or friend of the deceased who guided her to the abortionist is held guilty of being a party to the crime, if it can be shown that such person knew the purpose of the visit. The law emphasizes the illegal intent behind the act and regards all accessories to the crime as guilty as the principals. In this category also belong individuals who advise and prescribe drugs like ecbolic medicines or attempt to terminate the pregnancy by other means; if death ensues as the result of their administrations they are just as culpable under the law as though they attempted to induce abortion by instruments.

There is no distinction made in law between an expulsion of the fetus early in pregnancy or one late in pregnancy, as all of them are termed abortions. In most jurisdictions the fetus in the early stages before quickening is considered just as much endowed with life as in the later stages. An abortion is considered just as blameworthy in the early months as in the later months of pregnancy. In addition, if an abortion is attempted on a woman who is not pregnant but supposes herself to

* Liability of a Woman Who Has Abortion Produced on Herself. Under the New York Penal Law (New York Penal Code #81), a pregnant woman who takes any medicine, drug, substances, or submits to the use of any instrument or other means, with intent thereby to produce her own miscarriage, unless the same is necessary to save her life, or that of the child whereof she is pregnant, is punishable by imprisonment for not less than one year, and not more than four years. (From Herzog, *Medical Jurisprudence*, 1931.)

be pregnant, and death results from the attempt, the operator can be charged with homicide, and he would also be liable in a civil malpractice suit. The Penal Law in New York State places an added emphasis on abortion which is induced after quickening has occurred as indicated in the following quotations.

The Penal Law of the State of New York has the following sections on abortion:

‡1050. Manslaughter in the First Degree. The wilful killing of an unborn quick child, by any injury committed upon the person of the mother of such child, is manslaughter in the first degree.

A person who provides, supplies, or administers to a woman, whether pregnant or not, or who prescribes for, or advises or procures a woman to take any medicine, drug or substance, or who uses or employs, or causes to be used or employed, any instrument or other means, with intent thereby to procure the miscarriage of a woman, unless the same is necessary to preserve her life, in the case of the death of the woman, or of any quick child of which she is pregnant, is thereby produced, is guilty of manslaughter in the first degree.

‡1052. Manslaughter in the Second Degree. Woman producing miscarriage. A woman quick with child, who takes or uses, or submits to the use of any drug, medicine or substance, or any instrument or other means to produce her own miscarriage, unless the same is necessary to preserve her own life, or that of the child whereof she is pregnant, if the death of said child is thereby produced is guilty of manslaughter in the second degree.

The law specifically states that if an individual induces an abortion of the criminal type on a woman at any stage of pregnancy and her death occurs as a result, he would be guilty of manslaughter in the first degree. If the pregnancy has reached the stage where quickening has occurred, the defendant can be charged with manslaughter for causing the death or destruction of the child in utero quite apart from any harm which may occur to the mother. If the woman herself kills her child in utero after the stage of quickening, she can be charged with manslaughter in the second degree. The sensations of quickening usually are evident according to Eastman about the eighteenth to the twentieth week or roughly about the fifth month. If there is a prosecution based on the death of a quickened fetus, a post-mortem examination of the fetus is necessary in order to prove that it had reached that stage of intra-uterine development.

In New York City there is an ordinance of the Department of Health which requires physicians or hospitals to report to the department all cases of abortion regardless of their nature. In suspected criminal cases, the Police Department and District Attorney's Office are notified and they conduct an investigation. The Health Department is concerned with vital statistics of all fetal deaths regardless of whether they result from criminal abortion or not. At the same time, the requirement in the Sanitary Code that such fetal deaths be reported on special death certificates does tend to discourage the performance of criminal abortions in hospitals where they might otherwise be done under the guise of their being therapeutic.

The relation of the practicing physician to the question of abortions is a vexing one, and annoying problems may arise. For example, some women apply to their family physician for the termination of an undesired pregnancy in the expectation that he will either do it himself or refer them to some one who will. It is only by refusing to participate in the matter at all that the doctor can avoid complications with the law. Another type of problem occurs when an abortionist produces an incomplete abortion, and then sends the woman to her physician to be treated. The medical attendant is placed by this in an awkward position. But as soon as he recognizes the condition, he should have the patient transported to a hospital, or if that course is not possible, he should call in a consultant immediately, so that he can be protected in the event of an investigation. In New York City he would be obligated in addition to report the abortion to the Department of Health and to the Police Department.

It is important to remember that many women visit a gynecologic clinic and complain of symptoms which may lead an incautious surgeon to explore the uterus or curet it. Some may complain that their uterus is out of position, and this may influence the surgeon to pass a uterine sound into the corpus, thereby rupturing the membranes. The result is that the medical man unsuspectingly precipitates an abortion which might have been avoided if he had paid more attention to diagnosis. The corollary of this situation is one in which the physician knows the state of affairs, and wilfully performs an abortion while pretending to curet the uterus or to insert a sound for some fictitious diagnostic or therapeutic purpose.

Occasionally an abortionist, after he has bungled a curettage on a patient or has become aware that he has perforated the uterus, may call in a colleague to perform an abdominal operation on the woman, not only to repair any damage which might have been inflicted, but if possible to disguise the fact that an illegal abortion has been committed. The second physician, before starting the laparotomy, may pass a curet into the uterus ostensibly for diagnostic purposes, but in reality to confuse the case so as to hamper any subsequent investigation. In one instance the operating consultant actually assumed responsibility for the uterine and abdominal injuries probably produced by the abortionist, claiming that he, the consultant, caused them when he made his diagnostic exploration with the curet. If it could be proved in such cases that there was a conspiracy to cover up signs of abortion, the consultant could be subjected to criminal prosecution as an accessory to the crime. Even if he was acquitted of a criminal charge, he would expose himself to a civil action for malpractice, especially if he assumed responsibility for a grossly incompetent uterine curettage.

Nonfatal Cases of Criminal Abortion. It is important to remember that nonfatal cases of criminal abortion are classified in law as felonies, and those who are charged with the crime may be prosecuted in the criminal courts. In New York State if a physician is convicted of a charge of illegally inducing an abortion, his license to practice medicine in the state is revoked automatically.

The evidence necessary to establish the crime of nonfatal criminal abortion is proof which shows that the woman was pregnant and that the defendant terminated the pregnancy illegally. This evidence is gathered for the prosecution by the District Attorney and the Police Department who receive information about the activities of an alleged abortionist and then raid his premises at the time he is performing the illegal operation, thus obtaining visual proof of his connection with the case. If the raid is successful, the operator, his assistants and the patient are arrested as defendants, while the premises are searched for instruments, fetal remains and other confirmatory evidence. Medical testimony is necessary in order to establish the fact that the woman was pregnant and that an illegal abortion has been committed upon her. Accordingly the woman defendant is sent as a patient to a hospital in order that her condition can be diagnosed and the proper treatment given. The examination by the physician should include a general physical examination and a special investigation of the genital organs for any signs indicative of a recent abortion (page 559). In addition a watch must be kept for signs of intra-uterine bleeding, septic infections of the uterus, peritonitis and similar complications. If a laparotomy or other operation is performed, careful records should be made of the operative procedures and of conditions found during operation. All perforations of the uterus and of other abdominal viscera must be described. All pieces of tissue removed at operation or by curettage should be sent to the pathologist for histologic examination, and the urine of the patient preserved for the Aschheim-Zondek test, as both laboratory examinations may yield unmistakable indications of pregnancy. The attending physician has definite medicolegal responsibilities in this type of case, and he should compile his medical record carefully as his testimony will be needed to establish the proof of pregnancy and of illegal abortion.

Pieces of tissue found at the scene of an abortion must be collected and sent to the laboratory for histologic and serologic examination. The specimens should

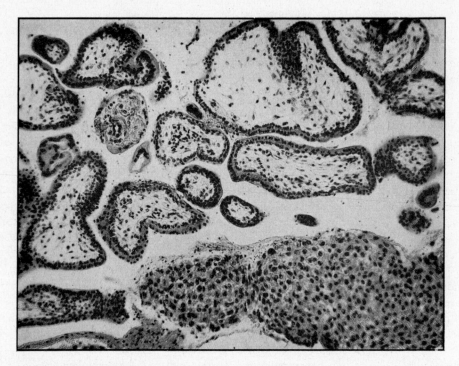

Fig. 22-1. Chorionic Villi and Syncytial Giant Cells About Third Month of Pregnancy.
Section of tissue recovered from abortionist's curet during police raid.

be identified to the examiner by the messenger who transports them so that they can be connected with the scene of the crime. If blood is present on the tissues it may be tested by the precipitin reaction to determine whether or not it is human in origin, and also examined in order to find out which blood groups are present; if the agglutinogens in the blood from the pieces of tissue are the same as those of the woman on whom the abortion was performed, that fact would be considered strong corroborative evidence in establishing the proof of the crime. In addition to decidua and endometrium, the histologic examination of the tissues may reveal chorionic villi and syncytial giant cells which are true fetal remains, and therefore strong confirmatory indications of pregnancy and abortion (Fig. 22-1).

If the patient is on the point of dying, and a police officer or district attorney is not present, the physician in attendance should take her dying declaration according to the rules noted on page 931. In abortion cases it is important that the patient tell of her condition at the time of her arrival at the office of the abortionist, especially noting whether she was bleeding or not, for if her testimony is negative on this point, it would contradict the allegations of the defendant who may claim that he was forced to operate on the deceased because she arrived at his office in extremis from loss of blood.

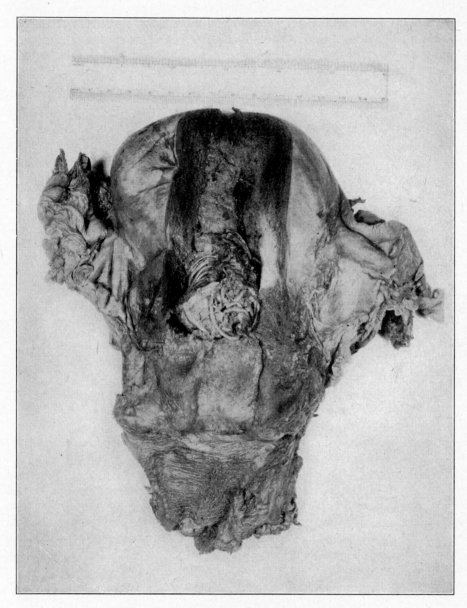

Fig. 22-2. Criminal Abortion. Fetal Remains in Uterus.

Traumatized fetus, about four months gestation, shown in cavity of uterus above internal os. Ribs of fetus exposed. Instrumental perforation through posterior wall of uterus shown in Figure 22-9.

Fatal Cases of Criminal Abortion. The fatal cases of abortion reported to the Office of the Chief Medical Examiner in New York City, are found in hospitals which have received the deceased in the last stages of her illness, or as deaths in doctor's offices, or as unexplained deaths which have occurred under a variety of conditions. The yearly number of abortion cases is about 106, taking the general average of the 24 years from 1918 to 1941, but in the 19 years from 1918 to 1936 the yearly average is 116, and in the 5 years from 1937 to 1941 the yearly average is 65. The reason for this sudden drop in numerical incidence cannot be determined with certainty, but it made its appearance about the time that the sulfonamide and similar antibiotic drugs began to be generally used. The different types of abortions occur as follows: criminal, by abortionist, 23 per cent; criminally self-induced, 16 per cent; spontaneous, 22 per cent; undetermined circumstances, 39 per cent; a few

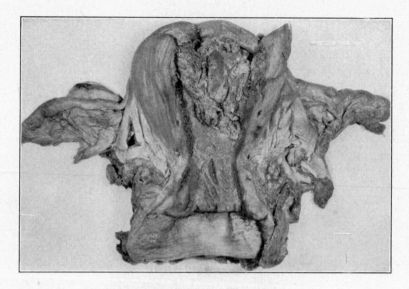

Fig. 22-3. Criminal Abortion Placental Remnants.

Septic endometritis with placental tissue on posterior wall of fundus and body of the uterus.

cases were classified as therapeutic. In all probability the undetermined cases as well as those which were allegedly spontaneous were criminal, but there was not enough evidence to justify their inclusion in this category. Rarely does a bona fide therapeutic abortion have a fatal outcome, and the same may be said for the spontaneous variety.

Two questions must be answered in every fatal case of induced criminal abortion and these are: (1) whether or not the deceased woman was pregnant when the attempt was made to induce abortion, and (2) whether or not death was the result of an induced abortion.

The Determination of Pregnancy. The question of pregnancy is determined at autopsy by discovering fetal remains and attempting to diagnose from them, and from the size and condition of the uterus and mammary glands, the probable month of pregnancy.

Fetal remains are not easy to find in many cases. If the woman has died during an abortion, the fetus, or parts of the fetus, may be found in the genital tract (Fig. 22-2). Rarely they are forced through a uterine perforation into the peritoneal cavity where they may be discovered at autopsy. Ordinarily, the body of the fetus is removed, and the placental site is marked by a circular raised area in the lining of the uterus near the fundus (Fig. 22-3) which may persist for days. The size of the placental site varies with the month of pregnancy and the number of days which have elapsed since abortion. After curettage parts of the placenta may remain in the uterine wall, in the form of stray chorionic villi and syncytial giant cells, and these may be demonstrated by a microscopic examination (Fig. 22-4) of the placental site. As they are part of the fetus they can be taken as a positive proof of pregnancy, in contradistinction to decidual cells which are tissues from the mother and are not, in themselves, a certain indication. The chorionic villi and syncytial giant cells may

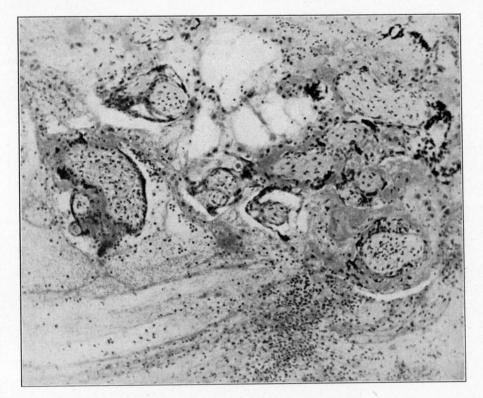

Fig. 22-4. Placental Tissue. Criminal Septic Abortion.

Histologic section through an infected placental site in the uterus. Note remains of chorionic villi and inflammatory exudate. 16 mm. objective.

last several days and then disappear except in the rare instance noted on pages 583 to 584. After that time the only criteria are the shape and size of the uterus, the state of the breasts and the corpus luteum in the ovary.

The finding of the fetus or parts of it is usually helpful in estimating the stage of pregnancy at which an abortion occurred. It is, therefore, of practical importance to be familiar with the progress of fetal development throughout all its stages. Roentgen-ray examination of larger fetal parts may reveal centers of ossification in the various bones and thus assist in estimating the age of such parts (page 574).

It is customary to designate the product of conception as an ovum during the first two weeks of pregnancy. From the third to the fifth week, during which period the various organs are developing and a definite form is being assumed, the organism is called an embryo. After the fifth week, it is spoken of as a fetus.

DEVELOPMENT OF THE FETUS IN THE 10 LUNAR MONTHS OF PREGNANCY. *First Month*. The fertilization, early cleavage stages and implantation of the human ovum have not as yet been observed. It is thought that the ovum probably reaches the uterine cavity and implants itself in the morula stage seven to eight days after fertilization. At this time it is about 0.2 mm. or $\frac{1}{125}$ inch in size. The youngest human ova observed have been found already embedded in the uterine decidua and were in the second to the third week of the development after fertilization. The youngest of these was described by Miller in 1913 and was estimated to be 10 to 11 days old. The recently embedded ovum appears as a minute elevated vesicular

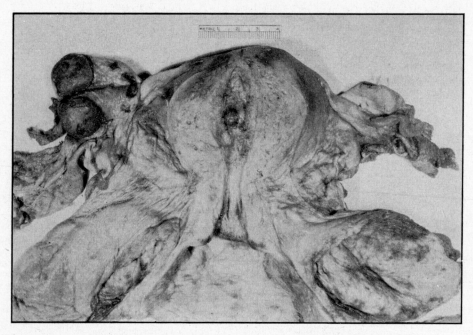

Fig. 22-5. Ovum of Early Pregnancy in Uterine Decidua. Estimated Age About 3 to 4 Weeks After Fertilization.

structure in the superficial portion of the decidua, separated from the uterine cavity by a thin layer of tissue. Figure 22-5 is a photograph of such an ovum found in the pregnant uterus of a woman who had been stabbed to death. A low power photomicrograph of a section through a young ovum or embryo estimated to have been in the third week of development after fertilization is shown in Figure 22-6. It was found by the authors in the uterus of a young woman who committed suicide by ingesting sodium cyanide. This ovum consists of a chorionic vesicle surrounded by young chorionic villi embedded in decidua basalis and covered by decidua capsularis which separates it from the uterine cavity. The embryonic tissue was not evident in the section.

During the first two weeks of development after implantation into the decidua, the ovum is a chorionic vesicle to the inside of which is attached the microscopic-sized future embryo. The latter has a conspicuous yolk sac and is covered with amnion. During the third week after implantation, the embryonic period begins. The medullary groove and canal are formed, followed by the appearance of the head folds. The abdominal pedicle comes off the tail end of the embryo which is concave on its dorsal surface and made up in great part of yolk sac. The heart begins to form, the cerebral and optic vesicles appear, and also the visceral arches and clefts. The yolk sac becomes constricted and connected by a broad pedicle to the ventral surface of the embryo. The limb buds make their appearance at the end of the third week. During the fourth week, there is considerable increase in size of the embryo which is flexed on its ventral surface. The rudiments of the eyes, ears and nose appear. At the end of the first four weeks of development after implantation,* the

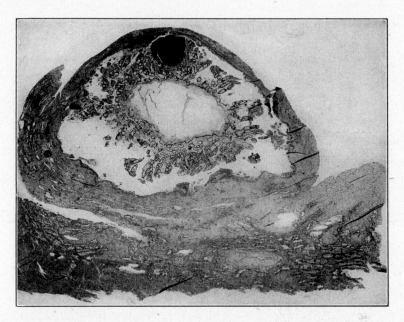

Fig. 22-6. Histologic Section of an Early Pregnancy.

This small ovum or embryo was found in the uterus of an unmarried woman who committed suicide by ingesting cyanide. It is a vesicle entirely surrounded by young chorionic villi and completely embedded in decidua. Beneath it is the decidua basalis and covering it is the decidua capsularis. The embryonic tissue was not evident in the section. Age about three weeks after fertilization. Magnification 8 times.

rudiments of all the organs have become differentiated and the embryo measures 7.5 to 10 mm. ($\frac{3}{10}$ to $\frac{2}{5}$ inches) in length. A series of early human embryos are illustrated in Figure 22-7. Since implantation occurs about 7 to 10 days after fertilization, and since fertilization occurs shortly after ovulation, and the latter about two weeks after the last menstruation, the development described at the end of the fourth week after implantation is more than seven weeks after the onset of the last menstrual period. If we consider the period of gestation as 280 days or 10 lunar months after the onset of the last menstruation, the development at the end of the first of these lunar months would correspond to that at the end of the first week after implantation.

Second Month. During the first half, the embryo is markedly flexed and the visceral arches and clefts are the most prominent features of the head region. The extremities are rudimentary. In the latter half of this month, the entire pregnancy is about the size of a pigeon's egg and the fetus measures about 2.5 cm. or 1 inch

* In the description of the development during the first four weeks, the interval is measured from the time of the implantation of the ovum.

in length. The amnion is filled with fluid and is in contact with the chorion. The placental site begins to differentiate and the umbilical cord and vessels to develop. The visceral arches, except the first, are closed. The brain develops considerably and the head is disproportionately large. The features can be distinguished. The extremities each show a division into three regions and the hands and feet are webbed. The external genitalia make their appearance. Ossification is beginning in the clavicle, lower jaw, vertebrae and ribs.

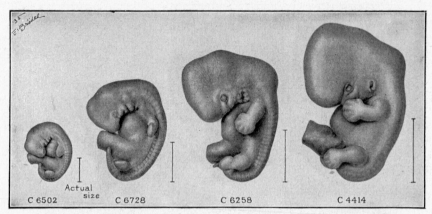

From Eastman, *Williams Obstetrics,* 10th ed., Appleton-Century-Crofts, Inc., 1950

Fig. 22-7 A. Human Embryos, 4 to 5.5 Weeks, Ovulation Age. × 2.5.

Ovulation ages: No. 6502, Carnegie collection, 28 days; No. 6728, 31 days; No. 6258, 38 days; No. 4414, 39 days (Streeter).

Third Month. At the end of the third month, the entire product of conception is about the size of a goose egg. The fetus is 7 to 9 cm. (2¾ to 3½ inches) in length. Most of the bones have ossification centers. The eyes are closed and the pupillary membrane appears. The fingers and toes are differentiated and supplied with nails. The external genitalia begin to differentiate. The placenta is formed and is small.

Fourth Month. At the end of the fourth month, the fetus is 10 to 17 cm. (4 to 7 inches) long and weighs about 120 gm. (4 ounces). The umbilical cord is about seven inches long and contains Wharton's jelly. The sex is revealed. Fine hair appears on the scalp and lanugo on the body. The cerebral convolutions develop. The head is about one-quarter the length of the body.

Fifth Month. At the end of the fifth month, the fetus is 18 to 27 cm. (7 to 11 inches) in length and weighs about 280 gm. (9⅓ ounces). The skin is less transparent and lanugo is found over the entire body. The umbilical cord is about 30 cm. (12 inches) long and the placenta about 180 gm. (6 ounces) in weight. The head and the viscera are well developed. The pupillary membrane persists but the eyes begin to open. The vernix caseosa appears.

Sixth Month. At the end of the six month, the fetus varies from 28 to 34 cm. (11 to 14 inches) in length and weighs about 635 gm. (about 21 ounces). The skin is wrinkled and has a red color. There is beginning deposition of subcutaneous fat. The head is relatively large. Meconium is found in the colon. The navel is placed slightly above the pubis. The testes begin to descend toward the inguinal rings. Ossification centers appear in the calcaneus and astragalus. A fetus born at this stage may attempt to breathe but usually does not survive.

Seventh Month. During this month the length varies from 35 to 38 cm. (14 to 15 inches) and the weight is about 1,200 gm. (2 pounds, 8 ounces). The body is thin and the skin is red and covered with vernix caseosa. The pupillary membrane has disappeared from the eyes and the lanugo from the face. The fetus born at this time has a feeble cry and may occasionally survive.

Eighth Month. At the end of this month, the fetus is about 42 cm. (about 17 inches) long and weighs 1,900 gm. (4 pounds). The skin has a reddened wrinkled appearance. An infant born at this stage may survive with proper care.

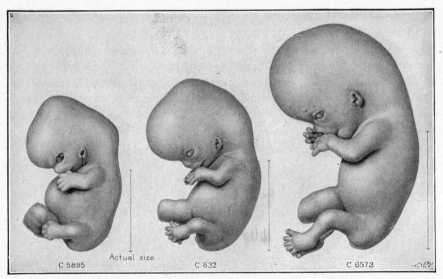

From Eastman, *Williams Obstetrics*, 10th ed., Appleton-Century-Crofts, Inc., 1950

Fig. 22-7 B. Human Embryos, 8 to 8.5 Weeks, Menstrual Age. × 1.9. Numbers refer to embryos in the Carnegie collection.

Ninth Month. At the end of the ninth month, the fetus is about 46 cm. (18½ inches) long and weighs about 2,500 gm. (about 5¼ pounds). The body is more robust because of the increase in subcutaneous fat. The face has lost its wrinkled appearance. An infant born at this stage may survive with proper care.

Full Term. Full term is reached at the end of the tenth lunar month. The fetus is fully developed. The average length of the full term child is 50 cm. (20 inches) with a sitting height of about 36 cm. (14 inches). The weight is about 3,400 gm. or 7½ pounds. The skin is smooth and covered with varying amounts of vernix caseosa. The lanugo has disappeared except over the shoulders, and the scalp is covered with dark hair about 2 to 3 cm. long. The features are well formed and the eyelids are open. The finger and toe nails project beyond the tips. In males the testes are usually in the scrotum. The meconium is present in the large intestine. The skull bones are well ossified and in close contact at the sutures. The anterior and posterior fontanelles are open. The eyes are slate colored. An ossification center about 0.5 cm. (⅙ inch) in diameter is found in the lower end of each femur and may also be found in the upper end of the tibiae and in the cuboid bones of the tarsus (page 594).

In measuring the lengths of the fetus, the sitting height (crown rump) is more accurately determined than the standing height. The weights and sitting heights of

704 human embryos at the end of each lunar month were determined by Streeter and compiled into the following table:

Month	Sitting Height (cm.)	Weight (gm.)
2	0.23	1.1
3	6.1	14.2
4	11.6	108.0
5	16.4	316.0
6	20.8	630.0
7	24.7	1045.0
8	28.3	1680.0
9	32.1	2478.0
10	36.2	3405.0

The length is considered a better criterion of the age of a fetus than its weight.

For practical purposes Haase has suggested that the approximate length of an embryo in centimeters, measuring from crown to heel, during the first five months of pregnancy can be obtained by squaring the number of the month to which pregnancy has advanced. In the second half of pregnancy, the number of the month is multiplied by 5. Thus:

Month	Length in Cm.
1×1	1
2×2	4
3×3	9
4×4	16
5×5	25
6×5	30
7×5	35
8×5	40
9×5	45
10×5	50

In a case of abortion which has survived for more than several days and in which no fetal parts remain in the uterus, it may be difficult to demonstrate the fact of recent pregnancy or the stage to which it had advanced before the abortion took place. The incomplete removal or expulsion of fetal parts, membranes or placental tissue, and the presence of intra-uterine infection may interfere with or delay the involution process of the uterus. Necrosis of fetal remains, membranes and placental tissue may make them unrecognizable on microscopic examination.

The dimensions of the uterus as measured at autopsy are often the only data available upon which the pathologist can rely in his estimation of the probable month of pregnancy. In the nonpregnant state the uterus is somewhat pear-shaped and usually 3 inches in length, 2 inches in width, and 1 inch in thickness. There is slight enlargement during the first two calendar months of pregnancy. At the end of the third month the uterus is 4 to 5 inches long, of which 1 inch is cervix and 3 to 4 inches is body; as the uterus enlarges, the corpus becomes more globular and the cervix becomes relatively shorter. At the end of the fourth month the uterus is 5 to 6 inches long; at the end of the sixth month about 6 inches long; at the end of the seventh month about 8 inches; at the end of the eighth month about 9½ inches; and at the end of the ninth calendar month 10½ to 12 inches.

After a full term delivery the uterus contracts and the wall becomes thick. After two days postpartum it is about 7 inches in length and 4 inches in width; at the end of one week it contracts to about 5 inches in length; after two weeks it is about 4 inches in length. After two months the uterus is about normal in size if involution is complete. The dimensions of the uterus after a case of abortion are more difficult to appraise; if the patient lives for a while after the expulsion of the fetus, the uterus will doubtless decrease in size, but there are no standards available by which its rate of involution after abortion in the different months of pregnancy can be measured. The examiner can only determine the dimensions of the uterus as accurately as possible and then draw his own conclusions in the light of his past experience with the same type of case.

The blood vessels and lymphatic vessels of the uterus increase in size during pregnancy and remain distended during the puerperium until involution is far advanced. This increased vascularity may explain the susceptibility of the gravid uterus to hemorrhage and infection.

The microscopic appearance of the chorionic villi changes as the pregnancy develops. In the first half of pregnancy the villi are large, ovoid on cross section and covered with the Langhans layer of cubical cells, while in the loose connective tissue core there are a few thin-walled blood vessels containing nucleated red blood cells; large ovoid syncytial giant cells with many centrally placed ovoid and circular nuclei, occur in between the villi. As the fetus reaches the second half of pregnancy, the villi become more numerous, circular on cross section and smaller, the Langhans layer is lost and are replaced by flattened syncytial giant cells; the blood vessels are much larger and contain red blood cells without nuclei for the most part. The chorionic villi and the syncytial giant cells usually disappear from the uterus after a few days of the post abortal period, but occasionally syncytial giant cells may persist longer. The authors saw a case which lived about three weeks after the abortion, and a few degenerated syncytial giant cells still persisted in the submucous layer even when the septic endometritis was healing (page 583).

The breasts enlarge during pregnancy due to hyperplasia of the mammary glands. In the nonpregnant woman the glandular tissue is represented by a few ducts with a small number of alveoli in a dense fibrous stroma, but with the progression of pregnancy the ducts branch and the glandular tissue proliferates and increases in amount. At the end of the second month the breasts are enlarged and have a nodular consistence on palpation. After a few months a watery milky secretion known as colostrum, can be expressed from the breasts on gentle pressure. At the end of gestation the secretion is so abundant, that when the breast is sectioned, a large amount of milky fluid oozes from the surface of the cut section. The nipple during pregnancy becomes more prominent, and the areola around it increases in extent and becomes more deeply pigmented; Montgomery's glands, the small sebaceous glands in the areola, increase in size during gestation and form small shotty subcutaneous nodules.

The presence of the corpus luteum in one ovary has been regarded as an important sign of pregnancy in the past, but in recent years has not been considered as pathognomonic of that condition, as it may occur in the absence of pregnancy, merely as a result of ovulation. The corpus luteum in pregnancy is usually larger than the one which is found after ovulation in a nonpregnant woman, but in a few instances it may even be inconspicuous in cases of pregnancy.

Some of the urine obtained post mortem from the bladder may be saved and used in the Aschheim-Zondek test for pregnancy, if it is collected within a week after the abortion (page 558). In some cases of abortion, death has been due to severe pyogenic infection and the urine may contain bacteria which will kill the animals used in the test and nullify the usefulness of the reaction.

Methods of Inducing Abortion. The methods of inducing abortion may be divided into three categories: general methods, use of special drugs, and operative methods.

GENERAL METHODS. The general methods used to induce criminal abortions are practically the same as those employed in self-induced abortions, the only difference being that in the criminal type the victim is helped by some other person. The procedures are all designed to encourage pelvic congestion and initiate uterine contractions which will expel the fetus, and include such means as baths, severe exercise, violence applied to the lower abdomen, application of the electric current to the uterine abdominal region, the ingestion of drastic cathartics like aloes or of strong emetics like zinc sulfate. In many cases, however, the attempt is not successful, and there is always the chance that the life of the woman will be endangered by the treatment.

SPECIAL DRUGS. A large number of drugs are used as abortifacients because of their effects on the uterus. They either produce congestion of the uterine mucosa and then uterine bleeding, followed by contraction of the uterine muscle and expulsion of the fetus, or they cause the uterine contraction by stimulating the myometrium directly. In some instances the fetus may be expelled and the pregnancy terminated.

A number of drugs exert their ecbolic effects by causing a pelvic congestion and engorgement of the uterine mucous membrane among which may be noted oil of pennyroyal, oil of tansy, oil of rue, oil of nutmeg, oil of savin, oil of turpentine, colocynth, cotton root bark, cantharides, methyl salicylate, black hellebore and laburnum. However, their most important action on the body is a severe gastroenteritis, irritation of the kidney and bladder, and a depressing effect on the central nervous system, so that while an expulsion of the fetus may follow their use, the woman may die of the toxic action of the drug before the abortion starts. White phosphorus, salts of arsenic and lead and other poisonous metals are sometimes taken internally as abortifacients and have a similar action on the body; they are discussed on pages 738 and 773.

Other drugs like nitrobenzol and apiol are occasionally taken as ecbolics, and cause gastroenteritis, renal irritation, hemoglobinuria and methemoglobinemia, often resulting in death. Quinine has the faculty of causing severe uterine contractions which may expel the fetus, but under certain conditions it is quite toxic, producing methemoglobinemia, hemoglobinuria and a toxic depressing action on the medullary centers.

Ergot and its preparations have been used as abortifacients, as they stimulate the uterine muscle to spasmodic contraction and may produce uterine hemorrhage. Such use is dangerous as ergot may cause an acute poisoning, marked by respiratory paralysis and collapse, or a chronic poisoning may develop, one type showing convulsions and dementia, and another type characterized by continued arterial spasm and gangrene of the extremities and other parts of the body. Oxytocin and pituitrin, both drugs which cause severe muscular contractions of the uterus, have been employed to produce abortion, and are dangerous because of this action.

Some drugs are injected into the vagina and uterus as abortifacients, and cause death partly by their escharotic action on the genital organs and partly by the toxic action of the poison after its absorption into the circulation. To this group belong corrosive sublimate (which is either placed in the vagina as a pastil, or injected as a solution), solutions of lysol and creosote, arsenic compounds, lead compounds, phosphorus, oxalic acid and alkalis. These preparations may produce a necrotic pseudomembrane in the vagina and the cervical canal. Death results from shock or toxemia, or is referable to a secondary infection from the damage inflicted on the genitalia.

In certain cases of abortion it is advisable to have a complete chemical analysis performed, and the proper organs should be saved for the purpose (Chapters 26 to 31).

OPERATIVE METHODS. The operative methods of terminating pregnancy are many, and practically all are attempted through the vaginal canal. They are designed to expel the ovum, either by causing muscular contraction of the uterus, or by removing the ovum mechanically with instruments. Some of these measures are used by the woman herself or by another amateur; others are employed by professional abortionists, whether midwives or medical men; and others are the means used by reputable gynecologists in therapeutic abortions.

One method of initiating uterine contractions is to dilate the cervical canal. This result may be effected by introducing a compressed sponge or a slippery elm stick (methods mostly favored by amateurs) into the cervix and leaving it there; the sponge or the stick swells from moisture in the uterine secretions, dilates the lower uterine segment, and may cause contractions of the corpus with expulsion of the fetus. Some abortionists attempt to dilate the canal by some form of dilator used in gynecologic practice.

Another method is to introduce a long thin sharp object into the uterus and lacerate the fetal membranes, thus allowing the amniotic fluid to escape, after which the uterus contracts and discharges the ovum. Many of these instruments are very crude, such as umbrella ribs or darning needles, and are employed in self-induced abortions. Others, like urethral sounds and catheters, sometimes are employed by abortionists and midwives. An elaboration of the catheter method is to attach a syringe or a bulb to the catheter and endeavor to inject some fluid like soapy water, abortifacient pastes or other chemicals into the uterus between its wall and the membranes. The separation of the membranes starts the abortion by causing uterine contractions.

Some abortions are produced by dilatation and curettage under general anesthesia. The woman is placed in the customary posture, on her back, a tenaculum is attached to the cervical lip, the uterus is pulled down towards the vaginal outlet, where it is dilated by a dilator and then emptied by a curette or ovum forceps.

All these operative and mechanical procedures give rise to serious or fatal complications in many cases, since the technic used by abortionists is most often crude and not aseptic. The morbidity and mortality rate of criminal abortions performed on healthy women is high in contrast to the low mortality rate of therapeutic abortions on women in poor health, when they are performed by reputable gynecologists in hospitals where proper aseptic surgical technic can be carried out.

Causes of Death. The fatal complications following induced abortions may be considered most conveniently by classifying such deaths in the following categories:

1. Deaths occurring at the time of or shortly after the abortion. The fatal complications in this group of cases are the toxic action of an anesthetic, hemorrhage from the uterus, perforating wounds of the uterus and abdominal viscera, and pulmonary air embolism.

2. Deaths which occur two or more days after the completion of the abortion. These include deaths resulting from septic infection of the uterus, perforations of

the uterine wall and abdominal viscera, oil embolism and similar delayed complications.

It is not possible to classify the fatal complication in every case exactly and fit it with precision into this scheme, but it has enough applicability to the facts to justify use of the two categories as a basis for discussing the subject, noting such exceptions that may occur.

EARLY DEATHS. Some of these cases die unexpectedly in the office of the abortionist at the time of the operation while the patient is under the anesthetic. Others are due to hemorrhage from the uterus, death usually occurring a few hours after the abortion has been induced. Still more rare are rapid deaths from shock or intra-abdominal hemorrhage, following perforation of the uterus or an abdominal organ during a curettage, or a sudden death from pulmonary air embolism following the injection of soapy water or air trapped under pressure in the tubing of an irrigation apparatus into the uterine cavity; these conditions will be discussed more fully under the later deaths.

ANESTHETIC DEATHS. An anesthetic death occurs occasionally when the abortionist attempts to terminate the pregnancy in his office by performing the operation under the influence of a general anesthetic. The patient may die suddenly in the midst of the operation, leaving the abortionist in an embarrassing position inasmuch as he must report the death to the authorities and find a satisfactory explanation for a situation distinctly dubious. As a recital of the plain facts would be disastrous, the defendant is forced to invent a narrative which will account for a strange occurrence without incriminating himself. Generally the story he concocts makes it appear that the deceased, whom he had never seen before, came into his office bleeding from her genital canal, and in order to save her life he was compelled to put her on the operating table in order to check the bleeding; while thus engaged, before he had any chance to use any instruments, the patient died. In the investigation of such a case the police and the medical examiner have their own duties to perform. The police are concerned in unraveling the circumstances of the case and establishing the connection of the dead woman with the abortionist. The medical examiner, in addition to helping the police search the premises for drugs and instruments used in the induction of abortions and for any fetal remains which may still be present in the waste receptacles, should obtain a statement from the defendant either as a written document signed by him or in the form of testimony taken under oath. Later if this account is compared to the autopsy report, discrepancies may be found which may cast doubt on the truthfulness of the defendant's statement, and thus be damaging to his defense.

Sudden death during the induction of the abortion is often due to an overdose of the anesthetic which is usually chloroform or ether. The autopsy discloses cyanosis, congestion of organs, dilated heart, and dark, red fluid blood in the cardiac chambers, signs characteristic of anesthetic deaths. If ether has been employed, the blood and viscera will exude the characteristic pungent odor of that drug. The lungs, brain and other organs should be preserved for toxicologic examination, as both chloroform and ether can be identified chemically and that evidence will be important in establishing the cause of death (page 796). Examination of the uterus and the other genital organs may show the marks of different instruments employed in the abortion, findings valuable as indications of the nature of the operative procedure. The tenacula used in grasping the vaginal portion of the cervix leave a pair of small circular punctures of pin-caliber size about one-quarter inch apart on the cervical lip. The curet may cause characteristic marks on the lining membrane of the uterus; the decidua may be scraped away in places and left intact in other places or it may be entirely removed; the placenta and fetus may be fragmented in different degrees, and the uterine wall may be lacerated. The more severe injuries will be discussed on page 587. The anesthetic deaths investigated by the authors in connection with induced abortion were few in number and occurred in women in the second to the third month of pregnancy.

HEMORRHAGE FROM UTERUS. Many abortionists, fearing that the patient may die in the midst of the operation, do not use an anesthetic, and also send her away as soon as possible after the curettage, thus increasing the danger of a fatal complication. A large proportion of the women so treated die at home or in a hospital. The cause of death rarely is a severe external hemorrhage from the placental site in the uterus; this complication occurs in less than 5 per cent of the total number of fatal induced abortions. In a study of six cases of this type, the victim died from three hours to six days after the illegal operation, showing clinically profuse bleeding from the uterine canal, signs of acute anemia such as pallor, cold clammy skin, reduced hemoglobin percentage, low erythrocyte count, and fragments of placental tissue in the body or the cervix of the uterus. The autopsy disclosed the uterus enlarged to about the third to the fifth month of pregnancy, containing blood clots, large distended vessels about the placental site, a hemorrhagic shaggy lining of the cavity, and such general signs of hemorrhage as loss of blood from the blood vessels, pallor of viscera, contracted heart and subendocardial hemorrhages on the left ventricle. In one case tenaculum marks were present on the external os, but in none were there any lacerations of the uterine wall. In one instance the victim lived six days and developed a septic endometritis in addition to the severe anemia occasioned by the hemorrhage. Another type of fatal hemorrhage after an abortion was illustrated by a case investigated by Dr. Charles Norris, in which the victim, a multipara advanced to the seventh month of pregnancy, bled profusely from a placenta previa when an attempt was made to terminate the gestation.

DELAYED DEATHS. The majority of cases of induced abortion die two or more days after the pregnancy is terminated. In most instances, the woman at the completion of the operation is not so badly shocked but that she is able to travel or to be conveyed away from the office of the abortionist, so that when serious complications set in, she dies in a hospital or in some other location far distant from the place where she was operated on. It rarely happens that the abortionist allows her to remain on his premises after the operation, if she can be moved at all, though exceptions have occurred under special circumstances. In this type of case the authorities must contend with a different situation than the one described under early deaths; the principal problem in the delayed deaths is to establish the connection between the operator and the induced abortion performed on the victim. In order to discover even the name of the abortionist, it is necessary for the police to rely on a dying declaration made by the deceased, or on information contributed by her relatives or friends. The next step is to obtain testimony which establishes the presence of the woman in the office of the abortionist, and the fact that an illegal operation was performed. If the deceased enters a hospital, the testimony of the attending physician and the clinical record of the hospital may, in addition to the autopsy report of the medical examiner, help to establish the fact of induced abortion.

The fatal complications which occur in the delayed deaths are septic infections of the uterus which occur without noteworthy injuries of the uterine wall, penetrating wounds of the uterus which cause death by abdominal hemorrhage and infection, external hemorrhage from the cavity of the uterus as discussed before, oil embolism following injection of abortifacient salves into the uterine cavity, and comparatively rare complications such as femoral vein thrombosis and pulmonary embolism.

SEPTIC INFECTION. The most common cause of death in induced abortion is a septic infection of the uterus, 76 per cent of the cases occur because pathogenic bacteria are carried into the cavity of the uterus during the operative procedure. After an induced abortion, the lining membrane of the uterus is especially vulnerable to infection by pathogenic bacteria, because it is vascular, lined by cellular spongy tissue and is covered by blood clot whenever the cavity is curetted. If bacteria gain entrance, their growth and spread are encouraged, sometimes in association with laceration and perforation of the uterine wall, but more frequently without any signs of gross intra-uterine injury. Within two to five days after an operation of this type, a septic inflammation develops in the uterus and gives rise to characteristic symptoms and signs.

Clinically the patient may show a febrile temperature, chills, sweats, vomiting, stupor, delirium, and occasionally jaundice and anemia; examination discloses tenderness of the lower abdomen, a slightly distended cervix, bleeding or foul purulent discharge from the external os, a tender and boggy uterus, and occasionally marks of tenacula and other instruments on the cervical lip. In the later stages the clinical manifestations vary, depending on the type of the septic invasion; in the event that the patient is developing a septic peritonitis, the chief complaint will be severe pain in the abdomen and marked ileus, but if a suppurative phlebitis and abscesses of the lungs are in the process of formation, dyspnea and pyrexia are the most prominent symptoms. The duration of the clinical course in cases of postabortal sepsis varies from 2 days to 30 days or over, and most of the patients die in the first 15 days after the operation. At autopsy the uterus is enlarged to about the third to the sixth month of pregnancy, a suppurative endometritis and other signs of sepsis are present, and in addition, a relaxed cervical segment, a soft uterine wall with distended sinuses, and occasionally tenacular marks or other minor signs of instrumentation are to be noted. Many criminal abortions in which instruments are known to have been used do not exhibit any other evidence of instrumentation than the infection. The clinical course of fatal postabortal infections has been considerably lengthened as the result of the use of the sulfonamides and other antibiotic drugs. For the same reason many cases now survive which formerly proved fatal.

Streptococcic Infection. A common pathogenic invader is the hemolytic streptococcus, probably the cause of fatal infection in about 54 per cent of the septic cases. Its most characteristic lesion is a suppurative endometritis. In some cases this is manifested by a purulent yellowish green or grayish brown pseudomembrane sometimes covering the inside of the uterus and sometimes localized at the placental site which may persist as a slightly raised plaque 2 to 4 cm. in diameter; in other instances the membrane is ragged, dirty red or red-black in color and gangrenous and there may be reddish brown, necrotic blood clot attached to the placental site. A phlegmonous infiltration of the uterine wall occurs in rare instances. Microscopically the pseudomembrane is composed of necrotic tissue, infiltrated with polymorphonuclear leukocytes and a few clumps of streptococci, while the adjacent submucous layer contains congested blood vessels, leukocytes, areas of hemorrhage and sometimes remains of uterine glands, decidua, syncytial cells and chorionic villi. From this site the streptococci spread to other parts of the body and produce different types of generalized septic infection. In about 58 per cent of the cases, there is a suppurative peritonitis which may or may not be associated with a septicemia, and in the remaining 42 per cent are to be found examples of streptococcic blood stream infection.

The cases of streptococcic peritonitis are associated with a suppurative endometritis, salpingitis and oophoritis in a little more than one half of the cases of peritonitis. The adnexal inflammation varies in degree from a swollen tube containing pus to a large tubo-ovarian abscess, and it may be unilateral or bilateral. Some of these lesions develop on the basis of a preexisting ovarian cyst or a chronic salpingitis. The infection is spread probably from the infected endometrium through the fallopian tubes to the peritoneum and in most cases is a mixed one. Some of the infections may spread through the lymphatics of the broad ligaments, and occasionally a septic parametritis is produced. Less than one half of the cases of peritonitis are associated with a septic endometritis alone and many of these are a pure streptococcic infection. The infection may spread also through the lymphatics or through the blood stream to the peritoneal cavity. Anatomically the peritonitis may be localized in the pelvic region or it may have a general spread, either in the form of yellowish green purulent abscesses walled off among the intestinal coils with a varying degree of ileus present, or in the form of a yellowish green membrane covering the entire peritoneum associated with an abundance of purulent fluid and a contracted intestine. In a few instances the pleurae may show a fibrinopurulent inflammation either generalized or restricted to the diaphragmatic surface of the lung and parietal pleura. Some of the cases of peritonitis may be associated with a streptococcic septicemia either in the form of a suppurative phlebitis and embolic lung abscesses or in the form of a vegetative endocarditis.

Sometimes the streptococci invade the endometrium, enter the lymphatics or blood vessels, and infect the blood stream without invading the peritoneal cavity. About two fifths of these cases occur in the form of a septic endometritis, an acutely hyperplastic spleen of 300 to 600 gm., and occasional petechiae in eyelids, bladder and kidneys. Another two fifths appear in the form of a septic endometritis, a septic vegetative endocarditis of the mitral, aortic and tricuspid valves, with a hyperplastic spleen, embolic abscesses and infarcts of spleen, brain, kidneys and lungs, petechiae in kidneys and intestines, myocardial abscesses, septic pericarditis and myocarditis. In about one fifth of the cases, in addition to the suppurative endometritis there may be yellowish septic thromboses in the veins of the uterine wall, brown-red thrombi or purulent exudate in the ovarian and uterine veins and in most cases septic infarcts and abscesses of the lungs and sometimes of the spleen; this type of septicopyemia is more common with staphylococcic than with streptococcic infections.

Occasionally the uterine inflammation in streptococcic septicemia subsides while the general infection is at its height. The authors have seen one case which survived the abortion about three weeks and showed a transitional stage in the restoration of an acute septic endometritis back to the normal state of the nonpregnant endometrium. On the surface a few remnants of the necrotic membrane still persisted, but in the submucous layer were large round cells, a few eosinophils, and large cells filled with granules of brown iron-containing pigment; the uterine glands were regenerating and a few degenerating syncytial giant cells were found here and there. Other cases of postabortal endometritis which have survived the infection for a longer period usually show a normal mucous membrane.

Staphylococcic Infections. Staphylococcus aureus is the infective agent in about 45 per cent of the septic postabortal cases, and produces a suppurative endometritis which is macroscopically similar to the streptococcus inflammation but microscopically shows a deep necrosis of the surface tissue permeated with numerous clumps of staphylococci, and a defense wall of polymorphonuclear leukocytes bordering the necrotic layer in the adjacent submucous tissue. In about three fourths of these cases the infection spreads to the veins of the uterine wall either in the

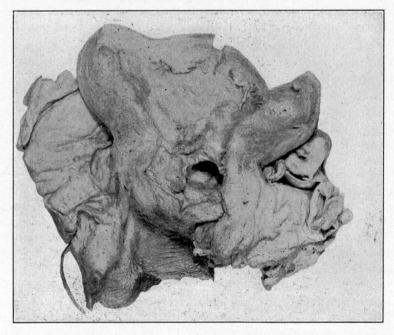

Fig. 22-8. Instrumental Perforation of Uterus. Criminal Abortion. The perforation is visible above internal os.

fundus or in the cervix, and these become the seat of a purulent thrombophlebitis, so that the myometrium is honeycombed with small purulent cavities. The process may extend to the ovarian and uterine veins, which contain a yellowish pus or purulent thrombi in their lumens, and on section their walls show a polymorphonuclear leukocytic infiltration. In cases where the patient has lived over two weeks, the acute inflammatory reaction may subside in the wall of the vein which may undergo fibrous thickening and a well marked round cell infiltration around the vasa vasorum may be found on microscopic examination. Emboli may spread from the infected veins to the lungs causing multiple abscesses and septic infarcts in these organs, and occasionally the septic processes may spread from the lung foci into the systemic circulation causing embolic abscesses in spleen, kidneys and other organs. In a few cases a suppurative peritonitis may be present varying in extent from a localized pelvic inflammation to a general involvement of the entire cavity.

A generalized septicemia, analogous to the streptococcic septicemia, occurs in one fourth of the staphylococcus cases, in which the infection invades the blood stream without causing a septic phlebitis of the pelvic veins and produces widespread emboli throughout the body. The most prominent lesions are exuberant vegetations on the mitral, tricuspid and aortic valves, an enlarged septic spleen and embolic abscesses and infections throughout the organs of the body.

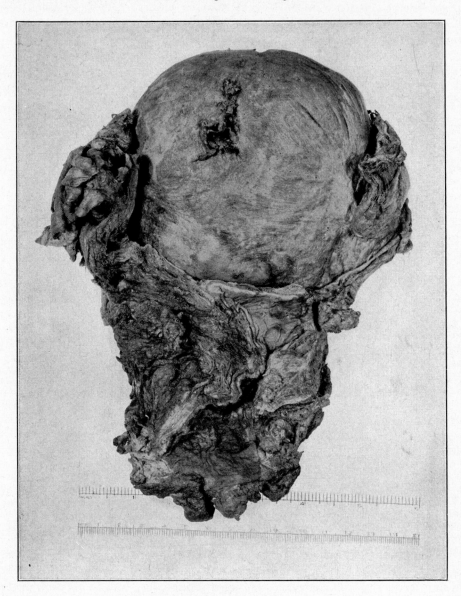

Fig. 22-9. Instrumental Perforation of Uterus. Criminal Abortion.

Same case as in Fig. 22-2. Perforation through posterior wall of body of uterus as seen from without.

Another bacterium which causes postabortal sepsis in rare cases is the *Bacillus welchii*. When infected by this organism, the uterus shows a marked gangrenous endometritis and myometritis, black-red in color, marked by necrosis, hemolysis, and gas bubble formation with slight leukocytic reaction in the tissues. If the bacillus enters the blood during life, the skin turns a bronze color and postmortem decomposition sets in early. An infection by the tetanus bacillus occurs in rare instances, and produces a moderate necrotic endometritis, and the bacilli and their spores are present in the uterine cavity. The victims die of the convulsions typical of the disease about two or three weeks after the abortion. Other organisms such as anaerobic streptococci, nonhemolytic streptococci and others are sometimes the cause of postabortal sepsis.

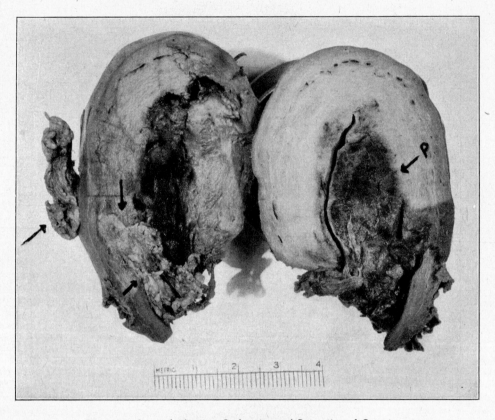

Fig. 22-10. Criminal Abortion. Perforation and Retraction of Omentum.

Specimen of uterus removed surgically after instrumental perforation of anterior wall by curet; piece of omentum pulled back into cavity of uterus (indicated by arrows). The uterus split sagittally to show remains of pregnancy in anterior wall of right half (indicated by letter P).

WOUNDS OF THE GENITAL TRACT AND ABDOMEN. Lacerations and perforations are produced when a curet or another instrument is forced into the uterine cavity against the uterine wall, sometimes causing a severe injury because the wall of the uterus during pregnancy is vascular, soft and easily penetrated. The lesions thus produced are the cause of death in about 21 per cent of the total number of fatal induced abortions. In a little over one half of these cases, the corpus uteri is involved, and the wall is perforated in the region of the fundus and the posterior surface (Figs. 22-8, 22-9, 22-10). The perforations are of different sizes and forms, varying from a small ragged stellate opening about 1 cm. in diameter to much larger tears of stellate, ovoid or irregular shapes and crater-like in appearance sometimes amounting to mangling of the uterine fundus. Occasionally two or more perforations may be present in the fundus, or the fundus and cervix may be injured by the curet. The uterus most easily perforated is the rare bicornuate type, because the operator, becoming confused, believes the uterine cavity to be longer than it really is and pierces the wall at the point where the cornua divide (Fig. 22-11). Wounds of the cervix uteri occur in a little less than one half of the instrumental injuries of the uterus, some of them being crateriform excavations into the cervical wall while others perforate into the abdominal cavity through any portion of the wall. These perforations are stellate and ragged and are directed in an upward direction; in one case the hole through the cervix was cylindric and was presumably made with an instrument like an auger (Fig. 22-8). Perforations of the vaginal vault are not common in abortions induced by an operator, but are most often seen in the self-induced

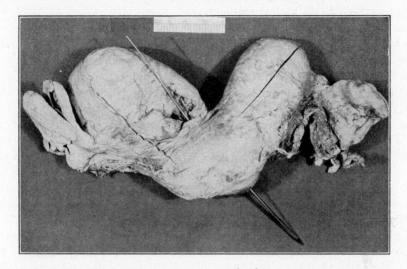

Fig. 22-11. Instrumental Perforation of Bicornuate Uterus during Attempted Abortion. The probe passes through the perforation.

type. One case was encountered by the authors in which the pregnant woman punctured her vaginal vault with a long darning needle, perforating her stomach and intestines several times causing a septic peritonitis.

The perforating instrument may pass through the corpus or cervix into the abdominal cavity, causing ragged stellate or irregular tears of the small or large intestine varying from small perforations to large lacerations which may cut the intestine across, and producing large stellate or ovoid tears of the mesentery or omentum. Any part of the small intestine may be involved, and the parts of the large intestine usually affected are the cecum, sigmoid and rectum. In some instances the curet when withdrawn from the abdominal cavity may pull a segment of the omentum, intestine or mesentery into the uterine cavity where it is severed by the operator; in one such case about 20 inches of the small intestine was stripped from its attachments and hung in the uterus. In a few instances the cause of death is a profuse intra-abdominal hemorrhage from the abdominal injuries, the patient dying soon after the operation or several days later. The most common cause of death is an acute suppurative peritonitis either because the infective organisms are carried into the abdominal cavity by the curet or because they invade the peritoneum by way of a perforated intestine. In two cases the curet perforated the lateral portion of the cervix, infecting the broad ligament and causing a fatal retroperitoneal abscess of massive proportions which extended as high as the kidney. In some cases where the laceration of the cervix did not perforate, a purulent phlebitis developed and numerous embolic abscesses appeared in the lungs, or a generalized septicemia resulted and was the cause of death.

Occasionally when the uterus is perforated, parts of the fetus may be left in the uterine cavity (Fig. 22-2), or forced into the abdomen, usually in a mutilated condition. During the autopsy on one case, the decapitated and mangled skull of a five months' fetus was found free in the pelvis in the midst of blood and blood clot. Several instances have occurred in which fetal bones and viscera were found in the cul de sac of Douglas; in one case of this type the victim was treated for an incomplete abortion by a physician who attempted to empty her uterus by giving her a dose of pituitrin, and the violent uterine contractions which ensued forced the fetus of three months into the cul de sac of Douglas through a cervical perforation which had been inflicted at the time of the induced abortion. In rare instances instruments causing the abortion are found in the uterus or free in the abdominal cavity, and should be preserved for evidence. In some of the cases, tenaculum marks may be present on the cervical lip and should be carefully noted as part of the evidence.

In the following case an abortion instrument was found at autopsy in the inferior vena cava of the victim. The history elicited was that a 16 year old girl went to an abortionist to terminate a pregnancy. A 10 inch stiff but flexible rubber catheter was introduced into the uterus to start uterine contractions; 1 inch of the instrument was allowed to project from the vulvar orifice for convenience in future handling. The following day the catheter was missed, and it was supposed to have dropped out and to have been lost. On the third day a second longer catheter was allegedly inserted into the uterus with considerable force, the operator introducing a stiff wire into the tube to insure its penetration. The patient was given a dose of quinine and bled from the uterus. On the fifth day she expelled a fetus of about five months gestation. On the ninth day of her illness she died with symptoms of sepsis. The autopsy disclosed a uterus 6 by 4 by 3 inches, with a wall about an inch thick, empty of fetus or fetal remains and the seat of a suppurative endometritis. There was no recognizable perforation of the uterine wall, but after a long search a ¼ inch slit was found on the right side of the cervix through the posterior lip about ¾ inch above the external os. The opening led backward and upward into the retroperitoneal tissues on the right side of the sacrum where it could not be followed. There was, however, a small retroperitoneal abscess on the right side of the sacrum midway between promontory and os coccyx. In the right iliac vein near the inferior vent cava there was a ³⁄₁₆ inch perforation which was sealed by a rusty colored thrombus. In the inferior vena cava extending from the iliac bifurcation to the diaphragm was a catheter 12½ inches long and slightly over ⅛ inch in diameter. There was a patchy septic thrombosis of the entire inferior vena cava. In some way the catheter had been forced from the cervix uteri through the retroperitoneal tissues on the right side of the sacrum into the right iliac vein and into the inferior vena cava. The fact that the catheter was introduced when the uterus was distended with the fetus and that shortly thereafter the uterus contracted to expel the fetus suggests the mechanism which moved the catheter to its final resting place but does not offer a complete explanation of this occurrence.

Cases of abortion in which the genital tract has been perforated and the abdominal organs lacerated may be admitted to a hospital for treatment of symptoms which compel the surgeon to perform a laparotomy. In many instances the operator may repair the wounds by suture, while in others he may remove the perforated uterus, or resect the intestine. If the patient dies, the surgeon should surrender to the medical examiner all organs, tissues, or foreign bodies obtained at operation (Fig. 22-12), and keep an accurate clinical record of the case. In this connection the question may arise as to whether or not the patient could travel after receiving the injuries under consideration, a problem which must be solved for each individual case. In general a curettage without complications would not incapacitate a woman seriously at the time of the operation, but if the uterus and abdominal viscera were severely lacerated, she would be prostrated by shock and probably could not travel unaided.

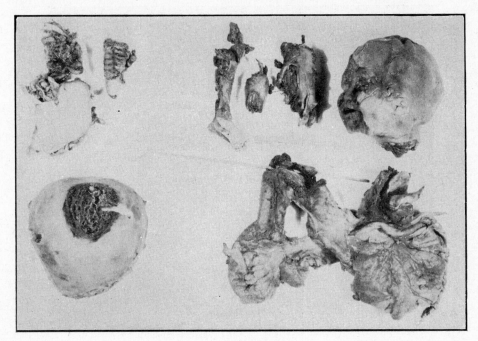

Fig. 22-12. Criminal Abortion Performed in Physician's Office. Perforation of Uterus. Dismemberment and Mangling of 5 Months Fetus.

Fetal parts forced into abdominal cavity during abortion. Freshly perforated uninflamed uterus and clean fetal parts removed during laparotomy shortly after abortion (left). Pus-covered, macerated fetal parts, including head, found in abdomen at autopsy (right). Death from peritonitis 10 days after abortion. Small intestine also perforated and not repaired.

RARE FATAL COMPLICATIONS. A rare fatal complication of an induced abortion is the formation of a bland thrombus in the femoral vein and sudden death by pulmonary embolism. This occurs more commonly after full term delivery than after abortion in the early stages of pregnancy.

When soapy water full of bubbles is injected into the cavity of the uterus just external to the fetal membranes, a fatal air embolism may occur (Fig. 22-13). The air in the soap bubbles enters the veins in the uterine wall and is carried to the right heart and lungs, causing sudden asphyxia and death. If the patient survives the attack, the air may enter the systemic circulation and produce a coronary or cerebral air embolism (page 173).

A method of injecting oily pastes through a syringe between the fetal membranes and the uterus for the purpose of stimulating uterine contractions in order to expel the fetus, was employed in Germany about the year 1932. The principal result of this method was to force the oil into the uterine veins and to cause death by pulmonary oil embolism, similar in all essential respects to fat embolism.

Similar injections of poisonous chemicals into the cavity of the uterus for abortifacient purposes have resulted in the death of the victim. Gander describes the injection of 750 ml. of an abortifacient mixture of soap, lysoform and alcohol into the pregnant uterus of a 19 year old girl, who had a fatal collapse shortly after the operation. The case of Straus and DeNosaquo was given an intra-uterine injection of a corrosive paste which penetrated the intra-uterine wall and caused a sup-

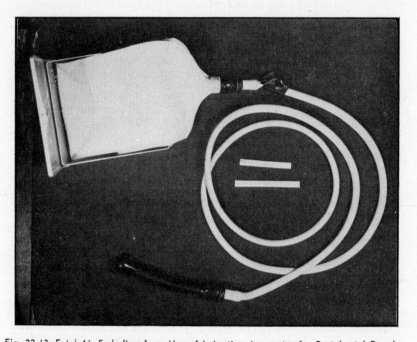

Fig. 22-13. Fatal Air Embolism from Use of Irrigation Apparatus for Postabortal Douche.

Note clamp at upper end of tubing which has volume of 40 ml. Air in tubing pumped into uterus by oncoming fluid.

purative peritonitis. Vance has reported a case in which Lysol was injected between amnion and uterine wall as an abortifacient, producing death without abortion by a combination of oil embolism and the systemic toxic action of Lysol itself. Dutra, Cleveland and Lyle have reported seven cases of criminal abortion including four fatalities induced by intra-uterine pastes composed essentially of a superfatted soap with added iodine, potassium iodide and thymol.

ATTEMPTED ABORTIONS ON NONPREGNANT WOMEN. An operation for abortion performed on a nonpregnant woman is in law just as culpable as a real abortion if the intent of the parties concerned was to terminate a pregnancy. Nonpregnant women occasionally apply to an abortionist for such an operation under the mistaken impression that they are pregnant, and in many cases the result of the procedure is not productive of trouble, as the nongravid uterus is tough and is resistant to perforation and infection. In some cases, a careless or inexperienced operator has perforated the uterus and torn the mesentery and intestines, producing injuries similar to those described on page 587, and causing death by abdominal hemorrhage or infection of the peritoneal cavity.

Sometimes an instrumental abortion is attempted on a case of ectopic pregnancy which has been wrongly diagnosed. The curettage of the endometrium may carry in pathogenic bacteria so that a septic endometritis results, or the pregnant tube may rupture under the manipulations incidental to the operation and fatal hemorrhage or sepsis may occur. In some cases an interstitial ectopic pregnancy may rupture and produce a crateriform lesion in the uterine fundus which may resemble an instrumental perforation. The differential diagnosis, however, does not offer much difficulty if the possibilities are considered.

Similarly an instrumental abortion may be attempted on a nonpregnant woman suffering from a pyosalpinx under the mistaken impression that she is pregnant, and the disturbance created in the genital organs by the curettage may spread the infection from the tube throughout the peritoneal cavity causing a fatal septic peritonitis.

In all of these cases the operator could be charged with criminal malpractice if sufficient evidence of his intent could be obtained, but in most cases this might be a formidable undertaking. However he could be charged with civil malpractice because of failure to diagnose the condition accurately and to institute proper treatment.

CONSIDERATIONS AT AUTOPSY

The pathologist in performing an autopsy upon an abortion case should make special notes in regard to the uterus and other genitalia in addition to the general description of the rest of the body.

The length, breadth and thickness of the uterus, the thickness of the uterine wall, the length of the uterine cavity, the circumference of the internal and external os, the length of the cervix, the diameter of the corpus luteum, and the measurements of the fetal remains, should be recorded. The examination should include the tubes, ovaries and breasts. Fetal parts should be searched for in the genital tract and the peritoneal cavity. Instrumental wounds and tenaculum marks must be identified. All organs in the abdominal cavity capable of causing a suppurative peritonitis, like the appendix, gallbladder or stomach, must be examined. All conditions in the body capable of producing a spontaneous abortion, like heart disease and hydatidiform mole, must be investigated. Septic conditions in the body must receive due attention. The uterine and ovarian veins should be carefully traced to where they empty into larger trunks for signs of purulent phlebitis. The spleen and other septic foci should be cultured to determine whether or not pathogenic bacteria are present. The therapeutic use of sulfonamides and other antibiotic drugs may in some cases inhibit the growth of pathogenic bacteria in postmortem cultures. A chemical examination should be performed on the brain and parenchymatous viscera when necessary.

Microscopic examination should be made of the uterine mucosa to determine whether or not chorionic villi are present. The other structures, such as tubes, ovaries, appendix, kidneys, spleen, liver, pancreas, heart, lungs and any other organ which seems abnormal should be sectioned.

If sufficient fetal remains are available, a roentgen-ray photograph can be taken to record the centers of ossification. This may be important in establishing the duration of pregnancy. Foreign bodies, like instruments, should also be preserved as evidence, if any are recovered from the body.

REFERENCES

Amreich, I.   Zur Ätiologie der von den Uterusvenen ausgehenden Luftembolie, Zentralbl. f. Gynäk., 48:521, 1924.

Dutra, F. R., Cleveland, F. P., and Lyle, H. I.   Criminal abortion induced by uterine pastes, J.A.M.A., 143:865, 1950.

Eastman, N. J.   Williams Obstetrics, New York, 10th ed., Appleton-Century-Crofts, Inc., 1950.

Gander, G.   Akute Vergiftung nach Einspritzung einer Losung von Seife, Lysoform und Alkohol in dem Uterus, Sammlung von Vergiftungsfallen, 8:65, 1937.

Gilbert, F. B.   Criminal Law and Practice of the State of New York, Penal Law, Albany and New York, Matthew, Bender and Company, 1943.

Herzog, A.   Medical Jurisprudence, Indianapolis, Bobbs-Merrill Co., 1931, section 916.

Kaufmann, E.   Lehrbuch der speziellen Path. Anat., Berlin und Leipzig, 1922, p. 1366.

Martland, H. S.   Puerperal infection, Am. J. Surg., 26:90, 1934.

Puppe, G.   Atlas und Grundriss der Gerichtlichen Medizin, München, J. F. Lehmann, 1908.

Reese, J. J.   Text Book of Medical Jurisprudence and Toxicology, 8th ed., revised by D. J. McCarthy, Philadelphia, P. Blakiston's Son and Co., 1911.

Reports of the Office of the Chief Medical Examiner in the City of New York from 1918 to 1951.

Reuter, C.   Uber gefahrliche Methoden der Schwangerschaftsunterbrechung, Med. Klin., 28:1338, 1932.

Smith, S.   Forensic Medicine, London, J. & A. Churchill, ltd., 1938.

Straus, R., and DeNosaquo, N.   Effects of an abortifacient paste ("Utra-Jel"), Arch. Path., 39:91, 1945.

Vance, B. M.   Intra-uterine injection of Lysol as an abortifacient, Arch. Path., 40:395, 1945.

23

Infanticide

Infanticide may be defined as the slaying of the newborn infant. The crime occurs in the period immediately after the child is born, up to the moment when the birth is reported to the authorities. In New York State, infanticide is classified as a form of homicide and legally no distinction is made between them.

The crime of infanticide does not include death of the fetus during labor when it is destroyed by craniotomy or decapitation. These procedures are employed by an obstetrician for the purpose of saving the life of the mother when the conditions attending the birth are such that it could not be completed without causing the deaths of both mother and child. For example, if a fetus is being forced through the genital canal in a transverse presentation, or if it is afflicted with a congenital hydrocephalus of excessive size, the medical attendant would be compelled to sacrifice the fetus for the sake of the mother.

About 14 cases of infanticide occur in New York City during a year and present themselves under a number of different forms. One large category includes infants who have been found dead in such places as garbage cans, furnaces, ladies' washrooms or parcel rooms. Another type is that in which the mother has been caught red-handed in the act of killing the infant, or through circumstances has had the crime traced to her.

The medical examiner who investigates a case of suspected infanticide should determine the answers to the following questions: (1) Is the infant viable? (2) Was it born alive as determined by the fact that it breathed after birth? (3) What is the cause of death? (4) Was death the result of an infanticide?

Is the Infant Viable? The first point to be determined is whether or not the newborn infant could have lived if it had been given the proper care. Generally, if it is normally formed and has had seven lunar months of development in utero, it may be considered capable of survival. On the other hand, when the period of gestation has been less than six lunar months, the infant is not able to sustain extra-uterine existence except in most extraordinary instances even though it may breathe for a short time. A description of the complete development of the fetus in utero has already been given in Chapter 22 and may serve as a guide for estimating the nonviability or viability of a fetus at any given stage. The months at which viability is achieved are indicated on page 575.

THE INFANT AT FULL TERM. The full term child has an average length of 50 cm. (20 inches) and weighs about 3,250 gm., or 7 pounds. The weight may vary from 2,500 to 5,000 gm. (5.5 to 11 pounds). The heaviest infant on record, cited by Eastman, weighed 11,340 gm. (25 pounds). The weight of male infants is generally about 100 gm. (3 ounces) more than that of females. There is considerable variation depending on race, size of parents, the number of children the mother has previously borne, the mode of life, nutrition and general condition of the mother during the later months of pregnancy. Eastman reports that among 18,160 full term white children born at the New York Hospital Women's Clinic, the average length was 50.8 cm. and the average weight 3,224.6 gm. The smallest infant was 1,660 gm. in weight and 49 cm. in length; the largest weighed 6,280 gm. and measured 62 cm. Colored infants generally weigh less than white infants; the average length of 915 full term colored infants in the New York Hospital Women's Clinic was reported as 49.9 cm. and the weight 3,078.1 gm., which is 146.5 gm. less than the average for white children delivered during the same period.

Eastman states that when the weight is below 2,500 gm., an infant should be considered premature. Excessive weight is suggestive of postmaturity. Generally, a

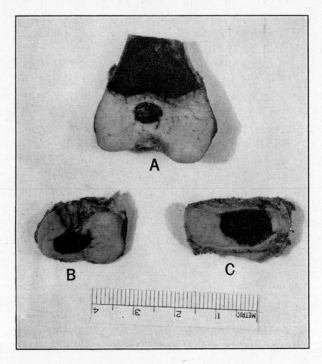

Fig. 23-1. Ossification Centers in the Full Term Infant.
A. Lower end of femur appears at nine months.
B. Astragalus appears at six months.
C. Calcaneus appears at six months.
Months (lunar) refer to intra-uterine development.

premature infant under 1,000 gm. has small chance of life but occasionally may survive when the weight approximates 1,000 gm.

A center of ossification in the lower epiphysis of the femur, about 0.5 cm. (⅕ inch) in diameter or slightly smaller, is generally found in infants at full term. In about 80 per cent of full term infants there is also a center of ossification in the upper end of the tibia, but in other cases it does not appear until shortly after birth. Centers are also found in the calcaneus and astragalus which usually have appeared towards the end of the sixth month of intra-uterine development (Fig. 23-1). The cuboid of the tarsus may show an ossification center at birth or not until shortly after. The absence of centers in the cuboid or in the upper end of the tibia does not necessarily indicate prematurity but their presence is usually indicative of maturity. The absence of the center in the lower end of the femur as well as in the tibia and cuboid would probably indicate prematurity.

The bones of the head are ossified and in close contact at the sutures at the time of birth in full term infants, and the frontal, sagittal, coronal and lambdoid sutures may be palpated through the scalp. The larger anterior diamond-shaped fontanelle and the posterior fontanelle are readily palpated as soft areas beneath the scalp.

CHANGES AFTER BIRTH. A number of changes take place in the body immediately after birth, and by a consideration of these it is possible to form some idea of how long the infant has survived the birth. The meconium in the large intestine is evacuated, and in the first 24 to 48 hours post partum is usually eliminated completely. The fetal blood contains nucleated red blood cells which ordinarily disappear during the first 24 hours of life; microscopic sections of the liver from a newborn infant reveal numerous foci of nucleated red blood cells in the sinusoids. The stump of the umbilical cord dries after birth and starts to separate from the navel region, and in about a week it drops off. Microscopic sections of the zone of separation show a slight inflammatory reaction which starts in the first 24 hours post partum; the first cells are usually polymorphonuclear leukocytes, but later lymphocytes and granulation tissue appear as the cord separates. The kidneys from the second to the fourth day after birth, develop an orange, fan-shaped deposit of uric acid salts in the pyramids of the medulla, but after the fourth day when the extra-uterine metabolism is established, these deposits vanish. At birth, the skin of a white infant is reddish in hue but becomes paler in the course of a week to two weeks; the skin of a newborn colored infant is a dusky bluish red but in a few weeks becomes a dark brown. The centers of ossification which develop after birth have been considered in Chapter 3 and are the most reliable criteria of age.

The fetal circulation changes immediately at birth, for as soon as respiration starts, the pulmonary circulation becomes established, more blood being pumped into the pulmonary artery and less into the ductus arteriosus. After the cord circulation is cut off, the umbilical vein stops functioning, less blood is returned to the right auricle by the inferior vena cava, and the increased flow of blood to the left auricle from the lungs closes the valve of the foramen ovale. The circulation in the umbilical arteries also is interrupted, and the distal ends of the umbilical vessels undergo atrophy and obliteration which is usually complete three to four days after birth; the same changes occur in the hypogastric arteries and the ductus venosus. The ductus arteriosus is not completely occluded until several weeks after birth. Permanent closure of the foramen ovale does not occur for some time, and in many cases it may remain anatomically but usually not functionally patent. The presence of air in the lungs and the significance of air in the stomach will be discussed under the next heading.

Was the Child Born Alive? When a baby is born, the birth is either a live birth and the child begins to breathe, or it is a stillbirth and the baby is born dead and therefore there are no attempts at respiration.

EXAMINATION OF THE LUNGS. Examination of the lungs at autopsy will determine whether the birth was a stillbirth or a live birth. The lungs of the stillborn baby are collapsed, have the consistency of a flaccid spleen and are dark purplish red in color. They are in the back of the chest and only a small portion is visible from the front. The diaphragm is high about the level of the third rib. The lungs of a live birth are distended, well aerated, fluffy, have a salmon-pink color, and are visible in the front of the chest when the sternum is removed. The chest is expanded and the diaphragm is at the level of the fourth to the sixth rib. When the case is a typical stillbirth or live birth the appearance of the lungs is pathognomonic. Unfortunately, in many cases the signs are not so characteristic, and it may then be difficult to decide the question of a live birth or a stillbirth.

A routine procedure which has been accepted as being fairly reliable is the hydrostatic lung test or the *docimasia pulmonum hydrostatica*. The basis for the test is that in the typical stillbirth the lungs are not aerated and will sink if placed in water, while in a live birth the child has breathed, the lungs are expanded with air and will float. The test is performed by removing the lungs at necropsy attached to the larynx, trachea and bronchi; the trachea may be tied before removal so that air will not be forced into the lungs post mortem. The entire specimen can now be placed in water at about room temperature (or in water cooled to 4° C. as insisted upon by the older authorities). After this, each lung may be separated and tested; finally pieces of tissue may be cut from each lung and put in the water. The sinking or the floating of both lungs, one lung or small pieces of lungs, will indicate the presence or absence of air in these organs, and may enable the examiner to form an opinion as to whether he is dealing with a stillbirth or a live birth.

Many cases are observed in which a whole lung or some parts of it float, but other parts sink. If pressure is applied to those portions which float, the air may be squeezed out of them and they will sink. The chances are that such lungs are from a stillborn baby and the presence of air is due to an artefact of some sort. If the lung has been aerated during life it is almost impossible to squeeze out the contained air so that the lung will sink.

Postmortem decomposition is present sometimes in cases which have been dead for several days, and gas bubbles may be present in the lungs. In the early stage of decomposition these bubbles may be seen in the interstitial tissue, and though they will interfere with the hydrostatic test, they can be recognized for what they are. They can be pressed out of the tissue in many instances, and the pathologist may distinguish whether or not the case is a stillbirth by application of the hydrostatic test. When decomposition is far advanced, it is often impossible to determine accurately the previous condition of the lung, as its tissue will be permeated thoroughly with gas blebs.

Pieces of tissue may be cut from different parts of both lungs and microscopic slides may be prepared from each specimen. This method has the advantage of providing permanent records of the case, and at the same time offering reliable but not infallible criteria indicative of aeration or lack of aeration of the lungs. In the typical stillbirth the alveoli and the bronchi on the microscope slide are collapsed. In the aerated lung the alveoli are more or less expanded, and the bronchi likewise. The microscopic section has the additional value of demonstrating pathologic processes in the lungs which may complicate the hydrostatic test (Fig. 23-2).

It is important to keep in mind the different possibilities which may occur during birth and to consider what effect they may have on the lungs of the newborn baby. For example, the fetus may be born with every expectation of breathing, but the cord may be wrapped around its neck so that it cannot breathe, and strangulation occurs during labor or just after it. Under such conditions the lungs are like those of a stillbirth, and such signs of asphyxia as cyanosis and subserous petechial hemorrhages may be present.

Many accidents are possible during an unassisted birth which the woman is attempting to conduct by herself. For example, the baby may present its head first, the head may be exposed to air in the birth canal, and breathing may take place there. Some have claimed that breathing has also taken place inside the uterus which can occur only when the membranes are broken, and the hand of the accoucheur has been introduced in utero to produce version, causing air to follow the hand and to stimulate the child to breathe, even inside the uterus; this condition is known as *vagitus uterinus*. After birth the child may suffocate by falling in the extruded membranes, or in the blood between the mother's thighs, or by accidental overlying of the mother. In other instances, especially after a difficult labor or a

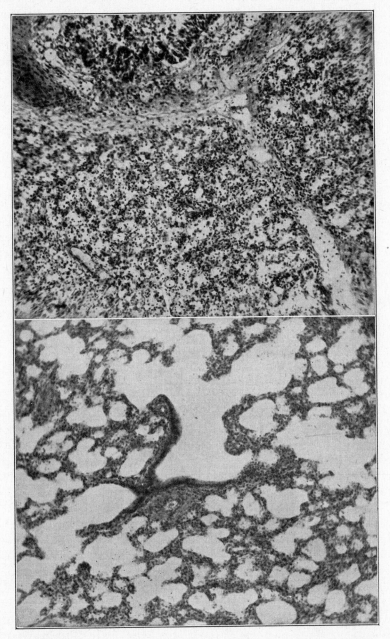

Fig. 23-2. Microscopic Sections of Lungs of Stillborn and Live Born Infants.
Top. Atelectatic lung of a stillbirth.
Bottom. Aerated lung of a live birth.

breech presentation, the infant may have received such severe treatment that it will breathe a few seconds after birth and die from the ordeal inflicted during delivery, even when there is no actual evidence of injury. The lungs, under such conditions, show aeration to a greater or lesser degree.

Partial aeration of the lungs does not always mean a live birth, as breathing may start before the infant is completely expelled from the birth canal, and the child may die before it is completely delivered. It is also possible in a case where artificial respiration was attempted that air may have been introduced into the lungs post mortem by the movements or manipulations applied to the baby's body by the accoucheur. The lungs of a stillborn child may be inflated with a catheter during attempts at resuscitation by a medical attendant and at autopsy may resemble those of a live birth.

Conversely, the lungs may be atelectatic and sink in water, even when the infant has breathed after birth. In a case of abandonment, a woman threw her newborn infant onto a heap of refuse, exposing it to the rigors of a cold winter day. After it had been there an hour, the baby was found and rushed to the hospital where it died 24 hours later. The pleural cavities at necropsy were filled with fluid, probably caused by internal congestion from the exposure to cold, and the lungs were compressed and airless. Pieces of the lungs sank in water, even though there was definite evidence that the child had breathed.

A confirmatory indication of breathing, when associated with definite aeration of the lungs, is the presence of swallowed air in the stomach and upper small intestine. The infant gulps during its attempt at respiration and air is introduced into the stomach, slightly distending that viscus and often forming bubbles in the swallowed amniotic fluid already present.

Cause of Death. The cause of death can be determined only by an autopsy, which must disclose whether the infant was stillborn, or died of natural causes, accidental birth injuries or criminal violence. The natural disease processes include such conditions as congenital cardiac malformations, malformations of other organs, constitutional diseases, erythroblastosis fetalis or adrenal hemorrhages of spontaneous type which may produce a fatal result after birth. Death of newborn infants often is referable to the strain of prolonged and difficult labor.

The child may die likewise of injuries inflicted accidentally by the process of birth or after birth. The lateral venous sinus and tentorium may be torn by the distortion of the child's skull in its passage through the birth canal and death results from intracranial hemorrhage. The obstetrical forceps may injure the head, and the bones of the extremities may be broken or dislocated during version. The liver may be ruptured by forceful flexion of the body and give rise to intraperitoneal hemorrhage. Sometimes the pharynx of the infant may be lacerated by the mother or by the obstetrician, from insertion of the finger into the month during delivery, especially in a breech presentation. A mother in delivering a child may grasp it in different ways, so as to injure it fatally; in some cases of infanticide this possibility is introduced as a defense.

Precipitate labor occasionally occurs, in which the baby is propelled forcibly from the uterus, especially when the woman is in the standing position, and it is possible for it to be hurled so violently to the ground that its skull is fractured, or the umbilical cord may be torn and death result from hemorrhage. Birth may take place also when the woman is straining at stool, and the child may be drowned in a privy or water closet. The question of precipitate labor is raised not infrequently as a defense but, as Herzog says, its presence does not disprove the theory of infanticide, and both may occur in the same case. An allegation of precipitate labor may be refuted by an autopsy on the child and by an examination of the mother. For if the infant is full term and presents a caput succedaneum or swelling of the scalp from a difficult passage through the birth canal, such a sign would indicate that the birth was slow and not projectile. In precipitate labor, the placenta usually emerges attached to the infant or the umbilical cord of the baby may be torn off near the navel and other injuries may be present. The mother also is likely to show a torn perineum or other marked birth lacerations unless she is a multipara with a relaxed genital passage and the infant is comparatively small in size.

Is Death Due to Infanticide? If the body of a newborn infant is found abandoned in such a place as a parcel room or a washroom without any previous history concerning its death, the autopsy must reveal that the baby was killed by criminal violence in order to substantiate a charge of infanticide. The methods of causing infanticide may be any of those employed in homicide, but certain methods of slaughter are common in infanticide because of the helpless nature of the victim and of the inherent conditions implicit in the act. Methods of destruction are used which would be difficult to accomplish successfully against an adult, such as choking the infant with a wad of toilet paper, or some other form of asphyxiation (page 482). From their nature these traumas could not be interpreted any other way except as an intent to kill on the part of another person. A consideration of the various forms of infanticide will indicate the types to which this interpretation is applicable.

The most common method of infanticide is some variety of asphyxiation employed usually in a hasty attempt to conceal the infant's cry. Many infanticidal deaths result from smothering after a hand or pillow has been placed over the face and the features may show signs of distortion or pressure. Sometimes a gag has been wrapped around the nose or mouth and may be still in place at the time of autopsy (Fig. 18-11). Infanticidal choking is caused by wads of paper, wads of gauze, and substances such as ashes or talcum powder which have been stuffed down the throat so as to block the larynx. Unless the foreign body is found in the mouth and air passages, the manner of death may be difficult to prove. Strangulation is produced ordinarily by a ligature around the neck, often with the cord still in place at the time of autopsy. Occasionally the strangulation is manual, and in such cases, the external marks are similar to the skin lesions produced in adults; the only difference is that the injuries in the deeper tissues are not so severe, because of the greater elasticity of the structures in the neck of the infant (Fig. 17-18). Fractures of the laryngeal cartilages and hyoid bone are rarely observed.

Sometimes the birth occurs in the bathtub or in a toilet bowl, so that the newborn child is drowned; the signs of drowning in such cases are often indistinct, especially when postmortem decomposition is present. The diagnosis cannot always be made positively on the evidence discovered at necropsy. Unfortunately, the free communication between the right and left sides of the heart in newborn children automatically eliminates the employment of the chemical test for drowning devised by Gettler, which has been described in Chapter 18. For these reasons a case of submersion cannot be pronounced definitely infanticidal, unless police investigation produces evidence which indicates the probability of the crime. These same considerations apply to asphyxial deaths such as smothering in the membranes or overlying by the mother, which may be produced accidentally during an unattended birth; usually there is not much to be seen at necropsy except cyanosis, petechial hemorrhages in the subserous tissues, or hemorrhages in the areolar tissues of the scalp. Unless the police investigation can prove that such smothering is intentional, it would be difficult to prove the death infanticidal.

Stab wounds of the head through the fontanels, stab wounds of the heart, incised wounds of the throat, or dismemberment of the body are encountered in some cases and cause death by shock or hemorrhage. Cutting of the umbilical cord and allowing it to bleed has been employed as a means of killing a newborn child, but it is not a certain method as the blood vessels become occluded soon after birth from

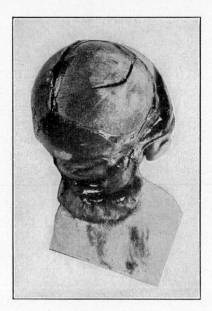

Fig. 23-3. Infanticide. Fracture of Skull.

Angular fracture of the right parietal bone in a newborn infant who lived 10 hours after the injury. Thrown from window.

shrinking of the cord. In all these cases if the necropsy discloses that death was the result of the injury, it can be classified as an infanticide.

Fractures of the skull occur as a result of repeated blows on the head or because the infant was thrown from a window. Other injuries are not common: the neck of the infant in some cases apparently was broken because the mother twisted it with her hands; fractures of the ribs and extremity bones occur occasionally. It is possible for many of these injuries to occur as a result of accidental traumas inflicted during birth, as already discussed on page 598. Furthermore similar lesions may have been produced after death, as, for example, extensive crushing of the head and trunk, and extensive burns, which are sometimes caused post mortem in an attempt to get rid of the body. In all cases in which death is due to blunt force, a history of the occurrence is necessary in order to sustain the contention that the violence is infanticidal in nature.

Fractures of the skull in the newborn are of a special kind inasmuch as the violence is applied to a skull composed of movable plates of bone, held in place by flexible membranes, and the injury is usually confined to the bones immediately struck. The parietal bone is most exposed and most frequently injured, the lines of fracture being directed as a rule between the striations in the bone; these radiate from the periphery to the central boss and the fractures converge toward the boss, taking a linear, angular or stellate form so that in the more extensive lesions the boss is in the center of the fracture (Fig. 23-3). In making a diagnosis of a linear fracture of the skull, care must be taken not to confuse a natural cleavage with a crack due to trauma. In addition some fractures of the skull may be caused by compression of the head in the birth canal or by obstetrical forceps. In severe violence more than one bone of the skull may be injured, but the brain is lacerated rarely by direct violence. Hemorrhages usually occur in the pericranium and in the scalp. Death occurs as a result of shock from the injury, and rarely does a laceration of the brain cause a subdural hemorrhage and death by cerebral compression.

Some cases of infanticide are due to exposure, where the child is abandoned to the inclemencies of the weather, starvation and the attacks of animals. In these cases the body may not show any marks, or antemortem and postmortem wounds inflicted by different animals may be present. Death may be caused without demonstrable change in the internal organs or the autopsy may reveal such lesions as hypostatic pneumonia or pleural effusions from internal congestion (page 598). In rare instances newborn infants who have been exposed are discovered before death has occurred, and their deaths are traced to the action of the mother; it is only under these conditions that the charge of infanticide from exposure has any chance of being prosecuted successfully.

Medicolegal Considerations. The prosecution in all cases of infanticide must assume the burden of proof which means that the medical evidence must establish these facts: that the infant had reached the period of intra-uterine development consistent with extra-uterine survival; that the infant was newborn and had breathed; and that death was due to a type of trauma which could be considered as a logical means of infanticide. The final part of the proof is to link the body of the infant with the defendant and to obtain medical evidence showing that the putative mother has recently been delivered of a baby of 7 to 10 lunar months gestation. This question has been discussed on page 560.

If the defendant is caught in the act of infanticide, the problem of identification is comparatively simple and may be established by witnesses who will testify to the proximity of the infant to the mother and to the circumstances of the crime. The medical examination of the mother and the autopsy on the body of the infant will then be sufficient to complete the proof.

Usually the investigation starts with the finding of the body of a newborn baby in a bundle deposited in a parcel room or in an ashcan, and in such cases it may be difficult or even impossible to follow the trail to the person responsible. This can be done in a few cases if objects such as newspapers, clothing or suitcases are found with the body and give some clue which indicates the defendant. In a large center of population like New York City, few cases of this type are solved. A large proportion of infanticides occur among unmarried mothers, for the motive in such instances is to conceal all signs of pregnancy.

It is essential for the prosecution to show that the uterine and abdominal signs on the defendant are compatible with the birth of the deceased infant. This may be accomplished as a matter of course if the defendant is in need of medical attention because of the birth and must be sent to a hospital. Otherwise the examining physician must either obtain the consent of the defendant or be authorized by an order from a court of record before he can examine her; this subject was discussed in Chapter 21. Serologic examination of the bloods of the deceased infant and the putative mother may reveal the same or compatible isoagglutination groups which is important confirmatory evidence of the mother-child relationship; in other cases the examination may reveal an incompatibility of blood groups which may exculpate an innocent defendant. It is desirable in all autopsies on bodies of abandoned infants to preserve routinely specimens of the heart's blood for serologic examination and determination of the blood group.

REFERENCES

Dorland, W. A. N.   Legitimacy, from Peterson, Haines and Webster, Legal Medicine and Toxicology, Philadelphia, W. B. Saunders Co., 1923, Vol. 1, p. 959.
Eastman, N. J.   Williams Obstetrics, 10th ed., New York, Appleton-Century-Crofts, Inc., 1950.
Herzog, A.   Medical Jurisprudence, Indianapolis, Bobbs-Merrill Co., 1931.
Puppe, G.   Atlas und Grundriss der Gerichtlichen Medizin, München, J. F. Lehmann, 1908.
Reports of the Office of the Chief Medical Examiner in the City of New York from 1918 to 1951.
Smith, S.   Forensic Medicine, London, J. & A. Churchill, ltd., 1940.

24

Virginity: Rape and Other Sexual Assaults: Examination of Semen

VIRGINITY

A virgin is a female who has not experienced sexual intercourse and whose genital organs have not been altered by carnal connection. An unruptured hymen is most often mentioned as the distinguishing feature of virginity, but it is not always a reliable indication. There are rare instances in which it is found intact after repeated acts of sexual intercourse, and on the other hand, this membrane may be destroyed by masturbation or physical trauma. The diagnosis of virginity is difficult and in many cases a physical examination of the genital organs may not help the examiner to decide this question.

The hymen appears after the fourth month of fetal life as two folds of mucous membrane which grow, one from the right and one from the left side of the uro-genital orifice, and fuse in the midline except at the hymenal opening. Thus a partial diaphragm is formed at the vaginal outlet and this forms the hymenal membrane. In the adult the hymen is generally thin and membranous but may be thick and fleshy, usually possessing one opening and rarely several (Fig. 24-1).

The different types of hymen are: (1) the infantile hymen which has a small linear opening in the midline; (2) the annular hymen in which the opening is ovoid and placed near the center of the membrane; (3) the semilunar hymen in which the opening is placed anteriorly so that the membrane has a semilunar shape; (4) the cribriform hymen which is perforated by several openings; (5) the vertical hymen which has a vertical opening in the form of a vertical linear slit; (6) the septate hymen in which two lateral openings occur side by side, separated partially or completely by a thin strip of tissue; (7) the imperforate hymen which completely closes the genital orifice. Other types occur such as the fimbriate hymen in which fine fimbria are present around the edge of the hymenal opening, or the lobate hymen in which the opening is stellate because of indentations in its edges. If care is not exercised, the fimbriate hymen may be mistaken for a ruptured one.

The hymen is usually ruptured by the entrance of the penis at the time of the first coition, and at first only presents a torn appearance. After repeated coitus the opening may be enlarged and small knobs of tissue known as carunculae hymenales are formed. In a few cases the membrane may be so tough and elastic that it will sustain coitus without rupturing, and it may be impossible to tell whether or not intercourse has taken place. In other instances the membrane may have been ruptured traumatically as a result of surgical operation or by masturbation.

The passage of the child through the birth canal obliterates the hymen, and small tabs of tissue known as carunculae myrtiformes are all that remain around the hymenal ring. Cases have been described, however, in which the hymen was so tough that it was intact when labor commenced and had to be sectioned surgically

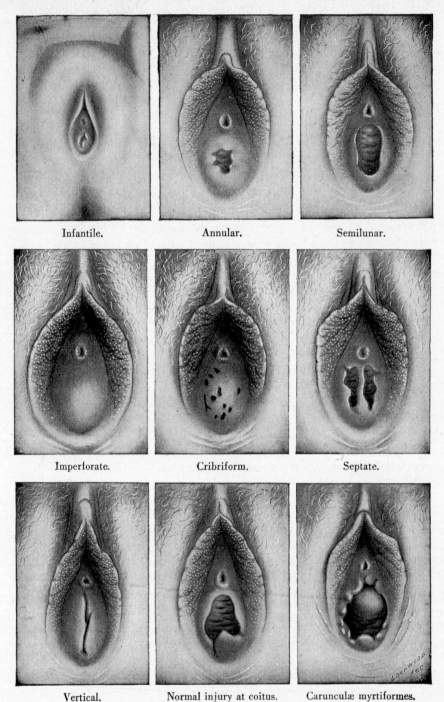

Infantile.   Annular.   Semilunar.

Imperforate.   Cribriform.   Septate.

Vertical.   Normal injury at coitus.   Carunculæ myrtiformes.

From Stander, *Williams Obstetrics*, 7th ed., Appleton-Century-Crofts, Inc., 1937

Fig. 24-1. Several Varieties of Hymen.

to allow delivery of the child. It is not possible to give a definite decision concerning virginity in a case, unless the individual presents characteristic signs. A small genital opening and an intact but fragile hymen are in favor of virginity. A large opening and carunculae myrtiformes would suggest absence of virginity. In other cases the signs are less clear and a diagnosis cannot be made.

RAPE

Rape is defined as the carnal knowledge of a woman by a male without her consent by compulsion through force, threats or fraud. In such cases it is not necessary to prove that the sexual act was completed; mere entrance of the penis into the vulva or between the labia majora is sufficient to constitute the crime.

The New York Penal Code, 2010, defines rape in the first degree by a man as "an act of sexual intercourse with a female not his wife, against her will or without her consent." It elaborates the definition by including cases in which the woman is of unsound mind; so weak that she cannot resist; overcome by force; overcome by fear of immediate and bodily harm; overcome by a narcotic or another drug; unconscious of the nature of the act and that this is known to the defendant; or when she is in the custody of the law in any place of lawful detention. The crime is not excused because the victim is a prostitute.

It is not a defense to urge that a man is so old that he is impotent to commit rape, as only a slight penetration of the genitalia is required to constitute the offense. Even if he did not accomplish his purpose he could be charged with the offense of assault with intent to commit rape. In some states a boy below a certain age cannot be considered as capable of this crime; the age varies with the jurisdiction and is from 14 to 16 years. However, he can be guilty of assault with intent to ravish.

The laws of some states fix a specified age for girls known as the "age of consent." If a man has sexual intercourse with a girl below this age, even if she is willing, he can be prosecuted for rape in the second degree, or statutory rape. In New York State, the age of consent is 18 years.

Rape is committed in secret and the statement of the victim backed by medical evidence is taken as proof of the crime. False charges of rape are common and medical evidence is necessary to establish or refute the accusation. The concern of the court is to sift the evidence and in doubtful cases to determine whether or not violation took place, and whether or not consent was given by the victim, questions often hard to decide. Accusations of rape are often unfounded and are brought against a defendant for the purposes of revenge or blackmail. A woman is supposed to exert her utmost resistance against an attacker and the evidence may throw doubt upon her claim.

Many cases of rape occur after the victim has been rendered insensible by force, strangulation, drugs or alcohol. The question sometimes arises whether or not it could be inflicted during natural sleep. A virgin or a woman with a narrow vaginal canal would probably be awakened by an attempt at coitus. Some writers, however, believe that a multipara with a spacious genital canal accustomed to intercourse might sustain coition during sleep and not be aroused.

Charges of rape are brought occasionally against dentists and physicians by women after a general anesthesia. The anesthetized person may experience erotic sensations and honestly, though erroneously, believe that she has been violated while unconscious. Similar experiences and charges occur during and after hypnosis.

Examination of Victim. Medical testimony is always necessary in a case of rape, and the victim should be examined as soon as possible by a physician. The date and hour of the examination should be recorded. The consent of the woman for the examination must be given either verbally in front of witnesses, or better still in writing, before the examination can be made; if she is an adult of sound mind, she alone is qualified to give such consent and the insistence of another party, even of a relative, does not authorize the examining physician to proceed. In the case of a minor or feebleminded person, the nearest adult relative may give consent. If the victim is examined without the proper authorization, the medical man can be prosecuted for indecent assault, and this applies in cases in which the examining physician is a woman. It is only when the examiner is acting on an order from a court of record that he can disregard the wishes of the victim (page 556).

The physician before starting his examination should question the victim concerning the alleged crime, and obtain a statement from her giving full particulars, in which such items as date, time of day, place, circumstances and resistance offered during the assault are all mentioned. The victim should be encouraged to elaborate upon her account in order that any important discrepancies in her story may be brought to light. The examination itself should be especially concerned with discovering (1) injuries on the body and genital organs of the victim; (2) disturbances of her clothing; (3) blood stains, spermatic stains, foreign hairs or other foreign substances on the body or clothing of the victim; (4) the existence of venereal disease; (5) the existence of pregnancy. The procedure of the examination may vary depending on whether the victim is a child or an adult.

CHILDREN. Many cases of rape are committed on children because of their comparative helplessness. In such instances the body and genital organs should be examined for scratch marks, abrasions, lacerations about the labia, dilatation of the vaginal orifice, tears of the vaginal wall and ruptures of the hymen. Sometimes the hymenal tears are absent, even with other injuries present; a ruptured hymen would not mean rape necessarily, nor would an intact hymen preclude rape. In the type of case where the assailant overcomes the child by force, the injuries may be severe. In another type of case there may not be any visible lesions as the defendant may have bribed the child with candy or some other lure and merely have taken liberties with the genital organs without causing physical damage. In any event the examination should take place without delay, because the signs may rapidly disappear.

If the assault has been recent, blood and seminal fluid or dried stains may be present on the person and clothing of the victim. The seminal stains should be taken to the laboratory and examined microscopically in order that spermatozoa may be identified, as their presence would constitute strong confirmatory evidence of the crime. If possible the group of the seminal stain should be determined and compared with the isoagglutination groups in the blood of the defendant, as discussed in Chapter 27. Blood stains should be removed to the laboratory for the precipitation and agglutination tests and for possible comparision with blood taken from the victim and the defendant, as discussed in Chapters 26 and 27. Foreign hairs and other material found on the victim should be examined microscopically and their nature determined as described in Chapter 28; these materials are sometimes valuable as clues as well as for evidence.

If several days or weeks have elapsed since the crime, the injuries of the genital tract may heal, but the child may show signs of a venereal disease like gonorrhea or syphilis. If the accused has a similar venereal disease, and if it is possible that he infected the child, such an infection would be evidence against him. The main difficulty is that a gonococcal vaginitis occurs in female children occasionally as as nonvenereal infectious disease. Similarly a nonspecific inflammation of the genitals occurs from dirt or pin worms.

False accusations are made occasionally against individuals by parents of a child who may influence the youngster to tell a circumstantial story of a rape. They may injure the genital organs of the child for the purpose of substantiating their accusations. It is necessary for the examining physician to keep these possibilities in mind before coming to a decision.

Some victims of rape are killed at the time of perpetration by strangulation, smothering, shock, blunt force injuries or anesthetics. Others may receive such mistreatment from the genital trauma that they develop a pelvic cellulitis and die of sepsis several days or weeks after the injury.

ADULTS. The examination of an adult female in a case of rape is similar to that described under the examination of children, but the injuries encountered may be different. A virgin who has been violated by force may show severe injuries of the genital tract in the form of abrasions and lacerations of the vaginal orifice, distension of the vaginal canal and ruptures of the hymen. Bruises and scratch marks may be present on the arms, thighs and elsewhere on the body. With a married woman, the chances are that the genital organs may show but little injury, but contusions and abrasions may be found on the other parts of the body. The implications in regard to blood stains, seminal stains and hairs are the same in adults as they are in children. The presence of venereal disease in the victim may be a matter of importance especially if the defendant has a similar venereal disease. In addition a woman may become pregnant as the result of rape, in which case the physician should look for the signs of pregnancy and consider the date of possible impregnation (Chapters 21 and 22).

Death may occur in the rape of an adult female as a result of blunt force, strangulation, smothering or poisoning by drugs. The genital tract may not show any injuries, but in other cases may be severely lacerated, and death may be caused by hemorrhage or sepsis. The most severe tears are produced not by the penis but by the hand of the assailant, as in the case of one victim, a virgin, whose vaginal outlet was lacerated and an injury like a birth tear was inflicted on the posterior commissure when the perpetrator attempted to force his hand through the opening. The victim was killed by strangulation during the assault. In some cases of rape death is caused by the shock of repeated blows on the head and neck probably from the fist. In three cases of this type seen by the authors, there was extensive discoloration and swelling of the left side of the head and neck; in one case there was a fracture of the neck of the mandible on the left, in another, fracture of the cranium, and in the third, fracture of the left superior process of the laryngeal thyroid cartilage. In none of the cases were the genital tracts injured, but spermatozoa were found in the vagina in two cases.

There were two cases of vaginal laceration which were the result, not of rape, but of sexual misconduct through cooperation. In one the defendant tore an ovoid opening about 4 cm. in the posterior wall of the vagina with his fingers, causing death a few days later from an infectious pelvic cellulitis. In the other case the defendant tore the vaginal vault with his fingers, introduced his hand into the pelvis and tore the left common iliac artery, causing death by hemorrhage.

Where death occurs at the time of the assault or shortly after, a chemical examination should be made of the viscera to determine the presence of any drug which might have been used to poison the victim. The vaginal tract should be examined for spermatozoa by means of a wet smear on a microscope slide as described on page 612. Seminal spots on the clothing or person of the deceased should be investigated as described on page 614. Blood stains on the clothing should be investigated as described on pages 625 and 628. Blood from the heart of the deceased should be tested for its agglutinogens and agglutinins so that it may be compared with other specimens. Foreign hairs and fingernail scrapings from the deceased should be examined microscopically for clues as described in Chapter 28.

Examination of the Suspected Perpetrator. The suspect should be examined for injuries of the penis and other parts of the body, for blood and seminal stains on penis and clothing, for foreign hairs, and for signs of active syphilis and gonorrhea. A specimen of his blood, about 5 ml., should be collected for the purpose of determining the isoagglutination groups present and for purposes of comparison with other blood specimens or spermatic fluid from the person and garments of the deceased. The consent of the suspect must be obtained for these procedures, unless the examining physician is acting by order of a court of record and examination must be begun without delay as the signs of the act disappear rapidly.

SEXUAL PERVERSIONS

Civilized and uncivilized people regulate sexual intercourse by law and custom. The problem of the law is to encourage the marriage relation and at the same time to discourage all abnormal variations connected with sex. Accordingly in the penal codes of communities there are statutes imposing penalties on sexual practices which are considered detrimental to society.

Heterosexual intercourse between man and woman with the organs intended for that purpose is the only normal means of gratification. All other varieties are abnormal. Even heterosexual intercourse is forbidden under penalties of the law to men and women closely related by blood. The technical name of the crime is incest, and mother and son, father and daughter, brother and sister, uncle and niece, or aunt and nephew are the relationships which come under the ban.

Some of the minor perversions of the heterosexual instinct occur in individuals who are victims of a compulsion neurosis or are psychologically abnormal and who frequently are impelled to display their aberrations openly. In men a common variety of such an impulse is exhibitionism or the exposure of the genitalia in public, often to children or persons of the opposite sex. Fetishism occurs when an individual obtains sexual gratification from a woman's clothing, hair or even her secretions, and is chiefly important because the sight of the fetish causes the victim to display his weakness. Necrophilia is the perverted desire of an individual for coitus with a dead body and has few legal complications, except defilement or mutilation of the cadaver.

Excessive sexual desire is known as satyriasis when it occurs in men and nymphomania when it occurs in women. It consists in an abnormal indulgence in sexual intercourse whenever possible, and is generally the expression of an advanced compulsion neurosis. The condition may occur in persons of any age. Occasionally precocious sexual development and practices are found in male and female children below the age of 10, and such individuals are a serious problem inasmuch as they corrupt other children. Elderly people, both male and female, sometimes lose their normal inhibitions, lapse into a libidinous state and commit many sexual transgressions. Most of them are cases of senile dementia and are especially troublesome because they try to pervert children or practice exhibitionism and for this reason run afoul of the law.

Other abnormalities of the sexual impulse are considered more culpable and incur more severe penalties under the criminal law. Most of the individuals who practice these perversions are psychopathic, even if they are not actually insane. An example of one type of such perversion is bestiality or the abnormal and unnatural carnal connection of human beings with animals. Cases have been reported in which both men and women have used many of the domesticated animals for such purposes.

Homosexual intercourse is a sexual relation between persons of the same sex. Between men coitus may occur in the anal region, in between the thighs or in fellatio; the same abnormal methods of gratification also may be practiced between men and women, and occasionally the man may practice cunnilingus. Homosexuality is punishable by law, and the legal proof requires that the crime shall be established, and that the penis of the active agent shall have entered the part concerned, emission of semen not being required. Both participants are equally guilty unless the passive agent was compelled to submit by force. The name usually given to male homosexuality per anum is sodomy. Pederasty is that variety of sodomy forced on a boy by a man.

Homosexual male persons are not all of the same type. Some of them are ordinarily heterosexual but become homosexual through such circumstances as being confined in prisons or asylums where there is no opportunity for normal sexual intercourse and latent homosexuality becomes manifest. Many homosexuals are innately vicious or depraved and are really bisexual rather than homosexual. Other types are men who lose their potency from senility or debilitating disease and drift into homosexual practices to satisfy their remaining infantile libido. Some individuals have a personal habitus more female than male with the exception of the genital organs, and many affect female attire and have feminine nicknames; they are generally termed fairies in common parlance.

Important medicolegal complications other than that of the act itself, may arise when homosexual persons are victimized by those whom they have solicited for their perverted practices. They are frequently assaulted, sometimes fatally, and then robbed. Some homosexuals become victims of blackmailers, or they are blackmailers themselves. Many are prone to commit suicide. A large proportion of them are chronic narcotic addicts.

Both participants in cases of homosexual perversion must be examined promptly by a physician who should obtain the consent of the examined or act under the order of a judge of a court of record. All injuries on the body should be noted, especially scratch marks, lacerations and contusions near the anal region of the passive agent. Spermatozoa should be searched for on the anal region and the clothing. The penis of the active agent should be examined for fecal fragments, semen and injuries, especially teeth marks if there is any suspicion of buccal coitus. Blood stains on the person or clothing of either party may be tested with the isoagglutination tests and the group compared with the blood groups of the active and passive agents. Spermatic stains may also be typed and the groups compared with blood groups of the active and passive agents. In a case of bestiality both animal and human participants should be examined in the same way; in addition the marks of teeth and claws and the presence of animal hairs should be searched for on the human participant. Such hairs should be examined microscopically and compared with hairs from the animal concerned (Chapter 28).

Occasionally a homosexual individual is killed by strangulation or some other form of trauma inflicted during the commission of the act. In a few cases the anal region is badly lacerated and the victim may develop a fatal sepsis. The authors have seen several cases in which the rectum of the victim was perforated through the anterior wall resulting in a ragged ovoid opening 1 to 1½ inches in diameter so that fecal content entered the abdominal cavity causing an acute suppurative

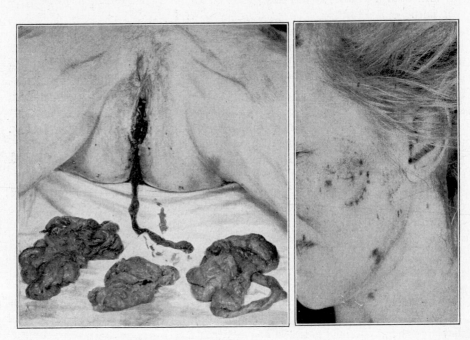

Fig. 24-2. Sadistic Murder.

A. Manual evisceration of small and large intestines through lacerated vagina. Three loops of intestine shown were found near body of deceased. Torn end of intestine protruding from vagina.

B. Impression of teeth of assailant on face of victim.

peritonitis; the method of perforation was not known but it was probably due to the introduction of the fingers or a foreign body through the anus into the rectum. In one case a glass tumbler, 5 inches long and 2½ inches wide, was forced through the anal region into the rectum, evidently while the victim was intoxicated, lacerating the anus, perforating the rectum and causing a fatal septic peritonitis. A gonococcal or syphilitic infection may be transmitted during the intercourse and may cause death later through various complications. If the patient lives, the presence of a syphilitic or gonorrheal infection in the anal region may be an important factor in the case. In cases of habitual sodomy a relaxed funnel-shaped anus has been described in the passive agent by some observers.

Female homosexuality is known as lesbianism or tribadism. This offense is not prosecuted by the law to any extent in the United States, as its devotees are not usually promiscuous. The methods employed are mutual friction of the genitals or cunnilingus, and the external genitals may show scratch marks, abrasions or teeth marks. The chief complication which attends lesbianism is that its practitioners, who are morbidly jealous of one another, when scorned may resort to homicide, suicide or both. This complication occasionally arises in cases of male homosexuality but not as frequently. Many lesbians are masculine in type, possibly because of endocrine disturbances, and are apt to affect male attire, but others are feminine and probably developed the practice from persistence of infantile conflicts.

Another of the varieties of sexual perversion is known as algolagnia. One of its forms is sadism in which the pervert obtains sexual excitement by the infliction of pain, and the other form is masochism in which satisfaction is acquired by the enduring of pain. Both sexes are affected but sadism is more likely to develop in males and masochism in females. Masochism in a male or sadism in a female are both considered as homosexual manifestations.

The sadist derives his satisfaction from acts of cruelty which he inflicts on his sexual partner, either by cuts with a knife, blows with a whip, strangulation, biting and scratching. The extreme occurs in the lust murders in which the sadist satisfies his libido by killing. He may cut the vagina, symphysis pubis and lower abdomen from below upward, as in the ripper cases. He may commit revolting acts on the body after death, such as stabbing the vagina or the tongue with a sharp instrument, or driving a stake of wood through the floor of the mouth into the neck. In one case (Fig. 24-2), the vagina was extensively torn and coils of the small and large intestine were pulled down and eviscerated through the lacerated vagina; in addition marks of teeth were present on the cheek of the deceased. It must be remembered that not all murders committed in the course of a sexual act are lust murders, for the homicide may have been perpetrated through anger, jealousy, fear of exposure, superstition or some other motive.

Masochism is the opposite of sadism in that the pervert obtains his satisfaction by being trampled upon, beaten, hurt or humiliated by the sexual partner. Its medicolegal complications are slight.

The law enforcement agencies are particularly concerned with those sexual perversions which disturb the peace or give rise to homicide. Some types of perverts are harmless, others are a potential source of danger, while others are a distinct menace. The descriptions given above will indicate the dangerous and the comparatively innocuous types.

EXAMINATION OF SEMINAL FLUID AND STAINS

The demonstration of semen is an important part of the routine investigation in cases of rape, adultery, sodomy, bestiality and sexual homicide. In such cases seminal fluid may be found fresh in the vaginal or rectal contents, or it may be noted as a wet or dried secretion on the hair and skin around the genitalia or as a dried stain on garments. The examination of the fresh material removed from the genital tract and the dried spots on clothing presents a number of significant differences.

Fresh Specimens. The seminal fluid deposited in the vagina after intercourse is soon altered by being mixed with a slightly acid matrix of mucus, cells and bacteria normally present in the female genital tract. After their arrival many of the spermatozoa spread in a few minutes through the slightly alkaline cavities of the cervix uteri, corpus uteri and fallopian tubes, if a female orgasm has taken place; in most cases of rape, the female orgasm is probably absent and the spermatozoic spread may take about six hours. Some spermatozoa remain behind in the vagina and are continually being removed by lysis, phagocytosis and other processes. Pollak believes that the acid nature of the vaginal secretion is not as detrimental to spermatozoa as some investigators have declared, and that many of these cells are acid and alkaline resistant. Some have claimed that spermatozoa may be demonstrated in the vaginal contents of nonfatal cases from 45 minutes to several days after the last coitus, but these considerations do not offer a satisfactory basis for estimating the duration of their residence in the vagina inasmuch as the time of the last coitus cannot always be determined with precision. The motility of the spermatozoa in the specimen may give a clue to their length of stay as they remain motile from 30 to 60 minutes after deposition in the vagina. If they are not motile, it might be difficult to determine the length of time they have been in the female genital tract. Motile spermatozoa are occasionally found in the uterus and fallopian tubes, but their presence in that location is not especially significant, as they could be the products of a coitus previous to the final coitus.

Spermatozoa may be found in the vagina in fatal cases of rape in which the death of the victim occurred at the scene of the crime, and may be demonstrated as motile cells in the first two hours post mortem, and as motionless cells up to 24 hours after death. Additional factors in the dead body operate to destroy these cells more rapidly than during life, as for example the postmortem growth of bacteria in the vaginal tract. In some cases of rape, spermatozoa may not be present in the vagina because the perpetrator had aspermia or azoospermia, or because he failed to have an emission of semen, or because he cleaned out the vagina or poured in antiseptic fluid so that the cells were destroyed. In the fresh specimens from the vagina, the presence of spermatozoa is the only reliable proof of the presence of semen, for though other cells of the male genital tract may be present they cannot be identified with certainty as they are often so altered by various factors in the vaginal secretion that they are indistinguishable from artefacts.

The high acid phosphatase content of its prostatic fluid component has provided the basis for new tests for semen. Kaye, and Benotti and his collaborators have utilized the acid phosphatase reaction to identify semen in vaginal secretions.

The first examination of a fresh specimen is best carried out in a wet smear in which some of the vaginal contents are removed on a round glass rod or a platinum loop to a microscope slide, mixed with a drop of water or 0.9 per cent saline solution, and covered with a cover glass. The examination is made with the high power objective of the microscope. Spermatozoa, if present, will be seen as small objects with a pear-shaped head about one third of the diameter of a red blood corpuscle, behind which is a short neck and then a tail about 10 to 12 times as long as the head. As a rule they occur in small groups of three to seven. Their appearance is characteristic. Occasionally a motile protozoan, the *Trichomonas vaginalis,* is found in the vagina, but it should not be confused with the spermatozoan as the two differ markedly in appearance.

If a permanent mount is desired, the wet specimen can be smeared carefully on a slide, allowed to dry naturally, and then fixed in methyl alcohol for three minutes, or fixed by passing the slide rapidly three times through a flame. It may be stained by Loeffler's methylene blue solution for a minute, washed in water, dried and examined with an oil immersion lens. Carbolfuchsin solution diluted 5 times, or Gram's aniline gentian violet without dilution, may be employed in place of the methylene blue. Spermatozoa in the fresh condition show a deeply stained posterior

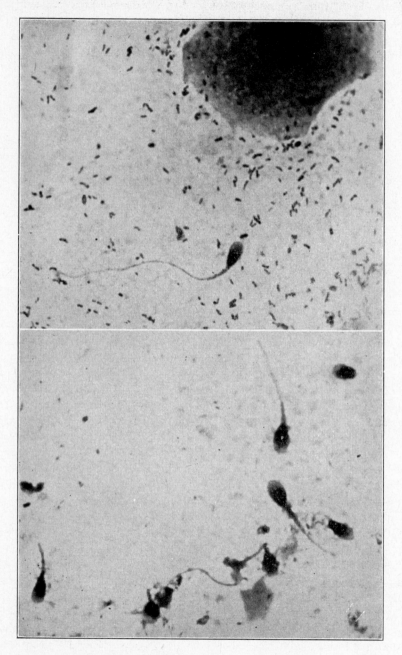

Fig. 24-3. Demonstration of Human Spermatozoa.

Top. Spermatozoon in smear of vaginal contents in case of rape and strangulation. Note bacterial flora and epithelial cell from vagina.

Bottom. Spermatozoa found in dry seminal stain on bed cover from same case. Oil immersion magnification. Note uneven staining of the head of each spermatozoon, the posterior half staining more deeply. The tails in the dry specimen are fragmented.

half of the head, while the anterior half of the head and the tail are either faintly stained or not stained at all (Fig. 24-3).

A useful stain for fresh specimens is the one recommended by Cary and Hotchkiss. It is of value in the study of sterility, where the specimens have been collected directly from a male subject, as this method brings out the degenerative changes in the spermatozoa. The procedure is as follows:

The secretion is smeared on a slide and fixed for 1 minute in Schaudinn's solution (mercuric chloride solution 7 per cent, 2 parts; absolute alcohol, one part) after which the following steps are carried out:
1. Place in 50 per cent alcohol for one-half minute.
2. Place in distilled water (which contains 2 drops of tincture of iodine for every 3 ounces) for one-half minute.
3. Wash in tap water.
4. Stain for one-half minute in 5 per cent aqueous eosin.
5. Place for one minute in 50 per cent alcohol contaning 2 drops of hydrochloric acid to every 3 ounces.
6. Wash in distilled water.
7. Stain in hematoxylin two and a half minutes.
8. Place in distilled water containing 2 drops of glacial acetic acid for every 3 ounces.
9. Wash in distilled water, dry and mount.

Dried Specimens. Seminal stains may occur on clothing from spontaneous emission or they may be smears on pieces of cloth which have been used in wiping the genital organs. Like fresh seminal material, the dry stains are easily eradicated by soap and water or destroyed by antiseptic chemicals. Sometimes they occur in large numbers in association with other spots and it is necessary to employ a macroscopic method to select those areas which are likely to yield the most promising results on microscopic examination. Ultraviolet rays directed on a dried seminal spot will cause the area to show a luminous fluoresence, and though the test is not specific, the rays help to localize a spot which is worth investigating. The same considerations apply in the use of a 0.01 per cent solution of alizarin sodium sulfate in distilled water, which on application to a suspected seminal spot produces a violet color if semen is present. These methods have the advantage of not interfering with further examination of the stains. The Florence reaction and the Barbiero reaction are reliable tests for substances normally present in semen and other organic material and so are not specific tests, merely serving to indicate suspicious areas. These procedures destroy that part of the seminal stain which is used for the reaction.

The acid phosphatase reaction as described by Kaye, and Benotti and his collaborators is also recommended as a test for identifying seminal stains. Walker more recently devised a rapid color test for such stains based on the histochemical technic of Seligman and Manheimer for demonstrating acid phosphatase. The fabric with the suspicious stain is immersed in a bath containing alpha-naphthyl phosphate as a substrate and a diazonium salt. The acid phosphatase in semen reacts with the phosphate ester to liberate alpha-naphthol which combines immediately with the diazonium salt to form a brilliant orange-red azo pigment. This procedure does not interfere with subsequent microscopic search for spermatozoa in the stain.

In the Florence reaction the following solution is used: dissolve 1.65 gm. potassium iodide in 30 ml. of distilled water and then dissolve 2.54 gm. iodine crystals. A small piece of the specimen is placed on a slide and a drop of distilled water is added. The preparation is allowed to stand for a minute or two. A drop of the solution mentioned above is placed near the edge of the dissolved specimen, and both are covered with a cover glass. Where the fluids meet, brown rhombic crystals form and indicate a positive reaction for choline, a constituent of semen.

The Barbiero reaction consists in adding a saturated solution of picric acid in distilled water to a drop of the suspected material as prepared above. Yellow ellipsoid and needle-like crystals of small size form and indicate the presence of spermine, another constituent of seminal secretions.

Microscopic examination of a dried specimen is done by teasing a small piece in a drop of distilled water on a slide. In cases in which the semen is adherent to a hard nonabsorbent surface the dried stain is scraped off with a sharp instrument and allowed to soften and disintegrate in the water. If the dried semen is incorporated in an absorbent fabric a small piece is cut away from the central portion and allowed to soak for several hours in the distilled water, and after teasing thoroughly, the preparation on the slide is allowed to dry overnight under a covered dish to exclude dust. Then it may be stained by any of the staining methods already described. In old specimens as a rule the entire spermatozoon stains more or less homogeneously. The presence of both head and tail is considered necessary for the diagnosis of a spermatozoon. Care must be taken in old specimens not to confuse them with bacterial spores.

Hektoen and Rukstinat have described a method by which the spermatozoa are stained in situ on a piece of cloth. A small piece of the suspected area on the fabric is allowed to stand in 1 per cent ammonium hydroxide solution in water overnight, after which it may be boiled for one minute in water. A single thread is selected and stained two minutes in 5 per cent aqueous solution of erythrosin, and then washed quickly in distilled water. It is placed in a 10 per cent aqueous solution of ferric chloride for two minutes, and it is then put directly in a 2 per cent aqueous solution of hematoxylin for two minutes. After washing quickly in distilled water the fiber is transferred to an 0.5 per cent aqueous ferric chloride solution and teased out to shreds. When the shreds are reddish pink or light brown it is washed in distilled water quickly, dehydrated in absolute alcohol, cleared in creosote and mounted in balsam. A good differentiation of the cell is obtained by this method.

Pollak has described a method in which the stained cloth is digested in concentrated sulfuric acid at 50° C. until the cloth is destroyed, and the material to be examined is left behind and may be mounted on a slide under a cover slip. The approximate number of spermatozoa in the specimen can be determined by this method.

Pollak also describes a method by which the cloth with the seminal spot is treated by boiling in water 15 minutes and then passing it through changes of alcohols from 70 to 100 per cent, through petrolatum and into paraffin in which it is embedded and then sectioned. The sections which should be 4 to 6 μ thick, are stained with erythrosin and iron-hematoxylin.

Farnum has devised a biologic test for semen which is a precipitin reaction like the corresponding process used to identify blood. Human semen is injected into rabbits over a period of three or more weeks at regular intervals, an antiserum is obtained, and the test is performed in a way similar to the blood precipitin test. The antisera for human blood will give a positive reaction for semen and may be used to identify a suspected seminal stain as one of human origin. The antisera for human semen will identify the stain as human semen, if it is strongly positive. These tests are useful when the question arises, as in a case of bestiality, as to whether the material is of human origin or derived from an animal. The group specific agglutinogen in a seminal fluid may be sought after by the method outlined in Chapter 27. It may be a matter of importance to see if the group specificity of the seminal fluid is the same as that of the suspect in the case under consideration.

REFERENCES

Benotti, M. S., Rosenberg, L., and Dewey, B.   Modification of the Gutman and Gutman method of estimating acid phosphatase activity, J. Lab. & Clin. Med., 31 (3), 1946.

Cary, W. H., and Hotchkiss, R. S.   Semen appraisal, J.A.M.A., 102:590, 1934.

Chaddock, C. G.   Rape and Sexual Perversions; Rape, p. 1033; Unnatural Sexual Offenses, p. 1047; from Peterson, Haines, and Webster, Legal Medicine and Toxicology, Philadelphia, W. B. Saunders Co., 1923, Vol. 1.

Farnum, C. G.   The biologic test for semen, J.A.M.A., 37:1721, 1901.

Hektoen, L.   Specific precipitin test for human semen, J.A.M.A., 78:704, 1922.

———— and Rukstinat, G. L.   Identification of human seminal stains, Arch. Path., 6:96, 1928.

Herzog, A.   Medical Jurisprudence, Indianapolis, Bobbs-Merrill Co., 1931.

Kaye, S.   Identification of seminal stains, J. Crim. Law and Criminol., 38:79, 1947.

Pollak, O. J.   Semen and seminal stains, Arch. Path., 35:140, 1943.

Seligman, A. M., and Manheimer, L. H.   New method for histochemical demonstration of acid phosphatase, J. Nat. Cancer Inst., 9:427, 1949.

Smith, S.   Forensic Medicine, London, J. and H. Churchill, ltd., 1940.

Walker, J. T.   A new test for seminal stains, New England J. Med., 242:110, 1950.

25

Impotence: Sterility: Hermaphrodism: Monstrosities

IMPOTENCE AND STERILITY

Impotence can be defined as the inability to have sexual intercourse. It can affect both male and female. Sterility is the inability of the male to beget children, and in the female it is inability to conceive children. Impotence and sterility are associated frequently, but are not synonymous. A person can be sterile without being impotent, and can accomplish coition without being able to impregnate or to be impregnated, as the case may be. Conversely, he can be impotent without being sterile though, obviously, the inability to perform the sexual act would have the same effect as absolute sterility.

The questions of impotence and sterility are sometimes important in criminal and civil actions. In criminal prosecutions for rape or seduction the defendant may claim that he is impotent, and thus could not have been guilty of the crime. In trials over a question of legitimacy or paternity, a man may aver that he is impotent, or sterile, or both, and so could not be the father of the child. Many actions for divorce are based upon impotence or sterility in either husband or wife. Where there has been injury to the genital tract, a claim may be made that impotence or sterility has resulted therefrom.

The age of the individual has a distinct bearing upon these questions. Normally, the male becomes fertile at the age of 14 to 16 years, and fertility may last until the age of 70 or 80 years. Each case must be decided individually, and it may be said that as long as live spermatozoa are present in the seminal fluid, the individual must be presumed to be fertile. Herzog mentions cases of abnormal sexual development in small boys of three and one-half to four years, and says that pregnancy has resulted from sexual intercourse with boys nine years old.

Impotence is either functional or organic. The functional causes include debilitating chronic diseases, masturbation, drug addiction, neurasthenia and various psychic disturbances. In such cases the physician may not be able to decide the question of whether impotence exists or not, especially since it can occur with apparently normal sexual organs. If an organic condition is present, however, the physician may discover enough evidence on which to form an opinion. The anatomic organic causes of impotence are castration, congenital deficiency of the testicles associated with infantilism, malformations and diseases of the external genitals, like epispadias, hypospadias, carcinoma of the penis, massive hernias, injuries, traumatic amputation and marked edema.

It is also possible for an impotent male to have normal or increased libido, so that he can commit an indecent assault even though he is not capable of coitus. This peculiarity is found especially in cases of senile dementia.

In the female a state of impotence may be the result of some organic defect of the genitalia, as an abnormal narrowing or a disease of the vagina, or lesions of other parts of the genital tract. Organic defects, as a rule, can be diagnosed without much trouble. Cases of functional impotence, on the other hand, may be hard to evaluate; most of these are essentially cases of frigidity and not impotence in the strict sense of the word.

Sterility is caused by debilitating diseases, diseases of the testicles, castration, traumas, gonorrheal inflammation of the genital tract or previous excessive coitus over a long period of time. As a rule the seminal fluid in such cases may not contain living spermatozoa, or it may contain a large proportion of malformed spermatozoa as described by Moench and Holt. A complete absence of spermatozoa in the semen is sometimes seen in sterile males who are otherwise healthy.

Sterility in women occurs normally with the menopause (Chapter 21). It can be associated with diseased conditions producing a hyperacid vaginal secretion, with obstructions of the genital canal, with an infantile uterus, with a bilateral gonorrheal salpingitis, or with an abdominal operation during which the genital organs have been removed.

In questions about marriage, a physician may be summoned to testify upon matters which may be concerned with its annulment or divorce. These matters comprise a wide range of subjects: impotence, sterility, paternity, virginity, proof of previous pregnancy, venereal disease, mental disorders, insanity, alcoholism and drug habits. He may be asked to testify on the subject of physical cruelty and mental cruelty of either the wife or the husband. The court, in cases concerning impotence, can order a medical examination of the parties concerned.

In divorce proceedings the examining physician may be asked to determine whether or not impotence or sterility was present prior to marriage, inasmuch as grounds for divorce exist if either partner conceals such defects at the time of wedlock.

The court rulings in these matters vary with the different jurisdictions, and it would not be profitable to try to unravel the various inconsistencies in judicial practice on the subject. The tendency is to end marital relationship in cases in which the spouse has a disease or a habit which makes married life for the other unbearable. The courts are not likely to grant a divorce or an annulment in instances where a defect was acquired after marriage and is not due to the fault of the defendant, unless, of course, it is of such a nature that married life would be impossible. They are prone, however, to declare for an annulment if the defendant, whether husband or wife, was guilty of fraud in concealing the true state of affairs from the plaintiff until after marriage. The testimony of a physician involved in such cases would be concerned largely with the nature of the diseased condition and what relation it would have to the considerations just mentioned.

When the spermatozoa of the husband are viable, but where obstacles to coition exist, the semen of the husband may be injected artificially into the uterus of the wife. This operation is termed artificial insemination and in many cases has resulted in pregnancy according to expectation. Herzog says that under such conditions the husband could be considered the father of the child.

Possible situations are mentioned in which the wife may be anxious to have a child and cannot because the husband's semen is not fertile. If she should resort to artificial insemination with the fertile semen of another man, a number of medico-legal complications would arise concerning the wife's and donor's adultery, the liability of the physician, the liability of the man from whom the semen was taken, inheritance and the legitimacy and paternity of the child. The subject has not received much attention from the courts in the United States, but it may in the future.

The prevention of conception is another phase of the problem of sterility. There are two ways of accomplishing this result.

1. One is by the methods of contraception which are intended to prevent each separate act of sexual intercourse from causing impregnation. There are various procedures, of greater or lesser efficacy, for producing this result, such as coitus interruptus, or the use of vaginal suppositories, tents, douches or condoms. The only legal complication likely to arise is concerned with the sale of such articles as contraceptives which is a criminal offense in some states. Other states allow their sale if the ostensible purpose of their use is the prevention of disease but their frank sale for contraceptive purposes is not permitted.

Occasionally more dangerous methods of preventing conception have been employed by the women concerned, or by physicians willing to oblige their patients, and the patients have died as the result of such treatment. Among these methods may be mentioned the injection of solutions of phenol, Lysol, or mercuric chloride into the genital tract to destroy spermatozoa, thus producing a corrosive effect on those organs which results in death. A case of this type investigated by Dr. Philip Goldstein was that of a woman whose family physician injected a solution of creosote as a contraceptive, and the victim died of the resulting pseudomembranous inflammation of the vagina and endometrium, combined with the general action of the drug. A doctor employing therapeutic measures of this type which result in death is guilty of criminal malpractice and could be charged with homicide.

2. The other method of preventing conception is by an operation which causes sterilization. In the male this is accomplished by resecting a portion of the vas deferens on each side, and in the female by resecting the fallopian tubes; the patient is usually sterilized permanently by this procedure, but the method does not diminish the capacity for sexual intercourse. Surgical sterilization has been performed therapeutically in women suffering from debilitating diseases. The surgeon who performs a sterilizing operation must be absolutely certain of his authority, for otherwise he would expose himself to a civil action for malpractice.

Compulsory sterilization for idiots and criminals has been enacted into law in some states. Some of these laws have been declared unconstitutional, and some have been sustained by the supreme courts of the various states. There is far from a unanimity of opinion on this subject in the various jurisdictions.

HERMAPHRODISM

By the term hermaphrodism is meant the presence of male and female gonads and sexual organs in the same individual. There is practically never a combination of perfectly developed and functioning male and female sexual organs in one person; one set or the other, or both, show faulty development. In some individuals the malformation may be so extreme that it may not be possible to determine the sex.

Normally the sex organs are laid down in embryonic life by the development of the genital ridge, the wolffian bodies and ducts and the mullerian ducts in a certain definite fashion for each sex. In the male the genital ridge forms the testis, the wolffian body and ducts form the epididymis, vas deferens and seminal vesicle, while the mullerian ducts atrophy and are represented by the prostatic utricle, and the appendages of the testes. In the female the genital ridge becomes the ovary, the mullerian ducts develop into uterus and tubes, and the wolffian structures form Gärtner's canal, paroophoron and epoophoron. The external genitalia form in similar fashion in both sexes; the male genitalia have their homologues in the female genitalia. Thus the male scrotum corresponds to the female labia majora, the labia minora in the female to the penile sheath in the male, and the penis and clitoris are homologous. In hermaphrodites disturbances of development occur and the genitalia are mal-formed because of faulty embryonic growth. Badly formed male and female organs are present in varying combinations.

1. True hermaphrodism includes those cases in which the gonads are combina-tions of ovary and testis forming an organ known as an ovotestis, or are ovaries associated with testes. There are several varieties: (a) Bilateral true hermaphrod-ism in which on both sides there is an ovotestis, or one testis plus one ovary. (b) Unilateral true hermaphrodism which is further differentiated into the complete and the incomplete types. The complete type shows on one side either one testis plus one ovary or an ovotestis, and on the other side either one testis or one ovary. The incomplete type shows on one side either one testis plus one ovary or an ovotestis, and on the other side no sexual gland at all. (c) Alternating true her-maphrodism in which an ovary is present on one side and a testis on the other. For the further elaborations of this classification the reader is referred to the works of Kaufmann and Young.

Helpern has reported a case of true unilateral hermaphrodism in an autopsy on a Negro of 37 years who had an ovotestis in the scrotum on the right side con-nected by the round ligament with the right side of the uterus, and a fallopian tube and ovary attached to the uterus in their usual position on the left side of the abdomen; a vagina extended from the uterus and communicated with the urethra. The external genital organs were of the male type with a short hypospadiac penis, and the physical habitus was masculine aside from distinctly female breasts and feminine hair distribution around the pubis. According to the previous history the libido was that of a male, the subject having been married and having had frequent carnal connection with his wife who, however, was never impregnated by him. There were indications that the deceased had menstruated, such as the corpora lutea in the ovary and the condition of the endometrium, but this could not be confirmed by history. For further discussion of this case the original article should be consulted.

2. Spurious hermaphrodism is associated with malformation of the genitalia to such a degree that the external organs apparently indicate one sex while the internal genitalia indicate the other sex. One variety is called pseudohermaphrodismus masculinus in which the individual has a pocket-like cleft simulating a vagina, a small penis and cryptorchid testes, so that while really a male, his external charac-teristics are those of a female. Another variety known as pseudohermaphrodismus femininus possesses a large clitoris and large labia majora so that the external appearance of the genital organs is that of a male, even though the internal gonads are ovaries. Some cases have large adrenal glands and small female genital organs, even though the body conformation is distinctly masculine.

When it is impossible to determine whether the individual is predominantly male or female, legal complications may ensue concerning sexual and marital relation-ships, in the matter of inheritance or in civil duties. A marriage, for example, be-tween a man and an individual who is supposedly a woman, but who really is a pseudohermaphrodismus masculinus, would be voidable from the beginning.

Herzog notes that hermaphrodites cannot bear children in the normal fashion, but that it might be possible for one to beget children. This would depend largely on the apparatus for seminal emission which the hermaphrodite might possess.

The decision of the sex in the case of hermaphrodites may be a difficult proposition, and a medical man should declare his inability to arrive at a decision, if he cannot see his way to make a positive diagnosis. If the case is a small child he can suggest that the matter be left open until puberty, when the sex may be determinable. In many instances, however, the true sex cannot be demonstrated except by operation or by a necropsy, and sometimes even these procedures do not supply the answer. Many hermaphrodites drift into sexual perversion and sometimes commit suicide. Because of the malformation of the genital organs and endocrine disturbances which often arise, hermaphrodites occasionally have difficulty in adjusting themselves to the society in which they live.

MONSTROSITIES

Monstrosities can be defined as malformations of the embryo, so deformed that they are unlike the normal human type. This subject is a subdivision of teratology.

Monsters occur with excess of parts, defects of parts or wrong position of internal organs. The definition of the law is a trifle vague concerning monstrosities, and probably each jurisdiction would have its own interpretation.

There are legal complications to be considered. In some jurisdictions the law denies the right of inheritance to monstrosities. The question of infanticide may arise, if a physician, nurse or midwife in attendance during the birth of a living monstrosity should destroy it. Fortunately, most monstrosities are not viable for any length of time after they leave the uterus. Slight deformities do not render an infant or a person a monster.

The only monstrosities which grow to adult life are some of the many varieties of Siamese twins, who are united in the umbilical region or at the pelvis. Some organs are shared in common, in several cases the vagina and the rectum. Interesting medicolegal complications may arise after the marriage of one or both of such twins especially if there are any offspring. Separation of the twins is rarely possible. Usually when one dies, the other dies also.

REFERENCES

Healey, C. E., and Gay, C. C.   Pseudohermaphroditismus masculinus externus, Arch. Path., 12:543, 1931.

Helpern, M.   True hermaphroditism, Arch. Path., 28:768, 1939. Trans. of New York Pathological Society.

Herzog, A. W.   Medical Jurisprudence, Indianapolis, The Bobbs-Merrill Co., 1931.

Kaufmann, E.   Lehrbuch der speziellen Pathologischen Anatomie, Berlin and Leipzig, Walter de Gruyter and Co., 1922, p. 1148.

Levinson, S. A., editor.   Artificial Insemination; Its Medicolegal Implications. Symposium of Medicolegal Problems, Philadelphia, J. B. Lippincott Co., 1948, pp. 43-87.

Moench, G. L., and Holt, H.   Sperm morphology in relation to fertility, Am. J. Obst. & Gynec., 22:99, 1931.

Seymour, F. I., and Koerner, A.   Medicolegal aspect of artificial insemination, J.A.M.A., 107:1531, 1936.

Young, H. H.   Genital Abnormalities, Hermaphroditism and Related Adnexal Diseases, Baltimore, Williams & Wilkins, 1937.

26

Examination of Blood

Tests for the identification of blood are employed as an important part of the routine investigation in many cases of violent death. Sometimes the specimen to be examined is fresh fluid blood or clotted blood collected at the scene of a crime. More often it is brought to the laboratory in the form of dried red or brown stains on weapons, clothing or other objects. Whenever such specimens are received, they should be formally identified to the examiner by the messenger who brings them, according to the procedure discussed on pages 11 and 95, so that the results of the examination can be connected with the other evidence in the case. The object of the examination is to determine whether or not the stain is blood which is usually accomplished by microscopic, chemical or spectroscopic examination, and then whether or not the specimen is human in origin which is done by the precipitin reaction. The significance of the findings will depend upon the nature of the individual case and upon the problems which may present themselves.

Whenever the examiner receives a weapon or other object, he should scrutinize it carefully, noting the distribution of the stain and its appearance. Sometimes hairs, fibers, fragments of tissues and other particles are adherent to the surface of the weapon or object, and these should be detached for microscopic examination. After this, parts of the stain should be prepared for blood examination. The examiner should mark the weapon or object with his initials and the date so that he can identify it at any future time if it is introduced as evidence in a homicide case.

Examination of the specimen should determine: (1) if the stain is blood; (2) if it is animal or human blood; and (3) if it is human blood, what blood groups are present. The methods employed to examine suspicious stains are visual inspection, microscopic examination, chemical analysis, spectroscopic investigation and serologic tests.

Inspection. Visual examination may determine whether or not a stain is blood or some other red substance like paint, vegetable coloring or aniline dyes. Ordinarily fresh fluid or clotted blood is easy to recognize, but when it is altered by age, high temperature or contact with other substances, identification may be difficult. Discharges from the body such as gastric secretion, mucus, urine or fecal matter, if mixed with blood may alter its appearance. Agencies such as fire or chemicals may destroy blood.

At the scene of a crime, the relation of the body of the deceased to blood which has been shed is important (Figs. 2-3 and 2-4). For example, a person stabbed in the neck may stagger away leaving a trail of blood on the ground in the form of large drops, or he may collapse where he was stabbed and shed a large pool of blood around him. If a small artery is cut, the blood will spurt in the form of small drops which may impinge against a smooth surface and form characteristic patterns. If the drop strikes at right angles, an irregularly circular stain with serrated edges is produced; if it strikes obliquely, the stain has a bowling pin shape, with the head of the pin pointing in the direction of the flight of the drop (Fig. 26-1).

Drops of spattered blood will form similar figures. In many instances it is possible to locate the source of these flying drops by the patterns which they form on surfaces. If a person has been bleeding profusely and a struggle has taken place, stains and smears of blood will be present over the floor walls and furniture.

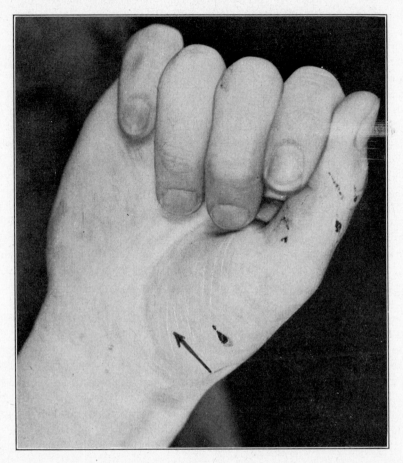

Fig. 26-1. Drops of Blood Spurted onto Thenar Eminence of Palm.

The tapering end of the drop indicates the direction toward which the drop was traveling when it struck the hand. Case of suicide by shooting in right temple. Gun was held in right hand which was splashed by blood from entrance wound.

Inspection may help in determining the origin of a flow of blood from the body orifices. If it comes from the lungs, numerous bubbles may be present. If it comes from the stomach, it may be brownish in tinge from the action of the acid gastric juice. The location of a stain on the clothing is important since hemorrhage from the mouth, nose or ears will stain the clothing on the upper part of the body, while blood from the vaginal or rectal regions will soil the nether garments.

The estimation of the age of a hemorrhage is based upon the appraisal of the postmortem changes present; these are regulated by the size of the effusion among other factors. A small drop clots and dries rapidly and the different changes are not easy to distinguish. With a large hemorrhage there may be distinct and visible separation of a red clot and serum. The pool of blood begins to dry at its edges and may be completely dry in from 12 to 36 hours, depending on its size and the external conditions. As it grows older it begins to darken and in from 10 to 12 days it is dark brownish-red in color. If the stain is present on a hard, nonabsorbent surface it becomes cracked and chipped, presenting a dark brown scaly appearance.

There are no criteria which enable the examiner to judge the age of different stains with any degree of certainty. The clotting time, for example, is altered by many circumstances or influences. Cold retards it and heat accelerates it. It is more rapid on a rough surface and slower on a smooth surface. Oily substances may not only increase the clotting time, but may alter the appearance of the blood. Even the peculiarities of the individual blood may affect the clotting time.

Microscopic Examination. Microscopic examination is useful for the demonstration and mensuration of the blood corpuscles, for making the distinction between mammalian, avian, piscine and reptilian blood, and for the investigation of menstrual, lochial and nasal discharges. On rare occasions blood abnormalities and parasites may be detected.

The microscopic examination of dried blood is made by taking two small fragments of the specimen and placing each in a drop of physiologic salt solution (0.9 per cent) on separate slides. The slides are put in a covered dish to prevent evaporation and the preparations are allowed to stand for an hour or two. One of the slides is examined as a wet preparation. It is covered with a coverslip and the cells observed with a high dry power. If the corpuscles are mammalian, they appear as characteristic, nonnucleated disks. The camel family have oval nonnucleated red cells. Bird, fish, and reptile corpuscles are larger, oval and nucleated; those of the lamprey eel are circular and nucleated.

The other preparation is spread evenly over the slide and allowed to dry. It is stained by one of the following methods:

The dried preparation is fixed in absolute methyl alcohol for three minutes. It is stained in a 0.5 per cent aqueous solution of water-soluble eosin for one to three minutes. Löffler's methylene blue is added for one to three minutes. The red blood cells stain with eosin, while the methylene blue stains the nuclei.

WRIGHT'S STAIN. The unfixed smear is flooded with the stain, and allowed to stand for one minute. Distilled water is added drop by drop until a metallic scum forms on the surface; it is allowed to stand three minutes, and then washed in water and dried.

GIEMSA'S STAIN. The stain is prepared by adding 10 drops of the full-strength Giemsa's solution to 10 ml. of distilled water. The dried smear is fixed in pure methyl or ethyl alcohol for three minutes. The alcohol is poured off and the slide is flooded with the prepared stain. It is stained for 15 minutes in a covered dish to prevent evaporation, washed in water, dried, and examined with a $\frac{1}{12}$ inch oil immersion lens.

The corpuscles in old blood specimens are likely to color deeply and it may be necessary to dilute the staining fluids. Wright's stain may be diluted with methyl alcohol. Giemsa's stain is diluted by using 5 drops of stain instead of 10 with the distilled water.

If the blood is mammalian it may be desirable to determine the average diameter of the red blood corpuscles. For this purpose, fresh and stained specimens are used and the cells selected for measurement should be well preserved. A micrometer eyepiece is employed in taking the measurements, and a large number of readings on different cells must be taken. The human red blood corpuscle has a diameter about $\frac{1}{3200}$ of an inch. The erythrocyte of the dog measures $\frac{1}{3500}$ inch, and of the domestic animals its size is the nearest to the human. Mensuration of corpuscles has only a limited value in any event, and the precipitin test has generally superseded it because it is more conclusive.

There are times when the blood corpuscles are observed as faint outlines or blood shadows because they have come in contact with water or some other hemolytic agent. The blood cells may be completely destroyed and the microscopic examination cannot be used. Under such conditions, chemical, spectroscopic and serologic tests must be employed to determine the nature of the specimen.

The microscopic examination of vaginal and nasal hemorrhages will show, as a rule, mucus, epithelial cells and bacteria. If nasal or vaginal inflammation is present, pus cells also may be found.

Vaginal hemorrhages, according to Smith, characteristically show numerous cocci and bacilli and large squamous epithelial cells, some of which give the iodophil reaction. This test is performed by dissolving a small amount of the blood specimen in a few drops of saturated sodium bicarbonate solution on a slide, adding a drop of Lugol's solution (iodine 2, potassium iodide 3, water 40), and examining under a coverglass. If the blood specimen is menstrual, red brown iodophil cells may be seen on microscopic examination.

A dried smear of the same specimen may be stained with carbolfuchsin in the same manner as for tubercle bacilli, except that the decolorizing fluid is an acid solution without alcohol. If this technic demonstrates smegma bacilli it would be strong evidence in favor of a vaginal origin of the stain.

Chemical Analysis. The chemical tests for blood are based upon the reactions of hemoglobin and its derivatives. They are used merely to demonstrate the presence of blood, and cannot be employed to differentiate the blood of different species.

The specimens of blood are usually prepared by dissolving them in normal saline solution or distilled water. The older the specimen, the longer it takes for it to go into solution; in some instances about 24 hours are required. If the blood to be examined has been subjected to heat or to any other destructive agent, it may be necessary to dissolve it in glacial acetic acid (Katayama test). When it is impregnated in cloth a small piece of the cloth should be teased in the diluting fluid. Where an attempt has been made to wash the stain from a garment or other absorbent material, the following method of concentration may be carried out before proceeding to the chemical tests.

A large piece of the cloth is placed in a porcelain dish and soaked in distilled water containing a few crystals of potassium iodide. The cloth may be folded and pressed with a glass rod to facilitate solution of the stain. The solution is filtered into a flask and the filtrate is acidulated with acetic acid. A saturated solution of sodium tungstate acidified with acetic acid is added and the solution is brought to a boil. The precipitate is collected on a filter, washed and dried. It may be tested then by Teichmann's hemin test.

TEICHMANN'S HEMIN REACTION. A drop of distilled water is placed on a slide and a crystal of sodium chloride is added. A small fragment of the blood specimen or of the residue from the method described above is mixed with the fluid. The mixture is gently heated to dryness and the spot covered with a coverglass. Glacial acetic acid is run under the glass; the preparation is warmed until a few bubbles indicate the beginning of boiling. It is allowed to cool and then examined under the microscope. If the specimen contains blood, dark brown rhombic hemin crystals will form. The test will not react with burned or heated blood.

GUAIACUM TEST (VAN DEEN). A fresh test solution is prepared by adding a few lumps of guaiac resin to 95 per cent alcohol, and then filtering. A small amount of the suspected blood specimen is diluted with water in a test tube. To this are added some drops of the test solution and a drop or two of hydrogen peroxide. If blood is present a blue color will result. As the test reacts with many substances other than blood, it is most valuable when it is negative and eliminates blood as a possibility.

BENZIDINE TEST. The test solution must be freshly prepared by dissolving a small amount of powdered benzidine in glacial acetic acid. A few drops of this are added to a solution of the suspected blood stain in a test tube, and then a few drops of hydrogen peroxide are added. A blue color indicates a positive reaction. This test is more sensitive than the guaiac test and is valuable as a negative test.

PHENOLPHTHALEIN TEST. The reagent is prepared by adding 1 to 2 gm. of phenolphthalein to 100 ml. of a 25 per cent solution of potassium hydroxide in distilled water. One gram of powdered zinc is added and the solution is heated in a reflux apparatus until it is colorless. A few drops of this reagent are added to a watery solution of the suspected blood stain, followed by the addition of a few drops of hydrogen peroxide. In the presence of blood a rose color develops. This test is delicate, and similar to the guaiac and benzidine tests in its applications. It is valuable in eliminating stains not blood when a large number of specimens must be examined.

HEMOCHROMOGEN TEST. This test is a positive indication of blood pigment and reacts with no other substance. The reagent is made as follows:

Sodium hydroxide (10 per cent solution)	6 ml.
Pyridin	6 ml.
Glucose (saturated solution)	6 ml.
Distilled water	14 ml.

This solution must be kept in an amber colored bottle.

A small fragment of the specimen to be tested is placed on a slide, a drop of the reagent is added, and the preparation is covered with a coverslip. Irregular rhombic crystals of hemochromogen gradually appear and form feathery masses as the slide is warmed. They change from a salmon color to a brown color and then to a pink color. An examination through the microspectroscope reveals the spectrum for hemochromogen.

Spectroscopic Examination. The spectroscopic examination, like the chemical examinations, can be employed only to detect blood, but not to differentiate the blood of one species of animal from another. The test is performed by means of an optical instrument known as a spectroscope, which is so constructed that the absorption properties of translucent colored fluids can be observed on the solar spectrum. There are several types of spectroscopes, the usual large laboratory spectroscope, the smaller direct vision spectroscope and the microspectroscope which can be attached to an ordinary microscope. The last two instruments are used when only a minute quantity of blood is available.

The blood stain is dissolved in water or physiologic salt solution and then placed in a small glass chamber with parallel sides so arranged that the rays of light will pass directly through it. This chamber is placed in the spectroscope and the instrument is so adjusted that the spectrum is clearly visible. The solution of blood must be dilute. It has the property of absorbing some of the rays from the spectrum, producing characteristic dark absorption bands, which vary with the type of blood pigment present (Fig. 26-2).

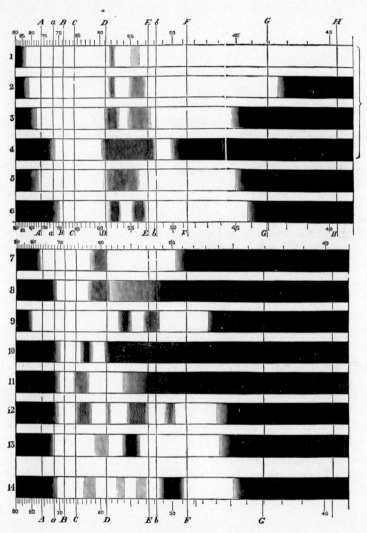

From Peterson, Haines and Webster, *Legal Medicine and Toxicology,* W. B. Saunders Co., 1923

Fig. 26-2. Various Spectra of Blood.

1, 2, 3, 4, oxyhemoglobin of various degrees of concentration; 5, hemoglobin; 6, carboxyhemoglobin; 7, 8, hematin in alkaline solution (dilute and concentrated); 9, hemochromogen (Stokes' reduced hematin); 10, methemoglobin; 11, acid hematin (blood treated with acetic acid); 12, acid hematin in alcoholic solution; 13, acid hematoporphyrin; 14, alkaline hematoporphyrin.

Oxyhemoglobin is marked by two bands in the yellow between Frauenhofer's lines, D and E. Hemoglobin shows a broad band, which lies between D and E with a small rim over D on the red side of the spectrum. Carboxyhemoglobin has a spectrum almost similar to oxyhemoglobin; it can be differentiated by the fact that its spectrum remains unchanged after the addition of ammonium sulfide, which reduces oxyhemoglobin to hemoglobin.

Methemoglobin is a derivative which contains the same amount of oxygen as oxyhemoglobin and is isomeric with it. Methemoglobin, however, is the more stable compound. Its absorption figure is a dark band in the red between C and D but nearer C. If the solution is diluted properly it splits into bands not unlike the bands of acid hematin.

Acid hematin gives several absorption bands. There is a sharp one between C and D but nearer C than D, while in between D and F is a broad band not clearly defined. By using alcoholic sulfuric acid solution in the test, several absorption bands may be formed.

Alkaline hematin is characterized by an absorption band between C and D. It also absorbs the violet end of the spectrum.

Hemochromogen gives a sharp and dark absorption band between D and E and a paler and broader band over E.

Hematoporphyrin in alkaline solution gives 4 absorption bands; a faint line between C and D, a broader band at D and extending towards E, a third band between D and E nearly at E, and a fourth broad band between E and F.

Hematoporphyrin in concentrated sulfuric acid gives a faint and narrow band between C and D but nearer D, and a dark, sharp and broad band between D and E.

Where the blood is fresh, the solution can be examined spectroscopically for oxyhemoglobin. A weak solution of ammonium sulfide is then added, and the absorption band of hemoglobin will be obtained. If a dilute solution of sodium hydroxide is added, the spectrum of hemochromogen appears. These reactions are proof of the presence of blood and also serve to eliminate substances of vegetable or animal origin which give spectra similar to oxyhemoglobin.

Older blood specimens, when diluted, may show methemoglobin as well as oxyhemoglobin. If a weak alkaline solution is added to one of these stains, alkaline hematin is formed. If a weak acid solution is added instead, acid hematin is produced.

If the blood specimen is old and decomposed, it is necessary to test for hematoporphyrin. This is done by adding strong sulfuric acid to part of the blood solution in which case acid hematoporphyrin will be obtained. The addition of a strong alkaline solution to another portion of the blood specimen will result in the formation of alkaline hematoporphyrin.

Serologic Examination. PRECIPITIN REACTION. Whenever an animal is injected with an antigen, like protein from another species of animal, an antibody called a precipitin develops in its serum and reacts specifically against that antigen. If serum of the immune or injected animal is brought in contact with a dilute solution of the protein or antigen in question, a whitish cloudy precipitate is formed. Thus when a rabbit is injected with human blood serum or whole human blood, the precipitins which develop in its serum will react with the proteins of human blood serum, other human body fluids and other human tissue extracts. The reaction is a specific one and, if positive, will identify blood proteins or any other protein as human in origin; the human antiserum will not react with protein from another animal species. The precipitin reaction will not identify a specimen as blood, except when the antiserum has been prepared specifically against human hemoglobin. As a general rule, whenever suspected blood stains are examined, the presence of blood is determined first by microscopic, chemical and spectroscopic methods, and then the precipitin reaction is employed to demonstrate the human origin of the specimen.

PREPARATION OF THE ANTISERUM. Rabbits furnish the most satisfactory antibodies, and the antiserum is prepared from them. Three or four of the animals are injected intravenously with 2 ml. of undiluted blood serum two or three times at five day intervals (Smith). Other workers supplement this course of injections with 4 or 5 ml. of whole blood given intraperitoneally six days after the last intravenous injection. Wiener uses a 1:10 dilution of blood serum in physiologic saline solution, 2 ml. of which is injected by the intravenous route on successive days for six or seven days; this course is followed by a rest period of one week after which a second series of injections is given subcutaneously, using the same amount of the diluted serum. Some animals develop potent sera after the second course while others require a third or fourth series. If time is a consideration, successive daily doses of 5, 10, and 15 ml. of undiluted serum or whole blood may be introduced into the peritoneal cavity, and the rabbits bled and the sera separated nine days after the last injection. In all these methods, the animals are bled in a week to 10 days after the last injection.

Regardless of the method which is used, the potency of the antiserum must be determined before the animal is finally bled. For this purpose, six clean test tubes, 0.5 cm. in diameter, are placed in a test tube rack. In the first and second tubes is placed 0.5 ml. of a 1:500 dilution of human blood serum in physiologic salt solution. To the diluted serum in the second tube is added 0.5 ml. of saline solution and the contents are thoroughly mixed; 0.5 ml. of this mixture is conveyed to the third tube and 0.5 ml. of saline solution is added and mixed. This procedure is continued to the three successive tubes, until the sixth tube contains 1 ml. of a very dilute solution, and 0.5 ml. of this last mixture is discarded. The tubes will then contain 0.5 ml. of the following dilutions: Tube 1, 1:500; Tube 2, 1:1,000; Tube 3, 1:2,000; Tube 4, 1:4,000; Tube 5, 1:8,000; Tube 6, 1:16,000.

The antiserum to be titered is drawn up in a fine pipet, and the point of the pipet is carried to the bottom of the first tube where the antiserum is allowed to flow slowly under the dilution until about 0.1 ml. has been delivered. The process is repeated in the other tubes, using separate pipets for each tube; as the antiserum is heavier than the dilution, it remains on the bottom. If desired, the antiserum may be placed in the six tubes first and the various dilutions of antigen layered over them, using a separate pipet for each dilution. If the antiserum reacts with a particular dilution, a white cloudy line will be observed at the contact point of the two fluids. A suitable antiserum should react immediately or within a minute on the 1:1,000 dilution; it will usually cause a reaction within 20 minutes on the 1:16,000 dilution. The serum of each rabbit must be titered separately and only those with the suitable titer should be reserved for the actual test. Such sera may be stored in the refrigerator in 1 ml. ampules or small bottles. As a further precaution a preservative may be added such as chloroform, 0.5 per cent phenol or a 1:10,000 dilution of merthiolate.

The specificity of the antiserum to human proteins may be determined by testing it in a similar manner with dilutions of 1:200 and 1:100 of sera from various domestic and food animals; the solutions should remain clear after 20 minutes. The rabbits are bled under sterile precautions when the serum for the test is prepared, as a satisfactory antiserum must be sterile and clear. Sterility may be obtained by passage through a Berkefeld or Seitz filter, and a clear serum is usually obtained if the animals are not fed for 18 to 24 hours prior to the collection of the antiserum.

Antisera against the blood proteins of other animals may be prepared in the same way as human antisera. It is desirable to have available sera of rabbits immunized against the blood proteins of other vertebrates, especially the more common domestic varieties or the more common food animals. For example, a defendant may claim that certain stains are from a piece of raw beef, and it might be imperative to test the truth of such an assertion by a precipitin test with bovine antisera.

PREPARATION OF SPECIMENS. Suspected stains may be submitted on a variety of objects such as weapons, wearing apparel, household furnishings or ornaments. Should the suspected stain be in the fluid state, a 1:1,000 dilution may be easily prepared. In most cases the stain is dry and only an approximate dilution can be made by dissolving a small amount of the material in a small quantity of 0.9 per cent saline solution. The resulting mixture should be clear, colorless and neutral in reaction, and if not it may be centrifuged or filtered through a Seitz filter; usually the dilution is neutral to litmus paper, but if it is acid or alkaline, it may be neutralized by 0.1 per cent solution of sodium hydroxide or hydrochloric acid respectively.

A sample of the diluted specimen at 1:1,000 should be tested for proteins by heating it in a test tube and adding a few drops of dilute acetic acid or a 25 per cent solution of nitric acid. A faint opalescence will indicate an approximately correct dilution. For further confirmation a part of the dilution is placed in one test tube and an equal amount of 0.9 per cent saline solution in another. If air is blown through each solution with a clean dry pipet, foam will appear on the surface of both fluids, and will persist in the tube containing the dilution, but will disappear quickly in the salt solution.

Old dried specimens of blood may be difficult to dissolve in 0.9 per cent of sodium chloride solution, and it may take a long time to extract such a specimen. If the process is over two hours in duration, the extraction should take place in the icebox, and a little chloroform should be added to inhibit bacterial growth.

The bloodless portion of the material from which the suspected specimen of blood is taken should be extracted with 0.9 per cent solution of sodium chloride, and the extract should be tested in some of the control tubes during the performance of the reaction. This is especially applicable to substances like cloth and leather which may have been in contact with human organic material and may contain elements which may produce false results with the precipitin reaction, and it would also apply to plaster which might be difficult to separate from the blood stain. In any event, it would be important to determine the presence or absence of organic matter which might react with the antiserum and thus interfere with the validity of the reaction of the antiserum on the suspected specimen.

TECHNIC OF PRECIPITIN REACTION. All glassware and pipets must be scrupulously clean and the saline solution uncontaminated. Six test tubes, 0.5 cm. in diameter, are prepared as follows:

Tube 1. 0.5 ml. of prepared dilution of suspected stain plus antiserum
Tube 2. 0.5 ml. of prepared dilution of suspected stain plus normal rabbit serum
Tube 3. 0.5 ml. of bloodless part of the material from which specimen was taken plus antiserum
Tube 4. 0.5 ml. of normal saline solution plus antiserum
Tube 5. 0.5 ml. of human blood serum at 1:1,000 dilution plus antiserum
Tube 6. 0.5 ml. of serum not human at 1:1,000 dilution plus antiserum

With a separate pipet for each tube, 0.1 ml. of antiserum is layered under the extracts in all the tubes except Tube 2, and in this tube the normal rabbit serum is placed under the antigen. A positive reaction for human proteins is indicated by the development of a white cloudy line at the contact points of the fluids in Tubes 1 and 5; this should appear immediately or within one or two minutes. If the test is negative only Tube 5 will show the white cloudy line, and the other tubes will remain clear at least 20 minutes or longer.

Antisera for other animal species should be kept on hand if it is necessary to test for the animal proteins of these species in blood sera or specimens. The antisera are specific for their respective antigens, and the test is performed as described above, substituting animal antiserum for human antiserum. It is also desirable to preserve bloods from different animal species as antigens, and the best method for storage is to keep them in a dried state on filter paper in the icebox, as under those conditions they are less likely to alter than if they are stored as liquids. They may also be preserved in dilutions of 1 : 100 in the icebox as fluids, a drop of chloroform being added to each container as a preventative of bacterial decomposition.

Other human proteins beside those of blood react with human antisera and may be detected by it. If a specimen of suspected tissue contains much fat, the fat must be extracted with ether before the tissue is prepared for the test. Other body proteins such as those from saliva, semen or mucus react with the antiserum formed against blood proteins of that species.

LIMITATIONS OF REACTION. The specificity and delicacy of the precipitin reaction is great, but the reaction may be inhibited or even destroyed by a number of factors. Chemicals such as acids, alkalis, alcohol, cresols, formaldehyde, corrosive sublimate or other germicides may alter the blood to such an extent that the reaction cannot be performed. Heat has the same effect; Hektoen and McNally mention that fluid blood loses its power of reacting with antiserum if it is heated from 60° to 90° C., while dried blood may withstand 150° C. Rust and postmortem decomposition may change blood so that the antiserum may react with it poorly. The age of the stain seems to have less influence, as old stains may be identified after a long period of time.

The specific sera not only produce a precipitin reaction with the blood proteins of a certain species of animal, but will react to a certain extent with the blood of closely related species of animals. Thus in the family of the ruminants, which includes kine, goats and sheep, antisera developed against the blood proteins of sheep will produce positive tests with the blood of cows and goats in high dilutions, and it may be difficult to differentiate the bloods of the different members of the family by the precipitin reaction. Human antisera acts similarly with the blood of apes and monkeys in low dilutions. To distinguish between them, the antiserum may be diluted 1:2 or 1:4, and the reaction may be carried out at these dilutions: under these conditions the homologous antigen alone will react with the antiserum. A more accurate method is to absorb the group precipitin in the antiserum with the heterogenous antigen; for fuller details of the method the reader is referred to Schiff and Boyd.

If the contention is advanced that a specimen of blood is not human but is from an animal like a dog, the precipitin reaction should be repeated, using dog antiserum in place of human antiserum. It would be important to determine whether or not dog's blood is present in the specimen. If both canine and human blood were combined in the same solution, they would react with their own specific antisera.

The precipitin reaction just described will not identify a specimen as blood, even though it determines that the specimen is human in origin. However, if the antiserum is prepared so that it acts specifically against human hemoglobin, it will demonstrate the presence of human blood in a stain. Extracts of this material are injected as described in the preparation of human protein antisera; washed human erythrocytes are used, the corpuscles are freed of plasma and laked in nine volumes of distilled water, after which the laked solution is made isotonic by adding one tenth volume of 10 per cent salt solution. After clearing by centrifugation or filtration, the solution is ready for use. The titer of the antihemoglobin serum must be carefully determined as hemoglobin has a relatively weak antigenic property (see reference to Hektoen and Schulhof).

An antiserum for human seminal fluid may be prepared by injecting rabbits with human semen and collecting the immune serum from the rabbits in the usual manner. The antiserum is not specific for seminal stains but reacts with other homologous proteins. According to Hektoen, these proteins can be prevented from reacting with the antiserum by absorbing the seminal antiserum with a 1:200 dilution of homologous blood serum; the antibodies for the homologous proteins are then removed, but the specific antibody for human semen remains and reacts with that antigen. This test is useful in cases in which spermatozoa cannot be demonstrated in a specimen by the usual microscopic methods.

The results obtained by blood examinations may furnish important links in a chain of evidence which is assembled to sustain a charge of assault or homicide. The demonstration of human blood on a weapon like a blunt instrument, hatchet or knife, which is suspected of having been used in the commission of a crime, is valuable confirmatory evidence which may support other testimony in the case, and is especially important if the instrument in question can be traced to the accused. If human hairs similar to those of the deceased are present in the dried blood on the weapon, or if the examiner can determine that the blood groups of the blood on the weapon are the same as those of the victim's blood, such evidence would be that much more significant. Police investigation, however, must connect the defendant with the crime and with the lethal weapon, otherwise the prosecution would not be able to introduce the results of the blood examination.

In other cases a defendant may attempt to explain the presence of blood stains on a weapon or on a garment by claiming that they are blood from some slaughtered animal and not human blood. The serologist must meet this problem by testing the stains with human antisera and antisera specific for the animal in question, and if these procedures prove the human origin of the specimen and the absence of animal proteins, these findings will be damaging to the defense case of the accused. If the defendant claims that a blood spot on his own clothing is his own blood from a nose bleed or an accidental wound, this problem must be solved through the isoagglutination reactions for the different blood groups (Chapter 27).

REFERENCES

Hektoen, L. The precipitin test for blood, J.A.M.A., 70:1273, 1918.
———— and McNally, W. D. In Peterson, Haines and Webster, Legal Medicine and Toxicology, Philadelphia, W. B. Saunders Co., 1923, Vol. II, p. 898.
———— and Schulhof, K. On specific erythroprecipitins, J. Infect. Dis., 31:32, 1922.
———— and Schulhof, K. Specific erythroprecipitins, J. Infect. Dis., 33:224, 1923.
———— and Rukinstat, G. J. Identification of human seminal stains, Arch. Path., 6:96, 1928.
Katayama, K. Vierteljahrsschrift f. gerichtl. Med., 49:269, 1888.
Nutall, G. H. F. Blood Immunity and Relationships, London, Cambridge University Press, 1904, p. 456.

Schiff, F., and Boyd, W. C.   Blood Grouping Technic, New York, Interscience Press, 1942, p. 163.

Smith, S.   Forensic Medicine, 4th ed., London, J. and A. Churchill, Ltd., 1934, p. 219.

Webster, R. W.   Legal Medicine and Toxicology, Philadelphia, W. B. Saunders Co., 1930.

Wiener, A. S.   Blood Groups and Transfusions, 3rd ed., Springfield, Ill., Charles C Thomas, 1946, p. 401.

27

The Human Blood Groups

Methods for the detection of human blood and for distinguishing it from the blood of other animals were described in Chapter 26. In this chapter the further differentiation of human blood is discussed, and due attention is given to its importance in solving problems of relationship in disputed paternity cases, or in investigating the source of blood stains in cases of rape, assault or homicide.

CLASSIFICATION OF THE A-B-O BLOOD GROUPS

A number of different groups of human blood are separated on the basis of the specific isoreactions which occur between the red blood cells and specific substances in the sera of different individuals. Furthermore, when human blood of a specific group is injected into another species of animal, a specific antibody for the group is formed in addition to the antibody for the human species. Such serologic reactions depend upon certain hereditary constant constitutional characters in human blood.

The most important isoreaction of human blood is isoagglutination in which the serum of one group agglutinates the red blood cells of another. Landsteiner in 1900 was the first to show that all human blood belongs to groups differentiated on the basis of the isoagglutination tests, and he described three distinct groups. Later a fourth and rarer group was recognized by Jansky and by Moss.

The groups are divided according to the following reactions:

Group O. Red cells are not agglutinated by sera of groups A, B or AB.

The serum of group O agglutinates red blood cells of groups A, B, and AB.

Group A. Red cells are agglutinated by sera of groups O and B.

The serum of group A agglutinates red blood cells of groups B and AB.

Group B. Red cells are agglutinated by sera of groups O or A.

The serum of group B agglutinates red blood cells of groups A and AB.

Group AB. Red cells are agglutinated by sera of groups O, A and B.

The serum of group AB is incapable of agglutinating the cells of any group.

The red blood cells of any one group, say group A, are not agglutinated by the serum of that same group, namely, group A, and this fact is the basis for using bloods of the same group in transfusion.

The classification just given was introduced by Landsteiner who named the four groups on the basis of the agglutinogen content of the red blood cells as indicated by the letters O, A, B, and AB. The agglutinins in the serum are indicated either by the Greek letters alpha and beta or by the terms anti-A and anti-B. The Landsteiner classification has superseded the designation of the groups by numbers, and it has been adopted by the Special Health Committee of the League of Nations and by the American Association of Immunologists.

Table 27-1 gives the Landsteiner classification and lists the percentage of each group in the white race. In eastern Europe and in Asia, the percentages of groups B and AB are higher than in western Europe.

Table 27-1.   Distribution of the four blood groups among Caucasoids

BLOOD GROUP	AGGLUTINOGEN PRESENT IN RED BLOOD CELLS	AGGLUTININS PRESENT IN SERUM	APPROXIMATE PERCENTAGE INCIDENCE AMONG CAUCASOIDS
O	O (none)	Anti-A or α and Anti-B or β	40 to 50
A	A	Anti-B or β	40 to 45
B	B	Anti-A or α	10 to 15
AB	A and B	none	3 to 6

The four blood groups differ merely because of the different distribution of the two agglutinogens A and B in the red blood cells and the two corresponding agglutinins anti-A (alpha) and anti-B (beta) in the sera.

The isoagglutination reactions which occur when the cells and the sera of the different groups are mixed are indicated in Table 27-2.

Table 27-2.   Isoagglutination reactions of the four blood groups

Group	SERA Agglutinins	CELLS (AGGLUTINOGENS) O	A	B	AB
O	(α) anti-A and (β) anti-B	−	+	+	+
A	(β) anti-B	−	−	+	+
B	(α) anti-A	−	+	−	+
AB	none	−	−	−	−

Individuals belonging to group O have been designated as universal donors because their red blood cells are not agglutinated by the sera of any of the other groups. Similarly group AB individuals are known as universal recipients, as their sera do not agglutinate the red cells of the other three groups. In some cases, donors belonging to group O were used to transfuse recipients, and individuals of group AB were transfused with blood of other groups. This practice, however, is not without danger inasmuch as the titer of the agglutinin in the serum of the injected blood might be high and work havoc with the cells of the recipient. In an infant with only a small total blood volume or in anemic or exsanguinated individuals, the transfusion of the blood of another group with a high agglutinin titer might prove fatal. Donor and recipient should belong to the same group, and their serum and red blood cells should be cross matched to establish further the individual compatibility of the bloods. A donor from a group other than that of the recipient should never be used except in a case of great emergency and when necessity demands it; even then only such donors who have low agglutinin titers in the serum should be employed.

The method of determining to which group a specimen of blood belongs, is simple, and can be carried out if the sera of group A and group B are available. A suspension of the red blood cells of the unknown specimen is mixed with each serum and the reactions will designate its group (Table 27-3 and Figs 27-1 and 27-2).

Whenever possible in medicolegal cases, the red cells from the unknown specimen should be typed against known sera possessing powerful agglutinins, and the unknown serum should be typed against known suspensions of red blood cells. Both of these reactions should be suitably controlled, using known cells against known sera.

Table 27-3. Blood grouping of cells

SERA	CELLS			
	O	A	B	AB
A (anti-B)	−	−	+	+
B (anti-A)	−	+	−	+

Group O cells are not agglutinated.
Group A cells are agglutinated by B serum.
Group B cells are agglutinated by A serum.
Group AB cells are agglutinated by A serum and by B serum.

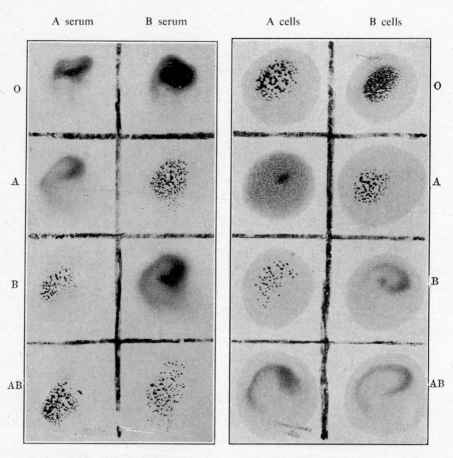

Fig. 27-1. Human Isoagglutination Reactions.

Fig. 27-2. Human Isoagglutination Reactions.

Unknown red blood cells typed with known group A and group B testing sera; O, A, B and AB are cells.

Unknown sera typed with known group A and group B testing cells; O, A, B and AB are sera. Typing reactions prepared by Dr. Kurt E. Landé.

CONFUSING AGGLUTINATION REACTIONS IN HUMAN BLOOD

The typing reactions are definite and strong for the most part. They will take place after considerable dilution and are stable for an appreciable range of temperature above and below 37° Centigrade. There are certain phenomena, however, which may cause confusion when the tests are carried out.

1. **Pseudoagglutination.** This occurs when undiluted testing serum and a thick undiluted suspension of red blood cells are used. The cells sediment out in rouleaux formation like stacks of coins. This reaction usually disappears when the testing serum is sufficiently diluted. Rouleaux formation is associated with sticky substances present in the sera during pregnancy and during active infectious diseases like tuberculosis, pneumonia or salpingitis.

2. **Cold and Autoagglutinins.** Some sera contain nonspecific agglutinins which at a low temperature, 0 to 5° C., will agglutinate human red blood cells of any group, including even those of the individual from whom the serum was taken. The name autoagglutination refers to this particular phenomenon. This reaction disappears as the temperature is raised and it is never demonstrable at body temperature. It does not occur often at room temperature except perhaps in certain pathologic conditions like paroxysmal hemoglobinuria, cirrhosis of the liver, hemolytic icterus, Raynaud's disease, trypanosomiasis, atypical pneumonia, and severe anemias in which the titer of these autoagglutinins may be high. When it does occur, it may be a source of error in blood grouping, especially if the tests are carried out at low temperature, since then autoagglutinins are absorbed by the cells and may cause clumping, thus masking the action of the testing sera. By washing the cells with warm saline, the interfering autoagglutinins can be removed, and then the correct blood group can readily be determined.

If the diagnosis of group AB is thought to be erroneous because of cold autoagglutinins, the serum of the specimen should be checked at 37° C. against known suspensions of red blood cells from all four groups. If the serum lacks agglutinins under these conditions this would support the diagnosis of group AB.

3. **Bacteriogenic Agglutination. Panagglutination (Huebener-Thomsen Phenomenon).** Certain specimens of blood if kept for some time become panagglutinable, that is, a saline suspension of such blood can be agglutinated by practically any animal or human serum including that of a person from whom the blood was derived. Thomsen noted that the property of panagglutinability could be transferred to fresh cell suspensions by the addition of a drop of panagglutinable cell suspension. Wiener also noted the property in menstrual bloods. The phenomenon was studied by Friedenreich and found to be caused by certain bacteria producing enzymes which activate a latent receptor in the red cells, for which a corresponding antibody exists in normal human serum. To distinguish bacteriogenic agglutination reactions from isoagglutination reactions a suspension of the cells can be tested with an AB serum which does not contain isoagglutinins. A positive reaction means panagglutination. The possibility of this phenomenon must always be borne in mind if fresh cell suspensions are not used for typing.

4. **Atypical and Irregular Isoagglutination.** Atypical and irregular agglutination is exhibited by about 3 per cent of all human sera. Errors in blood grouping undoubtedly have been made because the grouping sera had agglutinins other than anti-A or anti-B acting at room temperature on blood cells irrespective of the groups.

Certain atypical agglutinins occur spontaneously, and these while they may be specific as for example, for the subgroups of A (A_1 and A_2) or agglutinogens P and M, generally give much weaker reactions than typical isoagglutinins. These naturally occurring irregular isoagglutinins react only at low temperature, and are therefore of no importance for transfusions. Other irregular isoagglutinins resulting from isoimmunizations, especially the Rh-Hr antibodies (page 650) generally react at body temperature and may be quite potent, giving rise to dangerous hemolytic transfusion reactions (page 665).

Sera containing atypical agglutinins should not be used of course for preparing typing sera as the reactions may be confusing. Since the abnormality exists only in the sera while the red blood cells behave normally when agglutinated, it.is not difficult to determine the group of such sera by testing the corresponding red cells. The appearance of the atypical agglutinins provides the evidence for the assumption that there exists a great variety of individual blood differences aside from the classic four groups.

TECHNIC OF BLOOD GROUPING

Sera selected of group A and group B should be of high titer, avidity and specificity, so that they may react with cells of low sensitivity. Sera may be obtained commercially which have been certified by the Biologics Central Laboratory of the National Institutes of Health. Potent blood grouping sera are generally prepared nowadays by immunizing male donors with materials containing blood group specific substances.

1. **Collection of Testing Sera.** Collect blood in small test tubes and allow to clot. Rim clot with stirring rod. Separate by centrifugation or by allowing to stand in icebox over night. Transfer the serum to ampules using pipets. All operations must be made under sterile precautions. It is best to use 2 ml. ampules so as to avoid contamination by repeated withdrawals. The sera will retain their potency for years. Preservatives are unnecessary and undesirable.

2. **The Blood Cell Suspension.** The blood cell suspension should be fresh. It is prepared by allowing a few drops of blood from the ear lobe or finger to mix with several milliliters of normal saline solution to which a small amount of 3 per cent sodium citrate solution has been added. It is preferable to remove blood from an arm vein by needle and syringe under sterile precautions as it is less exposed to contamination. This suspension may be used directly or the cells may be washed once as follows: centrifuge suspension, and discard supernatant fluid. Suspend the sediment in normal saline solution to make a 2 to 5 per cent suspension.

If an examination of both serum and cells is desired, at least 1 or 2 ml. of blood is collected in a sterile test tube. The blood is allowed to clot, and then rimmed. The serum is centrifuged at high speed until clear serum can be pipeted off into another tube. The cells are collected by shaking up the blood clot with normal saline solution, and pipeting off some of the suspension into another tube. The blood cells are washed and resuspended as described above.

Known bloods may be kept for several weeks in the icebox by preserving with a solution recommended by Rous and Turner, as follows: mix 3 parts sterile whole blood with two parts of 3.8 per cent sterile sodium citrate solution and 5 parts of 5.4 per cent sterile glucose solution. Withdraw small amount as needed with a sterile pipet and suspend in normal saline.

3. **Landsteiner's Test Tube Method of Agglutination.** One drop of unknown cell suspension is mixed with 1 drop of saline and 1 drop of testing serum in a small test tube whose inside diameter is 7 mm. This is allowed to stand. The reaction is visible in a few minutes. The final reading is made after one hour.

The reaction can be intensified and hastened by centrifuging tubes at 2,000 revolutions per minute for three minutes. The tubes are returned to the rack and shaken until negative control bloods are evenly suspended. The reaction is read with the naked eye.

4. **The Glass Slide Method.** One drop of group A serum and one drop of group B serum are put on a glass slide. To each is added a suspension of red blood cells from the specimen. The slide is tilted back and forth for a few minutes (5 to 10) to mix the suspension thoroughly in the serum. The separate drops are covered with coverslips and read under the low power of the microscope. The tests should be performed at room temperatures inasmuch as low temperatures favor nonspecific reactions. The possibility of pseudoagglutination is always present as the serum is only half diluted.

5. **Titration of Serum.** Titration of a stock test serum is done to determine its strength. Different dilutions of the serum from the strength used in the tube agglutination tests to the highest dilution at which agglutination will occur, are tried against suspensions of sensitive red blood cells. The titer is the reciprocal of the highest dilution which still produces a definite reaction. For practical purposes, a good serum is one which will cause distinct macroscopic agglutination if it is mixed in dilutions of 1:20 on an open slide with an equal part of sensitive cell suspension. Lattes recommends that the testing serum be separated from the clot at icebox temperature, so that the cold agglutinins will be absorbed by the red cells of the blood before the serum is removed.

Newborn infants possess the expected agglutinogens in the red blood cells, but agglutinins may not have developed in the sera. These facts should be borne in mind, when testing such blood. After the infant is several months old, the agglutinins are developed and the agglutinogens become more sensitive.

HEREDITY OF THE BLOOD GROUPS

Ottenberg and Epstein in 1908 pointed out that the blood groups were hereditary properties and suggested that their inheritance followed hereditary principles. Von Dungern and Hirszfeld in 1910 established that the isoagglutinogens A and B were inherited as simple mendelian dominant characteristics. According to their theory, the heredity of the agglutinogens A and B depends upon the presence of two independent pairs of allelic genes (*A* and *a; B* and *b*), respectively located on two independent pairs of homologous chromosomes.

It will be necessary to define some of the terms used to describe the mendelian law as applied in the inheritance of blood groups. The gamete is the sexual cell; in the male it is termed the microgamete or sperm, in the female the macrogamete or egg. The fertilization of the egg by the sperm gives rise to the zygote. A gene is a factor occurring singly in a gamete and in pairs in the zygote; the genes determine the appearance of hereditary characteristics in the zygote. Alleles are pairs of contrasting genes which determine the expression of the inherited characteristics of an individual. One set of genes is derived from the maternal parent and the other set is derived from the paternal parent.

The genotype of an individual represents the composition of the somatic cells in terms of the paired allelic genes. If the paired genes are similar, the genotype is said to be homozygous or pure. If the paired genes are dissimilar, the genotype is heterozygous or hybrid. When more than one pair of genes are present, one pair may be homozygous and the other pair heterozygous; it is also possible for both pairs to be homozygous or both heterozygous.

The phenotype is a term used to denote the expression of the characteristics as found in the individual. In a heterozygous genotype, one of the paired genes may be dominant and the other is recessive. In that event, the phenotype will express the character of the dominant gene, while the character of the recessive will not appear. In a homozygous genotype of recessive genes, the recessive character will come out in the phenotype because the dominant gene is absent. Recessive phenotypes are always homozygous. Dominant phenotypes are either homozygous (pure) or heterozygous (impure). Generally, they cannot be distinguished, however, as the dominant character manifests itself in both the pure and the impure phenotypes. With some sera, especially anti-O, anti-N and anti-Hr there is a marked gene dose effect, as for example, homozygous Hr gives a stronger reaction with anti-Hr sera than heterozygous Hr. Similarly, type M blood is more agglutinable by anti-M sera than type MN blood.

The now obsolete theory of von Dungern and Hirszfeld lists the mendelian characteristics of the blood groups as follows:

Group O phenotype is determined by the presence in the genotype of two independent pairs of recessive genes, *aa* and *bb,* located on two independent pairs of homologous chromosomes and denoting the absence of agglutinogens A and B respectively. The genotype of group O has the composition *aabb*.

The phenotype of group A contains agglutinogen A as a dominant characteristic. The genotype may be homozygous or heterozygous for agglutinogen A, and is homozygous for the absence of agglutinogen B. It is expressed, therefore, either as *AAbb* or *Aabb*.

The phenotype of group B contains agglutinogen B as a dominant characteristic. The genotype is homozygous for the absence of agglutinogen A, and either homozygous or heterozygous for agglutinogen B, and is therefore expressed as *aaBB* or *aaBb*.

The phenotype of group AB contains both dominant agglutinogens A and B. The genotype may be homozygous for both pairs of dominant genes (*AABB*) or homozygous for one pair and heterozygous for the other pair (*AaBB* or *AABb*), or heterozygous for both pairs of genes (*AaBb*).

The theory of von Dungern and Hirszfeld did not conform to expectations when considered from a statistical point of view. In matings, O and AB, A and AB, B and AB, AB and AB, the theory calls for the appearance of offspring belonging to all four groups. Moreover, if A and B were independent, the following relationship between the frequencies of the groups should hold, O × AB = A × B; but as shown in Table 27-1 this is not true. Actually, certain groups never occur among the offspring of such matings. A new theory was therefore proposed by Bernstein in 1925.

Bernstein's Theory. Bernstein's theory postulates the presence of 3 allelic genes: *A, B* and *O*. According to him the blood group of any individual is determined by combinations of *A, B* and *O* in a particular pair of chromosomes. One gene is

PHENOTYPES	GENOTYPES	
O	*OO*	
A	*AA*	*AO*
B	*BB*	*BO*
AB	*AB*	

Phenotype A may be homozygous (genotype *AA*) or heterozygous (genotype *AO*).
Phenotype B may be homozygous (genotype *BB*) or heterozygous (genotype *BO*).
Phenotype AB is always heterozygous (genotype *AB*).
Phenotype O is always homozygous (genotype *OO*).

derived from the father, and the other gene from the mother. Genes A and B are dominant over gene O. A and B determine the presence of the corresponding agglutinogens, while O determines their absence.

The possible combinations of these three genes arranged in pairs give rise to six different genotypes corresponding to the four phenotypes or the blood groups.

The principles of the mendelian law governing inheritance apply to Bernstein's theory and are illustrated graphically in the following tables:

HOMOZYGOUS INHERITANCE

Parental phenotype } A   Parental genotype } $AA \rightarrow$ Gametes A

Parental phenotype } A   Parental genotype } $AA \rightarrow$ Gametes A

Genotype of children } $AA \rightarrow$ Phenotype of children { A

Similarly, parents of phenotype O (genotype OO) and homozygous phenotype B (genotype BB) display the same inheritance formula. The children are always homozygous and of the same group as the parents.

HETEROZYGOUS INHERITANCE

Parental phenotype } A   Parental genotype } $AO \rightarrow$ Gametes $\begin{matrix}A\\O\end{matrix}$

Parental phenotype } A   Parental genotype } $AO \rightarrow$ Gametes $\begin{matrix}A\\O\end{matrix}$

Genotypes of children { $\begin{matrix}AA\\AO\\AO\\OO\end{matrix}$ $\rightarrow$ Phenotypes of children { $\begin{matrix}A\\A\\A\\O\end{matrix}$

Seventy-five per cent of the offspring are phenotype A, of which 25 per cent are homozygous (genotype AA) and 50 per cent heterozygous (genotype AO). Twenty-five per cent are phenotype O (genotype OO).

Similarly when both parental phenotypes are heterozygous phenotype B (genotype BO), 75 per cent of the children will be group B and 25 per cent group O.

If one of the parents is homozygous A (genotype AA) and the other heterozygous A (genotype AO), all the offspring will be phenotype A but 50 per cent will be heterozygous AO and 50 per cent homozygous AA. The same formula applies to the mating of heterozygous and homozygous B parents (genotypes BO and BB). When one parent is homozygous A and the other is homozygous B, all the offspring are heterozygous AB. A heterozygous A parent matched to a heterozygous B parent will produce offspring in the ratio: heterozygous A, 25 per cent; heterozygous B, 25 per cent; group AB, 25 per cent; and group O, 25 per cent.

A mating between group O and group AB will produce children in the ratio of heterozygous A, 50 per cent; and heterozygous B, 50 per cent. Heterozygous A mated with group AB will yield offspring in the proportions of heterozygous A, 25 per cent; homozygous A, 25 per cent; heterozygous B, 25 per cent; and group AB, 25 per cent. The mating of homozygous A with group AB gives homozygous A, 50 per cent; and group AB, 50 per cent. The mating of homozygous B and heterozygous B with group AB follows the same formula.

If both parental phenotypes are group AB (genotype AB), the formula of inheritance is as follows:

Parental phenotype } AB   Parental genotype } $AB \rightarrow$ Gametes $\begin{matrix}A\\B\end{matrix}$

Parental phenotype } AB   Parental genotype } $AB \rightarrow$ Gametes $\begin{matrix}A\\B\end{matrix}$

Genotypes of children { $\begin{matrix}AA\\BB\\AB\\AB\end{matrix}$ Phenotypes of children { $\begin{matrix}A\\B\\AB\\AB\end{matrix}$

The offspring are therefore 25 per cent homozygous A, 25 per cent homozygous B, and 50 per cent heterozygous AB. It is readily seen that group O (genotype *OO*) offspring can never occur if one or both parents are AB.

Table 27-4 shows the offspring of all possible matings between phenotypes O, A, B and AB in accordance with Bernstein's theory. Filial phenotypes which are not possible for any combination of are also indicated.

Table 27-4. Heredity of the four blood groups (Bernstein theory)

PARENTS		CHILDREN		CHILDREN EXCLUDED
Phenotypes	Genotypes	Genotypes	Phenotypes	Phenotypes
O and O	*OO* and *OO*	*OO*	O	A, B, AB
O and A	*OO* and *AO* *OO* and *AA*	*AO* and *OO* *AO*	A and O	B, AB
O and B	*OO* and *BB* *OO* and *BO*	*BO* *BO* and *OO*	B and O	A, AB
A and A	*AA* and *AA* *AO* and *AA* *AO* and *AO*	*AA* *AA* and *AO* *AA, AO* and *OO*	A and O	B, AB
A and B	*AA* and *BB* *AO* and *BB* *AA* and *BO* *AO* and *BO*	*AB* *AB, BO* *AB, AO* *AB, AO, BO, OO*	O, A, B, AB	none
B and B	*BB* and *BB* *BO* and *BB* *BO* and *BO*	*BB* *BB* and *BO* *BB, BO, OO*	B and O	A, AB
O and AB	*OO* and *AB*	*AO* and *BO*	A and B	O, AB
A and AB	*AA* and *AB* *AO* and *AB*	*AA* and *AB* *AA, AB, BO, AO*	A, B, AB	O
B and AB	*BB* and *AB* *BO* and *AB*	*BB* and *AB* *BB, AO, AB, BO*	A, B, AB	O
AB and AB	*AB* and *AB*	*AA, AB, BB*	A, B, AB	O

A study of Table 27-4 emphasizes the following facts. When both parents are O, there can be no A, B or AB offspring. When both parents are A, there can be no B or AB children. When both parents are B, there can be no A or AB children. When both parents are AB, all the offspring are either homozygous A or B, or group AB, so that there can be no group O grandchildren. When one parent is O and the other is A, there can be no B or AB children. When one parent is O and the other is B, there can be no A or AB children.

The theory of Bernstein, in addition to upholding the theory of von Dungern and Hirszfeld concerning the dominance of agglutinogens A and B, explains why a group O parent cannot have AB children and vice versa.

When either parent is AB, half of the gametes of that parent must possess gene *A* and the other half gene *B,* so that a child of such a union will have at least one *A* or *B* gene and cannot belong to group O. Conversely, if either parent is group O, the offspring must have at least one *O* gene and cannot belong to group AB.

Table 27-4 gives every possible combination of mother and child, with the groups to which a father may belong and those to which he may not belong. According to Bernstein's theory, paternal exclusions are predictable in 10 out of 14 mother-child combinations. In the remaining four combinations it is not possible to exclude any of the groups except the homozygous state of A and B, which cannot be done unless it can be ascertained that the parents of the father were both group AB. As this group is comparatively rare, the likelihood of both paternal grandparents being group AB is small (Table 27-5). The incidence of group O and group A is much greater than B or AB which considerably reduces the percentage of cases in which paternity can be excluded below that which Table 27-5 might indicate if the incidence of all groups were the same.

Table 27-5. Summary of published studies on the heredity of the blood groups *

PARENTAL COMBINATION	NUMBER OF FAMILIES	NUMBER OF CHILDREN IN EACH GROUP †				
		O	A	B	AB	Totals
O & O	1,563	3,772	(14)	(9)	0	3,795
O & A	2,903	2,707	3,749	(10)	(1)	6,467
A & A	1,385	556	2,538	0	(2)	3,096
O & B	1,456	1,418	(7)	1,834	(1)	3,257
B & B	554	203	(1)	1,009	0	1,213
A & B	1,400	605	957	771	848	3,181
O & AB	530	(8)	633	646	(3)	1,290
A & AB	455	0	533	247	312	1,092
B & AB	323	(2)	183	406	232	823
AB & AB	59	0	28	36	65	129
Totals	10,628	9,271	8,643	4,965	1,464	24,343

From Wiener, *Blood Groups and Transfusion*, 3rd ed., Charles C Thomas, 1943.

* For the years 1924-1932 only those studies are included in which a total of 250 or more children were examined.

† Numbers in parentheses represent contradictions to the heredity theories of von Dungern and Hirszfeld and of Bernstein.

The Bernstein theory of the inheritance of blood groups has been confirmed in investigations on thousands of families carried out by independent investigators in many countries. Children from any combination of parents not expected on the basis of the theory may be considered illegitimate. The blood groups of children in a large number of families were compiled by Wiener (Table 27-5); discrepancies with the Bernstein theory, enclosed in parentheses, have been ascribed to illegitimacy or to errors in grouping.

These figures confirm the fact that the agglutinogens A and B are dominant characters and inherited through Mendel's law. They never appear in the offspring unless present in the blood of one or both parents. In exceptions in which A and B groups appear in the children of O group parents, the reasons are either illegitimacy or errors due to unreliable technic. Pseudoagglutination or autoagglutination is prone to cause a false reaction especially if whole blood is mixed with undiluted serum. Weak agglutinogens in the cell suspensions and weak agglutinins in the testing serum may lead to a wrong diagnosis; for example, another group may be mistaken for group O because of these factors. A test serum of high titer and specificity will obviate mistakes of this character. Since the technic of the agglutination tests has improved in recent years, the number of discrepancies has diminished greatly.

The other axiom of Bernstein's theory that if one or both of the parents is in group AB, the children cannot be in group O; or vice versa if one or both of the parents is group O, the offspring cannot be in group AB, is well established. Where discrepancies occur in such combinations they are due to illegitimacy, provided that they are not due to faulty serologic technic.

Independent confirmation of the hereditary transmission of the blood groups is furnished by the tests on identical twins who invariably have the same blood group. The groups in nonidentical twins vary as much as in ordinary brothers.

The blood group of an individual remains constant during his entire life and persists after death. This constancy is the basis of its medicolegal application. Disease and other influences do not seem to affect the integrity of individuality of the group. Sex does not play any part in the distribution of the blood groups, as the proportion is about the same in women as in men.

Superfecundation is a phenomenon denoting pregnancy with two or more children, the result of separate fertilizations of two or more ova liberated at the same ovulation by spermatozoa introduced during successive acts of coitus. In such cases, it is always possible that the father of each child may be different. Augsburger suggested that this obscure question might be cleared up in some instances by blood group determinations. For example, if a group O mother gave birth to twins, group A and group B respectively, and the father belonged to group A, the group B child would indicate the existence of a group B father. Lattes and Wiener, however, pointed out that in such a case superfecundation is not established, because adultery with a father of group AB would give rise to A and B offspring at the same coition. Wiener points out that to establish superfecundation by means of blood group determinations, it is necessary to have a group O mother give birth to triplets of A, B and O respectively in which case the existence of two fathers must be assumed. The likelihood of this occurrence, however, is remote.

Agglutinogens A and B with Animal Sera. Agglutinogens A and B in human blood may be demonstrated by the use of certain animal sera containing specific species heteroagglutinins for all human bloods and group specific heteroagglutinins for groups A and B. After preliminary absorption of the sera with group O human bloods to remove the species specific agglutinins, the sera may be used to test for the presence of groups A and B. On the other hand heteroagglutinins apparently specific for group O have been discovered in certain normal animal sera.

Group specific heteroagglutinins for agglutinogens A and B have been produced in the sera of rabbits immunized by injecting group A or group B human bloods. Before using, such sera must be absorbed after dilution by group O human blood to remove the species specific heteroagglutinin after which they may be used to diagnose the presence of agglutinogen A or B. The immune animal sera are more satisfactory than normal animal sera, but neither is as efficient as the use of the human isoagglutinins. The heteroagglutinins at times may serve as a check on the isoagglutinins and are indispensable when grouping blood from lower primates such as chimpanzees.

Subgroups of Groups A and AB. Von Dungern and Hirszfeld in 1910 demonstrated that after sera from group B and group O individuals had been absorbed by red cells from certain group A bloods, the following phenomena were observed: the absorbed sera did not agglutinate red blood cells of the type used in the absorbing blood, but did agglutinate most other bloods of groups A and AB. They suggested a subdivision of groups A and AB into those agglutinated by the absorbed B serum, now designated as A_1 and A_1B, and those not agglutinated, now designated as A_2 and A_2B.

Landsteiner and Levine were also aware that agglutinogen A is not a simple substance but is composed of two sorts of properties, A_1 and A_2. In addition they recognized that isoagglutinin alpha is composed of two agglutinins, one of which reacts strongly with agglutinogen A_1 and A_2, and is designated α or anti-A; the other component is designated a_1 or anti-A_1 because it reacts distinctly with group A_1 cells but hardly with group A_2 cells.

In a group B serum, the common anti-A agglutinin may be removed by absorbing with A_2 red blood cells, and only the specific anti-A_1 isoagglutinin is left. This absorbed serum may be used to identify group A_1 red cells by agglutinating them, and to identify A_2 red cells by not agglutinating them.

Occasionally the sera of individuals belonging to subgroup A_1 and A_1B agglutinate bloods belonging to subgroup A_2 but not to subgroup A_1, and is designated as anti-A_2 or a_2 agglutinin. This agglutinin also agglutinates group O red blood cells more strongly than it reacts on A_2 cells. The agglutinogen A_2 is weaker in its reaction to the group agglutinin than agglutinogen A_1.

The bloods of A_2 and A_2B sometimes possess an a_1 agglutinin, but the reaction is generally much weaker than the reaction of the absorbed B serum. For all practical purposes therefore the tests for A_1 subgroup are made with absorbed B sera. The tests for A_2 or O are made with normal animal sera especially of bovine origin which has been absorbed with human blood A_1 or A_1B. For further information the reader is referred to Wiener's book.

Some rare bloods of group A have been reported by Fisher and Hahn and by Friedenreich and are distinguished by the weak agglutination which their cells give to the strongest anti-A sera. Friedenreich believes that this characteristic is due to a third type of A agglutinogen which he designates A_3. A_3 is recessive to the other A subgroups but dominant over O. At present, subgroup A_3 is chiefly important because the feeble agglutination reactions of its cells may be a source of diagnostic error. With its discovery two additional subgroups A_3 and A_3B are possible, but further investigation is necessary. It is exceedingly rare and familial in nature.

Landsteiner and Levine in 1927 presented evidence for the hereditary nature of the subgroups of A and AB. As a result of this, the number of blood groups are increased and theoretically permit a greater possibility for the exclusion of paternity.

Thomsen, Friedenreich and Worsaae in 1930 proposed a theory of heredity for these subgroups postulating four allelic genes, A_1, A_2, B and O instead of the three allelic genes of Bernstein. Genes A_1, A_2, and B are dominant over gene O; A_1 is dominant over A_2. The genotypes corresponding to the phenotypes are as follows:

Table 27-6. Theory of heredity of the subgroups of A and AB

PHENOTYPE	GENOTYPE	
	HOMOZYGOUS	HETEROZYGOUS
O	OO	
A_1	A_1A_1	A_1O and A_1A_2
A_2	A_2A_2	A_2O
B	BB	BO
A_1B		A_1B
A_2B		A_2B

After Wiener, *Blood Groups and Transfusions*, 3rd ed., Springfield, Ill., Charles C Thomas, 1943.

The theory of the four allelic genes does not contradict the fundamental principles of heredity of blood groups.

The inheritance of these groups is as indicated in Table 27-6. The children excluded are in addition to those already given in Table 27-4 illustrating the Bernstein theory of inheritance as applied to the four major groups.

The following additional rules of inheritance should hold in addition to those derived from the Bernstein theory:

1. The agglutinogen A_1 cannot appear in the blood of the child unless it is in the blood of one or both parents. This rule depends upon the dominance of A_1 over A_2.

2. The combination A_1B parent with A_2 child, and vice versa, cannot occur. Conversely, the combination of A_2B parent with A_1 child, and vice versa, cannot occur.

3. In the special mating A_1B with B and A_1B with A_1B, A_2B children cannot result.

4. Where there are several children available in each mating, further special exclusions are possible in the following five crosses, A_1 with O, A_1 with A_1, A_1 with B, A_1 with A_1B, A_1 with A_2B. In these matings if there is a child belonging to either group O or group B, none of the remaining children can belong to subgroup A_2 or subgroup A_2B.

The genotype of the A_1 parent often can be determined if the groups of the grandparents are known. Thus if one of the two grandparents belongs to subgroup A_2B, the A_1 parent must belong to genotype A_1A_2. If one of the grandparents belongs to group O or group B, the genotype of the A_1 parent is A_1O. If both grandparents belong to subgroup A_1B, the genotype of the A_1 parent is A_1A_1. In all other cases the genotype of the A_1 parent remains uncertain. If the exact genotype of the parent is known the types of children possible are more limited and the value of the method is increased.

The available data of actual matings and offspring seem to indicate the correctness of the theory concerning inheritance of these subgroups. When the two parents and children were taken some exceptions were noted, but not when mother and child alone were considered and the question of illegitimacy did not enter. Because of certain limitations in the technic of testing for the subgroups of A, they cannot yet be safely applied in medicolegal cases.

Types M, N and MN. Landsteiner and Levine in 1927 reported that rabbits injected with human blood yielded immune sera which after absorption with certain samples of human blood still contained agglutinins capable of agglutinating most bloods in all four major groups but not capable of agglutinating other bloods in these groups. By these sera two additional agglutinogens, M and N, were identified which were independent of the agglutinogens A and B. Human sera, however, do not contain natural isoagglutinins for N, and very rarely isoagglutinins for M, so that these substances can be identified only by heteroagglutination reactions with appropriate immune rabbit sera. For this reason, the agglutinogens M and N do not play an important role in blood transfusion.

Very rarely, however, a type N individual transfused with type M or type MN blood may become sensitized to the M agglutinogen, so that a subsequent transfusion of blood of type M or MN may result in a hemolytic transfusion reaction.

Three distinct types of human blood are differentiated with respect to agglutinogens M and N, namely:

      M plus, N minus (blood possessing M but lacking N) designated M
      M plus, N plus (blood possessing M and N) designated MN
      M minus, N plus (blood possessing N but lacking M) designated N

There has not been a single instance of a blood which lacked both M and N. These additional agglutinogens occur in all the major groups and in both sexes with the same general incidence among Caucasoids of M approximately 30 per cent, N 20 per cent and MN 50 per cent. The types M, N and MN are present at birth and remain constant during life.

When the types M, N, and MN are combined with the four primary groups O, A, B and AB, 12 different kinds of blood can be differentiated. If the subdivisions of groups A and AB (A_1, A_2, A_1B and A_2B) are considered in addition, 18 different kinds of human blood can be differentiated.

The method of obtaining the sera to react with agglutinogens M and N is as follows:

Anti-M serum is produced by injecting rabbits with human blood belonging to group O and type M. Group O is used to avoid the formation of agglutinins against A and B. Similarly anti-N serum is produced by a group O blood of type N.

The sera from the immunized rabbits cannot be used directly for the tests inasmuch as human species agglutinins are also present. The latter are removed by absorbing them from the diluted immune serum with human red blood cells of the type which is not to be agglutinated. Thus if the serum is designed to agglutinate type M it is absorbed with blood cells of type N, and if it is to test for agglutinogen N, it is absorbed with cells of type M. The unabsorbed rabbit's serum will remain potent for many years, but the diluted absorbed serum is less stable.

The test is carried out by taking small amounts of the absorbed test sera for M and for N, and mixing each with a small amount of diluted washed cell suspension from the unknown blood. The agglutination can be observed both microscopically and macroscopically. The results are catalogued as follows:

Type M cells agglutinate with M antisera but not with N antisera

Type N cells agglutinate with N antisera but not with M antisera

Type MN cells agglutinate with both M antisera and N antisera

All bloods belong to one of the three types.

The technic for the determination of M and N is more delicate than for the four main groups and requires the services of an experienced serologist. For details of the principles and technic, the reader is referred to the papers of Landsteiner and Levine and to those of Wiener.

The heredity of the agglutinogens M and N, according to Landsteiner and Levine, depends upon a single pair of allelic genes, *M* and *N,* which gives rise to three genotypes *MM, NN* and *MN* corresponding to the three phenotypes M, N and MN respectively. Thus types M and N are always homozygous and MN is always heterozygous. Six different matings are possible between the three types as shown in Table 27-7.

Table 27-7. Heredity of the three M-N types

| | | PERCENTAGE OF CHILDREN IN THE DIFFERENT TYPES | | |
PHENOTYPES OF PARENTS	GENOTYPES OF PARENTS	M	N	MN
M & M	*MM & MM*	100	0	0
N & N	*NN & NN*	0	100	0
M & N	*MM & NN*	0	0	100
M & MN	*MM & MN*	50	0	50
N & MN	*NN & MN*	0	50	50
MN & MN	*MN & MN*	25	25	50

Table 27-8, compiled by Wiener, summarizes all the available data on the heredity of the agglutinogens M and N obtained by investigators in different countries up to 1943.

Table 27-8. Heredity of agglutinogens M and N

	TYPES OF CHILDREN			
TYPES OF PARENTS	M	N	MN	TOTALS
M & M	594	0	3 *	597
N & N	0	323	0	323
M & N	1 *	2 *	698	701
M & MN	860	5 *	988	1,853
N & MN	2 *	682	688	1,372
MN & MN	417	361	1,094	1,872
Totals	1,874	1,373	3,471	6,718

* Exceptions; probably denote illegitimacy.

Table 27-8 bears out the theory of Landsteiner and Levine concerning the heredity of agglutinogens M and N. In accordance with that theory the following rules for the inheritance of M and N hold:

1. Agglutinogens M and N cannot appear in the blood of a child unless present in the blood of one or both parents.

2. A type M parent cannot give rise to a type N child and conversely an N parent cannot give rise to an M child, since in either case the parent and child are homozygous but of different genotypes and this is impossible.

3. In matings where both parents are homozygous type M or homozygous type N, the children are always of the same type as the parents.

4. In matings where one parent is type M and the other type N, all children are type MN (heterozygous) and the parental types are excluded.

5. In matings where one parent is homozygous (M or N) and the other heterozygous (MN), the children are all of the parental types in a 50 to 50 ratio.

6. In matings where the parents are both MN, children of all three types are possible and none of the types can be excluded.

It is possible in many instances by using the factors M and N to exclude paternity merely from an examination of the blood of the child and the father. This is possible less often when factors A and B are used, namely, when one blood belongs to type O and the other blood to type AB.

Isoagglutinins for M and N agglutinogens have been reported in human serum, either occurring naturally or from isoimmunization of blood injected during transfusions. Such agglutinins are rare, and anti-M serum is encountered more often than anti-N serum.

A variant of agglutinogen N has been discovered, which has been found only in type MN (MN_2), and is named N_2. This variant is rare and is distinguished by the weak reactions it gives with anti-N sera. To avoid errors in determining blood types, the anti-N serum must be capable of detecting agglutinogen N_2.

An agglutinogen S, connected with the M-N system was detected several years ago, and demonstrated by isoimmune human agglutinins. It was found to be distributed as follows: in type M bloods, 73.4 per cent were S positive; type MN, 54.1 per cent were S positive; type N, 32.3 per cent were S positive. Later another agglutinogen, labeled s, was encountered, related to S. Nine M.N.S.s. types are known; M.S, M.Ss, M.s, N.S, N.Ss, N.s, MN.S, MN.Ss, and MN.s. The chief difficulty in the employment of the S-s types in the study of heredity is to obtain adequate antisera, especially anti-s, which is rare in human sera.

Agglutinogen P. In 1927, while experimenting with the first immune anti-M and anti-N rabbit sera, Landsteiner and Levine discovered sera which identified another agglutinogen in human blood and this they called P. Isoagglutinins against

P are sometimes found in normal human sera, and more rarely are formed by a process of isoimmunization in patients who have received P cells in numerous blood transfusions. In the presence of isoimmune isoagglutinins, the agglutinogen P could be the cause of a hemolytic transfusion reaction; with natural anti-P agglutinins which react only at low temperature, transfusion reactions do not occur.

There is a possibility that agglutinogen P may be used as another factor in individualizing human blood, and in solving cases of disputed parentage. The principal obstacle to its use is the difficulty of obtaining with any regularity immune rabbit sera of the proper potency and specificity which would give definite reactions with the red blood cells and distinguish type P blood (agglutination by sera) and type pp blood (lack of such agglutination). The original immune rabbit sera of Landsteiner and Levine gave a powerful agglutination with many bloods, but occasionally gave weak, inconclusive reactions with other bloods. The antisera since obtained by these investigators have been less satisfactory than the original serum. The anti-P isoagglutinins obtained by Landsteiner and Levine have given a more feeble reaction than the immune rabbit serum, but sometimes if the tests are made at icebox temperature, the isoagglutinins have differentiated between type P blood and type pp blood.

Anti-P agglutinins of fair titer have been obtained from normal animal sera, notably pigs and horses. To prepare the serum, Landsteiner and Levine suggest that it should be inactivated, then diluted with an equal volume of 0.9 per cent sodium chloride solution and mixed with half its volume of pooled, washed, packed type pp cells of groups O, A and B. This mixture is stored in the refrigerator over night, then the serum is separated and tested against P and pp red blood cells. In its hereditary transmission, P acts as a mendelian dominant and pp as a mendelian recessive. The P agglutinogen is distributed in the general population independent of the ABO blood groups, the M and N types, the Rh factor and also sex.

Landsteiner and Levine have noted that agglutination reactions on human blood with anti-P reagents derived from animal sera of different species sometimes produced many interesting variations. They are inclined to regard agglutinogen P not as a simple substance but as a series of related agglutinogens, similar in nature to the properties A and Rh.

The investigations of Furuhata and Imamura on human blood with an absorbed normal pig serum uncovered the so-called agglutinogen Q which is not related to A, B, M and N but showing marked similarities to P. Type Q is transmitted as a simple mendelian dominant, and qq is recessive. The Q property needs further definition.

Rh-Hr Groups. Landsteiner and Wiener in 1937 noted that the red blood cells of rhesus monkeys contained M-like agglutinogens and that injection of rhesus red cells into rabbits produced anti-M agglutinins. In some of these immune anti-rhesus sera, an antibody was found which agglutinated the red blood cells of 85 per cent of the white population independently of agglutinogens, A, B, M, N and P. This new property in human blood was designated as Rh from its connection with the blood of the rhesus monkey.

The Rh agglutinogen is therefore present in 85 per cent of white individuals and reacts to the immune anti-rhesus serum by agglutination; such bloods are designated Rh positive. The bloods not agglutinated by immune anti-rhesus serum are designated Rh negative. The heredity formula of the Rh groups at this stage, based on the reactions of the immune anti-rhesus sera is relatively simple and similar to that of the four original blood groups. The Rh property is a single mendelian dominant with a pair of allelic genes, dominant Rh positive (*Rh*) and recessive Rh negative (*rh*). The phenotypes and genotypes are:

Phenotype rh, genotype *rhrh* (homozygous Rh negative)
Phenotype Rh, genotype *RhRh* (homozygous Rh positive)
genotype *Rhrh* (heterozygous Rh positive)

Natural Rh isoagglutinins have not been encountered in human sera, but an immune isoagglutinin may be formed by injecting Rh-positive red blood cells into Rh-negative individuals. The first injection of Rh-positive blood would probably not cause any serious disturbance, but it may sensitize the Rh-negative recipient against the Rh factor. A second injection of Rh-positive blood into such a sensitized individual may precipitate a severe hemolytic transfusion reaction because of the development of immune antibodies. In similar fashion an Rh-negative woman may conceive an Rh-positive child, and during the development of the pregnancy become sensitized to the Rh property, thus creating an immunity against her own fetus. In hospital cases it is advisable to determine the Rh formula of the patient, especially if a series of transfusions is contemplated on a woman of the child-bearing age, so that if she is Rh-negative she can receive only Rh-negative blood and avoid developing an Rh sensitivity. Wiener points out that, while Rh is a good antigen, of those who are naturally exposed to the Rh factor by pregnancy only 1 in 25 have serious reactions. Deliberate injection of Rh-positive blood, as by transfusion, will on the other hand strongly sensitize most Rh-negative persons.

The complexity of the Rh agglutinogen formula was increased when sera from Rh-negative individuals, sensitized against Rh-positive erythrocytes, were studied and their agglutinations of human red blood cells were found to differ. Most of these immune human sera showed agglutinations similar to the immune anti-rhesus animal sera, reacting with about 85 per cent of Caucasoids; such sera were given the name of standard anti-Rh or anti-Rh_0. Then two other anti-Rh agglutinins were demonstrated in human sera by Wiener, one agglutinating 70 per cent of the positives and labeled anti-rh' and the other agglutinating 30 per cent of the positives and labeled anti-rh".

Table 27-9. The eight Rh blood types and their sera *

TYPES	BLOODS CONTAINING Rh_o REACTIONS WITH SERA			TYPES	BLOODS LACKING Rh_o REACTIONS WITH SERA		
	anti-rh'	anti-rh"	anti-Rh_o		anti-rh'	anti-rh"	anti-Rh_o
Rh_o	−	−	+	rh	−	−	−
Rh_1	+	−	+	rh'	+	−	−
Rh_2	−	+	+	rh"	−	+	−
Rh_Z or (Rh_1Rh_2)	+	+	+	rh_y or (rh'rh")	+	+	−

After Wiener, *Am. J. Clin. Path.*, 15:106, 1945.

* In this notation, R is used for bloods containing the Rh_0 property and r for bloods not containing Rh_0.

The three human antisera, anti-Rh_0, anti-rh', and anti-rh", have increased the number of Rh types from the two first identified by immune animal anti-rhesus sera, namely Rh-positive and Rh-negative, to eight different Rh types. The presence of Rh agglutinogens, Rh_0, rh' and rh" is determined by the red cells being agglutinated by their respective antisera and not by the other two antisera. Combinations of factors Rh_0 and rh', and the factors Rh_0 and rh'', add two new agglutinogens, increasing the number to five; thus factors Rh_0 and rh' are combined into agglutinogen Rh_1 (or Rh'_0), and factors Rh_0 and rh'' are combined into agglutinogen Rh_2 (or Rh''_0). Cells containing agglutinogen Rh_1 are agglutinated by sera anti-Rh_0 and anti-rh', and type Rh_2 cells are agglutinated by sera anti-Rh_0 and anti-rh''. There is evidence also for two additional complex agglutinogens rh_y (containing factors rh' and rh'') and Rh_z (containing all three factors Rh_0, rh' and rh''). The hereditary transmission of the Rh types rests on 8 major allelic genes, r, r', r'', r^y, R^0, R^1, R^2 and R^z and these determine the 8 Rh phenotypes and the 36 genotypes.

Table 27-10. The theory of multiple allelic genes for the Rh-Hr types

Gene	Corresponding Agglutinogen	Reactions of Serum			Rh Blood Factors Present in Agglutinogen
		Anti-Rh_0	Anti-rh'	Anti-rh''	
r	rh	—	—	—	none
r'	rh'	—	+	—	rh'
r''	rh''	—	—	+	rh''
r^y	rh_y	—	+	+	rh' and rh''
R^0	Rh_0	+	—	—	Rh_0
R^1	Rh_1	+	+	—	Rh_0 and rh'
R^2	Rh_2	+	—	+	Rh_0 and rh''
R^z	Rh_z	+	+	+	Rh_0, rh' and rh''

Red blood cells agglutinated by anti-rh' and anti-Rh_0 contain Rh_1 (or Rh'_0) agglutinogen in which the factors Rh_0 and rh' are united similar to the union of blood factors A and A_1 in the blood of subgroup A_1, rather than like the separate agglutinogens in blood groups AB. In the same way blood factors Rh_0 and rh'' are united in agglutinogen Rh_2 (or Rh''_0). The agglutinogens Rh_1 and Rh_2 are inherited as a unit. Thus Rh_1 homozygous (R^1R^1) mating with rh genotype rr would produce all offspring Rh_1, while heterozygous Rh_1 ($R'r$) mating with rh (rr) would produce 50 per cent R^1r and 50 per cent rr. Agglutinogen Rh_2 may be substituted for Rh_1 in these formulae. In rare instances, the factors Rh_0 and rh' in type Rh_1 may segregate in matings as types Rh_0 and rh' when the type Rh_1 parent belongs to genotype R^0r'; and Rh_0 and rh'' similarly may segregate as types Rh_0 and rh'' when the Rh_2 parent belongs to genotype R^0r''.

Bloods of types rh'rh'' and Rh_1Rh_2 most often contain separate agglutinogens and then the genotype is analogous to that of blood group AB.

Table 27-11. The eight Rh types and their thirty-six genotypes *

Phenotypes	Genotypes
rh	rr
rh'	$r'r'$ and $r'r$
rh''	$r''r''$ and $r''r$
rh_y (or rh'rh'')	$r'r''$, r^yr, r^yr', r^yr'', and r^yr^y
Rh_0	R^0R^0 and R^0r
Rh_1	R^1R^1, R^1r, R^1r', R^1R^0, and R^0r'
Rh_2	R^2R^2, R^2r, R^2R^0, R^2r'', and R^0r''
Rh_z (or Rh_1Rh_2)	R^1R^2, R^1r'', R^2r', R^0r^y, R^1r^y, R^2r^y, R^zr^y, R^zr, R^zr', R^zr'', R^zR^0, R^zR^1, R^zR^2 and R^zR^z

* Wiener's theory of multiple alleles.

Investigation of racial distribution of the Rh blood types shows that Chinese, Japanese, American Indians, Filipinos, Hawaiians and Australian aborigines are rarely Rh negative, and congenital hemolytic disease is rare among them. The incidence of Rh-negative blood in the whites is about 14.7 per cent, Negroes (New York City) 8.1 per cent, and among Asiatic Indians 7.1 per cent. Type Rh_0 is very common in Negroes as compared with the whites; in Negroes 41.2 per cent, in whites 2.5 per cent. Genes r^y and R^z are extremely rare among Caucasoids, but are less rare among mongoloids.

Statistical study of the Rh blood type in families, and employment of the gene frequency method supports the theory of multiple allelic Rh genes. In Negroes many individuals possess blood which reacts feebly or in intermediate fashion with one or more of the Rh antisera and these phenomena have suggested the presence of more Rh allelic genes, the intermediate genes.

Table 27-12. Summary of family studies on the Rh blood types

MATING	NUMBER FAMILIES	NUMBER OF CHILDREN OF TYPES [*]							
		rh	Rh_1	Rh_2	Rh_1Rh_2	Rh_0	rh'	rh"	Totals
rh & rh	4	14	0	0	0	0	0	0	14
rh & Rh_1	49	25	73	0	0	7	0	0	105
rh & Rh_2	16	10	0	20	0	0	0	0	30
rh & Rh_1Rh_2	15	(1)	18	14	0	0	0	0	33
rh & Rh_0	3	3	0	0	0	3	0	0	6
rh & rh'	2	1	0	(1)	0	0	1	0	3
rh & rh"	1	1	0	0	0	0	0	5	6
Rh_1 & Rh_1	26	5	62	0	0	4	1	0	72
Rh_1 & Rh_2	21	6	15	7	18	0	2	0	48
Rh_1 & Rh_1Rh_2	27	0	46	8	25	0	0	0	79
Rh_1 & Rh_0	1	1	0	0	0	0	0	0	1
Rh_1 & rh'	3	0	3	0	0	0	0	0	3
Rh_1 & rh"	4	1	2	0	3	0	0	0	6
Rh_2 & Rh_2	2	1	0	4	0	0	0	0	5
Rh_2 & Rh_1Rh_2	6	0	2	8	8	0	0	0	18
Rh_2 & Rh_0	2	0	0	1	0	4	0	0	5
Rh_1Rh_2 & Rh_1Rh_2	10	0	3	1	17	0	0	0	21
Rh_1Rh_2 & Rh_0	2	0	1	1	0	0	0	0	2
Rh_1Rh_2 & rh'	2	0	1	1	2	0	0	0	4
Rh_0 & rh'	1	0	0	0	0	1	1	0	2
Totals	207	69	226	66	73	19	5	5	463

After Wiener.

[*] Numbers in parentheses denote exceptions, and probably represent illegitimacy.

HR FACTORS. In the serum of an Rh-positive mother of an erythroblastotic infant, an agglutinin which could react on all Rh-negative bloods was detected by Levine and Javert. The corresponding blood factor thus identified was called Hr and the agglutinin was given the name anti-Hr. These investigators said that the anti-Hr serum reacted positively in about 30 per cent of cases, and that anti-Hr reacted with all Rh-positive bloods not agglutinated by anti-rh'.

In the serum of another Rh-positive mother of an erythroblastotic infant, Race and Taylor found in 1943 an agglutinin which agglutinated Rh-negative bloods, similar to the serum of Levine and Javert but stronger as it reacted positively in 80 per cent of the cases. The serum of Race and Taylor undoubtedly contained anti-Hr and the blood factor with which it reacts was Hr.

Race and his associates consider that Hr is a blood antigen present in agglutinogens in association with factors Rh_2, Rh_0, rh" and rh but absent in agglutinogens

Table 27-13. Nomenclature of the Rh-Hr types

Blood Factors	CDE * Equivalents	Agglutinogens	CDE Equivalents
Rh_o	D	rh	cde
rh'	C	rh'	Cde
rh"	E	rh"	cdE
(Hr_o)	(d)	rh_y	CdE
hr'	c	Rh_o	cDe
hr"	e	Rh_1	CDe
Rh Variants		Rh_2	cDE
rh^w	C^w	Rh_z	CDE
$\Re h_o$	D^u	Variants	
		Rh_1^w	C^wDe
		$\Re h_1^*$	CD^ue
		$\Re h_2^*$	cD^uE
		$\Re h_o^*$	cD^ue

From *J.A.M.A.*, 149:699-706, 1952.

* The introduction by British workers of the use of the letters C, D, E for the Rh factors was a new development. According to Wiener while incorrectly implying a relationship to the A-B-O group (C has already been used for a blood factor of the A-B-O system), and failing to indicate the special position of Rh_o, the C-D-E symbols do not present the serologic and genetic facts correctly. Wiener is critical of the failure to distinguish between blood factors and agglutinogens and feels the inadequacy of the C-D-E symbols is clearly evident from the failure to find satisfactory designations for the Rh-Hr phenotypes, and almost every writer uses different combinations of C-D-E symbols. For example, in the book by Race and Sanger the same Rh type is designated in as many as five different ways: in expressing the type Rh_1rh, there are enough C-D-E equivalents employed to be confusing. Wiener believes the only solution is to discard the use of the letters C-D-E entirely for his original Rh-Hr nomenclature which he insists is simpler to use, since it represents the facts accurately, tersely and unambiguously.

Rh_1 and rh', having the factor rh'. The genotypes of Hr-negative mothers can only be R^1R^1, R^1r' or $r'r'$; these mothers can only transmit genes R^1 or r', and cannot have any type rh children. Hr may be regarded as an allele of rh' and can be characterized as hr'. Later an allele of the rh" factor was found and designated hr". To date convincing evidence for the existence of the hypothetical factor Hr_0 has not been obtained.

Table 27-14. The reactions determined by the eight standard Rh genes

Genes	Corresponding Agglutinogens	Reactions with Rh Sera			Reactions with Hr Sera	
		anti-rh'	anti-rh"	anti-Rh_o	anti-hr'	anti-hr"
r	rh	neg.	neg.	neg.	pos.	pos.
R^o	Rh_o	neg.	neg.	pos.	pos.	pos.
r'	rh'	pos.	neg.	neg.	neg.	pos.
R^1	Rh_1	pos.	neg.	pos.	neg.	pos.
r"	rh"	neg.	pos.	neg.	pos.	neg.
R^2	Rh_2	neg.	pos.	pos.	pos.	neg.
r^y	rh_y	pos.	pos.	neg.	neg.	neg.
R^z	Rh_z	pos.	pos.	pos.	neg.	neg.

The anti-hr' serum may help to determine the homozygous or heterozygous nature of type Rh_1 fathers with erythroblastotic infants. There are five genotypes possible in agglutinogen Rh_1, and anti-hr' serum merely divides the Rh_1 blood into hr' negative and hr' positive types. The hr' negative Rh_1 blood is generally homozygous (R^1R^1) and the hr' positive Rh_1 blood is usually heterozygous and paired with gene r genotype R^1r.

The family studies of the rh' and hr' factors and the gene frequency method have justified the theory of Race and his co-workers. Blood cells negative for agglutinin rh′ are agglutinated by anti-hr′. The prevailing opinion is that there is a relationship between rh′ and hr′ serologically and genetically like M and N. Anti-hr″ agglutinin is difficult to obtain so that the genetics of rh″-hr″ have not been studied as thoroughly as rh′-hr′. Anti-Hr$_0$-agglutinin is not available at all.

Table 27-15. Rh-Hr types

8 Rh Types — Reactions with Anti-Rh serums				18 Rh-Hr Types — Reactions with Anti-Hr serums			Approximate Distribution in New York City, Per Cent *	
Anti-Rh$_o$	Anti-rh′	Anti-rh″	Designations	Anti-hr′	Anti-hr″	Designations	Caucasoids	Negroids
−	−	−	rh	+	+	rh	13.5	7.5
−	+	−	rh′	+	+	rh′rh	0.9	0.5
				−	+	rh′rh′	0.01	x †
−	−	+	rh″	+	+	rh″rh	0.5	0.5
				+	−	rh″rh″	0.005	x
−	+	+	rh′rh″ (or rh$_y$)	+	+	rh$_y$rh	0.01	x
				−	+	rh$_y$rh′	x	x
				+	−	rh$_y$rh″	x	x
				−	−	rh$_y$rh$_y$	x	x
+	−	−	Rh$_o$	+	+	Rh$_o$	2.5	42.5
+	+	−	Rh$_1$	+	+	Rh$_1$rh	33.5	26.0
				−	+	Rh$_1$Rh$_1$	20.5	2.0
+	−	+	Rh$_2$	+	+	Rh$_2$rh	12.0	13.0
				+	−	Rh$_2$Rh$_2$	2.5	2.0
+	+	+	Rh$_1$Rh$_2$ (or Rh$_z$)	+	+	Rh$_z$Rh$_o$	13.8	6.0
				−	+	Rh$_z$Rh$_1$	0.2	x
				+	−	Rh$_z$Rh$_2$	x	x
				−	−	Rh$_z$Rh$_z$	x	x

From *J.A.M.A.*, 149:700, 1952.

* These results do not take into account reactions for the rh^w factor.

† The blood types indicated by x are very rare and have not been observed in tests on a large number of persons, even several hundreds or thousands.

Rules of inheritance of Rh-Hr groups:

1. Agglutinogens Rh$_o$, rh′, rh″, hr′ and hr″ cannot be present in the children unless they are present in the blood of one or both parents.

2. An rh′-negative parent cannot have an hr′-negative child, and an hr′-negative parent cannot have an rh′-negative child.

3. An rh″-negative parent cannot have an hr″-negative child and vice versa. Due to the limited number of studies and certain irregularities observed in heredity studies, this rule is not ready to be applied in medicolegal cases.

Rh-Hr Variants. The so-called Rh-Hr variants, also named the intermediate Rh-Hr blood types are agglutinogens which react feebly with one or more of the Hr and Rh antiserums. Those variants connected with the Rh$_o$ factor are important in that their weak response to the antiserums may lead to an erroneous diagnosis of the types as Rh-negative. The injection of such blood into an Rh-negative patient may sensitize the patient to the Rh factor, or, in the event that the patient is already sensitized, it may precipitate a serious transfusion reaction. It is now possible to identify blood containing Rh$_o$ variants by special methods such as the use of antiglobulin serum or the treatment of the red blood cells with proteolytic enzymes.

Variants of the rh′ factor also occur, and for one of these variants, rh^w, an antiserum has been discovered. This anti-rh^w is potent and its reactions divide Rh$_1$ individuals into subtypes, Rh$_1$ proper and Rh^w$_1$. This serum also divides group Rh$_z$ in the same way. Variants of factors rh″, hr′ and hr′ have been identified. Most of them have been found among Negroes. At present the variants are chiefly important as complicating elements in agglutination reactions and possible sources of error.

Other Blood Groups. As already mentioned, some human sera are encountered which contain weak isoagglutinins acting on agglutinogens not related to the A-B-O system. Of these irregular isoagglutinins, most have an anti-P reaction, some are anti-M and others are not classified. They cause agglutination most strongly at low temperature in which interference from nonspecific agglutinins is a possibility. The Lewis system belongs to this group and in it two related factors, Le^a and Le^b, have been recognized. The difficulty is that specific and potent reagents for the group are not easy to obtain, so that knowledge of these factors is not sufficient to render them useful in medicolegal cases.

Occasionally mothers of erythroblastotic infants and persons who have had hemolytic transfusions contain in their blood an antiserum for a blood property found in about 10 per cent of white individuals. This antibody was detected first in the serum of a patient named Kell and given the symbol K. Then another antibody was found in the serum of a mother of an erythroblastotic baby, which had reciprocal reaction to the K factor, and was named the Cellano factor after the patient. Later when it was found that the Cellano factor occurs in 99.8 per cent of white individuals, it was given the symbol k. Using anti-K and anti-k sera, three blood types can be distinguished: KK, 0.2 per cent; Kk, 8.6 per cent; and kk, 91.2 per cent. The Kk system holds a promise for the future but at present is hampered by the difficulty of obtaining sera with satisfactory antibodies.

Wiener and others have reported a fatal hemolytic transfusion reaction produced by a hitherto unrecognized immune isoantibody in the blood of the recipient; to this factor they gave the name U. The red blood cells of 1,105 out of 1,110 individuals tested were agglutinated by the antibody, indicating that the reacting agglutinogen occurred frequently in the general population. There is not any relationship between U and A-B-O, MN, Rh-Hr, Kk or other blood systems.

Additional blood properties have been demonstrated but rarely produce isosensitization and so are not clinically important.

A number of blood properties are identifiable only by the antiglobulin technic, such as the so-called Duffy or Fy^a factor which has produced a definite number of serious intragroup transfusion reactions. It is not valuable for medicolegal problems because of its failure to give clearcut reactions with antisera.

GROUP SPECIFIC SUBSTANCES IN ORGANS AND BODY FLUIDS

Group specific substances based upon the four isoagglutination blood groups, (O, A, B, AB) are also present in the cells of most body organs and fluids. Landsteiner and Levine first reported them in spermatozoa. However, Wiener could not confirm this report and points out that it was not realized until later that the substances are present in solution in the seminal fluid (personal communication). Others have demonstrated them in liver, kidney, lung and pancreas. Schiff has noted that their proportion varies in different organs; for example the pancreas contains the greatest concentration of group A specific substance, whereas brain, aorta and muscle contain only small amounts. All tissues except the lens of the eye, hair, compact bone, cartilage and epidermal cells contain group specific substances. Thomsen has shown that the cells of benign and malignant tumors contain them.

The group specific substances can be demonstrated in the cells of organs, by their ability to absorb the specific isoagglutinin from human serum or the specific heteroagglutinin from immune animal serum. The agglutination titer of the test serum is determined first with a known suspension of red blood cells. Then the serum is absorbed with the tissue cells in question and the titer is determined again with the known suspension of red blood cells. If there is a significant difference in titer between the absorbed test serum and the normal test serum, a specific substance of the same group as the known suspension of red blood cells is present in the tissue cells and has removed the specific agglutinin from the serum.

Group specific substances can be extracted from the tissues in two forms, according to Schiff. One form is soluble in water, the other in alcohol and chloroform. These extracts have the power of specifically inhibiting agglutination and hemolysis according to their group specific content.

Group specific substances have been found in blood serum and, according to Schiff, are demonstrable by precipitin reactions with group specific immune rabbit's sera and also by inhibition of specific isohemolysins. These substances have been demonstrated also in spermatic fluid, saliva, tears, sweat, urine, digestive juices, bile, milk and fluids from pleura, pericardium, peritoneum, amnion, hydrocele sac and ovarian cysts. They are not present in cerebrospinal fluid.

Schiff and Sasaki have found that there are two types of individuals, the first having the ability to secrete group specific substances in the saliva, and the second type not having this ability. They believe that the first type possesses this trait as the expression of a dominant mendelian inherited characteristic. Secretors are characterized by the presence of water soluble blood group substances in tissues and organs, especially in salivary glands and gastric mucosa, and in secretions like saliva, gastric juice and semen. Such specific substances can be extracted from the organs of secretors by aqueous solutions. In nonsecretors, water soluble group substances cannot be obtained from body fluids or secretions. A-B-O-AB group specific substances are the only ones that can be demonstrated in the body and it is not possible to prove the presence of other group substances in the tissues and secretions, except the so-called Lewis factors. Le^a negative individuals are generally secretors of the A-B-O-AB group substances and Le^a positive individuals are almost always non-secretors.

The group specific substances in the fluids can be demonstrated by the specific inhibition of the isoagglutination reactions between known testing sera and known suspensions of red blood cells. The tests are conducted as follows:

Tube 1. Unknown fluid plus anti-A serum plus A cells
Tube 2. Unknown fluid plus anti-B serum plus B cells
Tube 3. Control, anti-A serum plus A cells
Tube 4. Control, anti-B serum plus B cells

Lack of agglutination of the red blood cells in a tube containing an unknown fluid, would indicate the presence of group specific substances in the fluid corresponding to the group of the known suspension of red blood cells. Titration tests may be tried to determine the amount of the group substances in the fluid, by diluting the unknown fluid and using constant amounts of the testing serum.

Isoagglutinins for red blood cells are found in body fluids rich in protein such as milk, lymph, exudates, transudates and cyst fluid, or, in other words, in fluids whose protein content corresponds most closely to the globulin fraction of blood serum. The titer of the antibodies in the fluid is less than that of the corresponding agglutinin in blood. Only traces of these substances are found in saliva, tears or spermatic fluid. None are found in normal urine, cerebrospinal fluid or amniotic fluid.

MEDICOLEGAL APPLICATION OF ISOAGGLUTINATION IN BLOOD AND OTHER STAINS

After appropriate tests have established that a certain specimen is human blood, the isoagglutination reactions are tested by the following procedures, which vary with the condition of the specimen.

If the specimen is fresh, cell suspensions are made and the agglutinogen content determined in the usual manner. If possible the serum should be separated and its agglutinin content determined. Blood at necropsy can be examined in the usual way.

The grouping of dried blood stains is difficult because of the alterations in the agglutinating factors produced by the exposure of the specimen to heat, sunlight or desiccation and contamination with bacteria and body secretions. Alterations vary from a slight weakening in the potency of agglutinin or agglutinogen to deterioration of these factors to the point where they fail to react at all. Many more considerations are involved in the typing of dried blood stains than in the tests on fresh blood. For example, the failure to detect an agglutinin in a dried blood crust does not necessarily mean that it was originally absent from that blood; the drying of the blood may have altered the antibody so much that it could not give a positive reaction.

The following hypothetical case illustrates the problems which an investigator must face in the typing of blood crusts. The extract from the crust is tested with known group B red blood cells and is strongly positive indicating an anti-B agglutinin in the specimen. On the other hand a known suspension of group A red cells was not agglutinated by the extract from the crust, so that anti-A is not demonstrable. These results simply indicate that anti-B agglutinin is present in the blood crust and that its blood group is a possible A. The inability to demonstrate anti-A agglutinin may mean that none was present in the original blood, and the blood is therefore group A, or it may mean that the blood is a group O whose anti-B agglutinin is still potent but whose anti-A agglutinin has deteriorated and does not agglutinate. In such a case, on the results of the agglutinin tests alone it would not be possible to make a definite diagnosis of the blood group. However, if an agglutinogen test is made and group specific substance A is demonstrated, the blood is certainly a group A. If group specific substances are not found the group is a possible O, but group A cannot be excluded for the specimen may have altered the reactions of an original group specific substance A so that it could not be demonstrated. It is desirable in identifying the type of a dried blood stain that both the agglutinin and agglutinogen content of the specimen should be determined in order to obviate or lessen errors of misinterpretation.

Agglutinin determination on dried blood may be performed by the slide method if crusts are available, but if crusts are not available, test tube extraction is the method of choice.

The *crust slide method* is used when a thin blood crust can be sliced from a weapon or a surface with a thin sharp blade; the crust should be so thin that the coverslip will not be raised much. Two per cent suspensions of fresh group A red cells, group B red cells and group O red cells are employed in the tests and should be sensitive.

Three glass microscope slides are used. On each one is placed a thin slice of blood crust from the specimen. Near but not touching the crust on the first slide one or two drops of group A_1 red cell suspension are placed. On the second slide a suspension of group B red blood cells is similarly placed near the crust. On the third slide a suspension of group O red blood cells is placed as described above. Each preparation is covered by its respective coverslip promptly and in such a way that bubbles do not separate the blood crust from the liquid suspension of cells. The agglutinins are slowly extracted from the stain by the fluid and agglutinate the specific red blood cells nearest them. The reactions should be observed at intervals for the next 30 minutes, so that a weak agglutination will not be missed. The coverslips should be pressed gently to break up rouleaux formation. The group A and B suspensions are used for diagnostic purposes and react with the appropriate agglutinin in the crust unless the agglutinin has deteriorated from desiccation. Only positive reactions should be considered and negative reactions which may be the result of agglutinin degeneration cannot be trusted. For example, one of the agglutinins in a crust of dried group O blood may degenerate and not the other thus leading to an erroneous diagnosis. The group O suspension of red cells is employed to detect nonspecific aggregation reactions and if such occur any agglutination of the A or B suspensions would not be diagnostically reliable. If the O cells do not agglutinate, and the A and B cells suspensions are agglutinated by the dilute crust agglutinins, a diagnosis is possible.

If blood crusts are not available, the *extraction test tube method* is employed. A blood stain on a solid object or clothing is dissolved in a small amount of saline and the fluid is centrifuged to remove debris. In each of three small test tubes are put 10 drops of the centrifuged extract. To the first tube is added a drop of A_1 cell suspension, to the second a drop of B cell suspension, and to the third a drop of O cell suspension. If the extract has a deep red tinge, a 2 per cent suspension of red blood cells is used, if the extract is dilute, the suspension of red blood cells is 0.5 per cent.

The three tubes are put in the refrigerator for 10 minutes. They are taken out and centrifuged for 2 minutes at 1,500 to 2,000 rpm. The supernatant fluid is poured from the three tubes, and a drop of saline solution is added to each tube. The tubes are gently shaken. If the cells go into suspension promptly the reaction is negative. If they form clumps which do not break up, the agglutination is positive. Occasionally the agglutination is intermediate between positive and negative probably due to the deterioration of the agglutinins.

Agglutinogen reactions are quite important. In dried blood the red blood cell is destroyed and cannot be agglutinated, but the group specific substances retain for a long time their ability to absorb their respective agglutinins. If a serum of known strength is in contact with an unknown blood stain, and then removed and retested to find that its agglutinating power is impaired or lost, it is reasonable to suppose that the antigen in the stain exerted a group specific reaction on the corresponding serum agglutinin.

The reagents required are: (1) saline suspensions of fresh group A_2 and group B cells at 2 per cent concentration for retesting respective antisera after absorption by unknown stain; and (2) anti-A and anti-B sera of high titer, 150, which are adjusted by dilution with saline to a titer of 10 to 15.

The controls required are known bloods O, A_1, A_2 and B which are allowed to stain a clean fabric and then dry. They play the role of control blood stains. The group O stain is used to show that the reagents are active under the conditions of the test when no strange antigen is present to interfere with the anti-A and anti-B sera. The A and B blood stains are used to show that the respective antisera will react with the proper antigen. The substrate or unstained part of the material is used to show that no group substance from saliva, sweat or urine which might interfere with the absorption reaction is present.

Twelve small test tubes of 2 ml. capacity are set up in two rows of six each.

The first tube in each row receives 1 square cm. of stained cloth or 5 mg. of blood from stain.

The second tube in each row: 1 square cm. of substrate cloth.

The third tube in each row: 1 square cm. of group O stained cloth.

The fourth tube in each row: 1 square cm. of group A_1 stained cloth.

The fifth tube in each row: 1 square cm. of group A_2 stained cloth.

The sixth tube in each row: 1 square cm. of group B stained cloth.

Anti-A serum is pipeted into each tube of the first row, and anti-B serum into each tube of the second row, in minimum amount so that in each tube there is an excess of two drops. The tubes are put in the refrigerator over night and carefully stoppered. On removal from the refrigerator a clean pipet is supplied for each tube. The serum may be centrifuged to remove debris.

One drop of serum is pipeted from the first tube of the first row into the first space on a well slide and the rest of the tubes in that row supply a drop of serum for the corresponding spaces. The second row of tubes also supplies a drop of serum for their appropriate spaces on the well slide. The spaces on the well slide repeat the pattern of the 12 test tubes. One drop of a 2 per cent suspension of known B cells is added to the absorbed anti-B sera in the space wells of the second row. One drop of a 2 per cent suspension of A_2 red cells is added to each well of absorbed anti-A sera in the space wells of the first row. After rocking or rotating the slides gently for five minutes they are examined visually and microscopically for signs of agglutination. A negative result shows the cells evenly suspended, and a positive result of the cells clumped; intermediate reactions of partial agglutination also occur.

If the substrate absorption tube changes the reaction of the serum from a potent positive agglutination to a weak or doubtful reaction, there is a possibility that the substrate contains group substances from saliva, urine or sweat, which inhibited the agglutinins. In this event it is not advisable to draw any conclusions concerning the group of the stain from the results of the absorption test.

A blood stain which is too old, or contains too little blood, or which has been in contact with a too powerful serum, may not be able to inhibit the action of the serum because the group factor is too weak. It may be advisable in some instances to retest the stain with a serum of lower titer, which allows a group specific substance of weak potency to develop its characteristic reaction.

If the tube containing the stain under investigation inhibits the antisera from an ordinarily potent reaction to a weak or negative agglutination, the group specific substance has abated the serum and has proven its identity, provided that nonspecific reactions can be eliminated as possibilities.

Theoretically group O is identified in dried blood by proving the presence of anti-A and anti-B agglutinins and the absence of group specific substances in the red blood cells. As already mentioned on page 657, deterioration of these agglutinins in the dried blood may lead to errors in diagnosis.

In dried blood, group A or B is identified by demonstrating the appropriate agglutinin which agglutinates known A or B red blood cells or by absorbing the appropriate agglutinin from known A or B antisera by group specific substances in the red cells. The possible errors in these examinations have been discussed above. If agglutination of A or B cells does not occur the specimen is either group AB, or the agglutinins may have disappeared from the dried blood. Group AB cannot be identified unless the agglutinogen content of the specimen is determined. Group AB can hardly ever be identified reliably in dried blood.

Landsteiner and Levine have demonstrated the presence of agglutinogens M and N in dried blood stains, by determining the absorbing capacity of the stain for the corresponding agglutinin in a known and prepared specimen of immune sera. In practice, however, this test has not proved to be reliable.

Lattes reports that he has been able to diagnose accurately the groups of many human stains on cloth, silk, stone, straw, wood, glass, cane-leaf and plaster. He was able to show that two blood stains about 18 months old belonged to the same group, and also to demonstrate the group of a blood stain on a piece of straw. In an important murder case, he determined the group of a small quantity of blood which had been recovered from a squashed flea.

The determination of the group of a blood stain in a criminal case may be a matter of considerable importance. For example, a defendant might claim that a spot on his shirt was his own blood, and not that of the slain man. If the iso-agglutination tests show that the group of the stain is the same as that of the blood of the deceased, this fact may be an important link in the chain of evidence. It cannot identify the blood as coming from a certain individual, because many persons belong to the same blood group, but it may disprove the allegation of a defendant. For this reason, it is important that routine examinations for blood groups should be carried out at the time of autopsy on the bodies of all homicide cases, so that comparison may be made with blood stains collected on weapons and clothing. If the blood group of the victim was group B, and the group of a blood stain on the suspected weapon was also group B, those items of proof would help to establish such a weapon as the means of the homicide especially if the wounds on the deceased were compatible with the type of instrument.

OTHER STAINS

Group specific substances in dried human secretions such as *saliva, semen* or *urine,* may be demonstrated by the absorption technic. These substances are said to occur in a highly concentrated form in saliva and semen so that relatively small quantities of such secretions would be sufficient for the purposes of the test. Schiff reports that the saliva present on the gummed edges of envelopes may be sufficient for a group determination, and Lattes reports a medicolegal case in which it was possible to determine the group from traces of saliva on cigarette stubs. Such tests, to be reliable, must be carried out with great care.

The fact that two classes of individuals have been recognized, namely, those who secrete and those who do not secrete group specific substances in the urine and saliva, is an item of considerable medicolegal importance. Thus if dried saliva stains contain group specific substances, they could not have been derived from an individual whose saliva does not contain such substances. If the dried stain is free of group specific material, three possibilities are present: (1) the saliva came from a group O individual, (2) the saliva came from an individual who does not secrete the group specific substances, (3) the specimen of saliva is free of the substances because of deterioration, and a definite opinion is not possible.

The following case from the Chief Medical Examiner in New York City illustrates the important role played by group specific substances in a medicolegal investigation. After midnight, a man was seen to carry a woman out of a tenement and deposit her on the sidewalk. He was observed and the police were notified. They found the woman dead, lying face up on the sidewalk in the supine position. Not far from the body were two knotted handkerchiefs. Then a man resembling the person who carried the body appeared with a bundle under his arm, which contained an empty wine bottle. He denied that he had ever seen the deceased before or that she had ever been in his apartment. His apartment was examined and on the linoleum was a dried shiny stain similar to that made by serous fluid. This stain, the handkerchiefs, blood and scalp hair from defendant and deceased were sent to the laboratory.

In the meantime an autopsy proved that death was due to strangulation, and in addition revealed postmortem lividity and pressure marks on the front of the body and face, which were not compatible with her supine position on the sidewalk. A large amount of alcohol was found in her brain on toxicologic examination. The stain on the linoleum by the absorption test showed the presence of group specific substance A. The blood of the deceased belonged to group A. The blood of the defendant was group B. The knotted handkerchiefs found near the body contained group specific substance B, probably from the nasal secretion. When confronted with this evidence and its implications, the defendant finally confessed that the deceased had been in his room drinking and that he had strangled her during a sudden quarrel. He had allowed the body to lie face down on the linoleum for several hours until he could find an opportunity to carry it out to the sidewalk. During that interval edema fluid oozed from her nose and dried on the linoleum. He also admitted ownership of the knotted handkerchiefs which, in addition to the group specific substance B, held some light brown hairs in the knots and these were similar to the scalp hairs of the deceased. The laboratory findings, the autopsy and investigation confirmed his confession in full.

THE ROLE OF THE AGGLUTINOGENS IN QUESTIONS OF ILLEGITIMACY AND RELATIONSHIP

Questions of illegitimacy and relationship in many cases may be solved by means of the blood groups as determined by the agglutinogens A, B, M, N and Rh-Hr. These have been shown to be constant factors, inherited according to definite mendelian principles independent of sex. Situations in which the blood group determinations may be of value arise frequently.

For example, a husband may deny that he is the father of a child born in lawful wedlock. The law presumes that a child born under such circumstances is legitimate, unless it can be proved definitely that the husband cannot be the father.

The most common situation is one in which a child is born out of lawful wedlock, and the mother accuses a man of being the father of the child, while the man disclaims the imputation of paternity.

There may be an interchange of newborn infants in a hospital by accident or design. A woman may simulate pregnancy and childbirth and obtain a child, claiming it as her own in order to compel marriage, or to obtain dower in the estate of her husband.

These situations must be solved in some way and the determinations of the agglutinogen content in the bloods from parents and children may be the only reliable way in which to clarify them. The parent-child possibilities have been discussed and the tables have indicated which combinations can be expected and which are impossible. The tests, however, have their limitations; they may exclude a certain individual as the possible father of a child but they cannot positively establish paternity. They can only indicate its possibilities. Another man with the same group as the father could be responsible for the child in question.

The most important laws which govern inheritance of groups O, A, B and AB are:

1. Agglutinogen A or B cannot appear in the child unless it is present in one or both parents (von Dungern and Hirszfeld).

2. An O parent cannot have an AB child and an AB parent cannot have an O child (Bernstein).

3. Parent A mating with a parent B is the only combination known, according to Bernstein, capable of producing children of all four groups, and this is only possible if the parents are heterozygous (AO and BO).

The chances of proving nonpaternity must vary with the group of the individual and to a certain extent with group distribution in the population. Wiener has calculated that the average chance of establishing nonpaternity is about 1 to 6. A European of group A has a chance of about 1 in 13; a group AB person has about 2 chances in 5 of establishing his innocence in a paternity case. In practice, fewer exclusions are made since many men accused are the actual fathers. In 6,665 cases, compiled by Schiff in 1932 from various European countries, the average exclusion percentage was 8.2 per cent or 1 in 12, whereas theoretically 16.3 per cent of exclusions or 1 in 6 was to be expected.

The tests may be carried out on the father and child alone and in 4.7 per cent of the cases, or 1 in 20, this procedure may be sufficient to establish nonpaternity. For example, a child of group O and a father of group AB or vice versa would be impossible. In other cases with a parent of group O and a child of group A or B the group of the mother must be determined before exclusion is established.

If it was possible to differentiate homozygous from heterozygous individuals of groups A and B the chances of proving nonpaternity by means of the four blood groups would be increased 10 per cent. This can be ascertained only if the blood groups of an individual's parents are known. For example, if a person belongs to group A or B, he is heterozygous if one parent is group O and the other A or B. On the other hand, if the individual is an A or B, he is homozygous if both parents belong to group AB (page 641).

If infants are interchanged in a hospital, a determination of the blood groups of the parents and children concerned may offer a solution in more than 50 per cent of the cases. A case of this sort occurred in Chicago in 1930 and the blood group determinations gave results which may be stated as follows:

Mr. B was group AB; Mrs. B, group O. Baby B was group O.

Mr. W was group O; Mrs. W, group O. Baby W was group A.

The babies imputed to the B parents and the W parents were not possible with these combinations and the results of the tests indicated that an interchange of babies had taken place.

If it is not possible to determine nonpaternity by use of the four main blood groups, tests should be carried out for the agglutinogens M and N. A man falsely accused has 18 per cent, or about 1 chance in 6, of proving his innocence by this method. If he belongs to type MN he has no chance of excluding his paternity, but if he is M or N he has more than 1 chance in 3. When all four agglutinogens, A, B, M, N, are used, the average chance of proving nonpaternity is doubled so that 1 out of 3 falsely accused men can be exonerated.

The following table represents the chances in per cent of establishing non-paternity:

Table 27-16. Chances of proving nonpaternity with agglutinogens A, B, M and N

Group	O			A			B			AB		AVER-AGE FOR ALL GROUPS
Percentage exclusion	23.5			7.7			14.6			39.9		16.3
Type	M	N	MN	M	N	MN	M	N	MN	M	N	MN
Percentage exclusion	50.0	54.6	23.5	39.6	45.1	7.7	44.1	49.3	14.6	60.7	64.3	39.9 31.9

After Wiener.

The chances of proving nonpaternity are least in group A, type MN, and greatest in group AB, type N.

The rules for the agglutinogens M and N are as follows: If a child possesses an agglutinogen of either M or N which is not present in the blood of one or both parents, nonpaternity is established. One third of the exclusions are of this kind. If the combination of type M parent with type N child or type N parent with type M child is found, nonpaternity is proved. These exclusions form two thirds of the M and N series. It is possible to prove them without examining the blood of the mother. In cases of the interchange of infants, if all four agglutinogens A, B, M, N, are employed, solution of 70 per cent of the cases is possible.

The mechanism of heredity is the same in the Rh-Hr types as it is in the A-B-O groups or the M-N types, but the details are more complicated because of the greater number of genes and antisera.

There are two conceptions of the inheritance mechanism of the Rh-Hr types as follows:

Wiener's theory of the inheritance of Rh-Hr is through a pair of chromosomes to each of which eight allelic genes stand in a position of possible relationship. Each chromosome has a single locus which contains one gene out of the eight principal possible ones:

Chromosome   8 principal genes (locus):(locus) 8 principal genes   Chromosome

The theory sponsored by Fisher and Race conceives of two chromosomes which have three loci each, while a pair of allelic genes stand in possible relationship to each locus; one pair is $Rh_0 - Hr_0$; a second, $rh' - hr'$; a third, $rh'' - hr''$. Each locus contains one gene out of the pair:

	Rh_0	rh'	rh''		rh''	rh'	Rh_0	
Chromosome	(locus)	(locus)	(locus)	:	(locus)	(locus)	(locus)	Chromosome
	Hr_0	hr'	hr''		hr''	hr'	Hr_0	

Wiener in 1942 found that the concept of separate genes for the factor pairs, $rh'—hr'$, $rh''—hr''$, and Rh_0 did not fit the facts which were available and he adopted the theory of multiple alleles.

These theoretic differences, however, do not interfere with the medicolegal value of the Rh-Hr tests in cases of inheritance or disputed parentage. It is only necessary to evaluate the eight allelic genes and their reactions with the three anti-sera of Rh and the two available Hr-antisera, and the fact that they are represented by 36 genotypes and 18 phenotypes. The serologic and genetic relationship between the Rh and Hr factors is similar to that between M and N and this simplifies to a certain extent their inheritance formula.

Table 27-17. Blood factors rh′ and hr′ in parents and children

MATING	PERCENTAGE OF CHILDREN TO EACH PHENOTYPE		
	rh′	rh′hr′	hr′
rh′ & rh′	100	0	0
hr′ & hr′	0	0	100
rh′ & hr′	0	100	0
rh′ & rh′hr′	50	50	0
hr′ & rh′hr′	0	50	50
rh′hr′ & rh′hr′	25	50	25

Table 27-17 is analogous to the inheritance table for the three M-N types, with rh′ in the place of M and hr′ in place of N. Similarly, tables can be devised to show the inheritance of rh″ — hr″, S-s, K-k and other paired contrasting factors.

The use of the Rh-Hr bloods in disputed paternity cases has greatly increased the bloods which can be differentiated, but at present it would be difficult to give an authoritative estimate of the exact number. Most studies on the heredity of the Rh-Hr groups have been concerned with factors Rh_0, rh′, rh″, and hr′ and only a few with hr″ and rh^w for the reason that their respective antisera are rare and difficult to obtain. So far, no convincing evidence for the existence of Hr_0 has been presented.

Precautions should be taken in medicolegal cases of ascertaining the identity of the individual who is submitting himself to the test. Finger prints, signature and photographs must be used as a means of identification. The date of the examination should be recorded. The tests should be carried out carefully with proper materials and controls; the determination of the M-N types and the Rh-Hr types requires the services of a reliable serologist.

The use of the agglutination reactions is to be recommended in paternity cases because it may exclude the accused as a possible father and save the courts the trouble of an involved and indecisive trial. It would discourage false accusations on the part of the woman who would be open to prosecution for perjury when her claims were proved false. It would not harm the chances of the accused as the tests cannot prove his paternity as a certainty but only as a possibility. Furthermore, it is possible that the result will eliminate him as a possible father. If a defendant refuses to submit to the test it would suggest that he was afraid of having his guilt disclosed.

The German courts in 1924 adopted the isoagglutination reactions of the four principal groups as a useful procedure in medicolegal cases. Since then they have been taken up by many of the other European countries. For the past few years the agglutinogens M and N have been employed similarly, and this is also true of the Rh-Hr types. In the United States in recent years, the tests have been used frequently in medicolegal cases.

In January 1934, Supreme Court Justice Steinbrink in New York State ordered blood grouping tests in a case of disputed paternity, thus setting a precedent. The New York Legislature passed laws empowering the courts to order blood tests in cases of disputed paternity, and many states have followed New York's example. Similar laws have been passed in Wisconsin, Ohio, New Jersey, Maryland, South Dakota, North Carolina, Maine and Pennsylvania.

Blood transfusions have caused a number of deleterious reactions on patients, and illness and death have resulted. Most harmful reactions have followed the use of (1) an incompatible blood for transfusion, or (2) the use of blood containing a harmful substance which affected the recipient unfavorably.

1. The injection of an incompatible blood is one of the commonest causes of hemolytic reactions following transfusion, and many cases result from diagnostic errors in blood typing or from carelessness on the part of someone who misread the label on the blood container. Most of these reactions occur after the administration of the wrong blood type of the A-B-O system, such as the injection of a group B blood into a group A patient or a group AB blood into a group O individual. Here the erythrocytes in the donor's blood are incompatible and there is severe and rapid hemolysis of the transfused erythrocytes by the antibodies in the recipient's serum.

Individuals of group O are known as universal donors because their blood is free of A and B agglutinogens and in cases of emergency can be used for transfusing an individual of other groups in the A-B-O series. The agglutinins in the group O donor's blood are the incompatible elements but they are introduced into the recipient in small amounts and are generally rendered harmless by dilution in the recipient's plasma and by absorption onto the recipient red blood cells. If the O donor has agglutinins of high titer, he may produce a transfusion reaction in an individual of another group, for the strong agglutinins coat the recipient's red blood cells and produce a slow hemolysis. This might be a danger in a recipient weakened by hemorrhage or suffering from a severe anemia, especially if the transfusion is given rapidly or in large amounts. A group O donor with weak agglutinins is preferable for transfusion into a person of another group. In this connection it has been found that when group O donors have received injections of tetanus antitoxin it seems to sharpen the action of the agglutinins in the donor's blood.

Of course if the donors are available, it is the best policy to transfuse the recipient with the blood of the same A-B-O group as his own. If this is not possible an O donor with feeble agglutinins may be employed, and the blood should be injected slowly and in small quantity. Both donor's blood and recipient's blood must be carefully typed, and the bloods should be cross matched for compatibility after the technic described by Wiener. With group O donors, the titer of the agglutinins in the donor's serum should be determined to see if they are too potent for use on a sick patient. The use of a universal donor is best reserved for an emergency case, when a donor of the same group as the recipient is not available.

If Rh-positive blood is transfused into an Rh-negative individual for the first time, a transfusion reaction is not likely to occur. Then after an interval, the patient may have been sensitized to the Rh-positive agglutinogens, and a second injection of the Rh-positive blood may cause a transfusion reaction of greater or less severity. If the patient is a woman who becomes pregnant with an Rh-positive fetus, her sensitization may cause the child to develop erythroblastosis, and sometimes produce a stillbirth. Conversely a woman not previously sensitized to Rh-positive blood, may develop that sensitivity if she becomes pregnant with an Rh-positive fetus. This subject will be discussed later.

It is highly desirable that an Rh-negative woman should be transfused with Rh-negative blood, and if such a donor is available and a member of the same A-B-O group the problem would be solved. Unfortunately transfusions on Rh-negative women in the child bearing age are often emergency procedures, and donors of the proper group are usually not to be found; there may not even be time to determine properly the Rh factor in the patient's blood. Some recommend that donors of group O, with agglutinins of weak titer, who are also Rh-negative should be available and that their blood could be given to Rh-positive and Rh-negative patients alike. There is not much danger in transfusing an Rh-positive individual with Rh-negative blood, and the possibility of sensitizing such a recipient to one of the Hr factors is remote. In rare instances an Rh-negative donor may contain powerful antibodies against Rh-positive bloods. If such blood is transfused into an Rh-negative woman, the strong antibodies may sensitize the recipient passively against the Rh-positive factor. A donor of this type would be dangerous to use on an Rh positive recipient and may cause a hemolytic transfusion reaction.

In an emergency, if an Rh-negative blood is not obtainable for an Rh-negative patient, a transfusion of Rh-positive blood may be undertaken, after a careful cross matching test has been performed to see if no other incompatibilities exist. As Wiener has pointed out, about 1 out of 2 Rh-negative persons become sensitized to Rh-positive blood after exposure to the antigen by injection, so that there is a chance that the recipient may escape those ill effects.

Irregular transfusion reactions are discussed under Other Blood Groups on page 655. Another type of hemolytic reaction is caused when blood is stored in a container and is damaged; if it is used for transfusion it will be destroyed by the recipient and produce a hemoglobinuric nephrosis.

The harmful effects of injecting a specifically incompatible blood into the circulation of a recipient may start during the transfusion with symptoms of oppressive precordial pain, a sensation of fullness in the head, tingling pains over the entire body and characteristic severe, sharp pains in the lumbar region. The face is markedly cyanotic, the respirations are labored, the pulse is rapid, and the patient may collapse with cold clammy skin, nausea and vomiting. In about 15 minutes to an hour, there is a chill, high fever ($103°$ to $107°$ F), urticarial rashes, delirium and shock. If he survives the attack, he may rally slightly. A somewhat light jaundice may develop, then hemoglobinuria, anuria and uremia. Stupor, convulsions and coma occur at the end. Death may take place in from a few hours to a few days. Some cases recover.

Some cases are reported who die suddenly of massive agglutination of the donor's cells with cardiac and cerebral embolism. Others develop a purpuric eruption.

Most deaths are due to the anuria and the kidney involvement. According to Witts, the anuria is caused by the blocking of the urinary tubules by the blood pigment and is only encountered when the urine is acid. The kidneys show a light brownish gray cortex and dark purplish pyramids. The cortex is swollen and the cortical epithelium shows parenchymatous degeneration. Microscopic examination discloses blood pigment, red blood cells, leukocytes and erythrocytes in the convoluted and collecting tubules (Fig. 27-3). This lesion is directly referable to the hemolysis of the transfused blood in the blood vessels and its attempted excretion through the kidneys.

The anaphylactic reaction is not so common. It is caused by a protein in the donor's serum which elicits an allergic response from the recipient. The symptoms start during the transfusion or shortly after with high fever, asthma from intense bronchial spasm, involuntary evacuation of urine and feces and death in a few hours from asphyxia. Hemolysis, hemoglobinuria and anuria are absent.

Infectious diseases sometimes transmitted from donor to recipient through a transfusion are homologous serum hepatitis which also may be transmitted by injection of stored plasma; malaria has been transmitted especially when the donor has acquired the disease in the tropics; syphilis is transmitted rarely; measles and influenza have been transmitted; stored blood may become contaminated by bacteria, especially the genus *Pseudomonas* and the coli-aerogenes group, and be toxic enough to cause death if used for transfusion.

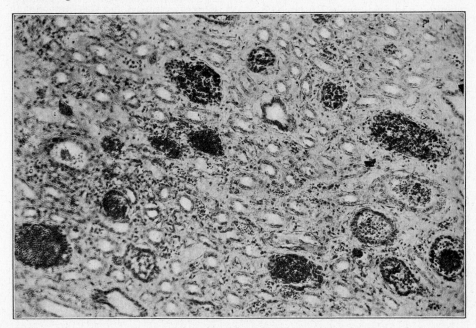

Fig. 27-3. Kidney Lesion after Transfusion with Wrong Type of Blood.

Collecting tubules of kidney are filled with agglutinated red blood cells and hemoglobin deposits.

Accidents following transfusion are pulmonary embolism from blood clots which have formed in the stored blood; air embolism caused by pumping air under pressure into the blood reservoir so that it enters the vein; infective thrombosis at the site of the vein used for injection. A transfusion given too rapidly or in too great quantity may cause death by heart failure or cerebral hemorrhage; if citrated blood is used and is given in excess it may cause hypocalcemia.

Deaths of patients following transfusions may result in a civil malpractice action against a hospital where the transfusion was performed, the physician who performed it, or both. Each case must be judged upon the circumstances which attend it; that in which the defendants would be most vulnerable would be where death resulted because the patient was transfused with an incompatible blood of the A-B-O series. Such a case would be a res ipsa loquitur which means that the law would require the medical defendant to exonerate himself by giving a satisfactory explanation for the fatality.

CONGENITAL HEMOLYTIC DISEASE

Levine and Stetson in 1939 reported the case of a woman, just delivered of a stillborn macerated fetus, who had a severe hemolytic reaction when transfused with a presumably compatible blood of the same A-B-O group. This intragroup reaction was considered to be the result of isoimmunization of the mother by some fetal antigen, acquired from the father and foreign to the mother.

In 1940 Landsteiner and Wiener reported the discovery of the Rh antigen, already discussed on pages 649 to 651. In 1940 Wiener and Peters demonstrated that the Rh factor in human blood was antigenic since repeated injections of Rh-positive red cells into an Rh-negative person produced an antibody which could hemolyze and agglutinate Rh-positive blood. These authors noted that pregnant or recently delivered women were especially liable to show severe hemolytic reactions after their first transfusion, and the theory was entertained that through microscopic breaks in the placenta fetal red cells passed into the maternal circulation and sensitized the mother to a fetal antigen of paternal origin. In 1941 Levine and collaborators reported statistic evidence which indicated that this theory was correct, and that the Rh antibodies formed in the mother were responsible for the hemolytic transfusion reactions and for the development of *erythroblastosis fetalis* or hemolytic disease of the newborn.

The bloods of mothers whose infants were suffering from congenital hemolytic disease were Rh-negative in 93 per cent of 153 cases, and in 30 per cent of 141 cases had anti-Rh agglutinins. The blood of the fathers and infants were invariably Rh-positive. The anti-Rh agglutinin in the mother's blood was transmitted through the placenta and caused congenital hemolytic disease in the fetus. Further studies indicated that Rh_0 is the most common and potent antigen in the production of isoimmunization in any maternal blood which is Rh_0 negative and is consequently common in congenital hemolytic disease.

In 1941 Levine reported the case of an Rh-positive woman whose infant had typical hemolytic disease of the newborn. An antibody was present in her serum which agglutinated the red blood cells of her Rh-negative husband and infant. Levine on the basis of the reversed immunologic pattern in the case gave the antigen found in father and child but absent in the mother, the name Hr. This Hr antigen of Levine was shown by the studies of Race and Fisher to be an allele of rh′ and could more properly be designated as hr′. Congenital hemolytic disease in an Rh-positive mother is not as common as in an Rh-negative mother.

The antibodies in the maternal circulation after entering the fetal circulation become attached to receptors on the fetal red blood cells and a small proportion remain free in the serum. These antibodies act with different intensity in different cases and produce a variable degree of hemolysis in the child's blood. Some of the newborn infants in these cases are stillbirths while others are born alive, either dying after birth or eventually recovering.

In isoimmunization to Rh, other varieties of antibodies are formed in addition to the anti-Rh agglutinin. They are the blocking antibodies or glutinins, which are more active than the agglutinins in causation of congenital hemolytic disease. These antibodies offer a means of demonstrating the sensitivity of the woman to the Rh antigen.

Agglutination Test. Rh-positive red blood cells and bivalent Rh-agglutinin give agglutination. A drop of a 2 per cent saline suspension of group O, Rh-positive red blood cells is mixed with a drop of the patient's serum in a small test tube. The mixture is incubated in a water bath for 30 to 60 minutes at body temperature. The sediment in the tube is examined; with a negative reaction the suspension is even and each red blood cell is separated from the others; with a positive reaction large clumps appear in the sediment; if the serum contains only a little Rh agglutinin it may be necessary to centrifuge the tube to bring out the reaction.

Like other antibodies, Rh agglutinins are conceived of as modified serum globulins. On each antibody molecule there are two combining groups for the receptors scattered over the surface of the red blood cells. When the antibodies combine with these receptors they link the red cells in a meshwork and agglutination takes place.

BLOCKING TEST. In some cases of congenital hemolytic disease it is not possible to show the presence of anti-Rh agglutinins in the maternal serum. Wiener points out that in such cases a special type of antibody is present which cannot cause agglutination perhaps because it is univalent. If enough of these join with the combining sites on the erythrocytes the univalent blocking antibody occupies the red cell receptors and prevents any combination by agglutinins. This can be demonstrated by the following test: A drop of group O, Rh-positive red blood cells is mixed with a drop of the patient's serum and incubated on the water bath. No agglutination occurs. Then add a drop of potent human anti-Rh serum and reincubate. If blocking bodies are not present, agglutination will occur. The absence of agglutination is diagnostic of the presence of blocking bodies.

Conglutination Test. Rh-positive red blood cells and univalent Rh-(blocker or glutinin) and conglutinin (X protein) give conglutination. This test is performed in two stages, and depends on a third component beside the Rh agglutinogen and the agglutinin. The third component is analogous to the complement in serologic hemolysis in that it is incorporated in the specially sensitized red blood cell where it accomplishes the agglutination. It is not precisely the same as complement as it is thermostable at 60° C., and is a colloid component in the plasma, a complex of albumin, globulin and phospholipid. It is known as the X protein. The Rh antibody in the conglutination reaction is univalent and is called the Rh glutinin. It seems probable that the Rh glutinin and Rh blocking antibody are the same, but conglutination is a more sensitive method of detecting the antibody than the blocking test.

If the plasma is diluted with saline solution the X protein is split into smaller molecules of albumin and globulin, and for this reason saline solution must be avoided and the red blood cells suspended in inactivated AB serum. Positive reactions in the conglutination test can be obtained when the agglutinins and blocking antibodies are present and when the other two tests are negative. More recently even more sensitive tests for detecting these antibodies have been devised, notably, the antiglobulin test (Coombs' test) or the use of test cells treated with proteolytic enzymes.

Complications During Pregnancy of Rh Incompatibility. Marriage between an Rh-negative woman and an Rh-positive man occurs in about 13 per cent of all marriages. To prepare for eventualities it is desirable that the Rh type of every pregnant woman should be determined. The physician should also ascertain if she has had a previous blood transfusion as there is a possibility that it was Rh-positive.

If the woman is Rh-negative, the husband's Rh formula should be determined. If he is Rh-negative there is no danger of congenital hemolytic disease in the offspring. If the husband is Rh-positive it is important to determine his genotype, whether homozygous or heterozygous. If his parents are alive and the gene formula of one is Rh-negative, he is a heterozygous Rh-positive. If both are positive he may be homozygous Rh-positive and if so, his offspring will then all be Rh-positive.

If there are indications that the mother has had an infant with erythroblastosis in a previous pregnancy, a high titer of Rh antibodies with a special rise in the last trimester of gestation, and a homozygous Rh-positive husband, there may be justification for an early delivery, at about the thirty-seventh week of pregnancy. If the woman has had previous pregnancies which were disastrous because of congenital hemolytic disease and the husband is a homozygous Rh-positive, it is obvious that future pregnancies will also be disastrous and it may be desirable to perform a therapeutic abortion before the third month after due consideration of the problem with a consultant. In a situation of this type it may be necessary to advise against future pregnancies.

Severe cases of congenital hemolytic disease show varied pathologic lesions. In one type the fetus in utero is affected and presents the form of hydrops fetalis in which the baby is swollen with massive subcutaneous edema and effusions in the serous cavities; the placenta is large, boggy and edematous with large swollen cotyledons. If the fetus dies before delivery it may show maceration. If the baby lives a few days after birth it may develop icterus gravis neonatorum, with intense jaundice sometimes accompanied by purpuric spots and petechiae. If there is much hemolysis, there is a red cell hyperplasia of the bone marrow and extramedullary hematopoiesis in the spleen and liver. Fatty degeneration of the liver cells, hemosiderin deposits and engorgement of the bile caniculae are noted. Spleen and liver may be enlarged. Pulmonary hemorrhages may occur. There may be yellowish pigmentation of the basal nuclei and other parts of the brain which may lead to neuronal degeneration and gliosis.

The hematologic changes in the disease in comparison with normal standards is as follows. The normal hemoglobin value during the first day of life is 16.0 gm. per cent and the normal red cell count is 5.5 to 6.0 millions per cubic millimeter. Cases of hydrops fetalis show a hemoglobin value of 4.0 gm. per cent and a red cell count of 1.0 millions per cubic millimeter. The blood smear in some cases shows an increased number of normoblasts and erythroblasts. A hyperbilirubinemia may be present. Agglutination tests on the maternal blood and also on the fetal blood show potent Rh antibodies.

One treatment of congenital hemolytic disease is to transfuse the infant with a type specific blood group, Rh-negative blood, when the proper indications exist. The preferred method at present is the so-called exchange transfusion. The reader is referred to Wiener and Wexler, and Diamond for further information.

Some infants at three to four weeks after birth show a severe anemia without jaundice accompanied by a slight splenic enlargement, which has been called congenital anemia of the newborn. In these cases the diagnosis is made by detecting specific antibodies in the mother's serum and in the infant's blood.

Other blood antigens may occasionally produce congenital hemolytic disease, such as group A or group B in heterospecific pregnancies, or the Kell-Cellano system as a result of isoimmunization. In such cases the serum of the mother must be investigated for antibodies which act on the red blood cell antigens of husband and offspring, as these are probably the stimulus for the antibody formation.

REFERENCES

Bernstein, F. Zusammenfassende Betrachtungen über die erblichen Blutstrukturen des Menschen, Ztschr. f. indukt. Abstammungs- u. Vererbungsl., 37:237, 1925.
────── Ergebnisse einer biostatistischen zusammenfassenden Betrachtung über die erblichen Blutstrukturen des Menschen, Klin. Wchnschr., 3:1495, 1924.
Bertinshaw, D., and others. The combination of blood groups in a sample of 475 people in a London hospital, Ann. Eugenics, 15:234, 1950.

Boorman, K. E., and Dodd, B. E.   The group specific substances A, B, M, N, and Rh. Their occurrence in tissues and body fluids, J. Path. & Bact., 55:329, 1943.

Boyd, W. C.   Genetics and the Races of Man, Boston, Little, Brown and Co., 1950, p. 453.

———— Present status of the Rh blood types and nomenclature, Am. J. Phys. Anthropol., 3:265, 1949.

Coombs, R. R. A., Mourant, A. E., and Race, R. R.   A new test for the detection of weak and "incomplete" Rh agglutinins, Brit. J. Exper. Path., 26:255, 1945.

Cutbush, M., and Mollison, P. L.   The Duffy blood group, Heredity, 4:383, 1950.

Diamond, L. K.   Replacement transfusion as a treatment for erythroblastosis fetalis, Pediatrics, 2:520, 1948.

———— and Abelson, N. M.   The demonstration of anti-Rh agglutinins: an accurate and rapid slide test, J. Lab. & Clin. Med., 30:204, 1945.

Epstein, A. A., and Ottenberg, R.   A simple method of performing serum reactions, Proc. New York Path. Soc., 8:120, 1908.

Fisher, R. A.   The rhesus factor, Am. Scientist, 35:95, 1947.

Furuhata and Imamura.   Reference to group Q in Japanese, Japanese J. Genetics, 12:50, 1936; 11:91, 1935.

Grubb, R.   Observations in the human blood group system Lewis, Acta path. et microbiol. Scandinav., 28(1):61, 1951.

Hooker, S. B., and Boyd, W. C.   The chance of establishing non-paternity by determination of blood group, J. Immunol., 16:451, 1929.

Landsteiner, K.   The Specificity of Serological Reactions, Rev. ed., Cambridge, Mass., Harvard University Press, 1945.

———— and Wiener, A. S.   Studies on an agglutinogen (Rh) in human blood reacting with anti-rhesus sera and human Isoantibodies, J. Exper. Med., 74:309, 1941.

———— and Wiener, A. S.   An agglutinable factor in human blood recognized by immune sera for rhesus blood, Proc. Soc. Exper. Biol. & Med., 43:223, 1940.

———— and others. On agglutination reactions observed with human bloods, chiefly among Negroes, J. Immunol., 27:469, 1934.

———— Forensic applications of serologic individuality tests, J.A.M.A., 103:1041, 1934.

———— and Levine, P.   Reference to group P, J. Immunol., 20:179, 1931; 18:87, 1930.

———— Newer Knowledge of Bacteriology and Immunology, in Jordan and Falk, Chicago, 1928, p. 905.

———— and Levine, P.   On individual difference in human blood, J. Exper. Med., 47:757, 1928.

———— and Levine, P.   On the inheritance of agglutinogens of human blood demonstrable by immune agglutinins, J. Exper. Med., 48:731, 1928.

———— Über Agglutinationserscheinungen normalen Menschlichen Blutes, Wien. klin. Wchnschr., 14:1132, 1901.

———— Zur Kenntis der antifermentativen, lytischen und agglutinierenden Wirkungen des Blutserums und der Lymphe, Zentralbl. f. Bakt., 27:357, 1900.

Lattes, L.   Individuality of the Blood, London, Oxford University Press, 1932.

Levine, P., and others.   The Kell-Cellano Kk genetic system of human blood factors, Blood, 4:869, 1949.

———— A Survey of the Significance of the Rh Factor, in Hill and Dameshek, The Rh Factor in the Clinic and the Laboratory, New York, Grune and Stratton, 1948, p. 3.

———— and Waller, R. K.   Erythroblastosis fetalis in the first born, Blood, 1:143, 1946.

———— and Wong, H.   The incidence of the Rh factor and erythroblastosis fetalis in Chinese, Am. J. Obst. & Gynec., 45:832, 1943.

———— Pathogenesis of erythroblastosis fetalis, J. Pediat., 23:656, 1943.

———— Isoimmunization in Pregnancy and the Pathogenesis of Erythroblastosis Fetalis, in Karsner and Hooker, Year Book of Pathology and Immunology, Chicago, Year Book Publishers, Inc., 1941, p. 505.

———— and others. Isoimmunization in pregnancy; its possible bearing on pathogenesis of erythroblastosis fetalis, J.A.M.A., 116:825, 1941.

———— and others. The role of isoimmunization in the pathogenesis of erythroblastosis fetalis, Am. J. Obst. & Gynec., 42:925, 1941.

———— and Katzin, E. M.   Isoimmunization in pregnancy and the varieties of isoagglutinins observed, Proc. Soc. Exper. Biol. & Med., 45:343, 1940.

———— and Stetson, R.   An unusual case of intra group agglutination, J.A.M.A., 113:126, 1939.

———— Blood groups, theory and medico-legal application, J. Lab. & Clin. Med., 20:785, 1935.

Mollison, P. L., Mourant, A. E., and Race, R. R.   The Rh blood groups and their clinical effects, Med. Res. Council (Great Britain) Spec. Rept. Ser., No. 19, 1948, Her Majesty's Stationary Office, London.

Morton, J. A., and Pickles, N. M.   Use of trypsin in the detection of anti-Rh antibodies, Nature, London, 159:779, 1947.

Mourant, A. E.   A new rhesus antibody, Nature, London, 155:542, 1945.

O'Hara, C. E., and Osterburg, J. W.   An Introduction to Criminalistics, New York, The Macmillan Co., 1952, pp. 412 to 424.

Race, R. R., and Sanger, R.   Blood Groups in Man, Springfield, Ill., Charles C Thomas, Publisher, 1950.

Rosenfield, R., and others.   The detection of weakly reacting Rh_o (D^u) factor, Blood, 6:1123, 1951.

Sacks, Milton S.   Hemolytic Disease of the Fetus and Newborn, in Eastman, Williams Obstetrics, 10th ed., New York, Appleton-Century-Crofts, Inc., 1950, pp. 1001-1025.

Sanger, R., and others. An antibody which subdivides the M-N blood groups, Heredity, 2:131, 1948.

Schatkin, S. B.   Disputed Paternity Proceedings, 2nd ed., New York, Matthew Bender and Co., 1947.

Schiff, F.   Die Technik der Blutgruppenuntersuchung für Kliniker und Gerichtsärtze, Berlin, Julius Springer, 1932.

Simmons, R. T. and others.   The A_1-A_2-B-O, M-N, and Rh blood groups in southern Chinese, Med. J. Australia, 2:917, 1950.

State of New York, No. 124, Int. 123, Jan. 9, 1935. Cited by Levine, above, also Nos. 167, 682, Int. 166.

Stiller, R. K.   A follow-up study of 35 erythroblastotic infants, Am. J. Dis. Child., 73:651, 1947.

Stormont, C., and others.   The B and C systems of bovine blood groups, Genetics, 36:134, 1950.

Strandskov, H. H.   Recent views on the genetics of the Rh-Hr factors, Bull. New York Acad. Med., 25:249, 1949.

Von Dungern, E., and Hirszfeld, L.   Ueber Vererbung gruppenspezifischer Structuren des Blutes, Ztschr. f. Immunitätsforsch. u. exper. Therap., 6:284, 1910.

Wallerstein, H.   Substitution transfusion: a new treatment for severe erythroblastosis fetalis, Am. J. Dis. Child., 73:19, 1947.

Waterhouse, J. A. H., and Hogben, L.   Incompatibility of mother and fetus with respect to the isoagglutinogen A and its antibody, Brit. J. Sociol. Med., 1:1, 1947.

Wiener, A. S., and others.   Blood group factors in anthropoid apes and monkeys, Am. J. Phys. Anthropol., 11:39, 1953.

——— and others. Fatal hemolytic transfusion reaction caused by sensitization to a new blood factor U, J.A.M.A., 153: 1444, 1953.

——— and others. Observations on isosensitization to the Kell factor, J. Lab. & Clin. Med., 42:570, 1953.

——— Terminology of blood groups, Am. J. Clin. Path., 23:987, 1953.

——— and others.   Medicolegal aspects of blood transfusion, J.A.M.A., 151:1435, 1953.

——— and others. Studies on the heredity of the human blood groups. I. The N-M types, Acta Geneticae Medicae et Genellologiae, 2:391, 1953.

——— Heredity of the M-N-S blood types, Am. J. Human Genetics, 4:37, 1952.

——— History of the rhesus blood types, J. Hist. Med. & Allied Sc., Vol. VII, No. 4, 1952.

——— and others.   Medicolegal application of blood grouping tests, J.A.M.A., 149:699, 1952.

——— and Wexler, I. B.   The mosaic structure of red blood cell agglutinogens, Bact. Rev., 16:69, 1952.

——— Heredity of the M-N types, Am. J. Human Genetics, 3:179, 1951.

——— The Rh-Hr blood types: serology, genetics, and nomenclature, Tr. New York Acad. Sc., 13:199, 1951.

——— and Wexler, I. B.   The management of the isosensitized pregnant patient and her erythroblastotic infant, M. Clin. North America, 35:749, 1951.

——— Treatment of erythroblastosis by exchange transfusion, Post-Grad. M. J., 7:1, 1950.

——— Heredity of the Rh blood types VII, Proc. Eighth Internat. Congress of Genetics, Hereditas, Suppl. vol., 1949.

——— Medicolegal aspects of the Rh-Hr blood types, Bull. New York Acad. Med., 25:255, 1949.

——— and Gordon, E. B.   Studies on the blood factor rh^w, Am. J. Clin. Path., 19:621, 1949.

——— Application of the Rh blood types and Hr factor in disputed parentage, J. Lab. & Clin. Med., 31:575, 1946.

——— and Wexler, I. B.   The use of heparin when performing exchange transfusions in newborn infants, J. Lab. & Clin. Med., 31:1016, 1946.

——— Conglutination test for Rh sensitization, J. Lab. & Clin. Med., 30:662, 1945.

——— and others.   Individual blood differences in Mexican Indians with special reference to the Rh blood types and the Hr factors, J. Exper. Med., 81:559, 1945.

——— Rh factors in clinical medicine, J. Lab. & Clin. Med., 30:957, 1945.

——— Theory and nomenclature of the Hr blood factors, Science, 102:479, 1945.

Wiener, A. S. A new test (blocking test) for Rh sensitization, Proc. Soc. Exper. Biol. & Med., 56:173, 1944.

——— The Rh series of allelic genes, Science, 100:595, 1944.

——— Blood Groups and Transfusion, 3rd ed., Springfield, Ill., Charles C Thomas, Publisher, 1943.

——— Genetic theory of the Rh blood types, Proc. Soc. Exper. Biol. & Med., 54:238, 1943.

——— Hemolytic reactions following transfusions of the homologous group: a further observation on the role of property Rh, Arch. Path., 32:227, 1941.

——— and Peters, H. R. Hemolytic reactions following transfusions of the homologous group with three cases in which the same agglutinogen was responsible, Ann. Int. Med., 13:2306, 1940.

——— Group P, cited by Zieve, Wiener and Fries, Ann. Eugenics, 7:163, 1938.

——— Determination of non-paternity by means of blood groups, with special reference to agglutinogens M and N of Landsteiner and Levine, Am. J. M. Sc., 186:257, 1933.

——— Lederer, M., and Polayes, S. H. Studies in iso-hemagglutination on the chances of proving non-paternity with special reference to blood groups, J. Immunol., 18:201, 1930.

Witts, L. J. A note on blood transfusion, Lancet, 1:1297, 1929.

Young, L. E., and others. Hemolytic disease in newborn dogs following isoimmunization of the dam by transfusions, Science, 109:620, 1949.

28

Microscopy of Hair and Other Material

The microscopic examination of hairs, fibers, fragments of tissues, and other minute objects from the scene of a crime is important as it may lead to the discovery of significant clues or vital evidence.

HAIR

Hair is a specialized epithelial appendage which occurs on the skin except on the palms of the hands, the soles of the feet, the nail areas, the vermillion border of the lips and similar regions. Anatomically the hair consists of a root, shaft and tip. The root is that part of the hair, buried in the subcutaneous fat below the dermis, and is the epithelial organ from which the hair develops; * it has the shape of an inverted goblet, its lower end being indented by a vascular connective tissue projection, the papilla, which carries nutrition and pigment granules to the hair. The shaft is the main part of the hair and grows from the root, extending through the dermis and onto the skin surface; in its passage through the upper layers of the skin, the shaft is enclosed in an epithelial canal, the sheath, which extends from the root to the surface epidermis. If the hair is undisturbed in its growth, the shaft tapers to a point, called the tip; in many instances the tip may be blunted because the hair has been clipped or the tip may be frayed because the hair has been brushed excessively.

The shaft of the hair is divided into three anatomic zones: medulla, cortex and cuticula. The medulla is the innermost zone, a central canal of varying size and shape containing cellular epithelial debris. Human hairs possess a medulla which is small in comparison with the shaft and frequently is not continuous; in many hairs it is absent. Usually the medullary canal in animal hairs is proportionally broader to the thickness of the cortex than it is in human hairs.

The cortex is the cornified zone of the shaft which surrounds the medulla. It develops from the polyhedral epithelial cells in the root, which project outward through the sheath and become flattened, elongated, spindle-shaped, non-nucleated horny plates; these overlap each other and cohere to form the cortical portion of the shaft. In some hairs pigment granules are not present in the cortex and the color of the hair is white. In most hairs the cortical cells contain pigment granules which give the hair its color; the microscopic pattern and distribution of the pigment granules in the cortex are important diagnostic criteria. In human hairs the pigment is concentrated in the peripheral portion of the cortex, while in animal hairs it is usually concentrated around the medulla.

The cuticula is the outermost layer of the shaft and surrounds the cortex; it is a single layer of flat, non-nucleated, pigment-free cells which overlap like the scales of a fish in such a way that the free edges of the scales point toward the distal end of the hair. The cuticular outlines form a distinctive pattern on the outside of a

* The rate of hair growth is given as one-sixtieth of an inch every 24 hours, but this is only an approximation because there is an individual difference between the functional activity of the roots of separate hairs, even in the same area, and therefore different rates of growth.

hair. On human hairs, they appear microscopically as fine, wavy, transversely-elongated, polygonal markings which are said by some to be narrower than similar markings on the hairs of other animals. The role of the cuticula in hair identification will be discussed later.

Hairs in different parts of the body increase in length until they reach their allotted growth after which they drop out. A new hair bulb develops from the remains of the old one, and from this another hair grows and drops out in turn. This process is continuous and is best observed in a region like the scalp where the hairs are closely crowded together. In a tuft of scalp hairs, the separate fibers will exhibit different lengths, thicknesses and degrees of pigmentation, because of the continual replacement and falling-out. Incidentally, the growth of hair stops at death; any apparent growth after death is due to postmortem shrinkage of the skin which exposes a little more of the hair shaft above the epidermis.

Examination of Hair. When a specimen is brought to the laboratory it must be identified to the examiner by the bearer, and then a record is made of the place, day and hour of delivery, the name of the person delivering the specimen, and the name of the person receiving it. This record is essential to establish the connection of the specimen with the other evidence in the case, for without such a link the result of the examination cannot be presented as testimony in court. Occasionally the bearer brings in a weapon such as a hammer, a monkey wrench or a pair of blacksmith's tongs, from which the examiner may recover a number of fibers. In such cases the examiner should mark the weapon with his initials and the date, so that he can identify the weapon in court at some future time.

The examination must be conducted systematically according to a procedure which is capable of modification so that it will meet the requirements of an individual case. The examiner should first scrutinize the fibers with the naked eye, and then examine them under a hand lens. Their number must be recorded and the length of each fiber actually measured; if a large number are present, enough fibers should be measured to determine the different variations in length. The color, texture and other characteristics of the fibers must be described and due record made of any abnormalities. Any foreign substance adherent to the fibers should be identified if possible. The fibers should be examined in the dry state under the low power of the microscope to check on the presence of extraneous substances.

The next procedure is to make permanent mounts of the specimens. The hairs or other fibers are washed with soap and water, alcohol, or any other solvent efficacious in removing dirt, dried, and finally mounted in xylol-balsam on a microscope slide as a whole mount. The treatment given the specimen will depend upon the problem presented in the individual case, and it would not be feasible to formulate a set of rules to apply to every conceivable contingency. If the fiber is a short hair, a whole mount is made, and the entire fiber may be photographed at a low magnification. If the hair is longer, a number of photographs may be taken of its entire length by photographing short segments in serial succession; after the films are developed and printed, the ends of the segments may be joined and an image of the hair in magnified form constructed. After the photographic record is made, the hair may be removed from the whole mount and prepared for cross section. With long hairs, the extremities and mid-portion may be mounted as whole mounts and the rest of the hair prepared for cross section. If the hair is small and minute, it may be sufficient to preserve it as a whole mount without sectioning it.

In most instances, microscopic examination of the whole mount should determine the nature of the fiber. If the specimen is hair this examination may determine the size, shape and characteristics of its longitudinal outline, the nature of the two ends of the hair, the type of pigmentation in the shaft, and the size and shape of the medulla (unless the shaft is opaque because of dark pigmentation). Some recommend measurement of the diameter of the hair by the micrometer eyepiece, but the authors agree with Glaister that such procedures are of doubtful value, because of the great individual variations in diameter between hairs from the same individual and even between different segments of the same hair.

Cross sections of hairs are made as follows: the hairs are placed in 95 per cent alcohol for 10 minutes, washed in water and then put in a 5 to 10 per cent aqueous solution of sodium or potassium hydroxide for 5 to 10 minutes, depending upon how soon the hair is softened. This interval is determined by the experience of the examiner and is usually considered complete if the hair shows signs of having lost most of its elasticity. It is washed in water, put in 95 per cent alcohol for 5 to 10 minutes and is ready for mounting. If the hairs are curly or kinky, they may be straightened out on a piece of blotting paper before their second immersion in 95 per cent alcohol.

The hairs are sectioned in cubes of liver tissue of about 3 mm. diameter which have been fixed in 10 per cent aqueous solution of formaldehyde, hardened in 95 per cent alcohol and then preserved in acetone. The cube is prepared for use by partially incising one surface at right angles to two of its parallel sides, then stretching out the prepared hairs in the bed of this incision, and trimming away excess hairs at each end with scissors. The cube and its load are placed in acetone one half hour, then partially dried and embedded 12 to 48 hours in celloidin dissolved in equal parts of absolute alcohol and ether. The cube is mounted on a wooden block so that the slit is vertical, and the mount is hardened in chloroform for one half hour or over. Cross sections of the hairs are made on the sliding microtome, the sections are mounted unstained on a microscope slide, cleared in oil of thyme, and preserved under a coverglass in xylol-balsam. The paraffin method of sectioning tissue can also be adapted to this procedure.

This procedure demonstrates the outline of the hair shaft on cross section, the relation of the cortex to the medulla and the distribution of pigment in the cortex. Cross sections are necessary when deeply pigmented hairs are to be examined, for such fibers are practically opaque when studied under the microscope in whole mount. The greatest advantage of cross sections is that it enables the examiner to see a number of individual hairs in the same field of the microscope, which is difficult to accomplish with whole mount preparations.

Many consider that the cuticular pattern on the outside of the hair is important diagnostically, and several methods are recommended for demonstrating these markings. In one, the hair either must be naturally colorless or must be bleached with a mixture of hydrogen peroxide and ammonia water so as to render it translucent; the markings are demonstrated by examining the dry hair microscopically on a microscope slide. In another method the colorless or bleached hair is stained in Gram's gentian violet, washed rapidly in 95 per cent alcohol without counterstain, cleared in oil of thyme and mounted on xylol-balsam; the cuticular markings appear as violet colored lines on the hair surface. These methods are disadvantageous in that the hairs are spoiled for other examinations.

Other methods consist in impressing the cuticular markings of hairs on some suitable material and then studying the pattern of the impression. Moritz has suggested that a plastic film made from a solution of cellulose acetate dissolved in an equal volume of amyl acetate, is excellent for this purpose. Chen Anliong has described a procedure in which the cuticular patterns are impressed on photographic plates. These methods have the advantage of not altering the hair appreciably so that it can be subjected to histologic and other examinations.

The patterns presented by the cuticula on the hairs of different animal species have been classified by Moritz as spinous, dentate, polyhedral, piscine, pavement polyhedral, annular and irregular annular. Human hairs are included in the irregular annular group. Moritz has pointed out that it is possible to identify some animal species by the cuticular patterns, but in other cases it is not possible because the diagnostic criteria are not well defined. For this reason examination of the cuticula should always be combined with other methods of investigation.

Identification of Hairs. Microscopic examination of hairs should: (1) differentiate hairs from other fibers; (2) distinguish human hairs from animal hairs; (3) determine if possible, the race, age and sex of the individual and the part of the body from which the hairs were taken; (4) identify any abnormality of the hair or any unusual treatment inflicted on the hair.

HAIR AND OTHER FIBERS. Several types of fibers may resemble hairs when seen with the naked eye but can be distinguished on microscopic examination. The most common of these are cotton fibers, silk fibers, linen fibers, wool filaments, felt fragments, straw fibers, wood fibers and feathers. All of these materials have a characteristic microscopic appearance and the chance of confusing them with hair is remote.

Cotton fibers are translucent, flat, tape-like, and colorless or dyed filaments which show a tendency to become twisted. Linen fibers are translucent, irregularly cylindrical, and under the microscope appear like miniature strands of bamboo, because of nodose markings at more or less regular intervals. Silk fibrils are fine translucent, cylindrical, smooth homogeneous filaments which may be dyed various colors. Wool is from the hair of sheep which has been treated to make it suitable for cloth manufacture, and its fibers, dyed or undyed, are translucent, smooth, cylindrical, curly and often show polygonal cuticular marks on the surface. Felt fibrils are hairs from rodents like beavers or rabbits, specially treated for the manufacture of felt articles, and microscopically present the typical appearance of wool hairs and smaller hairs found on the pelts of such animals. Fibers from straw and wood are easily diagnosed as they possess a longitudinal fibrillar structure with numerous elongated air spaces in between the fibrils. Feathers are of two types, down feathers and contour feathers; the latter have stiff and closely placed barbs which give them their trim shape and compact structure, while the down feathers have long, flexible barbs and have a fluffy appearance. Microscopically, feather fibrils have a branching appearance like the pattern of a fern leaf.

ANIMAL AND HUMAN HAIRS. When a fiber has been identified as hair, the examiner should determine whether the hair is of animal or human origin. Usually the diagnosis may be made without difficulty, if enough of the hair shaft is present to allow the animal or human characteristics to be discerned. Cross sections are especially valuable for distinguishing between animal and human hairs.

Human hairs possess a small medulla which is rarely continuous throughout the shaft, but is frequently interrupted like the dot and dash pattern of the telegraph code; it may be absent in some of the smaller hairs. The medulla is small in comparison with the diameter of the shaft, and is located in the center of straight human hairs, but has a slightly eccentric position in curly human hairs. On cross section, the straight hair is almost circular in outline while the curly hair is ovoid. In humans, the pigment in the shaft is concentrated near the outer rim of the cortex, and is not present to the same degree near the central portion of the hair.

In contradistinction to the human, most animal hairs possess a wide medulla in proportion to the diameter of the shaft, and the pigment in the cortex is concentrated near the medulla and not at the periphery (Figs. 28-1 and 28-2). Even the larger simians like the gorilla and the chimpanzee show these characteristics. The hair of the rhesus monkey possesses a small dot and dash medulla similar to

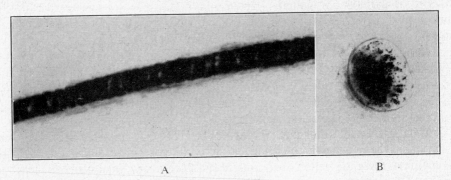

A   B

Fig. 28-1. Animal Hair. Dog.

A. Whole mount. Note prominent medulla.
B. Cross section. Note concentration of pigment near medulla. Contrast with Figures 28-3 to 28-5. Hair from a Pomeranian dog. High dry magnification, same scale as in Figures 28-2 to 28-6.

the medulla in human hair, but the cortical pigment is centrally located. Some of the tail hairs of the horse have a small medulla, but the hair shaft is much bigger and the pigment clumps in the shaft are larger and coarser than the corresponding structures in human hair. On cross section, the hairs of most animals are ovoid or circular in outline with an ovoid or circular medulla, extending most of the hair's length. Hairs from some species present bizarre characteristics on cross section; the rabbit family possess hairs which have an outline on cross section resembling a knuckle bone; water animals like the muskrat and seal have flattened ovoid hairs which, when closely applied together, form a water-proof covering; the deer family have a hair with a circular shaft, possessing a thin cortex and a wide medulla which contains a structure microscopically resembling wood pith. Some of the fur bearing animals possess principal coarse hairs and a fine down near the pelt known as wool hairs. Wool hairs have serrated edges and a relatively wide medulla which in some instances presents a peculiar stepladder pattern.

Human and animal hairs can usually be distinguished without much difficulty if typical specimens are presented for examination, but differentiation may be difficult if the specimen is not characteristic. For example, the examiner may receive a small segment of a light colored hair from a domestic animal like a dog, which if taken from near the tip or the pelt may not show a medulla; such a fragment may be similar to a human hair in whole mount or in cross section. Whenever the examiner is faced with a problem of this sort which cannot be solved with certainty, he should make it plain in his report that the material furnished him is not sufficient for him to make a positive identification.

The problem of identifying an animal hair as hair of a certain species may be difficult and cannot be solved by a few simple criteria. The best approach to the solution of such a problem is to compile an atlas of all animal hairs which are obtainable, including domestic animals, wild animals in the vicinity, furs and animals in zoologic gardens. Extensive studies of whole mounts, cross sections, and cuticular impressions should be made, and numerous microphotographs of typical specimens should be taken. In many instances the clue to the identity of a specimen sent in for diagnosis may be found by a comparison of its microscopic characteristics with those of known hairs in the slides and photographs collected by the examiner.

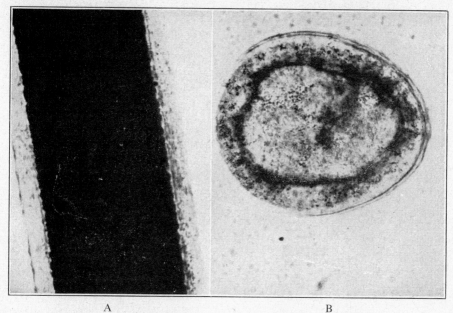

A   B
Fig. 28-2. Animal Hair. Cat.
A. Whole mount. Note very wide medulla.
B. Cross section. Note clumping of pigment near medulla characteristic of animal hairs. Coarse hair from a cat. High dry magnification, same scale as in Figures 28-1 to 28-6.

DIFFERENTIATION OF HUMAN HAIRS. After the fiber has been identified as a human hair, the next consideration is to determine if possible the race, sex and age of the owner of the hair and the part of the body on which the hair grew. This problem is not always easy to solve as the criteria used in diagnosis are frequently subject to qualifications, and the examiner must be guarded about expressing his opinion unless he is backed by the most unimpeachable evidence. As in the case of animal hairs, it is highly desirable that a large collection of human hairs should be made, including whole mounts, cross sections and cuticular patterns, and also an atlas of microphotographs.

Race. The human racial distinctions which can be determined by microscopic hair examinations are the white race, the black or Negro race, and the dark, straight-haired, brown or yellow races like the Chinese, other Asiatics and the American Indian. Of course, this is an oversimplified statement of the problem for there are many racial stocks which might be difficult to classify on this basis of hair characteristics, and there are hybrid combinations of the main stocks which offer the same difficulties in classification. Nevertheless the scheme mentioned above serves as a convenient working hypothesis and is capable of further elaboration if necessary.

Scalp hairs furnish the most reliable criteria for identifying the race inasmuch as they are better differentiated than hairs from other parts of the body; they grow more densely and may attain a length of 22 to 30 inches, much longer than hairs from other regions. In the white race the scalp hairs differ in texture, in size, in shape of shaft and in degrees of pigmentation from light to dark. The shaft may be

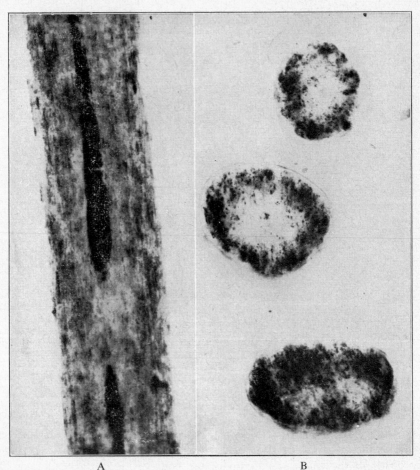

A   B

Fig. 28-3. Human Scalp Hair. White Race.

A. Whole mount. Note slender interrupted medulla.

B. Cross sections. Note ovoid shapes and peripheral concentration of pigment in cortex. Brown hair of a white man. High dry magnification. The hairs shown in this figure and in Figures 28-1 to 28-6 are all magnified and enlarged to the same degree.

straight with a fairly even caliber which gradually decreases near the tip, the cross section is circular or plump ovoid in outline, and the medulla is small, centrally placed, or is absent. Other hairs may be wavy or curly, showing an undulating gradual increase and decrease of its caliber alternately along their length, an ovoid shape on cross section, and a medulla of the interrupted type eccentrically placed in the shaft. In both types the pigment varies in intensity but is concentrated in the peripheral portions of the cortex; in most cases the pigment granules are dark, and the amount of such granules in the shaft determines the color of the hair to the naked eye, whether blond, reddish or dark; in some light haired individuals the pigment in the shaft may be an orange red color. In the white race the hirsute growth on the face or body may be profuse or scant (Fig. 28-3).

The American Indian, Chinese or other Asiatics have a moderate quantity of pigment in the skin, and possess long straight black scalp hair, circular or triangular on cross section, with a large diameter, and with a centrally placed medullary canal.

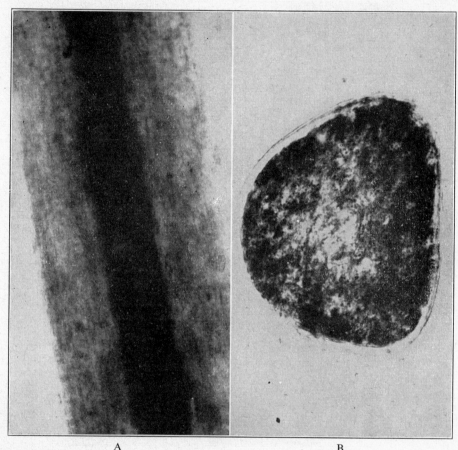

A   B
Fig. 28-4. Human Scalp Hair. Yellow Race.

A. Whole mount.
B. Cross section. Note large diameter of shaft and peripheral concentration of pigment in cortex. Black coarse straight medullated hair of a Chinese man. High dry magnification, same scale as in Figures 28-1 to 28-6.

The shaft is deeply pigmented and the granules of pigment are arranged with the greatest concentration just under the periphery of the cortex. The growth of the hair on the face and body is scant, and the hairs in the axillae and pubes are less curly and abundant than in the white and Negro races (Fig. 28-4).

The Negro races possess kinky black hair, the caliber of which alternately increases and decreases along the length of the hair. The hair when examined in whole mount is opaque and black, but on cross section has a narrow ovoid outline, while the medullary cavity is located slightly eccentrically. The dark pigment is arranged in clumps under the peripheral portion of the cortex. The beard and growth of hair on the body is usually scant but is occasionally profuse. Some of the Negro races possess curly or slightly wavy hair (Fig. 28-5).

Specimens of scalp hairs may show well marked characteristics which will enable the examiner to identify it as an example of one of the three main racial types. In other cases the specimen is not typical and may be difficult to identify. The hardest

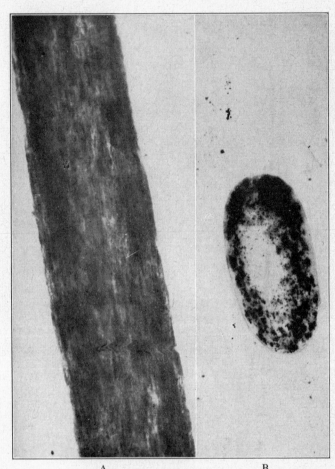

A   B

Fig. 28-5. Human Scalp Hair. Black Race.

A. Whole mount.
B. Cross section. Note flattened appearance and again peripheral concentration of pigment in cortex as in other human hairs. Black kinky hair of a Negro woman. High dry magnification, same scale as in Figures 28-1 to 28-6.

diagnostic problems are offered by scalp hairs which are coarse, dark and wavy, because such a specimen might have been taken from one of the darker white races, from a hybrid individual or from some colored person.

Age. Hairs from all parts of the body change during growth and senescence, but the age differences are most conspicuous in the scalp hairs. In the fetus, the lanugo hairs are fine, colorless and do not possess a medulla. In infancy and childhood, the hairs are larger, show pigmentation and racial characteristics similar to the adult, if not as well marked, and occasionally possess a medullary canal. At puberty, the hairs have increased in size, become darker, and a large number contain a medulla.

As a sign of the aging process, gray and white hairs appear in the scalp in gradually increasing numbers from about the fourth decade onward, and microscopic examinations of such specimens show hairs without pigment and hairs with sparsely scattered areas of pigment, as well as fully pigmented hairs. In other persons, the aging process occurs in the form of a bald area on the top of the scalp, and the hairs at the periphery may be dark with comparatively few gray. In some cases, hairs near an area of increasing baldness may exhibit a considerable variation in size, shape and pigmentation, because of the changes occurring in the scalp. Hairs of the pubis, axilla and the male chin are fine and downy during childhood but increase greatly in size during puberty. Changes due to age vary considerably in individuals, and the examiner should be cautious about drawing any conclusions as to age from the hair examination.

Sex. Sex variations are most plainly marked in the hairs of the face and scalp of adult individuals. The greatest differences occur in the hairs of the upper lip, jaws and chin, for in men a hirsute growth of thick wiry hairs may develop, while women usually display a fine downy growth; a few women of middle age who are suffering from a cortical adenoma of the adrenal gland or an arrhenoblastoma of the ovary may develop a visible beard but rarely one as profuse as that of the male. As a general rule the hairs of men are thicker, darker and more wiry than the hairs of women, but the variations between individuals are so great that these characteristics cannot be used successfully as reliable criteria of sex differentiation. The chief differences between the scalp hairs of men and women usually are artificially produced by popular custom. For example, women have been accustomed to allow their hair to grow long and to comb it continually so that the distal ends are frayed and brush-like, and men on the other hand cut their hair short so that the distal end is blunt and rounded. In some cases women may cut their hair short, and some adolescent males may allow their hair to grow so that they can brush it back; as a result the female hair would show the blunted end and the male hair would have brush-like tips. The presence of hair dye in the hair is not an indication of sex inasmuch as dye is used by both men and women. The determination of sex by hair examinations cannot be made positively except in rare instances.

Different Parts of the Body. Hairs from different parts of the body vary much in appearance. The varieties of scalp hairs have already been discussed; according to Belfield they vary in diameter from $\frac{1}{200}$ to $\frac{1}{1000}$ of an inch. The hairs of the male beard are larger and vary from $\frac{1}{150}$ to $\frac{1}{250}$ of an inch; their pigmentation is not so intense as the scalp hairs, their medulla is relatively large, they have a tendency to curl and on cross section their shape is ovoid, triangular or square with rounded corners. The hairs on the forehead are almost microscopic in size, are usually pointed, are free of medulla, but at the same time show pigmentation proportional to the intensity found in the scalp hairs. Hairs from the eyebrows, eyelashes and nasal apertures are about as large as the scalp hairs near the base, but are short, have a saber-like shape and end in a point. The medulla is comparatively large and may be continuous most of the length of the hair, the outline of the cross section is ovoid, triangular or square with rounded corners, and the degree of pigmentation is a trifle less than in the scalp hair.

Hairs from the axillae and pubis are wavy and curly, the caliber alternately increasing and decreasing throughout the length of the hair. The pubic hairs are about the same thickness as the larger scalp hairs and are larger than the axillary hairs; both pubic and axillary hairs have the same undulating outline in whole mount, have a flattened ovoid outline in cross section, and about the same degree of pigmentation. The trunk hairs and extremity hairs are less curly than the pubic hairs and are not so thick in diameter.

If the examiner is presented with typical specimens, it may be possible to identify the part of the body from which the hair came, but he must be careful about making a positive diagnosis unless the evidence is convincing.

Abnormalities of Hair. The more obvious abnormalities of hair may be recognized with the naked eye. Thus albino individuals who show complete lack of pigment in the hair, skin and retina occasionally occur in some races. More often localized white patches of hair may be present surrounded by dark hairs in the scalps of some persons. A rare case was observed of a colored woman of light skin who had no visible hairs in scalp, eyelashes and eyebrows or in any other part of the body, but microscopic sections of scalp, pubis and axillae showed fine hairs of microscopic size. Some scalp hairs are fragile and fracture when bent, probably because of some nutritional deficiency. Occasionally vermin and fungi may adhere to hair and may be easily recognized.

Microscopic examination of the whole mount may disclose any unusual treatment inflicted on the hair. If a hair has fallen out of the head naturally, the root end will show a cornified club-like structure. If the hair has been pulled forcibly away while still firmly attached to its bed, the root will be distorted and twisted into different shapes. The examination will disclose if the distal extremity has a natural point, or shows a flat sharp-edged surface from a recent cut, or a rounded extremity indicating an old cut, or frayed ends from excessive brushing. If flame has come in contact with the hair, the exposed portion may be swollen and blackened by smoke, bubbles may appear in the cortex, and in the later stages the hair may shrivel. Blunt force may split the shaft of the hair into its component fibrils, forming a spindle-shaped node at the point where the violence was applied, or it may sever the shaft leaving a brush-like extremity (Fig. 28-6).

Hair which has been bleached or dyed presents a characteristic appearance, best demonstrated by examining the hair under the microscope at the dividing line between the normal area and the bleached or dyed area. The bleaching is usually done by an agent which contains hydrogen peroxide and this removes the pigment from the shaft so that the treated portion is pale and translucent. Hair dyes when used on bleached hairs or white hairs either color the entire thickness of the shaft homogeneously or merely stain the outer layers of the cortex. Such dyes contain a number of different substances among which are lead salts, silver salts, bismuth salts, aniline colors, henna, pyrogallol and phenylene diamines. Hairs may be dyed adventitiously as when light-colored hairs come in contact with wet clothing and are stained by the dye in the cloth. Some workers in chemical plants may have their hair permeated and temporarily discolored by various chemical compounds. Chemical examination of dyed hairs is not satisfactory, unless metallic salts are present in the preparation, in which event the hairs could be subjected to spectrographic investigation. Organic substances in dyes are difficult to demonstrate chemically.

Medicolegal Considerations. Fibers are usually examined in the laboratory for the following purposes: (1) identification of the fiber, (2) evidence that the fiber or hair has received unusual treatment, (3) comparison of the specimen with the hairs of a certain individual.

1. In many cases if a fiber can be identified, the identification may furnish the police a needed clue or even important evidence. Such materials are sometimes

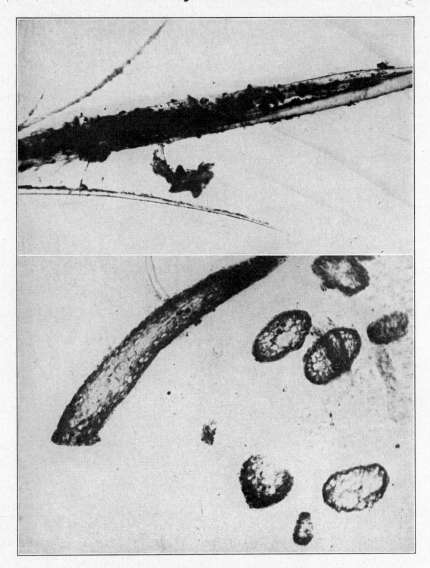

Fig. 28-6. Crushed and Burned Human Hairs.

Top. Whole mount of a crushed human hair removed from fender of a hit and run automobile. Note irregular longitudinal splitting of shaft.

Bottom. Scalp hairs of a Negro burned by flame of close-up pistol shot. Note vacuolated appearance in whole mount and in cross sections. High dry magnification, same scale as in Figures 28-1 to 28-6.

found in fingernail scrapings, on the heads or handles of weapons, or in the hands of victims of a crime.

Fingernail scrapings are examined to see if any objects are present which might give the police an important lead as to the most promising avenue of investigation. In most cases the microscopic examination brings to light such materials as minute hairs, cloth fibers, dust and other debris which are either nondescript or whose presence is explained logically by contact of the victim's nails with his own clothing, person or belongings. In rare instances the routine examination uncovers objects which are really significant. In one case a minute segment of pigmented human epidermis was found among the fingernail scrapings of a white woman killed by a Negro assailant during a robbery (Fig. 28-7); the defendant in this case displayed scratches on his arms which were probably the source of the specimen. In the fingernail scrapings of another woman who had been killed with a blunt instrument were two short thick hairs with clubbed ends at the roots and obliquely cut surfaces at the tips; later the defendant confessed that the victim had scratched his face, evidently digging out from his beard region two shaven hairs which were on the point

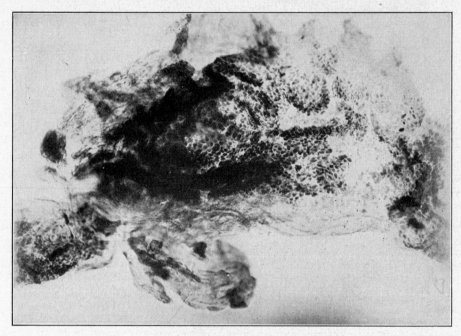

Fig. 28-7. Scrapings Removed from Fingernails of a Murder Victim.

Minute fragments of pigmented human epidermis found among fingernail scrapings of a white woman killed by a Negro during a robbery. When apprehended, the assailant had scratches on his arms which were probably the source of the specimen. Note characteristic mosaic of polygonal-shaped, pigmented epidermal cells. Unstained whole mount. Low power magnification, 16 mm. objective.

of separating themselves from their beds (Fig. 28-8). Microscopic examination of the fingernail scrapings of a woman who was killed by manual strangulation disclosed some fragments of wool fibers, dyed a vivid green and a light lemon yellow color, similar in appearance and size to the wool fibers on a plaid vest worn by the defendant. All such findings are important as clues for the guidance of the police in the conduct of their investigation; whether they can be introduced as evidence in court depends upon the problem presented in the individual case.

2. An examiner may be called upon to determine whether or not a hair has received unusual treatment. As an example, a woman was strangled during a struggle, and handfuls of long human hair apparently from her own head were found near the body; microscopic examination disclosed that the hairs had tortuous and deformed root ends, indicating that they had been torn from her head while still firmly attached to it. Figure 20-11 shows hair from a leg which was burned when the deceased was killed by a bolt of lightning. Figure 28-6 shows hairs burned by

flame from the discharge of a pistol, and a crushed hair recovered from an automobile involved in a traffic accident.

3. Hairs, usually from the scalp, are valuable as evidence when they are found
on a blunt instrument or automobile, especially if associated with blood. Whole
mounts and cross sections of such hairs are made and are compared with whole
mounts and cross sections of scalp hairs from the deceased or injured person. This
may be accomplished by using a comparison eyepiece which joins two microscopes

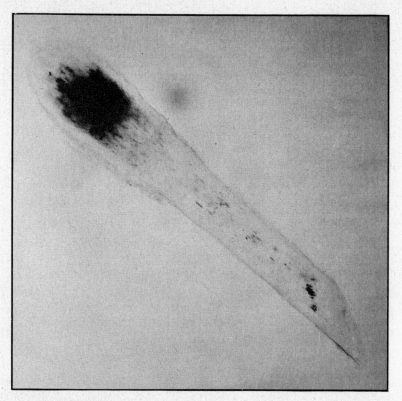

Fig. 28-8. Shaven Hair from Face of Assailant. Found under Fingernails of Woman Victim.

so that a slide on the stage of one microscope may be presented in the same ocular
field and at the same magnification as a slide on the stage of the other microscope.
A comparison may also be made by photographing both whole mounts and cross
sections at the same magnification and comparing the photographs. If the hairs are
similar in size, shape, degree of pigmentation and other characteristics, the examiner
is justified in testifying that the two sets of hair specimens are similar. The problem
in this case is not to identify an individual by his scalp hair, but to identify a
weapon; the presence of human hair on a blunt instrument, especially if it is in the
midst of blood stains, is significant in itself, and all the more so if the hair on the
weapon and the hair from the scalp of the deceased person possess the same characteristics (Fig. 28-9). In these cases the weapon must be connected with the
defendant by police investigation.

The following case illustrates how a fatal weapon was traced to a defendant by evidence
discovered at the scene of the crime. The deceased, an elderly woman, was found dead from a
depressed fracture of the skull evidently inflicted by a blunt instrument. On the floor beside the
body was a small triangular piece of wood, evidently broken off from a larger piece, and in the

wood was embedded a white hair, similar to the hairs on the head of the deceased. When the defendant was apprehended later, he had in his possession a revolver with a triangular piece of wood missing from the handle; the small flat segment of wood on the floor fitted exactly into the space in the handle.

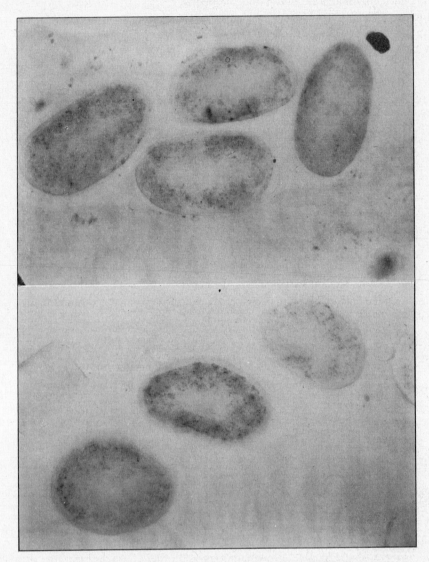

Fig. 28-9. Top. Cross Sections of Scalp Hairs of Victim. Bottom. Similar Hairs on Weapon.

Hairs are often found in the hands of women with long hair who are victims of physical violence inflicted during an altercation or an assault. Most of these strands come from the scalp of the deceased, as they are entangled in her hands and are torn away during the struggle. Occasionally in such cases, one or more hairs unlike those of the victim may also be found in her hands and after a microscopic examination has proved the presence of the foreign hairs, the police should be notified of that fact. If a defendant is apprehended, the next step is to compare his scalp hairs with the foreign hairs in the hands of the victim; if they are similar, such similarity would furnish the police with an important clue (Fig. 28-10). In this type of case, the results of the hair comparison are not admissible in court as evidence, for the implication would be that the microscopic characteristics of scalp hairs could be used for personal identification, which is not a permissible supposition. Hairs from the same scalp are similar to each other, but no two are identical and for the purpose of individual identification, mere similarity is not sufficient. In addition, other individuals may have scalp hairs similar to the specimen under consideration, which is always a complicating possibility.

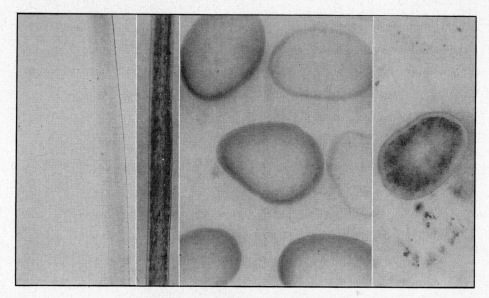

Fig. 28-10. Whole Mounts and Cross Sections of Gray Scalp Hairs of Victim and Brown Hair of Assailant.

HISTOLOGIC EXAMINATION

Pieces of tissues are sometimes removed from a blunt instrument, a motor vehicle, or from the scene of a crime, and brought to the laboratory for identification. The specimens must be delivered and identified to the examiner by the messenger as already noted on page 675. The tissue specimens usually consist of skin, subcutaneous tissues, fat, muscle, brain tissue and bone; blood and protein in this tissue should be tested by the precipitin reaction for the presence of human antigen as then its human origin will be specifically determined. Microscopic sections are made of the tissues, according to the technic described on pages 92 to 93; such sections will identify the type of tissue but will not determine its origin, unless definite human hairs are present in the skin sections. Uterine curettings are discussed in Chapter 22.

REFERENCES

Belfield, W. T.   Medico-Legal Examination of Hairs, from Peterson, Haines and Webster, Legal Medicine and Toxicology, Philadelphia, W. B. Saunders Co., 1923, Vol. II.
Chen Anliong.   Experimental Research as to the Possible Identification of the Individual on the Basis of Forensic Hair Examination, Inaugural Diss., University of Wurzburg, 1938.
McCarthy, L.   Histopathology of Skin Diseases, St. Louis, C. V. Mosby Co., 1931, p. 23.
Puppe, G.   Atlas und Grundriss der Gerichtlichen Medizin, München, J. F. Lehmann, 1908.
Smith, S., and Glaister, J.   Recent Advances in Forensic Medicine, 2nd ed., New York, Blakiston Co., 1939. Also including Moritz, A. R. The Cuticular Scales of Hair, pp. 110-118.
Vance, B. M.   The medicolegal examination of hairs, New England J. Med., 218:914, 1938.
Webster, R.   Legal Medicine and Toxicology, Philadelphia, W. B. Saunders Co., 1930.

29

Toxicology: General Considerations

A poison is a substance which acts on the body chemically and physiologically, consistently causing in toxic doses a disturbance of function which may result in illness or death. Toxicology is defined as the study of poisons, and is concerned with their detection, isolation, quantitative estimation, action on the organism, and the antidotes employed to counteract their toxic effects.

ACTION OF POISONS

Poisons harm the organism in two ways: (1) by local action; (2) by general action.

1. **Local Action.** Some poisons produce a marked irritation of the tissues to which they are first applied, or in other words cause a local reaction. This effect is usually intense with caustic alkalis, or mineral acids, or any inorganic or organic substances which have a marked affinity for water or some other constituent of protoplasm. The parts of the body usually affected are those which first come in contact with the toxic irritant such as the skin, conjunctivae, upper digestive tract or the upper respiratory tract, and less often the vagina, rectum, urethra, bladder, uterus and ureter. This type of poison produces local inflammation and corrosion of tissue inducing symptoms of pain, immediate or delayed symptoms of shock, and later signs of toxemia or septic infection; in most cases the poison is absorbed into the blood stream in varying amounts and produces general effects of greater or lesser severity. Other toxic substances which are weakly acid, weakly alkaline or neutral produce only a slight local reaction.

2. **General Action.** The general action occurs after the poison is absorbed into the circulation and is carried by the blood to the different organs and tissues throughout the body. It passes from the blood through the capillaries and small venules into the tissues and acts in different ways on the susceptible cells. Some toxic substances like hydrocyanic acid kill the vital neurons in the respiratory center of the medulla and cause death quickly after absorption without producing any visible anatomic changes in the affected tissue. Other poisons like the heavy metals act less rapidly causing acute and chronic degenerative and inflammatory changes in the blood, parenchymatous viscera, hollow viscera, skin, muscles and bones. Many toxic substances which harm the body by their general action may also have a marked irritant action at the site of absorption, which is usually of secondary importance in contrast to the local action of corrosive poisons.

Poisons are introduced into the body in various ways. Most of them are taken by mouth and are absorbed into the circulation after passing through the stomach and intestinal wall. Others are inhaled and enter the blood from the upper respiratory tract and lungs. Some are injected into the rectum, vagina, urethra, bladder or ureter. A few are introduced by hypodermic injection or intravenous injection, or are absorbed from the intact skin or from the surfaces of wounds. The rapidity with which a poison enters the system depends upon its solubility and method of administration. Absorption is rapid when the poison is given by intravenous injection or by inhalation, and more gradual when it is applied to the intact skin. The avenue of administration may determine the toxicity of a substance; for example, snake venom when injected hypodermically may be virulent, but if taken into the stomach it is altered by the gastric juice and is not ordinarily harmful.

The harmfulness of a poison usually depends upon the amount that has been introduced into the body, for the greater the quantity, the more potent the toxic action. For example, alcohol in small or moderate quantity may cause a pleasant sensation of well-being, but in larger amounts produces alarming symptoms of intoxication. This substance illustrates also the harmful effects of rapid absorption, for if alcoholic beverages are imbibed with food or in a manner which favors the gradual entrance of alcohol into the circulation, a much larger quantity will be tolerated than when it is ingested on an empty stomach in which case large amounts are absorbed rapidly and overwhelm the cerebral centers. Generally the more rapid the absorption of a toxic compound into the body, the more damaging will be the effects on the organism.

A number of factors may modify the action of poisons on the body. The age of the individual exerts a great influence, and younger persons as a rule are more susceptible to certain drugs than those more mature; given in proportional doses the opium derivatives are much more toxic to children than they are to adults. Disease may modify the toxic action of some medicines considerably, and persons suffering from conditions attended by great pain are less susceptible to the action of morphine and other hypnotics than normal individuals, so that a larger dose than the usual one is necessary to produce the desired analgesic effect.

Personal idiosyncrasy also determines the behavior of poisons in the system. Some people stand bromides, quinine and salicylates poorly. Others tolerate certain poisons fairly well, especially if they have become inured to the use of the drug by habit, as in the case of narcotic addicts who can take doses of heroin which would kill a normal individual. A previous exposure to the action of some chemicals, however, may make an individual hypersensitive to subsequent doses; thus, when the skin has been rendered susceptible to the action of formalin or chromate, a severe dermatitis may develop after contact with even dilute solutions of these poisons.

PATHOLOGIC LESIONS

Local Reaction. The pathologic lesions resulting from the local action of corrosive or irritant poisons will depend upon the way in which the poison is administered. In some cases the corrosive is ingested and, as a consequence, the mucous membrane of the mouth, gums, throat, esophagus, stomach, duodenum and small intestine shows irritation and necrosis of greater or lesser intensity or extent. Usually the corrosion extends as far as the upper portion of the small intestine, but in rare instances the entire intestinal tract is inflamed. Sometimes the poison may be regurgitated and spill over the face, producing reddish brown burns around the nostrils and mouth and inflammatory reddening of the conjunctivae. The regurgitated fluid may also be aspirated through the air passages, resulting in a necrotic pseudomembrane and edematous inflammation of the larynx, trachea and bronchi with a severe peribronchial inhalation pneumonia.

In other cases, corrosives like strong acids, strong alkalis or Lysol may be thrown on the face, producing burns of the skin and conjunctivae but rarely affecting the respiratory or digestive tract. Volatile irritant poisons like ammonia, mustard gas or lewisite may be inhaled causing an inflammation of the respiratory tract and an inhalation pneumonia; the skin and conjunctivae are usually inflamed, but the digestive tract may escape chemical injury. Injections of corrosive poisons into the bladder, urethra, ureter, rectum, wound cavity or subcutaneous tissues have occurred as a result of a therapeutic error. Corrosives have also been injected into the female genital tract to induce abortion or to prevent conception. Such procedures have caused a marked necrotic inflammation of the area involved, followed by death from shock, toxemia or septic infection. In addition to the local escharotic action, some of the poison is absorbed into the blood and produces a general systemic action on the organism, often causing definite pathologic lesions in different tissues. Both the local and general effects of corrosives are described in detail in Chapter 30.

General Reaction. Poisons after absorption circulate in the blood and attack tissues and organs susceptible to their action. Many chemical compounds like cyanides, alcohol, alkaloids and others paralyze the respiratory and other important centers in the central nervous system and cause rapid death without producing demonstrable anatomic changes. Similarly some of the suddenly fatal allergic reactions in humans following the injection of such organic chemical compounds as salvarsan or procaine, are the result of abnormal sensitivity on the part of the victim to the drug, and an autopsy in such a case may not disclose any obvious gross abnormalities. On the other hand, some inorganic or organic compounds after absorption have a destructive toxic action on the body and produce distinctive pathologic lesions. The liver which is the organ first to receive substances absorbed from the gastrointestinal tract, is one of the most important detoxifying agents in the body and is subjected to the toxic action of such poisons as arsenic, phosphorus, carbon tetrachloride and many others so that severe hepatic damage results. With similar exposure, the other glandular organs, the central nervous system, skin, myocardium, and other viscera and tissues may also suffer degenerative and inflammatory changes. Certain poisons may attack the blood, either by altering the hemoglobin to a physiologically, harmful variant like methemoglobin, as in the case of potassium chlorate poisoning, or by destroying the erythrocytes in the circulation as in the case of lead poisoning. For a description of pathologic lesions resulting from the allergic action of poisons like sulfonamides, see pages 830 and 831.

Poisons are excreted from the body unchanged, or excreted after they are transformed into other compounds by the metabolic activities of the liver and other organs. Elimination of such substances is carried out by the kidneys, lungs, bile ducts, gastrointestinal tract, skin and salivary glands, and many poisons produce their most destructive effects in these organs. Mercury bichloride, for example, is eliminated through the colon and kidneys, and there causes its most severe lesions. Other poisons like the radioactive compounds give rise to severe pathologic changes in the bones and bone marrow, because they are stored in these tissues and are in a position to cause harm. Lead and thallium compounds are stored and excreted slowly and may cause poisoning by cumulative action after a continuous and prolonged administration of small doses of the drug which, if taken singly, would not be dangerous.

LIVER. The liver as the principal detoxifying organ is damaged by such poisons as the corrosives, arsenic, phosphorus, heavy metals, ethyl alcohol, carbon tetrachloride, dinitrophenol, trinitrotoluene, cinchophen group, sulfonamides, *Amanita phalloides* and others. The mildest and least harmful lesion is parenchymatous degeneration or cloudy swelling of the hepatic cells by direct toxic action of the poison, characterized by enlargement of the cell, eosinophilic staining of the cytoplasm, congestion and polymorphonuclear leukocytic infiltration of the sinusoids especially at the periphery of the lobule. As this reaction is a reversible one, the cells may return to normal if the poison is eliminated from the body before actual destruction of the tissue occurs. It must be remembered that parenchymatous degeneration is not necessarily an indication of poisoning, but may occur as a result of bacterial infection.

Fatty degeneration and infiltration occur in the liver in conditions associated with deficiencies of oxygen metabolism which have a tendency to produce degenerative processes in parenchyma cells of organs. Poisons like phosphorus, arsenic compounds, carbon tetrachloride and alcohol, and such natural disease processes as primary pernicious anemia, severe tuberculosis, or diabetes mellitus, may derange the oxygen metabolism of the hepatic cells and give rise to fatty degeneration. In phosphorus poisoning, the fat appears in the form of fine droplets in the hepatic cells at the periphery of the lobule about 48 hours after administration. If the victim survives longer, the rest of the lobule may become involved, the individual liver cells become swollen, and the fat globules increase in size. The liver in such cases has a dull grayish red or yellow color, is slightly enlarged and shows rounded edges. In delayed poisoning with carbon tetrachloride, there may be localized areas of necrosis around the central veins in addition to the fatty degeneration, and the organ may present a spotted appearance. The process may be so severe that there is derangement of liver function, toxic jaundice and death from toxemia. In a condition of slow onset like chronic alcoholism, the fatty change in the hepatic cells develops more gradually with the formation of a single large globule which displaces the nucleus to an eccentric position. The fatty globules in the cell may be demonstrated by the histologic technics described on page 93.

Extensive necrosis and destruction of liver tissue may occur as a result of poisoning by arsenic compounds, salvarsan, carbon tetrachloride, the cinchophen group, trinitrotoluene, and many other substances. In delayed carbon tetrachloride poisoning, small areas of necrosis are observed around the central veins in cases which survive exposure to the drug for 36 hours or over, the liver showing a firm yellowish gray parenchyma regularly dotted with pin-head sized dark red areas of necrosis; microscopically the hepatic cells in the periphery of the central vein are eosinophilic, atrophic and even show disintegration, and may be replaced by leukocytes and large mononuclear cells containing brown pigment. Some of the hepatic cells bordering the lobule may show fatty degeneration. In some heavy metal poisonings, the destruction of the hepatic tissue is more intense and a condition like acute yellow atrophy is produced, in which the liver is small, has sharp edges and is deeply jaundiced; microscopically there is destruction of large areas of parenchymal cells, an infiltration of leukocytes and large mononuclears in the necrotic tissue, the presence of light yellow jaundiced nodules of hyperplastic liver cells, and an increase in the number of many small bile ducts. If the patient survives for a long period of time, fibrous tissue may replace the necrotic areas and a chronic interstitial hepatitis will develop. A toxic jaundice may follow the widespread necrosis of liver cells with bile pigmentation of all the body tissues.

Hydropic degeneration occurs when the hepatic cell is swollen and vesiculated from the accumulation of fluid in its cytoplasm, usually following the ingestion of poisons like potassium chlorate or diethylene glycol. Hydropic degeneration must be distinguished from the swelling of the liver cells in normal glycogen storage which is not related to any type of poisoning.

KIDNEYS. Degenerative changes similar to those just described in the liver may occur in the kidneys. Almost any type of irritant poison if severe enough will produce parenchymatous degeneration in the renal cortex. The kidney is slightly enlarged, the cortex is swollen, the markings are indistinct and the color is a dull yellowish gray; microscopically the epithelium in the convoluted tubules is swollen, is slightly eosinophilic, and the tubules may contain some albuminous exudate.

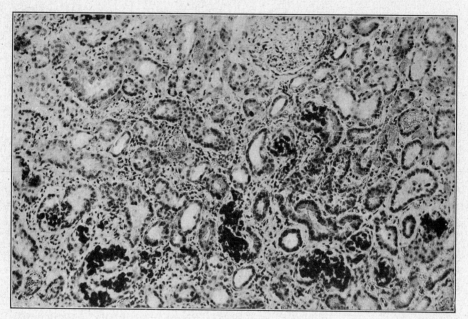

Fig. 29-1. Acute Nephrosis in Mercury Poisoning. Calcium Deposits in Tubular Epithelium.

Fatty degeneration may occur in chronic alcoholism or in phosphorus poisoning; the kidneys are enlarged with pale thickened cortex and the cells of the cortical tubules are thickened and contain fine fat globules which stain with Sudan III. Hydropic degeneration in the kidneys may follow poisoning with potassium chlorate or diethylene glycol.

Some poisons which produce hemolysis and secondary shock may be followed by a lower nephron or hemoglobinuric nephrosis. In this condition, hemolyzed blood passes out of the glomerular coil into the capsule of Bowman and encounters areas of necrosis in the tubules of the lower nephron segment; the formation of blood pigment casts in the tubules, occlusion of the lumens, and oliguria or anuria may result. This lesion has occurred in connection with poisoning by alkaline chemicals, phenol group, mercury bichloride, bismuth compounds, carbon tetrachloride, nitro aromatic compounds, sulfonamides, quinine and others. For further description see page 733. The formation of blue-staining, calcium bodies in the epithelium of the convoluted tubules (Fig. 29-1) is encountered in some cases of mercury bichloride and bismuth poisoning as described on pages 743 and 751. For kidney lesions in oxalic acid and fluoride poisoning, see pages 715 and 719.

The urine may show a variety of colors in different types of poisoning. After the administration of picric acid, naphthol or santonin, its hue is red or brownish yellow; in chronic sulfonal, barbital or antipyrine poisoning, the urinary color resembles that of port wine; in marked methemoglobin formation, the color of the urine is brownish red to brownish black; in poisoning by the phenol or salicylate group, the urinary hue is brownish green to dark green. Albuminuria may occur with almost any type of irritant poisoning. Hematuria is sometimes present after the administration of chromic acid, arsenic compounds, mercury compounds, strong acids, carbon tetrachloride, phenol group, turpentine, santonin, and other drugs. Hemoglobinuria occurs in cases associated with hemolysis as in poisoning by pyrogallol or quinine. Hematoporphyrinuria is one of the complications of sulfonal addiction. Oliguria or anuria may follow the administration of corrosive sublimate, arsine, carbon tetrachloride or any chemical substance likely to produce hemoglobinuric nephrosis. The urine is often used for toxicologic examination as it may contain some of the poison, either in relatively unchanged form as with lead compounds, fluorides or barbital, or transformed into other characteristic compounds as with methyl alcohol or members of the phenol group. The urinary bladder is occasionally irritated and inflamed by substances secreted in the urine as in poisoning with chromic acid, boric acid, potassium chlorate, anilin, santonin and cantharides. Bladder carcinomas have resulted from the continued excretion of noxious products in the urine of workers in anilin dyes over a number of years (page 810).

HEART AND BLOOD VESSELS. The same poisons which produce parenchymatous, fatty or hydropic degeneration in the kidney epithelium may be the cause of the same degenerations in the muscle cells of the myocardium. In such cases, the heart muscle is flabby, has a pale reddish or yellowish brown color, and the left ventricle is usually distended. Petri mentions degeneration of the myocardium followed by calcification, especially in poisoning by mercury or arsenic compounds. A consistent finding in arsenic poisoning is the presence of small flame-like hemorrhages in the endocardium of the interventricular septum of the left ventricle; these may also occur in phosphorus poisoning. The myocardium may show inflammatory infiltration in delayed carbon monoxide poisoning, especially in the papillary muscles of the left ventricle (page 506). Many of the degenerative and inflammatory changes in the heart muscle produce cardiac weakness and embarrassment of the circulation. The striated muscles in different parts of the body occasionally show degenerative and inflammatory changes similar to those in the myocardium.

Lesions are occasionally produced in the blood vessels by some poisons. Intravital clots may be formed in the small blood vessels during poisoning by mercury compounds, salvarsan, phosgene, carbon monoxide, strong acids, chloroform, ether, chloral hydrate, phenol and other substances (Petri). An acute dilatation of the finer branches with a high degree of capillary permeability is often observed in poisoning by arsenic compounds, salvarsan, sodium nitrite, nitroglycerine, alcohol and barbital, which is often instrumental in producing edema of the lungs and other tissues.

LUNGS. The lungs may show marked congestion and edema in poisonings by alcohol, chloroform, phenol, barbiturates, opium derivatives or other hypnotics, especially if the cardiac muscle is also weakened. With irritating gases like chlorine or nitric oxide, an acute emphysema may be produced as a result of cough, dyspnea and bronchial spasm. A hypostatic pneumonia may occur with almost any type of poisoning, but is most frequently encountered in cases which survive in coma for a prolonged period such as may be encountered after exposure to carbon monoxide, or after ingestion of alcohol or barbiturates. Degenerative changes in the lung tissue as a result of poisoning by phosphorus or arsenic compounds are mentioned by Petri. For putative connection of bronchial carcinoma and inhalation of poisonous dusts in certain ores, see page 890. For the action of beryllium compounds on the lungs, see page 769.

BLOOD. The condition of the blood in poisonings is either the result of non-specific factors, or is due directly to the toxic action of the drug on the blood. Nonspecific factors operate in rapid deaths from cyanide, alcohol, chloroform, benzol and many other chemicals to keep the blood fluid in the cardiac chambers and larger blood vessels, principally because the substances responsible for post-mortem clotting are not present in the blood in sufficient quantity at the time of death, and the sudden demise of the victim prevents their formation in the body. On the other hand, if the clotting elements are present in abundance at the time of death, as after a full meal, red and yellow clots are usually found in the cardiac chambers whether the manner of dying was rapid or delayed. If the victim dies after a long period of coma from a hypostatic pneumonia, clotting elements are prevalent in the blood, and yellow clots form in the cardiac chambers.

Some poisons produce their deleterious effects by direct toxic action on the cellular elements of the blood. A number of these drugs alter the hemoglobin in the red blood cells, changing the color of the blood and of the vascular organs and tissues. The cherry red hue of carboxyhemoglobin in carbon monoxide asphyxiation has been described on page 502. Some drugs like potassium chlorate, nitrobenzene, acetanilid, apiol and quinine transform hemoglobin to methemoglobin, thus reducing the oxygen-carrying power of the affected blood. If methemoglobin is produced in any quantity, a condition of anoxia occurs, the blood becomes chocolate brown or purplish brown, and the postmortem lividity, organs, muscles and bone marrow show a similar hue. In some cases of methemogloginemia, the red blood cells may be hemolyzed, and give rise to a hemoglobinuric nephrosis, jaundice, and the deposition of blood pigment in the reticuloendothelial cells in the spleen. Other poisons causing hemolysis are hydroquinone, pyrogallol, arsine, dinitrophenol, snake venom and similar substances, and may be accompanied by a dark reddish brown pigmentation in the blood and tissues and a dark reddish brown urine. Strong acids entering the blood may produce acid hematin and cause a brown color of the blood; strong alkalis similarly form alkaline hematin and give the blood a brown hue. Lead destroys the erythrocytes in the circulating blood, producing a severe anemia with marked pallor of the skin.

Drugs like aminopyrine, arsphenamine or sulfonamides may cause leukopenia or agranulocytosis by decreasing the white cells in the blood or disturbing their production in the bone marrow. Sedormid, a carbamide, causes destruction of the thrombocytes and may be followed by numerous purpuric hemorrhages throughout the body. For the discussion of purpuric hemorrhages in chronic alcoholism, phosphorus poisoning, benzene poisoning or dicumarol poisoning see pages 807 and 883. The chronic action of salvarsan, benzene, thallium compounds and radioactive substances may cause widespread changes in the bone marrow and produce aplastic anemia and other blood disturbances. Some poisons chronically act on the osseous tissues as well as the bone marrow: phosphorus, the compounds of mercury and radioactive compounds may give rise to necrotic changes in the jaw bone; osteosclerosis has followed the long continued administration of fluorides or radioactive compounds. For the association of multiple anaplastic sarcomas of bone with radioactive compounds, see pages 759 and 890.

GASTROINTESTINAL TRACT. The local action of corrosive and irritant poisons on the gastrointestinal tract has already been described on page 707. Other drugs, principally compounds of the heavy metals, act after absorption and cause an inflammatory reaction in the intestinal wall when they are excreted into the intestinal lumen. Rarely other types of inorganic and organic compounds produce similar lesions. The gross anatomic findings encountered at autopsy vary with the poison causing the inflammation. Arsenic compounds usually attack the stomach and small intestine, causing a cloudy red edematous infiltration in the submucous layer and rarely a pseudomembranous exudate on the mucous surface. Mercury compounds, excreted mainly through the large intestine, may cause a colitis varying in intensity from erythematous patches to ulcerative or gangrenous areas. For the gastrointestinal lesions in other types of metallic poisoning, see Chapter 31. Some inflammations of the intestine are caused by bacteria of the enteritidis group and other organisms which have been ingested with infected food, and whenever there is any doubt concerning the nature of the condition, bacteriologic, histologic and toxicologic investigations should be made on the autopsy material. In poisoning by phosphorus, benzene or other substances prone to produce hemorrhage the mesentery and intestines may show a widespread purpuric eruption.

SKIN. The local action of corrosives on the skin is described on page 726. The skin may also be inflamed by poisons absorbed into the blood and carried to the subcutaneous tissues. As an example, belladonna and its alkaloids may produce a marked generalized erythema of a scarlatiniform type. Numerous acute or chronic skin lesions such as urticaria, herpes, exanthemas, vesiculation, dermatitis of various types, ulcers, eczema and keratosis may follow the administration of such poisons as arsenic compounds, salvarsan, bismuth and other heavy metals, boric acid, phosphorus, iodides, bromides, chloral hydrate, sulfonal, salicylates, phenol group, nitro compounds, acetanilid group and many others. Hemorrhages may occur in the subcutaneous tissues in poisonings by phosphorus, benzol, sedormid, dicumarol, snake venom and others. Variation in the color of the skin may occur from the presence of abnormal pigments in the blood such as bile, methemoglobin or acid hematin (pages 734 and 772). A permanent discoloration of the skin may follow certain types of chronic poisoning: the continuous administration of silver salts results in a bluish gray discoloration of the skin and other tissues due to the deposition of black silver granules in the reticular and connective tissues; a melanosis may occur from the chronic use of arsenic, aniline colors or dichlorethyl sulfide; a type of ochronosis is reported to follow the continued use of phenol. For the putative connection of epitheliomas of the skin with arsenic compounds, see page 890.

Hair is often colored by chemicals and dyes externally applied. Argyrosis is said to produce a blue black color of the hair; the chronic administration of copper salts is reported to give a greenish discoloration of the hair (Petri). Alopecia has been described in thallium poisoning, chronic arsenic poisoning, mercury poisoning and borax poisoning.

CENTRAL NERVOUS SYSTEM. If the poison acts rapidly, killing the victim by paralyzing the respiratory and other vital centers in the medulla, it will not as a rule produce demonstrable macroscopic or microscopic lesions in the brain. If the patient lives a few hours or longer, a number of circulatory changes may occur: marked cerebral congestion has been described in poisoning by arsenic compounds, tetraethyl lead, phosgene, nitric oxide, alcohols, benzene, alkaloids and botulism; edema of the brain may result from poisoning with arsenic compounds, lead compounds, salvarsan, phosgene, fluorides, ether, barbital, botulism and others. Thrombi in the smaller vessels of the brain have been found in poisoning with lead compounds, salvarsan, phosgene, carbon monoxide and others. Small hemorrhages of petechial size or even larger have occurred with mercury compounds, lead compounds, nickel carbonyl, salvarsan, phosgene, carbon monoxide and nitrous oxide. A few poisons like lead compounds, arsenic compounds and phosphorus are said to produce fatty changes in the ganglion cells (Petri). Degenerative changes and inflammatory processes in the central nervous system may occur in chronic lead poisoning, chronic manganese poisoning, chronic alcoholism and carbon monoxide poisoning.

EYES. The conjunctivae and lids may suffer corrosion as the result of the local reaction of an irritant chemical (page 726). The chronic absorption of thallium compounds, naphthol or dinitrophenol over a long period may produce a turbidity of the lens. Lead compounds, arsenic compounds, methyl alcohol, naphthalene and others, if continually absorbed, may cause degenerative changes in the retina.

PERIPHERAL NERVES. Lead compounds, mercury compounds, arsenic compounds, ethyl alcohol and others if administered over a long period of time may cause degeneration of the peripheral nerves of the extremities and produce in such limbs paralytic or trophic lesions.

GENITAL ORGANS. Sterility in male and female may be produced if the genital organs are exposed to the action of radioactive compounds. In the male, azoospermia may occur in advanced cases of chronic alcoholism, chronic morphinism or lead poisoning. For the action of abortifacients on the genital organs of the female, see pages 578 and 579.

The fetus in utero may be killed by poisons which are absorbed by the mother and then enter the fetal circulation through the placenta. Among these are included the compounds of arsenic, lead, mercury and bismuth, phosphorus, iodine, oxalic acid, chloroform, ether, alcohol, salicylic acid derivatives, aniline, phenol group, Lysol, quinine, strychnine and ergot. Such drugs as phosphorus, lead compounds, potassium chlorate, oxalic acid, chloroform and Lysol have produced actual lesions in the different organs of the fetus after they had been administered to the mother (Petri).

The Autopsy. The pathologist in performing an autopsy on a suspected case of poisoning must describe the lesions carefully and interpret them with caution. Few pathologic conditions are pathognomonic of poisoning, and care must be taken to distinguish them from those caused by natural disease processes, traumatic injury, or even postmortem decomposition. The findings at autopsy are principally valuable when correlated with the investigation of the scene and the clinical history, for then the pathologist may be able to make a tentative diagnosis and to suggest to the toxicologist the most promising line of investigation (page 704). After he has received the toxicologic and other pertinent laboratory reports, the pathologist must appraise the significance and importance of different conditions in the body at the time of autopsy and base his idea of the cause of death on such considerations.

CLINICAL DIAGNOSIS

Cases of poisoning are not easy to recognize during life, and the attending physician must rely as much on the history and circumstances of death as on the signs and symptoms presented by the patient. Only a few clinical manifestations occur which are sufficiently pathognomonic to be employed as diagnostic criteria. Thus chemical burns around the mouth are reliable indications that a corrosive has been swallowed; a brownish discoloration of the blood suggests the presence of a toxic substance producing methemoglobin such as aniline, nitrobenzene, potassium chlorate, or acetanilid; a cherry red color of the blood indicates carbon monoxide poisoning (Figs. 4-3, 4 on page 53); but other clinical signs occur in natural disease conditions as well as in poisoning, so that they may not help very much in differentiation.

Cases occasionally occur in which the attending circumstances furnish the physician suggestive information. If an individual has enjoyed good health, and suddenly becomes ill after the ingestion of food, medicine or drink, poisoning must be considered among other possibilities. Unfortunately many natural disease conditions, such as heart disease, cerebral hemorrhages and abdominal inflammations may manifest themselves under similar circumstances with precisely the same symptoms. However, if several people are taken ill after eating the same meal, the suspicion would be justified that they had ingested some toxic substance in the food. In such cases, care must be taken to exclude the possibility that carbon monoxide from an unsuspected source has been absorbed by the victims, inasmuch as poisoning by this gas may produce gastrointestinal symptoms which may be attributed erroneously to the food.

The natural disease conditions which give symptoms simulating poisoning are many and varied. Haines has made an outline of these conditions which is given here in a modified form. The list is not complete, but is presented to indicate the problem faced by the physician in his treatment of a case.

Vomiting with diarrhea and abdominal pain is encountered in poisoning by such substances as arsenic, antimony, aconite, corrosives, wood alcohol, toxic foods, carbon monoxide and many others. Natural disease conditions such as acute gastroenteritis, cholera, uremia, eclampsia, coronary disease, Addison's disease and certain cerebral conditions may give the same symptoms.

Coma may result from the action of such drugs as opium, chloroform, chloral, alcohols, anesthetics, various hypnotics and cyanide. Many cerebral lesions and also uremia, eclampsia, and diabetes are attended by coma.

Dilatation of the pupil is produced by some of the alkaloids like atropine. Some diseases of the central nervous system cause the same sign.

Contraction of the pupil is caused by opium and a few other alkaloids; but also by diseases of the central nervous system such as tabes dorsalis or a spontaneous pontile hemorrhage.

Paralysis, either generalized or localized, is produced sometimes by the action of botulinus toxin or carbon monoxide; and also by such illnesses as cerebral hemorrhage and other brain lesions.

Slow respirations are caused by morphine poisoning; and also by uremia, or by any lesion which causes cerebral compression. Rapid respirations are caused by the action of atropine, cocaine and carbon dioxide; and by such respiratory infections as pneumonia, and by various cardiac and neurologic affections, including hysteria.

Delirium is often the result of poisoning by atropine, cocaine or *Cannabis indica;* and also may occur in natural diseases like insanity, infections, lesions of the brain, and in hepatic and renal conditions.

Cyanosis is caused by poisoning with nitrobenzene, potassium chlorate, acetanilid and morphine. Many cardiac and respiratory diseases are attended by both dyspnea and cyanosis.

The most reliable method of confirming the clinical diagnosis of poisoning is to send stomach contents, urine, spinal fluid, blood or feces to the chemical laboratory for analysis.

Chronic poisoning is more difficult to diagnose. A definite history of exposure to a noxious chemical should be elicited if possible. Many examples of chronic poisoning are encountered in industry in workers who are exposed to toxic fumes or dust.

TREATMENT

After the clinician recognizes that he is dealing with a case of poisoning, his chief efforts are directed toward the treatment of the patient as follows: (1) Removal of the poisonous material from the stomach; (2) Administration of antidotes; (3) Elimination of the poison by excretion; (4) Stimulation and other symptomatic treatment; and (5) Preservation of material for chemical examination.

1. The removal of the poisonous material from the stomach is occasionally brought about by inducing vomiting with emetics given by mouth such as soapy water, emulsion of mustard in water, or syrup of ipecac in doses of one-half to two teaspoonfuls—a method useful in children. One tenth of a grain of apomorphine hydrochloride given hypodermically produces prompt emesis by its action on the central nervous system, but because of the toxicity of the drug, the procedure is not devoid of danger. The stomach pump or the stomach tube may be used to empty that organ of its contents and accomplishes that purpose efficiently. It must be employed with care in cases of strong corrosive poisoning, for fear of perforating the stomach, and also with circumspection on unconscious persons who are apt to regurgitate and then aspirate stomach contents into the respiratory tract and die from asphyxia. In cases of strychnine poisoning, the stomach pump should not be passed until the convulsant action of the alkaloid has been somewhat abated by the intravenous injection of a short-acting, soluble barbiturate, for if the passage is tried before that stage, it may excite a convulsion.

2. Antidotes are given because of their mechanical action, chemical action or physiologic action.

The mechanical antidotes are fat, milk or egg albumen, which coat the mucous lining of the stomach and protect it. If the toxic material is soluble in oil, fat is contraindicated, as its use would then merely spread the noxious action of the poison. Powdered charcoal is efficient in the treatment of poisoning by organic substances as it absorbs such substances into its pores, delaying their absorption from stomach or intestines.

A chemical antidote is administered to form an insoluble or inert compound with the toxic material. The remedy varies with the individual poison; for example, ferric hydroxide is used as a specific against arsenic trioxide. In such cases the stomach is evacuated as rapidly as possible after the administration of the antidote because the compound binding the poison is only relatively inert and may be absorbed in time if allowed to remain. Gastric lavage should be repeated at intervals in order to make sure that any poison excreted into the stomach like an arsenic compound is removed. These measures should be attempted, even when treatment has been delayed and the case seems hopeless. When the exact poison is not known, a routine antidote consisting of a mixture of powdered charcoal, 2 parts; magnesia, 1 part; and tannic acid, 1 part, is mixed with water and given freely by mouth. The constituents are harmless, and neutralize some of the common poisons. Evacuation of the stomach should be carried out at the same time.

Physiologic antidotes are used after some of the poison is absorbed into the circulation, because their general action on the body counteracts the general action of the poison. Their use in treatment is somewhat limited and not devoid of danger. Such opponents are found most often among the alkaloid group as, for example, atropine and physostigmine, or atropine and morphine. In barbiturate poisoning, a recognized treatment is the intravenous injection of picrotoxin as a physiologic anti-dote, and more recently amphetamine sulfate has been used for the same purpose. The intravenous injection of a soluble short-acting barbiturate is employed as the antidote in cases of strychnine poisoning.

3. Attempts are made to favor the elimination of an absorbed poison through the excretory organs. The usual procedure is by enteroclysis, or by intravenous in-fusion of physiologic saline solution, or of dilute alkaline solution, or by a dilute solution of glucose. The poison is excreted generally through the urine, sweat, feces, vomitus or saliva.

4. Stimulation and symptomatic treatment is sometimes necessary and should be applied as occasion demands it. Thus, the following remedies are used as indicated: for excessive pain, morphine or another analgesic; for cardiac collapse, caffeine or digitalis; for convulsions, chloroform or intravenous injection of a rapid-acting barbiturate; for shock, oxygen inhalations and external heat; in morphine poisoning, atropine and caffeine.

5. It is desirable for the clinician, whenever possible, to preserve a large quantity of the stomach contents or the stomach washings for chemical examination, especially if he is dealing with a case in which the toxic substance is ingested. Other excretions and body fluids may be sent to the toxicologist as, for example, the urine in cases of barbituric acid poisoning, the urine and feces in lead poisoning, arsenic poisoning or mercury poisoning, the blood in carbon monoxide poisoning, and the blood or spinal fluid in acute alcoholism. Any materials supposed to be the source of the poisoning such as food, drink, cosmetics or medicine should be preserved and sent promptly to the toxicologist for examination, because the results of this investi-gation may help the clinician to arrive at an early diagnosis.

INVESTIGATIONS IN FATAL CASES

The investigations pursued by the authorities in fatal cases of suspected poison-ing are similar to those conducted in any other type of suspicious death. The medical investigator must visit the scene where the body was found, and he must determine the circumstances of death as far as possible. His next duty is to perform an autopsy on the body of the deceased, and withhold parts of organs and contents of hollow viscera for chemical examination by an experienced toxicologist. The toxicologic examination is necessary to prove or disprove the presence of poison in the body and, if positive, is an essential part of the corpus delicti. After receiving all reports which are pertinent to the case, the medical examiner determines the cause of death, and if it is due to poisoning, he classifies it as homicidal, suicidal, accidental, or as having occurred under undetermined circumstances.

Homicidal cases of poisoning are rare; about one to two a year occur in New York City, not including deaths from carbon monoxide. In the 33 years from 1918 to 1951, there were 45 homicides by poison as follows: burns by thrown corrosive, 8 (lye, 4, acids, 3; Lysol, 1); suffocated with chloroform, 5; ingestion of arsenic salts, 13; cyanide, 4; Lysol, 4; opium, 1; morphine, 2; and chloral, codeine, ergot, mercury, phenol, resorcin, sodium amytal and strychnine, 1 each.

Three of the poisonings in this list (ergot, 1; morphine, 1; resorcin, 1) were not homicides in the sense that a poison was administered intentionally for the purpose of killing the victim, but occurred because the drug was given by mistake or as the result of a therapeutic error.

Several varieties of intentional homicidal poisonings were encountered. In one type the toxic substance was used openly as a weapon under the stimulus of expediency, revenge, uncontrollable anger, or while the perpetrator was mentally deranged. Several cases occurred in children who were poisoned by their parents, the homicide usually being followed by the suicide or attempted suicide of the perpetrator; the poisons employed were arsenic compounds, Lysol, chloroform, cyanide and a mercury compound. In some instances, an assailant in a fit of passion threw concentrated mineral acid, lye or Lysol on the victim for the purpose of causing mutilation, and death followed as a result of severe chemical burns. In rare cases burglars have used chloroform or ether to stupefy a person and have killed him by causing him to inhale too much. In one instance a woman was killed because her existence was inconvenient to others, the method employed being the application of a towel soaked in chloroform to her nose and mouth so that she was compelled to inhale the fumes.

Other persons who employ poison as a means of homicide attempt to disguise its use so as to escape detection. Many of these perpetrators are distinctly low in intelligence or they are definitely psychopathic. As an example may be cited the case of a girl who fed her two brothers arsenic trioxide in coffee and caused their deaths. After the crime was traced to her, she confessed, explaining that she had desired to kill one brother but not the other, and not seeing how this could be accomplished, finally decided to poison both. In another case, the poisoner, a homicidal maniac, forced his victim at the point of a gun to drink coffee containing potassium cyanide, and his professed motive was simply to see the man die.

Other perpetrators, more clever in their methods, usually have an intelligible motive such as the removal of a person or persons who stand between them and an inheritance. A poisoner of this type may carry out his plans in such a manner that there is no direct evidence connecting him with the crime except the fact that he would be one of the routine suspects in the event of an investigation, inasmuch as he would be one of those who would benefit by the death of the deceased. In one case of this nature, the victim, a young woman seven months pregnant suddenly developed hypersensitivity followed by convulsions and was admitted to a hospital with a diagnosis of tetany. The following day she was pronounced out of danger. Consultants advised continued calcium treatment, and as the hospital pharmacy was closed at the time, the husband, a druggist, offered to supply the medicine (calcium chloride in elixir of lactopeptin). He delivered it to the hospital and a hospital nurse administered it to the patient who developed severe convulsions, dying inside of an hour. The body was buried under a diagnosis of tetany. Later, relatives of the deceased, suspecting her husband and the manner of her death, went to the district attorney with a complaint. The body was exhumed, and an autopsy and toxicologic examination several months after death disclosed a lethal amount of strychnine in the organs. It was then remembered that the mother of the deceased had died some time previously under dubious circumstances. Her body was also exhumed and autopsied, and toxicologic examination revealed the cause of death to be strychnine poisoning. The motive of this double homicide was financial gain through inheritance.

Suicidal cases of poisoning are more common, with a yearly average of 118 in which Lysol numbered 23; cyanides, 18; mercury bichloride, 12; barbiturates, 8; phenol, 8; arsenic compounds, 5; acid corrosives, 4; alkaline corrosives, 3; opium compounds, 3; iodine, 3; chloroform, 2 to 3; sodium fluoride, 2 to 3; strychnine, 1 to 2; phosphorus, oxalic acid and others, 1 or less. Carbon monoxide cases, the most common form of suicidal poisoning, are not listed in this group. In recent years the proportion of the different poisons has changed, for out of 178 suicidal poisonings in 1946, there were: barbiturates, 119; cyanides, 13; fluorides, 11; arsenic and phenol, 4 each; ammonium hydroxide and paraldehyde, 3 each; acetyl salicylic acid, iodine, mercury, phosphorus, sodium hydroxide and mineral corrosive acids, 2 each; acetic acid, borax, phenol, chloroform, codeine, methyl alcohol, paregoric and zinc sulfate, 1 each. Barbiturate poisoning is second only to carbon monoxide as a means of suicide by toxic substances.

Some of the substances employed as a means of suicide are comparatively painless in their lethal action, but others like the corrosives have a distressing effect which is apparently not a deterrent against their use. In some cases a person may be found dead, or overcome by the action of the poison, and the obvious circumstances at the scene of death, such as the presence of suicide notes, poison containers and signs of preparation for the act, may indicate suicide. Under other conditions, the family or friends of the deceased may discover the body first and remove incriminating evidence so that the diagnosis cannot be easily made. Even a victim, after taking a poison like potassium cyanide which usually produces its fatal action 2 to 4 minutes after ingestion, may be able to conceal all signs of the act before collapsing.

Accidental and undetermined poisonings occur at a yearly rate of 693 cases, of which the greater number are cases of alcoholism, 482; anesthetic deaths, 73; and opium and heroin poisoning usually associated with narcotism, 44. Other types of accidental deaths result from the therapeutic administration of some drug, the incautious exposure of individuals to some poisonous volatile substance as a result of their occupation, or the careless ingestion of toxic chemicals used in the household by a child, or an alcoholic individual, or by some one who has misread the label. Lysol, sodium fluoride in roach powder, or the phosphorus in roach paste have caused accidental deaths because they were taken by mistake. The presence of a large amount of alcohol in the body of a person apparently poisoned under such conditions may mean that the toxic substance was ingested accidentally while the victim was intoxicated, but of itself does not exclude the possibility of suicide or homicide. Some persons develop suicidal tendencies when in a state of intoxication and are most likely to kill themselves. Homicidal cases of poisoning are occasionally committed when the victim is under the influence of alcohol and thus in a condition in which he would be less likely to detect the presence of a poison in food and drink. The homicidal, suicidal and accidental poisonings will be discussed further under the different substances.

Fatal cases of poisoning are reported as (1) sudden or unexplained deaths which have taken place under questionable circumstances in the home, in hotels, furnished rooms, tenements, hallways or public places; or (2) deaths occurring after illnesses of equivocal nature which appear to the attending physician to be suspicious of poisoning.

1. The first type of case is investigated by the medical examiner who visits the scene of death, makes a careful record of all available history, and describes the condition of the corpse and the state of the surroundings in detail. Relatives and other witnesses should be questioned concerning symptoms, treatment, mental condition, and recent behavior of the deceased and as many pertinent facts as possible should be elicited. Medicines, food, drink, cosmetics or any other possible source of poison must be carefully investigated and if there is any suspicion that they contain a toxic substance, they should be sent to the laboratory for toxicologic examination.

The results of this examination are important to the police officials inasmuch as it is their duty to trace the source of poison found in such vehicles and the first step is to learn the identity of the toxic chemical.

The preliminary investigation should determine as far as possible, the nature of the suspected poison, the probable quantity administered, the method of administration, and what medication, if any, the deceased received during life. The medical examiner should search for clues which would enable him to determine whether death was homicidal, suicidal or accidental. A suicidal death is indicated by the discovery of notes in the handwriting of the deceased in which his intention of killing himself is declared. All due precautions should be taken to determine that all such notes are genuine, and not a blind to cover up a case of homicide. The notes must be preserved as evidence, for without them the proof of suicide is difficult and will necessitate more extensive investigation into the personal history of the deceased concerning mental condition, family troubles, business worries and similar points. In some cases of suicide, the poison may be in full view in a package of some sort, or remains of it may be present in a glass from which it was ingested. All such materials must be sent to the laboratory for toxicologic examination. Homicidal and accidental cases of poisoning can be determined only by sifting all the available evidence, including the nature of the poison, the circumstances under which it was taken, the amount in the body and other factors which might indicate the nature of the victim's death.

After the investigation of the scene, an autopsy is performed on the body to determine what pathologic conditions are present. It is important to identify lesions which are characteristic of toxic agents, and also to note the presence or absence of natural disease processes which might have produced clinical symptoms and signs similar to poisoning. Generous portions of the parenchymatous viscera and of the contents of hollow organs are preserved for toxicologic examination, and precautions are taken that they will not be contaminated by foreign substances which will vitiate the chemical analysis. After the organs and viscera have been examined and described, a step which should never be omitted even though chemical examination is contemplated, they are put in separate wide-mouthed glass jars, tightly stoppered and sealed to prevent the escape of volatile substances, and labeled with the name of the case, the date and place of examination.

The specimens for analysis, whether obtained at autopsy or at the scene of death, are delivered to the toxicologist as soon as possible and properly identified to him, for it is important to establish the chain of identification between the analytic laboratory and the source of the specimens. The toxicologist should be informed of the history of the case in order that he may know how to plan his analyses. The organs and tissues which are preserved for such analysis are listed in each subsection dealing with the individual poisons. If a complete toxicologic examination is desired, the brain, liver, kidneys, lungs, stomach contents, intestinal contents, blood, urine, skin, hair, muscles and bones are stored in separate receptacles.

2. If the victim has been treated by a physician, the duty of the doctor is to diagnose and treat the case, and also to search out the possible source of the poison, whether from food, drink, medicines, household preparations or other substances. All suspected materials and containers should be sent to the laboratory for analysis; adequate specimens of the patient's urine, feces, blood, spinal fluid, or stomach contents should also be submitted for examination so that the poison can be recovered in as large quantities as possible. The toxicologist should be furnished with

an adequate history of the case and the material should be properly identified to him. The physician should compile a careful clinical record, especially noting the medication given the patient, as this may have an important bearing on the interpretation of results obtained by toxicologic examination. When death occurs the medical examiner should be notified so that he can carry out his investigation. If the case is suspicious, the physician must notify the police and give them every possible assistance.

If the death of the victim presents features which indicate a homicide, it is the duty of the police to discover the identity of the perpetrator, the motive for the crime, where the perpetrator obtained the poison, and how he administered the poison to the victim. In order to establish the proof of the crime, the prosecution must piece all the evidence together so that the testimony offered will give a connected and credible account of the tragedy and its genesis. The duty of the medical examiner and the toxicologist is to inform the police of the identity of the poison as soon as possible, and to establish the corpus delicti by identifications which connect the body and the toxicologic examination with the scene of the crime. The testimony of the medical examiner and the toxicologist is necessary in all poison cases in order to establish the cause of death.

CLASSIFICATION OF POISONS

It is difficult to classify poisons satisfactorily, as the subject has many ramifications. For the purpose of forensic medicine, the most successful classifications are based on the physical and chemical properties of toxic substances. For example, Witthaus has divided poisons into five groups as follows: gaseous poisons; volatile poisons; acids, alkalis and salts; organic poisons; and mineral poisons. The classification of Webster is the most logical; it lists toxic substances in four categories: gaseous poisons; inorganic poisons; alkaloidal poisons; and nonalkaloidal organic poisons.

The authors have employed a classification based not only on the physical and chemical properties of poisons, but also on the effect of these substances on the body. It is designed to furnish the pathologist with a systematic guide which would enable him to correlate the pathologic lesions discovered at necropsy with the chemical properties of the toxic agent, and consequently to determine the organs and tissues most suitable for toxicologic analysis. The acumen which the pathologist displays in his conduct of the autopsy is an important factor in the success of the investigation, for unless a sufficient amount of the proper material is saved for chemical examination, the toxicologist may not be able to conduct his analysis to the best advantage. It is essential that the medical man performing the autopsy should understand the lesions produced by different poisons. The following classification is offered:

1. Gaseous poisons (poisons present in the gaseous state) already described in Chapter 19.
2. Inorganic poisons.
   (a) Corrosives (poisons characterized by an intense and destructive local action. A few organic corrosives are included in the group for the sake of completeness).
   (b) Metallic and nonmetallic poisons and salts (these chemicals are protoplasmic irritants, but their chief action is the deleterious effect produced after absorption).
3. Organic poisons.
   (a) Volatile poisons (volatile liquids or easily sublimated solids many of which are irritants; their chief effect occurs after absorption).
   (b) Nonvolatile, nonalkaloidal poisons.

  (c) Alkaloidal poisons (these substances are the toxic principles of plants, which characteristically act on some part of the central nervous system; they are a well-defined group).

 4. Miscellaneous poisons (including botulism and food poisoning).

REFERENCES

Haines, W. S. General Principles of Toxicology, from Peterson, Haines and Webster, Philadelphia, W. B. Saunders Co., 1923, Vol. II, pp. 17-69.

Lucké, B. Lower nephron nephrosis, Mil. Surgeon, 99:371, 1946.

Petri, E. Vergiftungen, from Henke and Lubarsch, Berlin, Julius Springer, 1930, Vol. X, pp. 486-563.

Reports of the Office of the Chief Medical Examiner in the City of New York from 1918 to 1951.

Webster, R. W. Legal Medicine and Toxicology, Philadelphia, W. B. Saunders Co., 1930.

Witthaus, R. A. Toxicology from Witthaus and Becker, New York, William Wood Co., 1911, Vol. IV.

30

Inorganic Poisons: Corrosives

The corrosives are poisons which intensely inflame and destroy tissues to such an extent that their local action dominates the clinical picture and produces the most prominent lesion found at autopsy. Most of the poisons of this group are also absorbed into the blood and cause a general reaction on the system.

A variety of dissimilar chemical substances is included under the name of corrosives and their effects on the body differ slightly. They may be classified as acid corrosives, alkaline corrosives and organic corrosives. Most corrosive substances are inorganic, but the organic types are discussed in this chapter because the pathologic lesions which they produce are similar to those caused by inorganic compounds.

ACID CORROSIVES

The substances which produce acid corrosion are: the mineral acids such as sulfuric, hydrochloric and nitric acid; the halogen group consisting of chlorine, bromine, iodine, fluorine and their compounds; organic acids such as oxalic, acetic, formic and citric acids; and salts or esters in which an overwhelming acid component is combined with a weak basic radical, as for example silver nitrate, zinc chloride or dimethylsulfate. The local action of an acid corrosive is to extract water from tissues, to coagulate protein and thus form an acid albuminate, and to transform hemoglobin to acid hematin. The effects produced will depend on the strength of the substance which comes in contact with the body.

If the corrosive is swallowed in dilute form, the mucous membrane of the stomach is irritated and thrown into folds by contraction of the viscus. The most intense action occurs on the top of the rugae, producing a bright red or brownish red barred pattern and small ulcerations may occur in the intensely injected rugal areas. The depressed portion in between is less intensely inflamed. With the weak acids, the skin around the mouth, the pharynx and esophagus rarely show corrosions, though the esophagus may be contracted into longitudinal folds. The duodenum and some of the small intestine may be inflamed due to the passage of the corrosive acid from the stomach, and the mucous membrane may be reddened diffusely or on the crests of the plicae. Merkel has mentioned instances in which the duodenum has been irritated and corroded by ingested acid which was not strong enough to produce inflammation in the stomach. In these cases of dilute acid corrosion, the chemical may be regurgitated into the pharynx and be aspirated into the air passages producing edema of the laryngeal mucous membrane, a suppurative bronchitis, and a peribronchial bronchopneumonia.

Microscopic examination of the stomach wall in a case in which zinc and lead chlorides were ingested disclosed changes characteristic of a mild grade of acid corrosion. The surface layer of the mucous membrane was necrotic and was colored brown from a heavy deposit of acid hematin. The adjacent submucosa showed engorged blood vessels containing pale erythrocytes with well defined borders, and dark brown granules of acid hematin. There was sharp demarcation between the necrotic area and the contiguous tissues. That part of the mucous membrane which was not corroded showed atrophy and granular degeneration of the chief cells, but good preservation of the eosinophilic, acid forming, polygonal, parietal cells. If the victim survives a few days, there may be a definite wall of polymorphonuclear leukocytes adjacent to the corroded mucous membrane, but rarely any extension of the process to the deeper tissues.

If the ingested corrosive is a concentrated mineral acid like sulfuric acid the effects on the stomach are much more intense and striking. The mucous membrane is converted into a wrinkled brown and black layer, dried and rough in appearance, which gives the impression of being charred; the process is known as carbonization and is attributable to the avidity of the acid for water and the conversion of the blood pigment in the affected area to acid hematin. Strong nitric acid differs in forming a firm corrosive layer which is yellowish green in color, the xanthoproteic reaction. The stomach wall is somewhat thickened and its lumen slightly narrowed, partly from the contraction of the muscular layers and partly from hemorrhage and inflammatory edema in the deeper tissues which may ensue if the patient lives a few days. The acid may diffuse post mortem into the larger blood vessels distending them with black plugs of acid hematin and at the same time staining the neighboring organs, the liver and spleen, brown and black from the same pigment. In some instances the mucous membrane is extensively ulcerated, and the wall of the stomach is softened, so that a stomach tube may easily perforate it and cause the corrosive material to spread into the peritoneal cavity producing a severe chemical peritonitis. In some cases the acid may pass into the duodenum and cause corrosion of the upper portion of the small intestine, but in other cases the pylorus may contract and attempt to keep the acid in the stomach.

The microscopic appearance of the corrosion produced by a concentrated acid is a formless necrotic surface layer permeated with granules and clumps of dark brown acid hematin, which extends to various depths in the stomach wall. If the victim lives, a polymorphonuclear leukocytic infiltration zone forms around the necrotic area and edema and hemorrhage occurs in the submucous layers, the blood cells showing different degrees of preservation. The blood cells in the blood vessels are usually destroyed and converted into formless clumps of eosinophilic material or dark brown acid hematin. In a few instances the ravages on the mucous membrane may produce an infectious cellulitis of the stomach wall and small intestine and lead to cicatrization and stenoses of the stomach and intestines. If the corrosive material enters the peritoneal cavity, it produces a gray necrotic membrane on the surface with a marked leukocytic zone in the adjacent tissues; this is replaced later by a subacute inflammatory reaction and a well-developed zone of fibroblastic proliferation. In the esophagus the same types of lesions occur with rather marked contraction of the tube which squeezes the mucous membrane into longitudinal folds. Cicatrization of the wall and stenosis of the esophagus may occur, a process which will be discussed further under the corrosive alkalis.

Dried reddish brown and black burns of geographic shape with small streaks running down the face may occur around the lips and mouth if the acid is ingested, sometimes as the result of spilling the corrosive on the face, sometimes due to regurgitation through mouth and nose. In other cases, acid may be thrown on the face and upper part of the body in an attempt to disfigure a person causing geographic splash burns of different size over chest and face. Microscopically the burned areas show the epidermis still present but discolored brown, and the dermis and subcutaneous tissues shrunken through loss of water, while the nuclei are poorly stained by hematoxylin and small bright granules appear in the epithelial layers (Strassmann). In rare instances, strong acids may be introduced into the rectum by mistake for some drug intended as a therapeutic measure, or into the vagina and uterus to cause abortion and the result is a fatal corrosion of these organs.

Occasionally the ingested acid may be regurgitated and inhaled into the air passages, causing a marked irritation of the larynx and edema of the glottis with death by shock. A pseudomembranous inflammation of the trachea and bronchi is produced with destruction of the superficial epithelium and necrosis which extends deep into the submucous layer. A pneumonia consisting of peribronchial inflammatory nodules may occur in some cases.

Severe acid corrosion may cause death by shock in a few hours. If the patient lives longer, a severe secondary infection may appear at the site of a skin burn or in the peritoneum as a result of a perforation of the stomach by a stomach tube, or as a bronchitis and bronchopneumonia from aspiration of the corrosive into the air passages. In some cases a large amount of poison may be absorbed into the blood and cause death by acidosis, due to the general action of the acid on the organism; fatty and parenchymatous degeneration of the liver and kidneys have been described as the result of this action. Stomach contents and a parenchymatous organ like the liver should be saved for chemical examination in recent cases. Stenoses of the esophagus and stomach may occur months after the acute inflammation has subsided and cause death by starvation.

Mineral Acids. The most common mineral acids are sulfuric acid, hydrochloric acid and nitric acid, and they cause the most intense corrosions. In the Office of the Chief Medical Examiner in the 33 year period from 1918 to 1951, there were 113 suicides from the ingestion of mineral acid reported, of which 21 were sulfuric acid, 68 hydrochloric acid, and 24 nitric acid. Accidental and undetermined cases of acid corrosion included 33 cases, mostly by ingestion. Homicidal cases were rare, 2 cases occurring as burns from acid thrown on the face and body.

SULFURIC ACID. Concentrated sulfuric acid, H_2SO_4, or oil of vitriol, is a chemical used in many manufacturing processes, and is also an important reagent employed for various purposes in laboratories. It is a heavy, odorless, colorless, nonfuming, oily liquid which has an avid affinity for water, and which has a tendency to carbonize organic substances. Another form, Nordhausen acid, is a brown, oily, fuming liquid with a formula of $H_2S_2O_7$; it is manufactured in Bohemia and is used in the preparation of indigo.

Sulfuric acid, due to its severe corrosive action, has rarely been given by mouth for homicidal purposes except to children. It is sometimes thrown on a person to disfigure the face, and it may cause death from the severe burns inflicted on the skin. Most of the cases are suicidal, due to the ingestion of the acid. Some cases are accidental, the acid having been ingested in mistake for a medicine, or mixed with food, or poured into the ear, or injected into the rectum by error instead of a therapeutic drug, or injected into the vagina for the purpose of causing abortion. Workers in chemical laboratories may receive burns from the accidental breaking of apparatus containing the concentrated acid. The occupational lesions produced by sulfuric acid will be described later.

The primary action of the acid is to produce a gray-white necrotic membrane with swelling of the affected surface, followed by a brownish or black discoloration.

The entire upper digestive tract after ingestion of the concentrated acid presents a black, swollen, dried and charred appearance of typical carbonization from the affinity of the acid for the water in the tissues (Fig. 30-1). The victim suffers pain in mouth, throat and stomach aggravated by swallowing and is unable to speak.

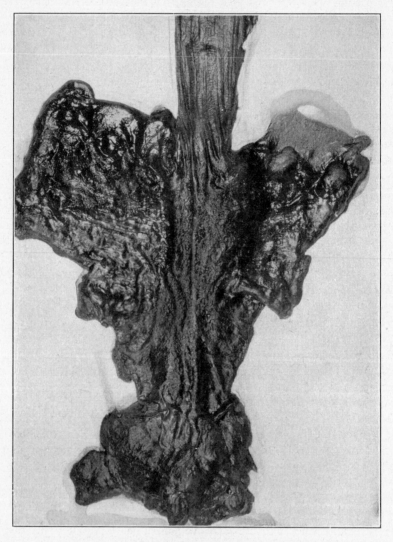

Fig. 30-1. Corrosion of Stomach After Swallowing Concentrated Sulfuric Acid. Suicide.
Note black carbonized necrotic appearance of entire stomach wall.

There are cold sweats, a feeling of anxiety and complete prostration. Death occurs usually in from 18 to 24 hours from a combination of severe shock and acidosis, but may take place after a much shorter interval as a result of shock following edema and spasm of the laryngeal mucous membrane if the acid is regurgitated and inhaled, or if the stomach is penetrated by the stomach tube and the acid enters the peritoneal cavity. In cases which survive the immediate effects of the corrosion, a terminal bronchopneumonia may supervene, or a toxic nephrosis may result from the excretion of the acid from the kidneys, usually manifested clinically by the appearance of blood, albumin and casts in the urine. Sometimes severe burns are present about the mouth, face and eyes. If severe external burns are present on the skin, death may result from shock, or from septic infection at the local site. Cicatrization of the stomach and esophagus occurs in a few cases and causes death much later as a result of starvation. Strassmann described a severe intercostal neuralgia as one of the symptoms which accompanies the lesions in the stomach and esophagus.

The fatal dose for an adult is small, and from the nature of its toxic action it would be difficult to determine what would be the minimal lethal dose in any one case. The treatment is the prompt administration of magnesia, chalk or other dilute alkali to neutralize the acid. White of eggs may be given to allay the corrosion. External burns on the face may be washed with water and sodium bicarbonate may be applied to neutralize the acid. The stomach pump must be used with caution for fear of perforating the stomach. Pain and shock must be treated symptomatically as described in Chapter 29.

Strong concentrated mineral acids like sulfuric acid destroy organic matter and rarely have been used by the perpetrators of a homicide to obliterate the body of the victim. The acids are generally applied in liquid form, and in large quantities, and act energetically especially if heated. The flesh, organs and even the bones are converted into a thick reddish, brownish or bluish liquid in the course of a few hours, and only such metal objects as gold dental fillings may remain behind. The same implications with regard to the corpus delicti exist as in the cases in which the remains are destroyed by fire. For fuller information on this subject the reader is referred to the work of Haines.

HYDROCHLORIC ACID. Hydrochloric or muriatic acid, HCl, is a pungent, colorless fuming liquid which has corrosive properties similar to sulfuric acid but not so intense. Most cases of hydrochloric acid poisoning are suicidal, produced by the ingestion of the concentrated acid. A few are accidental or homicidal. Occasionally the acid is injected into the vagina to produce abortion and may cause death by corrosion. One case is mentioned of hydrochloric acid solution injected by mistake into the anterior abdominal wall of a child as an infusion in place of normal saline solution; a fatal necrotic corrosive process followed.

The action of concentrated hydrochloric acid on the skin and mucous membranes is not as intense as that of sulfuric acid, and skin burns may not be present in some cases. On the mucous membrane of the stomach the acid causes a gray membrane to appear first, followed by a brown and black discoloration from acid hematin formation (Fig. 30-2), but not to the extent of causing carbonization. The symptoms, clinical course, complications and treatment otherwise are similar to those of sulfuric acid. The fatal dose varies; 4 ml. of the concentrated acid has been fatal. The corrosive effects of concentrated hydrochloric acid on the stomach are shown in Figure 30-3.

The authors have encountered an unusual complication following a concentrated hydrochloric acid corrosion of the stomach in an elderly man who died six hours after ingestion of the chemical. The autopsy disclosed a typical brownish black necrosis of the stomach wall, a stomach-tube perforation of the fundus of that viscus, and a localized chemical peritonitis over the viscera adjacent to the perforation; in the tributaries of the gastric veins near the perforation were homogeneous black-red clots which distended the vessels and extended into the branches of the portal vein in the liver. The liver was permeated throughout with dark red dendritic mossy figures, 3 mm. to 7 mm. in diameter, grouped characteristically near the islands of Glisson. Histologic examination disclosed that the dendritic areas were produced by localized, globular dilatations of groups of sinusoids to about 10 times natural size, forming a yeast-like pattern of cavities which were distended with laked erythrocytes and some polymorphonuclear leukocytes. The fibrillar walls of the sinusoids were preserved but the adjacent hepatic cells were necrotic, deformed and disintegrating. The larger radicles of the portal veins contained laked red blood cells, some brown pigment, a few leukocytes and fragments of necrotic fibrin. Evidently at the time that the stomach wall was perforated, some of the acid entered the ruptured tributaries of the portal vein and was conveyed into the liver producing the sinusoidal dilatations noted above.

NITRIC ACID. This acid, HNO_3, is used extensively in manufacturing processes and is an important laboratory reagent. It is a colorless, fuming, heavy liquid which develops a yellow color on exposure to light and air. In concentrated form it destroys organic matter by oxidation and produces a yellow discoloration of tissue, known

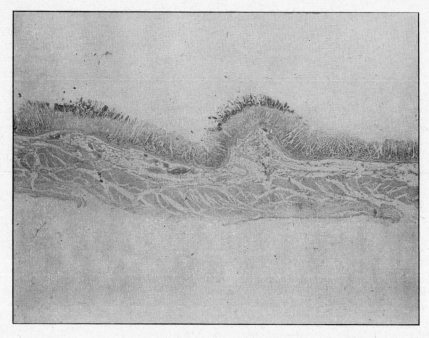

Fig. 30-2. Histologic Section of Stomach Showing Corrosion of Mucosa by Concentrated Hydrochloric Acid.

as the xanthoproteic reaction; in dilute solution this reaction does not occur. Aqua regia, which contains nitric acid, 1 part; hydrochloric acid, 3 parts, is similar in its action to concentrated nitric acid.

The cases of nitric acid poisoning are suicidal, accidental or homicidal in much the same manner and incidence already noted in the discussion of the other mineral acids. The corrosion on skin and mucous membrane is almost as intense as with sulfuric acid. The surface is at first whitish-gray and then the xanthoproteic reaction develops, with characteristic yellowish-green, citron and orange-yellow tints. Symptoms and treatment are the same as with sulfuric acid poisoning. Petri mentions a type of chronic poisoning from the continual ingestion of red fuming nitric acid, or nitric acid partly decomposed into nitro bodies, which was comparatively common in eastern Europe at one time; this substance was taken with the intention of producing abortion and after long continued administration caused anemia, fatty degeneration of the organs and enlargement of the spleen.

Organic Acids. The principal organic acids which produce corrosive effects on the tissues of the body are formic acid, oxalic acid, acetic acid and citric acid.

With the exception of formic acid, the corrosive action is not as intense as that of the mineral acids so that the principal lesions are found in the gastrointestinal tract and not frequently on the skin.

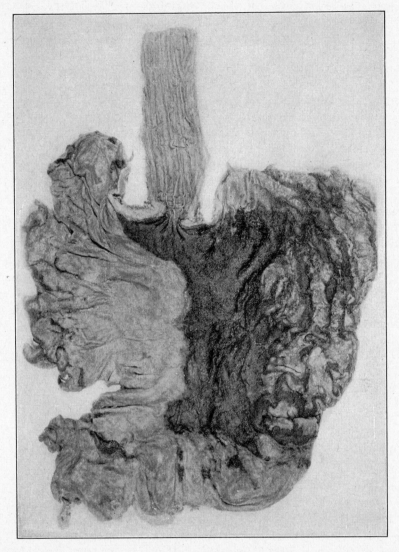

Fig. 30-3. Corrosion of Stomach After Swallowing Concentrated Hydrochloric Acid. Suicide.

The mucous membrane of the posterior wall is blackened by the formation of acid hematin. Death from laryngeal edema following aspiration of vomitus.

FORMIC ACID. Poisoning with formic acid, HCOOH, is not common. Its corrosive effects are intense, resembling those of sulfuric acid. Suicidal cases as a result of the ingestion of this compound have been described; a fatal poisoning has been reported in a worker who was distilling formic acid and was splashed over his face, neck and right forearm with the chemical, and died six hours later (Petri). At autopsy brownish red, sharply marked burns of the skin, swelling of the eyelids with hemorrhagic extravasation, gray-white corrosion of the air passages, a black-brown corrosive lesion of the stomach, necrotic areas in the intestines, hemorrhages and necroses in the lymph nodes near the corroded areas and red blood cell and pigment casts in the tubules of the kidneys have been described. The acid produces hemolysis, hemoglobinuria and methemoglobinuria after absorption. Formic acid is not found in the urine, stomach contents or viscera of fatal cases unless a large amount has been taken into the body. Necrotic local inflammation and severe general symptoms of formic acid poisoning have occurred in children who were bitten by ants or stung by hornets and bees.

OXALIC ACID. Oxalic acid, $H_2C_2O_42H_2O$, is a common corrosive organic acid which at times causes death. It is known as "acid of sugar" because it can be prepared by the oxidation of sugar with nitric acid. Oxalic acid is present in rhubarb and a number of other plants and is ingested in food in small quantities and is excreted as calcium oxalate in the urine under normal conditions. Commercially the acid occurs in the form of colorless, prismatic, foursided crystals which are similar in appearance to the crystals of magnesium sulfate and zinc sulfate. Oxalic acid crystals have a wide use as a bleaching or a cleansing agent and may be obtained easily from drug stores. Potassium binoxalate, KHC_2O_4, is similar in toxicity to oxalic acid and may cause poisoning.

The bitter taste of oxalic acid makes it easy to detect so that it is rarely used for homicidal purposes. Petri mentions a fatal case in which oxalic acid was injected into the vagina to produce abortion. In the Office of the Chief Medical Examiner in New York City from 1918 to 1951, there were no cases of this type reported. Suicidal and accidental cases occurring as the result of ingesting the acid, are more numerous, for during the same period there were 39 suicides and 14 cases of accidental and undetermined deaths. In rare instances because of the resemblance of the oxalic acid crystals to those of magnesium sulfate, some persons have taken oxalic acid by mistake with fatal results. If a pharmacist is responsible for putting oxalic acid crystals into a package labeled magnesium sulfate, and poisoning occurs as a result of his error, he is liable for civil damages and probably could be prosecuted criminally.

Oxalic acid differs from magnesium sulfate and zinc sulfate on four demonstrable points: The oxalic acid is acid in reaction, sublimes when heated, effervesces with sodium carbonate and bleaches ink. The sulfate salts do not sublime on heating, do not bleach ink, do not effervesce with sodium carbonate, and are neutral or only slightly acid.

Burns of the face and skin are rare in oxalic acid poisoning. After ingestion of the acid, the victim suffers from dysphagia, pain in the epigastrium, thirst, vomiting of a brownish fluid, low blood pressure, convulsions, tetanic spasms, coma, collapse and finally death. The clinical course varies from three minutes to several hours to a matter of days, depending on whether the patient succumbs to the local corrosive effects of the acid or dies of acidosis following its absorption into the blood. Anatomically the mouth, pharynx and esophagus show a grayish corrosion of various hues attended by a reactive inflammation in the neighboring tissues. The esophagus and stomach may be corroded especially on the top of the rugal crests with reddish streaks and dark brown necrotic areas of acid hematin formation (Fig. 30-4). The reaction may vary considerably—from marked congestion to surface necroses, detachment of the stomach lining, and acid hematin formation in the submucous blood vessels. Crystals of calcium oxalate may be present in the surface part of the corrosion or in the submucous tissues of the stomach, and are seen as elongated octahedral and dumbell-shaked crystals. The duodenum may show the same type of inflammation as the stomach. Rarely a phlegmonous gastritis develops as a result of the necroses in the stomach.

If the acid is absorbed into the blood, symptoms of shock, numbness and tingling over the body, tetanic convulsions, anuria and crystalluria appear, with death occurring in convulsions or in deep coma after an interval, depending on the action of the poison on the central nervous system. Oxalic acid when absorbed combines

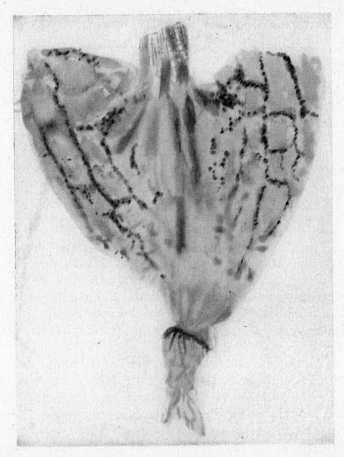

Fig. 30-4. Corrosion of Stomach Following Ingestion of Oxalic Acid. Suicide.

The brown barred pattern has resulted from the formation of acid hematin along the rugal crests.

with the calcium in the body so that the kidneys as the principal excretory organ contain calcium oxalate crystals in the forms already described, filling the tubules and appearing as whitish streaks in the medulla or as dots in the cortical tissues; the epithelium of the tubules show little anatomic change and the glomeruli are not involved. Occasional round cell collections around Bowman's capsule or some of the smaller blood vessels are to be seen. The crystals in the tubules may be an explanation of the clinically evident anuria and crystalluria and they may be demonstrated microscopically in unstained tissue fragments by the addition of a dilute alkali to the specimen in order to destroy the organic matter; they cannot be demonstrated with the ordinary histologic technic. Occasionally they are found in the blood and in some of the viscera.

The fatal dose has been as low as 4 gm., but in most cases is from 15 to 30 gm. The antidote is finely divided chalk or calcined magnesia which is given in a large amount of water, as this forms a precipitate with oxalic acid; sodium and potassium salts are not suitable antidotes as they form soluble and toxic salts with the acid. Vomiting should be encouraged, but the stomach tube must be used with caution, in spite of the fact that perforation is rare. The specimens to be saved for toxicologic examination are the stomach contents and parenchymatous organs like the liver and kidneys. Since the urine may contain oxalates under normal conditions, it would not be suitable for toxicologic use.

ACETIC ACID. Acetic acid, CH_3COOH, is the principal constituent of vinegar and is the end result of fermentation involving different organic substances. Glacial acetic acid is a 99 per cent solution used in chemical laboratories and it is a strong corrosive with a tendency to give off fumes.

Acute poisoning has been caused by the ingestion of the acid. In a few cases, it has been given for homicidal purposes; it has been swallowed with suicidal intent and has been ingested by children and alcoholics accidentally.

The action of the acid on the gastrointestinal tract is to cause a corrosive thickening and swelling of the mucous membrane, and a brownish discoloration due to the formation of acid hematin. Because of the fumes given off, inflammation and edema of the larynx, pseudomembranous inflammation of the air passages and aspiration pneumonia occasionally occur. Reddish brown burns about the face and mouth may be present and irritation of the conjunctivae is sometimes encountered. The symptoms are pain in the abdomen, vomiting, difficulty in swallowing, and a state of shock which follows any corrosive poisoning. After absorption the acid produces a marked hemolysis in the blood, hemoglobinuria, and generalized acidosis which may be fatal. In some cases the liver has been described as large and dark brown, and the kidneys as swollen, red and dark brown in color, and showing a nephrotic condition.

The fatal dose of acetic acid is hard to determine; the ingestion of 60 to 70 ml. of the glacial acetic acid has caused death from shock in about two hours. The treatment is about the same as for the other corrosive acids. Stomach contents and parenchymatous viscera are preserved for chemical analysis.

A chronic acetic acid poisoning has been described in workers in vinegar manufactories, in fat persons who drink vinegar to become thin, and in others who inhale the vapor continuously. These individuals are said to show a mild gastroenteritis, fetid breath, decay of the teeth, pallor, anemia, emaciation, weakness and chronic bronchitis.

CITRIC ACID. Citric acid has a corrosive action similar to the other organic acid corrosives but not so intense. Petri mentions the case of a 23 year old woman who drank about 20 to 30 gm. of pure citric acid as an abortifacient and died after two days of severe gastrointestinal symptoms. The corrosion of the upper digestive tract was manifested in a wrinkled rough mucous membrane of the tongue and esophagus, gray-white and yellowish green in color and the mucous membrane of the stomach was swollen and pale yellowish green and red, while the small intestine showed similar changes of slighter grade. Poisoning with citric acid is not common.

Halogens. The halogens include chlorine, bromine, iodine and fluorine. They act like strong acid corrosives and may produce fatal results when ingested or inhaled.

CHLORINE. Chlorine, Cl, is a yellowish-green gas, about two and one-half times heavier than air (specific gravity, 2.47). It has a wide use as a bleaching agent and as a disinfectant. It is pungent and irritating, and in World War I it was used as a lethal gas, causing numerous casualties. Some cases of poisoning have occurred in factories from its accidental inhalation. A number of alkaline preparations, such as calx chlorinata, sodium hypochlorite, Labarraque's solution, Javelle water, modified Dakin's solution, and dichloramine-T contain chlorine, and liberate it in the presence of a mineral acid, or on exposure to air.

Exposure to chlorine gas produces irritation of the conjunctivae and its inhalation causes laryngeal spasm, irritative cough, dyspnea, pain in the chest, cyanosis, asphyxia, weak pulse and collapse. Death may occur suddenly following the reflex spasm in the larynx. At necropsy the mucous membranes of the air passages may show a catarrhal inflammation associated with the exudation of stiff mucus; severe exposures may produce a pseudomembrane. Some of the mucus which contains a little chlorine may be swallowed, but under these conditions causes little irritation of the upper gastrointestinal tract. The lungs may show a massive edema, some of the alveoli may be hyperaerated, and there may be scattered pneumonic patches. The pulmonary edema causes some obstruction to the pulmonary circulation and the right heart is often distended. Chlorine gas is dangerous to life in dilutions of 40 to 60 parts per million in the atmosphere. The treatment is to remove the victim from the poisonous atmosphere and to combat shock and circulatory collapse. If death is due to inhalation of the gas, the lungs are saved for toxicologic analysis.

Occasionally some of the preparations which release chlorine are ingested and inflammation of the upper gastrointestinal tract results, due as much to the alkali in the disinfectant as to any chlorine which may be released. Petri mentions a case of fatal corrosion of the mouth, esophagus and stomach from a mixture of calx chlorinata and potassium chloride which was given orally to a child by mistake. A case of suicidal ingestion of sodium hypochlorite is recorded among the cases investigated by the Office of the Chief Medical Examiner in New York City.

BROMINE. Bromine, Br, is a dark reddish-brown liquid with a pungent odor. It is irritant and corrosive in its action on organic material. Poisoning by bromine is mostly accidental, but suicidal and homicidal cases have occurred.

The vapor of bromine may be inhaled, causing pain in the chest, severe cough, edema of the larynx and hemoptysis. The upper respiratory tract from the nasal passages to the finer bronchi are severely inflamed, showing swollen mucous membranes which are discolored reddish brown. Edema of the lungs may supervene and death occur in a few minutes from suffocation. If the liquid is splashed on the skin it produces an exceptionally severe skin burn which can cause death. Even the vapors may produce a marked conjunctivitis and burns of the face. When bromine is ingested, severe pain in throat and abdomen, dysphagia, vomiting and offensive dark brown eructations follow. The upper portion of the gastrointestinal tract is stained brown, showing intense necrosis, softening and exfoliation of the mucous membrane. The patient may die in a few hours of shock.

The fatal dose in a child may be small, in one case 0.2 gm. In an adult, death was caused by one ounce. If the poison has been swallowed, evacuation by emetics or the stomach pump is indicated, and starch emulsions from rice or flour may be given by mouth. Bromine after absorption is transformed into sodium or other bromides and is slowly eliminated in the urine over a number of days while a minute quantity is present in tears, milk, saliva and other secretions. The gastric contents, urine, blood and parenchymatous viscera are preserved for toxicologic analysis.

The bromides of sodium and potassium are given as sedatives in nervous and mental cases. When used in large amounts over a long period of time, they tend to replace the chlorides in the body, even to the extent of substituting hydrobromic acid for hydrochloric acid in the gastric juice. The bromides persist in the blood for a number of days and are eliminated slowly in the urine. A condition known as bromism may be produced, characterized by the appearance of large numbers of skin pustules over the body, resembling acne, or the formation of nodules on the legs known as nodose bromoderma, and in addition by stupor, fetid breath, digestive disturbances, muscular weakness, neurologic phenomena, and mental depression. If the bromides are given or taken injudiciously in large quantities, death from exhaustion or pneumonia may occur. A case of bromide poisoning has been produced by transmission of the drug from the mother to the infant through the milk. In bromide poisonings, the urine of living patients may be sent to the laboratory for toxicologic examination; in fatal cases, the urine and a large quantity of blood are reserved for chemical analysis.

IODINE. Iodine, I, is a crystalline dark purplish brown solid which produces a violet vapor when heated. It is a normal constituent of animal tissues and is closely associated with the physiologic activity of the thyroid gland. It is present in iodine liniment, tincture of iodine, Lugol's solution and many other preparations.

Poisoning may occur in susceptible persons when tincture of iodine or any other iodine-containing solution is applied to a large absorbing surface of the body. If the vapor of iodine comes in contact with the face, it may cause conjunctival inflammation, and if inhaled, it may cause a fatal inflammation of the respiratory tract When swallowed, the solution of iodine produces gastrointestinal lesions, causing pain, thirst, nausea and vomiting, and later delirium, collapse and finally death. Most of these cases are suicidal, or accidental and undetermined; homicidal cases are rare. In the 33-year period from 1918 to 1951, suicidal cases in the Office of the Chief Medical Examiner of New York City due to the ingestion of iodine numbered 109, and accidental and undetermined cases numbered 18, with no homicides.

At autopsy the upper digestive tract, and the stomach in particular are corroded, showing a firm, dry and dark brown mucous membrane. If a starch preparation has been used as an antidote, the contents and the lining of the stomach are stained a dark blue indigo. Microscopic section of the stomach wall corroded by iodine shows the surface epithelium swollen and transformed into goblet cells and apparently embalmed by the coagulating action of the iodine. Below this zone is an area of engorged blood vessels containing acid hematin, occasional submucous hemorrhages, varying degrees of necrosis of the glands with a predominance of the acid cells, and a wall of polymorphonuclear leukocytes which are most numerous in the deeper portions of the mucosa so as to suggest a defense wall (Fig. 30-2). The action of the iodine is like an acid corrosive except that it is not as destructive and has more penetrating power. In some cases reported in the literature cicatricial stenosis of the esophagus was described, probably as the delayed aftermath of an acute inflammation in the esophageal wall. If iodine is absorbed, the kidneys show a marked cloudy swelling of the tubular epithelium, the intestines are inflamed and suppression of urine and diarrhea may occur.

Death occurs in 24 hours to several days. Three to 4 gm. is generally considered a fatal dose. The treatment is to evacuate the stomach by lavage or emetics, using starch decoctions as an antidote. Stomach contents, urine and parenchymatous organs are used for toxicologic examination. The rate of elimination is slightly more rapid than that of the bromine compounds.

The persistent or excessive use of iodides in a person who is susceptible produces the condition known as iodism, marked by skin eruptions, anemia, malaise and loss of nutrition. Some individuals are abnormally sensitive to iodine and may develop a severe cutaneous inflammation when small amounts are applied to the skin.

FLUORINE. Fluorine, Fl, is a member of the halogen group, and is toxicologically important because of the compounds, hydrofluoric acid and sodium fluoride. These substances are strong corrosives and produce an escharotic effect on organic tissues.

Hydrofluoric acid is used in the manufacture of fertilizers and in gaseous form is employed in glass etching. When inhaled as a vapor it produces ulcerations of the conjunctivae, nose and mouth, and a marked escharotic inflammation of the air passages so that the mucous membranes are an intense red and brownish red from acid hematin formation. It occasionally causes painful burns about the fingers. When hydrofluoric acid is ingested in solution, the mouth and esophagus display a grayish-white eschar and the mucous membrane of the stomach shows a reddish-black corrosion on the top of the rugae with a dark crimson red in between. Whether swallowed or inhaled, the acid produces severe pain in the parts chiefly attacked and causes death by shock in from one to several hours.

Sodium fluoride is one of the constituents of different rat poisons or roach powders, and a number of cases of acute poisoning from these substances has occurred in the Office of the Chief Medical Examiner of New York City. In the 33 years from 1918 to 1951, there were 117 cases of suicidal poisoning and 57 cases of accidental or undetermined poisoning reported; homicidal cases are rare. Accidental poisonings are occasionally produced when a careless cook mixes roach powder by mistake in her cooking, and illness or death occur in those who eat the food; in one case a girl swallowed a fatal amount of sodium fluoride by mistake, believing it to be sodium bicarbonate. In the stomach the sodium fluoride is transformed into hydrofluoric acid by the gastric juice and a dark red corrosion of the mucous membrane occurs, with a milder reaction for mouth, esophagus and small intestine. The microscopic section of the stomach wall shows a moderately intense necrosis of the mucous membrane.

After ingestion of sodium fluoride, pain in epigastrium, dysphagia, nausea and vomiting follow, and after it is absorbed into the system, cardiac weakness, dyspnea, sensory and motor disturbances, epileptoid manifestations, renal irritation with albuminuria, anemia, and increased coagulability of the blood may appear. Death occurs as a result of shock in 45 minutes to 4 hours, or the victim may live longer and die of acidosis; the fluoride ion has a great affinity for calcium and extracts it from the tissues, so that calcium fluoride is found in the urine. At autopsy in addition to the acid corrosion of the stomach, there may be an irritative nephrosis with swelling of the cells of the convoluted tubules and dark red blood in the blood vessels. The fatal dose of sodium fluoride is from 5 to 10 gm.

When fluoride is ingested, the stomach should be evacuated by emetics or by the stomach pump, and washed out with weak lime water or magnesia in milk, because of the affinity of these basic radicals for the fluoride ion. Other alkalis are less suitable as antidotes. Intravenous infusion of normal saline solution is given to promote the elimination of the poison. Material vomited or recovered from the stomach of the victim, or the urine, may be sent to the laboratory for toxicologic analysis. At autopsy the stomach contents, liver, bones, kidneys and urine are preserved for analysis. The elimination of fluoride from the body is probably similar to excretion of the other halides.

Some organic fluoride compounds, such as sodium fluoroacetate (1080), methyl fluoroacetate, fluorethynol, Di-isoprophyl-fluorphosphate and B. fluorethyl-a-fluoro-butrate, are very toxic in small quantities. Sodium fluoroacetate no. 1080 is much more toxic than sodium fluoride and is a component of some rat poisons. Harrison and collaborators report an acute poisoning in a 40 year old man who ingested this substance for suicidal purposes and died in severe shock after 15 hours of coma, indicating a severe toxic effect on the central nervous system and the circulatory system. The autopsy disclosed a corrosion of the esophagus, stomach and duodenum, similar to that caused by sodium fluoride. A regulation of the New York Department of Health prohibits the use of sodium fluoroacetate as a vermin eradicator unless a permit is obtained from the Commissioner of Health for each separate use of the poison.

A minute quantity of fluorides is normally present in the body and is essential for the proper health of the teeth and bones. Children continually using drinking water which is free of fluorides, show a greater tendency to dental decay than other children who drink water with an average fluoride content of one part in a million. Conversely if an excess of fluorides is ingested in drinking water, or in beers or in baking powders over a period of months or years, a deposition of insoluble calcium fluoride may occur in the liver and the skin, but most strikingly in the bones and teeth. The clear pearly enamel of the teeth is mottled with dull opaque white areas, and the bones become brittle, more opaque to the roentgen ray, and the trabeculae become more thickened, sometimes to such an extent that a secondary anemia results from a narrowing of the bone marrow spaces. Impairment of growth, loss of weight, and symptoms of chronic intoxication are present in the more advanced cases.

Corrosive Metallic Salts. Many metallic salts and esters of acids and alkalis have a distinct corrosive action, because the acid or the alkaline radical is strong and predominates over the opposing radical in the combination. The result is that the salt has a strong acid reaction if the acid component predominates, as for example in the compound zinc chloride, in which the acid radical is more powerful than the basic. Conversely in potassium carbonate the base potassium overshadows the weak acid radical, and the salt is strongly alkaline in reaction.

SILVER. Metallic silver, Ag, is an inert substance, and its compound most important toxicologically is silver nitrate. It is used medicinally as a caustic, owing this property to the nitrate radical.

A few cases of suicidal and accidental poisoning have occurred after ingestion of the salt. The symptoms are those of pain in the throat and abdomen, vomiting and purging of black or blood-stained material, vertigo, spasms, coma and respiratory collapse. The mouth and lips are stained, first a gray-white color, and later black, from the precipitation of silver. The mucous membranes of the stomach and other mucous membranes are similarly stained and corroded.

The fatal dose is difficult to determine, varying from 30 grains to over an ounce. Death takes place in a few hours to a few days. For treatment the stomach is washed out, using a dilute solution of sodium chloride to neutralize the poison. The stomach contents and parenchymatous viscera are preserved for toxicologic examination.

When silver salts are given over a long period of time, silver is deposited in finely divided metallic form in the connective tissues, in the corium of the skin just under the epidermis, in the framework of different organs and in similar locations. This process is termed argyria, and it takes months and years to develop and is not reversible; it does not affect the general health. The prolonged application of colloidal organic silver preparations to the eyes or nose may result in a permanent bluish gray discoloration of the sclera.

ZINC. Zinc, Zn, is a bluish white metal, often used in alloys. Metallic zinc is inert, but some of the salts like the chloride and sulfate are poisonous. The human body under normal conditions contains a minute amount of the metal.

Vessels made of zinc are employed occasionally for the storage of foods, and it has always been a question whether or not enough of the metal would be dissolved by acids during the storage process to cause harmful effects when the material is eaten. Authorities advise against such use of zinc vessels, but claim that little zinc is dissolved in this fashion.

Zinc stearate has been employed as a dusting powder, and deaths have been reported from its use for this purpose on infants. There is reason to believe, however, that the fatal cases were caused by the mechanical action of the powder which was inhaled and produced a bronchopneumonia.

The sulfate of zinc or white vitriol is employed as an emetic and forms crystals similar to those of magnesium sulfate. When ingested in excessive doses or with suicidal intent, it causes vomiting, purging and prostration, usually from its depressing action on the central nervous system. It has been injected into the vagina and uterus as an abortifacient and has caused death. Homicidal cases are rare. Signs of gastrointestinal irritation of greater or lesser severity are found at autopsy. The fatal dose of zinc sulfate varies from 15.5 gm. to over 46 gm. This salt in dilute solution also is used as a mild astringent eye wash and for the treatment of gonorrheal urethritis, and if applied indiscriminately may cause a urethral stricture.

Zinc chloride is a soluble salt used in soldering fluid, disinfectants, preserving fluids for dead bodies, preparations for cauterizing ulcers and in the fluid employed to preserve railway ties from the ravages of insects. On the skin it causes a deep burn, sometimes incurred when railway ties covered with the solution are handled without gloves. Systemic poisoning may follow absorption of the chemical from the raw surface. Zinc salts are excreted by the large intestines and kidneys.

The cases of zinc chloride poisoning are mostly suicidal, accidental, rarely homicidal, and occur usually by ingestion. Under such conditions the substance exerts a powerful corrosive action on the gastrointestinal tract, producing a whitish membrane with exfoliation in places so that a reddish brown denuded area appears; softening, ulceration and even perforation of the stomach may occur. Pain in throat and epigastrium, excessive salivation, dysphagia, metallic taste in the mouth, vomiting of bloody material, purging and bloody fecal material occur, and collapse and death in coma may occur in a few hours. The fatal dose varies; in one case it was about 3.5 gm. If the person survives for a few weeks, extensive scar tissue formation occurs in the esophagus and stomach with stricture of these organs, and emaciation, and with occasional matting together of the stomach with liver, spleen, pancreas, diaphragm and omentum. Neurologic signs, such as muscular weakness, spasms, aphonia and disturbances of sensation occasionally develop. The chloride of zinc has been injected into the vagina and uterus as an abortifacient, causing death from corrosion.

Acute poisoning by zinc salts is treated by washing out the stomach and giving antidotes freely such as milk or the white of eggs. The materials examined toxicologically are the stomach contents and such parenchymatous viscera as the liver and kidneys.

A chronic poisoning is said to occur as the result of the vaporizing of impure zinc, or spelter, causing a syndrome among workers who inhale the fumes known as metal fume fever. It consists of shivering amounting to rigor, pains in the limbs and abdomen, metallic taste in mouth, nausea, diarrhea, cough, rapid pulse and high temperature. Exhaustion and somnolence follow the attacks, but in between the patient is normal. Brass founder's ague and brasier's disease are names given to similar attacks which occur in brass foundries (pages 767 and 893).

The corrosive effects of the compounds of copper, chromium, manganese, mercury and some of the other heavy metals will be discussed in the next chapter.

DIMETHYLSULFATE. This substance is a volatile liquid and is used to produce dimethlyaniline, an important compound used in dye manufacture. Its chemical formula is $(CH_3)2SO_4$. The vapor is corrosive, causing skin and conjunctival lesions and irritation of the upper air passages. In the severe cases, bronchopneumonia and degenerative processes in the liver and kidneys may occur. A case of suicide by the ingestion of dimethylsulfate with corrosion of the upper gastrointestinal tract, has been described by Boerner.

ALKALINE CORROSIVES

The principal corrosives of this group include such strong inorganic bases as the hydroxides and carbonates of potassium and sodium, lye, quicklime and ammonia water. In their action on the body, the alkalis pierce the cell membrane, form moist alkaline albuminates and soaps with the constituents of protoplasm, and produce alkaline hematin by their action on hemoglobin. The chemical effects of alkalis on living protoplasm is fundamentally different from that of acids, for alkalis produce a soft, moist, edematous, swollen eschar, red or brown from the imbibition of altered blood pigment, giving a soapy sensation when touched. In general the pathologic lesions caused by alkaline corrosion have about the same extent and distribution as those due to acid corrosives, even though the chemical nature is different. Strassmann has noted the fact that areas of alkaline corrosion which have been treated with dilute acids as antidotes, may acquire a reddish-brown dried appearance like the eschars due to acids.

When a strong alkali is ingested, the lips and the skin about the mouth may show burns of the geographic and rivulet form with areas of gray-white swollen epidermis interspersed in between reddish moist patches where the epithelium has been denuded. Similar burns occur on the face and upper chest when lye is thrown on the victim, a condition which will be described later. The same appearance is found also in the mouth and throat. The mucous membrane of the esophagus is often removed and the raw surface is soft, swollen, edematous and red in color often with a brownish tinge. In the stomach, the lining is swollen, edematous, slippery to the touch and crimson red, brown or black in color. The duodenum and upper jejunum may show inflammation of similar type but of lesser intensity in comparison with the lesion in the stomach, depending upon whether the pyloric ring has allowed a small or a large amount of the chemical to pass its portal. In some cases the alkali may be regurgitated and inhaled causing edema of the glottis, pseudomembranous inflammation of the air passages and a peribronchial pneumonia.

When a dilute alkaline solution is swallowed, the mucous membrane of the mouth, throat and esophagus may not show any obvious changes but the stomach is usually congested and crimson red or brown in color from the formation of alkaline hematin. The stomach and esophagus are not contracted to the same extent as in the cases of acid corrosion, and the inflammation is not confined to the crests of the rugal folds but usually involves the entire mucous surface. These changes are encountered typically in cases of potassium cyanide poisoning by ingestion in which

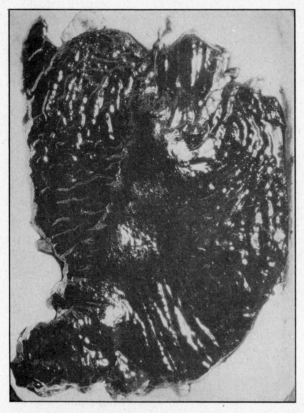

Fig. 30-5. Corrosion of the Stomach by Ingested Strong Alkali (Ammonium Hydroxide). Suicide.

the alkaline salt exerts a powerful but brief action on the gastric mucosa, but without demonstrable effect on the esophagus or mouth. Puppe describes a case in which an alkali containing ultramarine blue was ingested and at autopsy the lining of the esophagus and duodenum was comparatively intact but stained blue while the stomach showed a typical dark brown alkaline corrosion.

Microscopically, dilute alkaline corrosion is best studied in cases of sodium or potassium cyanide poisoning. In such rapid deaths the irritant action of the poison causes goblet cells to form in the superficial layer, the blood vessels in the adjacent layers are distended and in some the blood is changed to a fluid containing brown pigment dust. In a case in which potassium cyanide had been swallowed in solid form and death was delayed for about half an hour, there was destruction of the superficial mucous membrane, and exudation of mucus and cells on the surface, congested vessels, hemorrhage in the adjacent submucous tissues with dissolution of the red blood cells, an infiltration of leukocytes and large mononuclears in the affected area, while the mucosa and stomach wall beyond the penetration of the chemical were intact. Unlike the action of the acid corrosives, there was an infiltration of the chemical with destructive effects without a contraction of the corroded portion and without a strong defense reaction of leukocytes around the necrotic area.

Where a strong alkali like potassium hydroxide, lye or ammonia has been ingested, a formless necrosis extends deep into the tissues, the red blood cells are transformed into a fine pigment dust and stain the stomach wall, and there is a massive edema and leukocytic infiltration with the formation of cystic spaces in the

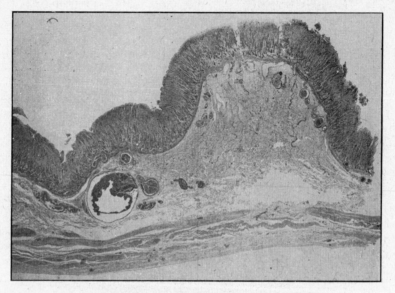

Fig. 30-6. Histologic Section of Stomach Showing Corrosion Pattern Produced by Strong Alkali (Ammonium Hydroxide).

Note marked edematous swelling of submucosa.

loose submucous tissues (Figs. 30-5 and 30-6). In some instances, if the patient survives the corrosion several days, the muscular layers of stomach and esophagus are infiltrated with polymorphonuclear leukocytes almost to the extent of pus formation. In some cases, as mentioned by Strassmann, the process may detach the epithelial layer, and casts of the esophageal mucous membrane may be regurgitated. If the patient recovers from the effects of the corrosion, the inflammation in the walls of the esophagus and stomach in the course of a few months may end in a fibrosis of the esophageal wall or of the stomach. In one case (Fig. 30-7) the esophagus was contracted into a tube of about 10 to 15 mm. in diameter with stenosis of the lumen to 3 mm. by 1 mm., with fibrosis and thickening of the wall, thickening of the epithelium and atrophy and disappearance of the submucous glands. Death in these cases occurs as a result of malnutrition consequent upon the stenosis of the esophagus which prevents the ingestion of food.

Potassium Hydroxide. Hydroxide of potassium, KOH, is a grayish-white solid, soluble in water, with a soapy feel and a bitter taste. A number of medicinal preparations contain this chemical such as caustic potash, potassa en calce (Vienna paste), and potassi carbonas impura. It is a strong corrosive and will inflict burns on the skin as well as on the gastrointestinal tract. Potassium carbonate has an action similar to the hydroxide but not as intense.

Most of the cases of poisoning are suicidal and accidental and as a rule the corrosive is taken by mouth. In the 24-year period from 1918 to 1942, suicidal cases numbered 84 of which 44 were caused by lye; the accidental and undetermined cases numbered 65. Few cases are homicidal and they are usually children on whom

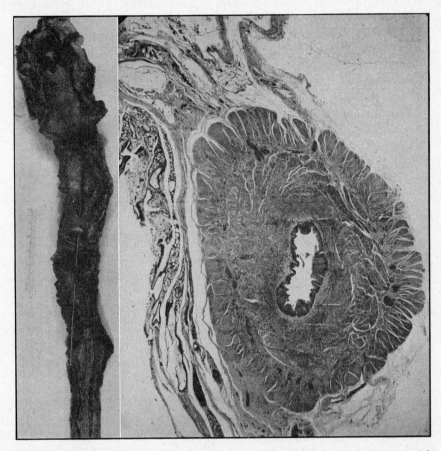

Fig. 30-7. Stricture of Esophagus Following Corrosion by Strong Alkali (Sodium Hydroxide).

Left. The lumen of the esophagus barely admits a probe.
Right. Histologic section reveals narrowed lumen lined by epithelium. Deceased drank lye several years before death.

the poison has been forced. The symptoms after ingestion are burning pains in the mouth, throat and epigastrium, and vomiting of slimy, blood-stained and brownish material which has an alkaline reaction. The pulse is fast and weak, the respirations are shallow and rapid, and the skin is cold and clammy. Death sometimes occurs in about three hours from shock, but occasionally the patient may live a few days and develop a bronchopneumonia.

The mouth and esophagus show a swollen and moist mucous membrane, which may be whitened or may be discolored brown. The stomach and upper intestinal tract show a swollen and moist lining which is stained red, brown and black, from the formation of the alkaline hematin in the stomach wall. In this type of case, care should be taken in introducing the stomach pump in order not to perforate the stomach wall. If the patient recovers from the acute effects of the corrosion, a fibrotic stricture of the esophagus may develop and eventually cause death by starvation.

The fatal dose varies; 30 grains to an ounce has caused death. The treatment is to wash the stomach out as soon as possible and give a weak acid like lemon juice as an antidote. The rest of the treatment is symptomatic. The vomitus, stomach contents, and the parenchymatous viscera are saved for chemical examination.

Sodium Hydroxide. Sodium hydroxide, NaOH, or caustic soda is similar in appearance and properties to caustic potash and the same description will apply to both. Sodium carbonate is also similar to potassium carbonate.

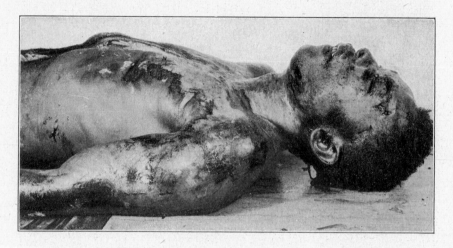

Fig. 30-8. Corrosive Effects of Strong Lye Solution on Skin. Homicidal Assault.

The skin of the face, chest and arms exhibits a corroded, slimy, swollen appearance as a result of the action of the concentrated alkali which was thrown on the deceased. See Figure 30-9.

Concentrated lye is a cleaning powder composed of a mixture of sodium hydroxide and sodium carbonate. This substance has been swallowed for suicidal purposes and has been ingested accidentally by children, causing death by severe corrosion of the gastrointestinal tract. In some instances, lye has been thrown on the face and body of an individual to cause mutilation, and burns of the face and chest and scarring of the cornea have resulted. Five such cases occurred in the period from 1918 to 1951. The eschars are reddish brown and have a corroded slimy swollen appearance, death usually resulting from septic infection and toxemia (Figs. 30-8 and 30-9). In one case of lye burns, a bland thrombosis developed in the left axillary vein and caused death by pulmonary embolism. An example of alkaline corrosion of the mouth and chin produced by concentrated lye solution spilled on the face when it was drunk with suicidal intent is shown in Figure 30-10. There was intense corrosion of the esophagus and stomach and perforation of the latter. Dilute solutions of sodium hydroxide or sodium carbonate have been injected into the bladder or ureter by mistake during roentgenography of the urinary tract and have produced death by corrosive inflammation and septic pyelonephritis.

Calcium Oxide. Quicklime or calcium oxide, CaO, acts in a similar fashion to potassium or sodium hydroxide, but less intensely. Corrosion of the skin, eyes, respiratory and gastrointestinal tracts have been described. The lime may be ingested accidentally or with suicidal intent. The dust from lime kilns or beds may also get into the eyes or be inhaled and cause irritation.

Ammonium Hydroxide. This compound, NH_4OH, ammonium hydroxide, ammonia water or spirits of hartshorn, is a common household article used mostly for cleaning purposes. Aqua ammonia fortior is a 28 per cent solution of ammonia gas in water, and aqua ammonia is a 10 per cent solution. Ammonia carbonas is

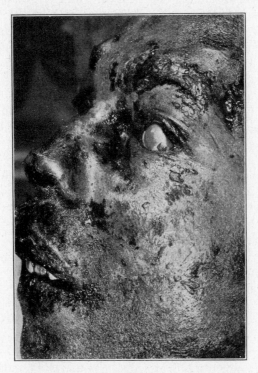

Fig. 30-9. Corrosive Action of Concentrated Lye Solution on Face.
Same case as Figure 30-8. Close-up view showing corrosion of skin and cornea by alkali.

a white caustic crystalline substance. Aromatic spirits of ammonia is a 10 per cent solution of ammonia gas in alcohol, with oil of nutmeg, lemon and lavender.

Gastrointestinal corrosion is caused by the ingestion of ammonia water. The symptoms are usually pain in the mouth, throat and epigastrium, salivation, vomiting, dysphagia and renal irritation with partial anuria, cylindruria, hematuria and albuminuria. The fatal dose is variable but has been as little as one dram of aqua ammonia fortior. The treatment is the same as for the other corrosive alkalis, and the postmortem lesions are also similar. A few cases are homicidal, some are suicidal and some are accidental. Ammonia water is often kept in the same closet as other drugs and may be swallowed by mistake. In rare instances ammonia water has been injected into the vagina and uterus with an intent to cause abortion. A case of corrosive proctitis, referable to the mistaken injection of ammonium hydroxide by rectum, was seen by the authors.

Ammonia gas is used in refrigerators and occasionally escapes through leaks in the pipes. If it is inhaled, a severe inflammation of the respiratory passages is produced, which results in a yellowish, purulent, pseudomembranous laryngitis, tracheitis, bronchitis and bronchopneumonia. The symptoms are pain in the chest, severe coughing, spasm of the glottis, and signs of a terminal lung infection. In a few cases, the same type of inflammation has been produced by allowing a prostrated individual to sniff strong ammonia fumes in an ill-advised attempt at resuscitation. The gas also comes in contact with the eyes and may cause severe conjunctival and corneal irritation.

The stomach contents are the only material which can be used for toxicologic analysis as ammonia compounds are usually present in the tissues under normal conditions, especially during decomposition. The characteristic pungent odor of the gas will serve to identify it in the stomach of a recently dead body.

Strong caustic alkalis like potassium hydroxide, lye or quicklime destroy organic material almost as rapidly as the acids and have been used either in liquid form or as a powdered solid by perpetrators of a homicide in an attempt to obliterate the body. They transform the flesh and organs except a few of the bones to a brownish soapy liquid or an amorphous mass. For fuller details see the reference by Haines.

ORGANIC CORROSIVES

Some organic compounds which are not acid, have a definite corrosive action on living tissue, ascribable to their ability to coagulate protein. The war chemicals yperite and lewisite belong to this group and have been discussed on page 719. At present the most common organic corrosives encountered in civil life are members of the phenol group and formaldehyde.

Phenol Group. The phenol group contains aromatic compounds which are hydroxyl derivatives of benzene, and are either obtained from coal tar or made synthetically. The simplest derivative is phenol, C_6H_5OH, popularly known as carbolic acid. Other compounds are the dihydroxybenzenes, $C_6H_4(OH)_2$, guaiacol, $C_6H_3(OH)_2(CH_3)$, the cresols, $C_6H_4(CH_3)OH$, and pyrogallol, $C_6H_3(OH)_3$.

PHENOL. Phenol occurs in the pure state as needle-like translucent crystals with a pinkish tinge. The drug is slightly soluble in water but quite soluble in alcohol, ether, chloroform or glycerine. Its principal uses are as an antiseptic or as a disinfectant. It is a definite protoplasmic poison and an appreciable number of deaths are ascribable to its toxic action.

Suicidal poisoning from the ingestion of phenol is encountered at about the rate of six cases a year according to the figures in the Office of the Chief Medical Examiner of New York City. Accidental deaths from phenol occur because alcoholics and children swallow the poison, mistaking it for a beverage, as a result of the practice followed by many individuals of keeping it in the same compartment with innocuous materials. Occasionally the drug is spilled upon the skin accidentally, and unless it is removed in a few minutes, it may cause a severe burn which may be the focus of a fatal septic infection. Its indiscriminate medical use in the rectum, vagina, wounds, abscesses or body cavities has resulted in poisoning. Accidental or undetermined deaths due to the action of phenol and related substances (but excluding lysol; see page 732) occur according to the statistics of the Office of the Chief Medical Examiner of New York City at the rate of about five cases a year. Sometimes phenol or similar drugs have been injected into the vagina and uterus to produce an illegal abortion, or for contraceptive purposes, and death has occurred. Phenol has rarely been used as a means of homicide (1 case between 1918 and 1941), and then it has mostly been employed against children and infants.

Sydney Smith has described toxic symptoms caused by the inhalation of phenol fumes from a large quantity of the chemical which had been spilled on the floor. The authors have seen two cases in which a phenolic preparation was applied to the face as a cosmetic treatment for the removal of acne scars, and a few minutes after the application the victims suddenly collapsed and died. The autopsy disclosed superficial phenol burns on the face, dark red blood and congestion of organs; toxicologic examination of lungs and brain showed a trace of phenol in both organs. Owing to the fact that other drugs were administered to the victims, it is difficult to appraise the role of phenol in causing death, but it probably contributed in these cases.

Locally phenol causes a precipitation or coagulation of the cellular protein and deep penetration into the tissues, followed by necrosis. Phenol forms with protein a loose combination which is easily dissociated, and the freed phenol penetrates deeper, combining with fresh protein and causing more necrosis. On the skin the sensory nerves are numbed, with a slight tingling sensation; then the superficial layers become grayish-white and necrotic, and slough leaving a brownish eschar. If the burns are extensive, shock, toxemia or septic infection may supervene and cause death.

When phenol is swallowed the victim complains of a burning pain in the throat, mouth and stomach; vomiting results and the ejecta usually reek with the characteristic odor of this substance. The symptoms, as a rule, are slightly delayed, because the corrosive action of phenol is not as immediately effective or as intense as the various mineral corrosives. It is understandable that phenol can be imbibed erroneously in mistake for an innocuous beverage, especially by a person who is intoxicated or by one who has not a keen sense of smell and is not able to detect the characteristic odor of the disinfectant.

Much of the phenol is absorbed from the gastrointestinal tract, skin or lungs and causes a severe general reaction, with depression of the central nervous system, a slight hemolysis and a severe irritation of the kidneys. Headache, muscular weakness, a dusky cyanosis of the face, rapid pulse, delirium, coma, irregular respirations, collapse, cold sweats, a pasty pallor and occasionally convulsions are produced by its strong toxic action. Internally phenol is oxidized to hydroquinol and pyrocatechol, and is excreted in the urine as phenol or as various combinations of glycuronic and sulfuric acids with phenol, hydroquinol or pyrocatechol; a large portion of the absorbed phenol is destroyed in the liver. The urine containing the substances becomes a dull dark and smoky green, especially on standing, and usually contains albumin and blood casts from the renal irritation.

Cases of acute poisoning through the ingestion of phenol show at necropsy brownish patches of corrosion about the mouth (Fig. 30-11). The upper gastrointestinal tract, especially the stomach and sometimes the adjacent small intestine, exhibit patches of bluish-gray and yellowish-gray pseudomembrane composed of necrotic tissue while the areas of mucous membrane in between are reddened and inflamed (Fig. 30-12). Histologic section in such stomachs shows a coagulation necrosis which extends deep into the mucous membrane but only a moderate degree of congestion and inflammatory reaction is present. The mouth, pharynx and esophagus are not so intensely involved. Laryngeal edema, inflammation of the air passages, and aspiration pneumonia may develop from the inhalation of vomitus. All the organs are markedly congested, due to the definitely depressing effect of the drug on the central nervous system, the myocardium and the capillary blood vessels. The kidneys show a nephrosis with cloudy swelling and necrosis of the cortical epithelium and occasionally extravasation of blood and blood pigment into the tubules but without any observable changes in the glomeruli. The urine is usually a dull gray green in color and smoky in appearance, and may be turbid from the presence of blood casts and free hemoglobin. The liver may show a few areas of focal necrosis.

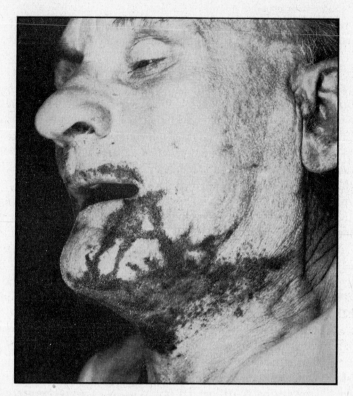

Fig. 30-10. Chemical Corrosion of Mouth and Chin by Lye Spilled Over During Suicidal Drinking of Concentrated Solution.

There was also strong alkaline corrosion and perforation of stomach.

The fatal dose of phenol is about one-half ounce when it is taken by mouth. If it is introduced into the cavity of the uterus, or into wounds or body cavities a much smaller amount may cause death. The average duration of the clinical course in a fatal case is from 2 to 12 hours, but may be shorter or longer. The treatment is to wash the stomach with warm water and add milk or egg albumin to neutralize the corrosive action of the phenol; the rest of the treatment is symptomatic. The stomach contents and the parenchymatous organs are used for toxicologic analysis. Phenol is probably eliminated from the body in the first 36 hours after the poisoning.

Phenol may cause chronic poisoning when absorbed over a long period of time, giving rise to symptoms such as nausea, anorexia, headache, diarrhea, skin eruptions, and renal irritation. If a dilute solution of carbolic acid is applied to a part continuously, gangrene of that area may result. In the early days of antisepsis when the carbolic acid spray was first introduced by Lister, many cases of superficial gangrene developed among patients and attendants in the surgical amphitheaters because of the vaporized phenol. Cases of carbolic acid ochronosis have been described, very

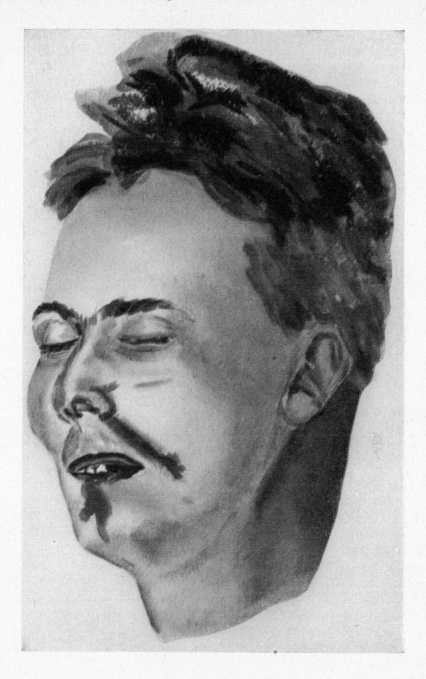

Fig. 30-11. Chemical Eschars Around the Mouth Following Suicidal Ingestion of Lysol.

much like the alkaptonuric variety, with the deposit of bluish-black or brown pigment in the skin, ear, tracheal and joint cartilages, heart valves, aorta and kidneys.

CRESOL. Cresols are phenolic compounds obtained from coal tar, and include ortho-, meta- and paramethyl phenols, $C_6H_4(CH_3)OH$. They are used as antiseptics and disinfectants in various mixtures, and most important of which are creolin (a mixture of phenols) and lysol (a mixture of cresols with alkali solution and linseed oil). The toxicologic action of cresol is similar to that of phenol as the same type of local corrosion is produced, and after absorption, depression of the central nervous system, hemolysis and parenchymatous changes in kidneys and

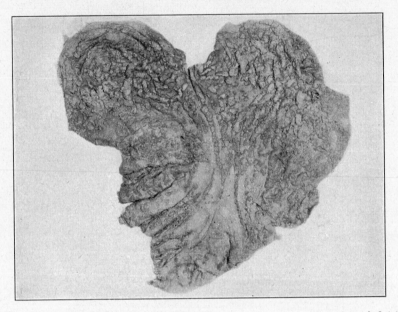

Fig. 30-12. Corrosion of Stomach Mucosa Following Ingestion of Concentrated Lysol. Suicide.
Note gray necrotic membrane formation especially along the rugal crests.

other viscera occur. The action of lysol because of the alkaline content varies slightly from that of the other cresol preparations.

LYSOL. Lysol is a clear yellow or dark brown liquid composed of a solution of 50 per cent cresols in potassium saponified linseed oil so that its reaction is markedly alkaline. It is valuable as a disinfectant because the mixture is miscible in water. Its action on the body is similar to that of phenol, but it is locally more immediately irritant because of the alkali in the solution, though its toxicity is not considered to be as great.

Poisoning with lysol is generally the result of suicidal ingestion of the drug, about 28 cases a year being recorded in the Office of the Chief Medical Examiner of New York City. In some cases it has been swallowed in mistake for an innocent substance; and fatal burns have been caused on the skin because lysol has been spilled on it accidentally. In the statistics of the Chief Medical Examiner of New York City the accidental or undetermined lysol cases are included in the group of phenolic compounds of which the yearly average is five cases. Like phenol it has been used as a means of homicide against infants and children. This disinfectant has been injected into the uterus as an abortifacient, a contraceptive or as an antiseptic, and into the rectum by error instead of a therapeutic drug; death has often followed such administrations. The authors have seen one case in which lysol was injected into a pregnant uterus between the amnion and the uterine wall and caused the death of the victim as a result of pulmonary oil embolism and systemic lysol poisoning before abortion occurred (Vance).

The symptoms of lysol ingestion are pain in the mouth, throat and epigastrium, followed by vomiting of material which has a penetrating lysol odor. Its action on the stomach is to produce a necrotic pseudomembrane of gray color not unlike the membrane in phenol corrosion, and in addition the marked alkalinity of the mixture causes edema and swelling of the tissues. The same type of lesion in varying intensity also occurs on the mucous membrane of the throat, esophagus, intestine, rectum, vagina and uterus. Dark reddish burns are found on the skin around the mouth, as in the case of phenol. Edema of the larynx, inflammation of the air passages, and scattered areas of bronchopneumonia may occur as a result of the inhalation of regurgitated lysol (Fig. 30-11).

After lysol is absorbed into the system, the pulse becomes small and weak, the respirations rapid and labored, marked cyanosis is present, and the patient develops headache, giddiness, convulsions and coma. Cresols have a marked affinity for the cerebral lipoids and are said to cause microscopic changes in the brain tissue and nerve cells. When the lysol acts on the blood in sufficient concentration, it destroys the red blood cells and produces dark brown alkaline hematin. In some cases the liver has been described as the seat of focal necroses. The kidneys are congested, enlarged and dull reddish brown in color, and microscopically show epithelial necroses in the convoluted tubules, and blood cells or blood-pigment casts in the lumen of the collecting tubules like a lower nephron nephrosis. The urine may contain albumin, casts, hemoglobin and red blood cells and be dark gray to black in color; occasionally oliguria may occur. Death is most often the result of the toxic action of the cresols on the brain and on the myocardium. In pregnant women, both lysol and phenols may be transported through the placenta and poison the fetus.

Microscopic section of the corrosive lesion in the stomach shows a formless necrosis of the superficial layers and a scant leukocytic infiltration if any in the adjacent tissues. In the necrotic area, some formless, brownish pigment may be present here and there. In cases which survive, a reactive inflammation develops and may progress to stenosis. In some of these cases granules of brownish yellow pigment may be present in the epithelial tubular cells of the kidney and collections of pigment may be found in the spleen (Petri).

The victim usually survives the ingestion of lysol a few hours to a few days. If an autopsy is performed on a case which has lived a few hours, the viscera and blood will usually have the characteristic lysol odor. The stomach contents and parenchymatous organs are used for toxicologic examination; to prove the presence of lysol it is necessary to demonstrate the cresols, fatty acids and alkali chemically. The fatal dose is variable, a teaspoonful causing death in a child, but much larger doses have been ingested with recovery. The treatment is similar to that of phenol.

DIHYDROXYBENZENES. The dihydroxybenzenes, $C_6H_4(OH)_2$, pyrocatechol, resorcinol and hydroquinol give symptoms similar to phenol, except that the action on the central nervous system is more stimulating, the hemolysis of the red blood cells is more pronounced, and the necrosis of the digestive tract less intense. Dr. Robert C. Fisher investigated the case of a soldier who took several spoonfuls of photographic hydroquinone crystals under the impression that they were Epsom salts. He went into a state of shock, developed vomiting and diarrhea and began to pass brown cloudy urine which contained large amounts of decomposed hemoglobin. Later he developed a brownish cyanosis of the skin and sclera, became severely anemic and toxic, and died six days later. At autopsy, there was a brownish cyanosis of the tissues, a marked hemolytic anemia, a severe nephrosis and hemoglobinuria; there were no obvious signs of corrosion of the intestinal tract.

Guaiacol (methyl pyrocatechol) gives much the same symptoms as the dihydroxybenzenes. This statement also applies to creosote, a mixture of crude phenols derived from the destructive distillation of wood tar.

PYROGALLOL. Pyrogallol, a trihydric phenol, $C_6H_3(OH)_3$, is used as a reducing agent in the dye and photographic industries, and in chemical and bacteriologic procedures, because it absorbs oxygen avidly. It is used in the form of a salve for the treatment of skin diseases, such as psoriasis. Most cases of poisoning are accidental; some cases are suicidal. Pyrogallol is a white, odorless crystalline powder which has the form of leaflets or fine needles; these melt at 134° C. In alkaline solution, it absorbs oxygen, turning a brown color.

The toxicologic action of pyrogallol consists in a mild corrosion at the local points of application, and severe systemic effects after gaining entrance to the system. It may cause poisoning by absorption from the skin when it is used as a salve, or from the stomach after it is ingested. It acts on the red blood cells causing a methemoglobinemia, followed by destruction of the red blood cells. The blood is reddish-brown in color, the corpuscles shrink, and many ghost cells are observed; the oxygen carrying power of the blood is inhibited. Jaundice, hemoglobinuria and signs of a nephrosis appear. Cyanosis, chills, vomiting, diarrhea, headache, weak pulse, dark colored urine, tremors and death by collapse constitute the clinical picture of the acute case, death occurring as a rule in a few days. In rare instances, death may occur with uremic symptoms. The body at necropsy shows reddish-brown blood coagula, congested nephrotic kidneys and blood-stained urine. The fatal dose varies from 4.9 gm. to 20 gm., but it cannot be placed at an exact figure. The stomach contents and parenchymatous viscera are used for chemical analysis.

The chronic cases last a few weeks and show an ashy gray cyanosis, hemoglobinemia, hemoglobinuria, submucous hemorrhages, ulcerative pharyngitis and stomatitis, and death usually occurs in coma. At autopsy, in addition to these lesions, there are hemorrhages in the submucous layer of the intestines and a terminal bronchopneumonia.

Formaldehyde. Formaldehyde, HCHO, is a colorless irritant gas made from the oxidation of methyl alcohol. Formalin is a proprietary name for a strong solution of formaldehyde in water about 40 per cent. This substance is often used as a disinfectant and because of its preservative action on tissues is frequently the chief constituent of embalming fluids or is employed as a tissue fixative in histologic technic. In strong solution it precipitates protein, and in weak solutions it is toxic to living cells.

The vapor of formaldehyde is irritating to the upper respiratory tract when inhaled, and with constant contact induces coryza, conjunctivitis, bronchitis and, with susceptible individuals, a marked dermatitis especially on the hands near the finger nails. Formaldehyde has been swallowed for suicidal purposes, five cases of this type being recorded in the Office of the Chief Medical Examiner of New York City between 1918 and 1951. Occasionally the chemical has been ingested by mistake for an alcoholic beverage. After swallowing, a marked local irritation occurs with pain in the throat, pain in the epigastrium, vomiting and diarrhea. In these cases the lower end of the esophagus and the stomach show a firm mucous membrane with a shrunken, gray, cooked appearance like the ordinary fixed tissue seen in preserved specimens and the lower end of the esophagus is contracted and thrown into longitudinal folds; the adjacent portions of the small intestine show lesions similar to the stomach but are not so intensely involved. In other cases, the corrosion has been described as being more pronounced (Petri). Regurgitation and inhalation of the fluid causes reddening and inflammation of the air passages and a scattered focal pneumonia.

Microscopically the stomach shows definite changes in the mucous membrane due to the chemically irritant action of the formaldehyde which kills and preserves the superficial cells of the mucosa and produces a reaction in the deeper layers. In one case investigated by Dr. Eugene Clark, a Negro man, 32 years old, drank some embalming fluid containing formaldehyde, entered the hospital in coma and died about 40 minutes later. Necropsy showed the typical gray shrunken appearance of the mucous membrane and the lower end of the esophagus was contracted and thrown into folds. Microscopic section of the stomach showed that the cells, in the superficial layer of the mucous membrane were swollen, elongated and the cytoplasm took a strong eosin stain. There was no postmortem desquamation of cells from this layer such as is usually seen in stomachs removed at autopsy. In the mid portion of the mucous layer, the blood vessels were engorged and there was a marked edema which compressed the glands in the deeper portion. Only a few polymorphonuclear leukocytes were present here and there.

In another case, a Negro woman, 37 years old, ingested 2 ounces of formaldehyde solution, and survived the acute attack 14 days, finally dying with signs of septic infection. The autopsy disclosed a thick-walled esophagus showing longitudinal wrinkling, a stomach with a softened mucous membrane stained greenish yellow probably from the regurgitation of bile, but without any involvement of the duodenum and the small intestine. Microscopic examination showed that the stomach wall was necrotic in all its layers without any cellular differentiation or any inflammatory reaction; the esophagus showed desquamation of the epithelial membrane and a diffuse infiltration of the wall with many polymorphonuclear leukocytes. There were abscesses in the upper left abdomen, probably extensions from the esophagus or through the necrotic stomach wall. There were no antemortem perforations of the stomach or esophagus.

After the poison is absorbed, a marked action on the central nervous system is produced, resulting in vertigo, convulsions, stupor and unconsciousness. Hemorrhages and areas of fatty degeneration have been described in the liver and areas of parenchymatous tubular degeneration have been described in the kidneys. The toxic dose varies from 1 to about 4 ounces, and death may occur in a few hours to several days from toxemia, or terminal pneumonia or from sepsis. After absorption some of the formaldehyde is oxidized to formic acid so that much of the treatment is concerned with combating acidosis. The stomach should be washed out and ammonium acetate administered as it transforms formaldehyde to hexanethylenamine. Stomach contents and parenchymatous viscera and brain are used for toxicologic analysis. There is no reliable information as to the rapidity with which formaldehyde is removed from the system.

Acetaldehyde. This compound, CH_3CHO, is one of the oxidation products of ethyl alcohol and is formed occasionally in the rectification of spirits. It is a colorless, volatile liquid with an irritant odor, and a boiling point of 20.8° C. Inhalation of its vapors may cause inflammation of the respiratory passages with cough and dyspnea, and an intoxication like alcohol. Corrosion of the exposed tissues, methemoglobin formation and hemolysis of the red blood cells may occur. In some respects its action is similar to that of formaldehyde.

REFERENCES

Accidents from zinc stearate, J.A.M.A., 84:750, 1925.

Dangers of zinc stearate dusting powder, J.A.M.A., 83:120, 1924.

Editorial. Chronic fluorine intoxication, J.A.M.A., 123:150, 1943.

Gettler, A. O., and Ellerbrook, L. Toxicology of fluorides, Am. J. M. Sc., 197:625, 1939.

Haines, W. S. The Destruction and the Attempted Destruction of the Human Body by Fire and Chemicals, from Peterson, Haines, and Webster, Legal Medicine and Toxicology, Philadelphia, W. B. Saunders Co., 1923, Vol. II, pp. 884 to 887.

Harrison, J. W. E., and others. Acute poisoning with sodium fluoroacetate (compound 1080), J.A.M.A., 149:1520, 1952.

Heiman, H., and Ascher, P. W. The aspiration of stearate of zinc in infancy, Am. J. Dis. Child., 23:503, 1922.

Holland, J. W. Inorganic Poisons, from Peterson, Haines and Webster, Philadelphia, W. B. Saunders Co., 1923, Vol. II, pp. 123-290.

Merkel, H. Die Magenverätzungen, from Henke and Lubarsch, Berlin, Julius Springer, 1930, Vol. X.

Petri, E. Vergiftungen, from Henke and Lubarsch, Berlin, Julius Springer, 1930, Vol. X.

Puppe, G. Atlas und Grundriss der Gerichtlichen Medizin, München, J. F. Lehmann, 1908.

Reports of the Chief Medical Examiner in the City of New York from 1918 to 1951.

Sollmann, T. Manual of Pharmacology, 4th ed., Philadelphia, W. B. Saunders Co., 1932.

Strassmann, F. Lehbuch der Gerichtlichen Medizin, Stuttgart, Ferdinand Enke, 1931.

Vance, B. M. Intrauterine injection of lysol as an abortifacient, Arch. Path., 40:395, 1945.

Webster, R. W. Legal Medicine and Toxicology, Philadelphia, W. B. Saunders Co., 1930.

31

Inorganic Poisons: Metals and Nonmetals

The inorganic poisons may be subdivided into metallic and nonmetallic groups which differ in chemical characteristics, and in toxicologic action.

METALLIC POISONS

The poisons in this group have a metallic element as the characteristic constituent in their molecular formula. With the exception of a few metals like mercury or lead, the pure substances are rarely toxic, but their chemical compounds may possess poisonous properties of varying intensity. A number of metallic compounds have an irritant or escharotic local action on tissues: a strong acid radical combined with a weak metallic base, for example, zinc chloride or copper sulfate, exerts an acid corrosive action; conversely a powerful base joined to a weak acid radical, for example, potassium carbonate, may produce a salt which will cause alkaline corrosion. The chief effects of metallic poisons occur after absorption, for they are carried through the blood and attack the parenchymatous and hollow viscera. Some substances, like mercuric chloride, not only cause corrosion of the stomach when ingested, but also produce inflammatory and degenerative changes in the kidneys and large intestine, the organs of excretion. Other metallic poisons, like the radioactive compounds, rarely cause disturbances at the points of absorption but exert their deleterious influences on the tissues in which they are stored such as the bones and the bone marrow. In some instances a poison like arsenic inflicts marked degenerative changes on the liver, the principal detoxifying organ of the body. Occasionally lead compounds may produce an anemia by destroying the red blood cells in the circulating blood.

Arsenic. The element arsenic, As, is a dark, steel-black metal which is often used with lead as an alloy in the manufacture of shot. Occasionally it is found in nature in the metallic state, and in that form is not toxic. Its compounds, however, are poisonous and many of them contaminate metallic ores, coke and lignite. Traces of arsenic are found in some soils, waters and plants. A few of its compounds are present as impurities in many chemicals used in industry, such as mineral acids, mineral alkalis, and metals such as tin, lead, iron and zinc.

The most important compound is arsenic trioxide, or arsenious oxide, As_2O_3, otherwise known as white arsenic or ratsbane, and sometimes erroneously as acidum arseniosum. It occurs in the form of a heavy white powder, or as a multitude of minute crystals of octahedral shape, and has a faint taste which is not particularly distinctive. Arsenic trioxide is poisonous and is present in many rat exterminators. Some official remedies such as liquor acidi arsenosi and Fowler's solution contain a small amount of arsenic trioxide.

Other toxic arsenic compounds are the trichloride, the triiodide, sodium arsenate in Pearson's solution, Scheele's green or copper arsenite, Paris green (Schweinfurt's or copper acetoarsenite), realgar or arsenic sulfide, Donovan's solution (1 per cent each of mercury iodide and arsenic iodide), Clemen's solution (potassium arsenatis et bromidi), and pigments like Brunswick green, Vienna red and mineral blue which contain various arsenites among other constituents. Arsine and some of the organic compounds of arsenic are also toxic.

INORGANIC COMPOUNDS. Arsenic compounds, more than any other class of poisons, have been used for homicidal purposes, the poisoner either giving them in one large fatal dose or administering them repeatedly in smaller quantities so as to evoke symptoms simulating a natural illness. Mass homicides, in which a number of persons have been poisoned by a single individual, occur frequently in the annals of murder by arsenic. In the past the lack of distinctive flavor of arsenic trioxide and the ease with which it could be disguised in food and drink favored its employment as a means of secret crime. At present this method of killing is not so common, as the poison is more likely to be detected and suspicion directed against the criminal than in former times. Some jurisdictions in the United States even require druggists to keep a record of all sales involving arsenic compounds. In a few homicidal cases, preparations containing arsenic have been introduced into the rectum, vagina and urethra, and similar deaths have resulted from the injection of such drugs into the vagina for the purpose of inducing abortion. In the Office of the Chief Medical Examiner, homicidal poisoning from the use of arsenic compounds is rare, 13 cases occurring between 1918 and 1951. One of these is described on page 702.

Cases of suicidal poisoning occur more frequently, and are usually the result of ingesting rat poison or Paris green. In the years between 1918 and 1951 inclusive, suicidal deaths from inorganic arsenic compounds numbered 145.

Accidental or undetermined cases of poisoning from inorganic arsenic are fairly common; in the interval from 1918 to 1951, there were 114 fatal cases of this type in New York City. Some of these are of the mass variety which is to be expected considering the widespread use of arsenic in fly papers, rat poisons, tree and garden sprays, paper glazes, cloth, dyes, pigments and wall papers. Poisoning of varying grades of severity may occur from eating fruit or vegetables from areas where a spray was used. Arsenic compounds have been found in drinking water, beer, tobacco, drugs, minerals, illuminating gas and coal products. From such sources many cases of poisoning in the household have originated, and even molds growing on wall paper containing arsenic have generated enough volatile derivatives of this metal to be dangerous to health. The therapeutic use of arsenic compounds may be attended by danger whether taken internally or applied in lotions, salves and powders to ulcers, tumors, or even the unbroken skin; toxic symptoms have occasionally resulted from the absorption of the drug. In some instances, arsenic trioxide has been sold for another white powder by mistake. Of the accidental cases listed above, in the Office of the Chief Medical Examiner, four occurred because the victims while intoxicated mixed rat poison in their food and ate it, and in another case a boy of 17 drank part of a bottle of insect poison under the impression that it was wine.

Inorganic arsenic compounds have little action on dead tissue, but they are protoplasmic poisons and when brought into contact with living cells produce degenerative changes. Usually their local irritant action is not pronounced, but after absorption they are carried by the blood to different parts of the body where they attack the tissues vigorously producing their most pronounced effects on the capillaries. The intensity of the toxemia depends on the amount of the drug administered and the rapidity with which it is absorbed. If the poison is in solution it may be absorbed rapidly, but if it is given in solid form the absorption may be slow. It is taken up and retained by the liver and some of the other organs for a number of days, but is continually eliminated through the kidneys and the gastrointestinal tract; in most of the cases that recover, the body is eventually freed of the drug.

Four types of poisoning occur:

1. The acute paralytic form in which the deceased has received a large quantity of inorganic arsenic compounds with rapid absorption into the system, is occasionally encountered. Nine cases of this type were studied of which six followed the ingestion of rat poison; one, the drinking of an insect spray containing arsenic; and two, the ingestion of Paris green. The most striking manifestations are a profound circulatory collapse with low blood pressure, rapid weak pulse, shallow or difficult respirations, a semicomatose or profound stupor, and sometimes convulsions. The patient may or may not show signs of gastrointestinal irritation. Death supervenes in less than 24 hours. The symptoms and signs are due to the depressing effect of a large amount of arsenic compound which overwhelms the central nervous system, especially the medullary centers.

2. The gastrointestinal type is the most common, and the symptoms which are characteristic of it are referable to the lesions in the stomach, intestines and parenchymatous organs. Soon after the ingestion of the arsenic compound, vomiting occurs followed by diarrhea after an hour or two. The prominence of the different clinical signs vary with the individual case. In some a profuse diarrhea is the most prominent symptom; vomiting, burning pain in the abdomen and abdominal cramps appear to be the chief complaints in other patients; a few may suffer from sore throat, urgent thirst and dryness about the mouth; various combinations of all these symptoms may occur. The vomiting may become persistent and distressing, the vomitus may have the appearance of rice water, and on occasion may contain blood-stained mucus and bile. The diarrhea may be profuse and the stools may be blood stained, or like rice water, similar to the ejections in Asiatic cholera. In the more marked cases the patient has a livid and anxious face, a cold clammy skin, cramps in the calves of the legs, delirium, albuminuria, suppression of urine, and dehydration from the loss of fluid from the blood caused by the persistent vomiting and diarrhea. It is significant in these cases that an attack of vomiting can occur after the primary ingested free arsenic in the stomach has been expelled; and this is doubtless referable to the presence of arsenic already absorbed which has been re-excreted back into the stomach. Death occurs in a few hours to several days. If the patient survives the initial attack, he has a chance of recovery.

The lesions found at necropsy are variable in degree. In the deaths which occur in a few hours from circulatory collapse, the mucous membrane of the stomach and intestines may not show any changes worthy of note. The stomach may be practically empty, or contain mucus or varying amounts of reddish or grayish fluid; sometimes in the folds of mucous membrane are octahedral crystals of arsenic trioxide, or flakes of Paris green or a yellowish deposit of arsenic sulfide formed by a chemical combination of arsenic in the poison with hydrogen sulfide generated in the stomach. In other cases the mucous membrane is a pale red, is congested and edematous while dark lines of slight corrosion are present on the top of the rugal crests, forming a barred and gridiron pattern from the local corrosion by the poison; the stomach may contain a dark tenacious mucus stained with blood. The intestines in the early stages may not show any changes worthy of note, though considerable arsenic may be present in the tissues.

The longer the poison acts on the body, the more pronounced are the lesions. The wall of the stomach and intestine may be swollen and show an edema and congestion of the submucous layer, and the color is usually a diffuse cloudy gray red with deeper red submucous hemorrhages of varying size here and there; in one case a grayish-yellow pseudomembrane developed on the mucous membrane of the upper jejunum. Some portions of the intestinal tract may be yellow from the formation of arsenic sulfide. The intestine may contain a large amount of rice-water contents, or they may be empty and contracted except for blood-stained thick mucus. The lesions are variable in distribution; sometimes the stomach and parts of the small intestine alone are inflamed and sometimes the entire gastrointestinal tract is involved. The mouth, pharynx and esophagus occasionally show the same process but less intensely. The skin also may develop blisters in areas where the poison has been applied. Edema of the face and eyelids has been described, occasionally hemorrhagic or purulent.

The gastric and intestinal inflammations occur mostly as a result of the excretion of arsenic through the mucous membrane and of its direct toxic action on the finer blood vessels in the submucosa, and less often from the direct corrosive action of the poison on the lining of the tract. In many cases where inorganic arsenic compounds were merely applied to ulcers or to the intact skin, gastrointestinal signs have followed because of the absorption of the drug, even though it had not been ingested by mouth. Microscopic examination of the lesions involving the stomach and intestines in arsenic poisoning, show the smaller blood vessels of the submucosa containing red blood cells and polymorphonuclear leukocytes while the vascular endothelium is sometimes swollen and enlarged; the extravascular portion of the submucous layer contains edema fluid, and a variable number of polymorphonuclear leukocytes and red blood cells.

If the victim survives a few days, parenchymatous and fatty degenerative changes occur in the cells of the myocardium, liver and kidneys which appear dull and gray-red or gray-yellow in color. In the liver the drug tends to accumulate, the parenchymal cells are swollen and icteric, and the body tissues show a varying degree of hepatogenous jaundice; after the poisoning has become subacute or chronic, an acute yellow atrophy may develop as a complication. Purpuric hemorrhages of different sizes may occur in the subserous or loose areolar tissues such as the mesentery, retroperitoneal tissues, epicardium, preaortic tissues and elsewhere; the subendocardial layer especially of the septal surface of the left ventricle may show discrete, small flame-like hemorrhages or a large broad hemorrhagic effusion (Fig. 31-1). These lesions are referable to fatty or other degenerative changes in the capillary endothelium, and microscopically there may be a slight infiltration of polymorphonuclear leukocytes in and about the hemorrhagic areas. In one case of acute arsenic poisoning, microscopic examination of the right adrenal disclosed a small area of cortical necrosis infiltrated by a sprinkling of leukocytes.

If arsenic is taken in solid form and death occurs in the early stages of the poisoning, most of the drug will be found in the stomach. If the clinical course is protracted, the quantity of arsenic in the stomach is diminished. After absorption, the poison is diffused through the organs, where most of it is stored in the liver, spleen, kidneys and other tissues for a few weeks, and then gradually eliminated in the urine and feces. The liver usually contains more arsenic than the other organs, but the amount is so variable that it is difficult to assign any specific amount in the tissues as a minimal lethal concentration. In 13 cases the amounts of arsenic compounds determined for 1,000 gm. of liver tissue varied from 7.2 mg. to 127 mg. for cases dying in 24 hours, and in cases which lived from 27 hours to 8 days, the amounts for the same bulk of liver tissue varied from 12 mg. to 52 mg. Moreover when different organs from the same case were analysed, the percentage of arsenic present in the separate organs was not the same. The fatal dose of inorganic arsenic compounds is difficult to determine, but most authorities have considered that 3 gm., approximately 200 grains, if absorbed into the system would kill a man of average weight.

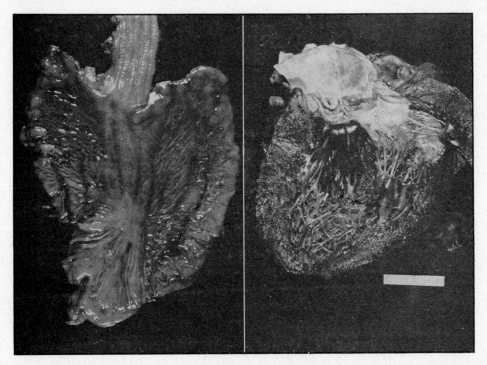

Fig. 31-1. Arsenic Poisoning; Hemorrhagic Gastritis; Subendocardial Hemorrhages on Left Side of Interventricular Septum.

The presence of a large amount of arsenic in a dead body may enable it to resist putrefaction. At one time arsenic compounds were important constituents of many embalming fluids, but at present their employment for this purpose has been prohibited in many states, including New York, on the ground that their presence in an embalmed body would interfere with a toxicologic investigation in a suspicious case.

It is evident from the foregoing that the significance of a minute amount of arsenic in the organs will depend upon the circumstances of the case. Unless the clinical history or the findings at autopsy are strongly suggestive of poisoning by this drug, the presence of a minute amount must be appraised with caution, inasmuch as arsenic compounds may reach the body as a result of medication. In embalmed or exhumed bodies, if the chemical analysis discloses that the poison is present in localized areas, as for example in the stomach and neighboring viscera, but not in other organs such as the liver, kidney and brain, it would not be conclusive that death was caused by arsenic poisoning. On the other hand if appreciable amounts of arsenic are discovered in different tissues and organs in the body, especially in conjunction with typical clinical signs and pathologic lesions, the results would be significant of antemortem absorption and toxic action. In the acute cases, the organs saved for chemical examination are the stomach and its contents, the liver, kidneys, and the brain; in some cases the intestinal contents and the urine may be of value. In autopsies on exhumed bodies buried in earth, samples of soil around the casket and part of the lining of the casket should be removed and tested for the presence of arsenic in order to eliminate possible sources of contamination.

The treatment of acute arsenic poisoning is to empty the stomach by the tube and wash it out with warm water and milk. An emetic of mustard, 1 part; salt, 6 parts; in a large amount of water may be valuable. A specific antidote is prepared by diluting one-half ounce of tincture of ferric chloride with a tumblerful of water, and then adding magnesia to saturation. Castor oil may be given to clear the intestines. The Council on Pharmacy and Chemistry of the American Medical Association recommends the early administration of BAL (British anti-lewisite, 2, 3,—dimercaptopropanol) which contains two unsaturated SH groups; these remove arsenic from the tissues and the resulting compound is excreted rapidly. BAL is administered intramuscularly in a 10 per cent solution of peanut oil every four hours in the proportion of 5 mg. per kilogram of body weight, until the symptoms of the poisoning are sufficiently alleviated.

3. A subacute type of poisoning may develop if the arsenic compounds are administered in small doses repeated at intervals, or it may even follow the administration of a single large dose which does not cause death rapidly but remains in the body, affecting it deleteriously during a slow excretion. The victims linger on from weeks to months: some may develop a toxic degeneration of the liver which progresses to an acute or subacute yellow atrophy accompanied by an intense toxic jaundice; multiple hemorrhages may occur in the subserosal layers or in the loose areolar tissues; the gastrointestinal tract may be chronically inflamed with a persistent diarrhea, cramps and dehydration; the kidneys may show a nephrosis with albuminuria and bloody urine; skin eruptions, eczematous areas, and keratoses appear on the skin in some instances. The patient loses weight, becomes emaciated and quite ill before death supervenes.

4. A chronic type of poisoning may develop in some cases after the acute symptoms subside, and it may display a number of different manifestations. In one form a chronic neuritis may appear with degeneration of the nerve fibers which starts at the periphery and extends toward the center; this lesion is characterized clinically by paralyses of the muscles of the hands and feet, anesthesia, and trophic disturbances such as muscular atrophy and falling out of the hairs and nails. In some cases a chronic gastroenteritis may supervene with anorexia, nausea and diarrhea. Progressive weakness, coryza, marked keratosis of the palms and soles, puffy eyelids, loss of weight, anemia, pallor and general ill health may occur. These syndromes may be evoked by the inhalation of volatile compounds formed by fungi on arsenic-containing wall papers, or by the exposure to vapors in industrial plants, or by the continual ingestion of small amounts in the food, or by the continual absorption through the skin of certain dyes in clothing. The chronic forms of poisoning may not be preceded by acute symptoms and may make their appearance insidiously.

The so-called arsenic eaters in India, Syria and lower Austria have been reported as habitual users of the drug, taking about ½ to 2 grains of arsenic trioxide a week. The popular belief is that endurance is increased by this medication, and, in any event, a large dose is taken without apparent toxic effects. Many have explained this immunity on the theory of increased elimination or decreased absorption. Others declare that toxic effects are produced, on occasion, even in such arsenic habitués.

Toxicologic examination in subacute or chronic cases of poisoning may show that only small amounts of arsenic compounds are present in the body. In appraising the significance of such findings, the duration of the illness and the attending excretion of arsenic during life must be taken into consideration. Rarely the toxicologic examination on the postmortem material may be negative, as in a case of chronic arsenic poisoning complicated by severe jaundice and numerous hemorrhagic lesions, in which arsenic was recovered from the urine during life by toxicologic examination, but at autopsy could not be detected in the organs of the deceased. In long continued cases of arsenic poisoning the metal is stored in the bones, skin and hair, where it is held in an inert form, and some of the hair, skin and bones should be preserved for chemical examination as well as other organs ordinarily set aside for that purpose.

Arsine (hydrogen arsenide, arseniuretted hydrogen, AsH_3) is a colorless gas which has a strong odor of garlic. It is extremely poisonous, and is formed whenever nascent hydrogen is liberated near a trivalent compound of arsenic, as in the Marsh test. Cases of poisoning by arsine occur in chemical laboratories, in industrial plants where ores are smelted, acids are manufactured and hydrogen is generated on a large scale. Numerous ores and chemicals contain arsenic as an impurity, and the processes to which they are subjected occasionally produce arseniuretted hydrogen. Some authorities mention the generation of this gas in submarines from the battery plates as a distinct hazard when this type of vessel was first put into operation.

The symptoms of the poisoning may occur immediately after exposure to the gas or they may not appear until a few hours have elapsed. The victim becomes ill or prostrated and complains of faintness, weakness, giddiness, headache, pain in the abdomen, nausea and vomiting. Arsine may act on the central nervous system and produce a narcosis and paralysis. An important effect of the gas is on the red blood cells, as it causes hemolysis, hemoglobinuria with port-wine colored urine and toxic jaundice, usually appearing about four hours after exposure. The destruction of the erythrocytes may be so intense that a severe anemia results. Death occurs in about 36 per cent of the cases either from cardiac collapse accompanied by edema of the lungs, or in a typhoid-like state with delirium. At autopsy the findings are an intense jaundice of all tissues, degenerative changes in the liver, enlargement of the spleen with deposit of blood pigment in the parenchyma, a toxic nephrosis and edema of the lungs.

The treatment is to remove the victim from the poisonous atmosphere and give oxygen by inhalation. Blood transfusions may be necessary to counteract the anemia. The rest of the treatment is symptomatic. The toxicology of arsine in the body is the same as that of inorganic arsenic inasmuch as the compound is oxidized to arsenic trioxide in the tissues. In acute poisoning the lungs and brain should be saved for analysis.

Chronic arsine poisoning is not a well-defined entity, but some believe that cases do occur when a person is exposed to minute doses, day after day; symptoms of multiple neuritis are said to be caused by this type of exposure.

ORGANIC ARSENIC COMPOUNDS. Therapeutic organic arsenic preparations are numerous, and the vast majority of them are synthetic. They belong to the aliphatic and aromatic groups, and contain either trivalent arsenic or pentavalent arsenic. The organic compounds are not as toxic as the inorganic, probably because they act less immediately on the organism. When taken into the system they are decomposed slowly and ordinarily do not cause serious trouble, but sometimes the disintegration is rapid and severe toxic effects may ensue. Many of the compounds of the trivalent type are used as parasiticides in such protozoan infections as trypanosomiasis and in spirochetal diseases like syphilis, yaws or relapsing fever. These compounds are stored in the different organs, especially the liver, and arsenic is released gradually, so that it acts on the parasites for a longer time than does in-

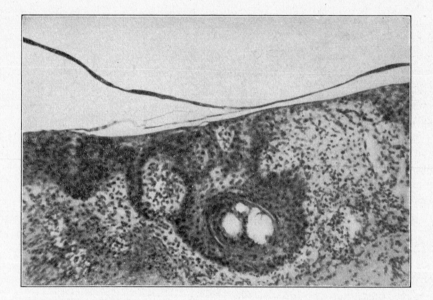

Fig. 31-2. Dermatitis Exfoliativa Following Administration of Arsphenamine.

Low power photomicrograph of skin showing inflammatory reaction in the corium and the desquamation of the epidermis.

organic arsenic. The organic compounds of pentavalent arsenic are not as efficient as the trivalent, and if used as parasiticides must be given in doses which may be dangerous to the patient. In the years from 1918 to 1951 inclusive, there were 230 deaths from the therapeutic administration of organic arsenic compounds recorded in the Office of the Chief Medical Examiner.

The trivalent organic arsenicals of most importance are derivatives of arsphenamine (salvarsan or 606, formula $HCl.NH_2.C_6H_3As:AsC_6H_3.OH.NH_2HCl.2H_2O$), among which are silver arsphenamine, sulfarsphenamine, bismarsen (bismuth arsphenamine sulfonate) and neoarsphenamine (mapharsen, arsenoxide, the basic radical of the arsphenamine group). These compounds are all efficient in the treatment of the spirochetal and protozoan diseases. They are given intravenously in slightly alkaline solution in doses of 0.3 to 0.6 gm., except silver arsphenamine which is given in smaller doses. In recent years a method of intensive treatment has been developed in which massive doses of mapharsen are given intravenously by various methods, such as the slow intravenous drip, the rapid intravenous drip and the multiple syringe injection. The injections of mapharsen are combined on occasion with bismuth compounds or with typhoid vaccine, which appears to improve the results of the treatment.

If the trivalent arsenic compounds are administered with due precautions, they are not harmful ordinarily, but in rare instances a fatality may occur. Occasionally a patient dies with symptoms of a sudden general collapse after a single injection of the drug, the autopsy showing little that is characteristic. In such instances the entire organic radical appears to exert a toxic effect and the reaction is probably an allergic one. In other cases death occurs as a result of chronic poisoning due to the dissociation of arsenic from the organic radical of the arsphenamine preparation in the body, and these effects may take days or weeks to develop. One of the most

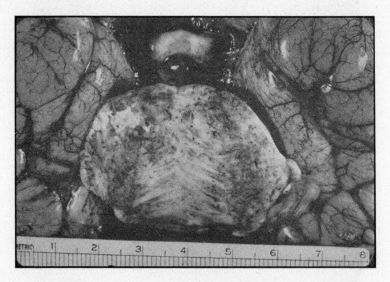

Fig. 31-3. Hemorrhagic Softening of Pons Following Arsphenamine Administration.

striking lesions is a marked dermatitis exfoliativa which may involve the entire body, characterized by desquamation of the epidermis and an infiltration of round cells and leukocytes in the corium (Fig. 31-2). In other cases an arsphenamine encephalorrhagia occurs and the patient dies in a fatal coma, the autopsy showing petechial and geographic hemorrhages distributed diffusely or in a patchy fashion throughout the brain in white matter and in some cases a hemorrhagic softening of the pons occurs (Figs. 31-3 and 31-4). A hemorrhagic diathesis may supervene and small hemorrhages occur in the subserous layers, especially in the mesentery of the small intestine and the heart muscle. Occasionally granulocytopenia, or aplastic anemia, or generalized thromboses may develop. As a late effect severe degenerative processes occur in the parenchymatous organs, and the liver may be involved, finally developing a fatal acute or subacute yellow atrophy with intense jaundice. Some cases which survive the acute effects may show a patchy fibrosis in the liver parenchyma and a chronic hepatitis as a late effect of the degenerative process. If the drug is injected carelessly and is allowed to infiltrate the tissues outside the vein, thromboses may result. Good results have been obtained with BAL in the treatment of some of the complications produced by the organic arsenicals of the salvarsan group, such as dermatoses, exfoliative dermatitis, encephalorrhagia and arsenical jaundice.

The pentavalent organic arsenicals include sodium cacodylate, $(CH_3)_2AsO.ONa$, arrhenal, arsacetin, acetarsone, tryparsamide and others. In poisonous doses they have the effect of causing subacute or chronic poisoning of varying intensity. Tryparsamide, among other effects, may produce an amblyopia.

Antimony. Antimony, Sb, is a grayish white, metallic substance which is used as an alloy in such combinations as bell metal or type metal. It is an industrial

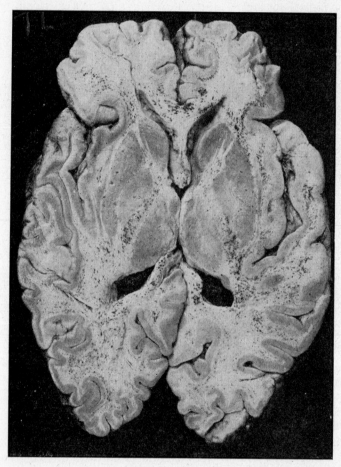

Fig. 31-4. Diffuse Encephalorrhagia Following Therapeutic Administration of Arsphenamine.

hazard in the printing trade, in the rubber industry and in the manufacture of paints containing antimony sulfide. In the metallic form it is tasteless, odorless and non-toxic, and when heat is applied it volatilizes, forming antimony trioxide. The compounds of antimony are toxic and two, the trichloride and tartar emetic, cause the most antimony poisonings. Antimony trichloride occurs as a liquid, composed of the salt dissolved in hydrochloric acid; it is employed externally as a medicinal application, and it is used in the treatment of protozoan diseases such as leishmaniasis, kala-azar and lymphogranuloma inguinale; it is also used in farriery and as a bronzing fluid. Tartar emetic or antimony and potassium tartarate, $K(SbO)-C_4H_4O_6$, is a substance much like cream of tartar in appearance. It is a white crystalline powder with a bitter metallic taste and is present in a number of pharmaceutical preparations, such as wine of antimony, syrupus scillae compositus, mistura glycerrhizae composita and unguentum antimonii. Pentavalent organic compounds of antimony are also used in medicine and are considered to be less toxic.

Poisoning due to antimony compounds is usually accidental, and few cases are suicidal or homicidal. Antimony salts are similar in toxic action to arsenic salts, evoke similar symptoms, and produce similar pathologic lesions after absorption. A single large dose may kill by involvement of the central nervous system without marked gastrointestinal manifestations. In most cases intense gastric and intestinal irritation occurs with epigastric pains, dysphagia, a metallic-like taste in the mouth, vomiting of blood-stained material, tenesmus, watery diarrhea, rapid pulse, profuse sweating, and spasms of the muscles of the arms, legs and fingers. In fatal cases cyanosis, subnormal temperature, delirium and collapse may supervene. The postmortem lesions are those of marked gastrointestinal irritation with reddening and edema of the submucous layer similar to the changes in acute arsenic poisoning. If the trichloride is used, the corrosive action of hydrochloric acid will be added to other noxious effects, and congestion, inflammation and ulceration of the pharynx, stomach and even the intestine may occur.

A chronic poisoning may occur when small doses are given at intervals over a long period of time. In a few cases of homicide in which the victims were invalids, the antimony compound was administered in this manner so that the symptoms of poisoning would simulate the clinical appearance of a natural disease condition. The victims usually complain of anorexia, nausea, vomiting, thirst, diarrhea, muscular cramps and cold sweats. In these cases the internal viscera such as heart, liver and kidneys may show fatty degenerative changes in the parenchymal cells and the nutrition of the body may be poor.

The fatal dose in antimony poisoning varies. In one case, a child died 45 minutes after the administration of ¾ of a grain. In adults, the action is so variable that it is difficult to fix a definite amount as a poisonous lethal dose. Three grains given in doses of 1½ grains caused death after a 24 hour interval but recovery has followed the administration of much larger doses. The drug causes its worst effects after absorption. The clinical course in a fatal case varies from a few hours to a few days.

The treatment is to evacuate the stomach by an emetic, such as mustard and water, or to wash it out with a stomach tube. The best antidote is tannic acid in hot water, which forms the insoluble tannate of antimony with the poison; the stomach should be washed out repeatedly so as to get rid of the poisonous material. The rest of the treatment is symptomatic. The material saved for toxicologic analysis is the same as for arsenic.

Bismuth. The official salts of bismuth, Bi, are the subnitrate, subcarbonate, subgallate and the subsalicylate. The subnitrate and the subcarbonate are heavy insoluble powders, and are often used as sedatives in gastric irritation, and as contrast meals in roentgen-ray photography of the stomach. Poisoning by the ingestion of such compounds is not frequent, as they are insoluble, but rarely they may be absorbed and cause toxic symptoms. Some believe that bismuth subnitrate is reduced to nitrite in the intestine by the action of bacteria, especially in children, and such symptoms as cyanosis, dyspnea and methemoglobinemia are attributable to the toxic action of this radical. Formerly many ill effects following the ingestion of bismuth preparations were blamed on impurities such as arsenic or tellurium compounds.

Many nonofficial organic bismuth preparations such as bismosol, mesurol, oleo-bi-Roche, potassium bismuth tartrate, or bismarsen are used in the treatment of syphilis, and are given by intramuscular injection; they may produce a fatal poisoning. The action may be cumulative and a toxic effect follow repeated small doses.

A number of pastes or salves containing bismuth have been used in suppurating sinuses or granulating wounds. Beck's paste, a bismuth petrolatum paste, is employed in suppurating sinuses and occasionally gives rise to toxic symptoms and death from the absorption of the salt from the raw surface. A preparation known as bipp, composed of bismuth subnitrate, 1 part; iodoform, 2 parts; and liquid paraffin, 1 part was used on suppurative wounds in World War I, with a few cases of bismuth poisoning. A preparation known as analbis, used in the form of a suppository for the treatment of upper respiratory inflammations in infants, has been accompanied in some cases by toxic degeneration of the liver, but whether due to bismuth in the preparation or to another toxic substance is difficult to determine.

The cases of bismuth poisoning are mostly accidental and are comparatively rare. In the Office of the Chief Medical Examiner, 5 accidental cases occurred in the 33-year interval from 1918 to 1951. The victims complain of a sore mouth with a metallic taste, salivation and foul odor to the breath. Vomiting, abdominal pain and diarrhea of a greenish black material, bismuth sulfide, may occur. The gums may show a bluish-black discoloration and some of the teeth are loosened. The urine may contain albumin, black deposits and tubular casts; in a few cases uremia supervenes. The clinical course is chronic; one case is reported to have died in about nine days after taking the drug but many of them live for several weeks. The fatal dose of bismuth is variable as a large portion of the poison is not absorbed but passes out through the intestine. In long continued treatment with bismuth compounds in luetic cases, jaundice and toxic hepatitis have resulted similar to the lesions described under arsenic poisoning.

Postmortem examination discloses spongy, hemorrhagic gums and loose teeth. Brown or sticky white membranous patches may line the mouth and throat. The mucous membrane of the small and large intestines may be covered by a gray or black false membrane, accompanied by ulceration and even perforation of the intestinal wall. The liver and kidneys may show parenchymatous or fatty degeneration, and microscopic, amorphous, basophilic deposits may occur in the epithelium of the convoluted tubules similar to those found in mercury poisoning. Some of the viscera, such as spleen, kidneys and mucous membrane of the large intestine, may contain hemosiderin deposits.

One case was seen by the authors among the routine autopsies in the Office of the Chief Medical Examiner in which a white girl, 19 years old, had taken for a stomach ailment some medicine which had been kept in her medicine closet for several years; vomiting and diarrhea developed, finally resulting in death after seven days. The autopsy disclosed a dull cloudy-red, edematous inflammation in the submucous layer of the stomach and intestines, parenchymatous degeneration in the liver and kidneys, and subendocardial hemorrhages in the septal part of the left ventricle. Microscopic section of the organs showed lesions similar to those found in cases of arsenic poisoning. The chemical examination of the viscera disclosed the presence of bismuth, and all other poisons including arsenic were absent. The bacteriologic examination was negative. In another case a baby of seven months developed vomiting and diarrhea five days prior to death, and at autopsy showed a fatty degeneration of the liver, marked parenchymatous degeneration in the kidney tubules, but no gastrointestinal lesions. Bismuth was recovered in large quantity by toxicologic examination, but no history could be obtained as to how the poisoning occurred.

The curative treatment is the same as that described under arsenic. If a bismuth salt is given by mouth, the best prophylaxis is to avoid administering it in acid solution. The poison is excreted through the gastrointestinal tract, urine and saliva. The material saved for toxicologic examination is the same as in the case of arsenic.

Mercury. Mercury, Hg, is a heavy, liquid metal with a silvery luster, which is quite volatile when heated. Metallic mercury is present in such medicinal preparations as hydrargyrum cum creta, blue mass and blue ointment. The metal itself is not poisonous, but it tends to form toxic compounds in the body, especially if it is retained in the system for any length of time. Cases have been described in which mercury, given as a cathartic, caused mild toxic symptoms because some of it remained in the body for a number of days after ingestion. Slight poisonous symptoms have followed the embedding of mercury globules in the finger by a wound from a thermometer. Umber, however, has reported a case of attempted suicide where an individual injected 2 ml. of mercury in the arm vein and caused the formation of metallic emboli in the right heart and lungs; the mercury in the pulmonary vessels was demonstrable for a long time by roentgen ray, but disappeared finally without any symptoms of poisoning. If inhaled in the form of vapor, the metal may be transformed into actively toxic compounds and cause symptoms of poisoning.

The inorganic compounds of mercury are either mercuric in type, usually soluble and actively toxic, or they are mercurous, insoluble and much less toxic. Official mercuric salts are mercuric chloride (corrosive sublimate), mercurammonium chloride, red mercuric iodide, yellow mercuric oxide and mercuric salicylate. Mercuric cyanide is another poisonous mercuric compound. The mercurous compounds are mercurous chloride (calomel), yellow mercurous oxide and the black oxide. Calomel, for example, is a white insoluble powder used as a cathartic; ordinarily it is harmless but under some conditions it may be changed in the body to mercuric chloride and cause poisoning when taken by mouth. Practically all of the official salts have caused fatal cases of poisoning.

A number of organic mercury preparations are in use at the present time as germicides, as diuretics and as agents against syphilis. These preparations include mercuric benzoate, mercuric oxycyanide, mercurochrome 220, salygran, mercurol, novasurol, mercupurin, merbaphin, esidrone, neptal and others. If they are given without proper precaution, death from poisoning may result. St. George has described five fatalities which followed the intravenous use of mercurochrome; they showed a marked nephrosis and colitis at necropsy. Mercupurin and salygran have been given intravenously as diuretics in heart disease and ordinarily are safe and efficient in their action. In a few cases death has occurred immediately after the injection with symptoms of orthopnea, dyspnea, sweating, pallor, bradycardia and syncope, and has been ascribed to an allergic susceptibility on the part of the victim to the entire chemical formula of the drug and not to any specific toxicity on the part of the mercury component. Some organic mercury compounds like merthiolate (sodium ethyl mercuric thiosalicylate) and merphenyl borate have been used as preservatives of blood plasma intended for transfusion and signs of mercury poisoning have followed the repeated injections of such plasma in individual cases. The authors have seen cases of this type in which the lesions in the colon and kidneys showed varying degrees of severity.

Mercuric chloride ($HgCl_2$), corrosive sublimate, is the compound of mercury which causes the most cases of poisoning. It is a crystalline solid which sublimes at 180° F., and is deposited in octahedral crystals. It is quite soluble, has a bitter taste, coagulates protein, and forms a precipitate with albumin. It is sold in tablet form for use as an antiseptic or disinfectant. Accidental cases of mercury bichloride poisoning occur when a tablet has been taken in mistake for some other drug. Rarely poisoning has resulted because an alcoholic solution of corrosive sublimate has been applied to the scalp to combat ring worm, or because the watery solution of the salt has been used to irrigate the field of a surgical operation. The ingestion of mercuric chloride is a fairly common method of suicide, though it is not used for this purpose at present as often as in the past. In several instances, fatal poisoning has followed the injection of a solution of mercury bichloride into the vagina to prevent conception or to cause abortion. Homicidal cases are rare. In the records of the Office of the Chief Medical Examiner of New York City, suicidal deaths due to mercuric chloride occurred at an average yearly rate of over 12 cases, and accidental and undetermined deaths at an average yearly rate of over 6 cases; poisoning from organic mercury compounds was rare.

The ingestion of mercuric chloride is followed in a few minutes to half an hour by symptoms of an acute gastrointestinal inflammation. The victim complains of an acrid, metallic taste in the mouth, thirst, retching, and soreness in the pharynx and abdomen. The most prominent symptom in the early stages is nausea, followed by vomiting of blood stained material and accompanied by severe abdominal pain. Later he complains of tenesmus and develops a bloody diarrhea, accompanied by continuous or intermittent suppression of urine, uremia and collapse. Death may occur inside of an hour or the patient may die of toxemia in from two to three weeks. The lethal dose is difficult to estimate because much of the material is vomited, but 3 grains have caused death.

At autopsy the mucous membrane of the mouth, pharynx and esophagus may show various degrees of corrosion, manifested in places by congestion and raw surfaces. A silvery gray, necrotic slough may cover the lining membrane of the stomach interspersed with areas of erosion; the stomach may be contracted and rugous, showing inflammation on the top of the rugae. If the bichloride is swallowed as a solid tablet, the corrosion may be localized in the fundus or some other part of the stomach; if the patient lives a few days the eroded area may take on a yellowish green color from the regurgitation of bile into the stomach. On the other hand if the poison is swallowed in a strong solution, the entire stomach is usually evenly involved. In the vaginal tract, a solution of bichloride produces a grayish pseudomembrane. In some cases of acute poisoning the mouth and teeth show a gingivitis and stomatitis of severe grade, usually associated with bluish discoloration of the gums, similar to, but not as intense as, the lesion described under bismuth.

After the poison is absorbed, whether the mode of administration is by mouth, vagina, unbroken skin, wound application, inhalation of vapor, hypodermic or intravenous injection, the principal effects are apt to occur at the points of excretion, the colon and kidneys. The colon shows inflammatory lesions, varying from superficial reddening of the mucous membrane to a thickened and swollen intestinal wall, lined by a gangrenous greenish-black and yellowish-gray pseudomembrane and occasionally associated with extensive ulcerations. The involvement of the mucous membrane may be patchy or continuous over a wide area. A small portion of the lower small intestine may be involved. In one instance, seen by the authors, the colon and lower small intestine were attacked rather intensely, but the appendix was not inflamed. Microscopic examination of the wall of the large intestine shows that the smaller blood vessels in the submucous layer have swollen intimal cells and contain numerous polymorphonuclear leukocytes, while the surrounding tissue is edematous and is infiltrated with leukocytes, and the surface tissue shows a varying amount of necrosis and leukocytic infiltration. Sollman attributes the lesions in the intestines to the formation of mercuric sulfide in the submucous layer and this acts as an irritant causing an inflammatory reaction.

The kidneys usually are swollen and have a characteristic appearance—a pale grayish-yellow thickened cortex with the markings obscured, which stands out in contrast to the dark purplish congested pyramids. In cases which die in from 24 to 48 hours, the cortical tubules are lined by swollen, necrotic cells which take the eosin stain intensely. In cases which live longer, the tubular cells are in part destroyed, and the tubules are filled with lumpy, eosinophilic albuminous material and a few polymorphonuclear leukocytes which may block the lumen; this lesion may be a cause of the suppression of urine already noted but it is only one among many theories advanced to explain this phenomenon. The epithelium may contain deposits shaped like microscopic coal cinders, known as chalk bodies, which stain a dark blue with hematoxylin; this lesion is not pathognomonic of mercury bichloride poisoning as was once supposed, for it is found, also, in cases of bismuth poisoning and of nephrotic calcinosis from other causes. In cases that recover, the tubular epithelium shows regeneration. The glomeruli and the interstitial tissue of the kidney are not affected as a rule by the poisonous action of corrosive sublimate.

The lesions in some cases of mercury poisoning may vary slightly from the above description. In one instance the deceased, a 34 year old Negro woman, was admitted to a hospital complaining of pain in the abdomen, rectal bleeding and vomiting of bloody fluid. She died two days later with signs of congestive heart failure. The autopsy disclosed an enlarged heart of the hypertensive type, a liver which was jaundiced and showed nutmeg markings, kidneys with swollen yellowish gray cortex and purplish pyramids, subendocardial hemorrhages on the left ventricle and a swollen edematous inflammation of the stomach and small intestines, or in other words lesions like acute arsenic poisoning. Microscopic examination showed a perilobular fatty degeneration of the liver and a fatty degeneration in the tubules of the cortical portion of the kidney, and an inflammation in the submucous layer of the small intestine. The only poison isolated toxicologically was mercury in large amounts. The nature of the mercury compound administered and the circumstances of the administration were not determined. In other cases, lesions similar to a lower nephron nephrosis were encountered.

The treatment of acute corrosive sublimate poisoning is to give albumin, such as the white of egg promptly and to wash out the stomach as soon as possible to prevent reabsorption of the mercury. Lavage of the stomach with a 5 to 10 per cent solution of sodium formaldehyde sulfoxylate is a good treatment as it forms an insoluble mercurous compound with corrosive sublimate; the stomach should be washed out promptly and milk and eggs administered. The rest of the treatment is symptomatic, and is designed to relieve the strain on the kidneys without overtaxing the circulation. Decapsulation of the kidneys has been resorted to in some instances, because of the swelling of these organs. The preparation BAL may be used for mercury poisoning, but is considered by the Council on Pharmacy and Chemistry not to be as efficient as in arsenic poisoning (page 742). Longcope and Luetscher recommend the use of BAL, giving an intramuscular injection of this substance—

300 gm. in peanut oil—and then following it in 1 to 2 hours by an injection of 150 gm. After 4 to 6 hours a second injection of 150 gm. is given, and before 12 hours have elapsed a third injection of 150 gm. is administered. By this method, Longcope reports that the mortality rate was materially reduced.

The best materials to save for chemical examination are kidneys, liver, stomach contents, feces and urine. The interpretation of the result depends on the amount of mercury present, and on the medication given to the patient prior to death. If the deceased had been receiving calomel or a mercurial diuretic just before he died, a small amount of mercury in his viscera would not be significant. Only an appreciable amount of the metal, combined with postmortem signs of poisoning would indicate a definite toxic reaction.

Workers who are exposed to the vapor of mercury, such as miners, mirror makers, thermometer makers, furriers and hatters, continually absorb the metal into their systems, and develop a chronic poisoning. The usual symptoms are anorexia, loss of weight, anemia, diarrhea, cerebral excitability, undue apprehension and timidity, fine tremors of face and extremities, insomnia and muscular weakness. The most characteristic sign is stomatitis, accompanied by tender gums, salivation, swollen tongue, fetid breath, ulcers in the mouth, and the development of a blue line in the gums near the teeth. The jaw bone may become necrotic from this process and undergo a spontaneous fracture. A peripheral neuritis may develop and palsies occur, but the muscles do not atrophy as a rule; the myelin sheath may degenerate but the axis cylinder is usually preserved.

Lead. Lead, Pb, is a flexible, heavy, steel-gray metal which is present in a number of alloys. Its salts are used for various purposes—in ointments (lead acetate and lead carbonate), with opium in external applications (lead acetate), and in some fabrics (lead sulfate). All forms of lead are dangerous if taken internally, even the metal itself. The basic carbonate, and especially the suboxide, Pb_2O, are extremely toxic. Litharge, PbO, and red lead, Pb_3O_4, have caused cases of poisoning. Lead sulfate, chromate and sulfide (galena) are insoluble in water and are consequently less toxic, but they are always potentially dangerous because of their solubility in gastric juice. The acetate, chloride and nitrate are soluble and more rapidly toxic. The types of lead poisoning are the acute and chronic.

ACUTE POISONING. Most cases of acute poisoning are suicidal and accidental, and only a few are homicidal; poisoning may occur following the use of lead compounds as abortifacients. Acute cases result from the ingestion of a large amount of a soluble salt like the acetate or nitrate, or by the intake of many small doses at intervals. The action of the drug is cumulative, and a sudden acute attack may occur after a long period of administration; the continued intake of small doses may abruptly give rise to a type of poisoning, similar to that which follows the ingestion of a large amount.

Symptoms may appear rapidly in acute cases. In some instances the lead salt is changed to lead chloride by the gastric juice and when it comes in contact with the fatty acids and bile in the jejunum, a compound is formed which is absorbed readily into the system. The victims complain of a metallic astringent taste in the mouth, a dry or burning sensation in the throat, cramps, retching and persistent vomiting. In some cases the mucous membrane of the gastrointestinal tract is covered with a firm crust as a result of the direct coagulant action of the lead salt, absorption is hindered and diarrhea may occur. The ejecta from the colon are bloody, or they are black from the presence of lead sulfide. Constipation is not a usual symptom in this type of case. The urine may be scant, the breath is fetid and the skin is dry. Cramps in the legs, numbness and local palsies may appear. The fatal dose is not known positively and is hard to estimate; a soluble salt like the acetate may be lethal in amounts over 10 gm., but cases of recovery have occurred when the dose was about 30 gm.

The patients may die on the second or third day from collapse, or they may live a little longer, and develop a few signs of the chronic type of poisoning. A blue lead line may appear on the gums; an anemia may occur with basophilic stippling of the erythrocytes; signs of a lead encephalopathy may appear with headache, delirium, maniacal excitement, epileptiform convulsions, blindness, paralyses, coma and sometimes collapse. At autopsy, a moderate gastritis and enteritis of the hemorrhagic type may be seen, sometimes covered by a black or gray crust and the intestines may be black from the formation of lead sulfide. Whitish gray or black erosions may be present in the mouth.

Lead is excreted in the urine and feces, and may be detected in those excretions by chemical examination. This fact has an important bearing on the treatment, inasmuch as the principal objective is to get rid of the poison before it is absorbed, and also to remove lead that is excreted into the gastrointestinal tract so that it will not be reabsorbed. The stomach should be washed out with the tube and magnesium sulfate should be given in order to form insoluble lead sulfate and also to clear the intestine. The rest of the treatment is symptomatic.

CHRONIC POISONING. The vast majority of the cases of lead poisoning are chronic, and are accidentally incurred, most frequently from exposure to lead compounds in industry. Workers around smelters or molten solder may inhale volatilized lead oxide (Pb_2O) which forms on the surface of the molten metal. Painters may develop plumbism from inadvertent ingestion of lead paint. Industrial lead poisoning is further described on page 892. In many cases lead compounds are derived from unsuspected sources and cause poisoning by being taken into the body continually in small amounts. For example, lead pipes are sometimes used to convey water in rural communities, and if the water is soft, soluble lead salts may be formed; people who use such water may develop symptoms of poisoning. Lead salts present in external applications, hair washes and dyes, or in food or drink may be a source of danger. Children may become poisoned by mouthing objects or surfaces covered with lead paint. Some individuals are said to have developed chronic lead poisoning from lead bullets which were embedded in the body. In the records of the Office of the Chief Medical Examiner, cases of chronic lead poisoning vary from year to year from 14 cases to none, but the average yearly rate for the period from 1918 to 1941 was about 4 cases.

Lead after absorption is carried in the blood to different organs where it produces the multiform symptoms and signs of chronic lead poisoning such as anorexia, loss of weight, weakness, abdominal colic, constipation, icterus and secondary anemia marked by pallor. Backache, arthralgia, gouty joint lesions, headache, hypertension, chest pains, a lead line on the gums, a metallic taste in the mouth, and numerous neurogenic phenomena also occur. These symptoms may be present in the individual case in different combinations, so that the clinical picture may be quite variable; some attribute many of these manifestations to spasm of the smaller blood vessels produced by lead compounds in the various organs (Petri). In most cases the greater proportion of lead absorbed into the system is stored in the bones where it is harmless as long as it remains in combination with the osseous tissue. In children absorbed lead is deposited in quantity near the epiphysial ends of the bones and may be demonstrated by the roentgen ray as a dark zone adjacent to the cartilage.

Secondary anemia, sometimes the most striking evidence of lead poisoning, is due to destruction of the red blood cells in the peripheral circulation. The victim shows a noticeable pasty pallor which, however, is not a true indication of the degree of anemia; generally the bone marrow is stimulated to produce more blood cells which rapidly replace those destroyed, and presents the picture of a moderate hyperplasia. The absorbed lead compounds combine with phosphates on the surface of the erythrocytes to form insoluble lead phosphate, the red blood cells become abnormally brittle and are demolished by trauma inflicted on them as they circulate through the blood vessels. During the absorption of the lead, dark blue granules appear in some of the erythrocytes and produce the spotted appearance known as stippling, a phenomenon believed to be the result of the degeneration of young reticulated erythrocytes. These stippled cells are considered diagnostic for though they may be found rarely in other conditions, they appear in the blood of those suffering from lead poisoning in large numbers, about 100 to every million of red blood cells.

A black lead line on the gums is a fairly reliable diagnostic sign, and is produced by the deposit of black lead sulfide in minute granules around the finer blood vessels at the tips of the gum papillae. This granular appearance is most obvious near the margin of the gums and can be demonstrated most clearly with a magnifying glass. In rare instances such granules may be deposited around the capillary vessels of the hair bulbs and other structures.

Abdominal colic may be an early sign of lead poisoning, and may appear when the victim has been exposed to a small quantity of lead. The pain of the colic is intense and often prolonged, and may be located about the mid-abdomen; it appears to be due to tonic spasm of the intestinal muscles.

Muscular paralysis of the extensor muscles of the forearm, especially the right, may develop rapidly and painlessly, and a definite wrist drop may appear. It is more likely to involve the right hand because it is used the more, but in some cases the paralysis may be bilateral. Occasionally there may be paralyses of the peroneal muscles with a foot drop. The opposing groups of muscles on both forearms and legs are not affected. The paralyzed muscles may atrophy and show considerable fatty infiltration. Degenerative lesions may occur in the anterior horn cells and the nerve fibers. In rare cases an optic neuritis and optic atrophy are noted as a result of chronic lead poisoning.

Lead has a particular affinity for the central nervous system and forms a fairly stable combination with nervous tissue. Various areas of the brain and cord may be affected. There may not be any gross changes, though neurologic and metal symptoms such as epileptiform convulsions, paralyses, headache, delirium, or melancholic mania manifest themselves. In other cases, general cerebral atrophy, or definite areas of softening and sclerosis of the brain and cord may occur, demonstrable by neuropathologic technic; the lesions are sometimes scattered resembling those of multiple sclerosis, or they may be spinal in distribution. Microscopically ganglion cell degenerations, microglial infiltrations around the smaller blood vessels in the white matter, perivascular regressive changes, and small perivascular hemorrhages have been described.

Chronic lead poisoning is thought to be an etiologic factor in the production of severe and precocious arteriosclerosis (especially in the brain arteries), arterial hypertension, cardiac hypertrophy and nephrosclerosis. According to some (Petri), the narrowing of the peripheral arterioles due to vascular spasm is the underlying cause of these changes. The evidence is not conclusive and others believe that the above conditions are not any more prevalent in persons exposed to lead than in other persons, although the cases reported by Nye seem to support the theory that the two conditions are related. Microscopically the kidneys show focal areas of round cell infiltration, interstitial hemorrhages, tubular degeneration, occasional fibrosis and indefinite glomerular changes. There is no evidence that chronic lead poisoning ever gives rise to a diffuse toxic glomerular nephritis. Some have attributed chronic gastric ulcer and chronic interstitial hepatitis to the chronic action of lead but the support for this theory is not convincing.

Lead compounds, like the other members of the heavy metal group, are protoplasmic poisons and damage various tissues of the body to a greater or lesser degree. They are toxic to the germ cells and chorionic epithelium, causing death of the fetus in the uterus, hence their occasional use as abortifacients. Degeneration of the male gonads has been described in some cases of lead poisoning. The poison is eliminated by the intestines, the urine and the bile. The intestinal excretion of lead exceeds the renal, even when the lead has entered by some other portal than the mouth.

Tetraethyl lead, a compound used in motor fuel, is poisonous if the fumes are inhaled in sufficient amount. In four cases described by Norris and Gettler, there were mental symptoms accompanied by delirium and convulsions, a hemorrhagic pneumonia of the influenzal type, jaundice, hemorrhages in the bone marrow, and red cell thrombi in the blood vessels of the brain. The fatal cases lived only a few days after the poisoning.

The best way to combat chronic lead poisoning is by prophylaxis. The principal ways of entrance of lead into the body are by inhalation and ingestion, so that workers in industrial plants should be guarded against the source of the poisoning, such as fumes and dust, by proper ventilation, by personal cleanliness and by the periodic use of magnesium sulfate as a cathartic. After the lead has been absorbed and is circulating in the system, the treatment of the attending physician should be directed toward storage of the compound in the bones where it will not do much damage. Accordingly the patient is fed a high calcium diet, milk, viosterol and calcium lactate. After the lead is stored in the bones, the symptoms of poisoning may subside and the metal is excreted slowly from the body. Any condition which provokes an acidosis in the body may liberate a large amount of lead from the bony depots and may cause a return of the acute symptoms. It is best to allow the excreting process to occur naturally rather than to stimulate it by the administration of acid substances like ammonium chloride or phosphoric acid. The constipation should be treated with magnesium sulfate, which is valuable in removing excreted lead from the intestines.

On the theory that lead stored in the bones is a potential menace to the victim, Belknap recommends a different type of treatment. He waits until the patient has been free of symptoms for a month. If the hemoglobin is 80 per cent or more, the red blood cell count 4 million or more, the counts of 50 fields yield less than 10 stippled cells, and a 24 hour specimen of urine gives less than 0.15 mg. of lead, he administers 15 drops of a saturated solution of potassium iodide twice daily to remove the storage lead from the body.

The lead is stored in various organs, chiefly the bones, liver, kidneys, brain and muscles, in decreasing order. For toxicologic purposes the organs, excretions and tissues most used in cases of suspected lead poisoning are stomach contents, feces, urine, liver, kidneys, bones and brain. The storage in the body depends to a great extent, on the route of absorption of the poison. If it is taken in by the gastrointestinal tract, more of the lead will be found in the liver than if the toxic compound is inhaled. The presence of lead in the bones in association with minute amounts in parenchymatous organs like the liver and kidneys, indicates that the individual has been exposed to the metal and has absorbed some of it, but does not necessarily indicate poisoning. On the other hand, fatal cases of lead intoxication generally reveal significant amounts of the metal in the parenchymatous organs. The toxicologic examination in seven cases of undoubted lead poisoning showed from 1 to 5 mg. of lead in 100 gm. of liver tissue, the amounts varying with the peculiarities of each individual case.

Thallium. Thallium, Tl, is a heavy metallic substance whose compounds are found in zinc salts and in the dust obtained by heating iron pyrites or raw sulfur. Thallium salts are used in the various industries and in vermin poisons as, for example, the sulfate which is a constituent of zelio paste. Thallium acetate was formerly given internally in medicine, and is used in salve form to treat fungus infections which involve the skin. It is a constituent of depilatory creams such as Koremlu cream.

Thallium poisoning occurs from the internal administration of the salts, either for suicidal or homicidal purposes, or as a result of accident as when a vermin poison has been ingested by mistake. In some cases symptoms have followed the external application of salves and creams containing thallium salts to the skin. Poisoning due to thallium has been described in workers who manufacture dyes or window glass.

There are a few cases of acute thallium poisoning from the ingestion of large quantities of the salts. Symptoms may develop in 12 to 24 hours, with metallic taste in the mouth, stomatitis, nausea, vomiting, diarrhea, abdominal colic and salivation. The cheeks and lips may be swollen and reddened from vasomotor disturbances, and edema and swelling of the eyelids may appear. Death may occur in a few days from the paralyzing effects on the central nervous system, with delirium, convulsions and death from respiratory failure. At necropsy, a stomatitis, gastritis and enteritis of moderately severe grade are present with swelling, reddening and blackened areas of thallium sulfide on the mucous membrane in some cases. The symptoms and signs are not unlike those caused by arsenic or mercury compounds.

If the poison is absorbed in repeated small doses over a long period of time, a sudden cumulative effect may occur, inasmuch as thallium is stored in the body, and released to act on the system in a manner similar to lead. The thallium salts are stored in the bones, muscles and in the central nervous system.

Chronic poisoning may occur as a result of repeated small doses, or it may be produced when a single large dose is stored up in the system and is released gradually into the circulation for excretion. The signs and symptoms of its toxic action are variable and depend to a certain extent on its action on the tissues where it is stored and on the sites of excretion. In some cases, nutritional disturbances with emaciation, fatigue, stomatitis, gingivitis, severe gastritis, enteritis, anorexia, vomiting and diarrhea are predominant; later parenchymatous and fatty degeneration of the liver and kidney follow and considerable albumin may appear in the urine. In other cases neurologic signs supervene such as trembling, incoordination, swelling of the legs, a multiple polyneuritis with motor and sensory disturbances of the legs, disturbances of vision associated with optic atrophy and turbidity of the lens, and symptoms resembling mild encephalitis and encephalomyelitis. The most suggestive symptoms and signs of chronic thallium poisoning are trophic changes in the finger nails, dermatoses, dermatitis and a falling out of hair amounting to alopecia, the hair follicles in these cases not showing any changes on microscopic examination. In animal experiments the continued administration of thallium salts may cause an osteomalacia, thickening of the endosteum, and a fibrous tissue growth in the bone marrow from which may ensue a secondary anemia with a relative increase in the lymphocytes, eosinophils and occasionally in the basophils.

The properties of thallium salts are like those of lead salts, and similarly are eliminated by the intestines and kidneys; the therapeutic methods used in lead poisoning may be applied in thallium poisoning. The clinical course is variable, lasting from a few days to several weeks. The fatal dose of thallium salts is estimated at 0.2 to 0.5 gm. The tissues to preserve for toxicologic examination are muscle, especially from lower extremities, brain, bone, liver and kidneys. The chemical detection is sometimes difficult as the chemical properties of the salts resemble those of lead. Spectrographic examination reveals a characteristic absorption spectrum by means of which the element may be identified.

Radioactive Compounds. Our present day conceptions regard the atom as a miniature solar system composed of a central nucleus with a positive electric charge, analogous to the sun, and a surrounding zone of moving negatively charged particles, or electrons, which rotate around the nucleus like planets. In the atoms of most elements, the central nucleus is stable and retains its structure regardless of the various chemical combinations which might involve that atom. In a few elements of high atomic weight, however, the nucleus is unstable, and the element is being slowly and continually transformed into energy by the emanations of small electrically charged particles from its structure. Such elements have been called the radioactive elements, and several of them, uranium, radium, thorium, polonium and actinium occur in nature.

Radium and Allied Substances. Radium and some of the other radioactive elements are found in nature in small quantities, radium occurring in a mineral known as pitchblende which is mined in Bohemia, southern Saxony, Colorado, Cornwall and the Belgian Congo. Radium is costly because of its rarity and the difficulty of its extraction. The demand for it exceeds the present supply.

The emanations given off by radium and similar substances are of three types: (1) Alpha particles which are high speed ionized atomic nuclei of the same size as the helium atom and are positively charged. These emanations form about 80 per cent of the total energy and are especially powerful, having the power to decompose organic and inorganic compounds. (2) The beta particles which are high speed electrons. (3) The gamma rays which are true electromagnetic radiations with a short wave length and a penetrating power similar to roentgen rays. The gamma rays are more penetrating than the alpha emanations but are not as powerful. The beta emanations are not as powerful as the alpha.

The disruptive action of the emanations has made radium and some of the other radioactive metals valuable therapeutically, as their radiations are destructive for certain types of neoplasms, but have little potency against other types. Some of their side effects are far from beneficial as the radiation may destroy normal tissue and produce untoward complications.

The therapeutic use of radium may cause lesions from the external or local application of a radium tube through the emanations of gamma rays. These have the power to inflict burns on the skin, which resemble those produced by the roentgen ray, in that they are deep and slow to heal. Even on external application, the emanations may act on the blood-forming organs and give rise to an anemia of

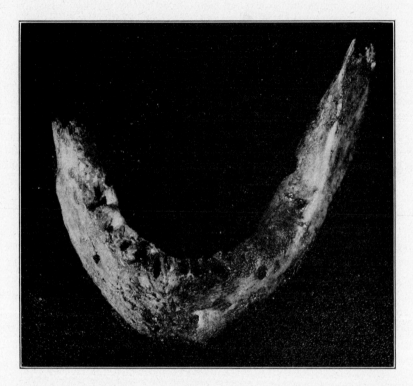

Fig. 31-5. Necrosis and Sequestration of Mandible from Excessive Therapeutic Application of a Radium Pack.

The deceased was a middle-aged white man who was treated with radium for a carcinoma of the tongue.

the aplastic type, or they penetrate and cause sterility by action on the germinal cells of the testes or ovary. In a case autopsied by the authors, a necrosis and sequestration of the mandible was found which followed the excessive application of a radium pack used in the treatment of a carcinoma of the tongue (Fig. 31-5). In another case a tube of radium was swallowed accidentally during its application to an ulcerative basal cell carcinoma of the face, resulting in burning of the cecum, perforation of the wall and a fatal suppurative peritonitis.

Radioactive substances may be taken internally, and cause a chronic poisoning which has peculiar features of its own. This occurs in three ways: (1) Through the inhalation of radium dust in operations requiring the tubing and retubing of partially aged radium, or in the handling of luminous paint. (2) Intravenous injection of soluble chlorides and bromides of radium, mesothorium, or radiothorium for therapeutic purposes. These two means of entrance into the system are not important. (3) The most common method of poisoning is caused by the ingestion of radioactive material.

Radioactive salts have in a few instances been ingested during the performance of industrial processes. The cases described by Martland, Conlon and Knef occurred in women who painted watch dials with a luminous mixture consisting of eight parts zinc pyrosulfide and one part of radioactive substances such as meso-thorium or radiothorium. The paint was applied with a brush which the operators often brought to a point by wetting with their lips, and in this way, a large amount accumulated in the system as a result of the continual ingestion of minute quantities over a long period of time. After absorption the radioactive substances are taken up by the wandering histiocytes and carried to the principal organs of the reticulo-endothelial system, namely, the bones, bone marrow, spleen and liver. There they are deposited and retained, continuously emitting alpha particles during their process of spontaneous disintegration which continues almost endlessly. The incessant bombardment of the surrounding tissues by the alpha particles and the lesions which result, are the basic factors in the pathogenesis of poisoning by radioactive material.

The emanations act on the blood-forming organs, first causing a stimulation, so that the patient enjoys a period of good health. Later degenerative processes occur, the blood forming organs are exhausted, and an anemia sets in, with decrease in the number of red blood cells and leukocytes, loss of weight, low blood pressure, bone pain and signs of neuritis. In the course of a few years, as the radioactive accumulations injure the bone marrow, a chronic pernicious anemia develops. In one typical case the blood examination was as follows: Hemoglobin, 33 per cent; red blood cells, 1,400,000; white blood cells, 400; polymorphonuclear leukocytes, 40; lymphocytes, 58; histiocytes, 2. A large-celled anisocytosis, and a few nucleated red blood cells were present, but only slight polychromatophilia and granular baso-philia were found. The jaw bone may become necrotic and an infection may occur around the teeth, so that an osteomyelitis develops and the victim dies as the result of a terminal sepsis. In some cases the bombardment of the alpha particles may produce a radiation osteitis in the cortex of the bone with thickening of the periosteum and bone and osteosclerosis, a condition most marked in bones subject to stress such as the head of the femur, acetabulum, spine, pelvis and tarsal scaphoid. In some instances, multiple anaplastic sarcomas of the oat cell or round cell type develop as primary growths in the different bones and in the liver, probably a direct effect of the bombardment by the radioactive particles. The cause of death in the chronic poisoning is the result of the severe anemia, or the neoplastic growth or an inter-current septic condition.

The best method of combating this condition is to prevent access of radioactive material to the system. Eradication of radium dust and insistence that care be used in handling the material are essential. The salts of radioactive substances should not be introduced into the mouth as in the cases described by Martland and his col-laborators. After the substances have entered the system, they will be deposited and cause harm, and once deposited in bone, the element cannot be dislodged or removed and will eventually cause the death of the victim.

Some cases have occurred as the result of the ingestion of water containing radio-active substances, which at one time was sold as an agent of therapeutic value. The case described by Gettler and Norris was that of a 52 year old man who had been drinking a water of this type continuously for five years, finally developing a necrosis

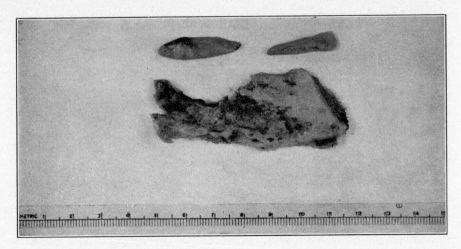

Fig. 31-6. Necrosis and Sequestration of the Mandible Following Prolonged Ingestion of Water Containing Radioactive Substances.

A piece of the mandible and two teeth are shown. The water was taken continuously for five years for its supposed tonic and rejuvenating qualities.

with sequestration of the mandible, progressive anemia and emaciation. At necropsy, a necrosis of the jaw bones with osteomyelitis, a brain abscess of the right temporal lobe, and a marked parenchymatous degeneration of the kidney cortex were described (Fig. 31-6). A few other cases of this type have occurred and have presented a similar clinical and pathologic picture (Figs. 31-7 & 31-8).

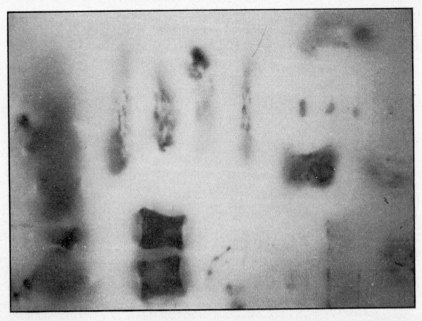

Fig. 31-7. Autoradiogram Prepared from Bones of Fatal Case of Radium Poisoning Following Ingestion of Radium-Containing Water Prescribed as a Tonic.

Death 13 years after administration from radiation osteitis and necrosis of mandible and bronchopneumonia.

Radium and its allied substances may be detected in the living and dead body by the electroscope. In making the test the time of the normal leak of the electroscope is determined, that is, the time it takes the gold foil to descend after an electric charge has blown it outward. If the apparatus is filled with the expired air of a patient who has radium emanations, these radiations will ionize the air and the rate of the leak will be quickened. In performing this test the expired air must be passed through phosphorous pentoxide to remove water.

In testing for the presence of radioactive substances after death, the bones and the parenchymatous viscera such as the lungs, liver and spleen are incinerated and

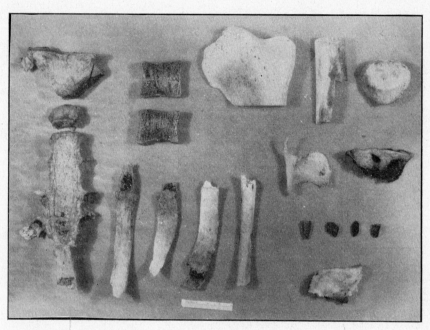

Fig. 31-8. Photograph of Various Bones from Which Autoradiogram Shown in Figure 31-7 Was Prepared.

their ashes are placed in a dark room on a photographic film, wrapped and sealed in black opaque paper. They are allowed to rest there for 10 days. If the tissues are radioactive, the films when developed show luminous areas corresponding to the ash. The bones usually give a greater luminosity than the soft tissues as they contain more radium and may be used without ashing. The electroscope may be used to test the ashes of the bones and the viscera, for by measuring the time of the leak and calibrating the apparatus with a definite radium quantity in an uranium ore, it is possible to determine the quantity of radioactive substance present in the ash.

URANIUM. Uranium is a radioactive metal which occurs in greater abundance in ores and may be isolated more readily from them than other radioactive elements. It is of high atomic weight, and several isotopes or nuclear variants of the atom occur in nature, namely U 234, 235, 236, 237 and 238. The radioactivity of uranium was recognized shortly after its discovery by Becquerel in 1896, as it was found that its salts have the power to ionize the air and remove the charge from an electroscope. The salts of uranium (the acetate, sulfate and nitrate) have not been important in human toxicology, but they have been used in animal experiments to produce a hemorrhagic gastroenteritis and a nephrosis similar to the degenerative changes in the kidney tubules produced by mercury bichloride and potassium dichromate. With the development of the atomic bomb and its use in 1945, the action of uranium on the human organism has become an increasingly important subject.

The basic principle of the atomic bomb is that atomic nuclei are shattered, causing the release of a fantastic amount of energy as a result of the sudden disintegration. According to Einstein the energy set free by this process equals the mass of the substance destroyed multiplied by the speed of light squared. In more graphic terms, a mass of one kilogram subjected to nuclear disruption would release 25 billion kilowatt hours of energy, in vivid contrast to 8.5 kilowatt hours of heat energy set free by burning 1 kilogram of coal. Atomic disruption is not a process which occurs naturally on earth, though it is believed to be a characteristic solar phenomenon; to take place under terrestrial conditions it must be contrived by human ingenuity. The major problem in the use of this power in an explosive, is to keep the process under some kind of control.

The disruption of atomic nuclei must be brought about by some method which renders them unstable or radioactive and this is accomplished by the employment of neutrons. Neutrons were discovered in 1930, when a few elements of light atomic weight and stable nuclei were bombarded with natural alpha particles from radioactive polonium, whereupon these substances (beryllium, boron, lithium) became secondarily unstable and radioactive, emitting particles of the size of hydrogen nuclei or protons. The particles in this emanation were free of electric charge, and for this reason were given the name of neutrons. It was soon discovered that there were two kinds of neutrons, the slow-moving and the fast-moving. The fast-moving neutron collides with other atomic nuclei but bounces off and does not penetrate them; as a result atomic nuclei are not affected by fast-moving neutrons. The slow-moving neutron, on the other hand, penetrates the atomic nuclei of other substances, especially those containing hydrogen, rendering them unstable, so that the bombarded atomic nucleus ejects protons in order to acquire stability.

Uranium was selected as a promising material for atomic explosion, as it is radioactive and occurs in considerable quantity in nature in comparison with other radioactive elements. Its isotopes, U 235 and U 238, make up regular metallic uranium, and their response to bombardment by neutrons is the basis for the production of atomic disruption.

If U 235 is bombarded by slow neutrons it undergoes fission, giving off four additional fast-moving neutrons which are unable to penetrate other uranium nuclei, so that the reaction does not continue beyond the uranium originally bombarded. If the speed of the fast neutrons can be retarded, they will act as slow neutrons and will penetrate other uranium nuclei, and the process will extend from atom to atom and a chain reaction would be produced. The establishment of a chain reaction is necessary to produce atomic explosion. Experiments have been tried of passing fast neutrons through substances rich in hydrogen atoms, like heavy water or paraffin, or rich in carbon atoms, like graphite, which reduce their speed to that of slow neutrons and thus establish the basis for a chain reaction.

U 238 when bombarded by slow neutrons does not undergo fission but is converted into a new isotope, U 239, which is not found in nature. U 239 is not stable but decays spontaneously into a new element called neptunium, and neptunium itself is transformed spontaneously into another new element called plutonium. Plutonium in small mass undergoes fission like U 235 when bombarded with slow neutrons, but if its mass is increased to a certain size, known as the critical size, an atomic explosion occurs. When a fissionable substance of this size is used as an explosive, the problem is to control the moment of explosion; this is done by placing separate pieces of the substance, all below the critical size, apart from each other in the bomb and then to bring them suddenly together in such a way as to make up the critical size at the moment of detonation.

The actual composition of the atomic bomb and the methods of causing the explosion are military secrets but some form of uranium and the principles outlined above are utilized in its preparation.

The blast of the atomic bomb has been described as similar to an infinitesimal explosion of the sun's substance on the earth's surface. The principal effects are: (1) a tremendous physical disruption which extends over a wide area and is sufficient in volume to create a high and destructive wind; (2) an intense and instantly produced heat; (3) an overwhelming and instantaneous release of radioactivity in the form of gamma rays which have unusual penetrating power and kill instantly or cause death in a few weeks. These rays travel with the speed of light and penetrate any barrier less resistant than a foot of concrete.

The description given by Warren and his collaborators of the effects of the explosions at Hiroshima and Nagasaki indicates that the injuries due to the blast were usually fractures or visceral ruptures produced when the body was struck by flying objects or when it was hurled against a fixed structure. The heat produced by the explosion was intense, evanescent and of instantaneous formation causing flash burn injuries and loss of hair. The radiation injuries were also instantaneously produced, many dying immediately, or in a few days with a high fever, complaining of weakness and anorexia. If they survived longer, symptoms characteristic of toxic exposure to roentgen rays supervened, such as loss of weight, diarrhea and loss of hair in a few cases. The radiation sometimes caused suppression of spermatogenesis, the tubules showing a thickened basement membrane, and containing mostly Sertoli cells, the interstitial cells were apparently not affected. The ovaries were apparently not affected to the same extent. The most damaging effects were inflicted on the bone marrow and three different types of reaction were noted: (1) An intense, rapid leukopenia (200 cells per cubic millimeter) with destruction of the leukocytes in the circulating blood simultaneously with deleterious effects on the bone marrow, death occurring in the first three weeks. (2) A marked thrombocytopenia caused by destruction of the megacaryocytes in the bone marrow with numerous hemorrhages, especially from the body orifices; death occurred in three to five weeks, the autopsies revealing large hemorrhages in the kidney pelves, multiple hemorrhages in the meninges and occasionally in the brain substance. (3) Some patients who survived the first few weeks developed an anemia with a low erythrocyte count of a million or less, accompanied by a hyperplastic or aplastic bone marrow as indicated by sternal biopsy. There was no sickness from residual radioactivity as persons who came into the bombed area after the explosion were not affected.

Gold. Gold belongs to the heavy metal group chemically, biologically and toxicologically. The metal is not poisonous. Gold salts are usually toxic and most cases of poisoning occur after their therapeutic use. A preparation known as sanocrysin which is employed in the treatment of tuberculosis, gold sodium thiosulfate which may be injected for lupus erythematosus or chronic arthritis, and other gold salts like gold chloride may cause toxic symptoms when administered.

Some gold compounds corrode the skin and mucous membranes, causing a yellow and violet necrosis which may turn black; occasionally gold is absorbed from this necrotic area. In the stomach the salts form a gold albuminate combination and may evoke such symptoms as pain in the epigastrium, vomiting, diarrhea and salivation. After absorption gold is carried in the circulating blood and may be found in the white blood cells as "transport gold", and then it is taken up by the reticuloendothelial system and is deposited in all the organs. There it can be demonstrated by the darkfield method as gold particles, the metal usually being separated from its compounds when it is stored in the body. It acts on the finer blood vessels sometimes giving rise to capillary hemorrhages in the brain and elsewhere.

The systemic effects, especially following the use of sanocrysin, are skin lesions similar to the salvarsan eruptions (dermatitis, keratosis, maculae and papules). The hair and fingernails may fall out. Fragments of gold may appear under the skin, causing a chrysosis similar to argyrosis, in cases where absorption has taken place over a long period. In some cases granulocytopenia may occur. Gold affects the capillary vessels, causing lesions in the mouth like mercury, and in the intestine like arsenic. Fatty degeneration of liver cells and nephrosis occur. The symptoms are headache, albuminuria, sleeplessness, pain in cardiac region and chills.

The authors have seen a case of gold poisoning in a white woman of 46 years, who received 300 mg. of gold sodium thiosulfate in three injections for chronic arthritis. Shortly after the third injection she developed a massive and widespread dermatitis exfoliativa, edema and subacute inflammation in the small intestine, and a marked parenchymatous degeneration in the cortical cells of the kidneys; and the blood vessels in the liver, spleen and kidneys contained numerous eosinophils. Death occurred on the twentieth day after the last injection.

The treatment after the ingestion of gold or after its application to the skin is similar to that used in any escharotic poisoning. Egg albumin may be used as an antidote to combat stomach corrosion. BAL has also been used to treat cases of gold poisoning. The treatment is otherwise symptomatic.

Osmium. Osmium is a black heavy metal, its principal compound being osmic acid which occurs as yellow prisms, soluble in water. This acid is escharotic and is used in histology as a tissue fixative. It gives off a vapor which is irritating, and inflames the mucous membrane of the eyes and of the respiratory passages, the osmic acid being reduced to osmium during the process. In the manufacture of incandescent lamps the vapor of osmic acid is produced and may cause ulceration of the eyelids, black discoloration of the body areas which are uncovered, inflammatory patches on the skin with dry gangrene, a chronic coryza of the upper respiratory passages and a mild nephrosis. Potassium osmate has been used in the treatment of neuralgia and neoplasms through hypodermic injection, and produces areas of black-green discoloration on the skin.

Platinum. The metal platinum is not poisonous, and is used to make bacteriologic and chemical apparatus because it can be heated in the flame without alteration. The soluble salts of platinum are poisonous. A salt like platinum chloride when coming in contact with the skin causes erythema and vesiculation, and when ingested causes a yellowish-brown corrosion of the stomach, accompanied by salivation, burning in the mouth, colicky pains, nausea, vomiting, headache, bloody stools and slight icterus. If a compound like sodium platinate is injected subcutaneously, a syndrome not unlike arsenic poisoning develops and kidneys, bladder and intestine show anatomic evidences of inflammation. The treatment is similar to that of any other heavy metal poisoning.

Nickel. Nickel, Ni, is a white metal used in many alloys and for nickel plating. It may be dissolved by acetic acid, lactic acid or butyric acid, and it may taint food. In human pathology nickel poisoning is of minor importance.

Workers in nickel develop sometimes a widespread eczema, nodular in type known as the nickel itch. This, however, may be due as much to the presence of alkali as to nickel compounds.

Nickel carbonyl is formed when nickel is extracted from calcined ores by carbon monoxide, and occurs in the form of a gas with the formula, $NiCO_4$. This may be inhaled during the extraction and cause poisoning, the toxic effects depending on the dissociation of the compound after absorption into nickel and carbon monoxide. The carbonyl produces cyanosis, difficult breathing, dilated pupils and vomiting. At autopsy there is usually inflammation and ecchymosis in the stomach and intestines. In the more chronic cases, kidney lesions may develop and small petechial hemorrhages may appear in the brain. The treatment is the same as for the other heavy metals.

Chromium. The compounds of chromium, Cr, which cause the most cases of poisoning are potassium bichromate, potassium chromate, and chromic acid. Potassium bichromate is a salt which occurs in the form of orange red crystals; it is employed as a constituent of battery fluids, and is used to stain furniture. Chromic acid is encountered in the form of needle-like crystals of crimson color, and is used in medicine as an external caustic, especially on growths of the skin or throat. Potassium chromate is a yellow salt used in the manufacture of chrome yellow or chrome red.

The fatal cases of poisoning are usually suicidal or accidental, and are comparatively rare, only one case of suicide by potassium dichromate occurring between 1918 to 1941 in the records of the Office of the Chief Medical Examiner. A few cases of homicidal nature are reported, and also a few where the compounds were used as abortifacients.

Chrome salts are irritants, causing escharotic changes in the gastrointestinal tract, since they are usually ingested. The victims complain of bad taste in the mouth, pain in the epigastrium, oliguria, hematuria, vomiting and bloody diarrhea; in addition the central nervous system is involved, and reacts with dilated pupils, coma, collapse and slow respirations, death sometimes occurring inside of an hour from respiratory paralysis and shock as a result of the action of the chrome salts on the capillaries. There is slough of portions of the mucous membrane and ulcer formation in the mouth, esophagus and pharynx, and the stomach may show a greenish-gray or a greenish-brown hardened pseudomembrane over its inner lining; the stomach contents are greenish yellow or blood containing. The chrome compounds coagulate protein and extract water from tissues in varying degrees. The rest of the intestinal tract shows varying degrees of inflammatory action.

The chromium compounds are readily absorbed from the stomach and raw skin surfaces, and cause changes in the internal organs. Parenchymatous and fatty degenerative changes are produced in the liver, kidneys and heart muscle, and inflammation of the intestinal tract and urinary bladder may occur, ascribed to the toxic action of the chromate ion. The organs may be bluish gray and the blood may be brown from methemoglobin formation, as a result of direct toxic action on the red cells and the other elements of the circulating blood and possibly on the bone marrow.

The period of fatal action varies from 40 minutes to several days. The fatal dose is about 3 gm. of the dichromate, but varies with the individual case. The treatment is to give chalk or magnesia to neutralize the acid ion of the poison, and to wash out the stomach with milk as a demulcent. The patient may be given infusions with normal saline solution in order to relieve the kidneys of some of the poison, inasmuch as it affects the organs of excretion. The rest of the treatment is symptomatic. Stomach contents, liver, brain and kidneys are saved for chemical analysis.

Chemical industrial processes like electrotyping, and plating may produce a state of affairs in which fine particles of chromium salts are inhaled by workers or brought into contact with their skin, with the result that chronic ulcerations of the skin occur on the face, eyes, arms and hands especially about the nails, and foul smelling inflammation and ulcers of the nasal and upper respiratory mucous membrane may occur. Complications may follow such lesions, such as perforation of the nasal septum, furuncles of the nares followed by septic thrombosis of the cavernous sinus, and occasionally asthmatic attacks, inflammation of the air passages and bronchopneumonia. Reports have been published indicating that the incidence of bronchogenic carcinoma in a number of American chromate plants ranged from

13 to 31 times the normal, confirming similar reports from Germany and suggesting by implication that chromates are carcinogenic agents.

Pascale and his collaborators have described a nonfatal poisoning of a worker in a chromium electroplating plant, who had continually inhaled spray from a chromic acid bath. After a while this individual became jaundiced and gave a positive test for chromium in the urine. Histologic section of a needle biopsy of the liver disclosed a toxic hepatitis with necrosis of the liver cells around the central vein varying from dissolution to eosinophilia of the cytoplasm and pyknotic nuclei. The sinusoids were dilated and contained lymphocytes. The Kupffer's cells were numerous and slightly enlarged. Bile pigment was present in the liver cells in the central vein area but was also noted elsewhere. There was an increase in the lymphocytes and other cells in the portal areas, and also an increase in the bile ducts and bile capillaries. Other workers in the plant had chromium in the urine, but did not present well defined signs of chromium intoxication.

Iron. Iron, Fe, is one of the frequently used metals in modern life, and is naturally present in the human body, especially in the red blood cells. It is ingested constantly in food, and is not inherently toxic to the human system. The two iron salts which have a reputation for being toxic are ferrous sulfate and ferric chloride, and they derive this noxious property from the acid ion in the molecule.

Ferrous sulfate is a compound which appears as green crystals, occasionally covered with brownish rusty incrustations. It is known as green vitriol or copperas. When taken internally it causes pain in the stomach, vomiting, diarrhea and other signs of gastrointestinal irritation.

Ferric chloride is present in tincture of iron, or tinctura ferri chloridi. This is a brown liquid with an acid reaction, used occasionally as an abortifacient and rarely for homicidal purposes. Taken internally, ferric chloride produces an inky metallic taste in the mouth, and vomiting, abdominal pain and diarrhea. In addition, paralysis of the extremities, convulsions, suppression of urine follow and death may occur. The feces are colored black by iron sulfide. The stomach is corroded in cases of acute poisoning and is covered with a greenish black or brown slough. The kidneys and the liver show congestion, ecchymotic spots and marked parenchymatous degeneration. The duration of the clinical course is from a few hours to several days. One and a half ounces of the tincture of iron has caused death. The stomach should be washed out with a stomach pump and flushed with abundant watery solutions of alkaline bicarbonates. The rest of the treatment is symptomatic.

Copper. Copper, Cu, is a heavy, reddish metal which is not toxic in the metallic state, but some of its salts in large quantities are occasionally the cause of a fatal poisoning. Copper is present in many ores and in minute quantities is a constituent of many soils and waters. A few plants and animals have a trace of copper in their tissues, and there is a minute quantity present in the human body. The copper salts of particular toxicologic significance are copper sulfate (blue vitriol), copper subacetate (verdigris), and copper acetoarsenite (Paris green).

Copper sulfate is a crystalline, blue salt with an astringent taste, occasionally used as an emetic in phosphorus poisoning. If it is ingested in large quantities it is toxic. Most cases of this type are suicidal, some are homicidal and a few are accidental. Isolated cases of poisoning have occurred from application of the copper salt to the scalp or from its introduction into the vagina.

The primary symptoms after ingestion are those of any gastrointestinal irritant, a coppery taste in the mouth, astringent action on the throat, vomiting of greenish material, pain in the stomach, thirst and purging with greenish stools. Later the urine becomes scanty, albuminous, inky and full of casts. Neurologic symptoms and signs appear with pains, tetanic spasms, delirium, paralyses and collapse. The liver may be affected by the poison and jaundice may appear.

Corrosive lesions are present on the mucous membrane of the upper gastro-intestinal tract, usually in the form of a firm, dried crust which is sometimes discolored green and occasionally reddish brown. Varying grades of ulceration and inflammation occur in the small intestine and the colon. The liver occasionally shows fatty or parenchymatous degeneration and the kidneys are congested and show varying grades of parenchymatous degeneration and albuminous deposits in the cortical tubules. The blood has been reported dark in color because of the formation of hematin.

Excretion of copper occurs through the bile, urine, gastrointestinal tract and skin. The fatal dose of copper salts is variable; in one case an individual died after taking a half ounce of the subacetate. Death has taken place as early as four hours after the ingestion of the poison but most cases survive a few days. The treatment is to evacuate the stomach and to use white of egg or milk as an antidote. Castor oil will favor the elimination of the copper salt from the intestines. The rest of the treatment is symptomatic. In fatal cases the materials to be preserved for toxicologic examination are stomach contents, parenchymatous organs and brain.

Chronic poisoning may result from the introduction of small amounts of copper in the food, but ordinarily toxic manifestations are not caused unless the doses are large. The copper compounds formerly added to maintain the green color of preserved vegetables are considered prejudicial to health by most investigators. Some metal workers inhale vapors which cause a condition known as copper colic, similar to lead colic, but differing from the latter in showing more diarrhea, more prostration and shorter duration. Many maintain that the poisonous symptoms are not due to the presence of copper but to lead and arsenic which are occasional impurities in the ore. In some chronic cases of poisoning, copper may be deposited in the tissues, giving rise to a greenish color of the hair and of the urine, and to a blue line on the gums. If large amounts enter the system, neurologic signs, anemia and cachexia may make their appearance. Some believe that chronic absorption of copper may produce hemochromatosis but this has been denied by others.

Cadmium. Cadmium, Cd, is a metal used in smelting; it is chemically similar to zinc but its compounds are more toxic. Cadmium sulfate causes gastrointestinal irritation if absorbed in toxic doses, and may produce a chronic enteritis, a nephrosis and degenerations of liver and heart muscle. Frank and Kleeman have described nonlethal poisoning by cadmium salts in individuals who drank lemonade or some other acid beverage which had been cooled in the metal compartment of an electric ice box; a few hours later they developed severe abdominal pain, vomiting and diarrhea, attributable to the metallic cadmium coating of the container which was dissolved by the acid in the lemonade and was transformed into toxic soluble salts of cadmium.

Poisoning is sometimes caused by the inhalation of fumes which occur when cadmium compounds are heated. Ross reports a case in which a workman "flanged" a cadmium-coated stainless steel pipe by heating it with a blow torch, and inhaled the fumes thus produced; he complained of irritation of the nose and throat, vomiting, chest pains, shortness of breath, and finally developed a serious inflammation of the air passages, dying in a few days of a pneumonia. There are also cases of chronic poisoning in which the victim inhales fumes over a long period of time and is affected with symptoms of epigastric pain suggesting lead poisoning except that the colic is absent.

Manganese. Manganese, Mn, is a metal closely related to iron and is often encountered in iron ore. It is present in the human body in minute quantities. Potassium permanganate ($KMnO_4$) is a dark purplish-red crystalline salt which oxidizes organic matter. In dilute solution it has slight action on human tissues, but in concentrated solution it is an irritant. On ingestion, a corrosive gastroenteritis with a brownish-black incrustation of the mucous membrane, and an acute pharyngitis with edema of the glottis are sometimes produced. Suicidal cases have been reported. The treatment of the condition is the same as in any other form of corrosive poisoning, that is, the stomach is evacuated, a gastric lavage is given and mechanical antidotes like raw eggs are administered. In fatal cases, stomach contents, parenchymatous viscera and urine are preserved for chemical examination.

A chronic industrial poisoning caused by the inhalation of fine dust containing manganese oxide gives rise to a definite syndrome of muscular weakness, languor, low monotonous voice, economical speech, a stolid mask-like facial expression, cramps in the calves of the legs, hand tremors and an unsteady slapping or festinating gait. Occasionally symptoms of mental disturbance, such as impulsive emotional displays of uncontrolled laughter or weeping, occur. This condition does not affect all workers but only those who are susceptible to manganese, and it rarely causes death. Necropsies fail to disclose any characteristic lesions. The treatment is mostly hygienic, and especially important is avoidance of dusty atmosphere. In these cases manganese may be isolated from the urine, parenchymatous viscera and brain.

Tin. Tin, Sn, occurs in the solder on cans of tinned food, and is occasionally dissolved in acid food mixtures. In rare instances, poisoning results for tin salts when ingested produce signs of gastrointestinal irritation such as nausea, vomiting, metallic taste in the mouth, pain in the abdomen, cyanosis, diarrhea and collapse. The salts of tin are slowly absorbed and slowly excreted through the gastrointestinal tract, while the renal excretion is secondary in importance. The treatment is to evacuate the stomach, using demulcent drinks, and to treat the case symptomatically. Stomach contents and parenchymatous viscera are used for chemical examination.

The authors have seen one case of tin poisoning in a 77 year old white woman who ate some canned cranberries and 12 hours later developed pain in the abdomen, vomiting and bloody diarrhea, finally dying after an illness of two days. At autopsy there was reddening of the stomach mucous membrane, a congested and inflamed intestine with pseudomembrane formation in places, subendocardial hemorrhages in the left ventricle, fatty infiltration of the liver (probably a result of obesity) and a terminal bronchopneumonia. Chemical examination of the viscera was positive for tin, and other poisons were not present.

Beryllium. Beryllium, Be, is used in the manufacture of beryllium copper alloy from which precision instruments, altimeters, carburetors, airplaine pipe lines and telephone switch boards are made. In the extraction of the inert crushed ore, beryl, by concentrated acids and fusion methods under high temperature, fumes and dusts are generated at different stages and constitute a distinct industrial hazard. The acid radical salts of beryllium, the sulfate, fluoride or oxyfluoride, are the most toxic and irritating products in these fumes. When they come in contact with the skin of exposed portions such as hands, arms, face and neck, an erythematous or papulovesicular eruption results, which tends to subside with desquamation if the victim is freed from exposure to the fumes. In some cases a small crystal of beryllium is deposited in the skin layers with the formation of a chronic ulcer with a caseous center; healing will not occur unless the crystal is removed. Conjunctivitis may result from exposure to the fumes.

Tenders of furnaces in which hydrous beryllium sulfate is heated to produce beryllium oxide, or where anhydrous beryllium fluoride and magnesium are processed to produce pure beryllium metal, may develop a chemical nasopharyngitis and tracheobronchitis. The chief manifestations of such exposures are soreness of the nose and throat, swelling and vascular engorgement of the mucous membrane, a mild epistaxis with blood clots, fissures in the nose, and later cough, rales in the lungs, blood streaked sputum, fever without chills, and a reduction of the vital capacity of the lung about 30 per cent. This condition usually clears up in 7 to 21 days.

The chemical pneumonitis has been described by Van Ordstrand and his collaborators as a complication of insidious development with cough, blood streaked sputum, burning substernal pain, dyspnea, cyanosis, anorexia, loss of weight and recovery in 2 to 5 weeks after cessation of exposure. More protracted cases occur which show discrete nodules of varying size on roentgenologic examination and these may not clear up for from one to four months. Autopsies on a few fatal cases showed that the lungs were heavy, and were the seat of an atypical pneumonitis with edema and hemorrhagic extravasation. Microscopic examination disclosed large, foamy mononuclear cells, lymphocytes and plasma cells in the alveoli and interalveolar septa, but no polymorphonuclear leukocytes. Occasionally fibroplastic proliferation was present in the septa and squamous metaplasia was seen in the lining of the alveoli and terminal bronchioles.

Some individuals exposed to beryllium have developed sarcoid-like granulomas in the lungs from six months to six years after the exposure. In a few instances the victim has been inflicted with sarcoid-like granulomas in the skin, similar histologically to the lung lesions. Beryllium has been demonstrated spectroscopically in the subcutaneous nodules. Cases have also been reported of sarcoid granulomas appearing after a number of years at the site of old lacerations sustained accidentally from broken fluorescent light bulbs which contain zinc beryllium silicate.

Vanadium. The compounds of vanadium, V, most in use are vanadic acid (HVO_3), vanadium chloride (VCl_3) and vanadium trioxide (V_2O_3). Vanadium compounds are used extensively in the manufacture of dyes, ferrovanadium is used in making nonductile steel, and many compounds are found in dusty ground ores. Poisoning occurs in workers who are exposed to dust and fumes generated in these processes. The trioxide is prone to produce a chronic intoxication, called vanadiumism, in those workers who inhale its fumes. They may display anorexia, nausea, diarrhea, anemia, cachexia, emaciation, dry paroxysmal cough, irritation of the eyes and throat, albuminuria, casts and blood in the urine; then headache, vertigo, tremors, retinitis and amaurosis appear. At necropsy there is congestion of the lungs, inflammation of the stomach and intestines, and a mild hemorrhagic nephrosis. The vanadium may be found in the urine and in the feces, and even in the saliva. The proper treatment is to prevent inhalation or ingestion of the fumes or dust by proper ventilation or by use of a respirator for those workers exposed during the process of dye manufacture or in the handling of ores. In fatal cases, the parenchymatous viscera, brain, urine and feces should be preserved routinely for toxicologic examination.

Alum. Alum, AlK $(SO_4)_2$ plus H_2O, is an astringent salt, white in color and crystalline in form; it is either potassium aluminum sulfate or ammonium aluminum sulfate. Alum and aluminum sulfate are sometimes constituents of baking powder, as they help to form carbon dioxide with the other constituent, sodium bicarbonate. It is a debatable point as to whether or not the aluminum compounds are safe substances to use for this purpose. Alum has occasionally been taken by mistake, for suicidal purposes or as an abortifacient and has caused gastrointestinal irritation, epigastric pain, vomiting of chocolate colored mucus, blood in the urine and signs of renal irritation. A grayish necrotic membrane may be found over the upper gastrointestinal tract, especially the stomach, and there may be necrosis of the cortical tubules of the kidneys and the liver may show some fatty degeneration. The treatment is that of any irritant poisoning. In the fatal cases, the stomach contents and the parenchymatous viscera are saved for chemical examination.

Alkaline Earths. Barium, Ba, has a number of salts which are found in some ores and are used in various processes. The more common salts are barium carbonate (a component of "Rough on Rats" with arsenic trioxide), barium sulfide, barium chloride, and barium nitrate. Barium sulfate is a heavy insoluble salt used as a water-color pigment and as a contrast meal in roentgen-ray examinations; it is nontoxic. Sometimes poisonous and soluble barium salts are substituted for the sulfate by an error of a druggist. The symptoms of ingestion of a barium salt of this nature are pain in the abdomen, vomiting, diarrhea and other signs of gastro-intestinal irritation. After absorption into the system there is a rapid respiratory paralysis, convulsions and collapse with dilated pupils, due to its action on the central nervous system. At necropsy, the stomach and the intestines are inflamed and show redness, swelling and erosion generally on the top of the rugae; the liver may show fatty degeneration, the kidneys may show necrosis of the cortical tubules, and there may be an acute cystitis of varying grade. Death may occur inside of an hour in some cases, but in others the victim may live for a few days. The fatal dose is variable. The treatment is directed to combating shock, and administering large quantities of magnesium sulfate to form insoluble barium sulfate and to remove it by catharsis. Stomach contents and parenchymatous viscera are saved for chemical examination.

Magnesium Sulfate. Magnesium sulfate, $MgSO_4$, given in dilute form with plenty of water acts like a purgative and is not absorbed in any considerable amount. However, if the dry salt is ingested, it may be absorbed from the gastrointestinal tract and enter the circulation. Repeated doses of magnesium sulfate may cause paralysis of the intestines and as a result absorption of the salt, so that symptoms of poisoning may develop.

Nausea, vomiting, pain in the intestines and stomach, and sometimes purging are caused from its toxic action on the intestines. After absorption, it produces suppression of urine, general anesthesia, relaxation of the muscles, convulsions and collapse; death takes place because of its action on the respiratory center. In some cases an enteritis, an irritative nephrosis, fatty infiltration of the liver and petechial hemorrhages of the serous surfaces are found at necropsy. The treatment is to use some other cathartic to rid the intestines of magnesium sulfate. An infusion of normal saline solution also combats the toxemia when the drug is present in the blood. Stomach contents, intestinal contents and parenchymatous viscera are used for chemical analysis.

Lithium Salts. Lithium salts, the chloride and carbonate, are constituents of mineral waters and some foods, and are also present in the human body in minute quantity. A dilute solution of lithium salts is sometimes used to treat uric acid diathesis. Until recently only experimental poisoning has been reported. Cleaveland ingested lithium chloride and suffered muscular weakness, blurred vision and ringing in the ears, all signs of its action on the central nervous system. He did not have any gastrointestinal symptoms. Good's experiments on animals, however, indicated severe gastrointestinal involvement and he reported a human case which showed similar symptoms. Elimination of lithium salts is by the saliva, urine and feces. The compounds are difficult to isolate. In the flame they give a red color, with two lines, a red and yellow, when seen through the spectroscope.

Fatal cases of lithium poisoning have occurred when the salt substitute, westsal, containing lithium chloride, citric acid and a little potassium iodide was used to give flavor to a salt free diet. After a variable period of a few days to a few weeks of this type of seasoning, the patients developed tremors, twitching of the muscles, hyperirritable reflexes, dizziness, apathy, confusion, difficulty in thinking, prostration, coma and death. The toxic action of the lithium ion on the central nervous system was the cause of death in these cases.

Potassium and Sodium Salts. These compounds are discussed more appropriately under the heading of the acids to which they are attached but a few salts deserve special mention because of their highly individual action. In general the sodium salts have an action similar to the salts of potassium, and many of the compounds of both metals, though toxic in their own right, do not play a great role in toxicology.

Sodium compounds are normal constituents of the body, and when present within physiologic limits are important factors in maintaining body health. An excess or deficiency of sodium salts may cause disturbances of metabolism which may be serious. Heat cramps (page 525) illustrate the condition which follows the lack of sodium chloride in the tissues. As an example of a dangerous excess, the ingestion of solid sodium chloride in large amounts has been noted by Petri as a means of suicide in China; it causes a severe gastroenteritis in the victim. Other important compounds of this metal such as the hydroxide, carbonate or fluoride have been considered while others are similar in their action to potassium salts and discussion of them would be repetitious.

Potassium salts are also necessary for body metabolism; if the tissues are deficient in the potassium ion, the health suffers. But if the ion is in excess, a cardiac collapse may result. As a rule, this action of the ion is not an important factor in poisoning inasmuch as the toxic action of different potassium salts is modified by the other components in the molecule in most cases. The effects of potassium hydroxide, potassium carbonate, potassium dichromate and potassium permanganate have been discussed. A few other salts remain which deserve mention because of their action on the body.

The bitartrate or sulfate of potassium when taken in large amounts may cause vomiting, purging, pain in the abdomen, exhaustion and collapse. The treatment is to empty the stomach and administer supportive measures.

Potassium nitrate is a white crystalline salt, much like oxalic acid and magnesium sulfate in appearance. It is sometimes mistaken for the latter and taken as a purgative. Saltpeter is used also to cure meats, and it is a question whether or not the salt is toxic in the proportions used. In doses from 8 gm. to 240 gm. the drug may cause fatal poisoning. The symptoms are those of gastrointestinal irritation and paralysis of the respiratory center; the clinical course is about 45 minutes or even longer. The therapeutic measures should be directed towards evacuation of the stomach, washing out of the stomach and appropriate symptomatic treatment. Windmueller reported a case of chronic poisoning in a farmer, 57 years old, who took a daily dose of potassium nitrate for 26 days for joint pains. He became emaciated, weakened and anemic (hemoglobin 50 per cent, red cells 290,000) with albuminuria and suppression of urine.

POTASSIUM CHLORATE. Potassium chlorate, $KClO_3$, is used in making explosives of various sorts, and in medicine is employed as a gargle or mouth wash. Poisoning occurs because it is swallowed by mistake for some other drug, or because it has been administered as a result of a therapeutic error. Some cases are suicidal, and a few are homicidal. In rare instances it is used as an abortifacient, the chlorate passing through the placenta and causing methemoglobinemia and fatal poisoning in the fetus. In large doses, from 15 to 46 gm., it may produce abdominal pain, vomiting, diarrhea, dyspnea, deep cyanosis, convulsions, coma, collapse and death. The patient dies in from one to five hours or he may live a few days. The therapy is to wash out the stomach and to treat the case symptomatically. The anoxia caused by the poisoning may be combated by blood transfusions.

The chief toxic action of potassium chlorate is from the chlorate ion which produces a direct irritation of the gastrointestinal tract, and after absorption, destruction of the erythrocytes, methemoglobinemia, methemoglobinuria and finally a fatal anoxia. The kidneys slowly excrete the chlorate unchanged, and develop a pronounced irritative nephrosis. The slow excretion of the chlorate may lead to cumulative poisoning if small doses of the salt are given over a long period of time.

The lesions at autopsy are an inflammation of the gastrointestinal tract with a grayish yellow or bluish gray color of the mucous membrane, congestion and small hemorrhages in the submucous layer, while the contents are usually dark. The blood may be a purplish brown color from methemoglobin formation, the internal organs are engorged and are colored different shades of brown, and in the lividity and suggillations have a purplish brown flush and in the paler areas the skin has a yellowish tinge. The liver, spleen and kidneys contain many of the decomposition products of hemoglobin. The lesions in the kidneys were illustrated in a case seen by the authors, as they were swollen, congested and brownish in color. Microscopically the cortical tubules showed the epithelium swollen and pale from an accumulation of fluid in the cells so that the lumen was narrowed to a small opening; other tubules showed flatter epithelium but contained an albuminous deposit or blood pigment or red blood cells undergoing dissolution; the tubules in the pyramids were largely filled with degenerating red blood cells, blood pigment and polymorphonuclear leukocytes, and the blood vessels in this area were injected and filled with leukocytes; the glomeruli were not remarkable but did not contain many erythrocytes. In some cases, the bladder may show a hemorrhagic inflammatory reaction and may contain reddish or brownish urine. Occasionally the gallbladder and the mucous membrane of the air passages may be congested and show a slight inflammation.

Stomach contents, urine and parenchymatous viscera are preserved for toxicologic examination. The stomach contents are important because potassium chlorate is recovered from them readily by dialysis through a dialyzing membrane.

The inorganic, nonmetallic poisons form a small and heterogenous group, both chemically and toxicologically. They act as local irritants in varying degrees, and after absorption into the circulation may produce an inflammatory reaction in various organs.

Phosphorus. The element phosphorus, P, is encountered in two common forms. One is the poisonous white or yellow phosphorus, which occurs often as white, waxy, translucent cylinders. It is oxidized readily in air, giving off fumes of the oxide, and is easily ignited at a temperature of 122° F.; in the dark it glows with a pale yellow light. It is usually kept under water from which all oxygen has been expelled by boiling. Yellow phosphorus has the taste and odor of garlic, and is freely soluble in ether, carbon bisulfide and many oils.

Red phosphorus is an allotropic variety of the element produced by heating yellow phosphorus in a closed vessel without air for 36 hours. It is a reddish-brown powder, which does not ignite spontaneously, and is not as toxic as the yellow form.

Phosphine, PH_3, a combination of phosphorus and hydrogen, is the most poisonous compound of phosphorus, most of the others having only a slight toxicity. Some of the phosphates are normal constituents of the human body.

Many rat poisons and other vermin poisons, such as J-O paste, contain as high as 1 to 4 per cent of white phosphorus combined with oil, flour, sugar, coloring matter and other materials. Medicinal preparations of phosphorus, including phosphorus pills, phosphorus cod liver oil, and other preparations were used at one time but now are not employed as frequently. Yellow phosphorus is used as one of the inflammable constituents of fireworks, and at one time was a constituent of lucifer matches, where it was mixed with potassium chlorate, sand and glue to form the composition for the head; such a match could be ignited by friction against any rough surface. At present, phosphorus sesquisulfide and red phosphorus, which are nontoxic, are substituted for white phosphorus by manufacturers. The safety match, on the other hand, has a head tipped with a mixture of potassium chlorate and antimony sulfide, and can be ignited only by scratching it against a special surface which contains nontoxic red phosphorus.

Phosphorus poisoning is suicidal, accidental or homicidal. The drug is rarely used as a means of homicide because its garlicky odor and taste cannot be disguised sufficiently to escape detection. It may be employed as an abortifacient, administered either by mouth or by vagina, as it has a rapid action on the fetus and placenta; when so used it may cause the death of the mother. Suicidal cases are more prevalent, 68 being recorded in the Office of the Chief Medical Examiner from 1918 to 1951. During that same period, 83 accidental cases occurred, especially in children and alcoholics. Children may suck the ends of lucifer matches, eat the contents of fireworks, or swallow rat poison which has been carelessly left around. Alcoholics have mistaken rat paste for some article of food and have died as a result of eating it. In the German literature, cases of intoxication have been reported from therapeutic use of phosphorus and cod liver oil as a cure for rickets. Else Petri mentions a reported case of mild phosphorus poisoning which occurred in a man who was wounded by a bullet containing the substance. When ignited, white phosphorus inflicts severe skin burns.

Phosphorus, after absorption, remains in the blood in its elemental form for a number of days, and then is slowly oxidized to hypophosphorous and phosphorous acids. It acts as a protoplasmic poison, which interferes with the normal processes of oxidation in the cells. The symptoms depend upon the rapidity with which the phosphorus is absorbed. As a rule, this process is slow and symptoms may not occur for two to six hours. However, if bile and fatty material are present in the intestines, the rate of absorption will be accelerated considerably.

1. *Acute poisoning* occurs in two forms. In one, the patient takes in a huge dose of phosphorus vapor or of phosphine by inhalation or by ingestion of the chemical, and dies of cardiac collapse in a few hours, after a stormy clinical course marked by delirium, stupor and coma. The poison evidently enters the blood in such huge quantities that it paralyzes the central nervous system and in such cases gastrointestinal symptoms are not ordinarily prominent.

The more common variety of acute phosphorus poisoning is characterized by severe gastric symptoms such as nausea, thirst, pain in the stomach and vomiting of material which is luminous in the dark. Diarrhea, occasionally phosphorescent, may occur, sometimes with and sometimes without the vomiting. The absorption into the blood is slower and is less overwhelming than in the type described above, and the duration of the clinical course is longer—from one to three days. The victim also shows a varying degree of stupor and prostration and may become unconscious toward the end.

If the patient dies in the acute stage, the necropsy will not show anything unusual, except dark blood and congested organs. The stomach is not corroded, though the folds of the mucous membrane may be reddened. Some consider that this organ is not harmed so much by the direct action of the phosphorus as by its excretion from the gastric mucous membrane. Occasionally the duodenum and jejunum appear reddened and irritated with excretion of a large amount of mucus. In acute cases the stomach contents are usually luminous, and phosphorus can be recovered from them and from the parenchymatous viscera by chemical examination.

2. In cases of *subacute phosphorus poisoning,* the patient may live a few days and survive the gastrointestinal involvement. The phosphorus is absorbed into the blood in fairly large amounts and acts as a protoplasmic poison on the tissues in general. The parenchymatous cells of the liver, kidneys, heart muscle, stomach, diaphragm, voluntary muscles, and other organs are attacked and undergo an intense fatty change. The same process affects the walls of the smaller blood vessels, and multiple small hemorrhages result. The degeneration may be so intense that lipemia occurs from the action of the poison on the liver. In one case glycosuria was present along with lipemia, and this condition was attributed to toxic effects of the poison on the pancreas.

As the victim develops symptoms of subacute phosphorus poisoning, he becomes weak, toxic, bilious, anemic and stuporous, showing many of the signs of an acute yellow atrophy. The liver may be enlarged or it may be smaller than normal, and severe jaundice is usually present. Delirium, convulsions, coma and sudden death from cardiac failure may result. The urine in this stage is decreased in amount, and contains many cleavage products of protein, such as leucine, tyrosine, sarcolactic acid and peptone, the lesion of the liver apparently deranging the protein metabolism in the body. The average duration of the clinical course in fatal cases is from 4 to 14 days.

The liver on postmortem examination is lemon yellow or grayish yellow in color and either smaller or larger than normal, with a marked but variable grade of fatty degeneration present. In some cases the organ is a homogeneous yellow in color with rounded edges, and on microscopic section the cells throughout are loaded with fine fatty globules and swollen, while the general architecture of the organ is preserved. In other cases the liver shows well-defined nutmeg markings, and microscopically there is fatty degeneration and destruction of the liver cells at the periphery of the lobule with many lymphocytes and large round cells containing a granular yellow pigment, while the other parenchyma cells in between show some fatty degeneration but are intact. In the literature, a chronic interstitial hepatitis has been described as the end stage of this type of degeneration. Some livers may show a condition resembling an acute yellow atrophy as they are jaundiced, smaller than normal and have sharp edges; microscopically there is an intense fatty degeneration of all parenchyma cells with varying degrees of destruction so that only the fibrillar framework of the organ is left in places.

The other viscera are grayish yellow in color due to marked fatty degeneration and jaundice; frozen sections of the kidney and heart muscle usually show the cytoplasm of the cells filled with fine fatty droplets. In one case the diaphragm was the seat of a fatty degeneration of the muscle fibers and there was an infiltration of lymphocytes and leukocytes in the interstitial tissue. Numerous small purpuric hemorrhages may occur in the subserous and submucous layers of different parts of the body, and also in the loose connective tissues such as the mediastinum or the periaortic tissues. Sometimes hemorrhages may occur from the pregnant uterus because of fatty degeneration in the placenta. In rare instances less frequent complications are noted such as toxic neuritis, localized gangrene of the skin, and indolent noncharacteristic ulcers in the intestines.

The fatal dose of phosphorus is hard to estimate, but 1.5 grains have caused poisoning in the case of an adult. The poison is mainly eliminated by vomiting or through the intestinal tract. The portion which is absorbed is oxidized into innocuous phosphates. The stomach contents, liver, kidneys or other parenchymatous viscera are saved for toxicologic examination. The intestine and its content may be valuable if the victim has died a day or so after the ingestion of the phosphorus. Phosphorus is more easily isolated and identified in the acute cases, but with the recently developed methods of analysis successful results have been obtained with the subacute cases, though the problem of toxicologic analysis is more difficult with that type.

The best treatment of phosphorus poisoning is to wash out the stomach with the stomach tube, using a solution of potassium permanganate of 0.5 to 1.0 per cent to speed the oxidation of the toxic element into innocuous phosphates. A solution of copper sulfate (0.25 gm. in half a pint of water, or 2 per cent of the official preparation of hydrogen peroxide may be used). All these mixtures should be removed from the stomach as soon as possible. The bowel should be evacuated with magnesium sulfate. Symptomatic treatment and stimulation should be used when necessary. The treatment should be started as soon after the poisoning as possible.

Phosphine, PH_3, is a poisonous, inflammable gas which has an odor of decaying fish. It is produced in small quantities in the manufacture of acetylene as the chief source of acetylene—calcium carbide—contains some calcium phosphide as an impurity. Most of the cases of poisoning have occurred from phosphine which was generated by the effect of moisture on ferrosilicon. A few instances were reported of chemists who were overcome during the process of generating phosphine in the laboratory.

The chief action of phosphine is on the central nervous system, which first is stimulated and then paralyzed. The patients usually show dyspnea, oppression of the chest, cough, headache, tremors, convulsions, vertigo, ringing in the ears, weakness and death. The blood is red in color and mainly fluid. Inflammation of the respiratory tract, edema of the lungs and fatty degeneration of the viscera are observed. The treatment and toxicology are similar to that of elemental phosphorus.

3. A *chronic type of poisoning* formerly was prevalent in match factories, which was probably the result of the continual inhalation of phosphorus vapor over a long period of time. The process would start in a carious tooth, and then spread, causing a severe necrosis of the jaw bone known as phossy jaw. Sometimes it was accompanied by other toxic manifestations such as anemia, diarrhea and jaundice. Prevention was the only means of combating this menace, and consisted mostly in employing general sanitary measures, such as dispelling the poisonous vapors in the workroom by a constant draft of air, and caring for the employee's teeth by the constant use of sodium bicarbonate as a mouth wash. Since nontoxic compounds of phosphorus have been used in place of the white poisonous form, phossy jaw has become rare.

Boric Acid and Borax. Borax, $Na_2B_4O_7$. 10 H_2O, is a white, odorless substance which is used as a cleanser and as an antiseptic in douches. Boric acid, H_3BO_3, is a white powder having a bitter taste, which in saturated solution is employed in medicine as an antiseptic wash for the conjunctival sac and abscess cavities. Borax and boric acid have been added to foods as preservatives but their continued use may be dangerous, since they have a cumulative effect on the system.

Most poisonings are accidental. Borax, for example, is kept in the household medicine chest with other white crystals and it may be mistaken for some other substance and swallowed inadvertently. It has been ingested with suicidal intent, and as an abortifacient. The symptoms of acute borax poisoning are salivation, diarrhea, vomiting, nausea, colic-like pain in the abdomen, and other signs of gastrointestinal irritation. Some of the poison may be absorbed and cause depression of the respiratory center with collapse. If the drug is absorbed in smaller quantities, it may produce a few symptoms which indicate that the organs of elimination, the skin and kidneys, are most affected. Blood, albumin and a large number of tubular casts appear in the urine. The skin may show a large variety of irritative lesions similar to eczema. There may be a toxic action on the central nervous system with depression, delirium, cyanosis and fatal collapse. The victim may live a few hours (in one instance 3½ hours), or he may survive several days. The fatal dose is difficult to estimate, but in one case death was caused by an ounce of borax.

Boric acid poisoning has occurred occasionally because of its medical use in flushing out abscess cavities or in lavage of the stomach. Seven fatal cases of acute boric acid poisoning are recorded in the Office of the Chief Medical Examiner of New York City. These occurred in dehydrated newborn infants from the accidental administration of saturated boric acid solution by hypodermoclysis, under the impression that it was normal saline solution; and in infants several days old from absorption of boric acid powder or salve used to treat a diaper rash. There was rapid, profound intoxication and death after two days. At necropsy large areas of exfoliative dermatitis were distributed over the body, and tubular degeneration of the kidneys was noted; the most striking lesion, which was found in all three cases, was a cystitis characterized by a severe hemorrhagic edema of the submucous layer of the bladder (Figs. 31-9 and 31-10). The fatal dose of boric acid is about 3 to 6 gm. in infants and 15 gm. in the case of an adult. The length of the clinical course is the same as for borax.

A subacute case of poisoning was encountered in an infant of four months who was treated for an extensive diaper rash over a period of weeks by local application of boric acid ointment; at autopsy fatty degeneration of the liver and parenchymatous degeneration of the kidney tubules was encountered, and boric acid was recovered by toxicologic examination of the liver.

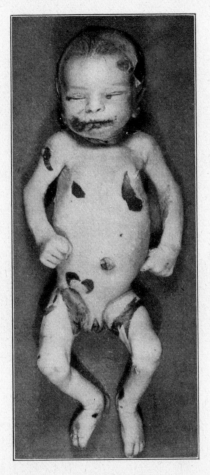

Fig. 31-9. Boric Acid Poisoning. Exfoliative Dermatitis.

Patchy exfoliation of epidermis in case of poisoning with boric acid, accidentally administered by subcutaneous injection. Death after two days.

The treatment of either borax or boric acid poisoning is thorough washing out of the stomach, general catharsis and symptomatic treatment. In fatal cases the stomach contents and parenchymatous viscera are used for toxicologic examination.

Tellurium. Tellurium, Te, is a substance allied to sulfur and is present in the ores of different metals such as copper, lead, iron or silver, either free or in the form of telluride. When such ores are purified, fumes which contain hydrogen telluride are formed and sometimes inhaled; or the dust from some of the ores may contain tellurates and tellurous oxide, and may also be inhaled. When they come in contact with living cells these compounds are changed into elemental tellurium and excreted in the feces. A small amount may be absorbed and be converted into methyl telluride which gives a garlic odor to the breath and is excreted in the urine. A toxic nonlethal poisoning is produced, the victim complaining of nausea, metallic taste in the mouth, fetid garlicky odor of the breath, dry skin, constipation, and suppression of saliva, sweat and gastric juice. Tellurium may be recovered from the urine and feces. Preventive measures should be taken to dispose of the injurious fumes and prevent their inhalation. The treatment is to promote elimination through the feces and the urine.

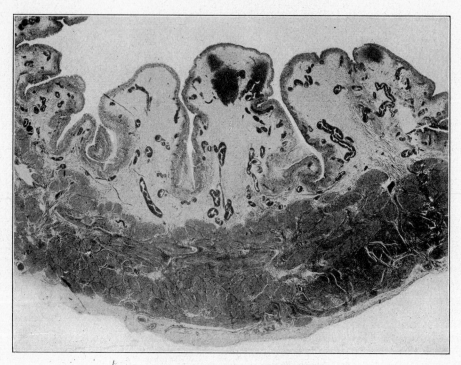

Fig. 31-10. Acute Cystitis in Boric Acid Poisoning.

The bladder shows marked edema and hemorrhage in the submucosa. Low power photomicrograph. A similar bladder lesion was found in two other infants who also received subcutaneous injections of boric acid solution in place of saline.

Selenium. Selenium compounds are used in glass manufacture, in making plastics, fireproofing for electric cables, pigments, chemicals and material used in many other industries. When inhaled or absorbed through the skin, in the form of dust or vapor generated in industrial processes, selenium is converted into methyl selenide, and produces nonlethal toxic symptoms with garlicky odor to the breath, pain in the abdomen and vomiting, symptoms suggesting hay fever, a metallic taste in the mouth, a coated tongue and a slight anemia. Selenium is found in the urine in these cases and is considered a sign of absorption of the toxic material, as it is not found normally in the urine in any appreciable quantity.

Selenium also occurs in some soils, most notably in the great plains of the western states, where it is taken up by the wheat and the other vegetation. Domestic cattle feeding on such provender develop alkali disease, characterized by abdominal pain, affections of the eyes, roughened coat, loss of hair, stunted growth, inability to reproduce, difficulty in walking and other signs. Selenium is also present in some insecticides and may find its way into plants through such sprays. While the domestic animals are affected in these areas, the human inhabitants do not develop selenium poisoning even though they excrete enough selenium in the urine to induce toxic symptoms in laboratory animals.

Sodium Silicate. Sodium silicate, $Na_2Si_4O_9$, known as water glass, is formed by the fusion of quartz, sodium carbonate in dry state and charcoal. The resulting produce is soluble in water and is used as a preservative. One case of poisoning is described by Eichhorst, concerning a man who drank 6.75 fluid ounces of this substance in solution mistaking it for wine. He recovered, but showed severe gastro-intestinal irritation and high temperature.

REFERENCES

Aub, J. C. Lead Poisoning, from Cecil's Textbook of Medicine, Philadelphia, W. B. Saunders Co., 1951, pp. 518-522.

—— Fairhall, L. T., Minot, A. S., and Reznikoff, P. Lead Poisoning, Baltimore, Williams & Wilkins Co., 1926.

Baker, M. H., and others. Sudden death and mercurial diuretics, J.A.M.A., 119:1001, 1942.

Belknap, E. L. Lead poisoning, Indust. Med., 9:505, 1940; J.A.M.A., 104:205, 1935.

Brandes, W. W. Nickel carbonyl poisoning, J.A.M.A., 102:1204, 1934.

Cleaveland, S. H. A case of poisoning by lithium, J.A.M.A., 60:722, 1913.

Corcoran, A. C., and others. Lithium poisoning from the use of salt substitutes, J.A.M.A., 139:685, 1949.

Council on Pharmacy and Chemistry, Report of the Council. "BAL" (British antilewisite) in the treatment of arsenic and mercury poisoning, J.A.M.A., 131:824, 1946.

DeGraff, A. C., and Nadler, J. E. A review of the toxic manifestations of mercurial diuretics in man, J.A.M.A., 119:1006, 1942.

Dudley, H. C. Selenium as a potential industrial hazard, Pub. Health Rep., 53:281, 1938.

Editorial. Chronic fluorine intoxication, J.A.M.A., 123:150, 1943.

Editorial. Deaths following the use of "Analbis" suppositories, J.A.M.A., 133:852, 1947.

Eichhorst, H. Ueber Vergiftung mit Wasserglas, Schweiz. med. Wchnschr., 1:1081, 1920.

Falconer, E. H., and Epstein, N. N. Purpura hemorrhagica following neoarsphenamine and bismarsen therapy, Arch. Int. Med., 65:1158, 1940.

Fisher, R. C. Metallic poisoning simulating acute surgical abdomen, Am. J. Surg., 26:175, 1934.

Frant, S., and Kleeman, I. "Cadmium" food poisoning, J.A.M.A., 117:86, 1941.

Gettler, A. O., and Norris, C. Poisoning from drinking radium water, J.A.M.A., 100:400, 1933.

Good. An experimental study of lithium, Am. J. M. Sc., 125:273, 1903.

Goodman, L., and Gilman, A. The Pharmocological Basis of Therapeutics, New York, The Macmillan Co., 1941.

Hanlon, L. W., and others. Lithium chloride as a substitute for sodium chloride in the diet, J.A.M.A., 139:688, 1949.

Holland, J. W. Inorganic Poisons, from Peterson, Haines and Webster, Legal Medicine and Toxicology, Philadelphia, W. B. Saunders Co., 1923, vol. II, pp. 123-290.

Longcope, W. T., and Luetscher, J. A., Jr. Clinical use of 2.3. dimercaptopropanol (BAL), J. Clin. Investigation, 25:557, 1948.

Martland, H. S., Brodkin, H. A., and Martland, H. S., Jr. Occupational beryllium poisoning in New Jersey, J. M. Soc. New Jersey, 45:5, 1948.

—— Radium Poisoning, from Cecil's Textbook of Medicine, Philadelphia, W. B. Saunders Co., 1947, pp. 582-587.

—— Conlon, P., and Knef, J. P. Some unrecognized dangers in the use and handling of radioactive substances, J.A.M.A., 85:1769, 1925.

Munch, J. C. Human thallotoxicosis, J.A.M.A., 102:1929, 1934.

Norris, C., and Gettler, A. O. Poisoning by tetra-ethyl lead, J.A.M.A., 85:818, 1925.

Oliver, T. Plumbism and nephritis, Brit. M. J., 1:284, 1934. A review of Nye, L. J. J. Chronic Nephritis and Plumbism, Sydney, Australia, Angus and Robertson, 1933.

Petri, E. Vergiftungen, from Henke and Lubarsch, Berlin, Julius Springer, 1930, vol. X.

Reports of the Office of the Chief Medical Examiner in the City of New York from 1918 to 1951.

Simon, S. D., and Iglauer, A. Death following mapharsen therapy, Am. J. Syph., Gonor. & Ven. Dis., 20:583, 1936.

Smith, M. I. Chronic endemic selenium poisoning, J.A.M.A., 116:562, 1941.

Sollman, T. Manual of Pharmacology, 4th ed., Philadelphia, W. B. Saunders Co., 1932.

Umber. Quecksilberemblien der lebenden Lunge, Med. Klin., 19:35, 1923; 22:1279, 1926.

Van Ordstrand, H. S., Hughes, R., DeNardi, J. M., and Carmody, M. G. Beryllium poisoning, J.A.M.A., 129:1084, 1945.

Walsh, E. N., and Becker, S. W. Use of bismuth compounds in syphilotherapy, J.A.M.A., 116:484, 1941.

Webster, R. W. Legal Medicine and Toxicology, Philadelphia, W. B. Saunders Co., 1930.

Weinstein, I. Fatalities associated with Analbis suppositories, Correspondence, J.A.M.A., 133:962, 1947.

Windmueller, E. Chronic poisoning from mixture of potassium nitrate and sulphur, J.A.M.A., 77:858, 1921.

ATOMIC ENERGY

Editorial. Effects of atomic bomb explosions at Hiroshima and Nagasaki, J.A.M.A., 131:598, 1946.

Le Roy, G. V. The medical sequelae of the atomic bomb explosion, J.A.M.A., 134:1143, 1947.

Ley, W. Inside the Atom, The Magazine of the American Museum of Natural History, 14:350, 1945.

Smyth, H. D. Atomic Energy, Princeton, N. J., Princeton University Press, 1945.

BERYLLIUM

Coakley, W. A., and others. Granuloma of skin at site of injury by a fluorescent bulb, J.A.M.A., 139:1147, 1949.

Grier, R. S., and others. Skin lesions in persons exposed to beryllium compounds, J. Indust. Hyg. & Toxicol., 30:228, 1948.

Hardy, H. L., and Tabershaw, I. R. Delayed chemical pneumonitis occurring in workers exposed to beryllium compounds, J. Indust. Hyg. & Toxicol., 28:197, 1946.

Martland, H. S., Brodkin, H. A., and Martland, H. S., Jr. Occupational beryllium poisoning in New Jersey, J. M. Soc. New Jersey, 45:5, 1948.

Nichol, A. D., and Dominguez, R. Cutaneous granuloma from accidental contamination with beryllium phosphors, J.A.M.A., 140:855, 1949.

Van Ordstrand, H. S., and others. Beryllium poisoning, J.A.M.A., 129:1084, 1945.

CHROMIUM

Editorial. Cancer of the lung in chromate workers, J.A.M.A., 138:823, 1948.

Hueper, W. C. Occupational Tumors and Allied Diseases, Springfield, Ill., Charles C Thomas, Publisher, 1942.

Machle, W., and Gregorius, F. Cancer of the respiratory system in the United States chromate producing industry, Pub. Health Rep., 63:1114, 1948.

Pascale, L. R., and others. Chromium intoxication, with special reference to hepatic injury, J.A.M.A., 149:1385, 1952.

32

Organic Poisons: Volatile

Many poisons are organic chemical compounds, or compounds derived from the different structural combinations of carbon, nitrogen, oxygen, hydrogen, sulfur and phosphorus which make up the constituents of the organic world. Toxicologically this category is divided into volatile poisons which are isolated from the organs and secretions of the body by distilling the material over or in steam and collecting the toxic chemical in the distillate, and nonvolatile poisons which are extracted from the organs and secretions by the means of immiscible solvents. Chemically organic compounds are subdivided into the aliphatic group in which the carbon radicals are joined in open chain combinations, and into the aromatic group in which the combination of carbon atoms, or carbon and nitrogen atoms are joined in the form of a closed ring. Both aliphatic and aromatic groups are subdivisions of the volatile and nonvolatile poisons.

VOLATILE ALIPHATIC COMPOUNDS

The volatile poisons of the open chain type are readily absorbed, exert a profound depressing and paralyzing effect on the vital centers in the medulla, and occasionally affect some of the other tissues in the body. The lower hydrocarbons possess only slight toxicity, but when other radicals such as the hydroxyl, aldehyde, acid, nitro and halogen groups are substituted for the hydrogen atoms, the poisonous properties of the chemical nucleus may be increased. The acid and aldehyde derivatives of the less complicated hydrocarbons are irritant and even corrosive, as for example, oxalic acid and formaldehyde. The addition of a halogen radical to the nucleus, as in methyl chloride or chloroform, enhances the toxicity of the resulting compound materially. With a few exceptions, the volatile aliphatic compounds are eliminated from the body in about 24 hours if the victim survives that length of time after the administration of the poison.

Methyl Alcohol. Methyl alcohol, CH_3OH, is a light colorless liquid with a faint aromatic odor, boiling at a temperature of 66° C. It is produced during the destructive distillation of wood or molasses. Purified methyl alcohol is marketed commercially as Columbian spirits, colonial spirits, eagle spirits or wood naphtha. The crude product contains many impurities such as furfurol, methyl and dimethyl acetate, allyl alcohol and ethyl dimethyl ketone. Methyl alcohol is used as an adulterant of ethyl alcohol in methylated spirit, as a solvent of varnishes, and has been used in the preparation of essences, in Jamaica ginger and in peppermint.

Poisoning by methyl alcohol before 1898 was uncommon, but since that time its incidence has increased, especially during the years of the Federal Prohibition Act. In that period a large number of cases resulted from the sale of beverages adulterated with this substance. This is a criminal offense according to the laws of New York State, and if death occurs from such a transaction, the vendor of the poisoned liquor can be prosecuted for technical homicide. In other cases the victim purchased methyl alcohol as such and drank it regardless of consequences. Such

781

poisonings are usually sporadic, but occasionally a large number of deaths occur when a group of individuals make a joint purchase and all imbibe it. Many of the indigent were accustomed to drink "smoke," a cloudy fluid obtained by mixing water and solid alcohol, a substance used for heating purposes, which contains a little methyl alcohol. After the repeal of the Eighteenth Amendment, there was a distinct decrease in the incidence of fatal methyl alcohol poisonings in New York City, except at those times when the lower grade of hard liquor beverages rose in price beyond the purchasing power of their users, many substituting wood alcohol for whisky during those periods. Inhalation of vapors from shellac, from the manufacture of essences, and from the application of rubbing solutions to the skin has also produced methyl alcohol poisoning. In the Office of the Chief Medical Examiner in New York City about 23 cases of methyl alcohol poisoning of the accidental or technical homicidal type are recorded per year, but with a wide yearly variation; for example 74 cases were recorded in 1930 as compared with 1 in 1934. Seventeen cases of suicide due to the ingestion of methyl alcohol were noted in New York City in the 33 year period from 1918 to 1951.

Methyl alcohol poisoning causes a primary depression of the central nervous system with weakness, nausea, vomiting, headache, epigastric pain, dyspnea and cyanosis. The symptoms may come on suddenly about one half hour after the poison is ingested, and may be followed by stupor, coma, delirium, convulsions, cold clammy skin, subnormal temperature and death from paralysis of the respiratory center; in this period a small quantity of the drug is excreted unchanged through the lungs into the expired air. In other cases the effects of the poison may not appear for 26 hours or more, at which time the patient is suddenly stricken and death may ensue. These effects are attributed in part to the depressing action of the drug on the central nervous system, in part to cerebral edema, and in part to acidosis produced by the slow oxidation of wood alcohol to formaldehyde and formic acid in the system. The toxic substances are retained in the body for a few days and explain the prolonged coma and other neurologic symptoms which are prevalent during that period. Methyl alcohol is more toxic than ethyl alcohol as its products of decomposition are more harmful to the human organism and their action more prolonged. In a clinical case the urine may be sent to the toxicologist, who may be able to demonstrate an excess of formic acid in that excretion; this finding would be good confirmatory evidence for suspecting methyl alcohol poisoning.

One of the most distressing sequelae of methyl alcohol poisoning is the bilateral impairment of vision, either as an early or a late complication of an acute attack or as the result of the chronic absorption of the drug by ingestion or inhalation. The symptoms start within a few hours or a few days with discomfort and photophobia, followed by blurred vision and even total blindness in 10 to 15 hours. After this, the patient may recover some of his sight but the blindness may return in a few weeks and be permanent. This condition is referable to the action of the poison on the ganglion cells of the retina with subsequent atrophy of the optic nerves. Where the blindness is not total, there is considerable contraction of the field of vision and an impairment of the color sense.

The signs at necropsy are those of any other depressant of the central nervous system. The blood is fluid and abundant and varies in color from a dark to a lighter red. The skin is cyanotic and the viscera are congested, especially the brain. The lungs are hyperemic and edematous. Congestion of the mucous membrane of the urinary bladder may occur. The mucous membranes of the stomach and duodenum may not show any noteworthy change, but in some cases are congested with small scattered hemorrhagic dots in the submucous layer; microscopically the blood vessels are engorged and contain red blood cells and polymorphonuclear leukocytes. Different stages of necrosis have been noted in the ganglion cells of the brain, spinal cord and retina by microscopic investigation. The pathologic lesions are not characteristic, and reliance must be placed on the toxicologic examination for establishing the diagnosis. As a rule there is no suggestive odor to the organs in cases of acute methyl alcohol poisoning, except occasionally a faint aromatic odor may be detected about some of the viscera or blood. The material usually saved for toxicologic examination consists of stomach contents, brain, parenchymatous viscera and urine. The elimination of methyl alcohol or its decomposition products, formaldehyde and formic acid, from the body is sometimes delayed, so that materials should be reserved for chemical examination, even when the victim has survived the administration of the poison several days.

The fatal dose varies in the individual case. Death has been caused by 30 to 60 ml., and blindness has followed the ingestion of 15 ml. of methyl alcohol. The patient may die in 24 to 36 hours or he may survive for two to four or more days.

The treatment is to wash out the stomach, and to introduce into that viscus a 4 per cent solution of sodium bicarbonate to combat acidosis and gastric irritation. Chew and his collaborators recommend intravenous injection of a sodium lactate preparation to alleviate acidosis. Shock should be treated by external warmth. Intravenous injection of normal saline solution or Ringer's solution may be employed to promote elimination. Stimulation with camphor or caffeine may be necessary on occasion. Cerebral congestion may be treated by the injection intravenously of hypertonic glucose solution, or the use of magnesium sulfate as a cathartic. The rest of the treatment is mainly symptomatic.

Ethyl Alcohol. Ethyl alcohol, C_2H_5OH, is formed by the fermentation of various carbohydrates in grain, fruit or flowers, and from materials subjected to this process it may be isolated by distillation. In the pure state, alcohol is a colorless, transparent, volatile liquid with an aromatic odor, boiling at 78° C. It is the principal constituent of alcoholic beverages, occurring in different proportions in each type: in beer, 2 to 6 per cent; in light wines, 7 to 12 per cent; in reinforced wines, 15 to 20 per cent; in brandy, whisky, rum and gin, 45 to 60 per cent.

Poisoning by ethyl alcohol is common and is usually accidental. It occurs when an individual drinks to excess and absorbs more than the system will bear. A few cases have been described in children who have imbibed from their parents' stock. Occasionally, toxic effects have followed the unintentional injection of an alcoholic fluid by clysis into a dehydrated patient. The authors have seen a case in which 120 ml. of 70 per cent ethyl alcohol was injected under the skin of a newborn infant in place of normal saline solution; death occurred 48 hours later and large amounts of alcohol were recovered from the organs.

In the Reports of the Office of the Chief Medical Examiner in the City of New York from 1918 to 1941 deaths from alcohol poisoning showed an average of 480 a year. Starting in 1918, the year in which the National Prohibition Amendment became active, the number of cases was 87 and the yearly total gradually mounted up to 794 in 1931. After the repeal in 1933, the yearly total sank to 424 in 1941. From 1941 to 1951 the average rose to 461. This yearly average includes cases of deaths from acute alcoholism and chronic alcoholism, for the two are frequently combined in the same case and are difficult to separate statistically. In many cases in which death occurred from other causes, alcoholism was present; it was observed in about 40 per cent of deaths from homicidal, suicidal and accidental violence. Homicidal and suicidal cases from ethyl alcohol are rare; homicidal cases were not present in the Reports, and five cases classified as suicides occurred in the 24 year interval from 1918 to 1941.

The local action of alcohol is that of an irritant to the skin and mucous membranes, and if swallowed in concentrated form and in sufficient quantity, it will cause an acute inflammation of the stomach. It is absorbed directly from that organ and produces a rapid general action on the system in a few minutes. First it is carried by the blood to the liver, where much of it is oxidized into carbon dioxide and water, while the remainder passes through to the rest of the organs. Most of it is changed by the tissues, but part is excreted unchanged in the urine and in the expired air. Its chief toxic effect is produced on the central nervous system by its absorption into the brain tissue where it acts directly on the neurons. The cerebrum first is affected, and then the cerebellum, spinal cord and medulla, with death resulting finally from paralysis of the respiratory center.

The symptoms of acute intoxication are ushered in by a primary stage of euphoria and exhilaration, soon followed by more advanced emotional manifestations, such as sentimentality, pugnacity or argumentativeness. As more alcohol is absorbed, muscular incoördination, ataxia, incoherence of speech, nausea and vomiting supervene. In the final stage, the patient passes into a stupor with complete relaxation, partial anesthesia, cold clammy skin, accelerated heart rate, pupils normal or dilated, slow and stertorous respirations, deep coma and finally death.

If the intoxication is not too pronounced, a patient may recover in a few hours In fatal cases the effects of the intoxication may be complicated by other conditions which may contribute to the death of the patient. If he is suffering from a pre-existing natural disease, like coronary arteriosclerosis, the added strain of an alcoholic debauch may be more than his system can sustain and he may die suddenly. Similarly if a surgical operation is necessary on a person in a state of acute alcoholism, the procedure is more hazardous than on a normal individual, especially if the patient is a chronic alcoholic; such people take general anesthetics poorly. An intoxicated individual also is likely to incur misadventures of all sorts, such as falling asleep in a cramped position and strangling or smothering himself inadvertently, choking on food which he has aspirated into his air passages, or blundering into some sort of injury (Chapters 10 to 20). Trauma is especially dangerous to an alcoholic person because his vitality is in a lowered condition and not in a fit state to overcome the effects of shock.

Death may occur in a number of different forms while the victim is in an acute alcoholic state. A few die suddenly, shortly after the start of the intoxication during the height of alcohol absorption, but most stop breathing about 5 to 12 hours after the coma begins when the peak of the absorption is passed and the alcohol is being eliminated from the system. Sometimes death is delayed for several days, the patient succumbing to a bronchopneumonia, or dying in the midst of convulsions. The fatal dose is difficult to ascertain, but a concentration of 0.7 per cent to 1.0 per cent in the blood is considered sufficient to cause death; in general, this amount is found after the ingestion of about 1 to 2 pints of whisky or brandy. In some of the fatal cases another toxic chemical may be present in the beverage, such as methyl alcohol, fusel oil, pyridine or carbon tetrachloride, and may be the lethal agent or at least may have contributed to death.

The postmortem findings are not characteristic. All the organs are congested and the blood is fluid, dark red in color and abundant. The stomach may be congested, reddened and inflamed, or it may not show any lesions worthy of note. The viscera, brain and blood usually have an alcoholic odor, sometimes characteristic of the beverage which has been imbibed.

The treatment is to evacuate the stomach by the tube or by emetics. Stimulation, usually by camphor or caffeine, may be required. In some instances, warmth should be applied to the body to combat shock.

The rapidity with which alcohol is oxidized in the system insures that it will disappear from the body during the first 24 hours after the ingestion of the poison. After that time, it would not be possible by toxicologic analysis to obtain any of the alcohol responsible for the intoxication. The organ most commonly used for examination is the brain, but the stomach contents or the liver should be kept for possible tests.

The criterion for intoxication is the finding of a considerable concentration of alcohol in the brain. In those cases in which the brain is not available, the liver may be used as its alcoholic content closely parallels that of the brain. The quantitative correlation between states of intoxication and the amounts of alcohol found in the brain is given in Chapter 46. The finding of alcohol in the stomach contents alone without its presence in the brain simply indicates its ingestion but does not prove that a state of intoxication necessarily existed; occasionally after injury, alcoholic beverages have been administered to counteract shock. In cases where death does not occur until more than a day after an alcoholic debauch, the organs will not reveal alcohol on chemical analysis.

CHRONIC ALCOHOLISM. The habitual use of alcohol to excess produces a slow degeneration of the organism which is manifested mostly in the parenchymatous organs and the central nervous system. Some cases develop a fatty infiltration of the liver to such a degree that this viscus reaches a weight of 3,000 gm. or more, is a light yellowish-red in color and has rounded edges (Fig. 32-1). On microscopic examination, the liver cells are loaded with fat droplets of large and small size which may displace the nucleus, and normal cells may not be demonstrable in the section. In some cases, the fatty infiltration may be accompanied by a growth of fibrous tissue and a chronic interstitial hepatitis of varying degree may supervene. Fatty infiltration is also evident in the wall of the right ventricle of the heart and may be accompanied by atrophy of the muscle fibers. There may be a disproportionate increase of adipose tissue in the retroperitoneal tissues and in the omentum and mesentery. The tubules of the kidneys and the myocardium in a few cases may show fine fatty granules in the parenchymatous cells. The patient shows indications of chronic ill health in a bloated face, reddened nose, and muscular atrophy especially of the upper extremities. Atrophy of the cerebral tissue, pial edema, relative widening of the ventricles of the brain and thickening of the meninges are frequent findings. At autopsy the diagnosis of chronic alcoholism is often made from the appearance of the organs, which show the above degenerative changes, the fatty infiltration of the liver being especially suggestive. A minor degenerative change which sometimes is present in advanced cases is atrophy of the tubules of the testes, the destruction of spermatogenesis, the appearance of vacuolized epithelial elements in the tubules and sometimes increase of the interstitial cells. In a few cases an acute hemorrhagic pancreatitis may develop (Fig. 32-1).

Patients suffering from chronic alcoholism are likely to develop hepatic insufficiency, attended by severe jaundice, and a prothrombin deficiency as indicated by a tendency to bleed readily in the subcutaneous tissues, and they are susceptible to various intercurrent infections, such as lobar pneumonia, acute enterocolitis and septic lesions of the skin. Many chronic cases show symptoms referable to the central nervous system even when degeneration of the parenchymatous viscera is not marked. Delirium tremens, Korsakoff's syndrome, polyneuritis with degeneration of the nerve fibers and atrophy of the muscles, beri-beri-like and pellagroid

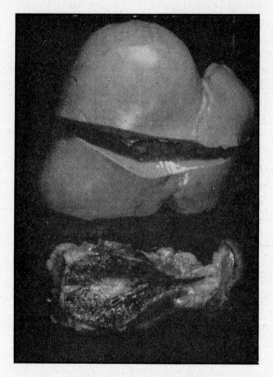

Fig. 32-1. Enlarged Fatty Liver and Acute Hemorrhagic Pancreatitis in Chronic Alcoholism.

Such a liver is a frequent finding. Acute pancreatitis is a not uncommon complication following an acute episode of prolonged drinking in the chronic alcoholic.

symptoms from vitamin deficiency (inadequate food intake because of alcoholic habits), epileptiform attacks and actual alcoholic insanity occur and cause death. Many of these cases die in the midst of a convulsion which accompanies an attack of delirium tremens, often precipitated after trauma or after a surgical operation. Chronic alcoholics are not good operative risks because they require a large amount of ether or other general anesthetic to obtain the requisite degree of anesthesia, often an amount dangerous to life.

Diethylene Glycol. Diethylene glycol is a volatile liquid employed as a constituent of antifreeze mixtures used in motor cars. Its chemical formula is HO CH_2. $CH_2.O$ .CH_2. CH_2OH. Rarely, accidental poisoning by this substance occurs when individuals drink antifreeze thinking that they are imbibing ethyl alcohol. Helpern has investigated two deaths of this type.

The victims were young Negro males in the early twenties, occupants of an institution for the treatment of drug addiction, who drank an undetermined amount of antifreeze mixture and after one to three days complained of headache, nausea, vomiting, generalized abdominal pain, pain in the kidney regions, anuria and uremia. A decapsulation of the right kidney was performed on both patients to relieve the pain. One patient collapsed at the time of operation and died 90 minutes later, about 11 days after he had taken the poison. The autopsy disclosed congested and succulent organs, a bronchopneumonia, and large swollen kidneys with a pale gray cortex and slightly darker pyramids. The liver appeared normal aside from the congestion. Microscopically the convoluted tubules of the kidney were lined by big hydropic cells which narrowed the lumen to a mere slit. Some tubules contained rusty blood pigment. Other tubules were filled with polymorphonuclear leukocytes, and some contained translucent fan-shaped or wheat sheaf-shaped crystals. There was an infiltration of round cells around the glomeruli and the glomeruli contained a few leukocytes. The pyramids were congested but otherwise not remarkable.

The other victim was operated upon 14 days after the poisoning and survived the operation 12 days, finally dying of uremia. The autopsy findings were similar to those in the other case with the exception that there were fewer hydropic cells in the convoluted tubules, many of which were lined by low epithelium. There was also a suppurative pyelonephritis involving pyramids and cortex. There was a fibrinous pericarditis, and hemorrhages on the septum of the left ventricle, a patchy hemorrhagic cystitis and a hypostatic bronchopneumonia. The liver did not show any noticeable pathologic changes.

Poisoning by Elixir of Sulphanilamide Massengil with 76 deaths occurred during 1937, shortly after the preparation was put on the market. Chemical analysis revealed that the elixir was a 10 per cent solution of sulfanilamide in 72 per cent diethylene glycol, to which coloring matter and flavoring agents had been added. These cases of poisoning were reviewed by Geiling and Cannon.

The elixir, in doses of 1½ to 6 ounces, caused nausea, vomiting, abdominal cramps, dizziness, attacks of diarrhea, and pain in the kidney region and abdomen. The onset of the symptoms occurred about 24 hours after medication in most instances, but in one case developed immediately after the drug was taken. Oliguria and anuria followed, then progressive unconsciousness, slight puffiness of the face, slight jaundice, varying degrees of pulmonary edema, subnormal temperature, slow pulse and respirations, edema of the dependent parts of the body, marked albuminuria with casts, a marked elevation of blood nonprotein nitrogen and death in two to seven days after the onset of the anuria.

The autopsy findings in 12 cases revealed enlarged pale livers with light colored areas around the central veins which microscopically showed a massive hydropic degeneration of the cells with shrunken pyknotic nuclei; around the margin of this area there was a slight amount of fatty degeneration and leukocytic infiltration. In one case the liver was small weighing 900 gm. and had a tawny appearance. The kidneys were enlarged, pale, swollen and flabby; in eight cases there were large areas of cortical necrosis, accompanied by recent hemorrhage, while hyaline thrombi were present in the smaller arteries and veins and a few of the glomerular coils. The cells of the convoluted tubules of the kidneys showed a massive hydropic degeneration with pyknotic nuclei, probably caused by glycol which is a hygroscopic agent. There was only a slight fatty degeneration of the kidney epithelium on the borders of the hydropic areas. Many of the collecting tubules contained hyaline casts, red blood cells and leukocytes. The other pathologic findings consisted of congestion and hemorrhage in the stomach and intestines, ascites, hydrothorax, hydropericardium, edema of the lungs, and a bronchopneumonia.

Higher Aliphatic Alcohols. Many of the higher aliphatic alcohols like propyl alcohol ($CH_2OH. CH_2. CH_3$) and isopropyl alcohol ($CH_3. CHOH.CH_3$) have a poisonous action similar to ethyl alcohol but are more toxic. Fatal cases are uncommon inasmuch as these substances are not used as generally as ethyl or methyl alcohol. One case was encountered of a 48 year old man who was found dead on a playground with a pint bottle of rubbing alcohol, or isopropyl alcohol, in his possession, one third empty. The autopsy disclosed fluid blood in the heart, congestion of the viscera, slight reddening of the gastric mucous membrane and a characteristic odor of the alcohol from the organs and blood. Toxicologic examination of the brain demonstrated the presence of isopropyl alcohol in large amounts. The general features of industrial poisoning from these compounds are discussed on page 897.

Amyl alcohol-tertiary or dimethyl ethyl carbinol, $(CH_3)_2:COH. CH_2 CH_3$, is a colorless liquid with an odor similar to camphor. It is employed occasionally in medicine as a hypnotic. In poisonous doses it produces deep coma and is a severe circulatory and respiratory depressant. Fatal cases have occurred; in one the drug was administered by rectum.

Fusel oil consists of iso-amyl alcohol, $(CH_3)_2:CH.CH_2.CH_2OH$, an isomer, methyl-ethyl-carbin-carbinol, and a number of the other higher alcohols. It is an oily mixture of bitter taste, and is about five times as toxic as ethyl alcohol. It occurs in many crude brandies and whiskies but rarely in amounts large enough to have toxicologic significance as far as such beverages are concerned. Fusel oil is one of the routine reagents in chemical laboratory work, and is used as a solvent for paint.

The vapors of fusel oil are unpleasant and when inhaled cause irritation of the respiratory passages, coughing, dyspnea and headache. If a large amount is ingested, severe intoxication occurs, with deep coma, cyanosis and respiratory collapse. In the presence of ethyl alcohol, the toxic action of fusel oil is enhanced because it is absorbed more rapidly.

Paraldehyde. Paraldehyde, $(CH_3CHO)_3$, is a colorless liquid, transparent, with a characteristic odor and a sharp taste. It is formed by adding sulfuric acid to acetaldehyde at ordinary temperature and polymerizing it into paraldehyde. This drug has a soporific and quieting effect on the central nervous system and is used extensively as a hypnotic in the treatment of acute and chronic alcoholism.

Occasionally, cases of acute poisoning are produced by a large overdose of the drug. Unconsciousness occurs rapidly and lasts for several hours. Nausea, vomiting, headache and dizziness are present in some cases. Death may supervene from paralysis of the respiratory center but fatal cases are not common. During the 33 year interval from 1918 to 1951 the records of the Office of the Chief Medical Examiner in New York City listed 49 cases of paraldehyde poisoning as accidental and 13 cases as suicidal.

The fatal dose is uncertain; in one recorded case, death was caused in about four hours by 25 ml., while in other instances large amounts have been taken with impunity. The drug is excreted in part by the lung and its penetrating odor may be detected on the breath, and it is excreted in part by the gastrointestinal tract and in the urine. The treatment is prompt gastric lavage, stimulation by coffee, strychnine and digitalis, and application of heat to prevent shock. Artificial respiration should be applied when needed.

The postmortem appearances are not characteristic, but there is a distinctive odor of paraldehyde in the various organs. The stomach may show a slight inflammation and the viscera are usually congested. The material to be preserved for toxicologic examination is stomach contents, brain, or liver. Paraldehyde is removed from the body if the patient lives 24 hours after absorption of the drug.

Paraldehyde is a habit forming drug, and the symptoms of chronic intoxication are similar to those of chronic alcoholism. Disturbances of digestion, emaciation, muscular weakness, mental confusion, hallucinations, delusions, tremors and a state not unlike delirium tremens are produced.

Methyl Chloride. This compound, CH_3Cl, is a nonirritating, colorless gas which has a peculiar aromatic odor. It is a constituent of many chemical processes and has a wide employment as a refrigerant. Its use for this purpose has been forbidden by law in New York State, a law passed after a series of poisonings had occurred in Chicago from the use of this gas. These cases were reported by Baker and Kegel, McNally and Pope.

Cases of methyl chloride poisoning are accidental and occur in plants where refrigerating machines are manufactured, or in households where leaks have taken place in the central refrigerating system. As the compound is not irritant, it is insidious in its action and may induce unconsciousness before the victim is cognizant of its toxic effects. The symptoms vary according to the amount of the gas which is inhaled. A small quantity will induce headache, dizziness and somnolence which usually disappears if the individual is removed from the dangerous atmosphere. If a larger quantity is inhaled, vertigo, anorexia, abdominal pain, diarrhea, staggering gait and a feeling of buoyancy occur. In popular parlance, this syndrome is spoken of as a methyl jag. Signs of depression then supervene, and weakness, cyanosis, labored breathing and profound coma develop. Just prior to death there may be convulsions of the clonic or tonic variety. The cases which recover may show mental disturbances and minor ophthalmic disabilities, like diplopia and slight blurring of the vision. Many of these symptoms are doubtless referable to the action of methyl alcohol and other decomposition products of methyl chloride produced in the body.

Methyl chloride does not tend to accumulate in the system, but is further decomposed into methyl alcohol, formic acid and hydrochloric acid. Formic acid may be found in the urine in amounts proportional to the severity of the exposure. The hydrochloric acid may produce a certain amount of acidosis. Methyl alcohol accumulates, and many of the after-effects of the gas are probably produced by the action of this compound. The poisonous concentration of the gas has not been determined specifically. With a high percentage in the atmosphere death may be rapid and take place in a few minutes. Many poisonings occur when the gas is present in small amounts in the air and is inhaled over a long period of time. Its action is insidious and the victim may be overcome without suspecting his danger. For this reason, even a small leak in the refrigerating system may have far-reaching effects. The treatment is to remove the patient from the poisonous atmosphere, administer oxygen and give artificial respiration. Dilute alkaline solutions, such as sodium bicarbonate, may be given by mouth or rectum.

The postmortem findings in cases of methyl chloride poisoning are not characteristic. The blood is fluid and there is marked congestion of the viscera. In a subacute case some of the parenchymatous viscera may show fatty infiltration. In a fatal case, toxicologic examination may be made on the brain, parenchymatous viscera, stomach contents and urine.

Methyl Bromide. Methyl bromide, CH_3Br, is a gas, with an odor like ether, which is employed in industry as one of the components in the manufacture of dyes and substances like antipyrine. Most cases of poisoning occur in industry from inhalation of vapor referable to leaks in the chemical apparatus.

The symptoms are headache, vomiting, visual disturbances, paralyses of the extremities, clonic spasms of all the muscles and later, coma and death. Convalescence in the nonfatal cases is slow, and ataxia, weakness, loss of memory and other neurologic phenomena may persist as complications for several months.

The pathologic changes, treatment and toxicologic considerations are similar to those described under methyl chloride. Methyl bromide is decomposed in the system into hydrobromic acid and methyl alcohol; many of the deleterious effects produced by methyl bromide are referable to the formation of methyl alcohol.

Anesthetics. Anesthesia is that state of the body in which the sensory impulses are inhibited so that pain is no longer felt and the conditions favorable for the performance of a surgical operation are produced. Many of the substances which cause this condition are derivatives of the aliphatic hydrocarbons. Anesthetics are classified as *local* and *general*.

1. *Local* anesthetics, represented in most instances by the derivatives of cocaine such as procaine, will be discussed later. They are injected subcutaneously to cause anesthesia in the area of injection, and intraspinally to produce anesthesia in that part of the body below the site of injection; in both instances the patient retains consciousness during the anesthesia. Some, such as nupercaine, produce analgesia by topical application.

2. *General* anesthetics are introduced into the system for the purpose of producing a loss of consciousness and with it complete anesthesia. The typical general anesthetic is given by inhalation in an open or closed system, usually in the form of a gas or a volatile liquid which is employed because it induces unconsciousness at a concentration well below the danger point and is not prone to produce serious after effects. There is considerable variation in the action of different general anesthetics. In addition, certain drugs are used as basal anesthetics, that is, they are administered prior to the operation to render the patient unconscious and partially anesthetized, and later during the operation are followed by a general anesthetic which is administered in reduced quantities to produce the required insensibility to pain. Morphine is not infrequently used as a basal anesthetic prior to operation, sodium pentothal and avertin also belong to this group.

Nitrous oxide is a common general anesthetic (pages 514 and 515). Two others, ethylene, $H_2C:CH_2$, and divinyl ether, $CH_2:CH-O-CH:CH_2$, have slight toxicity and have an evanescent anesthetic action on the central nervous system so that they may be used for short operations. Other general anesthetics give more prolonged and deeper anesthesia and are also more toxic.

TRIBROMETHANOL (AVERTIN). Avertin, CBr_3CH_2OH, is a white crystalline substance which decomposes into irritating cleavage products when heated. It is a bromine derivative of ethyl alcohol and is similar in many respects to the other halogen derivatives of the aliphatic hydrocarbons in its action on the body. When a dilute solution of avertin is injected into the rectum, it produces coma and general anesthesia by its action on the cerebrum. It is absorbed in about two hours and excreted from the body in a little over that time, except in cases in which the kidneys are functionally deficient, and then some of the drug may be retained in the system a little longer, possibly exerting a toxic action. Because of its rate of excretion, avertin is used as a basal anesthetic to induce unconsciousness before the patient enters the operating room and its action is supplemented by a general anesthetic when the operation begins. If administered with all due precautions the drug is comparatively safe and few deaths are traceable to its use. A large proportion of the fatal cases occurred in patients who were suffering from severe internal disease.

The toxic action of tribromethanol is a gradual depression of the respiratory and vasomotor centers in the medulla manifested by low blood pressure and slow respiratory movements. The patient may sink slowly downhill and death may occur in a few days from paralysis of the vital medullary centers, an eventuality which depends as much upon the poor physical condition of the victim as on the toxicity of the drug. Some of the lesions reported at autopsy are inflammatory reactions of varying intensity in the rectum and sigmoid, and slight degenerative changes in the parenchymatous viscera such as fatty infiltration in the cells of the liver and kidneys. Much of the drug is combined in the liver with glycuronic acid and in this form is eliminated by the kidneys and the large intestine. Any serious disease process, especially involving liver, kidneys, lungs or large intestine, would be a contraindication to its use. If toxic symptoms appear during the administration of tribromethanol, Goodman and Gilman recommend the use of a pharmocologic antagonist such as benzedrine, caffeine with sodium benzoate, or other drugs usually employed to stimulate the respiratory centers or to cause a rise in blood pressure.

ETHYL CHLORIDE. Ethyl chloride, C_2H_5Cl, is a colorless, volatile liquid with a burning taste, which boils at 12° C. It evaporates so rapidly that if a fine stream of liquid is directed against the skin surface, it freezes the surrounding tissues and induces enough local anesthesia to serve for simple operations. Sometimes the drug is administered by inhalation and is used as a general anesthetic.

Cases of poisoning have followed its use in anesthesia, and an appreciable proportion of them have been fatal. After absorption, the ethyl chloride is decomposed into ethyl alcohol and hydrochloric acid. Its toxic action is exerted, prior to decomposition, by the whole compound (C_2H_5Cl) which produces a depressing effect on the central nervous system, a derangement of the conduction of the cardiac muscle and the production of myocardial weakness. There is rapid anesthesia, myocardial fibrillation and depression of the respiratory center. If the drug is removed, recovery may be rapid. At necropsy, the blood is fluid and the organs are congested, but the findings are not characteristic.

ETHYL BROMIDE. Ethyl bromide, C_2H_5Br, is a heavy, colorless, volatile liquid, with an odor like chloroform. It is administered sometimes by inhalation as a general anesthetic, and it produces about the same effects as ethyl chloride. However, its action is uncertain, and its use in anesthesia has been discontinued. When inhaled in high concentration, it produces an irritant action on the respiratory passages, with congestion and edema. If small amounts of the gas are inhaled over a long period of time, a toxic nephrosis may be produced.

TRICHLORETHYLENE. Trichlorethylene, $CHCl\,CCl_2$, is a clear, colorless, volatile liquid with a sweet pungent odor. Therapeutically it is administered for the relief of pain in angina pectoris, in trigeminal neuralgia and in migraine, which it probably accomplishes by its depressing action on the central nervous system. It has also been employed as a general anesthetic, but in recent years it has not been used for that purpose as it is not as efficient as other compounds.

If this substance is inhaled in sufficient quantity, it may produce excitability, dizziness, nausea, palpitation of the heart, and finally somnolence, unconsciousness and death due to its depressing effect on the respiratory centers in the medulla. Most of the cases of poisoning have occurred in industry where this liquid has been used as a solvent for fats and oils, as in the airplane industry or as a cleansing agent for machine parts which have been fouled with grease. Two cases of poisoning originating in the same place of employment have occurred among the routine autopsies in the Office of the Chief Medical Examiner in the City of New York. The victims cleaned machine parts in an open tank containing trichlorethylene and had evidently breathed in a considerable amount of the vapor. One of them, when coming off duty, was observed to be a trifle sleepy; two hours later he suddenly collapsed and died on the street. The other victim showed signs of excitement and acted as if he was slightly intoxicated; a half hour later he died suddenly in a subway car. The autopsies on both bodies disclosed fluid blood and marked congestion of all organs; trichlorethylene was recovered from the viscera by chemical analysis. Chronic poisoning has not been described, and unlike chloroform and carbon tetrachloride, degenerative changes in liver, kidneys and heart muscle have not occurred as a result of the delayed action of trichlorethylene.

CYCLOPROPANE. Cyclopropane, C_3H_6, is isomeric with propylene, $CH_3\text{-}CH= CH_2$, but differs from it in that the carbon atoms are connected in closed ring form. It is a gas which has been extensively used as an anesthetic and is administered by inhalation in a closed system. It is comparatively safe inasmuch as 18 per cent concentration of the gas will produce deep anesthesia and it can be given with large amounts of oxygen so that anoxemia is not an immediate danger.

Serious complications are not common with this anesthetic, and the fatal cases reported are the result of the operation itself, or are due to postoperative pneumonia or to massive pulmonary atelectasis. This last complication is in part referable to the high oxygen content of the anesthetic atmosphere breathed by the patient, for the oxygen in the mixture may be absorbed rapidly in the lung alveoli, producing a rapid pulmonary collapse even in the absence of bronchial obstruction. Some have advocated the addition of a neutral gas like helium to the oxygencyclopropane mixture, which would resist absorption into the blood and prevent alveolar collapse. Another hazard of this anesthetic is the explosive nature of the mixture of oxygen and cyclopropane, for if the explosion occurs inside the mask the results are extremely unfortunate for the patient (Fig. 32-2). The authors have encountered two cases of death following the explosion of a cyclopropane-oxygen mixture in a closed anesthetic system.

Cyclopropane is excreted unchanged by the lungs and is rapidly removed from the system. It does not cause a chronic poisoning, nor does it produce degenerations of the parenchymatous organs like chloroform or carbon tetrachloride.

ETHER. Ether, $(C_2H_5)_2O$, is a colorless, volatile liquid with a pungent odor and taste. It evaporates rapidly at a temperature of 35° C., and is highly inflammable; when mixed with oxygen, an explosive mixture is formed.

Ether is used principally as a general anesthetic for the performance of surgical operations. It is administered by inhalation and is absorbed rapidly from the lungs, the drug having a moderate irritative action on the lining of the respiratory passages and producing an appreciable secretion of mucus. After absorption ether affects the central nervous system rendering the patient insensible in a short space of time, and if given in overwhelming amounts, it may cause death by paralysis of the respiratory center in the medulla. Sometimes ether is swallowed or given by rectum and it may cause a varying degree of gastrointestinal irritation at the point of application, but after absorption it causes unconsciousness by its action on the central nervous system. The drug is rapidly excreted unchanged through the lungs, without regard

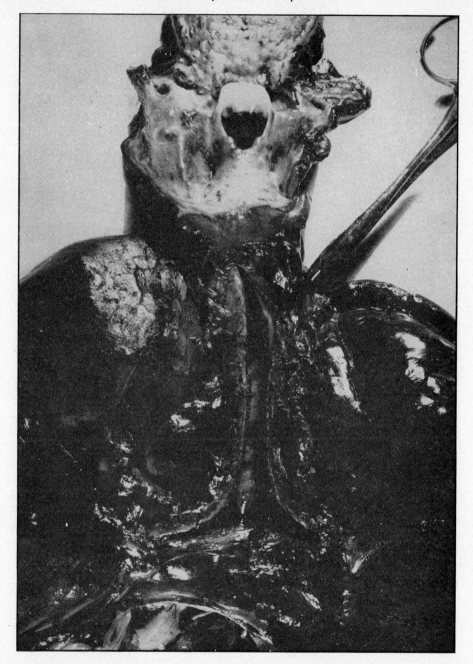

Fig. 32-2. Bursting Rupture of Membranous Portion of Trachea Extending into Main Bronchi Resulting from Explosion of Cyclopropane During Anesthesia.

to the method by which it was administered. The unconsciousness produced by ether is brief and the patient must be continually supplied in order to maintain anesthesia over an extended period of time. Sudden collapse of the patient under ether anesthesia is treated as described under Chloroform (page 795).

The fatal dose of ether is difficult to determine, but if the drug is administered by inhalation, the proportion of 11.2 per cent by volume in the inspired air is considered dangerous to life. When ingested, a fluid ounce or more may be sufficient to cause death. Death may occur early in the course of the anesthesia from the reflex irritation of the respiratory passages by the ether, or it may be induced later by the absorption of large amounts into the cerebral tissue with consequent paralysis of the respiratory center. Some patients, who resist the primary effects of the anesthetic, may die later of a secondary aspiration pneumonia which may become suppurative. Delayed degenerative changes in the liver, kidneys and heart muscle which are characteristic of some cases of chloroform or carbon tetrachloride poisoning occur rarely in ether anesthesia.

The postmortem findings in the fatal case are not characteristic. The blood is usually fluid, with cyanosis and congestion of the viscera, and the internal organs reek with a strong odor of the drug. The materials to preserve for toxicologic analysis are the lungs, brain, parenchymatous organs and stomach contents; the lungs are important because ether is absorbed and excreted from them, so that these organs usually contain large amounts of the anesthetic. Because of its volatile nature, ether is extracted from the tissues by a special process of distillation, as described by Gettler and Siegel.

Most of the fatal cases of poisoning by ether are accidental and occur during its administration as an anesthetic. In the Reports of the Chief Medical Examiner of New York City from 1918 to 1941, an average of 88 deaths from anesthesia occurred a year. For the year 1935 in the Borough of Manhattan, there were 58 deaths associated with the administration of anesthetics out of a total of 7179 deaths investigated by the Department in that borough. The anesthetics used and the number of deaths were as follows: ether (general), 22 deaths; gas-oxygen ether (general), 11 deaths; nitrous oxide (general), 6 deaths; ethyl chloride (general), 2 deaths; avertin (general), 1 death; procaine and other cocaine substitutes (spinal), 4 deaths; cyclopropane and spinal anesthesia, 1 death; procaine (local), 2 deaths; unascertained spinal anesthetics, 7 deaths; unascertained general anesthetic, 1 death. Ether was the anesthetic in slightly less than 57 per cent of the cases. It is not possible to appraise the responsibility of the anesthetic as the lethal agent in these cases inasmuch as other factors such as the severity of the operation and the general condition of the patient must also be considered. In rare instances ether is taken by mouth or inhalation for suicidal purposes. The drug is employed infrequently as a homicidal agent, as noted in one of the cases recorded in the Office of the Chief Medical Examiner of New York City, in which a woman was forced by burglars to inhale ether on a towel and died from its effects.

The pattern of general anesthesia administration in New York City has changed in recent years. Anesthetics are now used in different combinations in order to modify their action on the patient, and drugs are administered with them for specific purposes. In laparotomies under general anesthesia curare is given to relax the abdominal muscles.

The average yearly deaths from anesthesia in New York City from 1946 to 1951 were 215. In 1951 deaths occurred under the following anesthetics: cyclopropane alone, 19 cases; in combination with other anesthetics as ether, nitrous oxide or pentothal sodium, 27 cases; ether alone, 41 cases; ether in combination, 45 cases. There were 17 deaths in which curare was used.

Ether belongs to the group of habit forming drugs, and a few individuals have the practice of swallowing small doses of it constantly. When long continued, this vice is said to give rise to numerous signs of physical degeneration, and nervous manifestations such as trembling, muscular cramps, weakness and headaches. Chronic ether addiction is not commonly seen and has slight medicolegal significance.

CHLOROFORM. Chloroform, $CHCl_3$, is a clear colorless, volatile liquid, having a characteristic aromatic odor and sharp taste. It is not inflammable but when heated may be decomposed into phosgene, chlorine and hydrochloric acid.

Some cases of chloroform poisoning are accidental and occur during its use as a general anesthetic. It has been employed as a means of suicide, either by ingestion of large quantities of the drug or by inhalation of its vapors, emitted from rags soaked in chloroform and placed near the face. Homicidal cases, also, have been found in which a cloth wet with the anesthetic has been held forcibly over the face until enough was inhaled to cause death; in these cases slight abrasions and excoriations are present over lips, nose and cheeks, due in part to the trauma and in part to the irritant action of the drug. In other instances, chloroform has been used as an anesthetic in cases of criminal abortion, and sometimes has caused the death of the patient. In the Reports of the Office of the Chief Medical Examiner of New York City from the years 1918 to 1951, 53 cases of chloroform poisoning were listed as suicidal, 8 were diagnosed as accidental in addition to the numbers included among the anesthetic deaths, and 5 cases were noted as homicidal.

The action of chloroform is that of a depressant of the central nervous system. The first symptoms following its administration are dulling of the senses, weakness of the extremities, flushing of the face, rapid pulse and quickened respirations; in this stage, death may occur from a reflex stopping of the heart. After the initial symptoms, a stage of excitement follows which passes into coma and surgical anesthesia. The pupils become immobile and do not react to light, the muscles are relaxed, the respirations are slow and shallow, the pulse regular and weak. The patient may be kept in this state by judicious administration of the drug, and in favorable cases will recover without sequelae after the anesthetic is removed. The heart may stop beating during anesthesia, because of the toxic effect of the chloroform on the myocardium. If chloroform is administered in large quantities, the patient will go into collapse, with cyanosis, widely dilated pupils, blue lips, stertorous respirations, slow pulse, low blood pressure and death from paralysis of the medullary centers. If chloroform is swallowed, there is an irritation of the upper gastrointestinal tract with vomiting and diarrhea, and coma and death by respiratory paralysis may occur in a few minutes. Occasionally a few cases survive a few hours or days.

The fatal dose of chloroform varies. A concentration of 0.4 to 0.8 gm. per liter in the blood is considered dangerous to life. If the chloroform is ingested, an ounce is usually a fatal dose for an adult, but recovery has been described after larger quantities have been taken. Death may occur in any stage of the anesthesia or at any time during the first four or five days after the anesthesia. Other anesthetics have superseded chloroform because of their greater safety in cases where prolonged anesthesia is necessary.

If the patient collapses during the anesthesia, the treatment is to withdraw the anesthetic, administer artificial respiration, use warmth to combat shock, and use stimulants such as caffeine, strychnine and atropine. Care should be taken that the patient does not inhale any vomitus. If chloroform is swallowed the stomach should be washed out with warm water and milk. The rest of the treatment is symptomatic. The postmortem appearances of acute chloroform poisoning are not characteristic.

The blood is fluid, the face is cyanotic and the organs are congested. If the drug is ingested, the mouth, esophagus and stomach are congested and irritated.

The materials usually saved for toxicologic examination in cases of chloroform poisoning are the stomach contents, lungs, brain and some of the parenchymatous viscera. The lungs and stomach are the principal portals of entry for the drug, and the proportion of chloroform found in each is significant in certain cases. Like ether, chloroform is taken up by the alveolar epithelium in the lungs and thus enters the blood, and it is also excreted unchanged in large amounts through the epithelium into the alveoli. A little is excreted in the urine, the perspiration and the milk. Large amounts are found in the brain because of the affinity of this tissue for the drug. Chloroform is removed from the body within 24 hours after absorption.

Delayed chloroform poisoning occurs about 10 to 48 hours after the patient recovers from his unconsciousness. A toxemia is produced which effects the parenchymatous cells of the heart, liver and kidneys. The patient becomes restless, vomits, jaundice and liver tenderness sets in, and coma supervenes. The symptoms are much like those of phosphorus poisoning, and at necropsy degenerative changes are seen to have occurred in the cells of the liver, kidneys and heart muscle, similar to the lesions described in delayed carbon tetrachloride poisoning (see page 798).

Bromoform. Bromoform, $CHBr_3$, is a heavy, oily, colorless liquid which boils at 151° C. but volatilizes at a lower temperature. It has an odor similar to chloroform. At one time it was used as a sedative in whooping cough, and a number of deaths were caused by this treatment. The symptoms and postmortem lesions caused by bromoform are similar to chloroform, and treatment of the poisoning is identical with that of chloroform.

Iodoform. Iodoform, CHI_3, is a lemon yellow crystalline powder which has a penetrating odor and taste and distills readily in steam. It is used in medicine as an antiseptic. Practically all cases of iodoform poisoning have occurred because of its absorption from raw, ulcerated surfaces and wound cavities. One fatal case was encountered in which the drug entered the system from iodoform gauze packed inside a uterus in a case of placenta praevia. A few examples of accidental ingestion of the substance have been described. The molecule of iodoform when absorbed has a marked effect on the central nervous system; it is decomposed into iodides and iodine. These substances are slowly eliminated in the urine, saliva and perspiration.

Symptoms of poisoning may start with malaise, discomfort and anxiety and the patients suffer from insomnia, giddiness, headache, nausea, vomiting, mental confusion and hallucinations. The pulse is accelerated but the respiratory rate is not much affected. The patients pass into deep coma and die from paralysis of the respiratory center. In a few cases, the iodoform causes a distinct eruption on the skin resembling ivy poisoning.

Death may occur in 24 hours, or it may be delayed for days or weeks. The fatal dose is hard to estimate, because of the method of administration which is usually by external application. The treatment is to remove the dressings and to get rid of the iodoform. The rest of the treatment is symptomatic. If the iodoform has been taken by mouth it may be desirable to wash out the stomach with a dilute solution of sodium bicarbonate which is considered an antidote.

The lesions noted at necropsy in many cases are fatty degeneration of heart muscle, liver and kidneys, edema of the lungs and congestion of the viscera. The materials which are gathered for analysis in suspected iodoform poisoning are

stomach contents, kidneys, liver, brain, blood and urine. According to some observers, iodoform disappears slowly from the body, and iodides may be demonstrated in the urine for days after the poisoning.

A long-continued use of iodoform may cause a chronic eruption of the skin,
eczema, loss of weight, amblyopia, cardiac palpitation and paralytic manifestations.

Chloral Hydrate. This compound, $CCl_3CHO.H_2O$, is a colorless crystalline
substance with a slightly aromatic odor and bitter taste, and is split by alkalis into
chloroform, a formate of the alkali, and water.

Chloral hydrate is used in medicine as a hypnotic, but not as frequently as in
the past because of its depressing action on the heart. Most cases of poisoning are
reported as accidental, due mainly to mistakes in therapeutic administration. In
other instances the poisoning has been suicidal. Chloral hydrate also has been given
secretly in food or drink to render a person suddenly helpless for the purpose of
robbery or rape. Its action is so rapid under such conditions that it has been given
the name of knock out drops. In most cases the poison has been ingested, but occasionally it has been administered by rectal or intravenous injection. The Reports of
the Office of the Chief Medical Examiner of New York City from the years 1918 to
1951 indicate that 22 cases of chloral hydrate poisoning were listed as suicidal, 22
as accidental and undetermined, and 1 as homicidal.

The action of chloral hydrate, like that of chloroform, is to depress the cerebral
centers. In medicinal dose, it induces a natural sleep, with normal awakening. It
is absorbed readily from the intestine and the symptoms ensue in a few minutes,
especially if alcohol is mixtured with the chloral hydrate. The drug is decomposed
in the body and is excreted in the urine as urochloralic acid, a conjugated glycuronic
acid. When taken in toxic doses, signs of gastrointestinal irritation may occur, such
as a burning sensation in the throat, nausea, vomiting and epigastric pain. The
victim grows rapidly comatose, with low blood pressure, muscular relaxation, cold
extremities, convulsions, delirium and cyanosis, and may die of paralysis of the
respiratory center. Chloral hydrate produces vasodilatation and also has a depressing
effect on the heart muscle.

The fatal dose varies; in one case, 1.3 gm. has caused death in an adult, but as
a rule, larger quantities are required, such as 10 gm. Death may occur in from 15
to 30 minutes, or the victim may remain prostrated and die in about three days; the
usual period is from 8 to 12 hours. In the delayed deaths, jaundice of a light grade
may appear because of the toxic action of the drug on the liver. The treatment of the
acute poisoning is to wash out the stomach, keep the body warm and administer
oxygen and artificial respiration. Strychnine and strong coffee are valuable for
stimulation. Many of the measures employed in barbiturate poisoning can be used
in the treatment of chloral hydrate poisoning (page 822).

Examination of the body at necropsy shows a moderate irritation of the gastrointestinal tract, congestion of the viscera, fluid blood and edema of the lungs. The
findings are not characteristic. If death is delayed, fatty degeneration may appear
in the myocardium, liver and kidneys. The materials usually saved for chemical
analysis are stomach contents, brain and parenchymatous viscera. Because of the
propensity of chloral to decompose into chloroform and a formate in the presence
of an alkali the tissues should be tested as soon after death as possible. The drug
is excreted from the body within 24 hours after administration.

Chronic chloral hydrate poisoning follows continued use of the drug to the
extent of habitual addiction. The usual signs are indigestion, diarrhea, loss of weight,

insomnia, skin rashes, mental deterioration and occasionally jaundice. Fatty degeneration of the liver, heart muscle and kidneys may be found at autopsy.

Carbon Tetrachloride. Carbon tetrachloride, CCl_4, is a clear, colorless, mobile liquid with an odor like chloroform, boiling at about 76° C. It is not inflammable but, like chloroform, decomposes after long exposure to light or from the heat of a flame into phosgene, chlorine and hydrochloric acid; and poisoning may be produced by these substances. The tetrachloride is used as a solvent for fat and rubber, as a delousing agent, as an anthelmintic in hookworm infection, in the fire extinguisher Pyrene and in certain paints. In the Reports of the Office of the Chief Medical Examiner of New York City, 43 accidental and 4 suicidal cases of carbon tetrachloride poisoning occurred in the years between 1918 to 1951. Since that time one suicidal case has been reported, several cases of poisoning caused by its adulteration of alcoholic beverages, and one case caused by inhalation of the substance while used as a cleaning fluid.

The drug has a soporific and anesthetic action similar to chloroform but of briefer duration. When it is ingested in large amounts along with alcohol or fat, it is absorbed rapidly from the small intestine, and acute poisoning supervenes. A feeling of warmth pervades the stomach region, followed by inebriation, hiccup, convulsions, headache, abdominal pain, nausea, vomiting, diarrhea and death in a few hours from cardiovascular collapse or respiratory paralysis. A large portion of the compound is excreted unchanged by the lungs after absorption. The findings at autopsy in this stage are similar to those in chloroform poisoning.

Many cases of carbon tetrachloride poisoning show a latent interval of from 24 to 36 hours after ingestion, and at the end of that time drowsiness, dizziness, suppression of urine, jaundice, convulsions, cardiac weakness, intestinal hemorrhages, collapse and death may ensue gradually. Bile may be present in the blood and urine and hematuria has been described. The liver at necropsy usually shows fine nutmeg markings with necroses around the smaller central veins and some fatty infiltration in the periphery of the acini; microscopic examination of the necrotic areas may show numerous large phagocytic cells filled with yellow pigment and complete destruction of the parenchyma cells. Cirrhotic changes may occur in the livers of those cases which recover from the active stage of the poisoning (Fig. 32-3). Fatty changes often occur in the convoluted tubules of the kidneys and in the heart muscle. Lesions characteristic of a lower nephron nephrosis may be present in the kidneys. Necrosis has been described in the zona fasciculata and the zona reticularis of the adrenal glands. The skin, blood and internal viscera may show considerable jaundice. If the viscera are fatty prior to the administration of the drug, its toxic effects on the system are increased. The fatal dose is variable: a child of five and one-half years died after taking 1 ml. and an adult died after ingesting 3 ml.

In the acute cases the materials saved for toxicologic examination are stomach contents, brain and some of the parenchymatous viscera; practically the same organs which are used for the tests for chloroform. If the victim lives over 24 hours after the poisoning, carbon tetrachloride is usually excreted from the body and is absent.

The treatment in the acute cases is similar to the treatment described under chloroform poisoning. Because of the danger of delayed poisoning, carbon tetrachloride has been largely discontinued as an anthelmintic, and other remedies have been used. As carbon tetrachloride is prone to cause acidosis, the patient should always be watched for signs of air hunger, the usual preliminary indication of that condition, and appropriate treatment administered without delay.

Some cases of poisoning by carbon tetrachloride occur in industry under conditions which favor inhalation of fumes, usually manifested by irritation and inflammation of the air passages. The drug is a constituent of some dry cleaning fluids, often in association with a halogen derivative of the higher aliphatic hydrocarbons such as dichloropropane. Gonzales reported a case of acute toxemia and death produced by the fumes of this type of cleaning fluid in a domestic servant who was using it in a small, poorly ventilated room. A chronic poisoning is most apt to occur in workers who are continually exposed to the fumes of carbon tetrachloride, and

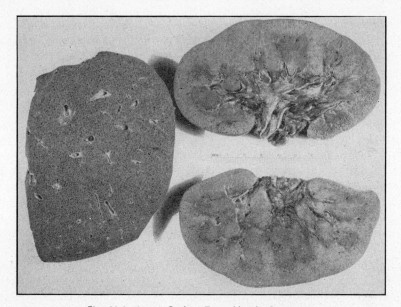

Fig. 32-3. Acute Carbon Tetrachloride Poisoning.

Acute central lobular liver necrosis following ingestion of carbon tetrachloride. Representative sections of liver and kidneys to show prominence of central veins and swollen kidney parenchyma.

coryza, dermatitis, nausea, anemia, toxic jaundice, loss of weight and chronic ill health are the prevailing symptoms.

Tetrachlorethane. Tetrachlorethane, $CHCl_2 . CHCl_2$, is a colorless, heavy, oily liquid which is not inflammable. It is volatile, gives off a vapor heavier than air and has an odor suggestive of chloroform. Tetrachlorethane is employed as a varnish solvent, as a solvent for cellulose acetate, in the making of lacquered goods, artificial silk, artificial pearls, airplane varnish, or "dope," and noninflammable cinematographic films.

Most cases of poisoning are acute or subacute caused by inhaling the vapors of tetrachlorethane during manufacturing processes. The sufferers complain of fatigue, drowsiness, nervousness, insomnia, anorexia and headache. In a few days, jaundice develops and gastric and nervous symptoms occur followed by mental confusion, delirium, coma and finally death. The liver during the period of jaundice is tender to pressure and palpable. On microscopic section, fatty changes appear in the parenchymatous cells of the liver, kidneys and heart muscle, similar to the changes which occur in phosphorous poisoning. Anemia and loss of weight are present in the later stages. Purpuric rashes, hematemesis and suppression of urine occasionally occur.

The treatment of this type of poisoning is to remove the worker from the poisonous atmosphere and enforce rest. Dilute alkalis given by mouth are often valuable in combating acidosis. The intestinal tract should be kept open by laxatives.

Organic Nitrites. The term nitrite is used here, according to the conception of Goodman and Gilman, to designate both nitrites and nitrates, whether inorganic or organic. Inasmuch as the pharmacologic and toxic action of these compounds is largely referable to the liberation of the nitrite ion (NO_2) in the body, this classification is justified. Some of the inorganic compounds belonging to this group have already been discussed, such as nitric oxide, bismuth subnitrate and potassium nitrate. Nitric oxide has already been discussed in Chapter 19. Bismuth subnitrate in the large intestine is decomposed by bacteria into nitrites which are absorbed and cause their characteristic toxic action. Potassium nitrate is not easily decomposed and may be given in large doses as a diuretic without causing nitrite action.

Sodium nitrite when given orally produces the characteristic nitrate reaction of causing the muscles of the smaller blood vessels to relax, and vasodilatation to ensue, and so is of value in relieving pain and discomfort in such conditions as marked hypertension and angina pectoris. The action of the nitrite may have a disturbing influence on patients with weak hearts as it causes a drainage of blood into the splanchnic circulation and thus creates a condition favorable for the onset of syncopal attacks. The toxic action of the drug is not potent and is only evoked when large amounts are administered, occasionally producing some gastrointestinal irritation and a variable degree of methemoglobinemia. Like the other inorganic nitrites the sodium salt must be decomposed into the nitrite ion in the small intestine and must be absorbed into the system before its action occurs, and as this process is not uniform the resulting nitrite action varies considerably. Two accidental fatal poisonings, investigated by the authors, occurred after the ingestion of pig's knuckles obtained by the victims from a vat in which the meat was being colored by sodium nitrite; a marked methemoglobinemia was found at autopsy and sodium nitrite was recovered from the stomach contents.

The principal organic aliphatic nitrites are amyl nitrite and nitroglycerine which are also employed in medicine for the relief of hypertensive states and angina pectoris. These compounds act more rapidly than sodium nitrite as they are rapidly absorbed, and they produce dilatation of blood vessels more quickly. Amyl nitrite is administered by inhalation and acts almost immediately. Nitroglycerine is absorbed as such and in the tissues is split into its nitrite component, and its effects are produced more slowly than those of amyl nitrite but more rapidly than those of sodium nitrite. Methemoglobin formation is not often encountered with these compounds unless the amount absorbed is large and the clinical course prolonged. The aromatic organic nitrites will be discussed later.

AMYL NITRITE. Amyl nitrite, $C_5H_{11}NO_2$, is a volatile yellowish liquid with a fruit-like odor. In large quantities it produces flushing of the face, vomiting, coma, dyspnea, cyanosis and death by paralysis of the respiratory center. The drug is administered by inhalation or ingestion. The postmortem lesions are not characteristic, aside from congestion of various organs.

NITROGLYCERINE. Nitroglycerine, $C_3H_5(NO_3)_3$, or glyceryl trinitrate, is an odorless, pale oily fluid which explodes when heated or when exposed to concussion. Its pharmacologic action is similar to amyl nitrite, but its effects are more prolonged. Most cases of poisoning are accidental, occurring in workers who manufacture explosives. Homicide by nitroglycerine has been described, and the drug has been administered in alcoholic drinks. In the Reports of the Office of the Chief Medical Examiner of New York City, one suicidal case of poisoning by nitroglycerine occurred between the years 1918 and 1941.

The most marked symptom in an acute case of poisoning is a severe headache, the so-called powder headache of workers in factories which manufacture explosives. In addition there are drowsiness, vomiting, colicky pains, diarrhea, flushed face, dizziness, dyspnea, cyanosis, convulsions, delirium, coma and death by paralysis of the respiratory center. If the course is prolonged, a certain amount of methemoglobinemia may supervene.

Most of the fatal cases are caused by taking an overdose of the drug for use as a cardiac sedative. A few drops may be lethal under some conditions, and death may occur in from two to six hours. At necropsy, the principal findings are congestion of the stomach, intestines and other viscera, and the mucous membranes of the respiratory passages are sometimes colored a reddish-brown. The treatment is to eliminate the poison by washing out the stomach, giving saline infusions, and to administer caffeine as a stimulant. Nitroglycerine is decomposed rapidly in the system and is hard to isolate from the tissues by toxicologic investigation. The stomach contents are more likely to yield it than any other material from the body, and should be preserved for examination along with one of the parenchymatous viscera.

Habitual use of nitroglycerine seems to induce a certain amount of tolerance for it, and a dose of 6 grains daily may be borne. A chronic form of poisoning has been described, characterized by skin eruptions, ulcers on the fingers and tachycardia.

Carbon Bisulfide. Carbon bisulfide, CS_2, is a volatile liquid with a penetrating, disagreeable odor like fecal material. This substance is used in the vulcanization of rubber, and most of the cases of poisoning are chronic, due to the inhalation of the vapors in factories. Many workers who are affected by the drug suffer from a chronic malaise and headache. The central and peripheral nervous system may be extensively damaged and the victim may show a parkinsonian syndrome, visual disturbances sometimes leading to optic atrophy, a peripheral neuritis occasionally accompanied by paralyses, and in some cases mental symptoms resembling manic-depressive insanity.

Sometimes acute poisoning occurs when the compound is taken for suicidal purposes, the ingestion of half an ounce occasionally causing death. The patient shows prostration, dyspnea, and cyanosis with dilated pupils and convulsions, finally lapsing into coma and dying in a few hours from paralysis of the respiratory center. The findings at autopsy are slight gastrointestinal irritation, congestion of the viscera, and the characteristic odor of the drug in the organs of the body. The treatment consists of evacuating the poison from the stomach by the tube and instituting artificial respiration and stimulation as required. Stomach contents, brain and parenchymatous viscera are the materials saved for toxicologic examination. In the Reports of the Office of the Chief Medical Examiner of New York City, one case of suicidal poisoning from the ingestion of carbon bisulfide occurred between the years 1918 and 1941.

Hydrocyanic Acid and the Cyanides. Hydrocyanic acid, HCN, is a colorless, transparent fluid with an odor like that of bitter almonds, is volatile and boils at 26.5° C. This compound is formed by the action of acids on alkaline cyanides and, when liberated in this fashion, is used to disinfect ships and warehouses. It is one of the most powerful poisons known. Hydrocyanic acid is present in many plants in combination with glucosides, as for example amygdalin which is in the different parts of the cherry laurel, and in the seeds of such fruits as cherry, peach, plum, apricot, apple and pear. Oil of bitter almonds contains 2 to 4 per cent of hydrocyanic acid and cherry laurel water contains 0.1 per cent. It occurs also in illuminating gases, in the distillates from coal tar and in the fumes from burning celluloid, but rarely in sufficient quantity to have a toxicologic significance.

Potassium cyanide is a deliquescent white salt which is used in photography, silver electroplating, gilding of metals and in blood chemistry as a reagent in uric acid determinations. Sodium cyanide is similar in most respects to potassium cyanide. These compounds are especially toxic in the presence of a dilute acid, as a chemical reaction sets in which results in the formation of salts of the acid and hydrocyanic acid. Other poisonous cyanides are ammonium cyanide, silver cyanide, zinc cyanide and mercury cyanide. Sodium nitroprusside, potassium ferrocyanide, potassium ferricyanide, cyanogen, cyanogen chloride and cyanogen iodide are less poisonous. The cyanates and the sulfocyanates are not as toxic as the other compounds as they are not decomposed as readily.

Hydrocyanic acid is absorbed from any mucous surface and enters the system just as easily by way of the nose and throat as by the stomach. Cases of poisoning are mostly suicidal and people who have access to the drug, like pharmacists, chemists and physicians, may take it for that purpose by mouth. Some deaths from ingestion of the acid are accidental, and occur when it is swallowed by mistake for something else. The eating of plants which contain cyanophoric glucosides sometimes proves fatal, because of the metamorphosis produced in the intestinal tract, which decomposes these compounds into hydrogen cyanide in quantity sufficient to be toxic. One frequent form of accidental poisoning is the inhalation of the vaporized acid during disinfection of ships or buildings. Homicidal poisoning occurs occasionally. In the Reports of the Office of the Chief Medical Examiner in New York City, poisoning by hydrocyanic acid is not differentiated from deaths caused by the other cyanides.

When hydrocyanic acid is ingested or inhaled in large amounts the victim collapses quickly, becomes insensible, has a convulsive seizure and dies in a few seconds or minutes from paralysis of the respiratory centers. If the dose is smaller unconsciousness is slower in onset, and is attended by collapse, cold sweat, rapid, weak pulse, gasping respirations, muscular spasms, coma and death. The breathing at the end becomes slow and shallow. Death may not occur until one to four hours have elapsed, and some cases may survive a matter of 12 days or more and in rare instances even recover. If the case is not a fatal one, hydrocyanic acid is excreted in the urine as sulfocyanides, and a small quantity is excreted unchanged from the lungs. It has been suggested that it may combine with the aldehyde group of the body sugar, or be hydrolyzed by ferments into ammonium formate.

The fatal dose varies. If the poison is inhaled the concentration of the gas in the air and the time of exposure are factors which must be considered. A concentration of 0.2 to 0.3 mg. per liter of air is considered by some to be almost immediately fatal, while 0.13 mg. is fatal if inhaled for a period of over one hour. Other investigators believe that higher concentrations than the foregoing may be withstood. The lethal dose of hydrocyanic acid by mouth is not known with certainty, as 1.87 ml. of a 2 per cent solution has caused death, but recovery has followed the ingestion of 15 ml. of a solution of the same strength.

The treatment in the cases of acute poisoning is to wash out the stomach and give a little ferrous sulfate in dilute solution as a chemical antidote. Artificial respiration, oxygen inhalation, stimulants and warmth to combat shock should be tried. Very few cases of cyanide poisoning recover or survive long enough to permit restorative measures to be applied. In cases which resist the immediate lethal action of the drug, intravenous injections of a dilute solution of sodium nitrite followed by an intravenous injection of a solution of sodium thiosulfate are recommended by Goodman and Gilman. The nitrite is injected to produce a methemoglobinemia which combines with the cyanide ion to form cyanmethemoglobinemia and by this the cyanide ion is rendered temporarily harmless. The solution of sodium thiosulfate is injected to combine with the cyanide ion and form with it a thiocyanate, when it is set free by the subsequent disassociation of the cyanmethemoglobin molecule. If the situation is urgent the patient may be given inhalations of amyl nitrite until the sodium nitrite and sodium thiosulfate solutions can be prepared.

The lesions produced by hydrocyanic acid are congestion of the viscera, edema of the lungs of greater or lesser intensity usually more pronounced where death has been delayed, and a distinct odor of bitter almonds about the viscera especially in the skull cavity and the brain. If the drug has been ingested, the mucous membrane of the stomach may not be much altered. Hydrocyanic acid is toxic for all forms of life, retarding the oxidation processes in the cells and preventing the tissues from absorbing oxgen from the blood. The cyanide ion also produces a brief but intense stimulation of the respiratory movements, thus increasing the amount of oxyhemoglobin. The blood is fluid and bright red in color and the postmortem lividity is bright red in many instances; sometimes, however, asphyxia may supervene, the blood may be dark and fluid and the suggillations dusky violet. In the few cases which survive the immediate effects of the poison and live a few hours or days, other lesions have been described such as hyaline thrombi in the small blood vessels of the brain, minute hemorrhages and necroses in the lenticular nuclei and the other parts of the brain, and changes in the ganglion cells and neurons; degenerative processes may occur in the peripheral nervous system. One case of acute yellow atrophy of the liver in hydrocyanic acid poisoning is described by Bein.

The materials usually saved for toxicologic examination are the stomach contents, lungs, brain and a viscus like the liver. If the poison is inhaled, the lungs will show a high hydrocyanic acid content and the stomach contents will contain very little. If the poison is ingested most of it will be in the stomach, and the lungs will yield only a small amount.

Chronic poisoning from the continual inhalation of hydrocyanic acid vapor has been described in gilders and silver polishers. These patients complain mostly of pallor, vertigo, gastrointestinal disturbances, dyspnea and oppression of the chest. Mental and encephalitic symptoms sometimes supervene.

Poisoning by the cyanides, especially potassium cyanide or sodium cyanide, is usually caused by their ingestion for suicidal purposes. Photographers, electroplaters and jewelers who use these salts in their work sometimes swallow it; and diamond dealers have been known to drink it in whisky. Accidental cases have occurred, as when a child drank it in white shoe polish; or when a cook inadvertently left some cyanide silver polish in a cooking pot in large enough amounts to poison a fellow worker who drank soup from that container. Homicidal cases have been encountered, as when a psychopathic individual forced a night watchman at the point of a gun to drink coffee containing potassium cyanide. According to the Reports of the Office of the Chief Medical Examiner in New York City, which do not separate the cyanides from hydrocyanic acid in the statistics, suicidal cases numbered 626; accidental and undetermined cases, 105; homicidal cases, 4 in the years from 1918 to 1951. Fifty-two of the accidental poisonings were due to fumigation by hydrocyanic acid.

The onset of the symptoms is frequently slower in poisoning by cyanides than in poisoning by hydrocyanic acid, inasmuch as an interval occurs during which the salt is decomposed by the gastric juice and hydrocyanic acid is formed and absorbed from the stomach. The time which elapses is long enough in most cases for suicides to dispose of the evidences of their act, or to walk a considerable distance before they collapse. The interval may be lengthened to a period of about 20 minutes if the salt is taken in solid form for then it is attacked with more difficulty by the stomach acids. If the compound is a complicated cyanide, the onset is also gradual because the compound is not easily decomposed. Potassium cyanide is fatal sometimes in amounts of 0.13 gm., but victims have recovered after doses of 3.25 gm.

Potassium or sodium cyanide after ingestion produce a diffuse crimson-red discoloration of the gastric mucous membrane (Fig. 32-4), which gradually changes to a rusty-brown and dark brown from the formation of alkaline hematin, changes referable to the strong alkaline component of the salt which produces a brief but intense alkaline corrosion (page 723). The findings at autopsy are otherwise the same as described above under hydrocyanic acid. The treatment and the materials preserved for toxicologic examination are the same as for hydrocyanic acid.

Thiocyanates, usually the sodium or potassium salts, are administered in hypertension to reduce the blood pressure or to relieve symptoms. The drug sometimes accomplishes this purpose effectively but in excess it has a definite toxic action so that its use would be contraindicated in patients with advanced heart and kidney disease. Toxic symptoms occur with only a small amount of thiocyanate in the serum and consist of anorexia, nausea, fatigue, hypothyroidism and depressed bone marrow function. Fatal excess of thiocyanate produces skin eruptions varying from purpura to exfoliative dermatitis, a hepatogenous jaundice and a toxic psychosis. The autopsy usually reveals marked cerebral congestion and edema especially of the brain stem, a degenerative nephrosis and a centrolobular necrosis of the liver with jaundice.

Paraffin Hydrocarbons. Petroleum, which has its origin in oil wells, contains a large number of constituents, some of them gaseous and some liquid. When the crude oils are distilled fractionally, the more volatile gases are removed, and liquids are separated which boil at different temperatures. The liquids are: (1) petroleum ether which contains the hydrocarbons pentane and hexane, and boils between 40° and 70° C.; (2) gasoline which is composed of hexane and heptane, and boils between 70° and 90° C.; (3) naphtha, consisting of heptane and octane, which boils between 90° and 120° C.; (4) benzine, made up of octane and nonane, with a boiling point of 120° to 150° C.; and (5) kerosene which includes the higher hydrocarbons from decane to hexadecane, and boils at 150° to 300° C.

The fractions which distill below 150° C. are poisonous whether taken by mouth or by inhalation of the vapor. In most accidental cases the vapor is inhaled because of the use of these substances in industry as solvents for paint, in rubber manufacture, in dry cleaning, in work on automobiles or in cleaning tank cars. Cases have been described of accidental poisoning from use of benzine to remove plaster from the skin, and from the use of gasoline as a hair wash. After inhalation the vapors may cause dizziness, constriction of the throat, nausea, vomiting, drowsiness, lack of self-control, staggering, headache and trembling of hands and arms, and the so-called naphtha jag is produced. The patient later becomes pale and shows livid lips, slow respirations, weak and scarcely perceptible heart action, convulsions and coma, finally resulting in death. The treatment consists in removing the victim from the poisonous vapors, in starting artificial respiration and in combating shock. The lesions found at autopsy are similar to those described in alcohol or ether poisoning.

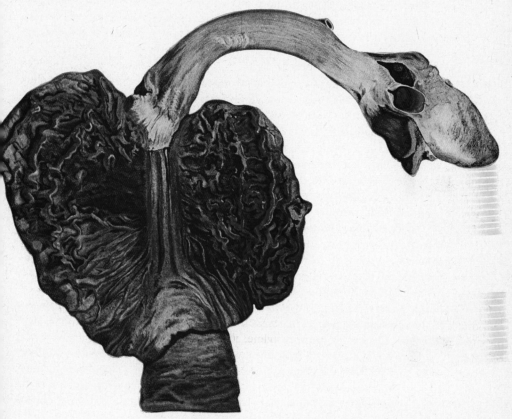

From Emerson, *Legal Medicine and Toxicology,*
D. Appleton-Century Co.

Fig. 32-4. Poisoning by Potassium Cyanide. Corrosion of the Gastric Mucosa.
Death occurred a few minutes after ingestion. The effect of sodium cyanide is similar.

Chronic poisoning occurs from continued inhalation with symptoms of nausea, vomiting, weakness of extremities and paresthesia. If the substances come in contact with the skin an acne-like or pustular eruption may develop, especially on the hands, arms and legs.

If benzine or some of the other fractions are swallowed, shortness of breath, cyanosis, cold clammy skin, coma and death by shock may occur. Most of the cases occur in children who take the material by mistake, or in people who swallow it for suicidal purposes. The Reports of the Office of the Chief Medical Examiner of New York City show 12 accidental deaths due to poisoning by paraffin distillates between the years 1918 and 1951. Autopsy on these cases show inflammation of the stomach and intestines, small hemorrhages in the submucous layers and an odor of benzine in the stomach. Irritative lesions of the kidneys, small hemorrhages in the lung tissue, slight hemolysis and methemoglobin formation may be present. The findings are not distinctive.

The kerosene or coal oil fraction, which distils between 150° and 300° C., causes poisoning in children who ingest it accidentally. There is an inflammation of the upper gastrointestinal tract, with vomiting, colic, thirst, painful urination, cyanosis, drowsiness, labored respirations and coma, occasionally resulting in death. Fatal poisonings are rare after coal oil ingestion. In these cases the stomach is washed out with warm water, and measures are taken to combat shock.

VOLATILE AROMATIC COMPOUNDS

This subdivision of volatile compounds is distinguished by the structure of their nuclei in which the carbon atoms, or the carbon and nitrogen atoms, are joined in the form of a ring. The substitution of different radicals for the hydrogen atoms in the ring produces other compounds with different properties, the process being analogous to similar substitutions in the aliphatic chain, but with many points of difference. As an example, halogen aliphatic compounds are toxic, but the halogen radicals added to the aromatic ring do not form a compound of greatly increased toxicity. An acid radical joined to the benzene ring does not always result in a compound which has a marked irritant action, unlike some of the caustic aliphatic acids. On the other hand hydroxyl derivatives of benzene are more corrosive than their aliphatic analogues, and the addition of nitro groups to the ring forms compounds of exceptionally poisonous quality far surpassing the compounds in the aliphatic nitro group. Most of the volatile aromatic compounds, with some exceptions, are absorbed readily and promptly eliminated from the system after absorption.

Benzene Series. The hydrocarbons of the benzene group are produced by the dry distillation of coal, and are found in the crude coal tars. The products distil over in fractions: at 170° C. benzene, toluene, xylene, pyridine and thiophene are collected, and are known as light oils; the distillate from 170° to 230° C. contains naphthalene and phenol, and is termed middle oil; the fraction which distils at 230° to 270° C. is composed of phenol, cresol and anthracene, or creosote, and is known as heavy oil. The products obtained at over 270° C. contain anthracene, phenanthrene and hydrocarbons. Some of the distillates of this last group contain carcinogenic substances which are derivatives of phenanthrene; a potent compound of this sort is dibenzpyrene. For a review of these carcinogenic compounds the reader is referred to the article by Francis Carter Wood in the literature.

BENZENE. This hydrocarbon, benzene or benzol, C_6H_6, is a light inflammable liquid, colorless and refractile, with an aromatic odor, which boils at 79.6° C. It is used in many industries as a solvent (rubber industries, artificial leather manufacture, shoe manufacture), as a constituent of varnishes and bronzing fluids, as a paint remover, in the manufacture of coal tar drugs, in aniline dye manufacture and in countless other processes.

Poisoning by inhalation of benzene fumes occurs in industry most often where benzene is used as a solvent, and especially when empty benzene tanks and stills are being cleaned. The laborer who is exerting himself physically on such a job may inhale some of the fumes and develop an intoxication which may make him resist all attempts to remove him from the poisonous atmosphere. He may complain of a burning sensation in the throat and irritation of the exposed parts of his skin, and show flushing of the face, cyanosis of the extremities, dizziness, restlessness, excitement, delirium, hallucinations, fever, convulsions and coma. Death may occur in a few minutes from respiratory failure and asphyxia. Sometimes the victim is pros-trated for a few hours and dies in coma.

Postmortem examination of such cases discloses abundant dark red fluid blood, an odor of benzene about the viscera, reddening and congestion of the mucous membranes of the air passages with formation of mucus, edema of the lungs, small scattered hemorrhages in the lung tissue and under the pleura, small hemorrhages in the submucous layer of the stomach and intestines, edema and congestion of the brain, small hemorrhages in the subarachnoid space and occasionally irritation of the exposed portions of the skin. If the case survives a few hours, the predominant signs are those of asphyxia.

Acute poisoning also occurs after the ingestion of benzene, either because of its therapeutic use in the treatment of leukemias, or because it has been swallowed with suicidal intent. The symptomatology and pathologic lesions are similar to those caused by the inhalation of the drug, with the exception that the victim exhibits more pronounced gastrointestinal irritation and inflammation in cases of ingestion.

The fatal dose of benzol is difficult to determine, but one ounce taken by mouth has caused death in 12 hours. The concentration in the atmosphere which might be fatal on short exposure is approximately 19,000 parts per million. The drug is eliminated from the lungs as benzene, or it is transformed in the body to phenol and excreted in the urine as conjugated sulfates and glycuronates of that compound where it may be detected by appropriate chemical tests (page 729). In the acute cases the materials preserved for chemical examination consist of stomach contents, lungs, brain, some of the parenchymatous viscera and urine. The results of the toxicologic investigation of the lungs and stomach contents may indicate the portal of entry of the poison, as more benzol is usually present at the point of absorption than at any other point. If the victim lives 24 hours the toxicologic examination may be negative.

The treatment of the acute case is to prevent further exposure of the victim, and to institute artificial respiration. If the drug is swallowed the stomach should be washed out. Stimulation may be necessary.

When the poisoning is caused by inhalation of fumes over a long period of time, or by continued ingestion of the drug therapeutically it becomes chronic in type with drowsiness, headache, purpuric eruptions over skin and mucous membranes, bleeding from the gums or nose, stupor and an aplastic anemia. The blood count shows erythrocytes, 600,000 to 800,000; leukocytes, 500 to 1,100; hemoglobin 8 per cent to 29 per cent; relative lymphocytosis, 50 per cent; diminution of platelets; anisocytosis; achromia, poikilocytosis; but with only a few nucleated red blood cells. In the early stages there may be a stimulation of the myelotic tissue so that there is an actual increase of the leucocytes and in rare instances a myeloid leukomia may develop. As a rule the drug attacks the bone marrow, especially the myeloid ele-ments and the platelets, preventing their formation; in mild cases the leukocyte count may be decreased to 1,200 as the only notable sign of the condition. In severer cases all the components of the bone marrow are attacked and the anemia may be severe, producing death in a few days to weeks from the severe tissue anoxia. Swelling of the upper jaw with periostitis and osteomyelitis and falling-out of the teeth have been described, much like the condition in phosphorus poisoning. At autopsy the bone marrow is aplastic in a few cases and may consist of fat with few, if any, blood forming cells; the blood may be pale. Numerous small hemorrhages may be present in the subserous tissues, in the subcutaneous layers, in the internal viscera and in the brain and its membranes, a condition partly referable to the diminution of the blood platelets and partly to fatty changes in the capillary vascular endothelium. Hemorrhages from the uterine cavity have been described. Heart muscle, liver, kidneys and adrenals may show fatty necrotic areas. The spleen is usually small and anemic. This condition of chronic poisoning is treated symptomatically, and blood transfusions and iron and liver extract may be administered for the anemia.

NITROBENZENE. The addition of the nitro radical to the benzene ring forms a number of poisonous compounds; mononitrobenzenes, dinitrobenzenes and trinotrobenzenes. The di- and trinitro-compounds are subdivided into ortho-, meta- and para-forms, depending on the arrangement of the NO_2 radicals on the ring. Though all these chemicals are toxic, mononitrobenzene and metadinitrobenzene are most important toxicologically.

Mononitrobenzene. This chemical, $C_6H_5NO_2$, is known as imitation oil of bitter almonds or oil of mirbane, and is a pale yellow oily liquid with a sweet taste and an aromatic odor like bitter almonds. It is used in the manufacture of aniline dyes and explosives, and formerly in the manufacture of shoe dyes, inks and flavoring extracts. Cases of poisoning have occurred from eating pastries and drinking alcoholic beverages into which such flavoring extracts have been introduced. Poisoning has been described in children who have worn freshly dyed shoes, and in an infant who came in contact with ink on a diaper, containing nitrobenzol. Similarly, this substance may cause toxic symptoms when applied to the skin in ointment form as a delousing preparation. Inhalation of vapors and the contact of the compounds with the clothing and skin of workers results in a large number of industrial disabilities because of the action of mononitrobenzene and metadinitrobenzene. Cases of poisoning by nitrobenzene have been described as a result of accidental ingestion of the drug, or as a means of suicide or as an abortifacient. In the Reports of the Office of the Chief Medical Examiner in New York City, 9 suicidal cases and 7 accidental cases of poisoning due to nitrobenzene occurred in the interval from 1918 to 1951.

The action of nitrobenzene depends upon the fact that it is a protoplasmic poison which first stimulates and then depresses the central nervous system and also effects profound changes in the blood. The red blood cells are damaged or destroyed, and the color of the blood is a distinct chocolate brown. The nature of transformation in the hemoglobin is not understood in all its details, but methemoglobin and a compound known as nitrobenzene hemoglobin are believed to be produced by the action of the chemical. In any event, the oxygen-carrying power of the blood is reduced both by the blood destruction and the transformation of the hemoglobin, and the tissue cells over the body suffer from a corresponding anoxia. Abnormal products like paramidophenol due to the decomposition of nitrobenzene in the body are found in the blood and in the urine.

If nitrobenzene is ingested, the sensations at first are numbness and tingling of the mouth and upper digestive tract, and then a quiescent period of a few minutes to about three hours may result. After this the toxic symptoms occur, the face becomes gray or gray-blue and a dark purple color of the lips and finger nails is present. The victim may display disturbed vision, fullness in the head, tinnitus aurium, dizziness, nausea, vomiting, and later weakness of the legs, muscular spasms in the face, an odor of bitter almonds on the breath, trismus, convulsions, fixed pupils, dark colored urine, chocolate colored blood. Cheyne-Stokes respirations, coma and death by respiratory paralysis in about one to seven hours. If he survives the acute symptoms, he may recover after a few days, or die from the damage inflicted by the compound on the blood and the central nervous system. If the nitrobenzene has been splashed on the skin and fumes have been inhaled, collapse and death may be sudden or supervene inside of an hour. Sometimes a dusky cyanosis is the only sign observable until the victim becomes suddenly prostrated and dies. Ordinarily the clinical course is longer in duration.

Postmortem examination reveals a grayish-blue color in the areas of lividity and a chocolate color of the blood. The viscera are congested, exude a strong and persistent odor of bitter almonds and are discolored a brownish purple as a result of the blood changes. Small hemorrhages may be present in the intestine, skin, brain substance and subserous tissues, and the spleen may be dark brown and contain pigment referable to blood destruction. There may be varying degrees of fatty degeneration and necrosis in the liver and heart muscle, and the kidneys may show fatty degeneration of the convoluted tubules, the collecting tubules may contain iron pigment, and the urine may be dark and almost black. Figure 4-7 illustrates the methemoglobinemia which results from poisoning by potassium chlorate; a similar picture is seen in cases of fatal nitrobenzene poisoning. The materials to save for toxicologic examination in acute cases are stomach contents, brain, lungs, liver and kidneys. Some of the blood may be saved for spectroscopic examination for the presence of methemoglobin.

The fatal dose of nitrobenzene is difficult to estimate, but small amounts like 8 drops or 15 drops have been credited with causing death. The treatment of the acute poisoning is to wash out the stomach, if the drug has been taken by mouth; if it has been applied to the skin, the source of contact must be removed. A saline purge may be efficacious in washing out the rest of the poison from the intestines. The ingestion of alcohol and fats should be avoided, as nitrobenzene is soluble in them and thus its absorption is favored. Blood transfusions and oxygen inhalations may be valuable in combating the anoxia.

A chronic form of poisoning occurs in some manufacturing processes which use nitrobenzene. It is marked by languor, somnolence, cyanosis, blindness, fatigue, anemia and dyspnea.

ANILINE. Aniline, $C_6H_5NH_2$, is a colorless liquid, oily and inflammable. It has a burning taste and a peculiar aromatic odor. It becomes brown on standing. Poisoning by aniline occurs in industrial plants where dyes, rubber solvents, shoe polishes and inks are manufactured, principally because its fumes are inhaled or because the liquid is splashed on the skin. An infant was accidentally poisoned because he wore a napkin stamped with ink containing aniline hydrochloride. Toxic symptoms followed the introduction of a dilute solution of the drug into the ear. Cases have been reported in which the aniline has been swallowed for the purpose of committing suicide.

The effects of aniline on the body are similar to those of nitrobenzene, in that it produces a primary stimulation followed by a secondary depression of portions of the central nervous system, a definite toxic action on the heart muscle and a brownish discoloration of the blood. There is a grayish-blue discoloration of the face, lips and nails. The changes in the blood are due to methemoglobin formation probably from the action of intermediate oxidation products of aniline in the body, namely paramidophenol and hydroxyphenylhydroxylamine. If the poisoning becomes subacute, the percentage of hemoglobin is reduced, the red blood cells are destroyed, and stippling, anisocytosis and poikilocytosis may develop.

The symptoms and signs of the acute poisoning are headache, giddiness, inebriation, somnolence, weakness, nausea, vomiting, small, rapid, irregular pulse, cyanosis and coma. The patient may die in about 12 hours as a result of toxemia and cardiac collapse, or he may live for several weeks. In the subacute cases, aniline may attack the liver and kidneys with the production of diarrhea and jaundice, and the urine may be dark from oxidation products, erythrocytes and hematoporphyrin. In non-fatal cases the illness is often prolonged from five to six weeks.

The characteristic postmortem findings in acute cases are the brownish discoloration of the blood and the tissues, and the strong odor of aniline in the various organs. In the subacute cases the appearances at necropsy may be those of blood destruction as described under pyrogallol on page 734. Stomach contents, blood, brain and parenchymatous organs are the materials used for chemical examination.

The fatal dose of aniline is not easy to determine but 25 gm. has caused death, though recovery has followed the ingestion of 75 ml. The treatment is to remove the victim from the source of exposure, and if the drug has been swallowed, to wash out the stomach. Warmth and inhalation of oxygen may be desirable. Infusions and transfusions may be indicated because of the condition of the blood.

Cases of chronic poisoning by aniline develop anemia, skin eruptions, nervous symptoms and amblyopia. In chronic cases which last a number of years, bladder carcinomas develop occasionally as a result of the continual irritation of that organ. In aniline workers there is a high incidence of papillomas and carcinomas of the bladder. These may develop several years after exposure.

COAL TAR DYES. Aniline dyes produce dermatoses and gastrointestinal lesions which are referable in part to the dye itself and in part to other chemicals such as strong acids, strong alkalis, bleaching powder, soaps, aniline, nitrobenzene and chlorine. The sodium and potassium salts of dinitrocresol known as Victoria yellow, dinitro-alpha-naphthol known as Manchester yellow, the phenylenediamines which are used on hair, and other dyes have caused fatal poisoning. The most prominent signs are dermatoses, gastrointestinal irritation, cardiac weakness and angioneurotic edema. Malignant tumors of the bladder have been described in aniline dye workers. The chemicals suggested as etiologic factors are some derivatives of the phenanthrene group which come over at about 300° C. in the dry distillation of coal.

PHENYLHYDRAZINE. Phenylhydrazine, $C_6H_5NH.NH_2$, is closely related to aniline and occurs as a yellowish-gray powder. It has been used in the treatment of polycythemia vera as it rapidly destroys red blood cells. The drug must be used with caution inasmuch as blood destruction may unduly tax the liver and kidneys. During its therapeutic use daily determinations should be made of the hemoglobin and leukocytes as undue increases in these factors are premonitory signs of the toxic action of the drug and indicate that the medication should be discontinued. Toxic signs caused by phenylhydrazine administration are jaundice and anuria, due to failure of the liver and kidneys to cope with the blood destruction.

BENZEDRINE. Benzedrine, or phenylisopropylamine, $C_6H_5.CHOH.CH.NHCH_3$. CH_3, is a volatile colorless liquid possessing a pungent odor and a burning taste. It is used as an inhalation for the purpose of shrinking the mucous membrane of the upper respiratory passages during a coryzal attack. Benzedrine sulfate (amphetamine sulfate) is sometimes given by mouth or by subcutaneous injection for narcolepsy and other similar disorders because of its stimulating action on the central nervous system. If excessive amounts are administered the patient exhibits irritability, restlessness, insomnia, delirium, mental confusion, a feeling of panic and may display such gastrointestinal and circulatory disturbances as vomiting, diarrhea, anorexia, palpitation of the heart and dyspnea. A fatal collapse has been reported following the use of benzedrine sulfate. Recently the drug has been used as an antidote for barbiturate poisoning.

Thymol. Thymol, C_6H_3 (CH_3) (OH) (C_3H_7), is an aromatic crystalline phenol which is present in the oil of thyme. It is used as an anthelmintic, especially for hookworm infections, and also as an antiseptic. Most cases of poisoning are caused by an overdose of the drug during therapeutic administration.

A poisonous dose may cause a burning sensation in the stomach and vomiting, but its local effects are slight. It has an action like phenol, but it is not so toxic. Vomiting, diarrhea, nausea, headache, giddiness, roaring in the ears and collapse may occur and death ensues in rare cases from its toxic action on the respiratory center. A dose of 6 gm. was said to cause death in the case of an anemic individual. For treatment the stomach is emptied and the patient is treated symptomatically. Stomach contents, parenchymatous viscera and urine are the materials preserved for toxicologic examination.

Pyridine. This coal tar derivative, C_5H_5N, is used to denature alcohol inasmuch as the disagreeable odor and taste of this volatile liquid render the alcohol unpotable. The local action of this compound is to cause irritation of the stomach, and its action after absorption produces cyanosis, dyspnea, prostration, edema of the lungs, delirium, coma and death in asphyxia. The signs at necropsy are not characteristic. The treatment and toxicologic indications are the same as for the other drugs of this series.

Naphthalene. Naphthalene, $C_{10}H_8$, is one of the coal tar hydrocarbons of the double ring type. It is a white crystalline mass, soluble in water and moderately volatile at ordinary temperatures. It melts as 80° C. and boils at 217.2° C. This compound is employed as an insect repellant, especially in the case of moths, and as one of the constituents in dye manufacture. In medicine it is used in dusting powders, as an intestinal antiseptic and as a vermifuge.

Continued inhalation of naphthalene vapor on bed clothes may be followed by toxic symptoms such as malaise, headache and vomiting. Most cases of poisoning occur in children who have eaten moth balls, or in individuals who have taken it as a vermifuge, or where the drug has been freely absorbed from the raw surface of wounds. If taken internally in toxic dose, naphthalene causes staggering gait, vomiting, abdominal pain, pain in bladder and kidney regions, a burning sensation in the urethra and strangury. A hemolytic anemia may develop and hemoglobinuric nephrosis and jaundice may follow. The urine is wine red or brown and contains albumen. The minimal lethal dose is difficult to determine satisfactorily. A fatal case occurred in a boy of 6 years who was given 175 gm. over a period of two days. The drug is absorbed slowly and may be removed; the treatment is to wash out the stomach and give purgatives, avoiding fats and castor oil in which naphthalene is soluble.

The postmortem findings in cases of naphthalene poisoning are the characteristic odor which this compound imparts to the blood and viscera, a dermatitis of variable intensity, an irritative gastroenteritis, a variable degree of methemoglobinemia as shown by dark violet or brown discoloration of the blood, a spleen which is enlarged and black-red in color, an enlarged dark-brown liver showing small foci of fatty degeneration and necrosis, congested kidneys with tubular degeneration and blood pigment casts in the lumen, and occasionally irritation of the cornea, chorioretinitis and degenerative changes in the retina.

Camphor. Camphor, $C_9H_{16}CO$, is a tough white translucent substance with an aromatic odor, derived from a tree, the *Cinnamomum camphora*. Chemically it is a ketone of the cyclic type. It slowly volatilizes at ordinary temperatures.

It is employed in medicine as a cardiac stimulant and a mild irritant. Most cases of poisoning are accidental, in which the drug has been given in overdose as a result of a therapeutic error. In a few cases it has been used as an abortifacient and death has resulted from this practice. Suicidal deaths occur, but are rare.

Toxic doses of camphor may cause irritation and a burning sensation in the throat and stomach, with thirst nausea and vomiting, and this is usually followed by blurred vision, ringing in the ears, dizziness and headache. A variable interval of a few minutes to hours follows, during which the victim develops symptoms similar to those of acute alcoholism, such as excitement, incoherence, hallucinations, delirium and convulsions. After this period of stimulation, the patient may lapse into coma and die from paralysis of the respiratory center in the medulla. Signs of renal irritation may occur, marked by albuminuria, strangury or suppression of urine. Dilatation of the pupil, cyanosis and irregular pulse may occur. The breath and urine may have an odor of camphor. Death may occur in a few hours to a day. The fatal dose of camphor in children has been about 15 to 30 grains. The fatal dose for an adult has not been determined; one individual took about 200 grains and recovered. The treatment is to wash out the stomach and administer saline cathartics to remove poison from the intestines. The body should be kept warm. The convulsions should be controlled by sedatives such as bromides, morphine and chloral hydrate.

The most striking postmortem finding is the odor of camphor about the viscera. Signs of gastric and renal irritation are occasionally present. The organs to preserve for toxicologic examination are stomach contents, brain and parenchymatous viscera.

Metrazol. This substance also known as cardiazol or pentamethylene-tetrazol is a complicated cyclic compound of formula $C_6H_{10}N_4$, closely related to camphor. It has a stimulating action on the central nervous system and is used as a stimulant in cardiac conditions and in the shock treatment for schizophrenia.

The toxicity of methrazol is not marked, and 2 mg. have been given without ill effects. The drug is rapidly absorbed and is rapidly detoxified by the liver, probably by conjugation. Fatal poisoning is rare, but has followed the oral administration of 10 gm. The drug causes a primary stimulation with tonic and clonic convulsions, followed by cerebral depression, anoxemia, coma, paralysis of the medullary centers and death. Convulsions are caused by the drug during the shock treatment of schizophrenia, and may occasionally produce compression fractures of the thoracic vertebral bodies. This drug is difficult to recover by toxicologic examination.

REFERENCES

Baker, H. M. Intoxication with commercial methyl chloride, J.A.M.A., 88:1137, 1927.
Barnett, H. J. M., and others. Thiocyanate psychosis, J.A.M.A., 147:1554, 1951.
Bein, G. V. Blausäurevergiftung und akute gelbe Atrophie, Zentralbl. Klin. Med., 45:970, 1924.
Chew, W. B., and others. Alkali treatment of methyl alcohol poisoning, J.A.M.A., 130:61, 1946.
Collins, J., and Martland, H. S. The result of poisoning by potassium cyanide, J. Nerv. & Ment. Dis., 35:417, 1908.

Esser, A., and Kuehn, A. Toedliche Cardiazolvergiftungen beim Menschen und im Tierversuch, Deutsche Ztschr. f. d. ges. Gericht. Med., 21:474, 1933.

Freireich, A. W., and Landsberg, J. W. Amphetamine sulphate for acute barbiturate poisoning, J.A.M.A., 131:661, 1946.

Geiling, E. M. K., and Cannon, P. R. Pathologic effects of Elixir of Sulphanilamid (diethylene glycol) poisoning, J.A.M.A., 111:919, 1938.

Gettler, A. O. Medicolegal aspects of death, associated with chloroform or ether, Am. J. Surg., 26:168, 1934.

———— and Freireich, A. W. The nature of alcohol tolerance, Am. J. Surg., 27:328, 1935.

———— and Siegel, H. Isolation of ether from human tissues, Arch. Path., 17:510, 1934.

———— and St. George, A. V. Toxicology in children, Am. J. Clin. Path., 5:466, 1935.

———— and St. George, A. V. Cyanide poisoning, Am. J. Clin. Path., 4:429, 1934.

Gonzales, T. A. Fatal inhalation of a dry cleaning fluid, J.A.M.A., 106:286, 1936.

Goodman, L., and Gilman, A. The Pharmacological Basis of Therapeutics, New York, The Macmillan Co., 1941.

Gordy, S. T., and Trumper, M. Carbon bisulphide poisoning, J.A.M.A., 110:1543, 1938.

Hunt, R., and Gettler, A. O. Non-Alkaloidal Organic Poisons, from Peterson, Haines and Webster, Legal Medicine and Toxicology, Philadelphia, W. B. Saunders Co., 1923.

Jones, O. R., and Burford, G. E. Massive atelectasis following cyclopropane anaesthesia, J.A.M.A., 110:1092, 1938.

Kegel, A. H., McNally, W. D., and Pope, A. S. Methyl chloride poisoning from domestic refrigeration, J.A.M.A., 93:353, 1929.

Kessler, D. L., and Hines, L. E. Hazards of thiocyanate therapy in hypertension, J.A.M.A., 138:549, 1948.

Lewin, L. Gifte und Vergiftungen, Berlin, Georg Stilke, 1929.

Mallory, T. B., Gall, E. A., and Brickley, W. J. Chronic exposure to benzene; pathological results, J. Indust. Hyg. & Toxicol., 21:355, 1939.

Norris, C. The lesions in wood alcohol poisoning, New York M. J., April 3rd, 1920.

Petri, E. Vergiftungen, from Henke and Lubarsch, Berlin, Julius Springer, 1930, Vol. X.

Polatin, R., Friedman, M. M., Harris, M. M., and Horowitz, W. A. Vertebral fractures produced by metrazole-induced convulsions, J.A.M.A., 112:1684, 1939.

Reports of the Office of the Chief Medical Examiner in the City of New York, from 1918 to 1951.

Rosenbloom, J. Chronic hydrocyanic acid poisoning, J. Lab. & Clin. Med., 8:258, 1923.

Smith, L. C. Collapse with death following the use of amphetamine sulphate, J.A.M.A., 113:1022, 1939.

Smith, S. Forensic Medicine, London, J. and A. Churchill Ltd., 1934.

Sollman, T. Manual of Pharmacology, 4th ed., Philadelphia, W. B. Saunders Co., 1932.

Webster, R. Legal Medicine and Toxicology, Philadelphia, W. B. Saunders Co., 1930.

Wood, F. C. A symposium on the etiology of neoplasms. Chemical factors, Proc. New York Path. Soc., Feb. 18th, 1936.

Zuelzer, W. W., and Apt, L. Acute hemolytic anemia due to naphthalene poisoning, J.A.M.A., 141:185, 1949.

33

Organic Poisons: Nonvolatile, Nonalkaloidal

A large number of organic poisons are not volatile and cannot be separated readily from the organs and secretions of the body by distillation. In such instances the poisonous agent is isolated by grinding up the organs, stomach contents or other material and extracting them with some selected immiscible solvent which dissolves out the poison but not the remaining organic constituents of the matrix. This process is described in Chapter 47.

The poisons which are isolated by this method of extraction with immiscible solvents are divided into two main groups: (1) Alkaloidal poisons, a homogeneous group of considerable importance, which are the toxic principles of certain plants and have distinctive chemical and pharmacologic characteristics, and which will be discussed in the following chapter. (2) Nonalkaloidal organic poisons which include a wide variety of chemical substances and which will be considered in this chapter.

Table 33-1. Nonvolatile Nonalkaloidal Organic Poisons

Aliphatic Hypnotics
    Barbiturates, hydantoins
    Carbamides
    Sulfonal, trional, tetronal
Aromatic Compounds
    Salicylic compounds, picric acid, dinitrophenol, trinitrotoluene, acetanilid, acetphene-
        tidin, antipyrine, aminopyrine, naphthol, cinchophen group, sulfonamides
Glucosides
    Digitalis, strophanthus, oleander, hellebore, scilla, gossypium, locust, *Cannabis indica*
Organic Purgatives
    Oils: croton oil, oleum ricini
    Anthracene group: aloes, rhubarb, senna, frangula, cascara sagrada
    Cathartic resins: colocynth, elaterin, jalap, podophyllum, gamboge
Essential Oils
    Aspidium, chenopodium, tansy, pennyroyal, nutmeg, savin, cedar, rue, thyme, apiol,
        saffron, turpentine
Picrotoxin Group
    Picrotoxin, cicutoxin
Miscellaneous
    Taxus, sparteine, abrus, laburnum, larkspur, heath family, santonin, cantharides

ALIPHATIC HYPNOTICS

The compounds in this group have a depressing effect on the central nervous system and are used therapeutically in induce sleep. If administered in overdose they may cause death by paralysis of the respiratory center.

Barbiturates. The derivatives of barbituric acid are white powders, usually crystalline, odorless and faintly bitter to the taste. They are only slightly soluble in water but are easily soluble in alcohol; the solution is slightly acid. The sodium salts of barbituric acid and its derivatives are crystalline, alkaline, bitter to the taste and dissolve readily in water.

The barbituric acid radical is a diureid formed from the combination of urea, $CO(NH_2)_2$, with malonic acid, $(COOH)_2 CH_2$, and the resulting compound is malonylurea, CO (NHCO)$_2$ CH$_2$, or barbituric acid which contains four atoms of carbon and two of nitrogen. The two H atoms in the malonyl component of barbituric acid are replaceable by different organic radicals, and a great variety of barbiturate compounds may be formed. Thus barbital or veronal, CO (NHCO)$_2$ C (C$_2$H$_5$)$_2$, is diethyl barbituric acid or diethyl malonyl urea; it is produced by the substitution of two ethyl groups for the two hydrogen atoms. In phenobarbital a phenyl radical is substituted for one of the ethyl groups, its formula being phenyl ethyl barbituric acid. Other barbiturate compounds of even greater complexity are manufactured. Among them are the thiobarbiturates in which the oxygen in the urea component is replaced by sulfur, as in thiobarbituric acid, CS (NHCO)$_2$ CH$_2$.

The barbiturates are depressants of the central nervous system, and are widely used as hypnotics, analgesics or anesthetics, usually in combination with other drugs. The depressant action is exerted on the cerebral cortex and the hypothalmic portion of the diencephalon; in the therapeutic dose little disturbance is caused in the brain or in any of the other organ systems of the body. The chemical structure of the barbiturate has a real correspondence with its pharmacologic behavior. Alkyl or aryl radicals must be substituted for the two hydrogen atoms attached to the carbon atom of the malonyl component if the barbiturate is to have a vigorous hypnotic action. If such an alkyl substitution chain is lengthened up to five radicals, the hypnotic potency of the compound will be increased but if the number of radicals in the chain is five or over, the sleep-producing effects are reduced and the resulting barbiturate may produce convulsions. A convulsant action may also be present in barbituric acid derivatives in which the alkyl groups are attached to the nitrogen atoms. When composed of alkyl groups, barbiturates of simple formula are relatively stable, resist destruction in the body and produce a protracted hypnotic action. Others with complex cyclic branches such as evipal, or the thiobarbiturates, are quickly destroyed after absorption and have a short action on the body. The stable long-acting compounds like barbital are usually excreted in the urine unchanged, while those easily destroyed like amytal or evipal occur in the urine in small amounts or not at all.

Table 33-2. Medicinal Doses in Grams of Various Barbiturates

Allonal	0.3	Ortal sodium	0.2 to 0.4
Sodium alurate	0.1	Pentobarbital sodium	0.1 to 0.2
Amytal	0.1 to 0.3	Pentothal sodium †	see below
Barbital or Veronal	0.3	Pernoston	0.2
Dial	0.3	Phanadorn	0.2
Evipal *	0.4	Phenobarbital (Luminal)	0.1 to 0.2
Ipral sodium	0.12 to 0.25	Sandopal	0.2
Nembutal	0.1	Seconal	0.2
Neonal	0.1	Vinbarbital sodium	0.1 to 0.2
Nostal	0.1 to 0.3		

* used as a hypnotic and also as anesthetic.
† used as anesthetic.
Other preparations used as hypnotics.

A barbiturate taken in a dose of 1 to 5 gm. may be dangerous to life, but recovery is possible if prompt treatment is applied. Pernoston is toxic and dangerous in amounts over 0.5 gm. The usual fatal dose of a barbiturate is 5 to 10 gm. or over; any amount over 15 times the therapeutic dose may be considered lethal. See Table 47-13 for structural formulas and melting points of various barbiturates.

Goodman and Gilman classify the barbiturates according to the speed of their therapeutic action into: (1) long-acting barbiturates (alurate, barbital, dial, ipral, neonal, nostal, phenobarbital), (2) action of moderate duration (amytal, ortal, pentobarbital, pernoston, phanadorn, sandopal), (3) short-acting (evipal, seconal), and (4) ultra short-acting used for intravenous anesthesia (evipal, pentothal sodium, thioethamyl). The rapidity with which barbiturates act on the body depends upon the method of administration and upon the nature of the derivative as to whether it is long-acting or short-acting.

Barbiturates are administered therapeutically by mouth, by rectum, by subcutaneous or intramuscular hypodermic injection, or by intravenous injection. Oral administration is by far the most common method, and the one of choice, unless contraindicated by some special consideration like persistent vomiting. The drug passes through the stomach and is absorbed from the small intestine readily, the hypnotic effect occurring in about 20 to 60 minutes on the average. A long-acting stable compound like barbital is probably absorbed in 45 to 60 minutes and in overdose produces a profound coma of several days duration; in fatal cases death usually supervenes after a protracted period of unconsciousness. The short-acting, more soluble barbiturates on the other hand are absorbed within 15 to 20 minutes and when a lethal quantity is injected death may be rapid.

Barbiturates are administered through the rectum in some cases, usually to patients who have persistent vomiting, or to infants. Injections, either subcutaneous or intramuscular, are given mainly when rapid barbiturate action is desired, using a 10 per cent aqueous solution of a soluble sodium salt of barbituric acid; the thiobarbiturates because of their irritant action cannot be used for this purpose. Intravenous injection of an ultra short-acting barbiturate is sometimes employed to induce a surgical anesthesia of short duration, and is usually resorted to only in emergencies inasmuch as such anesthesia cannot be controlled once the injection has been made. The method should only be employed by a competent and experienced anesthetist. As an example of this procedure, pentothal sodium is injected intravenously in quantities of 2 to 3 ml. of a 5 per cent solution over a period of 15 seconds, the injection is temporarily discontinued for 30 seconds, and if the desired anesthesia is not obtained, an additional 2 to 3 ml. is injected at the same rate. Intravenous injection of an ultra short-acting barbiturate is sometimes used in the treatment of strychnine poisoning.

Contraindications to the continuous therapeutic use of barbiturates exist when the patient has: (1) a severe liver disease which would interfere with the oxidation of the short-acting barbiturates so that their depressing effect is dangerously prolonged; (2) a renal disease which interferes with the excretion of the stable barbiturates so that they accumulate in the body and provoke an unwonted toxic action; (3) a personal idiosyncrasy to barbiturates which may be congenital so that on administration of the drug the patient suffers from arthritic pains, undue excitement and emotional disturbances, or an allergic idiosyncrasy acquired as a result of previous medication with such manifestation as swelling of lips, eyelids and cheeks and erythematous and bullous lesions of the skin.

Fatal poisoning as the result of the administration of barbiturates may be homicidal, suicidal or accidental; and usually occurs only with the ingestion of large amounts. Homicidal cases are rare and only one has been encountered among the cases investigated by the Office of the Chief Medical Examiner of New York City during the years from 1918 to 1951. Suicidal deaths from barbiturates have become increasingly numerous although the yearly average was only 8 cases for the period up to 1941, but in recent years the number has increased several fold, reaching 119 cases in 1946. The explanation may be the fact that these drugs are much more commonly prescribed than formerly and are easy to obtain; also they cause death painlessly as a rule. Many states and municipalities have passed laws regulating the sale of barbituric acid derivatives because of the increased use of these substances for the commission of suicide. In some instances a person contemplating suicide by submersion in the bath tub has taken a large dose of barbiturates evidently to dull the uncomfortable sensations produced by drowning. In many barbiturate suicides, large amounts of the drug are recovered from the stomach and internal organs by toxicologic examination.

Accidental and unexplained barbiturate deaths formerly were encountered in New York City on the average of 8 to 9 times a year, but in recent years the number of cases in this category have also increased so that there were 78 in 1946. Many of these result from the deliberate ingestion of barbiturates in large quantities while the victim is profoundly alcoholic, and in a state in which the toxic action of the barbiturates is enhanced by the synergistic action of the alcohol, both poisons having a depressant action on the central nervous system (see reference to Jetter and McLean). Most of the cases are probably suicidal, but the suicidal intent may be difficult to establish in the presence of coexistent acute alcoholism and in the absence of a suicide note or of a known prior suicidal attempt. An investigation of the circumstances of death in addition to a quantitative toxicologic analysis is necessary to establish how the poisoning came about. Accidental barbiturate deaths sometimes occur as a result of the intravenous injection of a barbiturate to induce anesthesia.

Barbital, $CO(HNCO)_2 C(C_2H_5)_2$, also known as veronal, is a slow-acting barbiturate, and, after it is ingested in toxic dose, causes premonitory signs of dizziness, headache, nausea, vomiting, ataxia, inarticulate speech and mental confusion, the patient gradually sinking into coma. The coma gradually becomes deeper, and either takes the form of a profound stupor, or is associated with excitement, delirium, restlessness and tonic spasms. There is a depression of the central nervous system, especially the cerebral cortex and diencephalon, and the respirations become slow and shallow and later Cheyne-Stokes in type. A marked vasodilatation of the smaller blood vessels is present, the blood pressure falls, and the pulse becomes rapid and weak. The temperature sinks, the skin is cold, clammy and cyanotic, anoxemia is favored, and a condition similar to secondary shock is produced. The urinary flow is decreased or suppressed, partly because of the depressant action of the drug on the diencephalon, and partly because of the low blood pressure. In some instances, the pupils of the eyes are dilated, in others they are contracted. The patient may regain consciousness after a few days and finally recover. If he survives the effects of a single massive dose, he may develop after effects, such as a neuritis with gangrenous areas on the feet, skin eruptions of various kinds and hematoporphyrinuria. Death may occur in from two to seven days on the average, from pneumonia, paralysis of the respiratory centers in the medulla, or uremia.

About 65 to 80 per cent of barbital is eliminated in the urine, and the remainder of the intake is changed by the liver through a process of side-chain oxidation. The absorption of the drug is gradual and its rate of excretion slow, reaching its height on the second day and continuing past the fourth day after ingestion. Because of the slow excretion of barbital, repeated small doses of barbital may accumulate in the system until it has reached a concentration which is capable of exerting severe toxic action. If a case of barbital poisoning is observed clinically, it is important to preserve some of the urine and stomach contents for toxicologic examination, for the drug can be isolated from these materials.

The quick-acting barbiturates are absorbed rapidly, usually within a few minutes after ingestion. In large overdose they may cause a rapid onset of coma and death. In several cases encountered by the authors, death occurred within a half hour. Medinal, seconal and amytal belong to this type of barbituric acid derivative. In cases where death has been rapid, the lesions found at necropsy are not characteristic, and consist mostly of congestion of the viscera and brain, fluid blood in the heart cavities, edema of the lungs and cyanosis. Gritty residues of unabsorbed barbiturate may be found in the stomach. In some cases the undisintegrated tablets of the drug or the partly dissolved colored gelatin capsules in which the drug is dispensed may be detected. In fatal cases which have survived a longer time, especially with supportive therapy, much of the more complex soluble barbiturate compounds are destroyed in the body, especially in the liver, and less is excreted in the urine. The longer the period of survival, the smaller the amount of barbiturate that can be recovered from the viscera. The survival period must always be taken into account together with the character of the barbiturate ingested in the interpretation of the toxicologic findings.

Medinal or sodium barbital, in addition to its solubility, prompt absorption and rapid toxic action, is alkaline and may cause an engorgement of the blood vessels and an intense crimson corrosion and reddening of the stomach mucous membrane, resembling the alkaline corrosion produced by cyanide. The following cases are typical of poisoning by quick-acting barbiturates and also show corrosion of the stomach mucous membrane like that caused by medinal:

A case of rapid barbiturate poisoning was encountered in a mentally depressed, middle-aged white woman who locked herself in her bathroom and refused to come out after a few minutes had elapsed. Alarmed by this, her maid summoned help, the bathroom door was forced after 10 to 15 minutes work, and the woman was found dead. In all, this death occurred in less than half an hour. The autopsy revealed a marked hyperemia of the gastric mucosa almost like a real corrosion such as one sees in potassium cyanide poisoning. However, the microscopic examination of the stomach did not show any corrosion but only an intense hyperemia of the mucosa. The toxicologic examination disclosed a considerable amount of medinal or sodium barbital in the stomach, brain and liver, and this substance by reason of its strong alkaline reaction produced an intense hyperemia of the gastric mucous membrane. The rapidity of the death gave reason to believe that the barbiturate was absorbed directly by the hyperemic stomach mucosa.

Another case of rapid barbiturate poisoning was encountered in a 30 year old white woman, living in a residential hotel, who was known to have been receiving symptomatic medication in the form of glandular extracts and sedatives for indefinite complaints, probably of neurotic origin. On the day of her death she was sitting on the edge of the swimming pool of the hotel with her feet dangling in the water, and she asked one of the attendants for a drink of water. After receiving this she collapsed and died within a few minutes, despite attempts at resuscitation. She was not submerged at any time. The autopsy disclosed an intense hyperemia of the gastric mucosa, and the toxicologic examination determined the presence in the stomach, brain and liver of a large amount of a barbiturate compound. The deceased probably ingested the poison just before she reached the pool or while she was sitting on the edge. The rapidity of her collapse and death indicated this. It might have been the purpose of the deceased to submerge herself in order to convey the impression of an accidental drowning, but if so her plan miscarried because of the rapid lethal action of the drug. A number of suicidal drownings have revealed the presence of barbiturates in the stomach.

Phenobarbital or luminal, $CO (NHCO)_2 C (C_2H_5) (C_6H_5)$, is a white colorless and crystalline powder and a long-acting barbiturate, but it is a more active sedative and hypnotic than barbital as its medicinal dose is smaller. More of the drug is oxidized by the liver, so that only 25 per cent is excreted in the urine. In toxic dose it produces practically the same symptoms and effects as barbital, but if used over a long period of time may cause a bullous dermatitis.

The principal pathologic lesion in delayed deaths from barbital and other barbiturates is a complicating hypostatic bronchopneumonia. A rare lesion was observed twice by the authors in such delayed barbiturate deaths, namely a bilateral

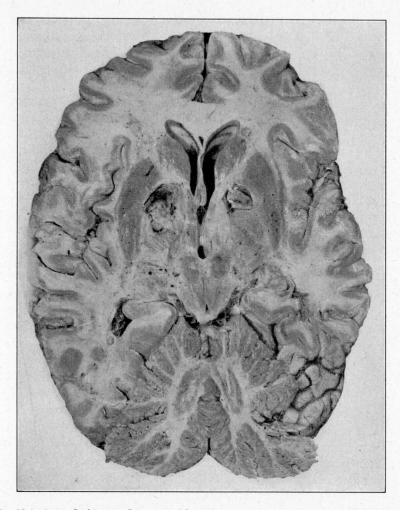

Fig. 33-1. Acute Barbiturate Poisoning: Bilateral Symmetric Softening of Globus Pallidus.

Death in coma four days after taking a large amount of a barbiturate. The lesion shown here is similar to that frequently seen in delayed carbon monoxide poisoning. It is very rare in barbiturate poisoning.

symmetric necrosis of the globus pallidus which in one case followed the ingestion of a fatal amount of dial with a survival period of four days (Fig. 33-1). De Groat has described a similar case. Other lesions described in the brain are small ring hemorrhages, degenerations of neurons and perivascular edema.

HYDANTOINS. A number of compounds chemically related to phenobarbital belong to the hydantoin group and are used in the treatment of convulsions arising from such disease conditions as epilepsy and chorea. Drugs like diphenylhydantoin sodium (dilantin), trimethadione (tridione), and methylphenylethyl hydantoin (mesantoin) are employed in the treatment of epileptic cases. Like phenobarbital they may be the cause of a pinkish or reddish rash accompanied by itching and burning which appears about 10 to 15 days after continued administration of the drug, and also may give rise to a granulocytopenia. Phenylethyl hydantoin (nirvanol), a highly toxic compound, is used in the treatment of chorea and may produce macular rash, eosinophilia, granulocytopenia, fever and stupor.

The authors have seen a bullous exfoliative dermatitis in a white man, 28 years old, who several months prior to death had been given tridione for lapses of consciousness diagnosed as petit mal, and 11 days prior to his admission to a hospital he developed a macular rash around the groin which increased in extent to huge moist, bullous, desquamative areas covering most of the body. A granulocytopenia appeared two days prior to death which occurred 15 days after the onset of the dermatitis. At autopsy an inflammatory reaction similar to the lesion in the skin was present in the mucous membrane of the mouth and buccopharynx but not extending to the nasopharynx or larynx. Ruskin described a similar case which followed the administration of mesantoin to a 10 year old white girl.

In fatal cases the brain, kidneys, liver, stomach contents and urine are preserved for toxicologic examination. The stomach contents are especially valuable in deaths which occur shortly after ingestion, for in this material the poison can be identified most conveniently. When the victim lives for two days or more, as in the case of barbital, the urine usually contains a large amount of the poison where it can be easily demonstrated; the stomach contents on the other hand may contain only a small amount of barbiturate. The brain, liver and kidneys generally show large quantities of the drug in most poisonings, and the muscles and bones contain much less. Webster has claimed that the concentration of barbiturates in the brain is greatest in the optic thalamus and corpus striatum but this has not been the experience of the toxicologic laboratory in the Office of the Chief Medical Examiner in New York City; investigations have indicated that the poison is fairly evenly distributed in different parts of the brain. In fatal cases, the concentration of barbiturates in the brain and liver usually varies from 2.5 to 8 mg. per 100 gm. of tissue. Smaller amounts may be found in cases in which most of the drug was destroyed or excreted during a long survival interval between the time the poison was taken and death which occurred from exhaustion or bronchopneumonia (Table 33-3).

Quantitative determinations of the amounts of barbiturates in the brain, liver, stomach contents and urine are quite important, because the investigator must calculate the quantity of poison which has been administered, checking his results with the body weight of the victim and the survival period after the poisoning. In cases which die soon after taking the drug, a large quantity recovered from the stomach contents and viscera would indicate that it was taken deliberately; if a homicidal poisoning can be eliminated as a possibility, a diagnosis of suicide is substantiated and doubt would be cast on the interpretation that an accidental overdose was taken. The synergistic action of alcohol with barbiturates has already been discussed. If the survival period is longer, over two days, the amount of barbiturate in the stomach and parenchymatous organs will be much less, as much of the drug will have been excreted or destroyed. The period of survival must always be considered in appraising the result of the toxicologic examination, and investigation of the circumstances of the poisoning is necessary for the classification of the case.

Table 33-3. Toxicologic Examination in Cases of Barbiturate Poisoning

Patient	Duration	Clinical Course	Autopsy	Toxicologic Analyses.* Amount of Barbiturate
Male white 43 yrs.	2 hours or more	Found in coma	Congestion of lungs	Liver, 11.6 mg. in 500 gm.
Male white 39 yrs.	2 hours	Found in coma Phenobarbital, amount not known.	Cyanosis Bronchopneumonia Congestion of viscera	Urine, small amounts Brain, 28.5 mg. in 1,000 gm.
Male white 49 yrs.	3 hours	Found in coma	Atelectasis of lungs	Liver, 28 mg. in 500 gm. Stomach, large amounts
Male white 45 yrs.	22 hours	Coma	Bronchopneumonia	Liver, 18.5 mg. in 500 gm.
Male white 24 yrs.	34 hours	Coma	Bronchopneumonia	Brain, 28 mg. in 1,000 gm. Liver, 25 mg. in 1,000 gm.
Female white 22 yrs.	2 days	Coma Probably took 9 gm. of barbiturate	Not described	Brain, 21.8 mg. in 300 gm.
Female white 45 yrs.	3 days	Coma	Bronchopneumonia	Brain, 15.9 mg. in 500 gm.
Male white 57 yrs.	4 days	Coma	Bronchopneumonia Symmetric softening of globus pallidus (Fig. 30-1)	Brain, 21.8 mg. in 500 gm. Liver, 18.9 mg. in 500 gm. Stomach contents, 31.5 gm. in total Urine (life), 25.0 mg. in 250 ml.
Female white 54 yrs.	8 days	Found in coma Urine positive for barbiturates.	Congestion of lungs	Liver, 8.8 mg. in 500 gm.

*Analyses performed by Dr. Alexander O. Gettler, toxicologist to the Office of the Chief Medical Examiner in New York City.

Death as a result of acute barbiturate poisoning cannot always be determined as a result of the autopsy findings even when supported by toxicologic analyses on material collected from the patient during life or from his body after death. First the autopsy must exclude other causes of death which would take precedence over the poisoning such as a spontaneous subarachnoid hemorrhage, a ruptured aortic aneurysm, a suppurative peritonitis from a ruptured abdominal viscus, or a bullet wound of the heart or aorta. In the absence of another cause of death, other than a secondary bronchopneumonia, the finding of barbiturates in the organs in significant amount would be sufficient to establish the cause of death as barbiturate poisoning. In determining what amounts are significant all due consideration must be given to the period of survival after the poison has been taken. In some cases the victim may survive long enough for almost all the barbiturate to be eliminated and death occur from exhaustion or bronchopneumonia. Even in cases with negative toxicologic findings at necropsy, death should be attributed to barbiturate poisoning if clinical observations and tests and investigation of circumstances substantiate the diagnosis.

The treatment of barbiturate poisoning depends on the dose and the severity of the symptoms. Most poisonings of minor grade that result from therapeutic over-dosage cause confusional states or coma from which the patients recover satis-factorily without treatment. The more severe cases of suicidal poisoning which are brought to the hospital have a mortality of about 25 per cent. The outstanding symptoms are deep coma, cyanosis, shallow respirations, rapid pulse, constricted pupils and sometimes fever. As the poisoning progresses, circulatory failure develops and bronchopneumonia may occur. Many fatal cases die unobserved and are found dead after an unknown period of survival. An important part of the treatment of severe barbiturate poisoning is the evacuation of the barbiturates from the stomach by lavage as quickly as possible; this must be carried out cautiously to prevent aspiration of gastric contents into the respiratory tract. Infusion of glucose and saline to combat circulatory failure, and high colonic irrigation to aid excretion are useful. The air passages should be kept clear and the tongue not allowed to drop back into the throat and mucus should be removed. Artificial respirations, inhala-tion of oxygen, or of oxygen and carbon dioxide, and the application of warmth to the skin should be employed. Intramuscular injections of ephedrine in doses of 10 to 30 mg., repeated 1 to 2 hours if necessary, may be given. Strychnine is doses of 2 to 10 mg., repeated every two hours was formerly employed but has been abandoned. Metrazol has been employed. Picrotoxin may be injected intravenously as a physiologic antidote in doses of 10 mg., repeated every 20 minutes, until the corneal and pupillary reflexes are restored. Signs of hyperexcitability may appear, and care must be taken not to produce convulsions; in such instances the amount of picrotoxin can be reduced and the interval between injections prolonged. If given cautiously, considerable total amounts of picrotoxin may be administered. Freireich and Landsberg recommend the intravenous injections of amphetamine sulfate in doses of about 20 mg. every half hour until the patient shows signs of returning consciousness.

Barbital and the other barbiturates are habit forming drugs and their long continued use may cause chronic poisoning. The most prominent symptoms are foul breath, nausea, mental confusion, ataxia, indistinct enunciation, emotional instability, skin eruptions of erythematous, urticarial, purpuric or scarlatiniform type, and trophic necrotic areas on the skin. Phenobarbital also may produce chronic poisoning with skin eruptions a marked feature usually of the urticarial, maculo-papular, scarlatiniform or bullous type; conjunctivitis and amaurosis have been noted in some cases. It is said that the barbiturates are responsible for about a third of the cases of drug psychosis admitted to mental hospitals. Chronic barbiturate addiction is frequently associated with chronic alcoholism and personality disorders. Many addicts have substituted barbiturates for heroin which for a time was un-obtainable and prohibitive in cost. In the absence of coma, chronic barbiturate poisoning may present a variety of symptoms such as delirium, disorientation, delu-sions and euphoria.

Carbamides. SEDORMID. Sedormid or allyl-isopropyl-acetyl-carbamide, $(CH_3)_2$ CH (CH_2CHCH_2) $(CONHCONH_2)$, is used as a hypnotic. In some individuals, small doses of sedormid cause destruction of blood platelets and thrombocytopenic purpura.

Sulfonal Group. Sulfonmethane or sulfonal, $(CH_3)_2C(SO_2C_2H_5)_2$, is a crystalline compound without odor, colorless and tasteless. Taken in medicinal dose it is a hypnotic which does not depress the circulation or respiration. It is eliminated slowly through the kidneys as sulfonal and ethylsulfonic acid. If repeated doses are given, the drug may accumulate in the system, and a dangerous poisonous effect may be produced.

Fatal sulfonal poisoning may result from the taking of an overdose. The drug is not very soluble and is absorbed slowly so that the soporific action is delayed. The medicinal dose is from 0.3 to 1.2 gm., the maximal dose is 2.0 gm. The fatal dose has been as low as 5.0 gm., but much larger amounts have been taken with recovery. Because of the cumulative action of the poison, death may follow the repeated administration of small doses. Sometimes the victim dies within a few hours after administration of the drug, or death may be delayed for many days. It is preceded by profound sleep and respiratory and circulatory failure. The acute poisoning is treated by washing out the stomach with warm water and encouraging the renal and intestinal elimination by infusion of dilute alkaline saline solutions. Stimulation and artificial respiration should be used according to need.

If sulfonal is administered over a long period of time a chronic poisoning may ensue. Toxic symptoms are headache, mental confusion, staggering gait, stupor and coma. The patient complains of varied symptoms; the paralyses, muscular cramps, ataxia, mental depression and signs of disseminated neuritis are referable to the continued action of the drug on the central nervous system; the vomiting, diarrhea, constipation and tympanites are gastrointestinal in origin. The chronic effect of sulfonal also produces methemoglobin and hematoporphyrin in small amounts in the blood, and hematoporphyrin, methemoglobin, pigment casts and red blood cells in the urine. In some cases erythematous and bullous eruptions appear on the skin, and edema of the eyelids may be present. Fatty change in the liver cells, fatty degeneration of the kidney tubules, cellular proliferation of Bowman's capsule and hemorrhagic extravasations from the glomeruli into the lumen of the tubules have been described. Recovery is slow and the outcome may be fatal if the urine changes develop. At autopsy congestion of all organs, especially the lungs, and signs of renal irritation may be present but the signs are not characteristic. Sulfonal resists putrefaction in the body, and may be found in the tissues a long time after death. The materials employed for toxicologic examination are the stomach contents, urine, brain, liver and kidneys.

Trional, $(CH_3)(C_2H_5)C(SO_2C_2H_5)_2$, and tetronal, $(C_2H_5)_2C(SO_2C_2H_5)_2$, are similar to sulfonal in some respects. They are bitter in taste, soluble in water and less toxic than sulfonal, though cases of poisoning have occurred. The symptoms, treatment, autopsy findings and extraction are similar to that described under sulfonal. Trional melts at 74° to 76° C., tetronal at 86° to 89° C., and sulfonal at 124° to 126° C.; the differences in the melting points are important criteria in the differentiation of these compounds during toxicologic analysis.

AROMATIC COMPOUNDS

These substances are nonvolatile derivatives of benzene and other hydrocarbon ring compounds. When given in fatal dose they paralyze the respiratory center in the medulla, and in many instances cause irritation of the gastrointestinal tract and kidneys, and exert a toxic action on the red blood cells and the liver.

Salicylic Acid. Salicylic acid, $C_6H_4OH\ COOH$, is a white crystalline substance which has a sweet taste when it first comes in contact with the tongue but later develops an acrid flavor. Most salicylic acid poisonings have occurred in connection with its internal use as an analgesic and antipyretic in acute rheumatic conditions or the external application of preparations containing it to raw wound surfaces or even the intact skin. At one time salicylic acid was added to foods as a preservative to prevent fermentation, but its use for this purpose has been forbidden by law in most jurisdictions. Suicidal poisonings occur occasionally. In the reports of the Office of the Chief Medical Examiner in New York City, there were 46 accidental and undetermined fatalities and 22 suicidal deaths from salicylate poisonings between the years 1918 and 1951; the individual salicylic acid compounds responsible were not enumerated.

When a moderately large dose of salicylic acid or a salicylate is given, ringing in the ears, perspiration, dimness of vision, confusion and mental dullness are produced in addition to the analgesic and antipyretic effects. In rare cases bullous or purpuric skin eruptions, deafness, renal irritation, acidosis with marked dyspnea and a condition resembling delirium tremens may develop; uterine hemorrhages may occur followed by abortion if the victim is pregnant. Some individuals are abnormally sensitive to the drug and react unfavorably to a small dose; a large proportion of these victims suffer from asthma or a similar allergic condition. Most individuals can take a large dose without apparent toxic effects. In some cases the application of a powder containing salicylates to an open wound causes local necrosis.

After excessive doses, pain in the throat and abdomen, dysphagia, vomiting, diarrhea, dyspnea, subnormal temperature, convulsions and death from respiratory center paralysis may occur within a few hours or after several days. The dose in acute fatal salicylate poisoning is variable; 4 to 10 gm. have caused death, while the ingestion of larger quantities has not been fatal. In some instances the patient has been suffering from a severe illness and it is difficult to determine whether death is due to the drug or to the disease. The principal therapy in acute poisoning is to wash out the stomach and to promote elimination of the poison from the intestines by administering magnesium sulfate as a cathartic. The treatment is otherwise symptomatic.

Salicylic acid is converted into sodium salicylate which is eliminated in the urine either unchanged or in the form of salicyluric acid; about 20 per cent or more is destroyed by the cells of the body. The elimination is complete in about 48 hours. In fatal salicylic or salicylate poisoning, autopsy may reveal a reddening and inflammation of the upper gastrointestinal tract, swelling of the renal cortex with small hemorrhages in the tubules, cloudy swelling and fatty degeneration of the tubular epithelium, fatty degeneration of the liver, pulmonary edema, and small hemorrhages in the heart, lungs and meninges. The materials saved for toxicologic analysis are the stomach contents, brain, liver, kidneys and urine.

Methyl salicylate, or artificial oil of wintergreen, is taken occasionally by accident, for suicidal purposes or to cause abortion. Its effects are similar to those caused by salicylic acid. Reddening and inflammation of the upper gastrointestinal tract, submucous hemorrhages in the kidney pelvis, small hemorrhages in the lumen of the renal tubules, congestion of viscera, and a characteristic odor of oil of wintergreen throughout the body were found in cases autopsied by the authors.

Salol, or phenyl salicylate, may produce combined symptoms of salicylic acid and phenol poisoning. In the body, salol splits into salicylic acid and phenol, and both compounds may be identified by toxicologic analysis. Fatal poisonings are rare.

Aspirin, or acetylsalicylic acid, is usually tolerated in large doses when used as an analgesic, but very large doses may cause poisoning, especially in sensitive individuals. The authors have seen three cases of suicide caused by ingestion of large quantities of aspirin which was identified by chemical analysis. At autopsy, aside from a generalized visceral congestion, the most striking lesion was a postmortem erosion of the stomach mucous membrane and a strong odor of acetic acid was detected in the gastric contents; much of the aspirin was decomposed after death into salicylic acid and acetic acid, and the latter produced a dull grayish white, reactionless necrosis of the gastric mucosa.

A chronic poisoning, known as salicylism, may follow continued use of the drug. Anorexia, diarrhea, constipation, mental depression, renal irritation and skin eruptions of erythematous, eczematoid and desquamative character may manifest themselves in such patients.

Picric Acid. Picric acid, $C_6H_2(NO_2)_3OH$, or trinitrophenol, is a bright yellow, odorless, crystalline substance with a bitter taste. It has a tendency to explode when heated or subjected to percussion. It is one of the constituents of certain high explosives, and is used in dye manufacturing processes. In medicine it is employed as an external application in the treatment of burns and skin diseases and for sterilization of the skin before a surgical operation.

Accidental poisoning by picric acid may occur as the result of its medicinal use as a salve or dusting powder in the treatment of burns, or it may be encountered in workmen who handle the substance. In a few instances this compound has been ingested for suicidal purposes. Rarely it has been used by malingerers to produce a yellow discoloration of the skin in order to simulate jaundice, but the yellow color produced by it can be differentiated from true icterus by the absence of bilirubin in the urine and blood.

When picric acid is ingested in large doses, abdominal pain, diarrhea and vomiting may ensue; the vomited matter and the fecal material are yellow. The urine does not contain bile, but at first is yellow in color and later turns a yellowish brown or reddish brown; anuria and strangury may develop. The blood may show hemolysis but does not usually contain bilirubin. Acute liver degeneration may occur and cause a true icterus. The skin and visible mucous membranes are colored yellow, and the patient may complain of yellow vision. Eczema and pruritus are frequently present. The compound is excreted slowly from the body, and the yellowish discoloration of the tissues may last for days. If the poisoning is severe, prostration, fever, stupor and convulsions follow, and the patient may have a fatal collapse due to the toxic action of picric acid on the central nervous system. In some cases death is due to anuria and occurs after several days.

The acute cases of picric acid poisoning are treated by washing out the stomach and evacuating the bowels with enemas. Cathartics are not to be recommended as they may increase the irritation of the intestinal tract. White of egg may be ingested as an antidote. The fatal dose of picric acid is not known, although 1 to 2 gm. may produce severe poisoning with recovery.

The postmortem findings in acute poisoning are an intense yellow discoloration of the skin and internal organs and signs of irritation of the upper gastrointestinal tract and urinary tract. Hemorrhages may be found in the tubules of the kidney, and, in rare cases, a toxic hepatitis. The materials used for toxicologic analysis are the stomach contents, brain, liver, kidneys and urine.

Chronic poisoning by picric acid occurs in laborers engaged in the manufacture of explosives. The poison may be applied to the skin, its fumes may be inhaled or its dust accidentally ingested. Dermatitis, yellowish skin, bronchitis, stomatitis, nasal catarrh, abdominal cramps, vomiting, diarrhea, strangury, dizziness and loss of weight may occur.

Dinitrophenol. Dinitrophenol, $C_6H_3OH(NO_2)_2$, is a yellow solid used in the manufacture of high explosives. It has been used medicinally as a weight reducer in cases of obesity, and this effect has been attributed to an increase of metabolic activity produced by the pharmacologic action of the drug. Cases of poisoning have occurred because it was not administered with sufficient care. Suicidal attempts by ingestion of dinitrophenol have been reported in the literature.

Acute poisoning, which follows the ingestion of large doses, may be attended by gastrointestinal distress, nausea, vomiting, flushed skin, sweating, high fever, restlessness and rapid deep respirations which become more pronounced as the accessory muscles are called into play. At this stage pain in the chest, abdominal cramps, marked fever, cyanosis, coma and failure of respiration may supervene and death may occur in a few days. Some individuals are abnormally susceptible to the drug, and a small dose may produce maculopapular or urticarial eruptions, itching of the skin, edema and joint pains.

In fatal cases the autopsy findings are not characteristic. Petechial hemorrhages are noted occasionally beneath the serous membranes. Marked pulmonary edema and congestion occur. The materials saved for toxicologic examination are the stomach contents, brain, liver and kidneys. The treatment is designed to speed the elimination of the poison from the body. The stomach is washed out with a solution of 5 per cent sodium bicarbonate and this antidote is allowed to remain to combat the dinitrophenol. Intravenous injection of a 5 per cent glucose in physiologic saline solution is recommended to promote excretion. The remainder of the treatment is symptomatic.

If dinitrophenol is used over a long period of time acute yellow atrophy of the liver, toxic nephrosis, agranulocytosis, anemia and cataracts may develop.

Trinitrotoluene. Trinitrotoluene, $C_6H_2(NO_2)_3CH_3$, is a crystalline yellow substance used as a high explosive. It is quite toxic and cases of subacute or chronic poisoning have occurred, incident to the handling of the material in ammunition factories. The poison is absorbed through the skin, the gastrointestinal tract and the air passages causing local irritation at the point of entry. If it is inhaled as a vapor, sneezing, coryza, epistaxis, nasal discomfort, watering of the eyes, sore throat, dry cough and pain in the chest may occur. If it is ingested, spasmodic gastric pain, anorexia, nausea, vomiting, diarrhea with griping, or constipation may follow. When the drug is applied to the skin, eczematous rashes may develop over the face and extremities with itching and yellow staining of the skin and hair. After absorption the red blood cells may be destroyed, and methemoglobin and hematin form in the blood; anemia and toxic hepatitis and jaundice may occur. The urine is dark in color and contains albumin. Trinitrotoluene is reduced in part in its passage through the body, and is excreted slowly in the urine as a chromogen in conjugation with glycuronic acid. This substance may be demonstrated in the urine if the examination is made a day or so after exposure.

The toxic symptoms are referable to the action of the poison on the blood, the victims complaining of dizziness, fatigue, dyspnea on exertion, headache, pains in the legs, drowsiness, frequency of urination and pain and tenderness in the right hypochondrium. The blood may show fragmented or fragmenting red blood cells, stippling, polychromatophilia, reticulated red blood cells, reduction of hemoglobin, leukocytosis and lymphocytosis. A true aplastic anemia may develop. Toxic jaundice occurs, first with liver enlargement, later with liver shrinkage, atrophy and necrosis similar to acute yellow atrophy. The kidneys may show a toxic nephrosis with parenchymatous and fatty degeneration.

The vast majority of poisonings occur in factories where the workers have been exposed to the poison for some time. In most cases symptoms appear about one to four months after employment has started, and the clinical course lasts from four to eight weeks. When symptoms develop the patients should be put to bed and given laxatives and alkaline substances such as sodium citrate and bicarbonate orally, and if necessary an intravenous infusion of dilute sodium bicarbonate solution. The workers should be protected as much as possible from exposure to the substance.

Acetanilid. Acetanilid, $C_6H_5NHCH_3CO$, is a colorless crystalline substance with a burning taste but without any odor. It is used in medicine as an analgesic and an antipyretic. For a long time it was sold under the name of antifebrin®.

Poisoning by acetanilid is mostly accidental and occurs when the drug is taken in overdose for the relief of headache. Numerous headache remedies contain acetanilid in combination with caffeine, and their indiscriminate use has been responsible for many cases of serious poisoning. Formerly this drug was used as an external application for burns and wounds, and toxic symptoms were caused by its absorption from the raw skin surface. A few fatal acetanilid poisonings have been suicidal.

Some people are more susceptible than others to the action of the drug, and the symptoms produced depend largely upon the dose and the idiosyncrasy of the patient. The most pronounced effect of the continued use of acetanilid is an intense cyanosis which is especially evident under the finger nails and in the lips. Some observers have attributed this to the formation of methemoglobin; others believe that it is caused by paramidophenol, a decomposition product of acetanilid in the body, which reacts with hydrogen sulfide to produce sulfhemoglobin after combining with some of the hemoglobin. Weakness, prostration, sweating, cold skin, feeble pulse and respirations, dyspnea, vomiting, subnormal temperature, dilatation of the pupils, delirium, convulsions and death may occur after overdosage. If the victim survives for a few days, destruction of the red blood cells, acute lower nephron nephrosis, hematuria and a progressive jaundice may supervene. Some believe that death is caused by the action of the drug on the respiratory center, but others think that it exerts a toxic action on the heart.

Deaths from the indiscriminate use of acetanilid preparations were formerly not rare. The fatal dose is variable, inasmuch as 5 to 10 gm. have caused death, and recovery has followed the ingestion of much larger amounts. Death may occur in a few hours or be postponed for several days. In recent years, acetanilid deaths have not been common. The Reports of the Chief Medical Examiner in the City of New York show 13 fatal cases of poisoning by acetanilid, acetphenetidin or antipyrine during the years 1918 to 1951; two of which were suicidal, one due to ingestion of acetphenetidin, and the other to acetanilid. The treatment of acetanilid poisoning is to wash out the stomach, and to administer purgatives in an endeavor to get rid of the unabsorbed drug. Blood transfusion may be of value in some cases. Otherwise the therapy is symptomatic.

The postmortem appearances are not characteristic. The blood is dark and fluid, and may be chocolate colored. The most suitable materials to save for chemical examination are the stomach contents, urine, brain, liver and kidneys. The drug is eliminated rapidly from the body, usually in 24 hours. Acetanilid is not excreted as such in the urine, but some of its products of decomposition, acetoparamidophenol or paramidophenol, occur as conjugated glycuronates or sulfates.

Acetanilid is habit forming and many individuals become addicts by the continuous use of patent headache remedies like bromo-seltzer® which contain it as an ingredient. The victim may show a syndrome of general weakness, anorexia, insomnia, mental debility and dyspnea on exertion. Chocolate colored blood, cyanosis and dark urine are usually present and are the result of methemoglobinemia and blood destruction. Reynolds and Ware have reported sulfhemoglobinemia in chronic acetanilid poisoning and have pointed out that this blood pigment unlike methemoglobin is not reversible and cannot be removed from the red blood cell even after the poison is eliminated from the body; as a result it produces a persistent cyanosis. A marked anemia similar to pernicious anemia may develop with progressive weakness, emaciation and collapse. In some cases of addiction forced abstinence from the drug may cause symptoms of acute mania, resembling the withdrawal symptoms in narcotic addiction.

Acetphenetidin. Acetphenetidin, $C_6H_4(OC_2H_5)NH(CH_3CO)$, or phenacetin is a white crystalline powder which has a bitter taste. Its effects on the system are similar to those of acetanilid, but the poisonous action is not so marked. Skin eruptions may develop when phenacetin is administered. Fatal poisoning is rare but can be caused by large doses as with acetanilid. Death may take place in a few hours or be delayed for days.

Postmortem examination shows no characteristic lesions. The treatment and toxicologic indications are the same as for acetanilid. Unless the drug is taken in large amounts phenacetin does not appear in the urine as such, but its cleavage products, paraphenetidin or paramidophenol, are present as conjugated sulfates or glycuronates. Chronic poisoning sometimes occurs, and occasionally a phenacetin habit is formed with withdrawal symptoms similar to those produced by acetanilid.

Antipyrine. Antipyrine, $C_6H_5NCO\ CH\ NCH_3CCH_3$, is a colorless, odorless, crystalline substance with a bitter taste. Its physiologic action is the same as acetanilid, but it rarely causes methemoglobinemia. Most poisonings have been caused by taking an overdose of the drug for medicinal purposes. One homicidal case has been reported. Symptoms and signs of poisoning are vertigo, delirium, auditory and visual disturbances, cold perspiration, cyanosis, rapid and feeble pulse, coma and collapse. Skin eruptions with itching occasionally occur, especially in individuals abnormally sensitive to the drug; they are apt to occur in chronic poisoning. Habit formation is not common. The fatal dose is large and variable. In other respects the action of antipyrine is similar to acetanilid.

Aminopyrine or pyramidon is a compound similar to antipyrine and produces about the same general effects toxicologically. Aminopyrine alone or in combination with barbiturates used medicinally has caused severe and fatal granulocytopenia; this condition may develop after long continued use of these preparations. The aminopyrine is believed responsible for the depression of the bone marrow in these cases.

Phenylbutazone (butazolidin) is a pyrazole derivative with a chemical structure similar to that of aminopyrine. Both drugs have been used in rheumatoid disorders and in psoriasis as analgesics and antihistaminics. With long continued use toxic reactions may develop such as edema, nausea, abdominal discomfort, skin eruptions, inflamed conjunctivae, mouth and throat, and agranulocytosis which is sometimes fatal.

Naphthol. Naphthol, $C_{10}H_7OH$, is a white crystalline powder with a faint phenol odor. There are two naphthol compounds, alpha and beta; the former is more toxic, is more powerful as an antiseptic, and exerts an injurious action on the blood and kidneys. Most poisonings are caused by the application of naphthol in ointment or in alcoholic solution to a raw skin surface for the treatment of scabies or other cutaneous disease. Some cases are produced by the ingestion of the drug as an anthelmintic or as an intestinal antiseptic. The beta compounds have been used as a therapeutic agent in hook worm disease and have produced toxic symptoms. Naphthol locally causes an irritation of the skin and mucous membranes, and its long continued application to such surfaces may bring about a brownish corrosion. The general symptoms of the poisoning are vomiting and stupor with such signs as anemia from destruction of the red blood cells, enlargement of the spleen and liver, changes in the retina, albuminuria, hematuria, and lesions of the skin which may be eczematous, icteric, variolar or hemorrhagic. The urine is dark from the presence of naphthol glycuronates and sulfates, and the products of blood destruction. At necropsy the stomach is reddened from irritation, the kidneys show a marked nephrosis with a yellowish gray cortex and dark red pyramids and microscopically reveal pigment masses in the lumen of the collecting tubules, there is evidence of anemia, jaundice is apparent and the spleen and liver are enlarged. The stomach contents, urine, brain, spleen, kidneys and liver are the most suitable materials to save for toxicologic examination.

The fatal dose is variable; 4 gm. of naphthol in ointment have caused death. The victim may die within 24 hours, or may survive the administration of the drug several weeks. The treatment is the same as in phenol poisoning.

Atophan and the Cinchophen Group. Atophan, one of the cinchophen derivatives, occurs as a white or grayish white powder with an astringent taste. It is sold in tablet form, mainly as a remedy for rheumatism. Some people are susceptible to this drug and degeneration in the liver may be produced after a long continued administration. The patients develop malaise, jaundice, indigestion, urobilinuria and enlargement of the liver. Usually if the drug is withheld the signs will disappear. In some cases a severe acute yellow atrophy of the liver occurs. Skin eruptions, such as scarlatiniform rashes, vesicles and edema have been described by Lewin as having followed the use of atophan. Neocinchophen is believed to be less toxic than some of the other compounds in this group.

Sulfonamide Compounds. These compounds are derivatives of an organic sulfur radical which is attached to the benzene ring in para combination with an amido group. Thus sulfanilamide is paramidobenzene sulfonamide, or $C_6H_4NH_2$-SO_2NH_2. A large number of similar compounds with more complicated formulas have been synthesized, of which the most important are sulfapyridine, sulfathiazole, prontosil and neoprontosil. All of them tend to combine with various proteins, including the bacterial proteins, and this property has made them valuable therapeutic agents in treating severe bacterial infections in animals and men. The sulfonamides have only a slight degree of toxicity for the patient, but they inhibit the invasive power of the bacteria, producing bacteriostasis. This enables the defensive antibodies and cells of the victim to attack the invading microorganisms successfully, but aside from this limited help, the drugs do not affect the bacteria more directly nor do they stimulate the protective forces of the body noticeably.

Sulfanilamide is an odorless, white, crystalline powder, slightly bitter to the taste, and its 0.8 per cent solution in water is neutral to litmus. It is a valuable therapeutic agent in the treatment of infections caused by hemolytic streptococci of group B, meningococci, gonococci, and *Clostridium welchii,* and in the treatment of different infections of the urinary tract.

The most desirable method of administering sulfanilamide is by mouth in the form of tablets and capsules, the drug passing through the stomach and into the small intestine before being absorbed. Subcutaneous injection may be used when it is not practicable to give the drug orally, as in cases of severe vomiting. Intravenous injection is not indicated and should not be used. Rectal administration may be accomplished through retention enemas of the drug as it is slowly absorbed from the large intestine. The object of the therapy is to maintain the concentration of sulfanilamide in the blood, spinal fluid and body tissues at the best level to deal with the infection adequately; in severe infections this is 10 to 15 mg. per 100 ml. and in less virulent cases from 4 to 10 mg. per 100 ml. This dosage is reckoned according to the weight of the patient and the desired concentration of the drug in the blood and body fluids; thus a person of 70 kilograms would be given 4.8 gm. of sulfanilamide as an initial dose, followed by 1.2 gm. every four hours in order to maintain a concentration of 10 to 15 mg. per 100 ml.

The early toxic symptoms produced by sulfanilamide are a transitory nausea, vomiting and diarrhea, accompanied by a state of mild inebriation and psychotic manifestations. The patient becomes cyanotic in a few hours to a day after starting the drug, and in some instances there may be a methemoglobinemia of 10 to 12 per cent which is partly responsible for the cyanosis. Fever, chills and headache may occur about the time that the fever due to the infection is brought under control, usually about the seventh to the tenth day after the treatment is started. Normally the kidneys are not much affected by the drug, but if they are diseased, they may excrete sulfanilamide so slowly that it accumulates in the body and gives rise to toxic symptoms. In some cases skin eruptions of different types ensue, including urticarial, erysipeloid, morbilliform, scarlatiniform and purpuric types, and occasionally a marked exfoliative dermititis. These are associated at times with various allergic conditions like bronchial asthma and eosinophilia, and occasionally with a toxic hepatitis either in the form of parenchymatous degeneration accompanied by a slight jaundice, or as a marked acute yellow atrophy. An acute hemolytic anemia may appear about 1 to 3 days after the administration of the drug and is most pronounced on the fifth to the seventh day; it is caused by a peripheral destruction of red blood cells, is attended by considerable pallor, and may be followed by a lower nephron nephrosis with urinary suppression and uremia. Severe neutropenia or agranulocytosis has been described and seems to be due to a personal idiosyncrasy on the part of the patient toward the sulfonamide. Rarer complications are symptomatic thrombopenic purpura, aplastic anemia, dyspnea, tachycardia and abdominal and chest pains.

Sulfanilamide is distributed throughout the body mostly unchanged, but about

10 to 20 per cent is conjugated in the liver to acetyl sulfanilamide. The greater part of the drug is excreted through the urine rapidly, provided that the fluid intake of the patient is adequate and the renal function is not impaired. A contraindication to the therapeutic employment of this sulfonamide would be the knowledge of a serious toxic reaction following a previous administration.

Prontosil and neoprontosil are sulfonamides sometimes employed in the treatment of infections, though less often than in former years. Both drugs are partially decomposed in the body into sulfanilamide, and it is this property which gives them their antibiotic power. Prontosil must be given by mouth and occurs as a white powder. Neoprontosil is a red powder and because of its solubility can be given by mouth or by subcutaneous or intramuscular injection; after absorption it stains the urine, skin and mucous membranes its own peculiar red color. The prontosil drugs are potentially capable of producing the same toxic symptoms as sulfanilamide but few cases have been reported.

The authors have seen one death following the injection of an ampule of neoprontosil intramuscularly into the gluteal muscle of a woman of 35 years for a limited and indolent cellulitis of the right forearm, the patient collapsing immediately, and dying inside of an hour. Previous medical history disclosed that the victim had had prior injections of neoprontosil without ill effects. The autopsy disclosed that there was a marked edema of the lungs, fluid blood in the heart, and a contracted heart muscle with flame-like subendocardial hemorrhages in the left ventricle. Microscopic examination of the tissues disclosed the infection of the right forearm, a moderate round cell infiltration of a nonspecific type in the subarachnoid space, numerous eosinophilic leukocytes in the bronchi, stomach, intestines and spleen, and some microscopic granulomas with foreign body giant cells surrounded by large mononuclear cells, lymphocytes and eosinophils scattered through the capsule of Glisson in the liver. The clinical and pathologic features of the case indicated that the reaction of the patient to the injection was an allergic one, either induced by previous injections of the drug or produced by some other cause. See page 832 for other allergic lesions following sulfonamide administration.

Sulfapyridine is 2-sulfanilyl aminopyridine and is a white, odorless, tasteless crystalline powder. It is about one thirtieth as soluble as sulfanilamide, and it is more slowly absorbed from the intestinal tract. It is more efficient than sulfanilamide in the treatment of infections due to the pneumococci, the Friedländer bacillus or the staphylococci. After the drug has been absorbed about 50 per cent of the sulfapyridine is conjugated in the liver to an acetyl compound, most of which is excreted into the urine; a large part of this is removed in 24 hours, but its excretion may be maintained from 50 to 90 hours. The acetyl compound tends to precipitate out in the kidney tubules, renal pelves, ureter and bladder and may occasionally obstruct the flow of urine, causing anuria, renal colic, hematuria and uremia. At necropsy the yellowish gray acetyl crystals may be present in the urinary passages, sometimes in the form of calculi, causing gross blockage of the lumen (Fig. 33-2). Many toxic effects mentioned under sulfanilamide may also occur with sulfapyridine.

Sulfathiazole is another one of the sulfonamides which is used in pneumococcic and in staphylococcic infections. It is poorly soluble in water and is given orally, but is absorbed readily from the intestines. Its sodium salt is soluble in water and may be given parenterally. It is able to cause most of the toxic reactions noted under sulfanilamide and sulfapyridine, but it most commonly produces skin eruptions, injections of the sclera and conjunctiva, and sometimes swollen and painful joints.

Part of the drug is conjugated by the liver into an acetyl compound, which is precipitated in the urinary passages and renal tubules, giving rise to oliguria, cylindruria and albuminuria. A few cases show renal colic hematuria.

Allergic lesions following the administration of sulfathiazole, and less often of other sulfonamides, have been described in fatal cases by More and his collaborators, by French, and by Lichtenstein and Fox. These pathologic changes appear a few days to a few weeks after the drug has been administered continuously over a long period of time, or after the administration of a few large doses; in some cases the lesions followed the resumption of sulfonamide therapy after previous administration of the drug. The principal lesions were necrotic areas in liver and bone marrow, microscopic granulomas composed mainly of large mononuclear cells with a lesser number of plasma cells, lymphocytes, leukocytes and eosinophils in the myocardium, liver, kidney, lung and other viscera, interstitial inflammatory lesions in the myocardium, liver, kidney and other organs, polyvascular necrotic inflammatory processes like periateritis nodosa in liver, kidneys, pancreas and elsewhere, fibrinoid necrotic areas in trabeculae of spleen, dermatitis exfoliativa, and nephrotic lesions in the kidneys.

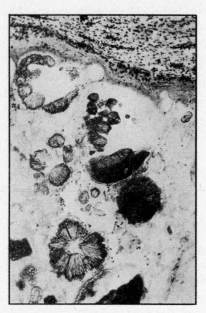

Fig. 33-2. Histologic Section of Ureter Blocked with Excreted Sulfadiazine Crystals.

Other sulfonamides are sulfadiazine, sulfaguanidine, sulfamerazine, and sulfapyrazine. These are generally less toxic than the compounds already described, but in rare instances may cause distressing reactions.

When a patient dies following treatment with a sulfonamide, it is difficult to appraise the role played by the drug, inasmuch as the disease treated is often a serious one and undoubtedly contributes to the death of the patient. The review by Sutliff, Helpern, Griffin and Brown analyzes 28 cases of death connected with sulfonamide toxicity in New York City in 1941; these cases were selected because they offered enough clinical and pathologic data for appraisal. In 13 of the cases the diagnosis was considered to have been satisfactorily established; and of these, 5 died as a result of sulfonamide toxicity. In the remaining 15 cases the diagnosis was considered acceptable and 5 of this group died as a result of sulfonamide administration. In the 28 cases of death, sulfonamide toxicity affected: blood cells and blood forming organs, 12 (agranulocytosis, 8; acute hemolytic anemia, 1; aplastic anemia, 1; purpura hemorrhagica, 1; thrombocytopenic purpura, 1); kidneys, 12 (uremia from renal obstruction, 5; and from failure of renal function, 7); other manifestations, 4 (dermatitis exfoliativa, 1; dermatitis with pneumonia, 2; convulsions with a complicating pneumonia in an 11 month old baby, 1). Acute toxic degeneration of the liver was not encountered in this series, but has been observed in other cases. Toxic myocarditis and vascular lesions resembling those of periarteritis nodosa have also been described as allergic manifestations of sulfonamide poisoning.

Glucosides are complex plant substances which yield glucose as a cleavage product, along with compounds belonging to the alcohol, phenol, aldheyde or acid groups. For example, salicin is a glucoside, found in willow bark which contains methyl salicylate among other constituents. Amygdalin is a glucoside, found in bitter almonds, which may be decomposed into glucose, benzaldehyde and hydrocyanic acid. Sinigrin and sinalbin in the mustard plant yield mustard oils and glucose. The reactions of the toxic glucosides on the body are similar to alkaloids.

Digitalis. The term digitalis is applied to the powdered leaves of the *Digitalis purpurea,* or foxglove. The drug is used therapeutically as a stimulant in cardiac decompensation resulting from disturbances in rhythm as in auricular fibrillation, or from exhaustion of the cardiac muscle incident to structural lesions. The preparations of digitalis most often employed are the tincture, the infusion and the powdered leaf in capsule or tablet form.

Toxic effects during the therapeutic use of digitalis frequently occur and are the result of overdosage. Most of these are mild, but severe and even fatal poisonings have been reported. Occasionally digitalis has been taken during military service to simulate the signs of cardiac disease for the purpose of malingering. It has also been administered to produce disturbances in cardiac rhythm and changes in the electrocardiogram simulating those of coronary artery disease for the purpose of fraudulently obtaining disability benefits from insurance companies. Homicidal and suicidal poisonings with digitalis have been recorded.

The action of digitalis is produced by a number of glucosides, digitalin, digitoxin, digitonin and digitalein, present in the leaves and also in the seeds. In medicinal doses they slow the heart and increase the power and completeness of its contractions. With toxic doses the heart is further slowed and partial heart block and a coupled rhythm occur. With excessive doses the heart action becomes rapid and irregular and fibrillation occurs prior to death. This action is due to a primary stimulation followed by a secondary depression of the cardio-inhibitory center, and an irritant action of the drug on the myocardium.

The symptoms of digitalis poisoning are slowing of the heart beat, 25 to 40 per minute, nausea, persistent vomiting, thirst, abdominal pain, suppression of urine, diarrhea, roaring in the ears, disturbances of vision, headache, hallucinations and delirium. Later the heart action becomes rapid and irregular, and is accompanied by dyspnea and collapse. Death may occur in convulsions and coma, or sudden cardiac failure may supervene. Digitalis is eliminated from the system slowly, and it is not uncommon for the administration of small doses of the drug over a long period of time to result in cumulative poisoning. Fatal cases of digitalis poisoning are rare with fractionated doses since vomiting and diarrhea would tend to prevent further absorption. Fatal poisoning may follow the administration of a single massive dose. The ingestion of 2.5 gm. of digitalis has caused death, although there has been recovery from a dose of 4 gm. The lethal dose of digitalis is variable and depends on the body weight. The authors have encountered a suicidal case in which a middle aged white man swallowed 60 one and a half grain tablets of digitalis leaf. Vomiting, cardiac arrhythmia, collapse and death occurred on the following day. Necropsy revealed a markedly hypertrophied heart weighing 700 gm. with extensive subendocardial hemorrhage on the left side of the interventricular septum. Fatalities are more apt to occur after intravenous injection of large doses of digitalis or strophanthin. In fatal poisoning death may occur after 1 to 2 days, or not until 5 to 13 days have elapsed. The treatment is to evacuate the stomach and intestines, usually by a cathartic, and to keep the patient in bed, giving symptomatic treatment as indicated.

The postmortem findings are not characteristic, except that occasionally the leaves or fragments of the drug are found in the stomach. In cases where the drug has been ingested, the stomach contents are saved for toxicologic examination. The recovery of digitalis from the organs is difficult, but the liver and kidneys should be saved for analysis. The determination of digitalis poisoning at autopsy presents great difficulties in the absence of a history revealing the quantity of the drug administered. The recovery of the drug by toxicologic examination might suggest poisoning in the absence of heart disease or any other natural disease process which in itself could be a sufficient cause of death. If death occurred as a result of an overdose of digitalis during its therapeutic administration for heart disease, this could hardly be established at autopsy.

The pharmacologic test for digitalis is carried out by injecting 1 to 2 mg. of the glucoside into the lymph sac of a frog and recording the heart beat. The contractions become slower and more complete after the administration of the drug and the heart finally stops in systole. The method of bio-assay, by observing the effect on the heart of the frog and also of the cat, is used to standardize preparations of digitalis for medicinal use. Text books of pharmacology discuss fully the action, uses and toxic effects of digitalis.

Strophanthus. The plant *Strophanthus kombé* contains as an active principle the glucoside strophanthin which, when purified, occurs in the form of a white crystalline powder. Its pharmacologic and toxic action is similar to digitalis but a great many times more powerful, and death may be produced in a few minutes to an hour. Treatment, toxicologic considerations, necropsy findings and pharmacologic test on the frog are similar to those of digitalis. Crystalline strophanthin, derived from *Strophanthus gratus,* is known as ouabain. The dose of strophanthin is 1 mg., or one sixtieth of a grain, and that of ouabain is one half of that amount.

Oleander. Glucosides similar to those of the digitalis series are contained in the leaves and bark of the shrub *Nerium oleander.* This drug has been used as an abortifacient and a rat poison in some of the south European countries. Many cases of poisoning have occurred among children who have eaten parts of the plant. The toxic symptoms are vomiting, vertigo, small slow pulse, abdominal pains, epileptiform convulsions, coma and death. The treatment, toxicologic indications and postmortem findings are similar to those of digitalis.

Hellebore. The powder obtained from the root of the black hellebore (*Helleborus niger*) contains two glucosides, helleborin and helleborein. This plant causes pharmacologic and toxic symptoms much like digitalis, and its other toxicologic features are the same.

Scilla or Squill. The sea onion, or *Urginea maritima,* possesses as constituents, scillatoxin, scillapicrin, and a glucoside, scillain, the action of which is similar to the glucosides of digitalis. Poisoning is rare but may be caused whenever any of the preparations is taken in toxic doses. The leaves of the plant are sometimes applied to wounds, and may cause a vesicular dermatitis and an eczema. Ingestion may produce pain in the legs, paralytic symptoms, convulsions, vomiting, watery stools, strangury, bloody urine, cyanosis and rapid paralysis of the respiratory center. Irritation of the gastrointestinal tract and urinary tract are encountered at necropsy. Treatment after emptying the stomach is symptomatic.

Gossypium. Some of the components of *Gossypium herbaceum,* or cotton root bark, when ingested cause symptoms of collapse with rapid weak pulse, dilated pupils, muscular relaxation, shallow respirations and death from paralysis of the respiratory center. These compounds may produce abortion and are occasionally used for that purpose.

Locust. The toxic substances in the leaves, bark, flowers and root of the common locust, *Robinia pseudacacia,* have caused poisoning when parts of the plant have been ingested. In the bark the poisonous principle is a protein called robin, while a glucoside, robinin, has been obtained from the flowers. The symptoms of locust poisoning are flushed face, vomiting, dryness of throat and mouth, dilated pupils, edema of the lids, epigastric pains, irregular heart action, convulsive movements and stupor. The skin in many cases may be desquamated. The effects are similar to those of belladonna poisoning.

Cannabis Indica. The Indian hemp, or *Cannabis indica,* is a plant, the dried flowering or fruiting tops of which are smoked in India, in other parts of Asia and in Africa under a variety of names. In India the preparation used is known as hashish, bhang, charas or gayah; in Africa as leainba and in Morocco as schira. The plant contains a number of active principles, such as cannabin, tetanocannabin, cannabinin and cannabisbalsam. Acute poisoning due to toxic doses of the drug makes its appearance about one-half to three hours after exposure. The symptoms are somnolence, cold skin, anesthesia, motor weakness, hallucinations, delirium, vomiting, cramps and, in rare fatal cases, death by respiratory paralysis. In nonfatal cases recovery may be delayed up to 48 hours.

The smoking of hemp must be classed among the drug habits and as a distinct social evil. The reputed attraction of the drug is that it causes dreams of a pleasant nature, a feeling of timelessness and wonderful visions which last until the dose can be renewed. Continued addiction may lead to mania or melancholia.

American hemp (*Cannabis americana*), sometimes known as marihuana, produces symptoms similar to the plant from India, but it is not so potent. A preparation from it, known as muggles, is smoked in Mexico and the United States, and produces at times partial inebriety, mental confusion and delirium. The name loco disease is given to it because the symptomatology is similar to an unrelated condition of that name which affects horses, cattle and sheep on western ranches.

The loco disease of horses, cattle and sheep has been attributed to the ingestion of certain plants of the *Astragalus* genus during pasture feeding. The animals show muscular incoordination, forced movements, hallucinations, stupidity, misjudgment of distance and death preceded by coma and convulsions. Chronic poisoning is marked generally by emaciation. Some dispute the significance of the *Astragalus* plants or the loco weed as an etiologic factor, and claim that the symptoms are often caused by malnutrition, parasites or some other cause.

The smoking of dried marihuana has become a fairly common drug habit during the past few years in the United States. The ease with which the plant is cultivated in vacant lots and other places has made it difficult to eradicate the source of supply.

The Marihuana Tax Act of August 2nd 1937 imposes a tax rate from one dollar to 24 dollars on various persons concerned with the importation, manufacture, production, compounding, sale, dealing in, dispensing, prescribing, administering and giving away of marihuana.

ORGANIC PURGATIVES

Many drugs, derived from different plants, are used as purgatives and cause poisoning if given in overdose. Chemically, these vegetable compounds belong to widely different groups, but their action on the body is similar, for they stimulate the intestines to greater contraction and cause them to expel their contents. Usually when taken in overdose, symptoms of gastric and intestinal inflammation develop, with colic, griping pain in the abdomen, purging, shock, collapse and sometimes death. Some of the drugs are also severe skin irritants. Vegetable purgatives are divided into three classes according to their chemical properties: purgative oils, anthracene purgatives, and cathartic resins.

Purgative Oils. CROTON OIL. Croton oil, or oleum tiglii, is present in the seeds of the *Croton tiglium*. It is a vesicant oil causing erythema, purulent vesicles and even ulceration when applied to the skin. On ingestion, it may cause salivation, a burning sensation in the mouth and throat, vomiting, bloody diarrhea, abdominal pain, straining and tenesmus. In severe cases there is shock with rapid feeble pulse, slow and shallow respirations, cold clammy skin, cyanosis, subnormal temperature, delirium and death may result from respiratory collapse in a few hours. At autopsy the mucous membrane of the stomach and intestines may be swollen and reddened and detached in places. Occasionally the postmortem findings at necropsy are negative. The oil is quite toxic, especially if it is old, and 2½ to 20 drops have caused death. Even swallowing or chewing the seeds of the *Croton tiglium* has been fatal. The poisonings have usually been accidental, from an overdose or from administration by mistake. The drug has also been taken as an abortifacient, or has been given in food for homicidal purposes. The treatment is evacuation of the stomach by the tube and the administration of demulcent drinks. Morphine is given for pain and stimulants are administered for shock. The stomach and intestinal contents are used for toxicologic analysis as there is little chance of recovering the drug from the parenchymatous organs.

OLEUM RICINI. Castor oil, or oleum ricini, is not poisonous in the pure state. The seeds of the castor bean contain also a phytotoxin called ricin which may cause fatal poisoning. The symptoms start about 45 minutes to several hours after ingestion, the victim manifesting weakness, vomiting, diarrhea, vertigo, pain in the abdomen, icterus, rapid feeble pulse and clammy skin; collapse and death may occur in three to five days or more. The stools may be like rice water or contain blood. Most of the poisonings are accidental and are occasioned by children eating the bean. At postmortem examination the mucous membrane of the gastrointestinal tract is inflamed, swollen and may show small submucous hemorrhages. Portions of the beans may be present in the contents of the stomach and intestines and are important diagnostic criteria. The stomach and intestinal contents may be extracted by water and the phytotoxin isolated in the filtrate. This substance causes agglutination of red blood cells, even in great dilution.

Anthracene Group. The anthracene group of purgatives contains glucosides composed in part of emodine and other derivatives of anthraquinone. These compounds include aloes, rhubarb, senna, frangula and cascara sagrada. The principal action is exerted on the large intestine.

ALOES. Aloes is derived from the dried juice or leaves of various aloe plants. It is intensely bitter so that it is usually administered in the form of pills. Poisoning has resulted from a too large dose of the drug, or from its employment as an abortifacient, the victim developing diarrhea, tenesmus, colicky pains and bloody stools 8 to 12 hours after administration. At autopsy pelvic congestion, colonic inflammation and renal irritation are sometimes noted. In rabbits, aloin, a derivative of the anthraquinone component in aloes, produces a tubular nephrosis with necrosis and calcification of the epithelium of the convoluted tubules, much like the kidney lesions in mercury bichloride poisoning. The treatment of aloes poisoning is similar to that used in croton oil poisoning. Stomach, intestinal and bladder contents are saved for toxicologic analysis.

OTHER ANTHRACENE CATHARTICS. Rhubarb, senna, frangula and cascara sagrada produce symptoms of gastrointestinal irritation if taken in excessive doses. Rhubarb administered over a long period of time evokes skin eruptions and a yellowish discoloration of the sweat and urine. These drugs are not as important toxicologically as aloes. Another drug is phenolphthalein which is used as a mild purgative and is not toxic even in large doses, very little of it being absorbed in the gastrointestinal tract.

Cathartic Resins. This group of active purgatives is toxic because of a number of resinous bodies, some of which are glucosides and some acid anhydrides. They act on the small intestine and cause violent diarrhea. The most important compounds are colocynth, elaterin, gamboge, jalap and podophyllum.

COLOCYNTH. Colocynth, or bitter apple, is the fruit of *Citrullus colocynthis* of the family Cucurbitaceae. It contains resinous bodies and an alkaloid, colocynthin, rather bitter in taste. It produces symptoms of marked gastrointestinal and renal irritation with prostration, irregular pulse, delirium and collapse. Poisoning may occur during the use of the drug as an abortifacient. Colocynth is excreted in the urine and in the milk. The toxic dose is 1 gm.; the fatal dose is 4 gm. Death may occur within 24 hours or may be delayed until after 40 hours. The stomach and intestines at necropsy are inflamed and may be ulcerated. Hepatic and renal congestion may be present. The stomach contents, kidneys and urine are used for chemical examination. The treatment is the same as for croton oil poisoning.

ELATERIN. Elaterin is the active principle of the fruit of the squirting cucumber, *Ecballium elaterium*. It is a powerful cathartic and causes symptoms not unlike those of colocynth. The toxic dose is 5 mg.; 0.6 gm. may be fatal.

JALAP. Jalap is a gum resin from the root of *Ipomoea orizabensis,* and is the mildest of the cathartic resins. The medicinal dose of powdered jalap is 0.3 to 1.2 gm. (5 to 20 grains).

PODOPHYLLUM. Podophyllum is the dried root and rhizome of the may-apple, mandrake or *Podophyllum peltatum*. It contains a resin, podophyllin, whose active principle is podophyllotoxin. Taken in therapeutic doses it acts in 12 to 24 hours. Poisonous doses act more rapidly; in severe cases vomiting and purging occur and then collapse with cold extremities, rapid weak thready pulse, coma, albuminuria, hematuria and finally death by respiratory paralysis. The fatal dose is 0.3 to 0.6 gm. Powdered podophyllum may cause skin irritation and conjunctivitis.

GAMBOGE. A gum resin found in *Garcinia hanburyi* has been used as a purgative and as an abortifacient. The effect is similar to that of colocynth and 4 gm. is considered a fatal dose.

ESSENTIAL OILS

Aspidium. The male fern contains a resin known under the name of oleoresina aspidii. It is administered to remove tapeworms and hookworms from the intestine. Poisoning has occurred from this use and was believed to be favored by the simultaneous use of castor oil which facilitates the absorption of the aspidium as the drug is soluble in oil; this effect of castor oil has been questioned. The symptoms of poisoning vary in severity and include gastrointestinal irritation, vomiting, abdominal pain, purging, muscular weakness, yellow vision, confusion, somnolence, convulsions, headache, dyspnea and finally death from respiratory paralysis. The drug stimulates and then depresses the central nervous system and violent convulsions may take place, especially in children. Glycosuria, albuminuria, hematuria, jaundice and blood destruction have been described. Blindness, either unilateral or bilateral, is a distressing symptom as it persists in many cases which survive. Congestion and inflammation of the stomach and intestines have been found post mortem. In children, severe and fatal poisoning may follow after the ingestion of 4 to 8 gm., and in adults after 20 gm. In fatal cases death can occur in from 6 to 24 hours. The treatment is evacuant and symptomatic with the use of demulcent drinks. The stomach and intestinal contents are used for toxicologic examination.

Oil of Chenopodium. Oil of chenopodium, or American wormseed, is a volatile oil used as an anthelmintic against hookworms. In large doses it can produce serious gastrointestinal irritation, convulsions and depression of the central nervous system and death after 2 or 3 days of coma. Deafness has complicated cases of chenopodium poisoning. The postmortem findings are not characteristic but fatty changes in liver and kidneys, and edema of the brain have been described. Daily doses of 0.5 ml. repeated for two or three days have caused death.

Abortifacients. Oils of tansy, pennyroyal, nutmeg, savin, cedar, rue and thyme have been used as abortifacients and have caused symptoms of gastrointestinal inflammation, renal inflammation, collapse, coma and death by respiratory center paralysis. The time of death varies from a few hours to several days after ingestion of the poison. The lethal dose is about 4 gm. or more.

Apiol. Apiol, oleum petrosilium and apiolum viride are all compounds obtained from the parsley plant. These drugs are used as abortifacients. They cause methemoglobin formation marked by a bluish-gray and brownish cyanosis, anemia, albuminuria, hematuria, hemoglobinuria, bilirubinuria, headache, dizziness, fever and ataxia. They are irritants to the skin and to the mucous membranes. Postmortem examination shows renal and gastrointestinal irritation and methemoglobinemia. The treatment consists of evacuating the stomach, administering infusions and transfusions and symptomatic remedies.

Saffron. Saffron, the coloring matter of the *Crocus sativus,* contains a glucoside, crosin, and an essential oil. It has been used as an abortifacient, and its toxic action is similar to the essential oils.

Turpentine. Oil of turpentine is obtained from turpentine or the oleoresin of various species of *Pinus.* It contains several terpenes, and is colorless, irritant and inflammable. It is used as a solvent for paint. Accidental poisoning has resulted when turpentine has been given by mouth as an anthelmintic, or when its vapors from freshly laid paint have been inhaled in a small closed room. It has been taken for suicidal purposes and has been used as an abortifacient. A few cases of poisoning are homicidal.

A large dose, taken internally, causes a sensation of warmth, abdominal pain, vomiting and diarrhea. The heart action becomes weak, and the respirations are slowed and become irregular. Incoördination, excitement, convulsions and coma occur; and death may supervene as a result of paralysis of the respiratory center. In some cases there is irritation of the kidneys, kidney pelves and bladder with strangury, hematuria, albuminuria and sometimes anuria; the urine may give off an odor of violets. Skin eruptions occur occasionally. When the drug is inhaled, symptoms of bronchitis also occur. Acute inflammation of the bronchi, stomach and urinary tract are found at necropsy, and the blood and viscera often have the odor of turpentine. Brain, liver and kidneys, lungs and stomach contents are used for toxicologic examination.

The lethal dose is not known exactly, but 6 ounces has caused death in an adult, and 1 dram to 4 ounces may be fatal for children. Death may occur in a few minutes to several hours after the drug is taken. The treatment is evacuation of the stomach with the tube, and the use of demulcent drinks and stimulation.

PICROTOXIN GROUP

This group is composed of nonnitrogenous nonalkaloidal poisonous plant compounds of unknown chemical structure which have the property of stimulating the medullary centers and causing convulsions in toxic dosage.

Picrotoxin. Picrotoxin, $C_{30}H_{34}O_{13}$, is a colorless, crystalline substance obtained from the dried fruit of the *Anamirta cocculus,* a climbing East Indian shrub. The fruit is known as grains of paradise, fish berries, or Levant nuts, and, when dried, is known as cocculus indicus. It has been used as a vermicide, and the dried berries have been thrown into streams in order to stupefy fish and thus facilitate their capture. The drug picrotoxin has been employed as a physiologic antidote in cases of barbiturate poisoning as it is a stimulant of the central nervous system and the respiratory centers in the medulla.

Most cases of picrotoxin poisoning are accidental, either the drug or the berries having been taken in mistake for something else. The berries occasionally have been added to rum to make knock-out drops. The drug has been employed occasionally as an abortifacient.

Picrotoxin has a strong action on the central nervous system, stimulating the medulla, increasing reflex excitability and giving rise to convulsions of the clonic type. After taking the poison by mouth, there is epigastric pain, nausea, vomiting, diarrhea and salivation, followed by weakness, perspiration, headache and coma. The pupils are dilated or contracted or partly so. The respirations at first are rapid, but later become slow. The clonic convulsions begin in about 20 minutes after administration of the drug, last about two minutes, with an interval of two minutes between attacks. Prior to each convulsion there is an outcry or twitching of the muscles of the face. Death may supervene in a half to several hours, or may not occur for several days. The usual treatment is to evacuate the stomach by tube or emetics, and to control the convulsions when necessary by inhalation of chloroform or the use of a quick-acting barbiturate. Twenty milligrams ($\frac{1}{3}$ grain) of picrotoxin probably is toxic, and death has occurred from 2.4 gm. of the powdered berries which is equivalent to 20 mg. or $\frac{1}{3}$ grain of the toxic principle.

The most common postmortem findings are mild gastrointestinal irritation, congestion of the lungs, meninges and other viscera. The stomach contents, brain or other organs are used for toxicologic examination. The pharmacologic test is to inject some of the suspected compound into a frog, whereupon the drug will cause convulsions of the clonic type, evidently of medullary origin; when the medulla of the frog is separated from the forebrain the convulsions persist, but when the medulla is separated from the cord, the convulsions stop.

Water Hemlock. The cicuta, or water hemlock, is toxic, especially the European variety or *Cicuta virosa.* The American varieties are the *C. maculata,* the *C. vagans,* the *C. bulbifera* and the *C. occidentalis.* The *Cicuta maculata* is considered the most poisonous plant in the United States, especially the root which is mistaken for an edible root. Most cases have occurred among children, and many deaths have been caused among cattle. The poisonous principle is cicutoxin which has an action similar to that of picrotoxin. The symptoms come on shortly after ingestion of the plant with dizziness, pain in the abdomen, and such signs as cold clammy skin, profuse perspiration, blood-stained vomitus, epileptiform convulsions, coma, weak pulse, dilated pupils and death by paralysis of the respiratory center. Death may occur in a few hours after eating the root. The postmortem appearances and treatment are similar to those of picrotoxin poisoning. The pharmacologic test and toxicologic considerations are also much alike.

MISCELLANEOUS GROUP

Taxus. Yew, taxus or *Taxus baccata* contains an alkaloid and an essential oil. The berries have been eaten by children with fatal results, and taxus has been used also as an abortifacient. After ingestion it produces symptoms of pain in the stomach, vomiting, diarrhea, coma, delirium, convulsions, collapse and asphyxia. At postmortem an inflammation of the stomach and intestine is seen and fragments of the leaves may be present. The treatment is evacuant and symptomatic.

Sparteine. An alkaloid from the broom plant, or *Cytisus scoparius,* is known as sparteine and causes a poisoning like coniine. It is particularly paralyzing to the phrenic nerves.

Abrus. A poisonous principle, abrus or jequirity, is present in the seeds of the *Abrus precatorius.* Abrus contains a phytotoxin known as abrin which is irritating and prone to cause conjunctivitis when used in the treatment of trachoma. It causes agglutination of the red blood cells in vitro. In man its action is somewhat similar to that of ricin.

Laburnum. An alkaloid, cystisine, is present in laburnum, which causes poisoning, especially in children who have sucked the plant. Salivation, thirst, vomiting, weakness, headache, rashes on the skin, cyanosis, chills, oliguria, delirium, hallucinations, convulsions and death by asphyxia may follow. The action is similar to nicotine.

Larkspur. Alcoholic preparations of *Delphinium staphisagria,* or larkspur, are used for purposes of delousing. They have an irritant action on the skin and cause a tingling of the tongue, salivation and symptoms similar to aconite, but not so powerful. The active principle of the drug is known as delphinine. Treatment in cases of poisoning, biologic tests and toxicologic considerations are similar to those in aconite poisoning.

Heath Family. The plants which compose the heath family are poisonous, containing a toxic principle andromedotoxin. In the United States the mountain laurel, or *Kalmia latifolia,* and the lambskill, or *Kalmia angustifolia,* are the best known members of the species. Some of the American Indians committed suicide by drinking concoctions of laurel. Poisoning has been reported from drinking homemade medicines made from laurel, and in other instances has been attributed to the ingestion of honey made from laurel flowers, or to eating the flesh of birds which have fed on laurel berries. Many cattle and sheep are poisoned by eating the laurel leaves. The symptoms of laurel and andromedotoxin poisoning are much like those caused by aconite. The stomach contents generally are used for toxicologic analysis.

Santonin. The chief toxic principle in the unexpanded flower heads of the *Artemisia pauciflora* is santonin which occurs as colorless and odorless prismatic crystals with a bitter taste. It is employed principally as an anthelmintic for intestinal round worms.

Most cases of poisoning are referable to the therapeutic use of santonin as an anthelmintic. There are disturbances of sight, and the victim sees all objects with a yellow tinge; disturbances of hearing, smell and taste also occur. The drug acts on the central nervous system, causing dizziness, ataxia, headache, dilated pupils, clonic convulsions and subnormal temperature. The patient passes into a state of stupor, with vomiting, pain in the abdomen, sweating, skin eruptions and fever. The urinary tract is irritated and strangury, hematuria, albuminuria and a yellow color of the urine develop.

Nearly all cases of santonin poisoning have occurred among children. The toxic dose varies and 2 to 3 grains may be fatal; death may supervene in from ½ to 14 hours. The treatment is to evacuate the stomach and intestines, to control the convulsions with a sedative, and to use warm applications to combat shock. The findings at necropsy are not characteristic, aside from signs of gastrointestinal, skin and renal irritation. In a fatal poisoning in a child who had been given two santonin candy cones for the expulsion of worms, autopsy by the authors revealed fatty changes in the liver. Urine, stomach contents, brain, liver and kidneys are used for toxicologic analysis. Santonin is excreted in the urine, either unchanged or as a decomposition product.

Cantharides. Cantharides, or Spanish fly, is the dried beetle, *Cantharis vesicatoria,* which contains cantharidin, the anhydride of cantharic acid $(C_{10}H_{12}O_4)$ in proportions of about 0.6 per cent. Cases of cantharides poisoning are reported in which individuals have taken the powdered drug or its tincture as an abortifacient, as an aphrodisiac, as a cure for tuberculosis or by mistake. Toxic symptoms have followed its absorption from the skin during its use as a vesicant or counterirritant.

The poison is locally irritant where it enters the body and also where it is excreted. Erythema, vesication and even gangrene follow its application to the skin. When taken by mouth vesication occurs in the throat and stomach accompanied by a burning pain, thirst and inability to swallow. This may be followed by vomiting of blood and fragments of mucous membrane, and later by bloody diarrhea, abdominal pains, weakness, collapse and death. The fatal dose is not positively known; 25 grains have caused death, but recovery has taken place after much larger doses. Death may occur in from 1 to 15 hours from shock caused by irritation. If the victim survives this stage he may die later from the damage inflicted upon the kidneys.

If the poison is absorbed from the skin, its action is not so intense and the principal symptoms and signs are referable to the organs of excretion, such as the intestines and the urinary tract. There is irritation of the bladder with desire to urinate, pain in the penis, hematuria, scanty urine and rapid pulse. The genital organs are inflamed and there is often, but not invariably, priapism and increased sexual desire. Abortion has been produced by the drug when it has been administered to a pregnant woman. Nephritis may occur and cause serious illness and death. Acidosis is a common result of the poisoning and concentration of the blood is fairly constant. Dyspnea and different types of convulsive seizures may occur. The treatment consists of gastric lavage with warm water, demulcent drinks and opiates. The use of oil is avoided. The bladder is washed out with warm water. Dilute intravenous infusions of alkalis are indicated in this type of poisoning.

At autopsy there are signs of inflammation of the digestive organs, urinary tract and skin. If the crude drug has been taken, green shining particles from the insect may be present in the stomach and the intestinal contents, and these are characteristic of the drug. Stomach contents, urine and parenchymatous viscera are used for toxicologic examination.

REFERENCES

Cogan, D. G., and Cogan, F. C. Dinitrophenol cataract, J.A.M.A., 105:793, 1935.

Conferences on Therapy. Treatment of poisoning by the barbiturates, New York State J. Med., 43:1, 1943.

De Groat, A. Symmetric necrosis of the globus pallidus in barbiturate poisoning, Arch. Path., 29:271, 1940.

Freireich, A. W., and Landsberg, J. W. Amphetamine sulphate for acute barbiturate poisoning, J.A.M.A., 131:661, 1946.

Goodman, L., and Gilman, A. The Pharmacological Basis of Therapeutics, New York, The Macmillan Co., 1941.

Guyton, W. L. Oil of chenopodium poisoning, J.A.M.A., 132:330, 1946.

Harrison, F. F., Johnson, R. D., and Ayer, D. Fatal aplastic anemia following use of triodone and a hydrastin, J.A.M.A., 132:11, 1946.

Harrop, G. A., and Westerfield, R. L. Sulfhemoglobinemia, J.A.M.A., 95:647, 1930.

Hoffman, A. M., Kahn, J., and Fitzgibbon, J. P. Thrombocytopenic purpura following allyl-isopropyl-acetyl-carbamide (Sedormid), J.A.M.A., 110:725, 1938.

Hunt, R., and Gettler, A. O. Non-alkaloidal Organic Poisons, from Peterson, Haines and Webster, Legal Medicine and Toxicology, Philadelphia, W. B. Saunders Co., 1923, Vol. II, pp. 602-772.

Jetter, W. W., and McLean, R. Poisoning by the synergistic effect of phenobarbital and ethyl alcohol. Arch. Path., 36:112, 1943.

Kracke, R. R. Relation of drug therapy to neutropenic states, J.A.M.A., 111:1255, 1938.

Lewin, L. Gifte und Vergiftungen, Berlin, Georg Stilke, 1929.

Mackay, R. P., and Gottstein, W. K. Aplastic anemia and agranulocytosis following triodone, J.A.M.A., 132:13, 1946.

McNally, W. D. Three deaths from T.N.T. (trinitrotoluene) poisoning, Industrial Med., 13:491, 1944.

Moody, A. M. Thrombocytopenic purpura following use of allyl-isopropyl-acetyl-carbamide (Sedormid), J.A.M.A., 110:726, 1938.

New and Nonofficial Remedies, Chicago, Ill., American Medical Association, 1946.

Petri, E. Vergiftungen, from Henke and Lubarsch, Berlin, Julius Springer, 1930, Vol. X.

Poole, F. E., and Haining, R. B. Death from dinitrophenol, J.A.M.A., 102:1141, 1934.

Reports of the Office of The Chief Medical Examiner in the City of New York from 1918 to 1951.

Reynolds, T. B., and Ware, A. G. Sulfhemoglobinemia following habitual use of acetanilid, J.A.M.A., 149:1538, 1952.

Silver, S. A new danger in dinitrophenol therapy, J.A.M.A., 103:1105, 1934.

Sollmann, T. Manual of Pharmacology, 4th ed., Philadelphia, W. B. Saunders Co., 1934.

Sutliff, W. D., Helpern, M., Griffin, C., and Brown, H. Sulphonamide toxicity as a cause of death in New York City in 1941, J.A.M.A., 121:307, 1943.

Tainter, M. L., and Wood, D. A. Fatal dinitrophenol poisoning, J.A.M.A., 102:1147, 1934.

Webster, R. Legal Medicine and Toxicology, Philadelphia, W. B. Saunders Co., 1930.

ALLERGIC LESIONS FOLLOWING SULFONAMIDE ADMINISTRATION

French, A. J. Histopathologic changes with sulphonamides, Am. J. Path., 22:679, 1946.

Lichtenstein, L., and Fox, L. J. Necrotizing arterial lesions following administration of sulphathiazole, Am. J. Path., 22:665, 1946.

More, R. H., McMillan, G. C., and Duff, G. L. The pathology of sulphonamide allergy in man, Am. J. Path., 22:703, 1946.

PHENYLBUTAZONE

Bershof, E., and Oxman, A. C. Agranulocytosis following use of phenylbutazone (butazolidin), J.A.M.A., 151:557, 1953.

Charet, R., and Siegel, I. Unusual reaction following use of phenylbutazone (butazolidin), J.A.M.A., 151:556, 1953.

Etess, A. D., and Jacobson, A. S. Fatality due to agranulocytosis following use of phenyl-butazone (butazolidin), J.A.M.A., 151:639, 1953.

Stifel, J. L., and Burnheimer, J. C. Agranulocytosis following administration of phenyl-butazone (butazolidin), J.A.M.A., 151:555, 1953.

34

Organic Poisons: Alkaloids

The group of alkaloids includes a number of toxic compounds present in various plants. Most of these substances are found among the Dicotyledones, especially in the Papaveraceae, Ranunculaceae, Solanaceae and the Rubiaceae. The only subdivision of Monocotyledones which contain alkaloids are the Colchicaceae. Similar compounds are found in some of the fungi, in the bacterial putrefaction of protein (ptomaines) and in uric acid products of animal metabolism (leukomaines).

Chemically an alkaloid is an organic base which is electropositive and can unite with acids to form salts. Its basic quality depends on the pyridine nucleus which is a ring of the fundamental benzene type, formed by five carbon atoms and one nitrogen, and is present in most of the common vegetable alkaloids; the individual compounds are simply complex elaborations and combinations of other organic radicals with the pyridine ring. For example, in the quinoline nucleus, which is an important constituent of the *Strychnos* alkaloids, pyridine is joined to a benzene ring. In some of the opium alkaloids the nitrogen component is united to the three-ringed phenanthrene nucleus. In one alkaloid, narceine, the nitrogen is embedded in an aliphatic chain which is joined to a benzene ring. The alkaloids of fungi, the putrefactive bases of ptomaines and the so-called animal alkaloids, or leukomaines, are composed mostly of open chains of carbon radicals holding a nitrogen base. In a few instances the nitrogen is held in closed chains of a type other than six-membered rings.

Alkaloids rarely are discovered in the pure state in nature, but are combined usually with certain acids to form salts. They are not distributed uniformly in the plant but are concentrated in different structures, such as the root, bark, leaves or seeds, which vary with the species. Members of the same family contain a number of similar alkaloids. It is rare to find compounds of the alkaloidal group which are alike chemically in unrelated families of plants.

Two categories of alkaloids are recognized on the basis of their physical properties. One large group is composed of odorless, nonvolatile, colorless or white crystalline solids which melt and sublime on the application of heat with a certain degree of decomposition. They contain carbon, nitrogen, hydrogen and oxygen. They cannot be distilled without alteration of their structure. The other category encompasses the volatile alkaloids and contains only a few members. They are odorless liquids which distill without change. They contain hydrogen, carbon and nitrogen without oxygen.

Pharmacologically the alkaloids produce their chief effect on some portion of the central nervous system. Each compound has its own individual action and, in some instances, this is so distinctive that the signs evoked by the poison on mice and frogs may be employed as a supplementary means of identification. As a rule the alkaloidal substances with a few exceptions affect the other tissues of the body as a secondary result of their action on the central nervous system.

VOLATILE ALKALOIDAL POISONS

The most important alkaloids in this group are nicotine in tobacco and coniine in poison hemlock.

Nicotine and Tobacco. Nicotine is the main alkaloid found in the leaves of the tobacco plant (*Nicotiana tabacum*). Other alkaloids, as nicotimine and nicoteine, are present in small amounts and are much like nicotine in structure. Nicotine is also the chief constituent of many plant insecticides.

Tobacco leaf is smoked in the form of cigarettes, cigars and pipe tobacco. In some places it is chewed. In earlier times it was used as snuff. A certain amount of nicotine is probably present in tobacco smoke, but the principal constituents are carbon dioxide, carbon monoxide, hydrogen sulfide, pyridine, hydrocyanic acid, furfurol and acrolein, which are in minute quantities and so are not toxicologically important. Inhalation of tobacco smoke may produce minor toxic effects, due to nicotine and the other constituents. Long continued smoking to excess has been attended by chronic irritation of the air passages, tobacco amblyopia and vascular reactions of a minor nature; some believe that smoking is an etiologic factor in the production of Buerger's disease or thromboangiitis obliterans.

Nicotine has the formula $C_{10}H_{14}N_2$, and it is a derivative of pyridine and pyrrolidine. It is beta-pyridyl-alpha-n-methylpyrrolidine. Physically it is an oily, sharp-tasting colorless fluid without odor when first isolated; after exposure it darkens to a deep brown and acquires a smell of tobacco. It can be distilled without decomposition in a vacuum or with steam.

Cases of nicotine poisoning are suicidal, homicidal and accidental. The accidental cases are numerous. Tobacco, in itself, has caused death; it has been either swallowed by mistake in food, taken as an enema in the form of an emulsion or applied to the body for a skin disease. In the Reports of the Office of the Chief Medical Examiner in New York City in the interval from 1918 to 1951, there were 20 suicidal deaths and 4 accidental deaths due to nicotine poisoning.

The action of nicotine on the body is both local and general. When it comes in contact with tissues, it is definitely irritant because of its alkalinity. After absorption it acts at first as an excitant and then as a depressant of the central nervous system, of the sympathetic and of the parasympathetic ganglia, where it blocks the nicotinic action of acetylcholine (as described under atropine, page 853), on the synapses and the terminal nerve endings in the skeletal muscles; on the latter the effect in the depressant stage may be a paralysis like that caused by curare. Death is due to the paralysis of the medullary centers and the specific curare-like action on the muscles of respiration. Much of the nicotine undergoes detoxification in the liver, while some is excreted in the urine.

Nicotine, when swallowed, produces a hot, burning sensation in the upper digestive tract from the mouth to the stomach. Immediately after there is salivation, nausea, vomiting, diarrhea and pain in the abdomen. After absorption the drug is a stimulant, then a paralysant of the central nervous system, causing muscular weakness, clonic convulsions, tetanic spasm, twitchings, vertigo and mental confusion. Later there is collapse and loss of reflexes. The respiration is rapid and death is due to respiratory paralysis. The pupils are dilated, the pulse feeble, the face pale and the extremities cold. If a large dose of the pure alkaloid is taken, death may occur without convulsions in a few seconds with complete paralysis of the central nervous system. When tobacco is ingested instead, death is usually delayed for a longer time.

The fatal dose is hard to estimate; 3 to 4 drops of the alkaloid are considered a lethal dose for an adult. Death has occurred after swallowing 0.8 gm. of snuff. An infusion of 2 gm. of tobacco in enema form has been fatal. The rapidity with which nicotine may cause death is only surpassed by that of the action of hydrocyanic acid.

At necropsy, if the drug has been taken by mouth, there will be congestion of the stomach and intestines and more or less acute inflammation. All the organs are congested and the blood is dark and fluid. A tobacco odor may or may not be present. The materials preserved for chemical examination are stomach contents, brain and parenchymatous viscera. Even in known cases of poisoning, this alkaloid is difficult to recover by toxicologic examination.

The treatment is to evacuate the stomach and administer powdered charcoal to absorb the alkaloid. Gastric lavage with tannic acid and dilute iodine solution is recommended. Warmth, artificial respiration and oxygen inhalation are used to combat shock.

Lobelia, or Indian tobacco, derived from the dried leaves and tops of the *Lobelia inflata* is employed as an expectorant and emetic in medicine. Its alkaloid, lobeline, is used as a cough sedative in doses of 0.015 and 0.03 gm. The action of lobeline is similar to that of nicotine but is not as powerful. At present it is not regarded as possessing much toxicologic importance.

Coniine and Poison Hemlock. The common or poison hemlock, *Conium maculatum,* contains six alkaloids: d-coniine, gamma-coniceine, methyl-coniine, conhydrine, pseudoconhydrine, and ethylpiperidine. D-coniine ($C_8H_{17}N$) is present mainly in the fruit. It is known, chemically, as alpha-n-propyl-piperidine. It is a colorless, oily fluid, but on standing it becomes yellow and resinous with a mousy odor. This is the typical active poisonous principle of the plant. Gamma-coniceine is even more toxic and is found in conium.

Most cases of poisoning are accidental, due to ingestion of the hemlock by mistake, or by taking an overdose of the alkaloid. There is a burning pain in the mouth and throat after ingestion. After absorption there is partial paralysis of the peripheral nerves and muscular weakness. Nausea, vomiting, profuse salivation, dysphagia and thick speech occur. The breathing is rapid and deep at the start, but it becomes weak and irregular. The heart is slow at first, but later accelerated. There is comparatively slight disturbance of the intellect. Death is due to asphyxia, in part caused by paralysis of nerve terminations in the respiratory muscles and in part by the depressing effect on the respiratory center. Dilatation of the pupil occurs at the end.

The treatment is to wash out the stomach, combat shock by stimulation and maintain artificial respiration if necessary. As a rule, if the patient does not die in the acute attack, recovery occurs.

The poisonous action is quite rapid, and death may occur from one-half to three hours. About 3 drops is a lethal dose. Coniine is excreted rapidly in the urine. At autopsy, the materials preserved for chemical analysis are stomach contents, brain and parenchymatous organs. The postmortem lesions are much like those produced by nicotine.

NONVOLATILE ALKALOIDS

The members of this group include the alkaloids which contain oxygen in the molecule and which decompose if distillation is attempted so that the poison must be isolated toxicologically by an immiscible solvent.

Opium and Morphine. The unripe capsules of the poppy (*Papaver somni-ferum*) yield a milky exudation which, when dried, is termed opium. Opium contains about 20 alkaloids which are united with various acids, such as sulfuric acid, meconic acid, acetic acid and lactic acid.

Opium occurs as rounded, somewhat flattened masses, gray-brown in color, plastic in the fresh state but brittle when aged, with a bitter taste and narcotic action. Powdered opium is a light brown powder made from the crude material. Many of the medicinal preparations are made from powdered opium. Some of the official preparations are tincture of opium or laudanum which contains 10 per cent of opium or 1 per cent of morphine in dilute alcohol; camphorated tincture of opium or pare-goric, containing 0.4 per cent of opium; Dover's powders or pulvis ipecacuanhae et opii, containing 10 per cent each of ipecac and opium. Pantopon is a purified mix-ture of opium alkaloids, containing 50 per cent of morphine and is soluble in water.

The alkaloids of opium are divided into two groups, one composed of morphine, codeine, narcotine, pseudomorphine, thebaine and a few others known as the morphine group which are important toxicologically. The members of the morphine group differ slightly in their action; in morphine proper the characteristic effect on the nervous system is narcosis, while in others, like thebaine, reflex stimulation is paramount and convulsions of the strychnine type are produced. The second group, known as the papaverine alkaloids, are not remarkably toxic.

Morphine is a complex alkaloid with a composition $C_{17}H_{19}NO_3$; it is the most poisonous ingredient of opium in which it is present in the proportion of 9.5 per cent. This alkaloid occurs as white, shining, rhombic prisms, as fine needles or as a crystalline powder. It is found also in the forms of morphine hydrochloride or mor-phine sulfate which are white crystalline compounds with a bitter taste.

The salts of morphine have an extensive use in medicine. The drug lessens pain, induces sleep, secures muscular quiet and facilitates the production of anesthesia. In addition, cough is suppressed, dyspnea is eased and intestinal peristalsis is checked. The pulse and respiration are slowed and the drug is used to control inaccessible internal hemorrhage.

Acute poisoning by morphine may be produced by oral or hypodermic adminis-tration. If the drug is ingested the symptoms appear in about 20 minutes, but if it is administered by hypodermic or intravenous injection its action is more rapid. By the time that the victim is seen by a physician, coma has usually set in. The cases are usually suicidal, accidental or homicidal. In the Reports of the Chief Medical Examiner from 1918 to 1941, there was a yearly average of 44 accidental cases of which about five were acute cases of poisoning and the remainder were deaths from chronic narcotic addiction; there was a yearly average of three suicidal cases; one case during the 24 year period was a case of homicide.

Morphine exerts its toxic action on the central nervous system, depressing the higher cerebral centers first and then the vital centers of respiration and circulation in the medulla. The action on the spinal cord in some cases is that of a stimulant and tetanoid convulsions are caused. Coma is usually the most prominent symptom, however, and, when toxic doses are administered, the coma is followed by a gradual paralysis of the respiratory center.

The first symptom of the poisoning is a sense of mental stimulation and physical ease with a quickening of the pulse which lasts a variable length of time. This is followed by dizziness, drowsiness, languor and nausea. The pulse is slowed and decreased in force. There is a distinct desire to sleep with gradual loss of muscular power and sensitivity. The pupils of the eyes become contracted. The breathing may be slowed to 3 to 4 times a minute and is accompanied by cyanosis, livid lips and cold extremities. The stupor grows deeper, the respirations become Cheyne-Stokes in type and finally death occurs in deep coma. The pupils, just before death, may dilate. In some cases the symptoms may vary slightly from the typical picture for in some susceptible persons, delirium rather than stupor may occur and the convulsions may be tetanoid in character.

The postmortem appearances in cases of morphine poisoning are not particularly characteristic. There is a congestion of the viscera, cyanosis and abundant dark fluid blood. When crude opium is taken by mouth the stomach may contain fragments of poppy, but nothing characteristic is found if morphine is ingested.

The fatal dose in a case of acute morphine poisoning in a person who is not an addict varies from 1 to 6 grains. Circumstances may modify this lethal dose, however, as an individual in severe pain can withstand the injection of a larger quantity of morphine than under normal conditions. On the other hand, some people are susceptible to the drug and succumb to a small dose. Children especially are likely to develop toxic symptoms after taking small amounts of the drug. Addicts develop a tolerance to large quantities of morphine which, however, is not constant, as it decreases whenever the use of the drug is discontinued for a long interval. The duration of the acute poisoning by morphine or opium is, on the average, from 5 to 18 hours. It may vary from 45 minutes to 4 days.

Some of the morphine is eliminated through the stomach and intestines, and this occurs irrespective of whether the drug is administered by mouth or by hypodermic. Some of it is oxidized by the liver and a little may be excreted in the urine. The alkaloid disappears from the system, as a rule, in the first 24 hours after ingestion. It is distributed over the body and is found in the stomach contents, parenchymatous organs and brain at the time of autopsy if the victim dies in the acute stage.

The treatment of acute morphine and opium poisoning can be divided into the following steps:

1. Repeated evacuation of the poison from the stomach by the stomach tube, as the drug is excreted continually and should be removed from time to time by gastric lavage. An emetic of powdered mustard in water may be given to promote vomiting. Goodman and Gilman minimize the excretion of the alkaloid into the stomach and intestine and do not recommend repeated gastric lavage.

2. The patient should be stimulated to breathe about 10 to 15 times a minute. Artificial respiration with inhalation of oxygen and carbon dioxide is useful. The Drinker respirator can be used if it is available. Slapping the face and neck with cold wet cloths and forcing the patient to walk are also measures of resuscitation.

3. Treatment with potassium permanganate (5 gm. per liter solution in water) is recommended to oxidize the morphine. This is given by stomach tube.

4. The patient can be given atropine, $\frac{1}{60}$ to $\frac{1}{20}$ grain, strychnine $\frac{1}{32}$ grain, and caffeine either hypodermically or as strong coffee to stimulate the circulation and respiration.

CHRONIC OPIUM OR MORPHINE POISONING. Chronic poisoning by alkaloids of the opium series is quite common and important from the point of view of public health inasmuch as these compounds are habit-forming drugs. The habitués find the effects of the physiologic dose pleasant and they gradually increase the amount until they can take enormous doses of the drug. Chronic poisoning may be caused by smoking crude opium, taking opium preparations by mouth or taking morphine by hypodermic or intravenous injection. The continued use causes mental and physical deterioration and also predisposes to chronic constipation and intercurrent infections. A definite proportion of morphine habitués die of pulmonary tuberculosis because of malnutrition referable to the fact that they spend their money for morphine instead of for food. Others who inject the drug subcutaneously develop indolent subcutaneous abscesses over the arms, the thighs and the abdomen. In a few cases these lesions have produced septicemia and bacterial endocarditis. Some of the abscesses become infected with the tetanus bacillus and cause typical wound tetanus.

Morphine or heroin addicts who take the drug by subcutaneous or intravenous injection present distinctive scars on the skin. Those using the subcutaneous method frequently dissolve the alkaloid in a spoonful of water by heating the spoon over a luminous gas flame and then aspirating the solution into the injection syringe. As this technic makes no concessions to the principles of asepsis, many impurities, including bacteria and soot, are injected subcutaneously with the result that small subcutaneous indolent abscesses form, slough on the skin surface and heal under a scab. Small circular or ovoid pitted scars about 1 cm. in diameter, similar to smallpox vaccination scars, result. In some instances, particles of soot are injected and form small subcutaneous nodules 5 to 10 mm. in diameter which are dark green or bluish green in color. These different lesions are present in large numbers over the shoulders, arms, hips, lower abdomen and thighs and strongly suggest chronic narcotic addiction.

Those addicts who inject the narcotic intravenously, usually heroin, make use of the superficial veins on the flexor surface of the forearm or the bend of the elbow. The scars appear as short tape-like thickenings of the dermis from $\frac{3}{8}$ to 1 inch in length and about $\frac{3}{16}$ inch in width. Sometimes minute dots appear on the area of thickening arranged seriatim or irregularly. These are caused by the penetration of the needle and are known as main line scars (Fig. 34-1).

Distressing nervous sequelae may occur in an addict when the drug is suddenly withdrawn. Addicts have been known to feign symptoms of such conditions as renal colic or biliary colic in order to obtain morphine to get relief.

CODEINE. The alkaloid codeine is present in opium in about 0.2 per cent to 0.8 per cent. Its formula is $C_{18}H_{21}NO_3$ and it is a methyl compound of morphine, according to its chemical formula. It occurs as translucent rhombic prisms, or as a crystalline powder. Codeine phosphate and codeine sulfate are the most common salts.

Codeine in its toxic action resembles morphine, but its depressing effects on the cerebral centers are more transient. The narcotic and sleep-producing effects are not so intense as morphine, but the respiratory center is depressed and the cough reflex is diminished. It does not produce as many constipating effects as morphine. Fatal cases are rare.

The signs of fatal poisoning are weakness, loss of consciousness, contraction of the pupils, delirium, irritation of the skin, muscular contractions, rapid heart beat, dyspnea and collapse. The lethal dose varies from 4.5 grains to 8 grains but much larger doses have been taken by adults without ill effects.

The postmortem appearance, elimination and treatment of the poisoning are similar to morphine. Codeine, however, does not belong to the drugs to which the system develops a tolerance and it is not a habit-forming drug.

HEROIN. Heroin is a synthetic alkaloid derived from morphine by replacing the hydrogen atoms of the alcohol and phenol groups of this alkaloid by the acetic radical. Its formula is $C_{21}H_{23}NO_5$, or diacetyl morphine. It is a white crystalline powder with a bitter taste, which becomes hydrolyzed by heating with water or acids. This process takes place, to a certain extent, in the body. The principal compound of heroin is the hydrochloride.

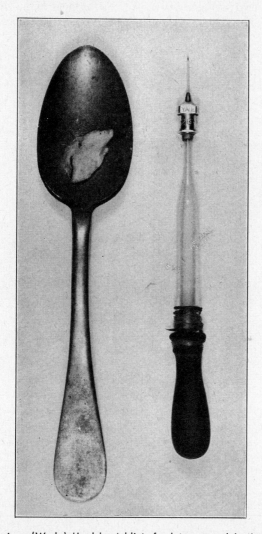

Fig. 34-I. Syringe (Works) Used by Addicts for Intravenous Injections of Heroin.

The solution of heroin is prepared in the spoon, sucked up, through the cotton to filter out coarse particles, into the improvised syringe made from a hypodermic needle and a medicine dropper. The apparatus is not sterilized and its common use between several addicts has resulted in the transmission of many cases of malaria, many of which have been fatal.

Heroin acts like morphine, but differs in that it is more stimulating, depresses the cerebral centers less, and the respiratory center more; the respirations are slower and deeper, as a rule. The toxic symptoms and signs usually are headache, restlessness, cyanosis, slow respirations, coma and finally death by respiratory paralysis. The postmortem findings and the treatment of acute heroin poisoning are practically the same as for morphine poisoning. The withdrawal symptoms in addicts resemble those of morphine addiction.

Heroin is an important habit-forming drug and is used more frequently than morphine by narcotic addicts. It is taken in the form of snuff by inhalation, and also is injected in watery solution subcutaneously and intravenously by syringe. In recent years many of the addicts have favored the intravenous method of administration, frequently improvising a syringe from a medicine dropper and a hypodermic needle. The apparatus is neither washed nor sterilized and sometimes is used for intravenous injection by several addicts in rapid succession; two may share the same heroin solution in one syringe. Usually, as the vein is entered during this process, a little blood flows back into the syringe and contaminates the contents. If it so happens that this blood contains malarial parasites, spirochetes or parasitic protozoa, a person who shares the use of the syringe will directly and artificially inoculate himself with the disease, which, in most instances, is malaria. In many parts of the world heroin

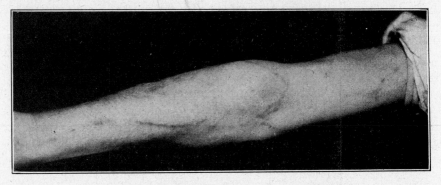

Fig. 34-2. Intravenous Drug Addict. "Main Line Shooter."

Note "tattooed" needle-scarred superficial veins on forearm. The injection apparatus used is illustrated in Figure 34-1.

addicts have transmitted malaria to each other in this manner. In New York City, during 1933 and 1934, an epidemic of fatal malignant estivo-autumnal malaria of the cerebral type broke out among the drug addicts, and since then the disease has become endemic among that group (Figs. 34-2 and 34-3).

A general blood infection by *Candida parakrusei* was transmitted to one addict by the intravenous injection of solutions of heroin. At necropsy an acute vegetative endocarditis, thromboses and multiple embolic lesions were found in the body, and these had caused the death of the deceased. The virulence of the organism was slight and the resistance of the patient to the invasion of the fungus was weak. The clinical course was a protracted one and while the disease spread gradually many of the older lesions in the body showed definite signs of recession and healing.

Apomorphine is a dehydrated morphine derivative which has only a slight toxicologic significance. It has no narcotic action, nor has it any habit-forming properties. It is used in medicine chiefly to induce vomiting by its action on the central nervous system. The drug, however, is toxic and may cause depression of the respiratory centers if not used with caution. Occasional fatalities have occurred after the therapeutic use of this drug.

Morphine, opium and its derivatives are under the jurisdiction of the Harrison Narcotic Act, which provides that every physician desiring to prescribe, dispense or own these drugs must register with the collector of internal revenue in his district and obtain a registry number on the payment of a fee. This gives him the authority to use narcotics in his practice for one year. The law is intended to curb illicit diversion of opium compounds. Prescriptions containing narcotics must be in writing and carry the signature, office address and federal registration number of the physician, along with the name and address of the patient. The druggist retains these prescriptions for two years, and the physician keeps duplicates of them for that time. A physician who dispenses narcotics must keep a record of the amount of his stock and when, and from whom, he received the drugs, for a period of three months, and give it to the collector of internal revenue on demand. Failure to obey this law exposes the offender to a fine of $2000, a prison sentence of not more than five years, or both.

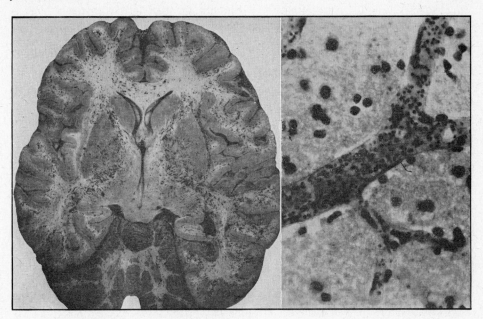

Fig. 34-3. Fatal Estivo-Autumnal Malaria Associated with Intravenous Heroin Addiction.

Left. Horizontal section through brain showing numerous punctate hemorrhages in white matter.

Right. Histologic section showing dilated capillary vessels containing red blood cells heavily infected with malarial parasites.

Regulation No. 2 of the Bureau of Narcotics, U. S. Treasury Department, relating to the importation, exportation and transshipment of opium or coca leaves, in effect January 1st 1952, stipulates that no crude opium may be imported for the manufacture of heroin or its compounds.

The report of the Chief Medical Examiner of the City of New York for the year 1950 indicates that among the suicidal deaths there were 3 cases of morphine poisoning; among the accidental poisonings there were 28 due to morphine and 22 to heroin. These figures do not indicate the total number of deaths associated with narcotic poisoning inasmuch as a large proportion of addicts die as the result of other conditions such as cerebral malaria, pulmonary tuberculosis or sepsis. Tetanus may result from infection of a hypodermic wound.

Aconitum and Aconitine. The root of the *Aconitum napellus,* or monkshood, contains the toxic alkaloid aconitine and a few other compounds not as toxic. The official preparation of the drug is the tincture, and this is used in medicine as a cardiac depressant.

Aconitine is the active principle of the plant and is a bitter, colorless, crystalline substance with the formula $C_{34}H_{47}NO_{11}$ denoting the chemical name acetyl-benzoyl aconine.

Most cases of aconite poisoning are accidental and are referable to errors in taking medicine on the part of patients, or to carelessness on the part of physicians or druggists. In some instances poisoning has occurred because an individual has eaten of aconitum root which he has mistaken for horseradish. Suicidal and homicidal cases of poisoning are not common. Two suicidal cases occurred in the reports of the Office of the Chief Medical Examiner of New York City from 1918 to 1951.

The drug is administered usually by mouth or hypodermic injection and is absorbed into the system readily. The symptoms come on rapidly and death takes place in three to four hours as a rule. A case of death in eight minutes has been reported; some have lived for a few days. The elimination of the aconitine takes place through the urine, intestine and saliva rather promptly.

A poisonous dose causes salivation, tingling and numbness in the mouth, burning in the throat and the stomach, nausea and vomiting, numbness and tingling of fingers, cramps in extremities, a few tetanic convulsions, dysphagia and signs of a general collapse. The pulse is slow, feeble and irregular, the respirations shallow and rapid, the muscles weak and the skin cold and clammy. There are few mental symptoms; delirium is unusual and coma only supervenes because of shock. The chief action is a depression of the medullary centers. The fatal dose is 1 to 6 mg. or more.

The postmortem appearances are not markedly characteristic. The blood is fluid and the viscera are congested.

The stomach is evacuated by the stomach tube, and tannic acid or charcoal may be used to render the alkaloid inert. Strychnine, digitalis and external warmth may be employed to combat shock.

Atropine and Related Alkaloids. Some toxic alkaloids are found in plants of the Solonaceae group. For example, atropine ($C_{17}H_{23}NO_3$) is present in the deadly nightshade or *Atropa belladonna,* scopolamine ($C_{17}H_{21}NO_4$) in *Datura stramonium,* also known as the thorn apple or jimson weed, and hyoscyamine ($C_{17}H_{23}NO_3$) in henbane or *Hyoscyamus niger.* Other alkaloids occur but they are not as important. The alkaloids are chemical compounds known as tropeins, with the exception of scopolamine which is a derivative of tropic acid. The tropeins are ester-like combinations of an aromatic acid with a base known as tropine ($C_8H_{15}NO$), and for this reason saponify readily. Homatropine ($C_{16}H_{21}NO_3$), or tropine mandelate, is an artificial or synthetic alkaloid similar to atropine, but is much less toxic.

The chief preparation of atropine is atropine sulfate. Hyoscyamine occurs as hyoscyamine hydrobromide. Scopolamine is present as the hydrobromide. All of these compounds are white, crystalline substances. Tincture of belladonna and atropine sulfate are the two most commonly used preparations.

Most cases of poisoning with the alkaloids of this group are accidental and few are suicidal or homicidal. In several cases overdoses of the various drugs were given by mistake, either by mouth or hypodermic. Two accidental cases of atropine poisoning were recorded in the Office of the Chief Medical Examiner of New York City between 1918 and 1951. Poisoning has been said to occur from eating the flesh of rabbits which have fed on belladonna leaves, or from the application of belladonna plaster to the skin. Children have developed toxic symptoms after eating the berries of the deadly nightshade, the root of *Hyoscyamus niger,* or the seeds of

Datura stramonium. A nonfatal poisoning in children who drank tea made of Datura seeds and developed transient signs of loss of self-control, exaggerated emotional displays and delirium was reported by Hughes and Clark.

Poisoning by atropine and its related alkaloids causes such symptoms as dryness of the throat, dysphagia, huskiness of the voice, dilated pupils, impaired vision, hallucinations, giddiness, delirium, excitement, choreiform movements and convulsions. The pulse may be full and bounding but later becomes feeble and rapid, and respirations at first deepened and quickened are depressed in the later stages. The skin becomes flushed and dry and shows a deep red eruption. Just before death, numbness and paralysis of the limbs, convulsions and unconsciousness supervene. The toxic action at this stage is due to a depressing effect on the respiratory center. In poisoning by atropine and the related alkaloids, the toxic action starts shortly after administration of the drug, but takes a few hours to develop fully. Death usually occurs within 24 hours and rarely after a few days. The fatal dose of atropine is about one twentieth of a grain, but it is difficult to determine the lethal dose of the other alkaloids. In nonfatal cases all of the atropine is eliminated in the urine inside of 36 hours, aside from a small portion destroyed in the body.

Secretory and neuromuscular signs such as dryness of the mouth, flushed skin and dilated pupils are due to the action of atropine which prevents the stimulating nerve impulses from acting on the salivary gland and the smooth muscles in the blood vessels and in the iris. The pupillary dilatation may be unilateral if a dilute solution of homatropine is applied to one eye, and for this reason it is used extensively by ophthalmologists.

The peripheral action of atropine on the salivary glands and smooth muscle is best understood by considering the normal neurogenic stimulation which controls these structures. The nervous impulse arises in the central nervous system and is first transmitted to the intermediate ganglion where it releases acetylcholine in varying amounts; if the acetylcholine occurs in low concentration, ganglionic activity is stimulated, but if a high concentration is present, a ganglionic depression occurs. The stimulating action in the ganglion is called the nicotinic action of acetylcholine. A similar effect is produced around the end organs of striated muscle by acetylcholine. Nicotine and related alkaloids block the nicotinic action of acetylcholine especially in the ganglia.

The nerve impulse is normally transmitted from the ganglion to the nerve termination in the gland or smooth muscle, releasing acetylcholine in these structures and thus stimulating the gland to secrete and the smooth muscle to contract. This effect is known as the muscarinic action of acetylcholine. Atropine acts directly on the gland cells and smooth muscle fibers and blocks the muscarinic action of acetylcholine, stopping the secretion of the salivary gland and paralyzing the constrictor muscles of the blood vessels. The nerve endings in these structures are not affected nor is the release of acetylcholine inhibited, but it is prevented from acting on gland or smooth muscle. Atropine does not affect the nicotinic action of acetylcholine.

Hyoscyamine has an action like atropine, but not so intense. Scopolamine or hyoscine acts like atropine, but depresses the central nervous system more markedly with symptoms of drowsiness, fatigue and stupor. In combination with morphine, scopolamine is used to produce twilight sleep during labor but its use is not devoid of danger.

The postmortem findings in fatal cases are not characteristic. All the viscera are markedly congested, and in a few cases faint signs of the red skin eruption may be distinguishable. In poisoning by ingestion of the plants, parts of the plants may be present in the stomach and intestinal contents. The materials preserved for toxicologic examination are stomach contents, brain and parenchymatous viscera.

The ptomatropines are substances formed in decomposing animal proteins, which cause mydriasis and other symptoms similar to belladonna constituents when they are taken into the system. They may be confused with the alkaloids if encountered during toxicologic examination, but they can be separated by careful analysis and distinguished because they do not give the reactions of atropine chemically.

The treatment is to remove the contents of the stomach by the stomach tube, to precipitate the alkaloid in the stomach by a dilute solution of iodine in water (6 drops to 4 ounces), or of tannic acid, and to treat the symptoms as they arise. The stage of excitement can be mitigated by administering morphine, and that of collapse by caffeine.

Ipecac and Emetine. Ipecac is the dried root of *Cephaelis ipecacuanha* or *Cephaelis acuminata*. Emetine is the principal alkaloid and is a colorless base which apparently cannot be crystallized. It is a quinoline derivative, having the formula $C_{29}H_{40}N_{20}O_4$. Its salt, emetine hydrochloride, a white or light yellow crystalline powder, is one of the common official preparations. Others are fluid extract of ipecac and Dover's powders (pulvis ipecacuanhae et opii). Cephaeline ($C_{28}H_{38}N_2O_4$) and psychotrine ($C_{28}H_{36}N_2O_4$) are other alkaloids which occur in the plant.

The marked toxicity of ipecac and its derivatives for amebas make it a valuable drug for the treatment of amebic dysentery. Its use is contraindicated if the patient is suffering from severe cardiac and renal disease. Most of the poisonings are accidental because the drug has been taken in overdose, or because it has been administered by mistake. Emetine has caused more cases than ipecac. Suicidal and homicidal cases are rare.

The symptoms are practically the same, whether the poison is given by mouth, subcutaneously or intravenously. The toxic effects may manifest themselves soon after the administration of the drug, or they may occur after a long continued treatment of a case of amebic dysentery in which a series of small doses has been given. The drug is slowly destroyed by the liver and slowly excreted over a number of days so that it often has a cumulative effect; for that reason large doses should not be administered nor should the treatment be long continued. The symptoms are salivation, abdominal pain, nausea and vomiting, frequent bloody diarrhea, vertigo, muscular weakness, lethargy, anuria, hematuria, cardiac weakness, low blood pressure, expiratory dyspnea and arrest of the heart in diastole. Death has occurred after ipecac in one and one half hours; its fatal dose is hard to determine because of the variation in toxicity of different preparations. Emetine chloride also is a cumulative poison and its clinical course may cover a number of days. Therapeutically the drug is usually administered in 10 daily doses for 10 days, the total dosage being 0.6 gm.

Ipecac and its alkaloids are marked depressants of the central nervous system, have a definite myotoxic action especially on the heart muscle, cause irritation of the gastrointestinal tract, and produce degenerative changes in liver and kidneys. At necropsy the mucous membranes of the stomach and intestines may be inflamed. The heart is distended and stops usually in diastole. Many cases exhibit a terminal pneumonia.

The remedy generally employed is tannic acid given by mouth and by rectum. The stomach is washed out by the tube and the large intestine by enemas. Stomach contents, brain and parenchymatous viscera are saved for chemical examination.

Cocaine and Allied Alkaloids. Cocaine, $C_{17}H_{21}NO_4$, is a constituent of the leaf of the coca tree, or the *Erythroxylon coca,* which is a native of South America. Cocaine is the methyl benzoyl ester of ecgonine, a base similar to tropine and, as a consequence, it saponifies quite readily. The official preparation of cocaine is cocaine hydrochloride which occurs in colorless, transparent, monoclinic prisms, or in the form of a white crystalline powder.

Most cocaine poisonings are accidental, a few are suicidal, while homicidal use of the drug is rare. The accidental cases are usually caused when habitués take an overdose, or because in therapeutic use the drug was applied too recklessly to a raw surface, or given too freely by hypodermic. In suicidal cases the drug may be taken by mouth or taken intravenously with an hypodermic syringe. In the records of the Office of the Chief Medical Examiner of New York City, 29 accidental cases and 2 suicidal cases occurred from 1918 to 1951.

Cocaine acts on the central nervous system, first stimulating the cerebrum, then the cerebellum and finally the medulla. Depression then follows the stimulation in the same order, cerebrum, cerebellum and finally medulla. Cocaine also has a local action on the nervous system, as it paralyzes the endings of the sensory nerves. It produces dilatation of the pupil. In poisonous doses the patient becomes talkative, restless, excited and gradually develops delirium, hallucinations and violent mania. There is a feeling of dryness in the mouth, mydriasis, suffocation, dysphagia, nausea, epigastric pain, headache, vertigo, numbness and tingling in the hands. The pulse is accelerated and feeble, respirations at first are rapid, then become Cheyne-Stokes in type and gradually weaken. Later, convulsions, collapse, cyanosis, clammy skin, shock and death occur. The symptoms appear promptly and are ordinarily over in two to three hours in nonfatal cases. In some instances a patient may die suddenly in shock immediately after injection, either as a result of a sudden toxic action on the heart or because of an allergic sensitivity to the drug itself.

The poison acts quickly after absorption and in most cases causes death within the hour. The fatal dose varies: by mouth 0.648 gm., by rectum 1.5 gm., by urethra 0.03 gm., conjunctival sac 0.04 gm. and by subcutaneous injection 0.3 gm. The toxicity of cocaine is increased if it is used in combination with adrenalin. Its use as a local anesthetic has been replaced generally by procaine and other substitutes.

After the cocaine is absorbed it is promptly detoxified by the liver, but if administered too rapidly as a local anesthetic the drug may accumulate in the system and be especially virulent in its action. When taken by mouth, a large proportion is hydrolyzed in the stomach and rendered inactive. That portion which is not altered is excreted in the urine. The treatment is to evacuate the stomach if the drug has been taken by mouth. In other cases the shock should be treated by warmth, artificial respiration and other appropriate methods, and symptomatic treatment must be given as the need arises. In some cases the intravenous administration of a relatively short-acting barbiturate is recommended as a valuable antidote to combat the effects of cocaine.

The postmortem appearances are not characteristic, but congestion of the viscera is present as a rule. The materials saved for chemical examination are the stomach contents, the brain, urine and the parenchymatous viscera like the liver and kidneys.

Cocaine is a habit-forming drug and chronic poisoning is fairly prevalent. It is taken by habitués in the form of snuff, and as it produces a pleasant, stimulating effect, many practice the vice. Many of these addicts develop hallucinations and paranoid delusions on which they may act, and so are dangerous characters. In time the habit causes serious disturbances of nutrition, pallor of the skin and mental deterioration. Like opium and its derivatives, coca and its alkaloids are under the control of the Harrison Narcotic Act. Heroin which is more easily obtained has superseded cocaine as the drug used by most addicts.

Synthetic alkaloids derived from cocaine are used for various purposes. Alpha-eucaine and holocaine are quite toxic while others are too weak in their action. Beta-eucaine and procaine hydrochlorides are used with adrenalin as local anesthetics or as spinal anesthetics. Both have caused toxic action similar to cocaine after injection. Procaine is readily destroyed in the liver and does not have a synergistic action with adrenalin, so that it is safer to use as a local anesthetic than cocaine. Deaths from the use of procaine as a spinal anesthetic have occurred. In all these cases, the findings at autopsy were not characteristic.

Efocaine is a local anesthetic preparation composed of procaine 1 per cent, procaine hydrochloride 0.25 per cent, and butyl-*p*-aminobenzoate 5 per cent, dissolved in a solution of 2 per cent polyethylene glycol-300, 78 per cent propylene glycol and water. This mixture has been injected for the relief of pain attending anal lesions, chest operations, neuralgia and similar conditions because it produces a prolonged local anesthesia. In some cases local inflammation with sloughing, postinjection neuritis, pain, and serious neurologic symptoms and signs have followed the injections. The fatal case reported by Angerer and others was injected for the relief of intercostal neuralgia with 1.5 ml. of Efocaine in the right eighth intercostal space near the posterior axillary line. The patient collapsed from pain and shock during the operation, and died 44 hours later.

The necropsy disclosed a thrombosis of the right eighth intercostal artery and vein near the site of injection and focal areas of necrosis and inflammation in the lower dorsal and lumbar spinal cord, both of which were considered to be a result of the Efocaine injection. In addition, there was a fibroid tuberculosis in the right lung, an empyema with pleurocutaneous fistulas in the right chest, and a bilateral bronchopneumonia.

Nux Vomica and Its Alkaloids, Strychnine and Brucine. Some of the plants of the *Strychnos* genus, belonging to the family Loganiaceae, contain certain alkaloids among which the most important are strychnine and brucine. Their principal source is the seed of the *Strychnos nux vomica,* but they are found also in varying proportions in the seeds of *Strychnos ignatii* or St. Ignatius' bean, in the root bark of *Strychnos tieute* or the deadly upas tree, and in the other trees of the same family.

The official preparations of nux vomica are the extract, the fluid-extract and the tincture. Strychnine is the most important of the alkaloids, with a chemical formula of $C_{21}H_{22}N_2O_2$. Its structural formula is not known, but the compound is stable and it resists decomposition well. It is a colorless, crystalline substance with an extremely bitter taste. The nitrate and the sulfate are the official salts of strychnine. Brucine, $C_{23}H_{26}N_2O_4$, is similar to strychnine both chemically and physiologically, but its action is much weaker.

Cases of strychnine poisoning are fairly numerous; most of them are suicidal, some are accidental and few are homicidal. In the Office of the Chief Medical Examiner of New York City, 46 suicidal cases, 40 accidental or undetermined cases are recorded from 1918 to 1951; and 3 homicidal cases were investigated. As a rule, the alkaloid or some preparation of nux vomica is swallowed or is taken by hypodermic injection. Strychnine stimulates the entire central and peripheral nervous system, especially affecting the spinal cord and the brain. The principal point of attack is the nerve cell body, and the result is to increase the susceptibility of the nerves to stimulation. The effect of even slight sensory impulses is to produce excessive generalized motor impulses which are expressed in the form of tetanic convulsions.

Symptoms begin about 15 to 30 minutes, on the average, after the oral administration of the poison, but they may occur immediately or after the delay of an hour, depending on the rate at which the alkaloid is absorbed. There is a premonition of impending calamity, shuddering, a sense of tightness of the chest, and then a sudden violent tetanic spasm, characterized by stiffness of the neck, extension of the legs, opisthotonos with the body resting on the heels and head, a stiff sardonic grin, staring eyes and stiffened muscles of respiration. The convulsion endures from a half minute to several minutes, accompanied by cyanosis, weak, rapid pulse and dilated pupils. After this a quiescent interval follows for a few minutes, marked by general relaxation, perspiration, weariness and somnolence. Before another paroxysm occurs there is a premonitory feeling of anxiety and the paroxysm may be precipitated by any sudden movement or sound. During the convulsion the body may be bent forward in the posture of emprosthotonos, or sideways in the posture of pleurosthotonos; at other times the arms are extended or flexed over the chest. The mentality of the patient during these convulsions is usually clear. Death occurs from exhaustion or, in the midst of a paroxysm, from asphyxia.

Tetanus and a few other diseases may simulate the symptoms of strychnine poisoning, but the history of the case and the nature of the convulsions will allow a differential diagnosis to be made. Usually, in the case of strychnine, there is an interval between the paroxysms, and the jaw and neck muscles are not affected until near the end. In tetanus the body is apt to be rigid most of the time and the jaw and neck muscles among the first to be involved.

Death usually occurs after 1 to 3 hours, but the period may vary from 10 minutes to 11 hours. The average fatal dose by mouth varies from 0.10 gm. to 0.12 gm., but recovery may follow the administration of larger quantities of the drug.

The treatment is to evacuate the stomach with the stomach tube and wash it out with a dilute solution of iodine, tannic acid and finely powdered charcoal to neutralize the alkaloid. Chloroform and chloral hydrate may be administered to control the convulsions. The intraspinous injection of Ringer's solution or saline solution may hasten the excretion of the alkaloid. On account of the convulsions it is often necessary to perform these operations under anesthesia. The patient should be kept as quiet as possible and free of disturbing influences for fear of starting fresh paroxysms. If the patient can be tided over the first few hours of the poisoning, he may recover.

One valuable method of treatment is the intravenous injection of soluble short-acting barbiturates. Sodium amytal is given in a 10 percent solution in doses of 0.4 gm. to 1.0 gm., and pentobarbital sodium is given in the same dilution in doses of 0.3 to 0.7 gm. The drugs are slowly injected until enough depression of the nervous system is obtained to combat the tendency to convulsions and cause sleep, but not enough to dangerously affect the respirations or the blood pressure.

The postmortem signs are not characteristic. Rigor mortis occurs soon after death, sometimes within the hour, and the body may remain in a condition of opisthotonos. The rigidity may continue even until postmortem decomposition is under way. The viscera are usually congested.

The materials usually preserved for chemical analysis are the stomach contents, urine, brain, liver or other parenchymatous viscera. The drug is readily absorbed, usually from the intestines, and readily destroyed by the liver; about 20 per cent of it may be excreted in the urine. The excretion starts soon after absorption, but in nonfatal cases may not be completed before from 2 to 5 days. It is isolated most easily from the stomach contents but may be difficult to detect in the brain and the parenchymatous organs.

Physostigmine. Physostigmine, or eserine, is the alkaloidal principle of the Calabar bean, or *Physostigma venenosum*. It is crystalline, colorless and almost tasteless. After exposure to light and air the crystals develop a rose color. The chemical formula is $C_{15}H_{21}N_3O_2$.

The cases of poisoning are mainly accidental, because children have eaten Calabar beans, or patients have been given an overdose of the drug. Only two fatal cases have been described. Suicide has been attempted with this alkaloid but without a fatal outcome.

The principal action of physostigmine is an inhibition of an enzyme in the tissues and body fluid called cholinesterase which continually destroys acetylcholine and thus prevents excessive stimulation of the muscles and glands. The action of the cholinesterase is removed by physostigmine, and this allows acetylcholine to exert its stimulation unchecked, both musarinic and nicotinic, so that characteristic glandular activity and muscular contractions are produced.

The symptoms are vomiting, epigastric pain, dyspnea, giddiness, muscular weakness and twitching, pupillary contraction, sweating and salivation. Its action is opposite to that of atropine, in that it stimulates vagus endings. The heart becomes slow and complete collapse occurs. The drug has a paralyzing effect on the central nervous system with paralysis of respiration. The peripheral action of the drug is to incite the smooth muscles to contract, especially promoting peristalsis of the intestine and excessive mucous secretion of the glands. Death occurs rapidly after the poison has been administered. The fatal dose has not been definitely determined.

The treatment is to evacuate the stomach as quickly as possible and wash it out with charcoal and tannic acid. Atropine or scopolamine in doses of 0.5 to 1.0 mg. may be used as a physiologic antidote.

The necropsies on physostigmine poisoning show congestion and reddening of the mucous membrane of tongue, throat and stomach, edema of the lungs, narrowing of the large intestine, hyperemia of the brain and subpleural petechial hemorrhages. The findings are not characteristic as a rule.

Stomach contents, brain and parenchymatous viscera are saved for chemical analysis. Physostigmine is excreted fairly rapidly in the urine, bile and other secretions. It is distributed evenly in tissues and is not changed by decomposition.

Alkaloids of the Veratrum Species. A number of different plants of the *Veratrum* genus contain alkaloids not toxicologically important. The term veratrine is applied to a mixture of several substances which has a variable pharmacologic activity, because its composition is variable. The *Veratrum sabadilla,* or *cevadilla,* has a seed from which alkaloids, known as cevadine, vertridine, cevadilline, sabadine, sabadimine, are formed. The white hellebore, or *Veratrum album,* contains a number of alkaloids, mostly found in its root. They are jervine, pseudojervine, rubijervine, veratralbine, protoveratrine and protoveratridine. The *Veratrum viride,* or green hellebore, or Indian poke, contains the same alkaloids as the *v. album.* The fluid extract and the tincture of the root are official preparations. Most cases of poisoning by these substances are accidental.

Cevadine and protoveratrine are the poisonous principles of the various species of *Veratrum.* The alkaloids act on the central nervous system and on the nerve endings of the sensory motor and secretory nerves much like aconite. Their effects are usually manifested in about 20 minutes to 1 hour.

The symptoms are similar to aconite poisoning with tingling in the mouth, burning pain in stomach, salivation, coryza, nausea, persistent vomiting, purging, tenesmus and abdominal pain of the colicky type. The skin is reddened, with an intense itching, and shows perspiration. The pupil is dilated and there is loss of vision. There are attacks of dyspnea, with shallow, gasping respirations. The pulse becomes feeble. Death may occur in from 5 to 24 hours from a respiratory paralysis or cardiac weakness. The vomiting may be distressing, and may be a factor in causing death by circulatory collapse.

The fatal dose is difficult to ascertain, but a teaspoonful of the tincture has caused death.

The treatment is to wash out the stomach with warm water and to control vomiting by an opium preparation per rectum. Strychnine, digitalis and atropine are used to combat the respiratory paralysis.

The postmortem appearances are not characteristic. There is congestion of the stomach, the intestines and the viscera in general.

The stomach contents, brain, parenchymatous organs, kidneys and urine are used for chemical analysis.

Gelsemium and Its Alkaloids. The jasmine (*Gelsemium sempervirens*) contains poisonous alkaloids: sempervirine, gelsemidine and gelsemoidine. There is a fourth, gelsemine, which is more or less inert. These alkaloids are not official. The official preparations are the extract, fluidextract and tincture prepared from the root. Practically all the poisoning by gelsemium products is accidental, through an overdose. Cases of poisoning also are reported from eating honey from jasmine flowers.

The symptoms of gelsemium poisoning are similar to those of coniine. They are disturbance and relaxation of the eye muscles, diplopia, pupillary dilatation, loss of accommodation, dropping of the lower jaw, muscular relaxation, collapse, low temperature, quickened and then slow and shallow respirations. Death is due to depression of the respiratory center and asphyxia.

The fatal quantity is from 12 minims to 3 teaspoonfuls of the fluidextract. The symptoms begin shortly after absorption into the circulation and death occurs in from 1 to 8 hours. The postmortem appearances are not characteristic; the viscera may show congestion. The treatment is to evacuate and wash out the stomach, apply warmth to combat shock, and to use stimulation as the symptoms may require. Chemical analysis is performed on stomach contents, brain, and parenchymatous viscera.

Colchicum and Colchicine. Colchicine is the alkaloid of the meadow saffron (*Colchicum autumnale*), and occurs in the seeds and root. The extract is prepared from the root, and the fluidextract and the tincture are prepared from the seeds. The pure alkaloid colchicine is also an official U. S. Pharmacopea preparation used in the treatment of gout. There is another alkaloid in the plant, colchicein, which is not very active.

Colchicine has the formula $C_{22}H_{25}NO_6$, and is the methyl ester of colchicein. This alkaloid may occur as pale yellow scales or as a pale yellow amorphous powder which easily saponifies and turns dark on exposure to the air. Ordinarily it is odorless, but if heated gently develops an odor resembling that of hay.

Poisoning by colchicum and its derivatives has been fairly frequent. Most cases are accidental, but a few have been suicidal and homicidal. One famous case of homicidal poisoning was that committed by Catherine Wilson who killed 4 people by administering wine or brandy containing seeds of colchicum. Cases of accidental poisoning have occurred because people have eaten colchicum leaves for salad, or have taken wine of colchicum by mistake for an innocuous beverage. Children have developed toxic symptoms after eating the seeds of the plant.

The symptoms of colchicum poisoning are those of an irritant, with a burning sensation in the throat, colicky pains, thirst, nausea, vomiting, purging, anuria, hematuria, cold clammy skin and symptoms of shock. The pulse is small and irregular, the respirations are shallow and death occurs from paralysis of the respiratory center in the medulla. Examinations of the blood may reveal an initial leukopenia followed in about an hour by a leukocytosis.

The onset of the symptoms is from one to three hours or more after the poison has been ingested. The alkaloid does not cause toxic symptoms until it is oxidized to oxydicolchicine $(C_{22}H_{25}NO_6)_2O$. As its excretion from the system is slow, repeated small doses may produce a cumulative effect on the organism. Death may occur in from 7 to 31 hours or it may be delayed for several days or weeks. The lethal dose of colchicine is about 20 mg., although death has occurred from lesser amounts, such as 3 mg. The fatal dose of colchicum is harder to estimate because the preparations are not uniform in strength.

The best treatment is to wash out the stomach and the large intestine with a dilute tannic acid solution. The rest of the treatment is symptomatic.

The gastrointestinal tract at autopsy may show marked congestion and acute inflammation. The blood is thin and dark in color. The kidneys are congested and may show parenchymatous degeneration; the other organs also are congested. The postmortem signs are not particularly characteristic.

Materials which should be preserved for chemical analysis are gastric contents, intestinal contents, urine, blood, brain, liver and kidneys.

Ergot and Its Alkaloids. Ergot is the compact mycelium of the parasitic fungus of rye, *Claviceps purpurea*. It is used extensively in obstetric practice and the official preparations are the extract and the fluidextract.

A large number of constituents are contained in ergot, and among them are a number of alkaloids; ergotinine, ergotoxine, ergotamine, ergotaminine, ergonovine, ergometrinine, ergosine, ergosinine, ergocristine and ergocristinine. Of these ergotoxine, ergotamine, and ergonovine are mainly responsible for the pharmacologic action of ergot and are the alkaloids used therapeutically.

Ergotoxine and ergotamine stimulate the muscle of the uterus directly, causing intermittent contractions followed by periods of relaxation with small doses, and powerful long-continued spastic contractions when large doses are given. The pregnant and postpartum uteri contract with these alkaloids much more readily than does the nonpregnant uterus. Both ergotoxine and ergotamine produce lesions of the capillary endothelium and cause a contraction of the smaller arterioles which is usually followed by a rise in blood pressure and a slowing of the heart; as they also inactivate cholinesterase, the slowing of the heart may be partly due to an action like that of physostigmine. The absorption of these ergot alkaloids from the digestive tract is slow and there is a delay between the administration of the drug and its action on the uterine muscle. When injected into a white leghorn rooster the alkaloids by their effects on the blood vessels produce bluish discoloration of the comb and wattles, and with repeated administration the appendage may become gangrenous and drop off.

Ergonovine causes uterine contractions and vascular effects like the other alkaloids, but it acts more quickly as it is more rapidly absorbed when administered orally or by injection and the action persists for several hours after absorption. Moreover it is not as toxic as ergotoxine and ergotamine. It is used extensively in obstetric therapy and may supplant the fluidextract of ergot, inasmuch as its action is just as powerful but much more certain.

The other constituents of ergot are histamine, tyramine, glucosides, acids, coloring matter, lipoids and putrefactive bases. Tyramine increases the blood pressure and slightly stimulates the uterine muscle. Histamine has a tendency to lower the blood pressure and to stimulate the uterine muscle. The pharmacologic effect of these constituents is less important than that of the alkaloids.

Most ergot poisonings are accidental and are due to taking an overdose of the drug internally or to eating a large amount of bread made from infected rye. Some have occurred from ingestion of a large quantity of an ergot preparation as an abortifacient. An excessive dose of the drug if administered to a pregnant woman will cause severe uterine contractions, abortion and profuse hemorrhage which may be fatal.

The symptoms of acute poisoning set in a few hours after the administration of the drug, with vomiting, thirst, burning pains in the abdomen, diarrhea, prostration and tingling of the extremities. The face and the limbs swell, abnormal sensations develop in the skin, and twitching and muscular contractions occur. After this there is a fall in temperature, with anuria, convulsions, coma, prostration and death from cardiac and respiratory paralysis, which may take place in a few hours or be delayed for a few days.

The chronic type of ergot poisoning is due to the long-continued eating of rye bread made from infected grain, or from the injudicious therapeutic administration of the alkaloids over a period of several days or more. The use of ergot derivatives is contraindicated in vascular disease, in septic conditions and in diseases of the liver, for in the presence of such lesions the blood vessels are abnormally sensitive to ergotamine. Vasoconstriction develops and is followed by lesions of the intima and thromboses of the smaller arteries; dry gangrene of the extremities may result, cataracts of the eyes may form and occasionally gangrene of the internal viscera may occur. Anginal pains, irregularity of heart action and disturbances of the blood pressure have been described. Other toxic manifestations have been described: gastrointestinal symptoms which include nausea, vomiting, diarrhea and weakness; cutaneous signs such as formication, itching and coldness of the skin; signs referable to the central nervous system such as drowsiness, mental confusion, convulsions, paralyses, tabetic phenomena and a persistent contraction of the pupil.

The fatal dose of ergot is difficult to ascertain, because the crude drug and its preparations vary so much in strength. A repeated administration of small doses is more likely to produce toxic effects than the absorption of one large dose. The fatal quantity in one case was 12 grains and in another was 30 grains, but in one instance, recovery followed after 150 grains were taken. The treatment of acute ergot poisoning is to wash out the stomach and evacuate the bowels by enemas and purgatives. Stimulants such as strychnine, coffee and others are recommended to combat collapse. Gangrene is treated by the usual procedures.

The postmortem lesions of ergot poisoning, aside from areas of gangrene, are not characteristic. Gastrointestinal inflammation and general visceral congestion occur in many cases. If fragments of the fungus are found in the stomach, they can be extracted for chemical analysis by chloroform in acid solution; failing that, the finely divided organs may be extracted in the same way. When the residue is obtained, it is tested by reactions which identify the combined ergot alkaloids.

Cinchona and Quinine. The bark of trees belonging to the rubiaceous genera, most notably *Cinchona* and *Remijia,* are the chief source of quinine and the other cinchona alkaloids. These trees were originally natives of the eastern slopes of the Andes mountains, but have also been successfully cultivated in Java, where the bark of a species, the *Cinchona ledgeriana,* has been the chief source of these drugs. More than 20 alkaloids are present in cinchona bark, but the two sets of isomers, quinine and quinidine, and cinchonidine and cinchonine are the principal ones.

Quinine is a white odorless crystalline substance, with an extremely bitter taste. Ten salts of this alkaloid are official, but the dihydrochloride and the bisulfate are the most commonly used because they are the most soluble. Quinine has not been synthesized, and can only be obtained from natural sources. New compounds, however, which are therapeutically valuable are formed in the laboratory in an attempt to produce drugs like quinine.

The action of quinine is that of a protoplasmic poison, and it is this property which determines the toxic action of the drug on the body and its efficiency as a destroyer of microorganisms. Its principal use is in the treatment of malaria for it successfully combats the invasion of the plasmodia, even though the way in which it eliminates these organisms is not fully understood. It does not destroy the plasmodia purely by its toxic powers because it has been proved that the highest concentration of quinine in the body compatible with the safety of the patient is not sufficient to kill the malarial organism in vitro. Goodman and Gilman have suggested that quinine may destroy some of the parasites, but may in some way stimulate the antibodies and the phagocytes to greater activity whereby the parasites are eliminated in greater numbers. The asexual stage of the malarial organism is successfully attacked by quinine, but it has only a limited efficiency against the gametocytes of the aestivo-autumnal type. Quinine can be used more efficiently when combined with the synthetic alkaloids plasmochin and atabrine which supplement its action. A dose of 1 gm. a day for five to seven days is considered sufficient to control a tertian or quartan infection, while from 1 to 2 gm. a day is considered necessary for an aestivo-autumnal infection.

The local effect of quinine on the body is that of an irritant, as it first causes pain and then anesthesia, followed by a reactive inflammation and fibrosis. If it is ingested in sufficient quantity it may produce an inflammation of the gastrointestinal tract. If it is injected subcutaneously or intramuscularly it may produce an abscess at the site of injection. One of the preparations, quinine and urea hydrochloride, has been employed as a local anesthetic, and has been injected into the site of varicose veins in order to produce sclerosis in and around the dilated blood vessels.

When the drug is absorbed it first stimulates and then depresses the central nervous system, causes spasms and rigor of the skeletal muscles, stimulates contractions in the uterine muscle and some of the other smooth muscles, and occasionally produces hemolysis and destruction of leukocytes. The mechanism of this last action is not clear as quinine in vitro at about usual therapeutic concentration has little effect on blood cells, and in the human body probably causes red blood cell and white blood cell destruction through factors not well understood. The absorption of the drug from the small intestine is rapid, but after absorption it is destroyed readily by the liver and to a lesser extent by the kidneys and muscles. About one third of the absorbed quinine appears in the urine, and lesser amounts appear in the bile, gastric juice, feces and saliva. Most of the drug is eliminated from the body in less than 24 hours, though traces of it persist longer.

Most cases of quinine poisoning are accidental, and occasionally occur when an overdose of the drug is taken by a mistake on the part of the patient. In the reports of the Office of the Chief Medical Examiner, four accidental cases of quinine poisoning occurred between the years 1918 and 1941. In one instance, an individual ate a box of chocolate pastilles containing a large quantity of quinine, under the impression that they were candy, and died soon after of acute poisoning. Sometimes a person develops toxic symptoms because he has an idiosyncrasy for the drug. In a few cases quinine has been ingested for suicidal purposes, or as an abortifacient.

When a large amount of quinine is ingested, the symptoms come on in from 15 to 30 minutes with headache, fever and vomiting, ringing in the ears, flashes of light before the eyes, contraction of the visual field, pain in the epigastrium and mental confusion; finally there is a fall of body temperature, cold clammy skin, lowering of the blood pressure, slowing of the pulse and respiration, marked cyanosis and loss of consciousness. Death takes place in from two to four hours because of the depressing action of the drug on the central nervous system. In some cases death may not occur for a few days.

Occasionally when the patient takes small doses of quinine over a long period of time, a subacute or chronic type of poisoning is produced. In some of these cases the patient is abnormally susceptible to the action of the drug. The chief manifestations are narrowing of the field of vision, ringing in the ears, insomnia and skin eruptions of various types. In some cases there may be a destructive action on the red blood cells with hematuria and hemoglobinuria so that the color of the urine varies from red to reddish brown.

The quinine may cause a degeneration of the retinal cells which may develop into an optic atrophy in severe cases. Some cases may recover with residual auditory and ophthalmic damage. Quinine therapy is contraindicated in individuals who are susceptible to its toxic action, in those who have optic neuritis, in pregnant women who are near the moment of delivery for fear of inducing uterine contractions and abortion, and in persons who are suffering from auricular fibrillation.

The fatal dose of quinine varies from 15 grains in adults to much less in children or susceptible individuals. The treatment for acute poisoning is to wash out the stomach, or empty the stomach by an emetic, and to combat collapse by the appropriate stimulation.

The chief postmortem lesions are a dusky skin lividity due to methemoglobin formation, rather dark blood, congestion of the organs, and, occasionally, collections of blood pigment in the tubules of the kidney similar to a hemoglobinuric nephrosis. The urine may be colored red because of the blood pigment present. The skin may show variable skin eruptions such as purpura and scarlatiniform rashes. The toxicologic examination is conducted on such materials as stomach contents, urine, liver, kidneys and brain.

Quinidine is one of the cinchona alkaloids which is dextrorotary, and is considered to be less toxic to protoplasm and less effective against malaria than quinine. It has been used to restore normal cardiac rhythm in cases of auricular fibrillation. In susceptible individuals quinidine may produce symptoms similar to those of quinine, such as nausea, vomiting, convulsions, palpitation, headache, faintness and flushing. In one case quinidine produced a thrombopenic purpura characterized by bleeding from the gums, petechiae in the conjunctivae and small hemorrhages over the trunk and extremities.

Plasmochin is a synthetic alkaloid derived from the quinoline nucleus, and its hydrochloride, a tasteless white powder, is used therapeutically. It is toxic to the gametocytes of all the plasmodia, and attacks all the asexual forms except those of the aestivo-autumnal variety. It is most valuable therapeutically when it is used in conjunction with quinine in the treatment of malaria. It is excreted slowly from the system, and is destroyed in a variable fashion in the body. A cumulative toxicity may develop if the drug is given over a long period of time. Its toxic manifestations are similar to those of quinine, but plasmochin has a propensity to cause methemoglobinemia, destruction of the red blood cells, cyanosis, hemoglobinuria and jaundice. In the fatal cases, central necrosis of the liver is a consistent lesion.

Atabrine, or quinacrine, is a synthetic alkaloid related to plasmochin, and is administered therapeutically as the dihydrochloride, a bitter yellow powder. It attacks all the plasmodia and is especially active against the asexual forms. In the treatment of a malarial case it is most efficient when combined with quinine and plasmochin. Atabrine is readily absorbed after ingestion and is slowly excreted. It has a tendency to color the urine and some of the other secretions a deep yellow, and the internal viscera and the skin are tinged a yellow color which disappears in a few days. In most cases the toxic symptoms are transitory, consisting of severe headache, mental depression, maniacal symptoms, stupor, abdominal pains and gastrointestinal disturbances. In a few instances the poisoning is fatal, with a marked exfoliative dermatitis and a chemical necrosis of the liver simulating acute yellow atrophy. Fatal cases of aplastic anemia following prolonged atabrine therapy have been reported.

Pilocarpus Jaborandi and Pilocarpine. The leaves of the *Pilocarpus jaborandi* contain two alkaloids: pilocarpine and pilocarpidine.

Poisoning by these substances is usually accidental, either because the drug has been taken by mistake or has been administered in an overdose therapeutically. Pilocarpine has been used in small doses over a long period of time for the purpose of improving the color of the hair, and sometimes causes mild toxic symptoms such as nervousness, insomnia, myosis and disturbances of visual accommodation.

The symptoms of acute poisoning are an increased salivation, lacrimation, secretion of mucus, perspiration, marked flushing of the skin, contraction of the pupil, disturbances in visual accommodation and vomiting. The action of the drug is a direct stimulation of the gland cells and the smooth muscle fibers so that the muscarinic effects of acetylcholine are produced. Later thirst, giddiness, hallucinations and convulsions occur, and in the last stages cardiac weakness, cyanosis, respiratory distress and death from collapse of the respiratory centers in the medulla. Albuminuria and other signs of renal irritation are often present. The treatment of the acute poisoning is to empty the stomach and to use atropine cautiously as a physiologic antidote.

In acute poisoning the lesions found at autopsy are those of asphyxia, cyanosis and pulmonary edema. The submaxillary and parotid glands are sometimes swollen. Death may occur at different intervals after the poison has been taken. In some instances the patient may survive the immediate effects, but dies later of a pneumonia.

Caffeine. Caffeine is one of the constituents of the coffee bean, and is present in appreciable amount in strong coffee. Poisoning by this compound is usually accidental and may occur from drinking large amounts of coffee. Caffeine is essentially a purine derivative and not properly an alkaloid, but it is usually described with the alkaloids because of its pharmacologic similarities with some of the members of that group.

Caffeine has been used in suicidal attempts and also to produce abortion. Sometimes it is taken by mouth and sometimes it is injected subcutaneously, a method which is prone to cause subcutaneous abscesses. Fatal cases have not been described in the literature because the lethal dose is large; it has been estimated at about 10 gm. Although doses over 1 gm. may produce distressing symptoms, cases of poisoning are rare.

The symptoms of acute poisoning are: burning in the throat, epigastric pain, nausea, vomiting, diarrhea, strangury, burning on urination, precordial pain, ringing in the ears, giddiness, irregular pulse and collapse. Consciousness is maintained throughout. The drug is primarily a stimulant of the central nervous system, but later a depressant. The treatment is to evacuate the stomach as soon as possible and administer such sedatives as bromides, chloral, morphine or barbiturates.

Curare. Curare is obtained from the bark and wood of plants of the *Strychnos* genus which occur in the tropics, and is used by the natives as a poison on the arrows of their blow guns. It contains an active principle, curarine, and a few other alkaloids. Curare usually acts on the body after its absorption from a wound by blocking the nicotinic action of acetylcholine on the skeletal muscles, and to a lesser extent on the autonomic ganglia by direct action on these structures. Efferent nerve impulses cannot reach the muscles, the muscles become inert and the individual is helpless and unable to move; consciousness and sensibility are retained. Death occurs from asphyxia, because the muscles of respiration are affected and breathing stops.

In recent years curare has been used in abdominal surgery conducted under general anesthesia to cause relaxation of the abdominal muscles; a few deaths have occurred in connection with its use. It has also been used in shock therapy for psychiatric patients to produce relaxation of the patient's muscles and thus mitigate some of the unpleasant features of the procedure. The drug is given intravenously in the form of d-tubocurarine chloride or purified chondodendron tomentosum extract and has a depressing effect on the muscles and on the autonomic ganglia thus tending to inhibit muscular spasm and convulsion. Unfortunately curare also has a depressing effect on the central nervous system and may cause a severe constriction of the bronchi with bilateral collapse of the lungs. A few deaths have resulted from this therapy. If the drug is ingested the harmful effects are not so likely to occur as its absorption from the digestive tract is limited, because of its alteration in the intestine.

Ephedrine. Ephedrine, C_6H_5. $CHOH.CH.NHCH_3.CH_3$, is an alkaloid found in the stems of various plants belonging to the genus *Ephedra*. Its principal salts are the hydrochloride and the sulfate which occur as white powders. These substances are used for the treatment of narcolepsy and bronchial asthma. When given in excess, nervousness, insomnia, sweating, cardiac palpitation and other toxic symptoms, similar to those produced by benzedrine, may occur.

Mescaline. Mescaline is one of four alkaloids in the cactus, *Lophophora williamsii*. This alkaloid has a depressing effect on the respiratory center, a stimulating effect on the rest of the central nervous system, a curare-like action on striated muscle and a slowing action on the heart. Repeated use of mescaline may cause auditory and visual hallucinations. Recently this alkaloid has been injected intravenously into psychopathic patients for diagnostic purposes. Deaths from such injections are rare, but may occur within a few hours with signs of cardiac collapse.

REFERENCES

Agress, C. M. Atabrine as a cause of fatal exfoliative dermatitis and hepatitis, J.A.M.A., 131:14, 1946.

Angerer, A. L., and others. Death following the use of Efocaine, J.A.M.A., 153:550, 1953.

Foregger, R. Fatalities following curare, J.A.M.A., 142:1344, 1950.

Goodman, L., and Gilman, A. The Pharmacologic Basis of Therapeutics, New York, The Macmillan Co., 1941.

Helpern, M. Epidemic of fatal estivoautumnal malaria, among drug addicts in New York City, Am. J. Surg., 26:111, 1934.

Hughes, J. D., and Clark, J. A. Stramonium poisoning, a report of two cases, J.A.M.A., 112: 2500, 1939.

Lewin, L. Gifte und Vergiftungen, Berlin, Georg Stilke, 1929.

Nudelman, P. L., and others. Thrombopenic purpura following quinidine, J.A.M.A., 137:1219, 1948.

Parmer, L. G., and Sawitsky, A. Fatal aplastic anemia following quinacrine therapy in chronic discoid lupus erythematosus, J.A.M.A., 153:1172, 1953.

Petri, E. Vergiftungen, from Henke and Lubarsch, Berlin, Julius Springer, 1930, vol. X.

Prescott, A. B., and Webster, R. W. Alkaloidal Poisons, from Peterson, Haines and Webster, Legal Medicine and Toxicology, Philadelphia, W. B. Saunders Co., 1923, vol. II, pp. 416-602.

Reports of the Office of the Chief Medical Examiner in the City of New York from 1918 to 1951.

Salan, I., and Carmichael, D. M. Hazards of curare, J.A.M.A., 138:205, 1948.

Smith, S. Forensic Medicine, London, J. and A. Churchill, Ltd., 1934.

Sollmann, T. Manual of Pharmacology, 4th ed., Philadelphia, W. B. Saunders Co., 1932.

Webster, R. W. Legal Medicine and Toxicology, Philadelphia, W. B. Saunders Co., 1930.

35

Miscellaneous Poisons

FOOD POISONING

People are poisoned occasionally by ingesting toxic substances which are present in different kinds of food. Such cases may be subdivided into illnesses or death produced by definitely noxious materials in the food, or those produced by some variety of individual hypersusceptibility to a normal constituent in the food.

Toxic Substances in Food. The definitely noxious materials in food will be discussed here under four classifications: (1) foreign inorganic or organic materials which have been introduced into foods during their preparation or preservation; (2) poisons which are present normally, or have been formed from chemical changes in the food; (3) pathogenic bacteria and parasites in food; (4) poisonous substances produced in food by bacterial activity.

1. FOREIGN MATERIALS. Poisoning from materials introduced accidentally or intentionally can be discussed briefly. Metallic salts of tin, copper or zinc have occasionally been present in canned goods because of some faulty technic during manufacture. Arsenic has been found in beer because the sulfuric acid used in brewing was not sufficiently free of that metal. Toxic symptoms have been caused by lead salts from the water in lead pipes, or have been acquired from food cooked in an utensil glazed with lead. Many preservatives, such as boric acid and its salts, or formaldehyde solutions (at one time used illegally in milk) are potential sources of poisoning, but are rarely ingested in sufficient quantity to cause serious results.

2. POISONOUS FOODS. Some animal and vegetable foods possess or develop substances which are poisonous. Thus fatal cases of oxalic acid poisoning are reported as occurring from eating rhubarb leaves. Ergot poisoning, caused by eating infected grain, has been described on page 861.

In Central America and Jamaica fatalities have been reported in children who, lured by the attractive appearance of fruit from the akee tree (*Blighia sapida Koen*), ate it raw while in an unripe or spoiled condition. The toxic principle is a glucoside or saponin which is made harmless by heating, and the cooked fruit is not poisonous. About 3 to 4 hours after eating the raw unripe product, vomiting occurs, and is followed a few hours later by cerebral vomiting, convulsions and coma; death occurs from one and a half to 12 hours after the start of the symptoms. An autopsy on a typical fatal case in Panama has been described by Kean, the principal findings being a marked fatty change in the liver and kidney tubules, congestion of the lungs and small terminal cortical and subarachnoid hemorrhages.

The habitual eating of certain types of peas in India and southern Europe produces a condition known as lathyrism in which pains in the lumbar region, girdle sensations, weakness of the legs, rolling gait, paralyses and tremors occur. The muscles of the upper part of the body do not appear to be affected. These disabilities have been ascribed to toxic compounds in the peas, among which the fruit of a weed which infests the pea crops has been mentioned by Damon as a probable cause.

Milk sickness is said to occur after drinking milk from cattle which have been feeding upon the white snake root, *Eupatorium urticaefolium*. The sick animals usually show a prodromal stage of two days, after which weakness, stiffness, a faltering gait, acetone on the breath, distended abdomen, constipation, a fetid odor and death by paralysis of the respiratory center ensue. In man there may be weakness, nausea, vomiting, low temperature, constipation and acetone, diacetic acid and beta-oxybutyric acid in the urine without glucose. Muscular paralysis is not present, nor is the central nervous system affected, except in fatal cases when death is preceded by coma. The prodromal stage is not constant, but the symptoms may come on in a few hours or after two days. The weakness may persist for a long time after recovery. There is no characteristic postmortem lesion; fatty degeneration of the liver and kidneys has been reported. The cause of the condition is not known definitely but has been attributed to some toxin in snake root, or to infection by the *Bacillus lactimorbus*.

Some bacteria which are found in milk are said to produce substances known as ptomaines, and these are reported to have caused poisoning in people ingesting the milk. While the possibility of intoxication from such a source cannot be overlooked, it is probable that most of these cases are due to infection of the person by pathogenic bacteria in the milk.

Poisoning from eating potatoes has been reported occasionally. Under certain conditions a potato which has sprouted contains a relatively large amount of a glucosidal alkaloid, solanine, which may produce toxic symptoms if it is eaten. Attacks come on a few hours after a meal with vomiting, colicky abdominal pains, diarrhea, tenesmus, suppression of urine, headache, jaundice, collapse, cold skin and coma. Deaths are rare and postmortem findings are not characteristic. The attack lasts from two to three days. The stomach contents or intestinal contents can be examined toxicologically in the fatal cases.

Fish poisoning, or ichthyotoxismus, occurs when certain fish are eaten. In some instances the flesh or other parts of the fish are toxic; some species like the tetradontidae or cluppea have toxic substances located in certain organs or over the entire body. After eating the fish, salivation, restlessness, nausea, vomiting, cyanosis, paralysis, dilatation of the pupils, dyspnea and death from paralysis of the respiratory medullary centers occur. Gastroenteritis of moderate grade is noted at autopsy. In other fish, infection with bacteria, such as the paratyphoid bacillus, may take place and give rise to symptoms when the fish is eaten.

Poisoning also occurs after eating shellfish such as crabs, shrimps, lobsters, mussels and oysters. The ingestion of some shellfish may cause nausea, vomiting, epigastric pain, tenesmus, rapid pulse, constriction of the mouth and a prickly feeling in the arms; later there is muscular weakness, dysphonia, dysphagia, a cold clammy skin, suppression of urine and death as a result of paralysis of the respiratory centers in the medulla. Ingestion of other shellfish may produce a sensation of heat and itching, a nettle rash, diffuse edema, asthma and convulsive movements of the extremities; these symptoms are allergic and may be manifestations of protein sensitivity rather than true poisoning. Cases of illness and death following the ingestion of mussels have been reported from parts of the California coast during the summer months when these molluscs feed on plankton washed ashore from the open sea. The presence of *Gonyaulax catenella* among the plankton makes the shellfish especially poisonous. Observations by Covell and Whedon and Sommer and Meyer indicate that the plankton is the source of the toxic substance in the shellfish of this geographic area.

Poisonous Mushrooms. Mushrooms are used for food frequently, and since there are large numbers of poisonous as well as edible varieties, an appreciable number of intoxications occur yearly from this source. The symptoms produced by the different fungi vary and the types of poisoning may be grouped into five categories.

Choleriform Type. Poisoning by *Amanita phalloides*. The *Amanita phalloides* is responsible for most of the cases of mushroom poisoning. This plant is quite toxic, and different writers have estimated the mortality at 41 to 75 per cent. It is especially fatal to children, and one third of a small plant has been known to cause death. The mushroom is on the average 4 to 6 inches tall and its expanded top is about 3 to 4 inches. The stalk is set in a vulva, or cup, in the ground and a small annulus or ring surrounds the stem about one inch from the cap, or pileus. On the under surface of the pileus are gills or radiating folds, and the top part of the pileus is dead white or smoke-colored with a delicate yellowish or slightly greenish tinge. The mushrooms are seen near the woods and roads during late summer and early fall. The cases of poisoning occur whenever the mushroom is gathered by mistake for an edible variety.

Symptoms start from 6 to 16 hours after a meal with acute abdominal pain, vomiting and diarrhea. The stomach contents contain pieces of fungus, food, blood and mucus. Constipation develops in some cases. Anuria has been described but, as a rule, the urine is not obviously abnormal. The patient has paroxysms of pain and vomiting, alternating with short periods of remission. After a lapse of 24 hours or thereabouts, cyanosis and cold clammy skin, especially of the extremities, supervene. The patient develops convulsions and coma and finally dies. Death occurs from the fifth to the eighth day in most cases.

On postmortem examination fatty degeneration of such internal organs as the liver, heart, kidneys, diaphragm and other voluntary muscles is encountered. The liver has an appearance not unlike that of phosphorus poisoning. The blood is fluid and postmortem clots are usually not present. Hemorrhages are noted occasionally in the submucous layer of the stomach and the intestines and in the subserous layer. Occasionally swelling and congestion of intestinal lymphoid follicles, Peyer's patches and mesenteric lymph nodes occur.

The toxic action of the fungus and its principle causes a widespread destruction of cells all over the body. The same effects also are produced in animals, though the manifestations in them are not precisely similar to those in human cases. The *Amanita phalloides* contains another toxin which hemolyzes red blood cells.

Neurotoxic Type. Poisoning by *Amanita muscaria*. This variety of *Amanita* is titled the *muscaria* because decoctions of the mushroom have been used as a fly poison. Human poisoning is fairly frequent, but death occurs only occasionally. Small quantities of the fungus produce some mental excitement and hallucinations, and the fungus has been used in beverages in certain parts of Russia to produce intoxication. Some cases of poisoning are referable to the fact that the *A. muscaria* has been mistaken for an edible mushroom, the *Amanita caesaria*.

The *muscaria* grows singly, usually in sandy soil and frequently among pine trees. It attains a fairly large size, with the usual *Amanita* cup and annular ring and with gills of pure white. The pileus has a deep yellow, orange or red cap covered by warty scales. The toxic principle of the fungus is muscarine which may be extracted from its substance by alcohol. Muscarine has a stimulating action on the gland cells and smooth muscle fibers similar to acetylcholine (see page 853).

The symptoms of *Amanita muscaria* poisoning occur in about two to six hours after the mushrooms are eaten. There is excessive salivation, lacrimation and profuse sweating, followed immediately by violent retching, vomiting and profuse diarrhea and watery stools. The patient becomes dyspneic, with rapid respiration and slow irregular pulse. Mental symptoms occur, manifested by confusion of ideas and hallucinations. The pupils are contracted but do not react to light or accommodation, a sign which is diagnostically important.

If a large amount of poison has been ingested, the irritation of the stomach may be of sufficient intensity to cause expulsion of the toxic material by vomiting. The mental symptoms come on early in intense form with delirium, convulsions, coma and finally death due to paralysis of the respiratory centers in the medulla about 48 hours after ingestion. The pathologic lesions are not striking. The heart is distended but degenerative changes are usually absent.

Gastrointestinal Type. A few varieties, the *Boletus satanas,* the *Boletus miniato-olivaceous,* the *Entoloma lividum,* the *Entoloma sinuatum,* the *Lepiota morgani,* and *Russula emetica* cause gastrointestinal signs such as thirst, vomiting, diarrhea, difficulty of speech and some ocular symptoms. The effects come on shortly after eating the mushrooms, either at once or in from two to four hours. The poisoning is not fatal in the vast majority of cases.

Anemic Type. The *Helvella esculenta,* or false morel, has a resistant hemolytic poison known as helvellic acid and, when ingested, may cause rapid jaundice and anemia, with a coffee-brown color of the blood due to methemoglobin formation. Death may occur in two to three days.

Cerebral Type. Two species of *Paneolus* contain a toxin which produces hilarity, mental confusion, dilated pupils and some cardiac depression. Gastrointestinal symptoms are absent. The cases recover in most instances.

The treatment of mushroom poisoning is to remove the fungi from the stomach as rapidly as possible by gastric lavage, and from the intestines by high enemas. In the *Amanita phalloides* type, the stomach is repeatedly washed out with dilute potassium permanganate, and after each lavage an ounce of a saturated solution of magnesium sulfate is left in the stomach. The same treatment may be applied in cases of poisoning by *Amanita muscaria,* and, in addition, atropine may be given as a physiologic antidote to muscarine.

3. PATHOGENIC BACTERIA AND PARASITES. Poisoning caused by pathogenic bacteria and animal parasites introduced into the system by food is fairly common and covers a wide range of different infections.

Protozoan and Parasitic Invaders. The protozoan and parasitic invaders will be mentioned briefly. The *Endamoeba histolytica* is carried into the gastrointestinal tract by drinking water. The different tapeworms are introduced by eating infested flesh which is not well cooked. The cysticerci and echinococci are taken in with food and other ingested material contaminated by feces from the host of the corresponding tapeworm. The same is true of intestinal infestations by other flatworms and by many of the roundworms.

An important parasite of this type is the *Trichinella spiralis* which is introduced through the medium of uncooked or poorly cooked pork. The larval forms of the worm are encysted in the meat, and after ingestion are set free in the stomach by the gastric juice. In the duodenum, these forms develop into adult males and females, sexual union follows, and the female deposits live embryos of microscopic size into the lymph spaces of the submucous layer of the intestine. From thence they reach the thoracic duct and the blood stream and are transported to the voluntary striated muscles in different parts of the body, where each embryo penetrates a muscle fiber and encysts itself. This invasion produces at first signs of gastrointestinal disturbance, followed by muscular pains, high temperature, swollen edematous features, eosinophilia and prostration which may result in death. The symptoms start usually from two to four days after ingestion of the infested pork. Not infrequently several persons are infected as a result of eating meat from the same source. At autopsy the parasites may be demonstrated by histologic examination of the muscles, though the gross appearance of the tissues is normal as a rule. During the acute stage of the invasion, there is an infiltration of polymorphonuclear leukocytes and round cells between the muscle fibers; the worms in various stages of development may be encountered inside the fibers either extended or partially coiled, sometimes flanked by giant cells derived from the cells in the muscle sheathes. At this period the myocardium is infiltrated with leukocytes and round cells but trichinae are not demonstrable here in most cases. If the patient survives the initial infection, the inflammatory reaction will disappear from the muscles, the worm will become fully coiled and will be encased in a fibrous capsule. Encysted trichinae are often discovered as accidental findings at necropsy.

Pathogenic Bacteria. Infection by pathogenic bacteria occurs frequently from the ingestion of food which contains such varied organisms as streptococci, staphylococci, tubercle bacilli, actinomyces, cholera spirilla, dysentery bacilli, typhoid bacilli, the brucelli of Malta fever and numerous others. Inflammations of the gastrointestinal tract of varying types and degrees are produced by such infective agents. However, the characteristic food poisoning infection is caused by members of the *Salmonella* genus of which the most common are *S. typhimurium, S. choleraesuis,* and *S. enteritidis.*

The sources of infection caused by members of the *Salmonella* genus are meats, frankfurters, fish, eggs, milk, milk products and vegetables, which may be contaminated in various ways. For example, the meat may have come from a diseased animal, or it may have been infected by the butcher, or by the droppings of rats and mice. Infection with these organisms may occur in cooked or canned food which was originally wholesome, the contamination occurring subsequently because of lack of cleanliness or faulty refrigeration.

Symptoms appear from 1½ to 72 hours after ingestion of the food. The average incubation period is approximately from 6 to 12 hours. The onset is sudden with chills and headache, followed by severe abdominal griping, nausea, vomiting and diarrhea. The stools are profuse, watery and foul smelling. The temperature rises to about 102° to 103° F., and prostration and collapse may occur. The severity of the clinical picture varies from mild cases showing slight malaise and diarrhea to fulminating fatal cases which die in 24 to 36 hours. The diagnosis is made by isolating the organism from the feces, urine or viscera of the patient, or from the suspected food, and identifying it by cultural characteristics and agglutination reactions. Isolated infections may occur, but the characteristic feature of food infections by the salmonella is an outbreak which involves a number of people and is referable to a definite course of infection. Such cases are reportable to the Department of Health.

The lesions noted at autopsy are gastrointestinal inflammations of varying intensity from simple congestion and swelling of the mucous membrane with petechial hemorrhages in the submucous layer to the formation of a yellowish-gray pseudomembrane on the mucosa of the small and large intestines. There are no characteristic ulcerations of Peyer's patches with enlarged spleen and lymph nodes. The kidneys and the liver usually show some parenchymatous degeneration.

4. BACTERIAL TOXINS. Another variety of food poisoning is produced by bacteria which elaborate a toxin in food before the food is ingested. The most common and the most important example of this type is poisoning induced by the *Clostridium botulinum,* a gram-positive anaerobic organism, very slightly motile and with its spores near the end. These organisms grow on vegetable and animal protein in food (usually home canned foods); whenever such food is eaten the toxin formed by the bacillus is absorbed from the intestine, affecting the central nervous system and exerting a curare-like action on the voluntary striated muscles. The toxin is highly potent, but is thermolabile and is easily destroyed by heat. After absorption the symptoms make their appearance about 48 hours after the intake of the poisonous food, but variations occur as some cases may react in about two hours and the onset in others may be delayed eight days.

After the ingestion of the poisonous substances, premonitory signs are caused by the absorption of botulinus toxin into the blood stream from the upper intestinal tract. In some cases there is a local gastroenteritis with vomiting, nausea and diarrhea. These symptoms pass and constipation may follow the diarrhea. After this, dimness of vision, paralysis of the third cranial nerve, irregularity and inequality of the pupils, diplopia, inability to accommodate, loss of the light reflex, mydriasis and blepharoptosis set in; there is no change in the retina. The patient has difficulty in talking and swallowing, as his voice has a nasal quality and he experiences a sense of constriction in the throat. There is functional involvement of the throat to such an extent that strangling spells occur whenever he attempts to swallow. Muscular weakness predominates and often there is distinct difficulty in coordinating the different muscles. Sensory functions and the mentality are not markedly involved. Sweat secretions, throat secretions and urine excretion are decreased slightly. Death is due to asphyxia from the muscular incoordination, or to the effect of the toxin on the heart. If the patient survives the immediate effects of the toxemia, he may die of a hypostatic bronchopneumonia. In the nonfatal cases, the nervous phenomena may persist for a few months before disappearing. The mortality of botulism is about 65 per cent. Deaths occur in about 3 to 9 days after eating the food.

At necropsy the organs are engorged, especially those of the central nervous system. There may be a few scattered hemorrhages in the base of the brain and in the cord. Areas of bronchopneumonia may occur in the lungs and the viscera may show some parenchymatous degeneration. There is no characteristic pathologic lesion discoverable, either on gross or on microscopic examination.

The predominant feature of the cases is their epidemic character, that is, a number of people are infected by eating poisonous food which comes from one source. The food may be olives, canned meat, fruit or vegetables usually of home preparation. Such food may be quite toxic without showing any sign of alteration in taste or appearance to arouse suspicion of its poisonous qualities.

The domesticated animals, cattle and chickens are occasionally affected by botulinus toxin. In forage poisoning from an infected silo the cattle are afflicted with typical symptoms of botulism. Chickens suffer from a fatal weakness of the muscles, termed limberneck, presumably the result of eating the larva of the green fly (*Lucilia caesar*) which is infected with the *C. botulinum.*

There are a number of strains of the *C. botulinum* which vary slightly, and are differentiated serologically. A suspected food or stool can be emulsified in saline and heated at 60° C. for one hour. It is then mixed with chopped meat medium, sealed and incubated under anaerobic precautions for about 20 days. The supernatant fluid is then removed, centrifuged and inoculated into guinea pigs, each protected by a different botulinus antitoxin. By this procedure, the pig which survives indicates the type of toxin produced in the culture. Complement fixation tests have been used and may be useful for identification of the toxin. The antitoxins made for each strain have sometimes been useful as a preventive, but not as a cure.

Hypersensitivity to Food. A number of individuals are hypersensitive to some normal constituent in a food, and react unfavorably whenever they ingest any of the material in question. Proteins in meat, fish, dairy products, eggs, vegetables or fruits may induce symptoms of nausea, vomiting, diarrhea, urticaria, coryza, sneezing and asthma in a sensitized individual quite rapidly. Fortunately these attacks are rarely fatal, though it is possible for such a result to occur.

POISONOUS PLANTS

A number of plants contain toxic substances which may inflict injury on the human organism in other ways besides ingestion. Different species of the *Rhus* genus belong to this category and they include a vine, poison ivy or *Rhus toxicodendron,* a tree, the sumac or *Rhus vernix,* and poison oak or *Rhus diversiloba.* The poisonous principles which they contain are toxicodendrols, nonvolatile irritant oils, soluble in alcohol and fats.

The mere contact of poison ivy with the skin causes a vesicular eruption over such oily areas as the face, hands and scrotum of any hypersensitive individuals who are exposed to the plant. The rash is irritating and itches considerably; it may be spread by the fingers to other portions of the skin if the patient is so ill-advised as to scratch the affected part. The treatment is to wash the inflamed skin immediately with soap and water or to apply a warm 2 per cent solution of potassium permanganate or hydrogen peroxide. Ointments and alcoholic solutions should be avoided as the toxic oil is soluble in these substances and may be spread by their use.

A few cases of poisoning have been caused by drinking tea made from the root of poison ivy in a mistaken attempt to secure immunity against the external action of the plant. This procedure has produced a skin rash with marked itching, suffusion of the eyes, pain in throat and stomach, renal irritation, albuminuria, stupor, drowsiness and delirium. The toxic substance may be isolated by extracting the suspected material with alcohol and then filtering. The filtrate is treated with an alcoholic solution of lead acetate which precipitates lead toxicodendrol. One test for toxicodendrol is to dissolve some of the ether extract in olive oil and apply it cautiously to the skin; if it is present, the skin will be inflamed. This test will not work if the person whose skin is tested happens to be immune to the toxic oil.

Plants which cause skin eruptions similar to rhus poisoning are varieties of buttercups and crowfoot (*Ranunculi*), the primrose (*Primula obconica*), rue (*Rhuta graveolens*), *Euphorbia corollata, E. marginata, E. lathyris,* arnica, *Daphne mezereum* and some species of *Cypripedium.* Magnesium sulfate on external application may relieve the itching of skin eruptions caused by these plants. If any of the plants are ingested, gastrointestinal, renal and neurogenic symptoms and signs occur like those which complicate cases of rhus poisoning.

POISONOUS ANIMALS

Many members of the animal kingdom manufacture poisons which occasionally become dangerous to man. Many jellyfish have nettle cells in their tentacles, and if these come in contact with the skin of swimmers, they cause reddened wheals with bluish-black edges, which may turn into deep wounds from necrosis of tissues. In addition to extensive skin involvement, inflammatory hemorrhagic changes in the nasal and laryngeal mucous membranes have been described. A few starfish secrete a hemolytic substance which may be toxic for humans under some conditions.

Arachnids. A number of spiders cause poisoning by their bite. The majority merely produce a local reaction with edema, suffusion of blood, inflammation and, less often, tissue destruction. Death may occur by secondary infection at the site of the bite. The general reaction depends largely upon the species of spider and the virulence of its toxin. The central nervous system, the blood vessels and blood may be affected by the poisonous secretion, and skin eruptions and hematuria may ensue. When the bite occurs on the eyelid, especially with children, it may be dangerous and even fatal. A tarantula bite on the eyelid of a child has been reported which caused death in four days as a result of a phlegmonous inflammation. An Asiatic spider belonging to the *Caracurtae* has a poisonous bite and death occurs in from one to two days with signs of jaundice, hematuria, pulmonary inflammation and motor paralysis. The *Latrodectus mactans,* or black widow, the most poisonous variety of spider in the United States, by its bite causes alarming general symptoms with dilated pupils, cyanosis, edema of the face and extremities, and neurotoxic and peritoneal signs; death occasionally occurs though the bite itself is usually small and insignificant.

Scorpions are a variety of arachnids which possess a long tail and a sting with poisonous secretion at the end of the tail. Poisoning from such a source can be serious, especially when the individual is stung by an African or Asiatic scorpion. Children are more susceptible than adults as a rule. In some cases lymphangitis and lymphadenitis develop near the wound, along with vascular lesions in different organs. The general symptoms are similar to those of strychnine poisoning with death by respiratory paralysis. In a few cases, palsies and severe leukopenia occur. At necropsy hemorrhages in the submucous layer of the mucous membranes and hemorrhagic effusions into the cavities of the body are noted.

Ticks may produce local skin lesions by their bites but rarely any general disturbances. Ticks harbor rickettsia organisms, some of which are pathogenic such as the organism causing Rocky Mountain spotted fever.

Centipedes. These arthropods are not particularly dangerous to man even in the tropics where the varieties are large. In rare instances, young children have died from the local gangrene following centipede bites.

Insects. A number of insects, such as bedbugs, ants, wasps, bees and hornets can introduce their toxic secretions into the human body by bites and stings and these lesions may be serious. Thus in one case, a wasp sting involved the base of the tongue, causing swelling and obstruction of the throat. An inflammatory edema of the wounded area almost invariably follows the injury, especially in the eyelids or in the ears and sometimes is attended by gangrene. A systemic reaction, consisting of a generalized urticaria and toxic signs of greater or lesser severity, may occur. Occasionally an ulcerative gingivitis, a hemorrhagic diathesis, and myeloblasts in the blood have been reported after the stings. The chemical nature of these poisons has not been fully determined. Some insects by their bites transmit infectious diseases to man; the louse spreads typhus fever and trench fever, the tsetse fly spreads African sleeping sickness and the mosquito transmits malaria, yellow fever, filariasis and other diseases.

INSECTICIDES. For a number of years a few chemicals have been used as insect toxicants or repellents and some of them, such as arsenic compounds, fluorides, phosphorus, naphthalene or tobacco have been the cause of fatal poisoning in humans. Their toxic properties have been described in previous chapters.

Since the end of World War II new insecticides have been developed and their uses have widened into complex ramifications. When a chemical substance has been found to be an efficient insecticide, information must be obtained about its effects on public health, farm animals, wild life, vegetation, soils, useful insects, such as bees, and similar considerations before it can be used on a large scale. The type of insect especially susceptible to the chemical must be known, and also the stage of development at which such an insect can be most efficiently attacked, whether as egg, larva or adult form. In any event the insecticide must be used at a dilute concentration when it is still toxic for insects but not for human beings or animals. The insecticide is employed as dust, powder, spray, vapor or aerosol, depending upon the problem which confronts the user.

There are three types of campaign waged against insects by the users of insecticides: (1) individual protective measures for humans and cattle, (2) premises treatment, (3) area control measures.

1. Individual protective measures refer to the application of insect repellents to the skin of human beings to ward off mosquitoes, black flies and similar pests and to the application of repellents and toxicants to clothing to counteract the infestation of lice, mites, ticks, fleas and mosquitoes. DDT and many other insecticides have been effective for this purpose.

Some insecticides have been used to control arthropod pests of cattle and other domestic animals. Sprays of DDT, benzene hexachloride, chlordane, toxaphene, methoxychlor, TDE and piperonyl butoxide with pyrethrum have been used for this purpose.

2. Premises treatment refers to the measures adopted to control the excessive propagation of insects such as mosquitoes, flies, sand flies, fleas, bedbugs, cockroaches and ants which invade dwellings. DDT has been used as a space spray and as a residual poison and has been effective. In recent years some strains of flies have developed a resistance to the toxic action of DDT, and such compounds as chlordane, methoxychlor, piperonyl butoxide plus pyrethrum.

3. Area control measures refer to the employment of sprays, and aerosols distributed from aircraft or ground equipment over an outdoor area especially around bodies of water. DDT in oil solution, TDE, benzene hexachloride, chlordane, and toxaphene are insecticides employed in this manner to keep such troublesome and dangerous arthropods as mosquitoes, black flies, chiggers and ticks under control. For a full discussion of the use of insecticides, see the reference to Knipling.

Insecticides are divided on the basis of their origin and chemical properties into (1) insecticides from vegetable sources, and (2) synthetic insecticides (see reference to Lehman).

1. Insecticides from vegetable sources are constituents of derris, pyrethrum and nicotine.

Derris. Derris is insecticidal because of its constituent rotenone. This drug is not absorbed from the skin; it is a mild irritant to the skin, the conjunctivae and the gastric mucous membrane. After absorption rotenone stimulates and then depresses the respiratory center, and it stimulates the emetic center causing vomiting. The inhalation or ingestion of finely powdered derris or rotenone may have serious consequences as these substances in this form are very toxic. Chronic experimental ingestion of rotenone or derris by animals produces necrosis of cells around the central veins and midzonal areas in the liver. The treatment of the poisoning is symptomatic.

Pyrethrum. Pyrethrum occurs as a 20 per cent extract in soy bean or sesame oil in which its active principles are pyrethrins. These substances are slightly sternutatory and have an acrid, bitter taste; they do not cause skin irritation. After absorption of pyrethrins there is hyperexcitability, incoordination and paralyses of muscles with death occurring from paralysis of the respiratory center. The drug is not especially toxic for humans; household preparations which contain about 108 mg. of pyrethrin in 100 ml. of kerosene are mostly toxic because of the kerosene.

Nicotine. For discussion of nicotine as an insecticide see page 845.

2. Synthetic insecticides include lethanes, DDT and its analogs, other chlorinated hydrocarbons, organic phosphates and insecticide activators.

Lethanes. The lethanes owe their toxicity to aliphatic cyanates and are usually dissolved in kerosene. Fatal doses cause dyspnea, cyanosis and respiratory failure. Much of the toxicity may be due to the kerosene. Death may occur in a few minutes or be delayed for 12 hours.

DDT and Its Analogs. DDT, or 4. 4'—dichloro diphenyl trichloroethane, has been used successfully as an insect destroyer because of its low toxicity for man and animals and its lethal potency against insects. It is a white crystalline, tasteless solid with an odor similar to chlorbenzene, soluble in oils and chemically stable. It may be applied over a wide terrain, either in the form of an oil solution spread by a spray, or in the form of finely divided dust mixed with talc. DDT is efficient in killing most insect pests, but is not so successful in disposing of such arachnids as ticks. As a powder applied to the human skin, DDT is innocuous but continual exposure of the skin or clothing to solutions representing 9 gm. of the substance is dangerous as absorption may take place. The fatal dose of DDT is estimated at 500 mg.

Poisoning by DDT occurs from accidental ingestion or inhalation of the insecticide during its use. In a few hours, nausea and vomiting occur followed by a feeling of apprehension, tightness of the jaws, muscular weakness and occasionally soreness of the throat; the victim recovers after a few days. Death is not common unless a large amount of the substance is taken. N. J. Smith reports a fatal case in a man, 58 years old, who ingested 120 ml. of a 5 per cent solution of DDT and survived six days; the lesions at autopsy were necroses around the central veins of the liver, parenchymatous degenerations in kidneys and other viscera and a peribronchial pneumonia. Animal experiments indicate that DDT in toxic dose acts on the central nervous system producing hyperexcitability especially cardiac, tremors, clonic and tonic convulsions precipitated by mechanical stimulation, and coma. Chronic poisoning by DDT in animals may produce necrosis of cells around the central vein in the liver, hepatic cell tumor formations and degenerative cerebellar lesions.

If DDT is swallowed, it should be removed from the stomach and intestines by appropriate methods. Oil cathartics should be avoided as the poison is soluble in oil. Phenobarbital may be used to combat convulsions.

Methoxychlor is slightly irritant to the skin and if a solution of this chemical in oil is applied to the skin in a dose of 36 gm. it may be absorbed and be dangerous to humans. The fatal dose is large and has been estimated at about a pound; fatal cases of poisoning are rare. Experimental poisoning in animals may cause atrophy of the glomeruli and kidney tubules.

TDE or dichloro diphenyl dichloroethane is slightly irritating when applied to the skin. Daily contact of oil solutions containing 6 gm. of the chemical may be harmful to humans. The fatal dose is about 10 times that of DDT. The symptom of poisoning is lethargy, the symptoms coming on in 24 hours, and death may occur 48 to 96 hours after ingestion. Central vein liver necrosis and atrophy of the adrenal cortex may be present.

Other Chlorinated Hydrocarbons. Chlordane is composed of several isomers and in pure form is irritating to the skin. In the usual insecticide dilution it is not an irritant and is capable of absorption from the skin surface. Exposure to 2.4 gm. in solution may be dangerous to humans. The fatal dose is from 6 to 60 gm. The symptoms of poisoning start in 45 minutes with irritation of the central nervous system, manifested first by convulsions and then by depression. Death occurs in from one to two days. Areas of central vein necrosis may be present in the liver.

Benzene hexachloride contains four isomers, alpha, beta, gamma and delta. Toxic effects are produced most readily if the gamma isomer is in excess of the others. The chemical is a skin irritant and if 1 gm. a day is absorbed it may be dangerous to humans. It is a marked excitant of the central nervous system and causes convulsions. The fatal dose is half an ounce of the pure drug. Symptoms occur in 30 minutes and death in 24 hours when the gamma isomer predominates, but the process is slower if the other isomers prevail. The pathologic lesions are similar to those produced by DDT. The treatment of the poisoning is also the same.

Toxaphene, a chlorinated derivative of camphene, is moderately irritating to the skin and is absorbed through it. A daily contact of 2.4 gm. is dangerous to humans. The fatal dose is 2.7 gm. Toxaphene acts like camphor causing epileptiform convulsions; the toxic symptoms occur within an hour and death in four hours. The treatment is to evacuate the poison from the stomach and give phenobarbital to control convulsions.

Organic Phosphates. Tetra ethyl pyrophosphate and parathion, the most important of this group, are very toxic, three to five times more toxic than nicotine. A daily exposure of 0.3 gm. is dangerous for humans. These compounds are not irritant and are readily absorbed from the skin surface. After absorption the toxic manifestations are the same for the two compounds in that both inhibit cholinesterase. The postganglionic cholinergic nerves which supply smooth muscles and glands are affected and the muscarinic effect is produced, resulting in lacrimation, salivation, sweating, gastrointestinal symptoms as nausea, vomiting and diarrhea, asthmatic distress from bronchiolar constriction, miosis and visual disturbances.

The organic phosphates may also affect the preganglionic and somatic motor nerves producing the nicotinic effect which is manifested by flushing of the skin, throbbing in the head, blood pressure disturbances, signs of heart block and peripherally excited muscular tremors. The acute poisoning does not cause visible pathologic changes. The cerebral cortex is not involved and any convulsions which occur are asphyxial in origin. The fatal dose is about 12 to 20 mg. Toxic effects are usually observed in 30 minutes and death 1½ to 4 hours after absorption.

The proper treatment is to remove the poison by the appropriate means from the stomach. Atropine may be given in 0.5 to 1.0 mg. dose to alleviate the muscarinic action of the organic phosphates, but it does not affect the nicotinic action of these compounds. Peripheral muscular depressants are valuable for controlling the tremors such as the parenteral administration of magnesium sulfate; here it is necessary to guard against respiratory failure by having ready a solution of calcium chloride or gluconate for intravenous injection.

Insecticide Activators. Insecticide activators are represented by N-propyl isome which is used to enhance the toxicant action of derris and piperonyl butoxide which is used to increase the potency of pyrethrum. Both of these activators are not by themselves markedly toxic except in very large dose.

Caterpillars. About the year 1790 it was claimed that small caterpillar hairs were put in drink to cause fatal poisoning. This theory cannot be dismissed summarily as improbable, but similar happenings have not been recorded in recent literature. Externally, caterpillar hair has caused urticaria, conjunctivitis and laryngopharyngitis.

Vertebrates. FISH. The poisonous varieties of fish, as far as edibility is concerned, have been described. Other fish have poison glands on the skin surface and occasionally inflict severe wounds with their spines, causing gangrenous necrosis, lymph vessel inflammation and even collapse and death. The sting ray is the most prominent member of this family of poisonous fish and is grouped among the elasmobranchii. The electric eel is a fish with a specially developed organ which can generate powerful electric charges.

AMPHIBIA. Some of the amphibia, like salamanders and toads, have glands on the skin which secrete an irritant poison. These secretions sometimes cause skin or conjunctival inflammation, but seldom produce lesions in man of serious import.

REPTILES. The heloderma, or gila monster, a large lizard native to Mexico and adjacent portions of the United States, secretes a hemolytic poison from its salivary glands. The bite is poisonous but it rarely produces symptoms of any consequence in humans.

The serpents or ophidae are an important group, for while many of them are harmless, others are quite poisonous. The difference resides in the fangs of the upper jaw, which are solid in harmless snakes, while in the deadly snakes two of the teeth in the front part of the upper jaw are hollow. These hollow teeth serve as conduits for venom which is secreted by glands near the base of the teeth. The poisonous serpents in the United States are the rattlesnake, copperhead, moccasin and coral snake. When striking, the head of the snake is thrown forward and down with the mouth open so that the upper jaw fangs are buried into the skin of man or animal, where they leave a characteristic paired set of perforations. The poison is injected into the subcutaneous tissues or into a superficial vein. The local effects are approximately the same for all species differing only in degree; there is edema and inflammation of varying severity about the teeth marks. The general symptoms depend mainly on the substances in the poison which are characteristic of the species of snake. There are two types of venom: the neurotoxic and the hemolytic.

The neurotoxic venom is encountered in *Naja tripudians,* or cobra from India. This snake is quite deadly, its glands secreting a neurotoxin which has a poisonous action like curare, in that it paralyzes the ends of the motor nerves. The principal symptom is difficulty in breathing which becomes progressively worse. The local action of the poisoning is not pronounced. The patient goes into shock, dying in from a few minutes to a few hours from paralysis of the respiratory center in the medulla.

The hemolytic venom is encountered in the snakes of the viperine type, such as the fer de lance. There is a marked lytic action on the red blood cells and the vascular endothelium, characterized by immediate swelling in the part that is bitten and extravasation of blood in the tissues. The lytic action is so great that oozing of blood occurs from mouth, conjunctivae and stomach. Blood is excreted in the urine and effusions occur in other parts of the body. Coma develops and death may take place in from 6 to 12 hours.

Most of the poisonous serpents in the United States possess both neurotoxins and hemotoxins. The rattlesnake, copperhead and moccasin have venom which is mostly hemolytic; the coral snake has a fairly powerful neurotoxin. Snake venom is a complex mixture and it is not completely known chemically. Its toxic effects are caused by such protein constituents as globulin, syntonin, seralbumin, protalbumose and heteroalbumose, according to Lewin. Petri believes that the poisonous components belong to the group of saponins.

The treatment is to remove as much as possible of the poison from the bitten part and to keep the remainder from being absorbed; the methods employed are incisions in the area of the bite, suction of blood from the wound, tourniquets applied above the wound, and injection of potassium permanganate into the wound and surrounding tissues to combat the venom. If possible, the specific antivenom for the species inflicting the bite should be injected intravenously or intramuscularly. The rest of the treatment is purely symptomatic.

BIOLOGICAL PRODUCTS

Biological products, serums, organic extracts and the like are used extensively in therapeutics at the present time. These preparations are ordinarily harmless, but may become toxic and lethal when used in cases in which the patient has a hypersensitivity to the material, whether congenital or acquired.

Hypersensitive individuals may display a distressing reaction after the injection of antitoxin or other foreign protein. In some cases, inflammation and even gangrene of the tissues is produced at the site of the injection; in other cases urticaria, colic and profuse diarrhea may develop and finally subside after an interval. The most serious complication of hypersensitivity to foreign protein is a sudden onset of shock symptoms which comes on a few minutes to hours after the injection and may result in death. The clinical signs may be manifested under several different forms: a common type is acute bronchial spasm in which the patient exhibits asthmatic wheezing, dyspnea and distension of the chest, and at autopsy shows ballooned and hyperaerated lungs. Other individuals become unconscious after the injection and show edema and swelling of the brain at necropsy. Some patients are prostrated and display a condition resembling delayed shock while at autopsy the lungs and the other viscera are found to be congested. Microscopic examination often discloses an exudation of eosinophil and other inflammatory cells into the submucous layer of the bronchioles, suggesting the hypersensitive nature of the reaction. In some instances the evidence indicates that the hypersensitivity is congenital and atopic, but in other cases the possibility that it has been acquired as a result of a previous injection of protein must be given consideration. For further discussion of this subject the reader is referred to the articles by Bullowa and Jacobi, Vance and Strassmann, and Werne and Garrow.

Examples of similar hypersensitivity to certain drugs have been discussed in the previous chapters on toxicology in connection with compounds containing organic radicals, such as arsphenamines, mercurial diuretics, sulfonamides and cocaine derivatives. Another drug which sometimes produces similar reactions is sodium morrhuate, a moderately irritant mixture containing sodium salts of the saturated and unsaturated fatty acids in cod liver oil; this is injected into varicose veins for the purpose of causing thrombosis and an obliterating sclerosis of the dilated vessels. In most instances the injection is not followed by ill effects, but a few individuals may collapse and show signs of shock with apnea, low blood pressure and coma. Death is rare and most cases recover under stimulation and artificial respiration. The authors have seen three cases which died shortly after administration of the drug, a result which is attributed in part to the action of the sodium morrhuate and in part to a natural disease process from which the deceased had been suffering. In other cases patients have been described as suffering from skin eruptions or intestinal disturbances which appeared after the treatment, indications which support the theory that the victim is hypersensitive to the drug.

Organic Drugs. Most of the organic drugs introduced during the past 15 years have the power to modify the activity of the body cells and sometimes produce beneficial results for the patient. Such power is not innocuous, however, for if the drug is given in excess or if the patient is hypersensitive to it, a distressing or a fatal complication may follow its administration. The mechanism of such untoward reactions is not completely understood at present because of the complex chemical formula of the compound and the complicated transformation which it undergoes in the body chemistry.

PENICILLIN AND RELATED ANTIBIOTIC DRUGS. Certain antibiotic drugs derived from molds or fungi are bactericidal or bacteriostatic in their action and are used therapeutically for that purpose. Penicillin is a product of a certain species of the mold *Penicillium,* grown on the proper medium and then extracted and purified. The amorphous form of penicillin occurs as sodium and calcium salts, and the crystalline form as sodium, potassium and procaine salts. The crystalline drugs may be given orally or by intramuscular or intravenous injection. Penicillin is excreted by the kidneys, 80 per cent from the tubules and 20 per cent from the glomeruli.

Streptomycin is extracted from the mold, *Streptomyceus griseus,* when grown on the proper media. The extract is purified and occurs as the sulfate, hydrochloride, trihydrochloride, calcium chloride and phosphate salts. There is also dihydrostreptomycin, another preparation derived from the mold. These drugs are administered by parenteral injection or by intravenous injection and are excreted through the glomeruli of the kidneys.

Chloramphenicol or chloromycetin is obtained from cultures of streptomyces in liquid media and is a neutral compound containing nitrogen and nonionic chlorine. The drug is administered orally and absorbed from the gastrointestinal tract or it is given by intramuscular injection.

Other antibiotic drugs related to penicillin are aureomycin, terramycin, neomycin, viomycin, tyrotricin, bacitracin and polymixin.

The toxic reactions to the antibiotic drugs may be classified as follows:

1. Allergic Manifestations. These may take the form of urticaria or angioneurotic edema and either appear promptly or two or more days after administration. In some cases mere contact of the drug with skin or mucous membranes may produce an inflammation. Injection of a solution of penicillin into the ventricles of the brain or into the cisterna magna caused convulsions and death by shock. Dermatoses of the maculopapular type, of the vesicular and bullous type, of the

erythema nodosum type and of the exfoliativa type may occur and cause death. Toxic erythema and purpuric hemorrhages have been described in the skin. In some cases the administration of the drug seems to reactivate latent fungus infections. At the site of the injection there may be an allergic inflammatory reaction which may even be necrotic or gangrenous. Deaths have been reported as the result of anaphylactoid shock, aggravation of a preexisting asthma, serum-like reactions, and a Jarisch-Herxheimer reaction with aneurysmal dilatation and bronchial occlusion. Such deaths have occurred as the result of sensitivity to penicillin, streptomycin, aureomycin and chloramphenicol.

2. Neurologic Phenomena. Streptomycin and dihydrostreptomycin may involve the otic nerve, causing vestibular dysfunction and even deafness. Such disturbances have also been reported after neomycin and viomycin administration.

3. Complicating Infections. The antibiotic drugs kill off all the bacteria in the body which are sensitive to their action but do not affect resistant organisms as *Proteus vulgaris,* some staphylococci, candidae, aspergilli, and the *Pseudomonas aeruginosa.* The resistant organisms freed of their competitors tend to increase and produce a fatal infection. If the process takes place in the intestine the results may not be serious, but in a bronchiectatic cavity or a lung abscess the spread of such organisms is disastrous. Even in the intestines strains of *Micrococcus pyogenes* var. *Aureus* which resist the antibiotic may replace the intestinal flora and produce a harmful diarrhea or a generalized infection.

4. Gastrointestinal Conditions. Sometimes after aureomycin administration a generalized gastrointestinal inflammation may occur, which is chemical in its nature, or fungal in origin, or due to lack of vitamin B. The organs involved are the tongue, pharynx, esophagus, stomach, colon and rectum. The change in the bacterial flora brings on a condition of hypovitaminosis B, resulting in a lack of folic acid, and paving the way for a growth of candidae on the mucous membrane. Sometimes the administration of terramycin in troches may produce a direct irritative action on the stomach mucous membrane.

5. Renal Complications. The renal function is sometimes disturbed by the administration of streptomycin as shown by the development of albuminuria, cylindruria, hematuria and azotemia. The disturbance may clear up, if the drug is discontinued, but if the kidney function is defective, the drug is not excreted and accumulates in the blood so that there is danger of a fatal azotemia. Bacitracin, neomycin, viomycin and polymixin are also nephrotoxic.

6. Blood Dyscrasias. After protracted administration of streptomycin or chloramphenicol, blood dyscrasias, including thrombocytopenia, granulocytopenia, pantocytopenia and aplastic anemia may appear. Some workers have thought the nitrobenzene radical in chloramphenicol to be responsible for the bone marrow depression, but, as Shoemaker points out, this theory will not account for all bone marrow dyscrasias, some of which are not connected with drugs. He believes that the antibiotics change the intestinal flora so that there is a diminished production of folic acid and other products necessary for the maturation of cells. The result is that the bone marrow fails to produce blood cells because of an intrinsic deficiency or because of an allergic suppression and the result is a fatal blood dyscrasia.

ANTICONVULSANT DRUGS. Many organic drugs if administered over a long period of time produce unfortunate reactions. Among these are the anticonvulsant preparations used for the relief of convulsions in epilepsy. Methylphenylethylhydantoin (mesantoin) has been reported as the cause of 2 fatal cases of pantocytopenia and a fatal case of bullous dermatitis. Trimethadione (tridione) has caused a fatal case of pantocytopenia. Phenacemide (phenurone) produced severe liver and kidney damage in one case and in another was the cause of a fatal aplastic anemia. There have been reports of four fatal cases of acute necrosis of the liver which followed a prolonged therapeutic administration of phethenylate sodium (thiantoin).

ANTIHISTAMINIC DRUGS. Agranulocytosis has followed the administration of antihistaminic drugs over a long period of time. The drugs were tripelennamine hydrochloride (pyribenzamine) and methaphenilene hydrochloride (diatrin hydrochloride). A fatal case of poisoning by methapyrilene hydrochloride produced marked cerebral edema and degeneration of the cells in the proximal convoluted renal tubules.

ANTABUSE. Tetraethylthiuramdisulfide (antabuse) is a drug used to sensitize a person to alcohol. If it is administered when the individual has alcohol in his system, his face feels hot and there is congestion of the surface vessels, especially in the sclera, with palpitation, dyspnea, nausea and vomiting. This reaction is due to the fact that antabuse converts the alcohol in the body to acetaldehyde in quantity sufficient to be toxic. Its use, therefore, is not devoid of danger. See reference to Jones for report of a fatal case.

AMINOPHYLLINE. Aminophylline (theophylline ethylenediamine) therapeutically dilates the finer bronchi and the coronary arteries and also acts as a diuretic. It is administered in asthmatic conditions, in coronary artery sclerosis and in renal disease. Bresnick and his collaborators report three cases of sudden death immediately following intravenous injection of aminophylline, probably the result of a too rapid injection of the drug.

ALLOXAN. Alloxan is a drug which has a specific action on the cells in the pancreatic islets and causes necrosis in those cells, thus giving rise to diabetes mellitus. It has been used to produce experimental diabetes in animals. The administration of alloxan to man in some cases has resulted in a temporary hyperglycemia, but in others has produced a true diabetes.

HORMONE EXTRACTS. Corticotropin (ACTH) and cortisone contain potent cortical adrenal hormones and have been used in the treatment of a great variety of disorders such as rheumatoid arthritis, rheumatic fever, disseminated lupus erythematosus, leukemias, ulcerative colitis and many other disease conditions. Corticotropin is given parenterally and cortisone is administered both parenterally and orally. In some cases the effects of such therapy have been beneficial, but in others, distressing side effects and complications of major or minor importance have followed the use of these drugs.

The good effects and ill effects of corticotropin and cortisone are caused by the potent cortical hormones which they contain. In physiologic amounts these hormones keep the salt and water in the tissues in balance, but in excess they cause a disturbance in the hemodynamics and kidney function of the organism resulting in retention of both salt and water in the tissues, followed by edema.

Under normal conditions the cortical hormones keep the metabolism of protein and carbohydrates working smoothly. If there is an excess of the hormones, an increased catabolism of protein is produced and an increased excretion of nitrogen from the system. Glycogen is deposited in the liver in large quantities. The utilization of carbohydrate is impaired and a glycosuria may result which in most cases is temporary, but may be permanent if the patient has a latent diabetes mellitus.

The cortical hormones cause a diminution of lymphocytes in the blood and an involution of lymphoid tissue in the body. Their physiologic action is to increase the resistance of the organism to stresses and noxious influences of all sorts. When they have induced a state of hyperadrenalism in the body, however, they may cause a decrease in the reactivity of the connective tissues to trauma so that healing is slow. There is also evidence that in some allergic conditions these hormones, especially cortisone, may have a definite effect on immune mechanisms.

Steinbrocker and his collaborators have reported the side effects and complications following the use of corticotropin and cortisone on their 128 cases of arthritis and locomotor disorders. This list gives an accurate impression of the harmful reactions of these drugs.

The metabolic disorders included glycosuria, 18 cases; peripheral edema, 16 cases; rounding of face and body, 12 cases.

There were 30 cases of hirsutism and various skin eruptions and other skin lesions.

There were menstrual disorders in 4 cases.

Gastrointestinal lesions comprised abdominal cramps (ACTH), 2; constipation, 4; perforation of duodenal ulcer, 1; unclassified, 2.

There were psychic abnormalities in 25 cases.

Cardiovascular conditions numbered 16 cases, mostly manifestations of cardiac insufficiency, except for 7 cases of thrombophlebitis.

There were neuropathic conditions in 6 cases.

Skeletal disorders due to osteoporosis, 2 cases.

In a few cases a patient may be allergic to corticotropin and develop alarming symptoms and signs after injection such as generalized urticaria, angioneurotic edema, probable edema of the larynx, signs of asthma and profound shock. In a case of this type reported by Feinberg and others the victim recovered after an injection of epinephrin and other appropriate measures.

Cortisone administered over a long period of time may cause atrophy of the adrenal glands which in turn is followed by a diminution of the body's capacity to meet trauma and stress. Fraser and others report the case of a man, 34 years old, who received a prolonged course of cortisone therapy for rheumatoid arthritis, and died at the end of a cup arthroplasty on the right hip from immediate postoperative shock. The autopsy disclosed a marked atrophy of both adrenals. The authors of this report are of the opinion that the adrenal atrophy meant adrenal insufficiency and a lessened ability to counteract trauma.

ANTICOAGULANT DRUGS. Dicumarol, or 3,3'-methylene bis (4-hydroxycoumarin), a compound originally discovered in spoiled sweet clover but now synthetically manufactured, is administered orally for the purpose of hindering thrombus formation. According to Barker the drug causes deficiency of prothrombin, slows up clot retraction, speeds the sedimentation rate of the red blood cells and interferes with the adhesiveness of the thrombocytes, so that thrombosis and normal clotting are inhibited. If the drug is given in excess, widespread hemorrhages and purpuric eruptions may occur; its administration in cases of renal or hepatic insufficiency, in any hemorrhagic disease, or in a surgical operation with big open wounds, is definitely contraindicated because of its tendency to cause bleeding. Lederer and Splevin have reported a case in a 79 year old woman who was given 100 mg. of dicumarol daily for 21 days because of a thrombosis of the right retinal vein.

Clinically her prothrombin and coagulation times were delayed, and bleeding from the gums and hematuria were noted. She finally died as the result of cardiovascular disease. At autopsy, in addition to chronic pathologic changes in heart and kidneys, there were subcutaneous hemorrhages over shoulders, hips and legs, retroperitoneal hemorrhages in left lower abdomen, subdural and subarachnoid hemorrhages and submucous ecchymoses in kidney pelvis and bladder.

Bacterial Cultures, Toxins and Viruses. Bacterial cultures, bacterial toxins and viruses have played the role of lethal poisons. A culture of plague bacilli was employed as a means of homicide in India. Klinger and Lauer report the case of a physician who attempted suicide secretly by injecting himself subcutaneously with tetanus toxin, but was revived by the administration of antitoxin when the nature of his ailment was revealed by clinical signs. The use of whole blood and plasma transfusions has caused an acute hepatitis with jaundice, post-transfusion hepatitis, ascribable to a virus present in the injected material (see list of references). Human cases of rabies occur when a victim has been bitten by a rabid dog or other rabid animal. After an incubation period of from 2 to 22 weeks, the patient develops a condition of excitability, restlessness amounting to mania, fever, convulsions and coma. Death occurs in a few days after the onset of symptoms. The cortical cells in Ammon's horn or in the cerebellum of a victim may contain characteristic inclusion bodies, known as Negri bodies, which are diagnostic of rabies. They are stained red and blue by a fuchsin-methylene blue mixture.

Glandular Extracts. Glandular extracts, like pituitrin, adrenalin, thyroxin and insulin, are often used in therapeutics and occasionally produce deleterious effects. For the most part, severe symptoms occur in susceptible individuals and minor inflammatory reactions are caused at the site of the injection, or elsewhere in the body. An overdose of pituitrin is reported to have produced a symmetric gangrene in the hands and feet of an infant as a result of its intense vascular constrictive action. In susceptible persons adrenalin has caused severe inflammatory lesions around the site of injection, but its general action which depends on vascular constriction and high blood pressure, produces few or indefinite toxic signs in humans.

Thyroxin has caused urticarial-like eruptions with amblyopia and lens turbidity in a few cases. Thiourea (NH_2C S NH_2) and its derivative 2-thiouracil are used in the treatment of hyperthyroidism, because they inhibit hormone production and produce hyperplasia of the thyroid gland. Thiouracil sometimes causes a fatal agranulocytosis, a granulocytopenia, drug fever, dermatitis, arthritis, arthralgia, swelling of the submaxillary glands, and toxic and obstructive jaundice with a marked cellular infiltration around the portal spaces and bile plugs in the biliary canaliculae. Methimazole, a related compound, is reported as having produced a fatal agranulocytosis.

Insulin, a derivative of the pancreatic gland, is used in the treatment of diabetes. If the administration of the drug is well controlled, the therapeutic employment of it is safe, but occasionally it is given in excess, causing a hypoglycemic state from which the patient may die; this condition is known as insulin shock. At necropsy small hemorrhages have been described in the subarachnoid space, and in the stomach and kidneys. Blood sugar determinations performed post mortem may be of value in ruling out insulin shock if a normal glucose value is demonstrated; its absence, however, is not positive proof of insulin poisoning. The findings in insulin death are not characteristic.

GROUND GLASS

The ingestion of finely ground glass does not cause poisoning, as the damage inflicted by the particles is mechanical and not chemical. A certain amount of enteritis is produced by the ingestion of the material, and is referable to minute and multiple small cuts on the mucous membrane of the pharynx, stomach and intestines.

On the other hand, larger particles with sharp edges may inflict considerable damage. A severe gastroenteritis is noted at autopsy, attended by some hemorrhage and mucus. Occasionally the stomach, esophagus and intestines are perforated and septic infection in mediastinum, peritoneum and chest may occur. Ground glass has been taken intentionally as a stunt by side show performers, and also for suicidal purposes; it has been administered for the purposes of homicide.

ASPIRATED OILS

The repeated aspiration into the lungs of oily substances like cod liver oil and mineral oil, if continued for any length of time, may result in the development of a characteristic pulmonary inflammation which may eventually cause death. Graef has been able to detect considerable quantities of the offending oil in the inflamed portions of the lungs of fatal cases. Aspiration of oil occurs frequently, especially in weak infants and in elderly paralyzed persons with a diminished gag reflex. The condition is apt to follow the careless or forced feeding of cod liver oil or the injudicious use of medications like nasal drops and sprays containing mineral oil as a base.

REFERENCES

FOOD POISONING

Dack, G. M.   Food Poisoning, Chicago, University of Chicago Press, 1949.
Damon, S. R.   Food Infections and Food Intoxications, Baltimore, Williams & Wilkins Co., 1930.
Kean, B. H.   Death due to akee poisoning in Panama, Am. J. Trop. Med., 23:339, 1943.
Lewin, L.   Gifte und Vergiftungen, Berlin, Georg Stilke, 1929.
Petri, E.   Vergiftungen, from Henke and Lubarsch, Berlin, Julius Springer, 1930, vol. X.
Rosenau, M. J.   Food Poisoning, from Cecil's Textbook of Medicine, Philadelphia, W. B. Saunders Co., 1933, pp. 585-596.

HYPERSENSITIVITY

Bullowa, J. G. M., and Jacobi, M.   Fatal human anaphylactic shock, Arch. Int. Med., 46:306, 1930.
Dobson, L.   Sodium morrhuate reactions, Ann. Surg., 111:645, 1940.
New and Nonofficial Remedies. Chicago, American Medical Association, 1945.
Staff Meetings of the Mayo Clinic. Sensitivity of sodium morrhuate and monoethanolamine oleate (monolate): report of a case, pp. 436-440, July 10, 1940.
Vance, B. M., and Strassmann, G.   Sudden death following injection of foreign protein, Arch. Path., 34:849, 1942.
Werne, J., and Garrow, I.   Fatal anaphylactic shock, J.A.M.A., 131:730, 1946.

POISONOUS ANIMALS

Covell, W. P., and Whedon, W. F.   Effects of the paralytic shell fish poison on nerve cells, Arch. Path., 24:411, 1937.
Ditmars, R. L.   Snake Venom Poisoning, from Cecil's Textbook of Medicine, Philadelphia, W. B. Saunders Co., 1933, pp. 596-599.
Sommer, H., and Meyer, K. F.   Paralytic shell fish poisoning, Arch. Path., 24:560, 1937.

INSECTICIDES

Council on Pharmacy and Chemistry.   Health hazards of electric vaporizing devices for insecticides, J.A.M.A., 149:367, 1952.
—————— Pharmacologic properties of toxaphene, J.A.M.A., 149:1135, 1952.

Council on Pharmacy and Chemistry.   Toxic effects of technical benzene hexachloride and its
    principal isomers, J.A.M.A., 147:571, 1951.
Haller, H. L.   Chemical aspects of some of the newer insecticides, Bull. New York Acad. Med.,
    25:374, 1949.
Hill, K. R., and Robinson, G.   A fatal case of DDT poisoning in a child, Brit. M. J., 2:845,
    1945.
Hill, W. R., and Damiani, C. R.   Death following exposure to DDT, New England J. Med.,
    235:897, 1946.
Klendshoj, N. C., and others.   Poisoning from tetraethylpyrophosphate TEPP, J.A.M.A., 149:
    1015, 1952.
Knipling, E. F.   Recent advances in medical and veterinary entomology, Bull. New York Acad.
    Med., 25:388, 1949.
Lehman, A. J.   The major toxic action of insecticides, Bull. New York Acad. Med., 25:382,
    1949.
—· — The toxicology of the newer agricultural chemicals, Bull. A. Food and Drug Officials,
    12:82, 1948.
Mackerras, I. M., and West, R. F. K.   DDT poisoning in man, M. J. Australia, 1:400, 1946.
Smith, M. I.   Accidental ingestion of DDT, J.A.M.A., 131:519, 1946.
Smith, N. J.   Death following accidental ingestion of DDT, J.A.M.A., 136:469, 1948.
Stone, W. S.   The role of DDT in controlling insect-borne diseases in man, J.A.M.A., 1946.
Pratt-Thomas, H. R., and Waring, J. I.   DDT poisoning, J.A.M.A., 131:1384, 1946.

ORGANIC DRUGS

Barker, N. W.   Anticoagulant Therapy, from Modern Concepts of Cardiovascular Disease,
    1946, vol. XV, No. 11.
Blanton, W. B., and Owens, M. E. B., Jr.   Granulocytopenia due probably to pyribenzamine,
    J.A.M.A., 134:454, 1947.
Bresnick, E., and others.   Fatal reactions to the intravenous administration of aminophylline,
    J.A.M.A., 136:397, 1948.
Brunschwig, A., and others.   Alloxan in the treatment of insulin producing islet cell carcinoma
    of the pancreas, J.A.M.A., 124:212, 1944.
Butscher, W. C., and Gallager, H. S.   Fatal hepatic necrosis occurring during therapy with
    phethenylate sodium, J.A.M.A.,148:535, 1952.
Conn, J. W.   In discussion on Bailey, C. G., Bailey, O. T., and Leech, R. Alloxan diabetes,
    Proc. Am. Diabetes A. (1946), 6:375-393, 1947.
Drake, T. G.   Agranulocytosis during therapy with the antihistaminic agent methaphenilene
    hydrochloride (diatrine hydrochloride), J.A.M.A., 142:477, 1950.
Editorial.   Diabetes due to alloxan, J.A.M.A., 138:891, 1948.
Flaxman, N.   Drug fatalities, J.A.M.A., 147:377, 1951.
Gargill, S. L., and Lesses, M. F.   Toxic reactions to thiouracil, J.A.M.A., 127:890, 1945.
Hilker, A. W.   Agranulocytosis from tripelennamine (pyribenzamine) hydrochloride, J.A.M.A.,
    143:741, 1950.
Jones, R. O.   Death following ingestion of alcohol in antabuse treated patient, Canad. M.A.J.,
    60:609, 1949.
Lederer, M., and Shevlin, E. L.   Postmortem findings after dicumarol therapy, Proc. New York
    Path. Soc., April 22, 1943.
Martland, H. S., Jr., and Guck, J. K.   Agranulocytosis after antihistamine therapy, J.A.M.A.,
    143:742, 1950.
Pryles, C. V., and others.   Acute hepatic necrosis and death occurring during phethenylate
    sodium therapy, J.A.M.A., 148:536, 1952.
Rives, H. F., and others.   A fatal reaction to methapyrilene (thenylene), J.A.M.A., 140:1022,
    1949.
Ruskin, D. B.   Fulminating dermatitis bullosa medicamentosa due to mesantoin, J.A.M.A.,
    137:1031, 1948.
Specht, N. W., and Boehme, E. J.   Death due to agranulocytosis induced by methimazole
    therapy, J.A.M.A., 149:1010, 1952.
Strecker, E. A., and Lathbury, V. T.   Tetraethyl thiuramdisulfide (antabuse) therapy, J.A.M.A.,
    148:463, 1952.

ANTIBIOTICS

Abbott, J. D., and others.   Pulmonary aspergillosis following post-influenzal bronchopneu-
    monia treated with antibiotics, Brit. M. J., 1:523, 1952.
Allison, S. T., and others.   Dihydrostreptomycin in the treatment of pulmonary tuberculosis,
    New England, M. J., 241-52, 1949.

References   887

Anderson, O. E.   Laryngeal obstruction due to antibiotic therapy, Arch. Otolaryng., 54:34, 1951.

Berne, R. M.   An unusual sensitivity reaction to penicillin, New England J. Med., 242:814, 1950.

Brown, R. L.   The gastro-intestinal tract and stool following aureomycin therapy, Internat. Rec. Med., 165:100, 1952.

Burleson, R. J.   Anaphylactoid shock due to penicillin, J.A.M.A., 142:562, 1950.

Claudon, D. B., and Holbrook, A. A.   Fatal aplastic anemia associated with chloramphenicol therapy, J.A.M.A., 149:912, 1952.

Crooks, H. M., Jr.   Chemistry of chloromycetin, Bull. New York Acad. Med., 25:794, 1949.

Curfey, T. J.   Report of two anaphylactoid deaths with autopsy in asthmatics treated with penicillin, Proc. Acad. Forensic Sc., 1952.

Diefenbach, W. C. L.   Fatal Jarisch-Herxheimer reaction with sudden aneurysmal dilatation and complete bronchial occlusion following penicillin therapy, New England J. Med., 241:95, 1949.

Duncan, G. G., and others.   Neomycin, J.A.M.A., 145:75, 1951.

Editorial.   Viomycin, J.A.M.A., 145:1138, 1951.

Farrington, J., and others.   Untoward reactions and cutaneous testing in penicillin therapy, South. M. J., 41:614, 1948.

Felder, S. L., and Felder, L.   Unusual reaction to penicillin, J.A.M.A., 143:361, 1950.

Flaxman, N.   Drug fatalities, J.A.M.A., 147:377, 1951.

Freeman, H. E.   Pigmented hairy tongue accompanying antibiotherapy, Arch. Dermat. & Syph., 65:99, 1952.

Geiger, A. J., and others.   Mycotic endocarditis and meningitis, Yale J. Biol. & Med., 18:259, 1945.

Gittell, G.   Unusual reaction to aureomycin, J.A.M.A., 147:1141, 1951.

Huber, T. E.   Exfoliative dermatitis due to penicillin and streptomycin, Mil. Surgeon, 105:4, 1949.

Hunnicutt, T., and others.   Fatal toxic encephalopathy apparently caused by streptomycin, J.A.M.A., 137:599, 1948.

Jackson, G. G., and others.   Terramycin therapy of pneumonia, Ann. Int. Med., 35:1175, 1951.

Kutscher, A. H.   Reactions following use of terramycin troches, J. Allergy, 23:177, 1952.

——— Oral manifestations of toxicity following antibacterial therapy, New York State Dental J., 17:261, 1951.

Langdon, E.   Exfoliative dermatitis following administration of penicillin, United States Armed Forces M. J., 1:210, 1950.

Lapin, J. H., and Mond, I.   Serum sickness-like syndrome from penicillin, Am. J. Dis. Child., 82:335, 1951.

Leibowitz, H., and Schwartz, E.   An unusual allergic reaction to penicillin, Ann. Allergy, 8:668, 1950.

Mayer, P. S., and others.   Penicillin anaphylaxis, J.A.M.A., 151:351, 1953.

McDermott, W.   Toxicity of streptomycin, Am. J. Med., 2:491, 1947.

Morginson, W. J.   Toxic reactions accompanying penicillin therapy, J.A.M.A., 132:915, 1946.

Patterson, D. B.   Anaphylactic shock from chloromycetin, Northwest M., 49:352, 1950.

Rabinovich, J., and Snitkoff, M. C.   Acute exfoliative dermatitis and death following penicillin therapy, J.A.M.A., 138:946, 1948.

Rich, M. L., and others.   A fatal case of aplastic anemia following chloramphenicol therapy, Ann. Int. Med., 33:1459, 1950.

Sachs, H. J.   Giant urticaria reaction due to chloromycetin, Ann. West. Med. & Surg., 43:249, 1949.

Shoemaker, H. A.   Untoward reactions to antibiotics, Proc. Am. Acad. Forensic Sc., 1953.

Spink, W. W.   Clinical and biological significance of penicillin resistant staphylococci, J. Lab. & Clin. Med., 37:278, 1951.

Thompsett, R., and McDermott, W.   Recent advances in streptomycin therapy, Am. J. Med., 7:371, 1949.

Weinstein, L.   The spontaneous occurrence of new bacterial infections during course of treatment with streptomycin or penicillin, Am. J. M. Sc., 214:56, 1947.

Wolff, F. W.   Moniliasis pneumonia following aureomycin therapy, Lancet, 1:1236, 1952.

Yater, W. M.   Penicillin, in Fundamentals of Internal Medicine, 3rd ed., New York, Appleton-Century-Crofts, 1949, pp. 1300-1310.

Yow, E. M.   Development of proteus and pseudomonas infections during antibiotic therapy, J.A.M.A., 149:1184, 1952.

Zimmerman, L. E.   Candida and aspergillus endocarditis, Arch. Path., 50:591, 1950.

CORTICOTROPIN AND CORTISONE

Baehr, G., and Soffer, L. J.   Treatment of disseminated lupus erythematosus with cortisone and adenocorticotropin, Bull. New York Acad. Med., 26:229, 1950.

Bordley, J. E., and others.   Preliminary observations on the effect of adrenocorticotrophic hormone (ACTH) in allergic diseases, Bull. Johns Hopkins Hosp., 85:396, 1949.

Feinberg, S. M., and others.   Allergy to pituitary corticotrophic hormone, J.A.M.A., 147:40, 1951.

Fischel, E. E.   The relationship of adrenal cortical activity to immune responses, Bull. New York Acad. Med., 26:255, 1950.

Fraser, C. G., and others.   Adrenal atrophy and irreversible shock associated with cortisone therapy, J.A.M.A., 149:1542, 1952.

Freyberg, R. H.   Effects of cortisone and ACTH in rheumatoid arthritis, Bull. New York Acad. Med., 26:206, 1950.

McEwen, C., and others.   The effect of cortisone and ACTH on rheumatic fever, Bull. New York Acad. Med., 26:212, 1950.

Pearson, O. H., and others.   The use of ACTH and cortisone in neoplastic disease, Bull. New York Acad. Med., 26:235, 1950.

Ragan, C., and others.   The effect of ACTH and cortisone on connective tissue, Bull. New York Acad. Med., 26:251, 1950.

Russell, J. A.   Physiology of the pituitary-adrenal system, Bull. New York Acad. Med., 26:240, 1950.

Steinbrocker, O., and others.   ACTH and cortisone as therapeutic agents in arthritis and some locomotor disorders, Bull. New York Acad. Med., 27:560, 1951.

BACTERIAL CULTURES

Blanchard, M. C., and others.   Serum hepatitis studies, J.A.M.A., 138:341, 1948.

Capps, R. B., Sborov, V., and Scheiffly, C. S.   A syringe-transmitted epidemic of infectious hepatitis, J.A.M.A., 136:819, 1948.

Grossman, E. B., Stewart, S. G., and Stokes, J., Jr.   Post transfusion hepatitis, J.A.M.A., 129:991, 1945.

Klinger, H., and Lauer, A.   Suicidversuch mit Tetanus-Toxin, Deutsche Ztschr. f. d. ges. Gerichtl. Med., 21:457, 1933.

London Letter.   Murder by plague bacillus, J.A.M.A., 106:933, 1936.

Mackenzie, G. M.   Serum Sickness, from Cecil's Textbook of Medicine, Philadelphia, W. B. Saunders Co., 1951, pp. 472-475.

Stokes, J., Jr., and others.   Serum hepatitis studies, J.A.M.A., 138:336, 1948.

GROUND GLASS

Haines, W. S.   Death from Pounded Glass, from Peterson, Haines and Webster, Legal Medicine and Toxicology, Philadelphia, W. B. Saunders Co., 1923, vol. II, pp. 888-898.

ASPIRATED OILS

Graef, I.   Pulmonary reactions to aspirated lipids, Proc. New York Path. Soc., Feb. 25, 1937.

36

Occupational Diseases and Toxicology

Most jurisdictions recognize that if a laborer suffers from a disability which is caused by his work, he should receive adequate compensation from his employer as a matter of justice. In most of the states, a special court is instituted to decide such questions; in New York State hearings are conducted before a referee of the State Workman's Compensation Board who passes on the validity of the employee's claim and makes the proper award if compensation is justified. Either the plaintiff or the defendant may appeal to a higher court against the decision of the referee, and his verdict is sustained or reversed by the higher tribunal. In most states compensation may be awarded if it can be shown that an injury incurred during work helped to shorten the worker's life, without requiring the plaintiff to prove that the trauma was the sole cause of death.

Conditions which develop as a result of occupation, and thus concern the compensation courts, may be classified as follows: (1) compensable injuries, (2) disabilities inherent in occupation, (3) occupational toxicology.

COMPENSABLE INJURIES

Many cases with a traumatic history appear before the compensation courts for appraisal. The referee must determine if sufficient evidence is present to justify the contention that the injury was inflicted while the claimant was pursuing his work, and was not received outside the sphere of his employment, for in the latter case the employer would not be liable for its consequences. If the worker incurred the injury while at work, the referee must judge concerning the effects of the trauma on the claimant and whether or not it was instrumental in causing the disability or death which ensued. Many of the cases presented to these tribunals are genuinely traumatic, as, for example, death due to a fracture of the skull and a laceration of the brain following a fall from a height; in such instances most of the questions at issue are easily decided by the referee. Other claims, however, are based on natural disease conditions whose connection with trauma is dubious, as for example, a sarcoma of the tibia which has arisen at the alleged site of a light bump on the shin. In other cases in which a natural disease process is the cause of death, the victim may also have sustained injuries of greater or lesser severity, and it is often difficult to determine the part played by the trauma. Such conditions as hernias, neoplasms, tuberculosis, diabetes, heart disease, septic infection, and thrombosis and embolism may be present in persons who have also sustained an injury, and it is not always a simple matter to evaluate the effect or the relationship of the injury to the disease process.

Inguinal hernias sometimes develop in workmen who lift heavy objects, and the question arises whether or not the lesion is a result of their occupation. The courts are prone to favor compensation for a disability of this sort, if the onset of symptoms can be shown to have followed an extraordinary muscular strain. If it can be proved that the hernia with its disability existed prior to the alleged strain,

889

especially if the employee persistently refused to submit to an operation, this fact might mitigate the liability of the employer.

The relation of malignant neoplasms to trauma has been discussed by Ewing and will be briefly mentioned here. Ewing's conclusions are, in effect, that neoplasms are autochthonous growths of tissue cells, and that traumatic influences, with certain exceptions, do not play any appreciable role in their etiology. The exceptions are such malignant tumors as may follow ingestion of radium (anaplastic sarcoma of bones) and of aniline (carcinoma of the bladder), exposure of skin to roentgen rays, dusts or vapors containing arsenic compounds and vapors from tar compounds (epitheliomas), inhalation of dusts and vapors containing arsenic or vapors and dusts containing chromates, or vapors containing tar compounds (bronchogenic carcinoma), or vapors and dusts in nickel-copper refineries (bronchogenic carcinomas or carcinoma of nasal sinuses). Long-continued chronic irritation by its action on certain of the body tissues may be one of the factors in the etiology of some neoplasms. A single physical trauma has never been convincingly shown to be the cause of a neoplasm.

Tuberculosis presents the same problem as neoplasms, in that it is a spontaneous infection caused by the tubercle bacillus, and that trauma plays a doubtful role as an etiologic factor. Conditions like silicosis or poisoning by a lethal gas like phosgene may be a predisposing influence in the progression of pulmonary tuberculosis. Physical injury probably has slight effect on the course of a tuberculous infection, though it has been claimed that it may cause localization of the disease at a certain site, or force it to disseminate through the body; these points are difficult to prove, and require the most convincing evidence.

Diabetes mellitus is a natural disease process which, in the vast majority of cases, is not related to trauma. Some individuals are potential diabetics in that they may not show any clinical manifestations of this malady but are on the threshold of developing the disease; if such persons are subjected to severe violence, the latent diabetes becomes an outspoken case and is probably precipitated by the traumatic injury. In such instances, the trauma is an aggravating factor which stirs the already existing disease condition into activity. Some injuries of the head and of the pancreas may be attended by a transitory glycosuria, but other phenomena of true diabetes mellitus are absent.

The relation of arteriosclerosis, cardiac disease, pulmonary disease, renal disease, alcoholism, embolism, thrombosis and septic infections to traumatic injuries has been discussed in Chapters 6, 7 and 8.

DISABILITIES INHERENT IN OCCUPATION

Many conditions which affect workers adversely are inherent in the environment of an occupation or industry. For example, tunnel workers are compelled to labor under high atmospheric pressure and sometimes develop caisson disease; sugar refiners and furnace workers are exposed to high temperatures and suffer from exposure to heat. These conditions are discussed in Chapter 20. Another type of occupational disability is a palsy produced by the habitual and monotonous use of the same groups of muscles in certain movements. Writer's cramp and cigar maker's cramp are examples of these affections; their medicolegal significance is slight.

Bacterial Diseases. A few bacterial diseases may result from following certain occupations. One of the most important is anthrax, caused by the *Bacillus anthracis*.

There are two industrial types of this infection, woolsorter's disease which is a pneumonia resulting from the inhalation of dust shed by infected hides, and malignant pustule caused by bringing the hide in contact with the skin. Glanders is an infection caused by the bacillus *Malleomyces mallei,* and is characterized by a generalized papular and pustular skin eruption; it is apt to attack stablemen who work around infected horses. Another pathogenic microorganism is the *Pasteurella tularensis* which may produce tularemia in butchers who handle infected wild rabbits. Laborers on tropical banana plantations often work under conditions in which they are exposed to attacks from anopheline mosquitoes and may develop aestivo-autumnal malaria of the malignant type. Pyogenic bacteria may cause sporadic septic conditions among industrial workers, but inasmuch as the infection is similar to nonindustrial varieties, and is not characteristic of any particular occupation, it is not truly occupational.

Pneumonoconiosis. The inhalation of finely divided dust particles is associated with certain occupations and if continued for a long period of time may give rise to a chronic inflammation of the lung tissue known as pneumonoconiosis, referable to the irritating physical properties of the various dusts. If enough material is aspirated, it is deposited in the lung tissues and eventually produces a chronic bronchitis, a chronic interstitial pneumonitis, and a pulmonary emphysema. The lung involvement may be severe enough to impede the flow of blood through the pulmonary vessels, which may result in secondary enlargement of the right ventricle of the heart and death from cardiac decompensation. In other instances, fatal pulmonary tuberculosis may be incited because of the irritating quality of the inhaled dust. The symptoms of pneumonoconiosis usually make their appearance after a long incubation period, sometimes a matter of years.

The different types of pneumonoconiosis are: (1) silicosis which is due to inhalation of silica dust by workers in granite quarries, anthracite coal mines, carborundum manufactories and in rock drilling. The silica particles, especially those of 0.5 to 10 microns in diameter are irritating to the lung tissue as the result of a physico-chemical reaction, and cause a widespread nodular fibrosis, often associated with a fatal pulmonary tuberculosis. (2) Chalicosis is produced by the inhalation of marble dust and is found among stone cutters. Some sufferers from this type develop a contracted chest. (3) Asbestosis is found among workers in asbestos and may produce a severe chronic fibrosis of the lungs; microscopically typical asbestos particles are found in the lung tissue. (4) Pneumonoconiosis also occurs in those who inhale metal dust (siderosis), coal dust (anthracosis), dust from dyes, and dust from vegetable material such as tobacco, cotton fibers, or bagasse. Some of these types have their own characteristic sputum, which may be colored by inhaled material; the sputum in anthracosis is black from the presence of coal dust and the sputum in that type of siderosis which accompanies mirror polishing may be red from ferric oxide. Byssinosis is the inhalation of dust thrown off by spun cotton and, as described by Bolen, workers in cotton mills inhaling such material become semi-invalids and complain of an irritating cough and a feeling of constriction in the chest. Bagassosis is caused by the inhalation of dust from bagasse, the dried stalks of sugar cane from which sugar has been extracted; workers who handle bales of this material and inhale the dust develop cough, dyspnea, rapid heart action and miliary granulomas in the lungs.

OCCUPATIONAL TOXICOLOGY

Most occupational diseases are caused by poisons which are generated as a part of the industrial process or are present as accidental by-products, among which are included heavy metals, corrosive acids, sulfur compounds, cyanogen compounds, aliphatic organic compounds, aromatic organic compounds and carbon monoxide. Many of these substances cause cases of poisoning not associated with the industrial process, but others, such as brass, manganese, carbon disulfide, nitro compounds, aniline, tetrachlorethane and amyl acetate are described as producing their toxic effects mostly in connection with manufacturing. The subject of occupational toxicology covers an extensive field and will be discussed briefly in outline. For more complete accounts, the reader is referred to the writings of Alice Hamilton and the other references at the end of this chapter.

Occupational poisons enter the body through the air passages as a result of the aspiration of noxious gases or dust, and less often from the contact of volatile liquids with the skin. Ingestion by mouth is neither frequent nor important in industrial cases, but it is not unknown, a few cases occurring from the ingestion of the poison on food or tobacco as a result of careless or untidy habits of the laborer. Contact with the skin is to be feared in the case of aromatic volatile liquids such as aniline or dinitrobenzene, especially in hot weather when perspiration is increased and the surface blood vessels are dilated. The chief hazard in a factory is inhalation of toxic substances in dust and fumes and the vast majority of cases of industrial poisoning occur as a result of entrance of the noxious substance by way of the respiratory tract.

Most cases of industrial poisoning are chronic, due to a long-continued exposure to the toxic chemical or to the delayed action of a large dose on the system. In the United States, cases of acute poisoning have occurred especially in industries using lead, arsenic, benzene or wood alcohol, as workers in these industries are unduly exposed to heavy concentrations of toxic chemicals. Occasionally cases of industrial intoxication are produced by the combination of two different toxic products and may present atypical signs. For example in the smelting of zinc, lead and arsenic compounds may be present in the ore, and if absorbed may give rise to a combination of lead and arsenic symptomatology, so that it may be difficult to determine which poison is most responsible for the deleterious effects on the worker.

Inorganic Poisons. *Lead.* Lead is considered the outstanding metallic poison encountered in industry, and produces many cases of illness and death. Mining of lead sulfide ore or galena does not result in plumbism ordinarily, but during the smelting and refining processes, dusts and fumes are evolved with the result that 18 to 23 per cent of the workers may develop lead poisoning. Melting of the metal causes volatilization of the newly formed oxide, so that solderers, lead temperers, lead burners, welders and workers who make lead objects such as pipes, wire, storage battery plates, printer's type, sheets, solder or bullets may suffer intoxication. If the contents of a lead pot, heated to 310° C., are agitated, fumes may contaminate the air and be a source of danger.

Chronic lead poisoning may even occur in individuals who handle the heavy metal or its alloys, because of the tendency of lead to form compounds when exposed to other substances. Printers are said to have acquired plumbism by contact with type containing lead, though it is possible that many of these cases were due to some other variety of metallic poisoning. Plumbers at one time complained of lead poisoning when they routinely worked with lead pipes, but as such pipes are no longer in general use, only a few sporadic cases of lead poisoning have occurred from this source in recent years. Magnuson and Raulston report cases of lead poisoning in roofers who were accustomed to hold galvanized nails in their mouths during work; the nails were coated with zinc containing an impurity of 3 per cent of lead, and enough lead was absorbed by mouth from this source to cause plumbism in victims who had been indulging in this practice for a number of years.

The basic carbonate of lead is toxic, and is the chief danger in the dust produced during the process of manufacture. It is one of the constituents of paint and is responsible for the poisoning which occurs in painters and in those who glaze pottery by flame. Red lead is used in glazes on tiles, storage battery plates, paint and enamel for sanitary ware; and litharge is used for storage battery plates, in glass compounding and in glazes. The making of storage battery plates and the enameling of sanitary ware are dangerous processes because the heat may cause some of the compounds to volatilize. Cases of plumbism also may occur in the use of powdered lead paints and in the dusting of paper with a lead compound for lithograph purposes.

The clinical picture of lead poisoning is varied, and a physician in a manufacturing plant should be alert to detect atypical forms of the disease. If a worker is known to have been exposed to lead, and develops indefinite symptoms of indigestion, abdominal distress, loss of strength, muscular pains, and vague nervous disturbances, a beginning case of industrial plumbism should be suspected and the patient treated accordingly.

Zinc. Brass poisoning, or brass founder's ague, is a syndrome produced in those who work in foundries around the molten alloy, in brazing, in smelting of zinc, and in the galvanizing or the smelting of zinc sheets. It results from the exposure to the fumes of zinc which volatilizes at 300° C. The affected workers complain of irritation in the throat, painful cough, lassitude, weariness and pain in the limbs. If the body is cooled, the victim develops a severe chill, a rise in temperature and an increase in the pulse and respiration rate; as a rule the attack does not last overnight. The nature of the syndrome is puzzling inasmuch as inhalation of zinc fumes alone produces the ague, and zinc compounds administered in other ways do not give rise to similar effects. The resemblance of the symptoms to an acute bacterial throat infection or to an allergic reaction is striking, and some believe that the irritation of the mucous membranes produces a protein compound which causes the above syndrome. Zinc is found in the urine in these cases.

Cadmium. Cadmium poisoning is caused by the inhalation of fumes which occur when cadmium compounds are heated. Ross reports a case in which a workman inhaled smoke as he flanged a cadmium-coated stainless steel pipe by heating it with a blowpipe. He complained of irritation of the nose and throat, vomiting, chest pains, shortness of breath, and finally developed a serious inflammation of the air passages, dying in a few days of pneumonia. There are also cases of chronic poisoning in which the victim inhales fumes over a long period of time and is affected with symptoms not unlike lead poisoning without the colic.

Mercury. The vapors of heated mercury which are generated in such processes as the manufacture of thermometers, gold or silver amalgam or soft solder, cause a rapid subacute toxemia in those who are exposed to them. Stomatitis, combined with tremors, psychic disturbances, loss of memory, depression, timidity, insomnia and irritability, characterize this particular type of poisoning. Any occupation in which mercury is scattered over the floor, such as the making of instruments containing the metal, exposes the workers to the same dangers, but in a less intense form. Acid nitrate of mercury which is used to mat fur into felt in the manufacture of hats, also produces a chronic mercurialism in hatters, characterized by anemia, emaciation, fine tremors of the lips, tongue, eyelids and fingers, and the mental symptoms noted above; stomatitis is not a prominent feature of this variety of mercury poisoning.

Arsenic. The compounds of arsenic used in industry are arsenic trioxide, Paris green and lead arsenate. The trioxide is a constituent of sheep dip, a preservative for hides, an ingredient for glass compounding and a component for the antifouling paint on ships. Cases of poisoning have occurred in workers who handle skins and hides, apply sheep dip, work in copper mines, smelt lead or copper ore, and labor in Paris green or lead arsenate works.

The dust or vapor containing arsenic compounds produces skin affections like scleroderma, warts or horny patches with diffuse brown pigmentation. Dust may fall on vulnerable surfaces such as edges of lips, nostrils, eyelids, and folds of skin in axilla, groin and scrotum, the pressure of the skin favoring the irritation of the dust by keeping the skin warm and moist. Some of the cutaneous lesions may develop into carcinomas. Many argue that the chimney sweep's cancer was so prevalent in England because the coal contained considerable arsenic which was given off in the smoke, thus affecting the skin of the scrotum. It is pointed out that this tumor is uncommon outside of England, where much less arsenic is present in the coal. Others, however, believe that this cancer is caused by vapors of coal tar derivatives which contain the phenanthrene nucleus.

The inhalation of arsenic compounds in dust over a period of time produces hoarseness, drying of the throat, cough, and in some instances perforation of the nasal septum. The patients also complain of colic, vomiting, loss of strength, peripheral neuritis and neuralgic pain. Later bronzing of the skin occurs in the eyelids, temples, neck, axilla, nipples, and may involve most of the body surface. In the Schneeberg region of Saxony, where cobalt arsenite is mined, carcinoma of the lung is prevalent, and this is attributed by some to the constant inhalation of dust containing this compound.

The most serious type of industrial arsenic poisoning is that caused by hydrogen arsenide or arsine. It is mostly accidental and unforeseen, because it is produced by arsenic compounds which contaminate the ores of iron, zinc, lead, copper and antimony. Some commercial sulfuric acid contains arsenic because it is made from iron pyrites in which arsenic compounds occur as impurities. If such sulfuric acid is used to make hydrochloric acid from common salt, arsenic will be transferred to the hydrochloric acid. Many industrial processes bring such acids and the heavy metals together, and when this occurs, arsenic impurities are liberated in the form of arsine; arsine fumes, when inhaled, usually produce a toxic reaction. Sometimes the true nature of the poisoning is overlooked, or attributed to such vague causes as acid fumes. In all cases of mysterious illness among workers in metals or acids, a careful search for arsine should be made. Such fumes are most likely to be given off in storage battery manufacture, in the production of hydrogen for balloons from zinc and hydrochloric acid containing arsenic, and in repairing and cleaning tanks used for that purpose. The symptoms and lesions produced by arsine poisoning have been described on page 743.

Antimony. Antimony is used in the making of printer's type and in compounding rubber, and is said by some to be the cause of nervous symptoms affecting printers, and of eczema affecting stereotypers. Others are inclined to blame these ills on arsenic which is often present as a contaminant. Antimony and its compounds are not important industrial poisons.

Other metallic compounds which cause industrial poisoning have been described in Chapter 31, and include those of beryllium, chromium, manganese, nickel, radium, thallium and vanadium. Some nonmetallic inorganic compounds also cause industrial disability, as for example, phosphorus, selenium and tellurium, and have also been described in Chapter 31.

Gaseous Poisons. Sulfuric acid and sulfur dioxide may be considered together, inasmuch as the gas SO_2 is converted to H_2SO_4 when it acts on the mucous membranes of the body, and the effect is practically the same whether the workmen breathe sulfur dioxide or a fine spray of sulfuric acid. Irritation of the eyes and respiratory passages begins at low concentrations, but in time the workers seem to establish a tolerance for the fumes. On excessive exposure, the fumes may produce a croupous inflammation of the bronchi and a lobular pneumonia. If small quantities are constantly inhaled over a long period, a chronic catarrh may result. Liquid sulfuric acid is used in a large number of processes, such as refining sugar, starch, linseed oil, in nitrate processes, and in cleaning metal, but aside from causing a few acid burns, it is not an important source of poisoning.

Dimethyl sulfate is used to produce dimethylaniline, an important compound used in dye manufacture, and is locally caustic, causing skin and conjunctival lesions and irritation of the upper air passages. In severe cases bronchopneumonia and degenerative processes in the liver and kidneys may occur. A similar compound is metol which is the trade name for monomethyl paramido metacresol sulfate; this is used by photographers and may cause a trade dermatitis, an inflammation of the eyelids and a bronchial irritation.

Nitric acid is used extensively in the manufacture of explosives, celluloid films, airplane dope and dyes, and in etching and similar processes. The poisoning usually occurs when a leak in the apparatus allows escape of the acid or of nitric oxide. The workmen do not realize their danger and inhale the fumes which cause inflammation of the nares, pharynx and larynx. If the gas reaches the finer air passages, there is marked bronchial spasm with choking, burning pain in the chest and a strangling spasmodic cough. A mild case may become severe after a few hours. Some cases may recover but show distressing aftereffects, such as dyspnea, cough, pain in the chest, gastrointestinal disturbances and nervousness.

Hydrochloric acid produces irritating fumes during its manufacture, which are caustic to the mouth and the upper air passages and may cause erosion of the teeth. Chlorine fumes are encountered in the manufacture of nitric and hydrochloric acids, in the electrolytic production of chloride of lime from common salt, in one of the methods of producing soda, in the bleaching of paper and in some of the processes of dye manufacture. Occasional cases of acute asphyxia occur from this gas, but it does not produce much industrial poisoning. Similarly phosgene is formed in the manufacture of certain dyes, and in rare instances causes acute poisoning.

The employment of cryolite in the preparation of aluminium and in the manufacture of certain artificial fabrics, or of enamel, or of some ceramic products have caused the emanation of fumes containing fluoride compounds, with the result that in some instances the chronic effects of fluoride absorption such as mottled enamel on the teeth and chronic osteomyelitis of the skeleton have resulted. Acute poisoning from such sources is rare.

Hydrocyanic acid is formed during the manufacture of Prussian blue, the burning of celluloid, in blast furnace gas, and is liberated in disinfecting processes, occasionally causing fatal accidents. Chronic poisoning from these sources is not common, but occurs when workers in galvanoplating are exposed to small amounts for a long period of time. The symptoms are headache, vertigo, pallor, loss of appetite, dyspnea and offensive breath.

Calcium cyanamide is produced at one of the stages in the fixation of atmospheric nitrogen, and is also used as a fertilizer. The powder is caustic and causes severe abscesses and even cellulitis when it falls on a sweating skin. Severe ulcers may occur on the mucous membranes of the nose, mouth and throat.

Hydrogen sulfide is a danger in certain industries which manufacture sulfur dyes, epecially browns and khakis, or sulfur monochloride or the trisulfide of barium which is a parasiticide. In sufficient quantity the gas causes a sudden acute poisoning which has been described in Chapter 19. If small amounts are inhaled continually, mental disturbances, a chronic headache, conjunctivitis, cough, pallor and furunculosis may occur.

Carbon monoxide in industry is found around blast furnaces, in flues, in the manufacture of illuminating gas and in any place where it is used for fuel. It is present in mines and in the exhaust gases from gasoline engines. Cases of acute poisoning have occurred in steel works and in mines where blasting is taking place. During the process of removing the dust from the mains of steel mills, the accumulated carbon monoxide may affect the workers who inhale it. The acute cases of industrial poisoning are usually nonlethal.

The exhaust gases from gasoline engines seem to be more toxic than illuminating gas, and may cause definite changes in the brain and cord which are said to result in mental impairment, paralysis and other sequelae. The greater toxicity of exhaust gases has been attributed to other constituents, such as benzine, which are not found in illuminating gas.

Organic Poisons. The organic industrial poisons are divided into aliphatic or open chain compounds, and aromatic or ring compounds. The aliphatic hydrocarbons are usually increased in toxicity when other radicals are joined to the chain. The aldehyde and acid groups have a tendency to make the resulting compound irritant and halogen combinations create poisons of definite virulence. The aromatic hydrocarbons are toxic in their own right and the addition of certain radicals enhances the toxicity; hydroxyl ring compounds are especially irritant and a nitro radical attached to the ring forms a virulent poison, but the halogen derivatives though harmful are not as toxic as derivatives of other radicals.

Volatile solvents are used in industry in large quantities and cause many cases of industrial poisoning. These chemicals are employed to dissolve cellulose and gums used in synthetic finishing materials, lacquers, dyes, cements, plastics, and grease and other waste products fouling containers and machinery. As the solvents are easily vaporized, most of the poisoning occurs after they have been inhaled into the air passages and lungs. Some of the vapors are fat-soluble and may be absorbed through the intact skin, often causing irritation at the point of contact. In a few instances inflammation of the conjunctivae may occur. Occasionally the poisonous substance is ingested, but then its action is less virulent as more of it undergoes detoxification by the liver.

The conditions under which volatile solvents are used may favor their inhalation. For example, when quick drying lacquers are applied to a container, the solvent vaporizes rapidly and may fill a confined space with toxic fumes. Similarly the use of a spray gun to apply the solutions may generate a poisonous concentration of the vapor, and the employment of large quantities of the solvent in large open tanks as a cleaning fluid will produce the same dangerous conditions. Acute and chronic poisoning is prone to follow inhalation of such toxic fumes.

ALIPHATIC SOLVENTS. The principal aliphatic solvents are the petroleum distillates, alcohols, carbon disulfide, esters, ketones, glycols, glycol ethers, furfural and the halogen derivatives.

The petroleum distillates are used in a number of processes, the heavier oils being employed in the preparation of bindery twine and the cleaning of printing press rollers, and the volatiles, naphtha and benzine, being used for dry cleaning, for the cleaning of tank cars, and as solvents for rubber and fats. Inhalation of the vapors first produces stimulation and inebriation which is followed by collapse and depression of the respiratory center in the medulla. Chronic exposure produces malaise, vomiting and muscular weakness, and in those places where the oil comes in contact with the skin, acute dermatitis, acne-like lesions and skin abscesses may result.

The different alcohols are used extensively as solvents. Ethyl alcohol is employed to dissolve gums, resins and other compounds, but is not markedly toxic in this role. Methyl alcohol is used in the manufacture of pyroxylin plastics, as a solvent for varnishes, and in the preparation of essences. It is toxic and produces poisoning, not so much during its manufacture, but in other processes such as the application of shellac or airplane dope. Formerly, when it was employed in the stiffening of felt hats, toxic effects were frequent, but since this process has been abandoned the number of cases has decreased. The symptoms were produced by the inhalation of fumes or absorption through the skin; blindness and death have occurred in a few instances. The incidence of poisoning has fallen when denatured alcohol is employed in its stead, but as this mixture contains a little methyl alcohol its use is not unattended by danger. Some of the alcohols of higher molecular weight are employed as solvents, such as isopropyl alcohol which is used in the preparation of perfumes and toilet articles, or butyl alcohol which is used in the manufacture of nitrocellulose lacquer. These substances are quite toxic, but as they are less volatile than the alcohols of low molecular weight, they cause fewer cases of industrial poisoning.

Carbon disulfide is used in the vulcanization of rubber and in the manufacture of artificial silk. A chronic type of poisoning occurs if the worker is exposed for a long time to low concentrations of its fumes, and both the central and peripheral nervous system are affected. The victims complain of sleepiness, persistent headache, muscular weakness, symptoms of polyneuritis, tremors, ataxia, mental confusion, psychoses of varied types and visual disturbances such as anesthesia of the cornea. In some cases there may be an anemia with a leukocytosis.

Some of the organic acetate esters, ketones, glycols, glycol ethers, and furfurals, are used to dissolve cellulose acetate and nitrocellulose. Inhalation of the vapors of amyl acetate, or banana oil, causes irritation of the respiratory passages, the upper gastrointestinal tract and the conjunctivae. The victim may complain of headache, dizziness, and show anemia and leukocytosis, while in fatal cases fatty changes occur in the liver and kidneys. Methyl, ethyl, propyl and butyl acetate are also solvents, especially ethyl and butyl which are the most used; all are depressants of the central nervous system if absorbed in high concentration. Another group of solvents are the ketones, among which is acetone, a compound prone to produce narcosis if inhaled in high concentration but not likely to cause a chronic poisoning. Pentanone (methyl-propyl ketone) and hexanone (methyl-butyl ketone) have an irritant action on the conjunctivae and upper respiratory passages but rarely produce more serious effects. Glycols and their ethers, as for example the monoethyl ether of ethylene glycol, or cellosolve®, are used as solvents for nitrocellulose and resins; diethylene dioxide, or dioxan, is a solvent of lacquer; furfurals are also classified as industrial solvents. Irritant vapors emanate from these substances which warn the exposed worker of his danger so that fatal poisoning is usually avoided. Fatal cases of dioxan poisoning have been described in which there was necrosis around the central veins of the liver and a hemorrhagic nephrosis.

Some of the halogen derivatives of the aliphatic hydrocarbons are efficient solvents but also very toxic compounds. Carbon tetrachloride or tetrachlormethane is the chief ingredient of noninflammable cleansing fluids, of some chemical fire extinguishers and of certain solvents for rubber. When inhaled this compound has an anesthetic action on the central nervous system like chloroform but less intense, and, at the same time, produces more profound delayed degenerations in liver, kidneys and heart muscle. Inhalation of the vapors causes irritation of the upper respiratory passages, acute bronchitis, bronchopneumonia, toxic jaundice and anuria. See page 798 for more complete description. If the vapors of carbon tetrachloride come in contact with naked flame, the compound may be broken up into chlorine and phosgene, and these, if inhaled, may cause symptoms of poisoning as described on pages 518 and 717.

Tetrachlorethane is employed as a solvent for cellulose acetate which is used in airplane dope, in the manufacture of artificial silk, noninflammable photographic films, lacquer and artificial pearls. Tetrachlorethane is toxic, producing effects similar to carbon tetrachloride.

Trichlorethylene is employed as a solvent for fats and oils, as a thinner for varnishes and as a rubber solvent. It is a depressant of the central nervous system, as described on page 791, but does not cause such severe degenerative changes in the parenchymatous viscera as tetrachlormethane or tetrachlorethane. Dichlorethylene is used as a solvent for lacquer, and when inhaled causes a severe narcosis. Tetrachlorethylene is used as a solvent for the same type of materials, and while it is not as depressant for the central nervous system as the other two ethylene derivatives, if it is inhaled repeatedly it produces giddiness, headache, drowsiness and a narrowing of the visual field.

OTHER ALIPHATIC COMPOUNDS. Some of the organic aliphatic compounds are formed as products or by-products of industrial processes or are used in the manufacture of certain chemicals, and occasionally produce cases of poisoning. Nitroglycerine is formed during the manufacture of some explosives, and workmen may inhale its fumes or absorb it through the skin. In an acute attack, the victim complains of severe headache, flushed face, a feeling of anxiety, transient blindness, nausea, vomiting and polyuria. Poisoning by nitroglycerine has been discussed on page 801. Methyl bromide is used in Germany in the manufacture of antipyrine and certain dyes, and if inhaled may cause such symptoms as muscular cramps, mania and psychosis, and even result in death. Aldehydes such as formaldehyde and acrolein are irritating substances which may cause dermatitis, conjunctivitis, respiratory irritation, abdominal pain and diarrhea. Formaldehyde is used as a disinfectant, in the manufacture of bakelite and as one of the components in the vulcanization of rubber. Acrolein is an irritating gas which is formed when fats are heated, as in candle making, soap manufacture or the melting down of old type.

AROMATIC SOLVENTS. Aromatic compounds derived from the distillation of coal tar such as benzene, toluene and allied compounds, have been used extensively as solvents since 1914, though prior to that date they were employed infrequently for that purpose. For the most part they have replaced the petroleum derivatives, naphtha and benzine, inasmuch as the coal tar derivatives, though more toxic, are less expensive and more powerful solvents. They are employed in the manufacture of explosives, in the production of coal tar dyes and aniline, in the manufacture of rubber, and as solvents for shoe dyes, varnishes, quick drying paints and cements for artificial flowers. Workers are exposed to the toxic action of this solvent, when paint containing benzene is applied with a spray gun.

Benzene or benzol causes both acute and chronic types of poisoning. In mild acute cases there is a condition resembling early alcoholic intoxication with excitement and headache. If the exposure is more intense, the victim may become delirious, maniacal and resist rescue from the poisonous atmosphere. Loss of consciousness, rapid shallow respirations, rapid weak pulse and convulsions precede death.

Cases of chronic benzene poisoning are characterized by leukopenia, bleeding from the gums, nose and gastrointestinal tract, and generalized purpura. A diminution of the antibodies in the blood like the lysins and precipitins, a diminution of the phagocytic power of the leukocytes and a leukopenia may be produced. There are also severe lesions in the bone marrow and an aplastic anemia may develop. Recent investigations of chronic benzene poisoning in industry have indicated that the blood and bone marrow changes are quite variable; polycythemia, leukemic blood pictures both lymphocytic and myelocytic, eosinophilia, megalocytosis and microcytosis occur as well as anemia and leukopenia; the bone marrow may show marked hyperplasia as well as hypoplasia and aplasia.

Toluene is a solvent fully as toxic as benzene but less volatile, and for that reason is less dangerous as a source of poisoning. Exposure to this compound may cause a slight enlargement of the liver, a low red blood cell count, macrocytosis and an absolute lymphocytosis without leukopenia. As a rule the clinical effects are not alarming.

Cyclohexanol is a hydrogenated phenol which is used as a solvent in preparing pyroxylin lacquers. It is a distinct toxic depressant of the central nervous system but as it is not especially volatile it is not likely to cause many cases of poisoning. The tricresyl phosphates are employed as plasticizers and while potentially toxic are not important as an industrial menace. Orthotricresyl phosphate is more toxic than the meta or paratricresyl phosphates which are used in industry; the ortho compound was the poisonous component which was responsible for a widespread peripheral nerve paralysis occurring in individuals rash enough to drink bootleg Jamaica ginger during the last years when the eighteenth amendment was in force.

Turpentine is used as a solvent for paints, and painters who inhale its fumes develop a mild grade of intoxication with irritation of the conjunctivae and upper air passages, headache, mental confusion, dizziness, a sense of intoxication, strangury and a characteristic odor of violets about the urine.

OTHER AROMATIC COMPOUNDS. Aromatic compounds like nitrobenzene, picric acid, dinitrophenol and trinitrotoluol are used in the manufacture of explosives and may cause severe and fatal cases of poisoning as described on pages 808 and 826. The poisonous nitro and amino compounds of benzene and toluene employed in dye manufacture are discussed on pages 809 and 810. A substance known as tetryl is formed in the manufacture of some explosives and if inhaled causes an erythematous dermatitis on the face like sunburn, with sneezing, epistaxis, anorexia and rapid secondary anemia.

Some substances of greater or lesser toxicity are formed in the manufacture of synthetic rubber, of which the most important are butadiene (methyl allene), styrene (vinyl benzene), and acrylonitrile (acrylonitrylvinyl cyanide). Butadiene when inhaled causes conjunctival, nasal and bronchial irritation with coughing, a sense of fatigue and drowsiness, but does not produce cumulative effects as a rule. Styrene causes the same type of symptomatology, but also shows a tendency to inflict damage on the liver and kidneys. Acrylonitrile is dangerous as hydrocyanic acid may be liberated from its molecule, and inhalation of the vapor induces vomiting, weakness, diarrhea, headache, oppressive sensation in the upper respiratory tract, jaundice, liver tenderness and a slight anemia.

The chlorine derivatives of the aromatic ring hydrocarbons are not as toxic as the derivatives of some other radicals combined with the ring, but they are poisonous enough to cause trouble if a person is exposed to their action. Berliner has described toxic symptoms following continued exposure to the fumes of a moth repellant, paradichlorobenzene; the victims show jaundice and loss of weight, and months later may develop cataracts in the lenses of the eyes. Cotter has reported the poisonous action of pentachlorinated naphthalenes which are used to coat wire cables for the purpose of rendering them water repellant and heat resistant; workers handling such wires incautiously, develop a papular rash on the hands and face from the irritant local action of the compound, and also drowsiness, indigestion, polyuria and a marked jaundice. If the vapors are inhaled in sufficient quantity, death occurs, the liver showing lesions similar to those found in acute yellow atrophy.

Sanitary Problems. The conditions produced by the emanation of poisonous fumes and noxious dusts during manufacturing processes are among the problems postulated for physicians and sanitary experts employed by industrial corporations. One of their aims is to determine the maximum amount of the various atmospheric contaminants to which the average workman can be exposed during a working day without impairing his health. For this purpose an examination of the atmosphere of the factory for chemical poisons and microscopic dusts is necessary, and an attempt is made to set a standard for the maximum allowable concentration of the individual contaminants.

One group is composed of volatile poisons and gases whose toxicity in the atmosphere is reckoned in so many parts of gas or vapor to a millon parts of air by volume. In the following listing compiled from Lewman, the more important members of the group are given, the figure opposite each representing the number of parts of the contaminant per million parts of air by volume which would be considered the maximum allowable concentration:

Acetone, 1,000	Carbon tetrachloride, 50	Methyl alcohol, 200
Acrolein, 1	Chlorine, 1	Nitrogen oxides, 39
Aliphatic acetates, 500	Ether (diethyl ether), 500	Perchlorethylene, 100
Ammonia, 100	Ethylene dichloride, 100	Petroleum vapor, 500
Benzene, 75	Formaldehyde, 10	Phosgene, 1
Bromine, 1	Hydrogen chloride, 10	Sulfur dioxide, 10
Carbon dioxide, 5,000	Hydrogen cyanide, 20	Toluene, 200
Carbon disulfide, 20	Hydrogen fluoride, 3	Trichlorethylene, 100
Carbon monoxide, 100	Hydrogen sulfide, 20	Turpentine, 200
		Xylene (xylol), 100

A second group is composed of harmful dusts whose noxious properties are reckoned in terms of so many million particles per cubic foot of air (standard lightfield count). The maximum allowable concentration according to this standard is asbestos, 5; silica, 5; and ordinary nuisance dust free of silica, 50 (Lewman).

The third group is composed of metallic compounds whose toxicity is reckoned at so many milligrams per 10 cubic meters of air. The maximum allowable concentration for different members of this group is:

Cadmium, 1	Iron oxide fume (Fe_2O_3),	Magnesium oxide fume, 150
Chromic acid, 1	150	Manganese, 60
Fluorides, 25	Lead, 1.5	Mercury, 1
		Zinc oxide, 150

Lewman points out that these figures are not unchangeable standards but are subject to constant revision as further investigation is pursued in determining the toxicity of various substances. As an example, carbon tetrachloride at one time was considered to have a maximum allowable concentration of 100 parts per million parts of air by volume, until it was found that 50 parts per million is a more accurate determination. For further information the reader is referred to the literature at the end of the chapter.

The best method of combating industrial poisoning is to protect the workers against poisonous fumes and dusts by hoods, masks or the proper ventilation to dispel the fumes. Care should be taken that dust is stirred up as little as possible in order to diminish the chance of inhalation of noxious substances. Vacuum cleaners should be used whenever possible.

In New York State, compensation is payable for disabilities sustained or death incurred by an employee resulting from the occupational diseases compiled in Table 36-1.

Table 36-1. Compensable Occupational Diseases

Anthrax infection	Epitheliomatous cancers from tar, etc.
Lead poisoning	Glanders infection
Zinc poisoning	Compressed air illness
Mercury poisoning	Miner's disease, bursitis, tenosynovitis, etc.
Phosphorus poisoning	Glassworker's catarrh
Arsenic poisoning	Radium poisoning
Wood alcohol poisoning	Methyl chloride poisoning
Benzol poisoning	Carbon monoxide poisoning
Carbon bisulfide poisoning	Poisoning by sulfuric, hydrochloric and hydro-
Poisoning by nitric fumes	fluoric acids
Nickel carbonyl poisoning	Infections from petroleum products
Poisoning by "dope" or tetrachlormethane	Disabilities from blisters and abrasions
Poisoning by formaldehyde	Bursitis and synovitis
Ulcerations by chromic acid salts	Dermatitis venenata

From McKinney.

REFERENCES

Bolen, H. L.   Byssinosis, J. Indust. Hyg. & Toxicol., 25:215, 1943.
Braunstein, L. E.   Subacute yellow atrophy of the liver due to solvent, J.A.M.A., 114:136, 1940.
Cotter, L. H.   Pentachlorinated naphthalenes in industry, J.A.M.A., 125:273, 1944.
DeJong, R. N.   Methyl bromide poisoning, J.A.M.A., 125:702, 1944.
Editorial.   Chronic industrial benzene poisoning, J.A.M.A., 114:587, 1940.
Emerson, C.   Pneumoconiosis, from Cecil's Textbook of Medicine, Philadelphia, W. B. Saunders Co., pp. 907-909.
Ewing, J.   Modern attitude towards traumatic cancer, Arch. Path., 19:690, 1935.
Gordy, S. T., and Trumper, M.   Carbon disulphide poisoning, J.A.M.A., 110:1543, 1938.
Greenburg, L., Mayers, M. R., Heimann, H., and Moskowitz, S.   Effects of exposure to toluene, J.A.M.A., 118:573, 1942.

Hamilton, A.   Industrial Toxicology, New York, Harper and Brothers, 1934.

—— Industrial Poisoning in the United States, New York, The Macmillan Co., 1925.

—— Industrial Toxicology, from Peterson, Haines and Webster, Legal Medicine and Toxicology, Philadelphia, W. B. Saunders Co., 1923, Vol. II, pp. 772-802.

Jacobs, M. B.   The Analytical Chemistry of Industrial Poisons, Hazards and Solvents, New York, Interscience Publishers, Inc., 1941.

Kaufmann, C.   Handbuch der Unfallmedizin, Stuttgart, Ferdinand Enke, Vol. I, 1919; Vol. II, 1925.

Lehmann, K. B., and Flury, S.   Toxicology and Hygiene of Industrial Solvents, Translated by King, E., and Smyth, H. F., Baltimore, Williams & Wilkins Co., 1943.

Lewman, M. B.   Occupational Chemical Hazards in Industries of Louisville and Jefferson County, Ky., M.S. thesis, University of Louisville, 1945.

McConnell, W. J.   Volatile solvents as a problem in industrial medicine, J.A.M.A., 110:762, 1938.

McKinney.   Consolidated Laws of New York, in Workmen's Compensation Law, Northport, N. Y., Ed. Thompson Co., 1935, Book 64 suppl., pp. 59-61.

McNally, W. D.   Three deaths from T.N.T. (trinitrotoluene) poisoning, Indust. Med., 13:491, 1944.

Machle, W.   Gasoline intoxication, J.A.M.A., 117:1965, 1941.

Magnuson, H. L., and Raulston, B. O.   Lead poisoning in roofers, J.A.M.A., 114:1528, 1940.

Ross, P. Cadmium poisoning, Brit. M. J., 1:252, 1944.

de Senarclens, F.   Contribution à l'étude de l'ostéopathie fluorique, Helvet. med. acta, 8:379, 1941.

Sodeman, W. A., and Pullen, R. L.   Bagasse disease of the lungs, Arch. Int. Med., 73:365, 1944.

Spolyar, L. W., Keppler, J. F., and Porter, H. G.   Cadmium poisoning in industry, J. Indust. Hyg. & Toxicol., 26:232, 1944.

U. S. Public Health Service, Division of Industrial Hygiene. Threshold Limits Established, Industrial Hygiene News Letter No. 3, 1943, p. 2.

Wilson, R. H.   Health hazards encountered in the manufacture of synthetic rubber, J.A.M.A., 124:701, 1944.

Witkowski, L. J., Fischer, C. N., and Murdock, H. D.   Industrial diseases due to tetryl, J.A.M.A., 119:1406, 1942.

OCCUPATIONAL DISEASES

Anderson, N. P.   Management of common occupational skin diseases, J.A.M.A., 139:912, 1949.

Belknap, E. L.   Differential diagnosis of lead poisoning, J.A.M.A., 139:818, 1949.

Foulger, J. H.   Physiologic effects of industrial solvents, J.A.M.A., 139:826, 1949.

Greenburg, L.   Diagnosis and treatment of occupational metal poisoning, J.A.M.A., 139:815, 1949.

Hamlin, L. E.   The pneumonoconioses, J.A.M.A., 139:909, 1949.

Wilentz, W. C.   Treatment of lead intoxication, J.A.M.A., 139:823, 1949.

Wilson, R. H.   Diagnosis and treatment of industrial solvent poisoning, J.A.M.A., 139:906, 1949.

37

The Government and the Physician

The relation of the physician to the government will be discussed as it occurs in New York City, for the principles which determine his status in that community are valid for other municipal or county units. The basic principles are that the professional life of the doctor in New York City or any large municipality is subject to the government of the state in which he resides, to the government of the United States and to the municipal or county government.

STATE GOVERNMENT

The New York State government, as in all other states, decides whether or not a license to practice medicine in that state will be issued to the individual physician. Formerly in the light of the common law and the old civil law, opportunity to treat the sick or injured was considered a property right which belonged in the natural course of events to anyone who desired to exercise it in a community. With the growing complexity of social conditions, the state was forced to protect the community against those not qualified to be practitioners of this important profession. At present in all states a person is only allowed to undertake the practice of medicine after he has satisfied the requirements of the State Department of Education.

The practice of medicine in the New York State law is defined as "the ability to diagnose, treat, operate, or prescribe for any human disease, pain, injury, deformity or physical condition." Those qualified to pursue this profession in New York State are practitioners who obtained legal authorization prior to September 1st, 1891, or were issued a license under Article 8, Chapter 661 of the laws of 1893, or obtained the license to practice by passing the examinations of the National Board of Medical Examiners or the New York State Board of Medical Examiners.

The individual who intends to obtain a license to practice medicine in the State of New York by passing the state board examinations must make a formal application for this purpose to the State Education Department and pay a fee of 25 dollars. In his application he must submit sworn evidence which must be satisfactory to the Board of Regents, that he is over 21 years of age, that he is of good moral character, and that he has the proper educational requirements. An applicant who has been convicted of a felony in any court or of any offense which is considered to be a felony according to the laws of the State of New York is not acceptable as a candidate for a license to practice medicine. The educational requirements consist of a degree of Doctor of Medicine or Bachelor of Medicine from a registered medical school whose standards are satisfactory to the Board of Regents and this includes the general education needed for admission into such a medical school. If the application is accepted, the applicant is given written examinations in anatomy, physiology, pathology and bacteriology, chemistry, hygiene, surgery, obstetrics and gynecology, and the practice of medicine. When he passes these examinations successfully, he receives the license and registers in the office of the county clerk in his county, sets up an office, prescribes medicine and collects compensation for his services. Every year the practicing physician pays a registration fee of two dollars to the New York State Department of Education at Albany, New York. Dental practitioners also have similar educational requirements and are required to pass state board examinations much like those of physicians. This is also true of osteopaths who are granted a license to practice osteopathy but not to administer drugs or to perform surgical operations.

The State Department of Education has the power to revoke the license of a physician to practice, if he has been guilty of improper conduct. If he has been convicted of a felony such as the performance of an illegal abortion or the perpetration of a fraud, he is debarred automatically from the practice of medicine. If the offense is less serious, the accused is given a hearing and a chance to prepare a defense before the actual revocation proceedings are started.

Other limited practitioners, such as chiropractors, naturopaths or therapists of any type who either treat one particular part of the body or who minister to all ailments by a special method, are allowed to practice their form of therapy but are forbidden to practice medicine under the penalty of violating the medical practice act. If a person has sustained injury at the hands of this type of therapist, his recourse is either to bring a civil action against the practitioner for damages in an attempt to prove that the defendant was indulging in malpractice according to his own system of healing, or have him prosecuted for wrongfully attempting to practice medicine. In New York City if a person should die while under the care of a limited practitioner, the death would be referred automatically to the Office of the Chief Medical Examiner as an example of a death occurring "while unattended by a physician." If it so happened that death was caused by diphtheria or similar communicable, infectious disease, the limited practitioner could be prosecuted in the criminal courts because he would have violated the regulations of the Department of Health governing the reporting and treating of these diseases and thus endangered the safety of the community.

There are also other types of irregular unqualified practitioners such as those who base their therapy on fortune telling, spiritualistic seances or magic formulae. They are forbidden to practice by statute and, if they disobey this law, they can be prosecuted in the criminal court for violation of the medical practice act.

Thirteen cases of death following chiropractic treatment are listed in the reports of the Chief Medical Examiner from 1918 to 1941. In these cases death resulted from aggravation of a pre-existing disease, probably by the manipulation of the chiropractor. For example, in one case an elderly woman, following the manipulation, died from a rupture of an ascending aorta weakened by medial necrosis which produced hemorrhage in the pericardial sac. In another case a boy was treated by a chiropractor for abdominal pain and died a few days after the treatment from a suppurative peritonitis secondary to acute appendicitis. In these cases it is difficult to prosecute the practitioner in the criminal courts because evidence necessary for conviction is hard to obtain. In rare cases such as one which occurred more recently than the above mentioned series, a chiropractor in manipulating the neck of a slightly built boy fractured the cervical spine and caused death. Pratt-Thomas and Berger describe similar cases.

FEDERAL GOVERNMENT

The Federal Government imposes the Harrison Narcotic Act upon the general practitioner, in effect requiring the practicing physician to obtain a license from the

Director of Internal Revenue in order to prescribe narcotic drugs such as cocaine or the opium derivatives. This subject is considered at greater length in Chapter 34. During the days of prohibition, the same restrictions, embodied in the Volstead Act, were applied to alcohol; this law was repealed in 1933.

MUNICIPAL OR COUNTY GOVERNMENT

The following branches of government come into intimate contact with the practicing physician: (1) the Department of Health, (2) the Office of the Chief Medical Examiner, or the Office of the Coroner in counties where that institution exists, (3) the Office of the District Attorney and the Courts.

The Department of Health. The chief purpose of this department is to safeguard the health of the community by combating the spread of disease. In New York City, its governing body, the Board of Health, enacts rules and regulations for this purpose embodied in the Sanitary Code which cannot be violated without the violator incurring the danger of being prosecuted for a misdemeanor. These regulations are concerned with the sale of food, with the control of smallpox vaccination, with the administration of quarantine regulations and other activities, some of which have a distinct relationship to the professional life of the physician. For example, a doctor is required to report to the department as soon as possible all cases of contagious and communicable disease, and food infections and poisonings which he may encounter in his practice. In this way the department obtains information of a threatened epidemic and can prepare to deal with it adequately. There are well equipped bacteriologic laboratories and diagnostic experts in the Department of Health are concerned with the diagnosis of infectious diseases and their prevention. The physicians and laboratories furnish bacteriologic and medical diagnostic aid to physicians who request it.

Doctors and hospitals are also obliged to report to the Department of Health all cases of abortion, whether spontaneous or induced. This subject is discussed in Chapter 22. Cases of criminal abortion are also referred to the Police Department.

An important function of the Department of Health is to compile vital statistics, or in other words to keep a record of births and deaths. The doctor who delivers an infant must file within 10 days a certificate of birth on which appears the name, sex, date and place of birth of the infant along with the name, age, nationality, race and other pertinent data regarding the parents. The physician who has a natural death in his practice must also issue a certificate of death promptly and deliver it to the undertaker who in turn must file the certificate with the Department of Health before he can obtain a permit to bury the body. The death certificate contains the name, social security number, sex, age, color, nationality, civil condition, occupation, birthplace, residence of the deceased, whether or not a citizen, whether or not a veteran of a war waged by the United States, father's name, father's birthplace, mother's maiden name, mother's birthplace, place, day and hour of death of the deceased, and the diagnosis of the cause of death. This document is not only important for the purpose of vital statistics, but it is also an indispensable governmental record of the death of an individual and on it are based the settlement of estates; payment of insurances, pensions and social security benefits; and the decision in liability suits and cases of disputed inheritance. A physician must fill out the death certificate correctly and never deliberately falsify it for then he would be liable to criminal prosecution for a misdemeanor.

The Department of Health in New York City groups certificates of death into two classes: (1) the ordinary death certificate and, (2) the medical examiner's death certificate.

ORDINARY DEATH CERTIFICATE. These are certificates recording the death of individuals who have died naturally of a disease condition not associated with trauma of any sort, while under the care of a physician. In cases of this sort, the attending physician, whether he is in private practice or in a hospital, issues the death certificate giving the disease condition most compatible with the clinical course as the cause of death. The Department of Health also stipulates that the medical attendant must have attended the deceased for a definite period prior to death and must have paid him a professional visit in the last 24 hours of his life, otherwise the death certificate is not accepted, and the death is referred to the Office of the Chief Medical Examiner.

The present classification of the causes of death for the purposes of vital statistics is the one found in the International List of the Causes of Death. This list includes congenital defects, infectious diseases, parasitic diseases, intoxications, poisons, traumas, and diseases of the separate systems of the body as the circulatory system, central nervous system, and the rest. The diagnosis on the certificate must conform to the nomenclature in the International List and should convey the idea of a specific pathologic lesion, as for example coronary arteriosclerosis, or of a definite disease entity like diabetes mellitus. Mere symptoms or symptom complexes, as for example cardiac decompensation or hypertension are by themselves not admissible though they may be used to qualify an underlying primary cause, as, for example, chronic mitral valvulitis, mitral stenosis, cardiac decompensation.

A number of pathologic lesions, such as acute or chronic inflammations like peritonitis or pleuritis, thrombosis, embolism, abortion or hemorrhage are not by themselves acceptable as causes of death because they are immediate and not primary but must be qualified further, since they may occur either as the result of trauma or natural disease. When they arise out of trauma the attending physician should not fill out the certificate but should refer the case to the Office of the Chief Medical Examiner or the Coroner's Office. On the other hand if the lesion was caused by a natural disease process entirely, the doctor in filling out the death certificate should give the underlying cause and qualify the primary cause with the terms spontaneous, or nontraumatic. For example a septic infection of the abdominal cavity due to natural causes would be properly signed out as follows: acute suppurative peritonitis, acute suppurative appendicitis, spontaneous.

If another pathologic process besides the main or primary cause of death is present and has contributed to death, that should be recorded in the place set aside for it on the certificate. Thus the primary cause of death may be chronic duodenal ulcer, the immediate cause of death stemming from the primary cause may be hemorrhage into the gastrointestinal tract, spontaneous; and if a primary carcinoma of the lung were present, that may have played a role in hastening death, that should be entered as a contributory cause in its proper space. Considerable misunderstanding exists as to the meaning of primary cause of death, immediate cause of death, and contributory cause of death. The primary cause is the process principally responsible for death; the immediate cause is the fatal complication which kills the individual and is always derived from the primary cause with which it must be linked on the death certificate. The contributory cause is an independent process which plays an accessory role in producing the death of the patient, and it must not be linked with the primary and immediate causes of death.

An autopsy may be performed on a case of death due to natural causes, in which the attending physician issues the death certificate; the nearest relative of the deceased must sign a written consent for this type of postmortem dissection. The nearest relative in the case of a married individual is a wife or husband; with a widowed individual the children who are not minors in order of seniority; with a minor, a single, or a childless widowed person, the father, mother, brothers and sisters and relatives in next degree of kinship have the right to permit an autopsy. When a deceased has no living relatives, an executor of the will may authorize the autopsy. The nearest relative has the power to limit the extent of the autopsy and to insist that all organs be returned to the body for burial. If the autopsy is performed without the consent of the nearest relative, a liability suit for damages can be brought against the hospital, or the pathologist performing the autopsy, or both. Autopsies performed by a hospital pathologist must be properly protocoled, and the report attached to the hospital history. In the event of a consent autopsy, the death certificate should not be filled out until after the autopsy, and the cause of death recorded should be based on the autopsy and not on clinical impressions.

MEDICAL EXAMINER'S DEATH CERTIFICATE. If a person in New York City dies as a result of "criminal violence, casualty, suicide, suddenly while in apparent health, while in prison, or while unattended by a physician or in any suspicious or unusual manner", the certificate of death must be issued by a medical examiner from the Office of the Chief Medical Examiner. The medical examiner may release the body after an investigation and an external examination of the remains, but if he forms the opinion that an autopsy should be performed in order to determine the cause of death, he has the power to do this without requesting consent from the relatives of the deceased. After the autopsy he issues the death certificate on the basis of his findings at autopsy. In the performance of this duty he must be certain that the case is really under his jurisdiction because, if it is not properly a medical examiner's case, he is just as vulnerable as any other pathologist to a damage suit brought by the relatives of the deceased for performing an unauthorized autopsy.

When the medical examiner issues a certificate on a case which has died as a result of a natural disease process, in stating the cause of death he follows the principles which were discussed under the heading of Ordinary Death Certificate. If the death is the result of trauma or any other external cause, the certificate must contain the principal lesion produced by the trauma, the fatal complication, the place where the injury occurred, the time when it occurred, and the manner in which it occurred. The following would be examples of such death certificates: fracture of the skull, epidural hemorrhage, cerebral compression, accidental fall on the street at Times Square, January 9th 1944; or acute corrosive gastritis following ingestion of sodium fluoride, January 10th 1946, suicidal; or bullet wound of heart and lungs, hemorrhage into the chest, homicidal.

The Office of the Chief Medical Examiner. The deaths which come under the jurisdiction of the medical examiner include those which are the result of criminal violence, suicide, casualty and so on, and so are a matter of concern to the police and district attorney. In such instances the investigations of the medical examiner are concerned with the proper administration of justice and are also as important as the investigations of the police. The doctor who has treated a case of this sort is obliged to cooperate with these authorities and to furnish them with whatever pertinent information he may have at his disposal.

The police must be informed of any bullet wound, stab wound, blunt instrument laceration or any other injury of a suspected criminal nature which a doctor might encounter in his practice, especially if he has treated the case in his office or in a private home. Any bullets or fragments of other lethal weapons recovered from the body of the patient during the operation should be turned over to the police as part of the evidence of the crime. The doctor should keep a careful clinical record of the case and accurately describe, measure and even make a diagram of the various injuries especially if there is any likelihood that a surgical operation will obliterate these lesions. If a wound heals or has been obliterated, it may be necessary for the doctor to testify in court as to his findings since he would be the only physician who saw the injuries in their original state. This subject has been discussed at greater length under the various forms of trauma.

The following case is an example of the importance of such testimony by an attending surgeon. An elderly white man, 67 years of age, was struck over the head with a revolver butt during a hold-up and was admitted to a hospital in coma, suffering from a compound depressed fracture of the skull in the right parietal region. A craniotomy was performed and the surgeon in removing the depressed bone noted that the indentation in the skull was in the form of a pyramid ⅝ inch deep, with a triangular base about ⅝ inch in diameter. Two weeks later the patient died of a suppurative meningitis which developed from the skull injury. At autopsy the medical examiner noted the suppurative meningitis but was unable to describe the original injury because that had been obliterated by the surgical operation. The surgeon was called into court to testify to the nature of the depressed fracture and thereby furnished important testimony, linking the revolver with the homicide for as it happened the revolver butt was defective and presented a triangular corner which was capable of having caused the pyramidal depression in the skull.

Occasionally the doctor may be the only person present who can take the dying declaration of a patient succumbing to a homicidal injury, and this procedure should be carried out according to the precautions discussed under that heading in Chapter 38.

If an attending physician reports any case of death to the Office of the Chief Medical Examiner it is his duty to furnish the medical examiner with a clinical history which contains all essential information. The form issued to the hospitals in New York City by the Office of the Chief Medical Examiner gives a brief outline of the information which is really desirable.

1.   The first section contains the patient's name and the other items necessary for vital statistics as already noted on the death certificate, and in addition the date and hour of his admission to the hospital, the place from which he came, or was brought, and how he was transported to the hospital whether by ambulance or by other means.

2.   In this section is given the clinical signs and symptoms which the deceased presented during his stay in the hospital. Enough of the clinical record should be inserted to indicate clearly the ideas of the physician about the case.

3.   The injuries from which the deceased was suffering at the time of his admission are described and, if possible, the time and place of their occurrence and the manner in which they were received are also mentioned. It is important for the surgeon to describe accurately the original appearance and character of the wounds on the patient, because if the patient survives the trauma for a week or more the area of injury may be altered by the processes of repair, or by a septic infection or by operation. The character, size, location and number of the wounds should be designated accurately.

4.   Any operations performed must be described in sufficient detail to indicate their purpose and nature. The surgeon should give particular attention to internal

and external injuries which would probably be altered as a result of the operation. Any tissue removed from the body should be sent to the laboratory for safekeeping or histologic examination, for example, a uterus which was removed at a laparotomy in a case of criminally induced abortion. Such specimens must be produced for the medical examiner if he requires them to complete his case. Any bullets or parts of a lethal weapon removed at operation must be preserved and delivered to the police and this fact should be recorded in the report. Bullets located by roentgen ray or other means in the body, but not removed during an operation, should be mentioned.

5. The date and hour of death must be accurately stated.

6. The space entitled "Remarks" is intended for statements not otherwise included.

7. The physician who fills out the report must sign his name at the bottom of the page. This is important as this report becomes a government document and the doctor by his signature automatically makes an affidavit that the statements contained therein are true to the best of his knowledge. These reports must never be compiled carelessly or irresponsibly or falsified in any particular for that would be a misdemeanor and punishable by law. The information contained in the report does not belong in the category of privileged communications, but on the contrary the physician is required to furnish to the medical examiner all the information which is pertinent to the case. In filling out this report it is desirable that the doctor make a clear distinction between facts which he has obtained from his own observation and statements which have reached him by hearsay. The latter should be properly qualified, for example, "according to police, patient was struck by an automobile," or "the family claims that deceased was struck with a blackjack".

The Office of the District Attorney and the Courts. Any physician, whether he is practicing medicine in a city like New York City or in any other municipality or county may be subpoenaed into a criminal or civil court to give testimony concerning some case which he has treated. It is desirable, therefore, to give a brief description of the different types of criminal and civil courts and outline the ways in which they operate.

The criminal courts are closely connected with the Office of the District Attorney. The public prosecutor officially connected with that office prepares evidence to substantiate the charges brought against individuals arrested for various crimes. Representatives from the District Attorney's Office are present in all criminal courts from the highest to the lowest, prepared to present the case against a defendant, who, in turn, is represented by a lawyer, technically known as "counsel for the defense." In all courts the testimony of witnesses is recorded verbatim by a court stenographer and is taken under oath, with the liability of incurring a severe penalty if the testimony can be proven to be perjured.

When a person is arrested, the arrest is first recorded in the police precinct where it occurred and the charge against him is entered on the files. The first tribunal which the defendant encounters is the magistrate's court. These are of various kinds; the ordinary district courts which are distributed in different parts of the city and are mainly concerned with misdemeanors; the traffic court which deals with traffic violations; the felony court in which more serious crimes receive a preliminary hearing; the homicide court in which those charged with the crime of homicide are first arraigned.

The defendant in a homicide case is brought before the magistrate shortly after his arrest and is charged by the arresting officers with the crime. This first hearing is usually brief as the magistrate hears the charge, asks the defendant if he pleads guilty or not guilty, fixes bail for the prisoner or refuses it depending on the circumstances, and postpones the principal hearing for a later date so that the defendant may have a chance to employ counsel. At the principal hearings, the magistrate hears testimony presented by the district attorney and the counsel for the defense and then decides in the event of a felony whether the defendant shall be discharged or held for the decision of the Grand Jury. If the magistrate finds the prisoner guilty of a misdemeanor, he may impose a fine or a short jail sentence. The magistrate in the homicide court has judicial powers similar to those of a coroner. In some instances the defendant may waive examination in the magistrate's court and in major crimes is held automatically for the Grand Jury. In certain types of crimes, the magistrate may hold the defendant for the Court of Special Sessions.

The Grand Jury is an empowered special body of 23 men, carefully selected, who are presented with the evidence against the defendant by the district attorney and who decide, after hearing the witnesses, whether the defendant shall be discharged or indicted for a felony, that is, held for trial before the Court of General Sessions or the County Court. In certain types of cases, the defendant may be held for the court of Special Sessions (page 911). The witnesses for the defense are not heard by the Grand Jury but on certain occasions the defendant may be allowed to tell his story under oath after he has signed a waiver of immunity, in which he agrees to the stipulation that his testimony before the Grand Jury may be used against him at a future trial. He cannot be forced to testify before the Grand Jury. Dismissal of a case by the Grand Jury merely means that the evidence is not sufficient to warrant indictment and it does not forbid reopening of the case later if additional evidence is unearthed by the prosecution. In addition to this duty the Grand Jury has the power to hold an investigation on any existing condition which may bring the administration of justice into discredit.

A true bill of indictment brought by the Grand Jury charges a defendant with one of four degrees of homicide:

1. Murder in the first degree, in which the killing was premeditated. The penalty is death in states with capital punishment.

2. Murder in the second degree in which the homicide is intentional but not premeditated. The penalty is 20 years to life imprisonment.

3. Manslaughter in the first degree in which the guilt is considered to be of less degree than the guilt in murder cases, in that there may have been intent not to kill but only to inflict bodily harm. It covers a wide range of homicide cases, including assaults with deadly weapons, and a few cases of technical homicides, that is, cases in which the defendant did not have any intention of killing the deceased but caused his death by inexcusable negligence in operating a machine like a motor vehicle or an elevator. The penalty for this degree of homicide is 5 to 20 years in prison.

4. Manslaughter in the second degree implies a lesser degree of guilt than first degree manslaughter as it includes cases in which death followed an assault without use of a deadly weapon, and most cases of technical homicides. The penalty for this degree is 1 to 20 years. The other types of homicides are the justifiable homicide which occurs when a police officer kills a person who attempts to resist or evade arrest; and the excusable homicide which occurs when a defendant has been shown to have killed an assailant in self defense.

The final court which determines the guilt or innocence of the accused charged with and indicted for felony is known as the Court of General Sessions in the Borough of Manhattan and as the County Court in Brooklyn, Bronx, Queens and Richmond. Here the defendant is tried before a judge and a petit jury of 12 men plus two alternate jurors who hear the testimony but only serve if any of the original 12 become sick during the course of the trial. The proceedings start with the opening statement of the district attorney who informs the jury of what crime the defendant has been accused, and gives an outline of the evidence which he expects to present and a brief statement of what he hopes to prove. In similar fashion the defense counsel makes his opening address or he may postpone that formality until he is ready to present his own evidence. The prosecution then introduces its witnesses who are put under oath and their statements taken down verbatim by the court stenographer; each witness is then cross examined by the counsel for the defense. After this the defense presents its witnesses and they are in turn cross examined by the district attorney. The prosecution may call in witnesses for rebuttal of testimony offered by the defense and the defense in turn may call in new witnesses to counteract any new testimony offered by the prosecution. At the end of the testimony the counsel for the defense first sums up his case, and he is followed by the district attorney who sums up the case of the prosecution. Finally the judge charges the jury enumerating the significant points in the testimony and outlining the legal considerations which should influence their decision on the verdict. After this the jury retires and decides on the guilt or innocence of the accused.

If the district attorney agrees, the defendant may plead guilty to any degree of homicide except murder in the first degree, either before the trial actually starts or at any time during its progress. In such cases the proceedings do not continue but the defendant is held automatically for the imposition of sentence at some future date, just as though he had been found guilty by a jury. If the case is one of first degree murder the defendant is not allowed to plead guilty but must stand trial in order that the jury may decide his fate.

After a conviction, the defendant in a criminal case has the right of appeal through his attorney to the Appellate Division of the Supreme Court, and then to the Court of Appeals of the State. The judges in the higher courts review the evidence, especially noting instances where the defense counsel has registered an exception to a ruling of the trial court. If they decide that the rights of the defendant have been infringed, the higher court may set aside the verdict and order a retrial. The district attorney, however, in New York State cannot register an exception to any ruling of a trial judge and a defendant found innocent of a charge is automatically freed of that charge at the end of the trial.

Other courts associated with criminal cases are the Childrens Courts, in which violations of the law by individuals under 15 years of age are fittingly disposed of and settled. The Court of Special Sessions deals with offences such as petit larceny, prostitution, illegitimate paternity, illegal possession of firearms and other serious misdemeanors; the cases in this court are heard and decided by three judges sitting together. Such cases are referred to the court by a magistrate or by the Grand Jury.

The medical testimony in the criminal courts trying homicide cases is generally given by physicians employed by the municipal government in an official capacity; as, for example, the medical examiner in homicide cases who testifies to the cause of death of the victim and thus establishes the most important part of the corpus delicti. Occasionally a surgeon in practice may be called in as a witness before the criminal courts if he has given medical attention to the victim of a homicide or if he has treated a victim who has been criminally assaulted. He would be summoned by the prosecution if he has operated upon the wounded man and has destroyed the wound by his surgical procedures, or if he has found a fragment of the lethal weapon in the body during the operation, for in such cases his testimony would be necessary to complete the proof of the crime. The surgeon might also be subpoenaed by the defense if he had observed that the victim was suffering from alcoholic intoxication at the time of his admission to the hospital for this fact might be in favor of the accused.

The testimony given by the doctor in the criminal courts is governed by the same rules of evidence which are in force in the civil tribunals and will be discussed later. The chief differences may be summarized by stating that the medical witness in a criminal trial is usually subpoenaed because he has had some previous professional connection with the case; the hired expert who testifies to his opinions without previous professional connection with the case, is rarely seen in jurisdictions where the medical examiner is independent of the police department and prosecuting office. In the civil courts both types of medical testimony are common. Unlike the civil tribunals where the medical man cannot be compelled to assume the role of an expert witness, the doctor who testifies before a criminal court must not only be prepared to give factual testimony but must also give his professional opinion to the best of his ability concerning the subjects about which he is qualified to speak, if in the opinion of the judge such testimony is essential for the purposes of justice.

The different varieties of civil courts are concerned with the right of a claimant or plaintiff to money compensation in any suit which he may bring against a defendant. In New York City, the principal courts are the Municipal Courts where the claim is below 1,000 dollars, the City Courts where the claims are between 1,000 and 3,000 dollars, and finally the Supreme Court of New York State which considers litigation involving any sum above 3,000 dollars. In these courts the types of civil cases which may require medical testimony are claims brought against an insurance company for accident insurance or double indemnity benefits, or damages sought for physical injury suffered by a plaintiff resulting from an alleged wrongful action on the part of a defendant. Among this last-mentioned group may be included malpractice suits brought against physicians (Chapter 38). Other types of Civil Courts are the Workmen's Compensation hearings of the State Labor Commission which decides the compensation of laborers injured or killed while at work (page 889); the Surrogates Court devoted to the probating of wills; and Federal Courts and Federal Compensation Courts which are concerned with cases analogous to those presented before the State Labor Commission and the State Supreme Court. The procedure in these different tribunals is similar to that described under the criminal courts, the principal difference being that in civil cases both plaintiff and defendant have the power of appealing a verdict to higher courts.

Medical Testimony in Court. The doctor who testifies in court in his professional capacity does so as an ordinary factual witness, or as an expert witness. As a factual witness, he must observe the rules of evidence, testifying only to those facts which he knows through his personal experience and avoiding hearsay evidence, or information communicated to him by some other person or agency. The ordinary medical witness is served with a subpoena and is only entitled to a nominal subpoena fee, usually fifty cents to a dollar and fifty cents which is presented at the time of service of the subpoena. The physician so served is obligated to attend the court at the time mentioned on the subpoena or at whatever date he is able to arrange with the attorney who desires his testimony. As an ordinary witness, the doctor is only required to testify to facts which he discovered in his examination of a patient or to the findings of an autopsy, but he is not required to express any opinion regarding such facts or findings, unless he is duly qualified by the attorney as an expert in that branch of medicine. In a civil case a physician is not obliged to testify as an expert if he does not desire to assume that role. The relation of confidential communications to medical testimony will be discussed in Chapter 38.

If a medical witness is to assume the character of an expert, he is entitled to a fee for his services from the attorney who desires his testimony. It is desirable that the medical man should have a clear understanding with the attorney about the remuneration for his testimony before he takes the stand. Without a previous agreement the witness might not be able to collect after the testimony the fee of an expert in the amount to which he believes himself entitled. The physician must obtain from the attorneys all pertinent facts in the case and he should make plain to them that he must be absolutely honest in expressing his opinion on the stand and what his opinion will be and that he will not give expert testimony unless he is satisfied concerning the merits of the case. It is the right of the medical witness to demand all the information available from the attorneys and it is his duty to tell them beyond any possibility of misunderstanding the content of the testimony which he expects to give, including what admissions he will have to make on cross examination.

Needless to say a medical witness before accepting the role of an expert should have sufficient professional experience with the disease conditions under discussion that he can form his own valid opinions about the case independently of other authorities. Opinions based on his own observations are more credible and less easily attacked by the opposing counsel than if they are based only on the writings of the accepted authorities. However in preparing his testimony, the witness should consult the important literature on the subject in order that he may know the viewpoints of the various authors and clarify more exactly his own ideas about the points at issue. In any event he may be compelled to meet the contentions of opposing counsel who may quote these authorities against him and he must be prepared to face such eventualities.

The expert witness whether or not he has had any previous professional connection with the case must study the medical record thoroughly and arrange all the facts systematically in his mind. He must familiarize himself with the important points of the medical history and ascertain exactly dates, measurements and medical observations in the matter under discussion. If the witness is testifying from his own professional record he is allowed to refresh his recollection from his original notes but he may not be permitted to read his notes verbatim.

After he takes the stand and is sworn in, the medical witness must be qualified as an expert by the attorney before he can be allowed to testify in that role. Accordingly he is asked his name, age, educational background, professional experience and any special qualifications which he may possess apposite to the subject under discussion. The presiding judge then rules on whether or not the medical witness is qualified to testify as an expert. In giving his testimony the doctor must present his observations concisely and in clearly understandable, nontechnical language as much as possible. He should be careful to avoid hearsay statements. The terms which he uses should be exact and not be capable of being misinterpreted or twisted by the opposing counsel into meanings other than those he intended.

The opinion of the expert witness should be expressed with due regard to scientific correctness and without any undue bias in favor of either plaintiff or defendant. It has been correctly said that a physician on the witness stand should never express opinions which he would not be willing to express before a reputable medical society. Furthermore the doctor should not give his opinion on a subject with which he is not familiar but should simply say that he is not an expert in that particular field, or should merely say that he does not know. The physician should bear in mind that he is expressing his opinions with reasonable certainty and not simply suggesting a speculative possibility.

Not infrequently the expert medical witness has had no previous connection with the case but is engaged by the attorneys because of his special knowledge and his willingness to testify favorably for the side which employs him because he believes in the merits of the case. The testimony of such an expert cannot be introduced unless the hypothetical question is employed. After he has established the doctor's qualifications, the attorney then proceeds to ask the witness the hypothetical question which assumes all the facts in evidence. At the end, the medical expert is asked, that: "if, given these facts, he is able to form an opinion about the case?" and to this he replies either yes or no. If the answer is yes, the attorney requests the witness to state his opinion, and then the witness is delivered over to the opposing counsel for cross examination.

The cross examination may merely be designed to bring out additional facts not previously mentioned or it may be an attempt to discredit the testimony of the witness. The doctor should answer all questions responsively on cross examination but must be absolutely certain that he understands the question before he replies to it. The success with which he weathers the cross examination will depend largely on how well and how truthfully he has presented his case in the direct testimony and how clear an impression he has made by his behavior on the stand. The expert who is really qualified to speak about the subject in question, and can draw his ideas from his own professional knowledge, can prepare an opinion which is not easily assailed, provided of course that the conclusions which he expresses are justified by the premises. The utmost that the opposing counsel can do is to find fault with some interpretation of a symptom or sign expressed by the witness on direct examination, especially quoting various authorities and text books which disagree with the witness. Such attempts need not cause the expert any great concern, especially if his experience is extensive enough to allow him to speak authoritatively in his own right. A medical expert in turn should be cautious in quoting another authority in support of his own opinion, inasmuch as it gives the opposing attorney an opportunity to search through the writings of the quoted authority until he finds some statement which disagrees or seems to disagree with the opinion of the witness so that he can embarrass the witness with this on cross examination.

The medical expert on cross examination must not take offense or display annoyance at the manner of the opposing attorney. He should answer all questions without attempt at evasion. If the question requires an answer of yes or no, the witness should reply directly if the answer will not be misleading. If a question is framed in a way that the reply of either yes or no would be incorrect, the witness can only appeal to the judge to allow him to qualify his answer so that he will not be forced into making a false statement. The judge may or may not grant such a request depending on the circumstances attending the individual case.

REFERENCES

Emerson, R. L.   Legal Medicine and Toxicology, New York and London, D. Appleton and Co., 1909.

Herzog, W.   Medical Jurisprudence, Indianapolis, The Bobbs-Merrill Co., 1931.

Pratt-Thomas, H. R., and Berger, K. E.   Injuries after chiropractic manipulation, J.A.M.A., 133:600, 1947.

Reports of Office of Chief Medical Examiner in the City of New York from the years 1918 to 1941.

38

The Rights and Obligations of Physicians: Malpractice

The legal status of a physician in the practice of his profession is a matter of considerable complexity. The laws and court decisions on this subject are so numerous that it would be difficult to present it adequately in a short chapter. The most that can be attempted is to outline briefly the problems of law which the practitioner of medicine faces in order that he may be prepared to cope with them.

The fundamental relationship in law between the physician and his patient is simply that of a contract, in which the doctor agrees to furnish medical care to the patient. In the vast majority of cases this contract is an implied one, which means specifically that, whenever a doctor is summoned or engaged by a patient and accepts the assignment, he is pledged automatically to observe the following conditions:

1. He shall treat the patient with an ordinary or reasonable degree of skill, such as would be expected to exist in the community in which he is practicing.

2. He shall exercise due care and diligence in his treatment of the case. This means that he shall not only avoid negligence in the administration of his curative measures, but that he shall use prudence in discontinuing his attendance on the patient. As long as the patient requires aid, the physician must continue to render his services. He cannot quit the case unless the patient consents, or unless he gives the patient timely notice so that another physician can be engaged in his place, or until he pronounces the patient as no longer in need of medical attention, a responsibility which he, the physician, must assume.

3. He shall use his best judgment at all times for the benefit of the patient.

As soon as the doctor agrees to treat the patient this implied contract is legally in force, even though it is not specifically mentioned by either patient or physician. The contract does not guarantee that the patient will be cured or necessarily benefited by the treatment of the doctor, but it does promise that the doctor shall use his best efforts to effect a cure or alleviate the patient's condition.

The above contract also implies that the physician is entitled to fair compensation for his services. He may recover such compensation by law-suit if it is denied him, even though the patient has not been benefited by his treatment. The law and the judicial practice vary considerably on this point; in any event, the physician who seeks to recover his fee through the courts should have his case well defined as regards his employment, the number of his visits and the condition for which he treated the patient.

If a physician is summoned to treat a minor or an individual, such as the employee of a corporation, who does not assume the financial responsibility himself, care should be taken to ascertain who is legally bound to compensate the medical attendant for his services. Ordinarily, a father is liable for the medical care of his minor children, or a husband for the medical care of his wife. If a couple are separated or divorced, the courts may adjudicate the matter and may decide that the financial arrangement in the case of a separation, or the alimony in the case of a divorce may be sufficient to cover medical expenses and may direct payment of the medical bill.

Industrial organizations are responsible for the welfare of their employees insofar as injuries, poisonings and diseases which are directly connected with employment are concerned. It is customary for the employer to carry workmen's compensation insurance for this eventuality, and in the great majority of cases, medical fees are paid to the physician by the insurance carrier, representing the employer. An employer is not responsible in law for the medical expenses of an employee who is suffering from a disease or injury unconnected with his employment. The workman's compensation laws in most states and in federal jurisdictions have provisions regulating the medical care of employees in industry. Some organizations provide emergency medical care in their plants and a few others voluntarily assume the medical expenses of their employees. The bureaus of industrial hygiene of the state and federal labor departments are concerned with conditions safeguarding the health of employees in industry.

If a physician responds to the call of some one who is not legally responsible for the patient, he may not be able to collect his just compensation for his services, unless the person who summons him, or the patient, declares his responsibility for the fee. In this connection a physician is not required by law to undertake the treatment of any case, even if an emergency exists and another medical man is not available.

If the physician signs an expressed contract which differs from the customary implied contract with the patient, he obligates himself to fulfill all the conditions set forth in that document. He must be very careful to understand what sort of obligations he assumes before he enters upon such a bargain, because the law will hold him strictly to the terms of the expressed contract. For example, if he agrees to heal a patient or forfeit his pay, the courts will deny him his compensation unless he effects a cure. If he enters upon such a contract with the purpose of obtaining an unfair advantage over a patient, the courts may set the contract aside. As a general rule, expressed contracts are not desirable, unless special circumstances justify their existence.

MALPRACTICE

Malpractice is the term applied to the wrongful or improper practice of medicine, which results in injury to the patient. For malpractice a physician may be liable under the criminal or civil law.

Criminal Malpractice. Criminal malpractice occurs whenever a physician, by his management of a case, has violated the penal law and has subjected himself to prosecution by the state. For example he is required to report to the police all cases of criminal violence which he is called upon to treat, and if he fails to do this, he commits a misdemeanor. It is also unlawful for a plastic surgeon to alter the features or destroy the finger prints of criminals for the purpose of making identification difficult. A doctor may be prosecuted if he wilfully falsifies a birth or death certificate, or prepares a fraudulent affidavit for any purpose, or wilfully attempts to conceal the nature of a criminal case.

A charge of criminal malpractice may be brought against a doctor because he has inflicted injury or death on a patient by methods of treatment which are wholly unjustified and dangerous. In such instances the prosecution is required to prove that the physician was cognizant of the dangerous and unjustifiable nature of his treatment at the time he administered it. Because of the difficulties in assembling such proof, many of these defendants escape conviction in the criminal courts, but they can be and usually are sued in the civil courts for civil malpractice. One variety of criminal malpractice occurs when a patient incurs injury or dies as the result of treatment given by a doctor while in a state of alcoholic intoxication; such treatment is usually the performance of a major surgical operation, the administration of a dangerous drug, or a bad mistake in therapy. If the patient dies the doctor can be charged with manslaughter in the second degree, the interpretation being that even though the intention of the physician was not to cause the death of the patient, his inexcusable negligence produced the same result (Section 1052 of Penal Law of New York State). Other types of criminal malpractice cases occur in the induction of illegal abortions, or the use of contraceptive measures, already discussed in Chapters 22 and 25.

Civil Malpractice. Civil malpractice is that type in which the physician has inflicted death or injury on the patient by his treatment, but at the same time has not violated any statute of the criminal law. While the state cannot prosecute him, the physician is liable to be sued for malpractice in the civil courts by the injured patient or his relatives who endeavor to obtain a money award as compensation for his suffering. The liability of the medical man is not decreased in such instances by the fact that the plaintiff is a charity patient or a nonpaying patient.

In most states there is a statute of limitations denoting the length of time after alleged malpractice in which a plaintiff may file an action against a defendant physician. Such statutes do not give a right of action, but restrict the period within which the right may be asserted. In New York, a malpractice action must be commenced within two years after the cause of action has accrued (Section 50 of the Civil Practice Act), and in other states the period varies from one to five years. The object of the statute of limitations is to suppress fradulent and stale claims and keep them from springing up long after the occurrence of the alleged event, when evidence may be lost, when facts may be obscured from defective memory or lapse of time, or when essential witnesses may have died or moved away. There is also a statute of limitations on the period in which a physician may file suit in order to obtain compensation for his professional services; in New York State, this is six years after the last service (Section 48 of the Civil Practice Act).

The case of Conklin vs Draper, 229 Appellate Division 227, affirmed without opinion 254 New York 620, illustrates a suit for malpractice which was barred because the action was not commenced within the statutory period. The defendant operated upon the plaintiff for appendicitis on May 27th 1925, leaving a pair of forceps in the plaintiff's abdominal cavity. In July 1927, the plaintiff was appraised of the instrument in her abdomen as the result of a roentgen ray picture, and had the forceps removed by a second surgical operation during July 1927. The attorney for the plaintiff filed a malpractice suit against the defendant on July 5th 1929, within two years after the discovery of the forceps, but more than two years after the operation during which that instrument had been enclosed in the abdomen. The ruling of the court was that the malpractice action was not filed within the statute of limitations and that the plaintiff was not entitled to recover damages as the result of unskillful treatment. In that same case, however, an action was brought against the defendant, based on the breach of an expressed contract in which the defendant was to furnish proper medical care to the plaintiff; the statute of limitations for breach of contract is six years and the court allowed that cause of action to stand. On the basis of the breach of contract, the plaintiff could sue to recover the sum paid to the operating surgeon and to recover such other medical expenses as were inflicted on the plaintiff as a result of the defendant's breach of contract.

A plea of malpractice must be established by the plaintiff patient who must offer proof to sustain his allegations. According to Hubert W. Smith, a valid court action for malpractice must prove the four following points: (1) that there was a duty due the plaintiff from the defendant physician (**duty**), (2) that a breach of that duty occurred (**dereliction**), (3) that the breach of duty was responsible for the damage (**direct causation**), and (4) that physical damage actually occurred (**damage**). If the plaintiff fails to prove any one of the four parts, his plea cannot be sustained. All malpractice suits are susceptible of being analyzed by this formula and their strengths and weaknesses discovered.

1. The idea of **duty** refers to the obligation in force whenever a physican treats a patient under the usual implied contract or under a special expressed contract. To prove **duty,** the plaintiff must show that the relationship of physician and patient existed between the defendant and himself at the time of the alleged malpractice. An example of the failure to prove **duty,** is the hypothetical case of a plaintiff who meets the defendant on a train, discovers accidentally that he is a doctor, and in the course of a casual conversation asks him to recommend a medicine to relieve headaches. The defendant mentions a certain drug as effective for that purpose. Later the plaintiff obtains the drug on his own initiative, uses it, and after a period of benefit, suffers untoward effects. He brings a malpractice suit against the defendant for the damages which he suffered, but is unable to prove **duty,** for the defendant had not been engaged by the plaintiff as a physician and had not accepted the responsibilities attached to that relationship. Under these circumstances the attorney for the defendant is justified in making a motion to have the plea dismissed after the plaintiff has presented his case, and the court would in all probability grant the motion for dismissal.

If the defendant on the other hand has accepted the role of a physician and is bound by the implied contract, he automatically assumes responsibility for any deleterious effects which might result from his treatment, and the question of **duty** is a proven fact. This conception would apply even in the case of a doctor who is near at hand during a highway accident and administers first aid to a badly injured victim; if he is so unlucky as to convert a simple fracture into a compound fracture by his manipulations, he assumes responsibility for that result because he undertakes to treat the victim. In spite of the urgent nature of the injuries and the humanitarian intentions which would inspire the medical man, the law holds that he would be bound by the implied contract in such a case. In the event of a malpractice action, the court and jury would consider each case according to the circumstances which were present at the time, and which might be sufficient justification for the doctor's treatment. When presented with an emergency of this sort, the doctor must decide what is the right thing to do, and certainly if he considers himself unable to cope with the problem presented, he should not offer his services and should refuse to take the responsibility if summoned. A doctor cannot be compelled by law to undertake the treatment of a case, even though an emergency may exist and no medical aid is available.

(2) The question of **dereliction of duty** is concerned with whether the

defendant applied to the treatment of the patient, the knowledge, skill, care and judgment which the average physician in that community would use under the same circumstances. The legal authorities must decide whether or not the defendant has shown deficiency in any of these necessary professional qualities while treating the case under consideration, because if proof of this deficiency is forthcoming, the physician can be charged with **dereliction of duty.** Deficiency in professional knowledge and skill must be proven by expert medical testimony which must show that the defendant disregarded established principles, held by the majority of the profession as necessary for the treatment of the disease under consideration and that such disregard produced the disability; also that proper adherence to the principles would have prevented the untoward result. The defendant of course may produce expert medical testimony to justify the method of treatment that he used.

Whether a proper amount of care was used or not, depends on whether the defendant was guilty of an error of commission, such as administering the wrong medicine through negligence, or of omission, such as neglecting to warn the patient against dangers which should have been foreseen, or in declaring a patient cured without taking due precautions. In the errors of omission belong also a number of considerations which are sometimes difficult to appraise properly; such as charging a doctor with negligence because he failed to order a roentgenogram to aid him in his diagnosis, or because he failed to refer the patient to a specialist or send him to a hospital when a complication developed which was difficult for the defendant to treat successfully, or because he failed to reveal to the patient or his relatives the real nature of the illness as a precautionary measure against future complications. The plaintiff must prove negligence by showing that the defendant was guilty of an error and that this error harmed the patient, which must be done by introducing expert medical testimony. If the defence can introduce testimony to show that contributory negligence on the part of the patient, such as his failure to cooperate in the treatment, was responsible for the damage, the case for the plaintiff may be weakened or even defeated. The burden of proof in this connection is on the defendant and must be introduced in his part of the testimony; such proof might not absolve the defendant of responsibility if the plaintiff can show that the damage to the patient was originally the result of the negligence of the defendant.

Contributory negligence may be defined as the failure of a patient to use reasonable care for his own welfare so that his ill-considered behavior while under a doctor's care is a real factor in producing an unfortunate therapeutic result. Thus if a surgeon, summoned to treat a fracture of the radius, desires to have a roentgen ray picture taken as a necessary aid in diagnosis and treatment, but is prevented by the patient who refuses to give his consent, such refusal could be claimed by the defense to be an example of contributory negligence on the part of the plaintiff. In the event that a poor result followed the doctor's treatment, the defense of contributory negligence would probably defeat the plaintiff's plea of malpractice.

The allegation that a physician failed to use his best judgment for the welfare of the patient, is encountered rarely as when a medical man adopts wrongful methods of treatment through gross carelessness, ignorance, malice or while intoxicated. This question has been considered under the heading of criminal malpractice.

The following hypothetical case illustrates a malpractice suit which fails to prove dereliction of duty. A concert violinist falls and sustains fractures of the bones of his left wrist and forearm. The defendant physician sets the fractures, and after they are firmly knit, the plaintiff finds a disability of the left hand which interferes with his playing of the violin. The plaintiff files a malpractice suit against the defendant, offering testimony from his fellow musicians that he has lost the delicate fingering necessary for playing his instrument successfully, and also medical testimony of the actual damage inflicted on the left hand. In the event of a motion by defense counsel, the court would dismiss the claim against the defendant, as dereliction of duty was not proved by the testimony offered by the plaintiff, for there was no expert medical testimony indicating that the damage to the left hand was the result of any wrongful treatment on the part of the defendant. The mere fact that the disability is present is not sufficient, because a doctor is not required to guarantee that his treatment will be successful, only that he will use proper methods of treatment.

The question of the liability of a physician for the acts of persons associated with him arises not infrequently. If nurses and attendants employed by a surgeon, are negligent in the performance of their duty and harm results to the patient, the surgeon is liable for their dereliction. Thus if a laparotomy is performed, and a nurse employed by the surgeon fails to make a correct sponge count, and as a result a sponge is left in the abdominal cavity, the surgeon must accept the responsibility for her acts. The same rule applies if the physician is operating a private hospital and employs nurses. However if a surgeon performs an operation in a hospital which is not owned or controlled by him, and is assisted by nurses employed by the hospital and not by him, he is not responsible for errors made by the nurse. Thus in the performance of a laparotomy, just before the abdomen is closed, the surgeon is required only to be sure that there was a correct sponge count and that all sponges were accounted for. If he was properly reassured on this point and in spite of this precaution a sponge was left in the abdomen due to the error of a nurse not in his employ, the surgeon cannot be justly charged with negligence.

If a physician treats a case with another physician jointly, he is responsible for any mistakes of his colleague, if he has agreed with him concerning the course of treatment. If he sends a substitute to a case he is treating himself, he must take the responsibility for the therapeutic measures administered by the substitute. On the other hand, if he recommends another physician who treats the patient independently, he is not liable for that physician's negligence.

(3) **Direct causation** means that a direct connection is established between the damage sustained by the patient and the lack of adequate skill or by the negligence displayed by the defendant in his diagnosis and treatment. Medical evidence given by duly qualified experts must establish the direct causation in any malpractice case. The chief difficulty in judging the proof showing direct causation lies in the proper evaluation of the causes assigned for the damage sustained by the patient. In some instances the cause is obvious as when a corrosive drug is injected into the rectum in mistake for a nonirritant enema, and causes a corrosive proctitis. In other cases the connection between an unfortunate result and an alleged fault in therapy cannot be decided so surely, for example, when a person who has been anesthetized previously a number of times with nitrous oxide for minor surgical operations without ill effects, dies suddenly under the same anesthetic. In such a case it would be difficult to prove faulty methods of treatment unless the anesthetist made an egregious blunder.

The following case is a good example of a plea which does not prove **direct causation.** A person was knocked unconscious in an automobile accident, and was examined later in coma by a police surgeon who, though he had been informed of the accident, made a diagnosis of acute alcoholism. Because of this the victim was kept in the police station overnight, and was not sent to the hospital for proper care. The next day he was released and was given medical treatment, but died seven days later as a result of a head injury. The plaintiff was the widow of the deceased who sued the police surgeon for malpractice and negligent treatment. Dereliction of duty was proved in this case, but what was not established was the fact that the damage occurred as the result of such dereliction of duty, for no expert medical evidence was introduced to prove that there was causal connection. Moreover the severity of the injury was such that there was no assurance that the wounded man would have recovered even if he had been given promptly the best care available.

(4) A few cases of malpractice are not proven because there is no proof that **physical damage** has been sustained. The hypothetical case given by Hubert W. Smith to illustrate this point is that of a pregnant woman who, feeling labor pains, summons an obstetrician. He arrives and finds that the case is progressing slowly. He says that he will be away for an hour and a half, and leaves, staying away for four hours. On his return he delivers the baby without any complication to mother or child. Later the mother, as plaintiff, sues the defendant for mental anguish sustained because of his unjustifiable absence. Inasmuch as mental anguish without **physical damage** is too unsubstantial a condition to warrant a reasonable judgment against a defendant, the court would probably dismiss the complaint against the defendant.

The question might arise in this type of case especially if there is an expressed contract between doctor and patient whether the dereliction of duty is a breach of contract, in which event the defendant might be assessed nominal damages and court costs even though actual injury to the patient was not proved. According to Smith, most courts would try all malpractice pleas based on the implied contract as torts, and disregard the conception of breach of contract; in these cases actual injury to the patient must be proved by the plaintiff, and if he wins his case he is entitled to exemplary or punitive damages. If the malpractice suit is based upon a special expressed contract, the dereliction of duty is a technical matter and the defendant can be judged guilty of breach of contract and assessed nominal damages. On the other hand if the plaintiff can prove dereliction of duty, direct causation and damage, the defendant would be guilty of a tort as well as of a breach of contract and may be assessed an exemplary award.

The plaintiff must plead to all four parts of the malpractice claim, and he must offer proof at the trial of what he actually pleads and not attempt to bring out any evidence additional to his plea. The court may refuse to allow such evidence to be offered if defense counsel objects. Unless the plaintiff can obtain from the court permission to file a trial amendment to make his plea conform to the proposed proof, he can lose his case because of an insufficient original pleading in advance of the trial. The practice of the courts in these matters varies considerably.

Some malpractice suits are brought by the patient because the physician has brought a civil action to recover the amount of his medical bill. The patient then brings a countersuit alleging malpractice, and attempts to recover damages and defeat the suit of the physician. This purpose can only be accomplished by the patient if he has a real case of malpractice and can prove it. Most courts consider the medical contract in its entirety and the proven dereliction of the physician at any time during the treatment will defeat his chance of collecting his fee.

The testimony offered by either side in a malpractice suit, if it is based on a claim of negligence, must fulfill its burden of proof. If the evidence offered by the plaintiff is so insufficient that reasonable men could not find a verdict on it, the trial court by a timely motion of the other side can prevent consideration of the case by the jury and instruct a verdict for the defendant. On the other hand, if the plaintiff presents strong proof which the defense cannot contradict in its evidence, so that a reasonable person cannot hold a contrary opinion, the judge is empowered to instruct a verdict for the plaintiff. If a presiding justice concedes having made an error in a trial, he can rectify the error by ordering a new trial. In court actions in which the verdict is appealed, the appeal court can also set aside the verdict, or reverse it and remand the case for a new trial, if the evidence was not substantial enough to justify the verdict.

A prima facie case in a malpractice action is one in which the direct evidence as presented and not contradicted or rebutted by the defense is sufficient to prove the claim of the plaintiff. As an example, if the plaintiff's testimony shows that the doctor-patient relationship was valid and that the doctor performed a laparotomy and left an instrument in the abdominal cavity of the patient, a prima facie case is established, and unless the defense can controvert the evidence the plaintiff would be entitled to a favorable decision. In some malpractice cases of this type, the doctrine of *res ipsa loquitur* or, the thing speaks for itself, is held to be applicable; thus, the evidence put forward by the plaintiff, showing that a surgical instrument was left in the abdomen has advanced the plaintiff's cause to the point where the case will not be dismissed at the end of the evidence, and the burden of proof is put on the defendant who must explain or controvert the plaintiff's testimony. The types of cases to which *res ipsa loquitur* applies are: (1) leaving instruments or sponges in a body cavity; (2) administering a poison mistakenly; (3) failure to use roentgen rays or to require their use before setting certain types of fracture; (4) causing burns by the use of roentgen rays; (5) causing burns by heat or electric treatment.

The doctrine of *res ipsa loquitur* is not necessarily helpful to a plaintiff, its efficacy depending on the evidence in the individual case. Before the doctrine can apply, it must be clear that the cause of the injury was solely under the control of the physician or his employee. Usually a physician can explain most of his acts, or he may find his best defense in showing contributory negligence on the part of the patient. For example, a patient undergoing baking treatment for disease of a joint was cautioned to notify the doctor or the attendant if the treated area felt too hot; but the patient having formed an idea that heat was good for the joint failed to follow instructions and received a bad burn. In such a case the failure to notify the operator would be considered contributory negligence which might invalidate a plea of malpractice.

In some malpractice actions, when the evidence on both sides is not conclusive, the plaintiff and defendant may reach an agreement on a settlement, after which the plaintiff signs an instrument in writing known as a release, absolving the defendant from all claims brought in that particular suit.

Most civil malpractice suits are included in the following categories: treatment of a fracture giving a bad result; surgical treatment attended by an anesthetic death, or a postoperative death, or a bad result due to instruments or sponges left in a body cavity; obstetric treatment; serum injection followed by death; administration of toxic drugs in mistake for nontoxic drugs; negligent use of roentgen rays, of thermic or electric apparatus, or of radium.

Fatalities Following Surgical Operations. The Reports of the Chief Medical Examiner from 1918 to 1941 indicate that a yearly average of 65 cases die as a result of postoperative shock combined with the toxic effect of the anesthetic; an average of three cases a year die as a result of some form of postoperative hemorrhage; an average of one to two a year die of some form of postoperative sepsis. Isolated cases of other postoperative complications occur such as pulmonary embolism, delirium tremens, massive collapse of the lung or hyperthyroidism following a goiter operation.

Fatalities following surgical operations are routinely reported to the Office of the Chief Medical Examiner when the patient dies during the procedure or within a few hours after the operation, because during that period the toxic action of the anesthetic is effective and may be a possible cause of death. If the patient survives the operation 24 hours or over, the toxic action of the anesthetic is less likely to be an important factor; comparatively few postoperative deaths of the delayed type are reported to the Chief Medical Examiner, and the death certificate is issued by the attending doctor. The statistics of the Chief Medical Examiner thus include only a portion of the total number of operative and postoperative deaths; furthermore they are limited to surgical operations performed for the purpose of alleviating or correcting natural disease conditions and do not include abortions of any type, illegal operations, or operations performed because of complications following traumatic injury.

One uncommon type of operative fatality is that due to a **surgical procedure** which creates a condition directly responsible for death. For example, faulty use of the esophagoscope may produce a perforation of the wall of the esophagus near the tracheal bifurcation, circular or ovoid in shape, about 8 to 10 mm. in diameter, through which pathogenic bacteria invade the surrounding tissues and give rise to a suppurative mediastinitis. Similarly the passage of a sound or catheter into the bladder may perforate the fundus and cause a suppurative peritonitis. Sometimes during the administration of an enema, the anus or rectum may be lacerated and result in the development of a suppurative infection of the pelvis or abdomen. The dangers of trocar perforations of the brain during craniotomy, and of the perforation of the cribriform plate and of the laceration of the brain during a nasal curettage have been described on pages 303 and 351 respectively. Asphyxia from the aspiration of food into the air passages during anesthesia, and asphyxia due to the impaction of a piece of gauze in the larynx following a tonsillectomy are described on page 480. Fatal effects produced by the mistaken injection of corrosive or toxic drugs into the subcutaneous tissues or various body orifices is discussed on pages 619 and 711. Accidents connected with the administration of anesthetics are discussed on pages 792 and 793.

The majority of operative and postoperative deaths are not so much ascribable to faults of omission or commission on the part of the surgeon or anesthetist, as to **ordinary dangers inherent in all surgical procedures.** Any type of operation may be a definite hazard to the life of the patient, but those involving the chest, abdomen, head and neck are especially dangerous because of their length and severity. Most cases of death in the operative or early postoperative stages are the result of **surgical shock** combined with the **toxic action of the anesthetic;** in some cases one factor may predominate, in other cases the other, but they must be considered together as it is impossible to separate their action.

In addition the patient may be the victim of disease processes which may be so serious as to reduce his vital resistance and render him susceptible to operative shock and the other noxious influences attending the operation. Some of these disease processes are (1) surgical conditions which demand operative intervention for their alleviation, and (2) severe constitutional diseases not connected with the need for surgical operation.

1. The surgical conditions which may be a contributory cause of death in abdominal operations are perforated duodenal ulcer, suppurative conditions of the gallbladder or appendix, acute pancreatitis, calculi impacted in the common bile duct, calculi impacted in the ureter, incarcerated hernias, intestinal obstruction, mesenteric artery thrombosis with gangrene of the intestines, malignant neoplasms in the abdomen, and other processes. A laparotomy performed upon a patient with a severe lesion of the above-mentioned types may result in the sudden death of the patient at the time of the operation because of the lowered resistance induced by the disease. Similarly operations on the chest for such conditions as lung abscesses, areas of tuberculosis, or bronchial carcinomas may result in an operative death. Occasionally the removal of the thyroid body in a case of Graves disease may bring about a fatal attack of hyperthyroidism. Craniotomies performed on cases of intracerebral neoplasm, brain abscesses or chronic subdural hematomas may be attended by an operative death because the intracranial pressure induced by the disease had reached a dangerous height when the operation was undertaken.

2. A serious constitutional disease of cardiac, pulmonary, hepatic or renal origin may render an individual susceptible to the various stresses of a surgical operation, so that a patient may die during or after a comparatively uncomplicated surgical procedure. A well-developed case of chronic alcoholism is also a poor operative risk inasmuch as the patient requires a large quantity of a general anesthetic such as ether to produce proper narcosis, and he may succumb to its toxic action. Another postoperative complication which may develop in cases of chronic alcoholism is an attack of delirium tremens, often fatal.

Post operative hemorrhage may occur as the result of an accidental injury to a large blood vessel during the manipulation, or it may occur as a delayed hemorrhage due to the slipping of a ligature from a large blood vessel, or from the erosion of a blood vessel by secondary infection and inflammation. Sometimes in tonsillectomy operations on middle aged individuals, the raw area in the throat may ooze blood in sufficient quantity to cause death, most of which is usually swallowed into the stomach. Other postoperative gastrointestinal hemorrhages may occur as a result of lesions already present in the tract, such as duodenal ulcers, or esophageal varices accompanying liver cirrhosis, or from blood dyscrasias of temporary or constitutional nature.

Individuals who survive the immediate effects of the operation may develop a secondary infection, usually in the area of operation. If a laparotomy is performed for a suppurative appendicitis or cholecystitis, an acute suppurative peritonitis may occur about two days after operation from the septic process in the viscus. In other cases, the infection may enter the abdomen either before or after the laparotomy through an opening or ulceration in a hollow viscus; in a few cases the infection may enter the abdomen from the skin surface. In similar fashion operations on the chest or cranial cavity may cause a fatal septic infection in these spaces, either because they have encouraged the spread of microorganisms already present, or carried pathogenic bacteria into the cavity.

In a few instances, the connection of the postoperative infection with the surgical procedure may be explained only on the basis of an area of lessened resistance, created by the operation. In one case an enlarged thyroid of the Hashimoto type was removed from a white woman of 48 years, and in less than 24 hours she developed an acute septic laryngitis from which she died 48 hours postoperatively. In this case the operation cannot be ignored as a possible factor in the development of the laryngeal infection. In another case, a man of 45 years had an inguinal hernia corrected under intraspinal anesthesia with procaine, and in three days developed a fatal pneumococcic meningitis for which there was no apparent source. It was believed that, as a result of the intraspinal injection of procaine, the meninges were rendered less resistant to pathogenic microorganisms in the nasal or otic bony sinuses and so allowed the meningitis to develop by invasion from those foci. It was not considered probable that the pneumococci were injected with the procaine. In all postoperative septic infections, the connection of the infection with the operation must be reviewed carefully in determining the question of causal relationship.

Postoperative pneumonia may follow the administration of a general anesthetic, and usually occurs a few days after the operation. It may take the form of a simple hypostatic pneumonia, or it may be an inhalation pneumonia with abscess formation following the aspiration of food or other foreign material into the air passages. In some cases a hypostatic pneumonia may develop in individuals who have a lowered vitality because of a severe chronic disease condition.

Some postoperative deaths of patients who are severely ill of a chronic disease condition may simply be due to the failure of the patient to react successfully against his chronic illness because of the shock of the operation so that he dies from complications naturally produced by the disease. Thus a patient with chronic cardiovalvular lesions may develop a fatal cardiac decompensation, or a patient with diabetes mellitus may sink into diabetic coma, or a chronic alcoholic patient may be afflicted with delirium tremens.

The formation of bland thromboses in the femoral and pelvic veins with fatal pulmonary embolism is another postoperative complication which develops in from one to three weeks, usually after abdominal and pelvic operations. This complication may be referable to a generalized slowing of the venous circulation from such a condition as cardiac or pulmonary disease, or is referable to a local interference with the venous circulation in the lower extremities, both of which conditions predispose to bland thrombus formation. Coronary artery thrombosis or cerebral artery thrombosis may develop in a few postoperative cases as in traumatic ones (page 156). The possibility of air embolism or fat embolism after operative procedures is discussed on pages 106 and 172.

Deaths following other therapeutic procedures, such as thermic therapy, electric therapy, roentgen ray therapy, injection of foreign protein, injection of drugs, blood transfusions and many others have been discussed in previous chapters devoted to those subjects. Surgical operations on traumatic cases have been discussed in the chapters on physical trauma.

Thoracotomy for cardiac massage is performed on individuals who suddenly collapse during an operation with cessation of respiratory movements and heart beat. The left chest is entered by a lateral transverse incision through the fourth or fifth interspace, the pericardium is incised and the hand is introduced into the chest and massages the heart rhythmically. In most cases the patient remains dead but in a few instances he may be revived for a few hours. He finally dies of anoxemia from deficient oxygenation of the blood which produces necrotic lesions in the brain.

The authors have seen a case of this type in a white woman, 57 years old, who fell and sustained a depressed fracture of her left tibia near the knee. Two weeks after the injury an operation was performed to clean up the area of fracture and the patient collapsed during the anesthesia. Cardiac massage and other restorative measures were applied and the heart and respiration began to function once more. The patient remained in coma for 77 days, finally dying of a bronchopneumonia. The autopsy disclosed wide spread anoxic lesions in the brain, appearing as patchy glioses and areas of atrophy in the cerebral and cerebellar cortex, ill-defined areas of softening, vascularization and glioses in the white matter of the cerebrum, distention of small vessels and occlusion by hyaline thrombi, and vascularization and softening of the basal nuclei. The cerebral arteries, pons, medulla and spinal cord were natural. The brain lesions were similar to those described by Courville in delayed nitrous oxide poisoning. The heart showed a moderately severe coronary arteriosclerosis and an obliterative fibrous pericarditis. A necrotic cystitis, a suppurative pyelonephritis and a terminal bronchopneumonia were also present. There were no decubital skin lesions.

Tracheotomy is an emergency operation performed upon an individual who has developed an obstruction in his upper air passages, and consists in an incision into the trachea and the introduction of a cannula to allow air to reach the lungs. This operation is sometimes necessary in natural disease conditions such as syphilitic laryngitis, laryngeal diphtheria, or carcinoma of the larynx which may close the air passages, and also in some traumatic injuries of the larynx when asphyxia is imminent (pages 309 and 474). In some of these emergency cases, the immediate danger of asphyxia may be averted and the patient may eventually recover; in others the victim may succumb to asphyxia. In rare instances the condition has been wrongly diagnosed by the physician who has mistaken a pneumonia complicated by cyanosis for an obstruction of the air passages and has performed a tracheotomy on such an erroneous assumption.

The duty of a pathologist or medical examiner in an operative death is to perform a complete autopsy and pursue such additional investigations of toxicologic, microscopic, serologic or bacteriologic nature as are necessary for that particular case. It is wise for such an investigator to be reticent in expressing his opinion about a case of this type, and to base it strictly on his objective findings at autopsy or on the results of the additional investigations mentioned above.

Other Legal Liabilities of Physicians. As a result of his professional activities a physician may incur liabilities which, strictly speaking, are not malpractice. Most of these liabilities are torts, some requiring the physician-patient relationship for their commission, while others might occur either outside or inside that relationship.

One variety of tort is the negligent behavior of a doctor during his professional duties toward a person not the patient, as a result of which the third person suffers damage. As an example, a doctor is called in to treat a patient with an infected wound, and he requests the patient's wife to assist him in dressing it; he not only fails to warn her that she might become infected but on the contrary tells her that there is no danger. The wife assists the doctor, and, because of contact with the wound, develops an infected hand through a scratch on her finger. The physician is liable for this untoward outcome because he neglected to warn her of the dangers involved in dressing an infected wound.

The tort of battery or of touching another without consent occurs when the physician performs an unauthorized operation on a patient or conducts a physical examination against the patient's expressed desire. Such an act is considered an invasion of another's personality, and this is not sanctioned by the law. A physician cannot call a consultant, order a roentgen ray examination or other laboratory test, send a patient to a hospital, or perform an operation without the consent of the patient. In all cases where an operation is considered necessary, the written consent of the patient to the operation must be obtained, or if the patient is a minor, the written consent of his parent or guardian. This permission allows the surgeon to perform only a necessary operation, and if he performs an unnecessary or even an additional one, he exposes himself to a legal action for damages. The only exception is when an emergency arises with an unconscious or helpless individual, and the medical man must assume responsibility for the patient's welfare; then he can operate without the consent of the patient.

The tort known as false imprisonment occurs when an individual is put under duress and detained against his will without legal justification. This is a situation which is not often encountered, but it is conceivable that it might arise if a person in the early stages of insanity is put into a mental institution for observation. Unless he was held there by a court order or by regular commitment papers, and was obviously in need of restraint or medical attention, he could not be detained if he desired his freedom.

The question of slander or libel would arise if a negligent and incorrect diagnosis of such a condition as gonorrhea, syphilis, drug addiction, alcoholism or pregnancy is made by a doctor and communicated to others. The competent, well-intentioned physician is not liable to make such a blunder, but it is well for either a clinician or a laboratory worker to consider carefully the evidence which supports a diagnosis of this type in any given case, and to be very cautious about committing himself unless he has the fullest possible proof for his opinion. If a medical man gave a wrong diagnosis of a venereal disease through negligence, he could be sued for slander if he expressed his opinion verbally, and for libel if he put it in writing.

Interference with custodian or property rights of a person refers to the performance of unauthorized autopsies and will be discussed under that head. It may also include failure to preserve an amputated arm or leg for the family of the deceased who have a right to bury such a limb with the body of the patient if he dies shortly after the amputation. In New York City, if the patient survives, the leg is buried under a special certificate, unless the patient gives written consent for the hospital to dissect it, and then dispose of it.

Failure to disclose pertinent facts about his illness to a patient or his nearest relatives would constitute breach of trust or actual fraud, depending on the conditions present in the individual case. Commission of such a tort lays the physician open to a charge of negligence or one more serious. The doctor who committed an act of criminal malpractice against a patient would also lay himself open to a liability action for the tort involved in such an act.

Other civil suits against the physician are brought because his behavior has caused the patient pain or distress. The physician occupies a privileged position in relation to his practice, and it is one which requires tactful handling. It is safe to say that if he displays a proper consideration for the patient's feelings, he will not often incur this type of legal action.

The precaution should be taken of having a woman nurse present at the examination of a woman patient. If circumstances do not allow this, then a female relative of the patient, or a woman friend will serve the purpose. In conducting gynecologic examinations or operations under general anesthesia on a woman, it is necessary to have a woman nurse present, not only to reassure the patient of the regularity of the procedure, but also to protect the physician's reputation. Some woman under general anesthesia may experience erotic sensations and bring sincere though erroneous charges of misconduct against the doctor.

A minor act which is occasionally a source of a liability suit is the introduction without the consent of the patient of any person not a qualified physician, nurse or medical student into the room where the patient is being examined. A similar infringement of the patient's rights is the publication of a case report in a medical journal without concealing the identity of the patient. This would apply especially to the publication of a recognizable photograph of the subject. In the majority of instances the photograph can be rendered unrecognizable without materially affecting the demonstration of the lesion in question.

The physician should keep accurate and clear records of his cases, carefully noting dates of visits, symptoms, signs, diagnoses and courses of treatment. Needless to say, these records should be kept in a private receptacle accessible to the physician alone, and should not be disclosed without the consent of the patient, unless they are subpoenaed by court order. These considerations are pertinent to the subject of privileged communications.

Any doctor entering into practice should safeguard himself against civil suits, not only by observing the obvious precautions against them as far as his professional conduct is concerned, but also by taking out liability insurance. If he is threatened with a malpractice action, he should engage competent legal advice. In New York City and in most other jurisdictions, the County Medical Society furnishes legal defense for its members, and gives them an opportunity to obtain liability insurance from a reputable company at reasonable rates.

PRIVILEGED COMMUNICATIONS

Information furnished a physician by a patient, which is intended to serve as a guide for treatment, is considered confidential, and is technically known as a privileged communication. In many jurisdictions of the United States, New York among others, privileged communications are declared inviolable by statute, and they must not be revealed by the physician. The prohibition also applies to dentists, to nurses, to internes who are treating a patient under the direction of a licensed physician, and to hospital records. The patient, or his personal representative if he is deceased, has the power to waive the restrictions implied by confidential communications if it serves his purpose, but the physician cannot exercise that right nor can a third person. The privileged communication cannot be waived by contract, as in waivers which were formerly inserted in life or accident insurance policies, but later were made invalid by statute.

The prohibition in privileged communications is against disclosure of information acquired while attending a patient, and embraces statements made by the patient, and facts obtained by observation or physical examination. Privilege may only be claimed where the physician-patient relationship exists; it is in force, however, in cases in which a doctor attends an unconscious person in an emergency, even when he has not been formally employed by the patient. A plaintiff can only urge the question of privileged communications if the physician is duly licensed to practice his profession.

A physician cannot reveal any facts told to him by a patient, if the treatment is based on those facts, but in the event that the patient is unconscious and a third person relates the same facts to the doctor, the communication is not considered privileged. Information related by the patient which has no connection with the curative treatment is not privileged. For example, if the patient has a tibial fracture, it is not necessary for the surgeon to know how the fracture was sustained in order to treat it successfully, so that if the patient tells the surgeon how he was injured, that communication is not privileged and may be disclosed. In a criminal trial a court may compel a doctor to reveal a privileged communication, if its content is necessary to serve the ends of justice. In any trial, the question of privileged communications is determined by the legal authorities, and if no objection is raised the physician may answer the question with propriety. The proper objection is that the witness is incompetent to testify to the facts demanded, not that his testimony is incompetent. In any event it is not the duty of the medical witness to assert an objection.

It is often to the advantage of a plaintiff to sign a release waiving the right of privileged communication, especially in claims against insurance companies where the medical evidence favors the plaintiff's case, for then such a waiver may expedite a settlement. In some instances the plaintiff may waive the privilege in open court and call in a doctor as witness; by this the privilege in this particular case is waived permanently for all purposes and any physician may testify in the case. However, the plaintiff may prevent the introduction of testimony which would disgrace the patient, especially in a death case.

Public records relating to the illness of a patient are not privileged. The information obtained at autopsy is not privileged and can be disclosed by any physician except the doctor who has treated the patient; this is because the information acquired at autopsy may have pertinent relationship with the therapeutic measures of the attending physician. Privileged communications are legal in the United States only in jurisdictions where they are established by a definite statute, while other jurisdictions do not recognize them. They are not mentioned in the common law. Privileged communications are not recognized in the laws of foreign countries.

LIABILITY OF HOSPITALS

The liability of a hospital for injuries sustained by a patient because of the negligence of a hospital employee depends on whether the hospital is operated for profit or is a charitable institution. Generally the hospital operated for profit is responsible for torts committed by its employees. In the case of a charitable institution the theory has been, that it is not liable for negligence of its employees, which has resulted in harm to paying patients or to charity patients. Usually the only redress for the injured patient is to bring suit against the negligent employee as defendant. Civil actions for damages, however, based on injuries which resulted in the deaths of patients, have been entered against charitable hospitals in New York City, and some of them have been won by plaintiffs.

A hospital conducted for profit, whether incorporated or not, is liable for ordinary care towards its patients, and it can be sued for any injuries to them, resulting from negligence of its employees. If a physician or a surgeon has charge of a hospital employee, such as a nurse for one of his cases, he, as well as the hospital, is liable for any negligence of the nurse. Whether or not the hospital is liable for the negligence of a physician in its employ depends upon the contract of the physician with the hospital or the relation of the claimant to the hospital. In some jurisdictions, these matters of liability are decided, either by a referee in a preliminary hearing or by the court at the time of trial.

A hospital is liable if persons not patients have suffered injury because of the negligence of hospital employees. Such injury may result from an unauthorized autopsy on a deceased patient which caused mental anguish to his relatives. In order to protect themselves against civil actions of this nature, hospitals should obtain a written consent from the nearest relative of the deceased before performing the autopsy.

Liability for an Autopsy. Autopsies are divided into two categories.

The first includes autopsies performed by a medical man acting in an official capacity, such as a medical examiner or a physician appointed by a coroner. This procedure has the sanction of the law, and the official in charge has the power to overrule the objections of the relatives of the deceased. Such an official, however, cannot perform an autopsy on a case which does not come under his jurisdiction without exposing himself, like any other pathologist, to the dangers of a legal action for damages.

The second group includes autopsies undertaken for scientific purposes by any qualified physician or pathologist, and such dissections are performed only when the nearest relative of the deceased has given consent in writing. The relative can limit the extent of the autopsy and insist that all organs be returned to the body for burial. If the autopsy is performed without the consent of the relative, a civil suit for damages can be brought against the hospital or the pathologist or both. The plea usually alleged in suits against the person or persons performing the supposedly unauthorized autopsy is that the property rights of the plaintiff in the dead body have been invaded wrongfully. Special emphasis may be put on the mutilation of the remains and on the retention of the organs by the pathologist after the autopsy as a further aggravation of this offense.

DYING DECLARATIONS

Dying declarations are statements made about the cause and circumstances of a homicide by the victim, under the conviction that he is about to die and cannot recover. Such allegations, if properly witnessed, may be used as evidence in criminal trials for homicide. The statement is introduced by testimony of the individual who took the dying declaration and who is subject to direct and cross examination on this point. A dying declaration cannot be used in a civil action and is not admissible if the patient recovers.

Occasionally a doctor may be the only person available who can take a dying declaration, and it should be his responsibility to put the statement in the proper form. The doctor should have the patient state, in so many words, his belief that he is about to die and cannot recover, and then the exact words of the dying man's story should be taken down. If the patient is too weak to talk, his story may be given in answer to questions by appropriate signs indicating yes, or no. A dying declaration may also be obtained in writing and should be signed by the declarant.

Dying declarations are admitted on the ground that belief in impending death is equivalent to the sanction of an oath, and the persons making them are considered in the light of witnesses and stand in the same situation as if they were sworn. It is essential that the declarant be in extremis at the time of his statement and that he fully expects to die and is without hope of recovery. The statement is not invalidated by the fact that death is postponed longer than had been anticipated. However if the declarant had the slightest hope of recovery at the time he made his statement, the declaration would not be admissible as evidence. It is also necessary that the dying declaration should be competent testimony of the homicide itself, made by a victim who would be competent to testify if he were alive. Any narrative of past events or statements not concerned with the actual crime are not admissible as evidence.

A woman dying as the result of a criminal abortion may give a dying declaration, in which case specific information should be obtained from the patient as to whether or not there had been any vaginal bleeding immediately prior to the time that she submitted herself to the abortionist. A statement that there had been no prior bleeding would then refute the false allegation frequently made by an abortionist that the deceased was already bleeding when she arrived at his office.

A dying statement made by a person not a victim cannot be considered a dying declaration, as in the case of People vs. Becker, 215 New York 126, when one of the defendants who shot Rosenthal for hire declared immediately before his execution, that as far as he knew Becker had nothing to do with the homicide. The Court of Appeals held that this statement was not admissible.

REFERENCES

Herzog, A. W.   Medical Jurisprudence, Indianapolis, the Bobbs-Merrill Co., 1931.
Reese, J. J.   Textbook of Medical Jurisprudence and Toxicology, 8th ed., revised by D. J. McCarthy, Philadelphia, P. Blakiston's Son and Co., 1911.
Smith, H. W.   Legal responsibility for medical malpractice, J.A.M.A., 116:2670, 1941.
Weinmann, G. H.   A Survey of the Laws Concerning Dead Human Bodies, National Research Council, Bull. No. 73, December 1929.

39

Insanity

Insanity can be defined as a disease of the mind or the personality which discloses itself in the form of a derangement of the mental or emotional processes. The intelligence is weakened or perverted, but the insane person may not show physical deterioration. The condition is of medico-legal significance because an individual who becomes insane may be a danger to the community.

The question in cases of insanity is whether or not the suspected individual is able to manage his affairs or, in other words, whether or not he is capable of civil responsibility. Each case must be considered by itself. Mere eccentricity and the belief in things which are palpably not true are not necessarily signs of insanity, and many persons of that description can perform their civil duties satisfactorily. However, the mental disorder may lead the individual into courses full of peril and distress for himself and his friends and cause him to commit antisocial acts against the community. Under these circumstances, it is desirable that such a person should be restrained in some way, inasmuch as he is liable under the civil law for any torts which he may commit, even when his mind is unsound.

In cases concerning business contracts, marriage, divorce and the making of wills and testaments, insanity may be a factor. The questions involved are complicated and hinge on whether or not the individual can be proved to have been of unsound mind at the time he assumed the contract, made his will or married.

There are times when it becomes necessary to commit a person to an insane asylum. The method for accomplishing this varies in different states, but the principles involved are the same.

If an individual develops signs of insanity in New York City, the Psychopathic Division of the Department of Hospitals through the agency of the police will send an ambulance to remove the insane person promptly to the psychiatric division of Bellevue Hospital or Kings County Hospital. He is held for a period of observation limited to 30 days, during which time the mental condition of the patient must be diagnosed and a decision made as to whether he is to be discharged or committed to an institution.

Sometimes a complaint is made to a magistrate concerning the actions of a psychopathic individual and, if sufficient evidence is offered, the magistrate issues a commitment sending him to the psychiatric hospital for observation. A relative or a roommate of a suspected insane individual, or a licensed physician, or a peace officer, or a representative of an incorporated charitable society may apply to the hospital for his commitment. The alleged insane person and also his relatives must be notified of this petition.

The patient must be examined jointly by two licensed physicians of three years' standing duly qualified as examiners in lunacy, neither of whom is a relative of the patient or in any way connected with the state hospital of commitment. If they find the patient mentally sick they file a certificate of lunacy which states explicitly that he is mentally sick and a proper subject for custody in an institution. The petition and the certificate are then taken before a Justice of the Supreme Court or a Judge of a Court of Record, who orders the individual committed to an appropriate hospital or to the care of his friends or his relatives. If the alleged insane person demands a hearing it must be held before the judge or a referee appointed by the judge who, when he has heard all the evidence, gives his decision.

The documents in the case—petition, certificate, order directing a hearing, decision of judge and order of commitment—must be presented to the superintendent of the hospital when the patient is committed. He forwards copies to the State Department of Mental Hygiene.

The superintendent of the hospital can refuse to admit the patient if the papers are not in order or if the person is not mentally sick within the meaning of the statute.

Needless to say, it is a serious proposition to declare an individual insane and relegate him to an asylum. The medical man who undertakes this task should be conversant with the subject and extremely careful in making his diagnosis.

The question of insanity also arises in criminal trials when a plea is advanced that the defendant, charged with a certain crime, committed it while insane. The defendant, in such instances, must be shown so unsound of mind that he is incapable of distinguishing between right and wrong for this contention to carry any legal weight. Generally, whenever this plea is advanced, the courts appoint alienists to examine the prisoner for sanity. Alienists may be called by both sides, and in such cases the expert testimony is conflicting. It is to be noted that this criterion is not a medical one, and is radically different from the considerations leading to a hospital commitment.

The following description of the different forms of mental derangement is intended merely to outline the problem for the practitioner.

TYPES OF INSANITY

Idiocy and Imbecility. Idiocy is a state of arrested mental development amounting in many cases to a complete lack of understanding. It is not a mental disease or insanity, but a lack of native endowment. The condition is congenital and its basis is an original defective structure of the brain. The behavior level of the idiot is below that of an animal in many cases, and he is not able to care for himself without aid. Due to the fundamental defect of the central nervous system the idiot is capable of only slight improvement if any.

Imbecility is due to the same factor as idiocy, but the defects are not so marked. The mentality of the imbecile is a trifle higher than that of the idiot, but not sufficient to permit him complete freedom of action. Aside from a certain amount of habit training the imbecile is not improvable.

Both idiocy and imbecility can be classed as entirely irresponsible mental states, and unless such cases can be individually supervised they belong in a separate institution for the care and training of mental defectives.

A moron is a feebleminded person of considerably higher intelligence than an imbecile or an idiot, but his intellectual faculties and judgment are not so well developed as in normal individuals. He can carry on the routine duties in civilized society as long as the demands made upon his mental capacity are not too discretionary. Morons are generally amenable to the customs of the community and they do not present any problem, unless their age discrepancy or emotional instability makes them sex delinquents or the tools of others.

Idiots and imbeciles at necropsy, show in the central nervous systems malformations of greater or lesser degree, such as smallness of the brain, porencephaly, absence or faulty development of different parts of the brain, or congenital hydrocephalus. Malformations of face or eyes, tongue, palate, nose and ears occasionally occur. Many of these individuals die sooner or later of secondary bronchopheumonia or other terminal infections.

Morons, on the other hand, do not necessarily show abnormal lesions of the central nervous system, and the findings at necropsy generally are not distinctive of the mental condition.

Dementia Praecox. Dementia praecox is an insanity which becomes apparent in individuals from the stage of adolescence to about the age of 30. It may occur sporadically in families whose history is not peculiar in any way, but it is more apt to develop in a person who has a family with a history of similar mental disease. This type of insanity is also called schizophrenia, a term which signifies the splitting or dissociation of the personality; this is a characteristic feature of the disease.

The basis of the process is an arrest of mentality on the childish adolescent plane. The individual's ego is ill developed, he regresses to a dream world and is thus not robust enough to stand the stress and strain of adult life. It is more a lack of vitality of the personality than anything else; some cases of dementia praecox deteriorate in mental power, but others possess brilliant mental attainments. In all of them, however, the mental equipment is ill-balanced and unstable.

The manifestations of dementia praecox are variable. Some of the patients show a dementia, with decay of the mentality, lack of concentration, moodiness, loss of memory, mutism, and the stuporous condition known as catatonia.

Others have hallucinations, delusions, suicidal tendencies, maniacal excitement alternating with depression, and a general state of mental dissolution known as hebephrenia.

Another type is the paranoid type, in which the progressive dementia is associated with egomania and delusions of grandeur. It is similar to true paranoia, except that the delusions are not as well systematized.

The danger of dementia praecox is that some individuals suffering therefrom are irresponsible and commit various crimes. Most of them should be confined to an asylum. A few may recover, but they do not, as a rule, attain normal mental health.

Manic-depressive Insanity. In this variety of insanity periods of maniacal excitement of varying intensity occur in between severe or mild periods of depression or complete well being. In some instances these phases alternate more or less regularly, and the name circular insanity is given to the condition.

The maniacal stage may be severe, characterized by struggling and raving, or it may be mild in which the patient merely has a rapid and uncontrolled flow of ideas due to excessive mental activity. The reasoning power is not lost, but ungoverned. The patient is seized with wild impulses, even homicidal in type, and he may act upon them.

In the depressive stage the subject is depressed or even stuporous. He is attacked by delusions and may commit suicide under their influence.

Paranoia. Paranoia, or monomania, is a chronic insanity characterized by systematized delusions of personal grandeur, but showing little or no mental impairment. The patient believes himself to be an exceptional personage, even divine, and his ideas are founded on complex and systematic reasoning which is built on false and erroneous assumptions. Paranoiacs frequently have delusions of persecution and grandeur. If they imagine themselves wronged, they may descend to violent action.

The lesions found at necropsy in cases of dementia praecox, manic-depressive insanity and paranoia are not characteristic. The central nervous system may not yield any well-defined evidences of disease. In many cases death occurs from exhaustion or intercurrent infection.

Senile Dementia. Many other types of insanity occur which can be assigned to definite causes, and some of these show distinct pathologic processes in the brain.

There is, first of all, the so-called senile dementia caused by the onset of old age and cerebral arteriosclerosis. The patient loses his memory, becomes childish, silly and sometimes perverted in his behavior; later he sinks into a condition of complete deterioration.

The lesions at necropsy are chiefly those of arteriosclerosis, atrophy of the brain and conditions associated with vascular disturbances.

General Paresis. General paralysis of the insane, or general paresis, is an organic disease of the brain, occurring in the later stages of syphilis, which gives rise to a disturbed mental condition combined with physical disease. The patient shows progressive decline of mental and physical powers, with lack of concentration, poor judgment and delusions of grandeur. The deterioration continues, with periods of remission when the patient may seem quite normal. Neurologic signs become manifest even before the disease develops, such as Argyl-Robertson pupil (lack of sensitivity to light), difficulty in speech, convulsions and paralysis. The disease progresses gradually to a fatal conclusion if untreated.

At necropsy a chronic inflammation of pia arachnoid and cerebral cortex is noted, especially in the frontal region. This may be visible macroscopically in the form of a thickened membrane and atrophic convolutions. The microscopic sections of the brain show, as a rule, a chronic inflammation which is characteristic. Spirochetes may be demonstrated in the brain tissue.

Alcoholic Dementia. Alcohol used habitually may produce a great variety of mental conditions, such as mania, delirium and alcoholic paranoia. The signs at necropsy are those of chronic alcoholism. The brain may not show anything unusual, except pial edema and a slight atrophy of the cerebral convolutions.

Puerperal Insanity. Puerperal insanity is the condition of insanity which follows childbirth and it is doubtless referable to the action on the brain by the toxemia of pregnancy. A woman with puerperal insanity may manifest the condition after childbirth, and it may take a great variety of forms, the most common of which is mania, sometimes of the homicidal type. This may express itself by suicidal or homicidal acts.

Epilepsy. Epilepsy is a mental disease characterized by recurring motor paroxysms or their equivalent, such as spells of amnesia or of irresponsibility. True epilepsy has no demonstrable anatomic basis. Some pathologic conditions, however, such as brain tumors, or pachymeningitis interna hemorrhagica and cerebral injuries produce symptoms similar to true epilepsy. Epileptics, sooner or later, show mental deterioration. Their chief interest, forensically, is that during the epileptic fit or its equivalent, the epileptic may commit some crime.

Minor Types. There are, in addition, other forms of mental aberration which are simply complexes with characteristic manifestations which may complicate some of the foregoing insanities.

Kleptomania is the involuntary and neurotic compulsion to steal.

Pyromania is the uncontrollable impulse to set fire to structures, and may occur without frank mental disease.

Dipsomania is a periodic compulsion to alcoholic drink.

Suicidal mania is the insane impulse to kill one's self.

Somnambulism is the unconscious state known as sleep-walking.

Amnesia is the loss of memory for various periods, most commonly associated with epilepsy, but also occurring in alluminating gas poisoning or concussion of the brain, or as a manifestation of true hysteria.

Examination of Patients. Each separate case of alleged insanity and its degree of civil or criminal responsibility must be judged on its own merits with reference to the problem under consideration.

The Department of Mental Hygiene of New York State issues instructions for the examination of patients who are proper subjects for commitment to an institution for the insane. Some of these instructions are worth quoting.

PREPARATION OF CERTIFICATE OF LUNACY

The certificate of lunacy must be made out by two qualified examiners after a joint examination of the patient within ten days next before the granting of the order of the commitment.

The history of the patient obtained by the examiners should be as complete as possible. The statements regarding legal residence are of great importance, as they may suggest proceedings for the deportation of aliens or the removal of residents of other states. In giving the birthplace of the patient the state should be mentioned if possible. All answers to the questions should be definite and complete. For example, in answering the question, "Has patient been considered as of normal mental standard?" instead of merely answering "No" give details, as, "Has been considered an imbecile, or idiot, or not bright, queer or eccentric, etc.," as the case may be.

Examining physicians must certify to the fact that the person examined is insane and a proper subject for custody and treatment in an institution for the insane.

EXAMINATION OF THE PATIENT

The examination of the patient must be made jointly by the qualified examiners and the findings recorded in detail on the blank.

Physical Examination. State whether the general physical condition of the patient is good, fair or poor. If the physical condition is such as to prevent the removal of the patient to the hospital, the fact should be stated. If the patient is confined to bed, the commitment should be deferred. No commitment should be considered if death is impending. The existence of any contagious, infectious or other physical disease should be mentioned. A brief neurological examination should be made, showing the condition of the pupils and patellar reflexes and mentioning any defect of speech, and gait, and any paralyses, etc., which may be present.

Mental Condition. In describing the mental condition the following lines of inquiry, which for the sake of clearness have been grouped under different headings, are suggested, and the different possibilities to be thought of are mentioned under each heading:

I. Behavior, Attitude and Emotional State
   Natural, distant, suspicious, bashful, elated, depressed (sad or anxious), perplexed, apathetic, etc.

II. Motor Condition
   A. General motion
      a. Normal
      b. Overactivity; excitement
      c. Diminished activity; slowness of motion, complete inactivity, catalepsy, resistiveness, etc.
   B. Speech
      a. Normal in amount
      b. Increased in amount; shouting, singing, loud talking, etc.
      c. Diminished in amount; slow speech, complete mutism.

III. Train of thought
   Clear, logical, jumping from topic to topic, yet so that it can be followed (flight of ideas), disconnected, fragmentary, etc.
   Give short examples.

IV. Content of thought
   Peculiar ideas, delusions, hallucinations, ideas of being observed, ideas that the acts of those about the patient refer to him (ideas of reference), etc.
   Give examples.

V. Orientation
> Does the patient understand his environment, *i.e.*, know the place, time, persons present, understand the situation?

VI. Memory
> Memory for old events: Best tested by determining whether the patient can give an account of his life.
> Memory for recent events: Best tested by determining whether the patient can give an account of his recent activities.

VII. Insight
> Does patient know that he is mentally abnormal?

HOSPITALS FOR MENTAL DISEASES

Hospitals for the insane, because they are under the necessity of restricting the liberty of their inmates, are subject to the same disabilities as prisons. This not only applies to difficulties of administration, but also to the possibility that deaths which occur within their jurisdiction may be the result of violence or other external means. The prisons in New York City must report to the Office of the Chief Medical Examiner all cases of death within their walls, regardless of whether the cause of death is natural or traumatic. On the other hand the hospitals for the insane in the City are not governed by such a rule but report only traumatic or suspicious cases to the Office of the Chief Medical Examiner, the chief exception being a hospital for the mentally deficient which operates under the same rule as the prisons.

The causes of death which occur among the inmates of hospitals for mental disease include: (1) Those resulting from natural disease conditions, some of which like cerebrospinal syphilis, idiopathic epilepsy, or chronic alcoholism may be the basis of the psychosis, while others like coronary arteriosclerosis may be an independent disease. In some instances death may be due to the psychotic state itself as when a manic-depressive patient after prolonged excitement sinks into a state of exhaustion and dies of a terminal pneumonia. (2) Those due to violence, which might occur if a patient commits suicide by jumping from a window, hanging himself or incising his neck or wrists. The violence may be homicidal as when a patient attacks an attendant or another patient, and inflicts manual strangulation or fatal blunt force injuries. Figure 15-41 illustrates a cause of death in which an insane patient killed an attendant by gouging out both eyeballs. In some instances injuries may be inflicted by attendants on patients while attempting to restrain them, death sometimes resulting from strangulation or blunt force injuries (Fig. 11-32). All these cases are technical homicides, and are investigated by the Office of the District Attorney as well as the Office of the Chief Medical Examiner. A civil action for the death of the victim may be brought by his relatives against the hospital, and in some cases the hospital has been judged liable.

REFERENCES

Hamilton, S. W., and Haber, R.   Summaries of State Laws Relating to Insane, from Peterson, Haines and Webster, Legal Medicine and Toxicology, Philadelphia, W. B. Saunders Co., 1923, Vol. 1, pp. 843-857.

Reese, J. J.   Text Book of Medical Jurisprudence and Toxicology, Revised by D. J. McCarthy, Philadelphia, P. Blakiston's Son and Co., 1911.

State of New York.   Department of Mental Hygiene, Instructions to Qualified Examiners.

40

Insurance and Survivorship: Malingering

INSURANCE AND SURVIVORSHIP

Insurance is a form of contract. One party, the insurer, guarantees to recompense the other party, the insured, in the event of a certain contingency, and for this protection the latter pays a definite sum of money known as a premium. In most instances, the payment of the premium is made periodically.

There are many varieties of insurance contracts, but the types in which medical men are interested primarily are the following: life insurance, accident and health insurance and insurance for workman's compensation.

Life Insurance. The contract in life insurance arranges for payment of the policy to the beneficiary on the death of the insured; in some instances it allows for payment of an annuity to the latter person after he reaches a certain age. Other policies contain a clause of double indemnity which guarantees that if the insured meets his death as the result of accidental violence, the beneficiary will be paid double the face value of the policy.

An insurance company is careful about formulating its contracts, in order that it may not be defrauded or assume damaging obligations. Its principal concern before issuing the policy is to have the applicant questioned and examined by a medical representative of the company, in order that it may ascertain whether or not he is a good risk.

The prospective insured submits a written application on which he gives the following data: name, residence address, occupation, date and place of birth, social condition, amount of insurance already in force on life, previous rejection or postponement of an application for insurance by any company, amount and kind of insurance desired, name of beneficiary, the former health of the applicant, (especially in regard to the dates and subject matter of consultations with physicians, the presence or absence of certain diseases, the results of previous medical examinations and surgical operations, and his use of alcohol and narcotics), and the family history. These questions must be answered truthfully and accurately to the best of the ability of the applicant. Many individuals believe that they can omit mention of previous illnesses, but this course is not advisable inasmuch as it may result later in rendering the policy void.

Some insurance policies are issued for amounts below 1,000 dollars, and a physical examination of the applicant is not required. In most cases, however, a questionnaire relative to the previous health of the applicant must be filled out and the answers must be as accurate and as truthful as though the policy was for a much larger sum.

These questions help to determine how good a risk the applicant would be for the company. The items of greatest significance are the occupation, age, previous health, personal habits, family history, and previous medical examinations. For example, certain dangerous and hazardous occupations, such as working with explo-

939

sives, aviation and the military or naval services in times of war, are not accepted for life insurance as a rule. The age is important, as the older the insured, the less desirable he is as a risk. Questions concerning the previous health, personal habits, family history, and the results of other medical examinations, are intended to discover whether or not the prospect is suffering from an insidious disease like tuberculosis, malignant tumor, alcoholism, narcotism, cardiorenal disease or syphilis.

The medical representative of the company after this questioning, examines the applicant, paying special attention to the condition of heart and lungs, the state of the blood pressure and the contents of the urine. Tests are made especially for glucose and albumin, in order to discover whether or not diabetes mellitus or renal disease is evident. Sufferers from these conditions are considered bad life insurance risks.

The examination may uncover serious ills, but it will not always bring to light the most common cause of presenile death, which frequently is manifested only by subjective symptoms, namely, coronary artery disease. At present, there is no reliable method of examination which will diagnose some of these cases before death, and many of them die without warning, only a short time after they have received the policy.

Sometimes a number of insurance companies receive information concerning applicants from a central bureau. A person whose application has been rejected by one company will be catalogued in the central bureau, and as a consequence the fact will be known to all the other companies.

Some companies require in the terms of the contract that the insured must be in his accustomed good health on the date that he receives the policy. If it can be proved later that the insured was in a parlous state of health on that date, and that he died soon after the policy was issued, this may be sufficient to void the contract when the claim is made. If the insured in his application states that he never consulted a physician, but does so between the date of his application and the date of the delivery of the policy, it is his duty to disclose the consultation or reject the policy; otherwise it will be void.

Information given in the application for insurance may be included in the contract and is known as a warranty. This means that it must be truthful and accurate, and that if it is found to be a misrepresentation, even though it is not an intentional one, the contract will be void. In other policies the information given on the application is not included in the contract and is known as a representation. An erroneous statement in a representation will not void a contract necessarily unless it is given for the purposes of fraud and has a direct bearing on the aim of the policy. Facts in an application are considered to be representations unless there is an express stipulation in the policy that they are warranties. In most states now no distinction is made between a warranty and a representation. Even if a statement in an application is incorrect, whether termed a warranty or a representation, the insurance company cannot take advantage of it unless it proves that the misstatement was made with intent to defraud or is material to the risk to be assumed by the company.

A physician who is an examiner for an insurance company must question an applicant thoroughly and record facts accurately. The examiner must be careful not to ignore items which may be important. When the contract is drawn up, a copy of the application is attached to it, and the applicant is supposed to read them both before he signs them. If he finds that the medical examiner has misstated his answers, the applicant must call attention to the matter promptly. After his death, his beneficiary will not be able to raise any question of error in the application.

If there has been an attempt at fraud by the company physician and the applicant, and proof can be produced to that effect the policy can be voided. Under such circumstances the physician could be subjected to criminal prosecution.

After the insured dies, the burden of proof is on the beneficiary of the policy, who must prove that the last premium has been paid and must establish the proof of death. The attending physician of the deceased, who issued the death certificate, fills out an insurance form stating the cause of death and answers pertinent questions relative to the previous health of the deceased. All answers should be accurate inasmuch as the beneficiary presents this statement as part of the proof of his claim, and it may be used as evidence in a court of law.

The company may not allow a claim for a number of reasons, some of which are based on false or fraudulent representations given on the application form. If the deceased has committed suicide within a year after paying his first premium, many policies are rendered void. A claim may be disallowed if the insured has died from the use of alcohol or drugs. The substance of the contract will determine to a great extent when the contract becomes void. In all these instances the burden of proof is on the insurer.

Presumption of Death and Survivorship. Presumption of death is a question closely connected with life insurance. If a person is absent from his usual haunts and has not been heard of for seven years, the law presumes him dead. However, if evidence is forthcoming that he probably perished in a calamity, or was suffering from melancholia with suicidal tendencies, or was in an advanced stage of a chronic disease like nephritis, he may be presumed dead after a much shorter interval. Medical evidence is offered sometimes to substantiate points of this sort. A direct proof of death is not required in all cases. The courts usually base their decisions less on the medical evidence offered than on questions of fact elicited by direct testimony.

The question of survivorship arises after calamities of different kinds in which two or more persons from the same family perish. These calamities include disasters at sea, train wrecks, highway accidents, conflagrations, carbon monoxide poisoning, exposure to cold, exposure to tropical heat, starvation or thirst. The settlement of an estate and the disposal of insurance policies will depend often on which member of a family died first.

The following case which came up for solution in a New York court illustrates clearly the problems which attend any legal action complicated by the question of survivorship. A man, 45 years of age, while driving in an automobile with his seven-year-old son, crashed into a post and wrecked his car. When medical help arrived both father and child were dead.

The problem of survivorship was important in this case because there was a question concerning the rightful heir of the father's estate. One claimant was the divorced mother of the boy, and the other claimants were the kinfolk of the father. If it could be proved that the boy died first, the property would revert to the relatives of the father. If the man died first, the mother would inherit the property through the boy.

The medical testimony disclosed that the man had a severe laceration of the neck with severing of both carotid arteries, a fracture of the cervical spine and crushing of the cord. The child had an injury of the lungs and traumatic hemorrhages in the brain; death was apparently due to shock. The lay witnesses who first reached the car after the accident claimed that the child was still breathing, but that the father was dead. The court was unable to solve the question of survivorship in this case at the time of the trial.

The law does not hold any presumption concerning the type of person who would likely survive the longest in a calamity involving a large number. It tries mainly to determine the probabilities in each individual case from the facts in evidence. Expert medical testimony may be sought as a useful adjunct, but is never considered in the light of a deciding factor. However, if it is probable that all persons who perished during a catastrophe were afflicted alike, it is reasonable to conclude that a healthy adult male would live longer than a child, an elderly person, a woman, or a sick individual. This reasoning may be fallacious. In some calamities, the strong may endeavor to protect the weak, so that the weaker party may actually survive the stronger. Young children, as a rule, succumb easily to most adverse conditions, but are said to resist the action of the sun's heat fairly well. A hard case to decide would be that of a mother and her newborn child, both of whom perished during childbirth, especially if medical care was not available.

Accident and Health Insurance. The contract in health insurance stipulates as a rule that the insurer shall pay the insured if he suffers such loss of health that he cannot pursue his occupation. Some contracts provide for partial disability. An affidavit of a physician is required before the insurance company will pay its obligations under the policy.

The contract in accident insurance calls for payment to the insured for disability resulting from an accident, or payment to his beneficiary if death occurred from accidental violence. The chief question is whether or not disability or death was the result of accident. Unlike tort or compensation cases, the question of negligence is not a factor unless the policy so states. The liability of the company depends upon the contract, and many policies definitely eliminate cases in which alcohol, drugs, suicide, and the commission of a crime by the insured caused his injury or death.

Court decisions concerning accidents are varied and depend upon the wording of the policy as to whether death results by accidental means or from an accidental event. In the latter instance, an unexpected death resulting from means which were deliberate and not accidental, has been considered accidental; in one recorded instance in the State of Utah, the courts on appeal have upheld the payment of the claim. Thus the case of Whatcott v. Continental Casualty Company (Utah) 39P. (2nd) 733 was concerned with the death of the insured under spinal anesthesia from procaine hydrochloride during an operation for chronic appendicitis. The Supreme Court of Utah ruled in effect that though the means were not accidental, the beneficiary was "entitled to recover benefits for injury or death from the unusual or unexpected results of an intentional act even though such results occur without mischance, slip or misstep."

The policies of accident insurance vary in their provisions. Some disclaim liability unless injury or death was due solely to the accident. Some insure only for immediate and total disability, while others insure for partial disability. Some policies refuse liability unless there is a visible sign of injury. Others refuse to pay if death was due to a poison, disease or infection.

The application forms, physical examinations, warranty and representations are similar in the case of accident and health policies as in life policies.

Some policies provide for a medical examination of the body after death. Where appropriate language has been used, this means the right of autopsy, including dissection. If the insurance company learns of the death before interment and also knows that there is a question as to the cause of death, it must demand the autopsy before interment. Of course, if it does not learn about the matter until after interment, it has the right to an autopsy within a reasonable time after burial. Most courts require the company to prove that an autopsy would serve some useful purpose and that the demand for autopsy is not made arbitrarily. In a large proportion of the cases, however, the company cannot compel an autopsy of the remains unless the family of the insured consent.

Insurance for Workman's Compensation. Laws have been passed in different states enabling workmen who have been injured in the course of their employment to present a claim for compensation before the State Labor Commission. If the referee appointed by that body decides in their favor and his decision is upheld by the higher court, the injured employee can collect suitable compensation. If the employee was killed in an accident arising out of his work, his family similarly will be allotted compensation for his death. Many firms and employers of labor sign contracts with insurance companies who underwrite this form of liability.

In order for the compensation court to grant an award to an employee the evidence must clearly show a causal connection between an injury which was incurred during employment and the disability or death which followed. It must be reasonably clear also that the casualty was not occasioned by the carelessness of the employee. Many medicolegal tangles occur in fatal cases when the plaintiff attempts to prove causal connection between the accident and the death, when the latter often is due to a natural disease condition. This question has been discussed in Chapter 6.

The problems which arise in workmen's compensation cases are not always easy to decide. The hardest decisions to make are those concerned with medical conditions which have become manifest during employment. They are divided into two categories:

1. Occupational disease which might be anticipated logically from the continued application of the patient to certain kinds of work, as for example, lead poisoning from work as a painter. Formerly compensation was not considered for diseases of this type, but in most states the law has been amended to include them.

2. Nonoccupational ailments which are affected by unusual conditions of work, such as a fatal attack of bronchial asthma, which was precipitated by inhalation of ammonia fumes from a leak in a pipe. A decision in such a case is likely to favor the claimant, if the available evidence indicates that the irritating gas actually was inhaled by the deceased.

ACCIDENTAL TRAUMA AND HYSTERIA. Claims have been made for damages in many cases of accidental trauma, not on account of physical injury to the body, but because of nervous shock and fright. The legal decisions vary in different jurisdictions so that it is difficult to make a definite statement regarding this type of case. In general, however, it may be said that in most states shock and fright do not entitle one to money damages unless they accompany some type of trauma. In other states, however, damages are awarded for shock and fright even though there has not been any physical injury.

MALINGERING

Malingering is defined as the feigning or the simulation of a disease or injury. The motives for malingering are usually to escape military service, naval service, jury duty, or to avoid the punishment for a crime, to obtain the verdict in a liability action, to pass as a disabled beggar, or to acquire notoriety.

The disability in some cases of malingering may be built up out of pure imagination and not have the slightest basis in fact; this type is termed feigned or fictitious. For example, an able-bodied man may simulate paralysis by pure acting, or pretend to have an attack of epilepsy. Some individuals will claim that they have a disease without making any attempt to feign it, and will present a certificate from their physician to that effect; their purpose is usually to avoid such a minor unpleasant duty as serving on a jury. In other circumstances, a person suffering from some disease or disability will cover it up for the purpose of passing an examination for life insurance.

Other cases of malingering are termed factitious, inasmuch as they are exaggerations of a real complaint; there is a basis in fact which is converted into a more serious disability by the efforts of the claimant. For example, a person receives a broken arm in an accident and claims that it is a permanently crippling injury, even after the fracture has healed.

Sometimes insanity is feigned by individuals desirous of avoiding the consequences of a criminal trial. In such instances, the prisoner is examined by alienists and an attempt is made to determine his real mental state. Often this is not easy to accomplish and it may be necessary to observe him over a long period of time. If he can be surprised while off guard, the fraud can generally be brought to light.

Malingering occasionally is encountered in cases of civil action for liability. The plaintiff may allege that his disability is due to a certain accident, when in reality all his symptoms are the result of an injury which was incurred a long time before. Sometimes the plaintiff may declare that he is suffering from pain, headache, lameness, loss of vision and paralysis, all of which are symptoms difficult to controvert. In such cases the only way to establish the reality of the malingering is to prove the claimant a liar.

The court may order a physician to examine the patient and to report upon the truth or falsity of his allegations after one examination. This may be impossible in all but a few instances. Besides the possibility that the doctor may be dealing with the wiles of a clever faker, there is also the consideration that the claimant is suffering from hysteria or neurasthenia resulting from shock or somatic disease. The best plan to pursue is to examine the patient carefully, especially the affected area, and give him plenty of opportunity to elaborate on his deception. Sometimes the claims that he makes will be so at variance with the circumstances that the fraud will come to light.

If neurologic symptoms, such as epilepsy, amnesia, aphonia, catalepsy or paralysis are claimed, some recommend the method of taking the patient off guard and exposing him to a weak but sudden electric shock, as if by accident. The patient may forget himself and reveal himself as a faker if he is surprised suddenly in this fashion. General anesthesia or the scopolamine morphine treatment may be employed if the patient gives consent; these methods may be useful for detecting a malingerer, but their use is not without danger and their real value is questionable.

Ankylosis of the joints sometimes is simulated, but is easily detected. If steady traction is put against the supposedly fixed joint, the muscles will begin to tremble with the strain, thus disclosing the lack of ankylosis. General anesthesia will remove the ankylosis without difficulty.

Alleged deaf-mutism or blindness may be exposed first, by examination of the affected organs, and second, by catching the patient off guard and demonstrating that he can see or hear. If the patient claims blindness in one eye, the fraud can be detected by a great variety of tests. One is to order the patient to keep both eyes open and place a prism of 6 to 8 degrees' strength in front of his good eye; if the alleged affected eye is sightless, he will see a single object, but if it is not blind he will see a double image, as the prism produces just enough refraction of the line of vision in the good eye to cause diplopia. The disabling symptoms and signs claimed by litigants not infrequently clear up after the liability action has been decided one way or the other. Undoubtedly, many of these cases are definite malingerers, but others are probably examples of hysteria.

Irregularity of the heart beat caused by the use of veratrum or digitalis; contusions; bleeding from the nose, mouth, rectum or bladder; ulcers; abrasions; hernias; hydroceles; discharges from the nose or ears; jaundice; skin diseases and diarrhea have been simulated on occasion, especially in military organizations. Such frauds, however, are uncovered by a little investigation.

REFERENCES

Armstrong, S. T.   The Medical Jurisprudence of Life Insurance, in Peterson and Haines, Legal Medicine and Toxicology, Philadelphia, W. B. Saunders Co., 1923, Vol. 1, p. 1096.
———— The Medical Jurisprudence of Accident Insurance, in Peterson and Haines, Legal Medicine and Toxicology, Philadelphia, W. B. Saunders Co., 1923, Vol. 1, p. 1161.
———— Accident insurance: death under spinal anesthesia and appendectomy, an "accidental event," J.A.M.A., 105:1298, 1935.
Herzog, A. W.   Medical Jurisprudence, Indianapolis, The Bobbs Merrill Co., 1931.

ANALYTIC TOXICOLOGY

41

Introduction

Toxicology has been defined as the science dealing with the properties, physiologic action, detection and estimation of, and antidotes for, poisons. A poison is any material which, if introduced into the living body or brought into contact with any part thereof, will produce ill health or death.

The wide variety of substances which constitute poisons and the large number of sciences involved in toxicology make it necessary to break down the field into separate subjects for the purpose of discussion. Symptoms, antidotes, treatment and pathologic findings are phases of medicine. Physiologic activity is covered in the field of pharmacology, while the matter of industrial hazards is a subject for special treatment. The detection and estimation phases of toxicology are entirely chemical and, in order to differentiate the chemical aspects from the other branches of the subject, we have used the term analytic toxicology for them. Analytic toxicology differs from pharmacologic analysis in that the substances to be analyzed are contained in organs, tissues and body fluids.

The analytic toxicologist is concerned primarily with the isolation, detection and estimation of substances that are not normal components in the biologic material obtained at autopsy to aid in establishing the cause of death or in elucidating the circumstances of the death. Less frequently, material from a living patient such as urine, blood, hair, fingernail clippings or tissue from biopsy is submitted to the analyst for diagnosis in a case of suspected poisoning.

The material collected at autopsy for chemical examination is selected on the basis of the case history and the pathologic findings. The pathologist should send as much of the material to the laboratory as circumstances permit, for an inadequate amount will seriously hamper the analysis. If the toxicologist is compelled to work with an insufficient sample, the limitations imposed in the testing process are the responsibility of the person who selected the material. It is an easy matter for the analyst to dispose of unused material but, if the quantity supplied is inadequate, the size of the sample tested must be reduced in order to conserve material for further testing and the difficulties connected with the analysis mount proportionately.

Brain tissue is the material best suited for analyses involving volatile and nonvolatile organic poisons. Liver is the next choice but the purification of liver extracts requires considerably more labor than those from brain tissue. Blood and urine are seldom submitted in quantity but are very good sample material for certain nonvolatile organic poisons. Extracts from blood are easier to purify than those from the brain. Sulfa drugs, salicylates and some barbiturates can often be detected in blood filtrates after protein precipitation. Many drugs or their degradation products concentrate in the urine in delayed deaths from overdoses. For this reason, hospitals should be alerted to save the urine in fatal cases in which the patient is received in coma.

946

Recent information concerning the detoxification mechanisms for drugs indicates that certain compounds are stored in relatively large amounts in the fatty tissue. This type of tissue has not been studied sufficiently to warrant its examination in toxicologic analyses but it might well be examined for its scientific value.

The kidney and the liver are the most important organs to examine in acute heavy metal poisonings. The blood should be examined in cases of chronic poisoning and bone, hair and nail clippings should be included particularly when thallium or radium poisoning is suspected.

Blood and lung tissue are the materials of choice when gaseous poisons are involved and in cases of death from inhalation of volatile solvents. Lung tissue is the only material needed for chemical analysis in suspected silicosis. Lymph nodes should be analyzed when the pathology indicates a possible berylliosis.

The presence of a toxic substance in the parenchymatous organs or blood is proof that it has been absorbed into the system during life and has exerted its poisonous action. Toxic substances found in the stomach contents do not possess this significance unless the agent is a corrosive chemical. Nevertheless, the stomach contents should always be submitted for analysis along with the other organs in acute cases and in fact should be the material to receive first attention by the analyst. Although the unabsorbed poison in the stomach contents is in a pharmacologic sense outside the body, it is more likely to be found in larger quantities there than in the organs. The isolated material will be obtained in an unchanged form so that reactions to specific tests are more characteristic than when the material has undergone absorption with subsequent alteration due to the detoxification mechanisms. If a drug is found in the organs and large amounts are not present in the stomach contents, a quantitative analysis is important to rule out the possibility of a medicinal dose.

The stomach contents are the only materials adequate for analysis in poisonings by corrosives such as inorganic alkalies, acids and salts. The pathologic findings will indicate the particular analysis for this class of compound. When corrosion of the gastrointestinal tract is reported, a small amount of the stomach contents should be reserved for pH measurements and for acid or base titrations.

Isolation is best accomplished by dialysis and in fact, even in the absence of corrosion, it is good practice to reserve some of the stomach contents for this purpose. Mixtures of some drug preparations can be more conveniently separated by dialysis than by extraction.

With the exception of fluorides and cyanide, corrosive chemicals can seldom be detected in the organs. After absorption, these substances are so altered that their original composition cannot be determined from the analysis. Moreover, the ions of most corrosives are normal components of tissue and, after their distribution in the body, the difference between normal and toxic levels is not significant.

After the pathologist has removed and examined the organs and other substances, he seals them in properly labeled jars without delay in order to prevent the escape of volatile poisons. The sealed specimens are transported to the laboratory where the analyst receives them, recording the date and hour of their receipt, the name of the person making the delivery and any history or information concerning the death.

The time of death in relation to the onset of symptoms is a major factor in planning a procedure for the analysis. Many persons overcome by carbon monoxide die after 24 hours. The gas cannot then be demonstrated in the blood. Tests on victims of accidents who have lived for some hours do not give alcohol values indicative of the degree of intoxication at the time of the accident and after 18 to 24 hours may fail to show any evidence of having ingested alcohol. Death from ingested carbon tetrachloride may occur in a few days from extensive degenerative processes in the parenchymatous viscera, but by the time of death all of the poison may have been eliminated.

The analyst should be informed whether or not extraneous evidence was found at the scene of death. Medicinals or a prescription submitted as evidence in suicides may reduce the analysis to a single determination. The contents of unlabelled pills or capsules or an apparently empty drinking glass are much easier to identify than the same material extracted from the organs, and they serve as a convenient starting point in the examination. The analyst should be informed concerning treatment if the deceased was under the care of a physician; if death occurred after hospitalization, he should be furnished with any records of drug therapy. In barbiturate suicides in which the body comes to autopsy from a hospital, the analyst can expect to find a stimulant such as amphetamine, picrotoxin or nikethamide as well as the barbiturate.

The importance of obtaining all available information about the circumstances of the poisoning and particularly about the drugs administered therapeutically to the deceased cannot be overemphasized. There are many cases in which much time has been spent in identifying an isolated drug only to find that this substance had been given as a therapeutic agent. In medical examiner's laboratories located in heavily populated areas, the large volume of work would be impossible to handle if short cuts in analytic procedure had not been suggested to the toxicologist by information available in the different cases.

The material obtained at the autopsy should be placed in a deep freeze prior to storage in a cooler. Specimens that cannot be delivered quickly to the laboratory should be kept in a frozen condition. The toxicologic examination should be started as soon as possible, but since only a part of the material submitted for analysis is utilized at one time, the toxicologic laboratory should have adequate facilities for storage under conditions which prevent putrefaction. The difficulties encountered in the isolation and purification processes increase with the degree of postmortem change, and more of the toxic compound is lost with each added purification step.

Postmortem decomposition, embalming and burial introduce conditions which seriously interfere with the toxicologic examination. Postmortem changes are likely to vitiate tests for the poisons, either by altering the structure of the drug or by forming substances which simulate it chemically. If ptomaines are produced by degradation of the tissue they will be isolated along with the basic organic poisons and will give a positive reaction with many of the reagents used to detect alkaloids. Most of the volatile organic poisons will escape detection. Results of quantitative analyses for many substances will be unreliable, although heavy metals and relatively stable organic compounds such as strychnine and some barbiturates can be isolated and identified satisfactorily.

Embalming nullifies the tests for most volatile poisons and interferes with the isolation process for all of the nonvolatile organic compounds. Formaldehyde undergoes condensation with cyanide and many other compounds so that even when isolated in quantity the material does not respond characteristically in the identifying reactions. Formaldehyde-fixed tissue is much more resistant than untreated tissue to the action of solvents with the result that recoveries of organic compounds from it are invariably low. Methyl alcohol in the embalming fluid makes analysis for ethyl alcohol in questionable intoxications so complicated that the findings are difficult to interpret. The embalming fluid may contain substances other than formaldehyde and methyl alcohol and should always be examined prior to analysis involving embalmed tissue.

Exhumed bodies present the problem of postmortem imbibition (Vaughan) and contamination. In those cases in which heavy metals are suspected, portions of the surrounding soil and wrappings of the corpse should be examined in order to eliminate the possibility of contamination from the outside.

Cremation which reduces the corpse to a fine ash nullifies most toxicologic tests. The destruction of the body by corrosive acids or alkalies also interferes with toxicologic analysis for all poisons but a few metallic ones.

After the analytic toxicologist has recorded all of the available information on the case, the course of his analysis is guided by the material at his disposal and the evidence at hand as to the possible cause of death. Case history, clinical symptoms, testimony of witnesses, extraneous evidence found at the scene or pathologic findings may suggest a particular substance as the toxic agent. Such information, therefore, centers his attention on one particular poison, and he can refer to the literature for the physical and chemical properties of the compound. A specific isolation method can be developed and identifying reactions applied to the isolated substance. The analytic approach in this type of case is a direct one in that the analyst has a lead as to the nature of the poison. The presence of the suspected substance will be verified or ruled out as effecting the death by application of direct chemical testing.

When the case history is not known and pathologic findings are absent, the analytic problem confronting the toxicologist is quite different. The negative pathologic report does serve to eliminate those poisons which produce definite pathologic evidence. On the request from the pathologist for toxicologic examination, this type of case is listed as "general unknown." A case is so labeled when any poisonous substance may have been the cause of death, and a complete examination is indicated.

Unfortunately there is no existing literature describing a systematic method for attacking this type of analytic problem. Publications and texts in the field of analytic toxicology approach the problem on the assumption that the analyst has been furnished some knowledge of the cause of death. All existing toxicologic literature lists the physical and chemical properties of poisonous substances under the name of the compound; tabulations of toxic substances according to their properties have not yet been published. In the general unknown type of case the identification process is outside the realm of toxicologic literature.

Few analytic toxicologists agree as to the best method of carrying out the analysis on a general unknown. Each relies on his own experience and knowledge of the chemical behavior of the common drugs. The general method of attack has been to carry out spot testing until a reaction is found pointing to a particular substance. This positive reaction serves as a lead; the analyst then follows the standard pattern in which the literature is consulted for tests which will confirm the identity of the substance or eliminate it as the toxic agent. However, even when clear-cut positive reactions are obtained for a substance isolated from the tissues, if it is an uncommon poison or a new drug that has not come to the attention of the analyst, he cannot get a further lead as to its identity from the literature.

A systematic method of attack is a prerequisite for the identification of unknown substances. Because of their diversified nature, toxic substances cannot be classified into a system in which related properties such as structure, chemical behavior and pharmacologic action are correlated. The most convenient classification places the toxic substances in five major groups based on the methods for their analysis in biologic materials.

1. *Gaseous poisons* may be demonstrated in the atmosphere or in the blood, lungs and body fluids of the deceased.

2. *Inorganic poisons* include the metals and most of the nonmetals, which require the complete destruction of the organic matrix for their analysis. This class may be subdivided into four groups determined by structure and physical properties.

a. *Nonvolatile metals* are the metallic poisons that are not volatile at temperatures of 450° to 500° C. and can be detected in the residue after ashing the tissue in the muffle furnace.

b. *Volatile metals* are the metallic poisons that are partially or completely volatilized at muffle furnace temperatures. The destruction of the organic matter must be accomplished by a "wet digestion" with strong oxidizing agents.

c. *Nonmetallic inorganic poisons* include the small number of toxic anions that are not normal constituents of tissue. Each requires a special analytic procedure in which both a qualitative and quantitative determination can be conducted at the same time. Analysis is performed by direct aeration of the macerated tissue or by tests on the tissue ash made alkaline prior to the ashing process.

d. *Corrosive nonmetallic poisons* are distinctive in that death from them is due in part to corrosive action on the gastric and intestinal walls as a result of the acidity, alkalinity or oxidizing action of the compound. They include those acids, bases and salts that are elemental constituents of normal tissue. Toxic action can only be established by demonstrating the presence of abnormal amounts in the stomach. Isolation is accomplished by dialysis or extraction of the stomach contents.

3. *Inorganic and organic poisons volatile with steam* may be isolated by steam distillation of the finely ground tissue. Tests for most of the volatile poisons are sensitive enough to permit detection by direct testing on the distillate. Isolation may be accomplished by fractional distillation or rectification.

4. *Organic poisons not volatile with steam* include all of the organic drugs met with in pharmacology that can be separated from tissue by extraction with organic solvents. Even relatively nontoxic organic pharmaceuticals must be included in this classification since they may appear as a residue in the isolation process and unless the identity of the isolated material is established it cannot be excluded as the toxic agent. Unfortunately, no reliable tests exist for distinguishing between toxic and nontoxic organic substances.

The general separation and purification procedure for organic substances is the basis for a tentative classification determined by solubility and the relative acidity and basicity of the compound. Solubility in the isolation process creates five major classes of nonvolatile organic poisons: (1) alcohol, water and solvent soluble compounds; (2) water and alcohol soluble, solvent insoluble compounds; (3) water insoluble, alcohol and solvent soluble compounds; (4) water soluble, alcohol and solvent insoluble compounds; (5) alcohol and water insoluble, special solvent soluble compounds.

Noncorrosive toxic substances, if ingested, must be absorbed through the gastric and intestinal walls in order to exert their toxic action. Most of the toxic organic compounds are therefore water and alcohol soluble, and this class comprises the major compounds met with in toxicologic analysis. Compounds falling into classes (2), (3), (4), (5) are few enough in number to be considered as exceptions in the isolation and purification steps for the nonvolatile organics. The water and alcohol soluble compounds may be further classified into three major groups with three subgroups. The classification scheme depends upon the fact that salts of organic compounds are more soluble in water than in nonpolar solvents whereas the free organic molecule is more soluble in organic solvents than in aqueous solution. Although the divisions are not sharp, the degree of overlapping of a compound in adjacent groups is not so great that its position in the scheme becomes questionable. Alcohol and water soluble poisons may be classified as follows:

1. Acid ether or acid chloroform soluble compounds
   a. acids
   b. phenols (intermediate acids)
   c. neutrals
2. Basic ether soluble compounds
3. Ammoniacal chloroform-alcohol soluble compounds

The three major groups are those of the conventional Stas-Otto procedure.

The acid ether or chloroform soluble compounds are either neutral organic molecules or acidic compounds which form salts with alkali. Addition of mineral acid to an aqueous solution liberates the organic acid, and upon extraction with the immiscible solvent, the free organic molecule passes into the solvent in proportion to its distribution coefficient.

The subdivision of the acid group is based on the relative acidities of the compounds. Organic acids are defined as those compounds whose degree of ionization in aqueous solution is sufficient for formation of a sodium salt in sodium bicarbonate solution. Most organic acids contain carbonyl or sulfonic groups. However, the division is without regard to functional groupings. Saccharin, an imide, and picric acid, which is a phenol structurally, act as strong organic acids and appear in this fraction.

The class labeled phenols might better be termed intermediate acids. The term phenol here designates a degree of acidity rather than a type. Phenols are those compounds which are sufficiently acidic in nature to form water soluble sodium salts in sodium hydroxide solution, but whose degree of ionization in aqueous solution is not great enough for the formation of a sodium salt at the pH of a sodium bicarbonate solution. All barbiturates are imides and fall into this category.

Neutrals are those compounds that are neither acidic nor basic in reactivity and hence pass into the organic solvent phase in any extraction with water and an immiscible solvent.

The basic ether soluble compounds are primary, secondary or tertiary amines which form water soluble salts when added to mineral acids. In the first step of the extraction process, when the aqueous solution is made acidic with mineral acid, the water soluble salts of the bases that are formed remain in the aqueous phase upon extraction with a nonpolar solvent, while the free organic acids and the neutrals pass into the organic solvent phase. When the acid aqueous solution is then rendered alkaline, the liberated base becomes more readily soluble in organic solvent and passes into the nonaqueous liquid phase in the extraction process.

The ammoniacal chloroform-alcohol fraction comprises the small group of basic organic molecules that are amphoteric or else ether insoluble. The amphoterics are bases with weak acidic properties. At higher alkalinities they act as weak acids and form water soluble sodium salts, which remain in the water layer during the extraction of the basic compounds. Ammonia is a weaker base than sodium hydroxide, and when the aqueous alkaline solution is made acid and then just alkaline with ammonia, the pH is not sufficient for salt formation and the free compound passes into the solvent phase upon extraction with the chloroform-alcohol solution. Morphine is the most common drug in this class and the use of 10 per cent alcohol in the chloroform is primarily to increase the solubility of the morphine in the chloroform.

5. *Nonvolatile organic poisons other than alcohol and water soluble compounds* are relatively few. The number of drugs that are not sufficiently soluble in both alcohol and water to be removed in the isolation process in amounts sufficient for identification is small. These comprise classes 3, 4 and 5 under the classification of *Nonvolatile Organic Poisons.* They may therefore be grouped into a separate class whose main characteristic is that a special isolation procedure is required. The search for each compound in this group is an individual examination and is carried out only after completion of tests for class 1 or when a particular member is indicated as a possibility by the case history or pathologic findings. Fluoroacetic acid and *alpha*-naphthylthiourea are typical examples. Due to the limited number of possibilities, the conventional approach in which an examination is conducted for individual compounds becomes a practical procedure even when the case is of the "general unknown" type.

When all the available information concerning the death has been evaluated by the toxicologist, the method of attacking the analytic problem is outlined. In the general unknown type of case, those determinations should be started first that are most affected by postmortem changes. A logical order is to set up the volatiles for distillation and to make an examination to eliminate the gaseous poisons while the distillation is being carried out. The organs to be tested for nonvolatile organic poisons should be prepared for extraction before proceeding with the analysis of the distillate. Since isolation and purification difficulties for organic poisons increase in proportion to the degree of postmortem decomposition, the safest practice is to set up the analytic processes as soon as possible. Distillates and tissue extracts may be stored in the icebox until the analyst is ready for the examination. Precautions to prevent putrefaction are not necessary in samples to be analyzed for metals. When corrosive acid, bases or salts are suspected, the stomach contents should be examined without delay by titration for acidity or basicity as well as by measurement of the hydrogen ion activity.

The size of the sample used in a particular analysis is determined by the amount of material submitted by the pathologist and by the lead, if any, which has been given to the analyst concerning the nature of the poison. It is easier to work with small individual quantities of tissue and, in analyses for substances with high lethal dosages, a small sample will simplify the processes of purification. In the analyses for potent drugs or for general unknown cases, the use of one large sample is preferable to a number of determinations on smaller samples. In the analysis for organic compounds, final identification is made more certain by isolating a large quantity of the drug, along with a large amount of normal tissue extractives, rather than by attempting to shorten the process of purification by reducing the size of the sample.

Regardless of the nature of the analysis, a cardinal rule in toxicologic analysis should be that a reasonable sample be saved for examination by an independent analyst in the event the case comes to trial. For this reason it is extremely important for the analyst to see that the pathologist has recorded the weights of the submitted organs, particularly when insufficient material is sent to the laboratory. It is inexcusable for a toxicologist to report positive findings and later to testify that all of the material was used up in carrying out the analysis. In a medicolegal case, evidence is frequently requested when it is known to be missing. Rarely is an independent toxicologic examination requested when ample material has been held as evidence.

In outlining the method of attacking the analytic problem for a particular poison, there are three phases to be considered: the isolation process, the identification or qualitative procedure, and the quantitative analysis. In the analysis for certain specific poisons such as the fluorides, cyanide and many of the metals, it may be practical to select an isolation procedure that will permit the qualitative and quantitative phases to be carried out simultaneously. However, the analyst must not overlook the fact that the history may be misleading or that components other than those indicated may be present. If analyses carried out for a specific poison are negative, the sample has been wasted. In the "general unknowns," the chances for a successful analysis will be greater if each phase is treated separately. The isolation process should include the maximum number of possible poisons, even at the expense of decreased chances of recovery of certain common members of the group. The identification process should include all possibilities with emphasis on the purity rather than on the yield of the individual substances. Once the qualitative phase has been completed, the analyst can refer to the literature in order to select a special isolation procedure for quantitative recovery on a new portion of the sample.

The final report of a toxicologic examination usually includes the positive findings only. However, a complete record of the case including the tests performed and the conclusions drawn should be on file. An expert witness who does not recall the negative tests or his source of information may be put to considerable embarrassment on cross-examination. Conversely, when the positive analytic findings cannot stand up under cross-examination they deserve condemnation.

The analyst should be prepared to interpret results with regard to possible deviation in values and percentage of error. He needs to have a knowledge of lethal doses and, the more complete his knowledge of symptoms and of the use of drugs in specific diseases, the greater the number of short cuts he can take in proceeding with the analysis. However, the analytic phase of toxicology is concerned only with the substance found and its concentration in the organs. Establishment of the cause of death is the duty of the pathologist; it is his problem to evaluate the amount of poison reported in relation to his autopsy findings in order to determine whether or not that substance was the cause of death.

In the chapters which follow, methods used and developed in the Microchemical and Physical Laboratory of the Chief Medical Examiner of the City of New York for the analysis of materials received from autopsy will be described. Emphasis will be placed on the general unknown type of case. Space does not permit inclusion of all procedures. Newer methods will be given preference and many of those determinations that are standard in current texts will be omitted. Since quantitative methods for all of the common poisons can be found in the literature, the general scope of this discussion will be limited to qualitative identification. Although many of the methods to be described have not been published, they have been tested and found reliable in our hands. Every toxicologic method has limitations with regard to sensitivity and specificity. If there is any secret in toxicologic analysis, it is the knowledge of the limitations of the tests when applied to a toxic substance contaminated with normal tissue components. Our procedures or, in fact, other published toxicologic methods are not recommended for the novice with no previous experience in the analysis of substances isolated from biologic materials.

In a field devoid of standard practice one is always open to criticism concerning the choice of a modus operandi. The aim is not to set up hard and fast rules for toxicologic analysis, but, rather, to introduce a pattern that will warrant extension by independent workers or else to stimulate interest toward the development of something better.

In setting up procedures for toxicologic investigations involving general unknowns, it is assumed that adequate personnel and equipment are available. The expansion and increased scope of the field of pharmacy and therapeutics have made it imperative for the toxicologist to have access to expensive equipment such as the spectrograph, the ultraviolet and infrared spectrophotometers and X-ray diffraction. Toxicologic laboratories with limited facilities therefore need access to university centers, not only to supplement their equipment, but also for consultation with specialized scientists.

REFERENCES

Vaughan, V. C.   The Postmortem Imbibition of Poisons, from Peterson, Haines and Webster, Legal Medicine and Toxicology, Philadelphia, W. B. Saunders Co., 1923, Vol. II, pp. 861-875.

42

Gaseous Poisons

The circumstances surrounding a death will, in most cases, indicate whether a gaseous poison was a possible cause of death. With the exception of carbon monoxide poisoning, death from this class of toxic substances is usually accidental. Pathologic findings indicative of acute asphyxia with varying degrees of cyanosis are sufficient evidence to initiate a search for toxic gases if the circumstances of death support this theory.

Chemical diagnosis of deaths from these poisons is obtained by tests performed on the blood and lungs of the deceased, or indirectly by analysis of the poisonous atmosphere. In suspected gaseous poisoning, collection of samples of the surrounding atmosphere should be the first step in the investigation. In order for the samples to be representative, this duty should be delegated to some agency other than the Medical Examiner. By the time he has been notified of a death suspected to be from gas, the area in which the body was found will have been ventilated by the emergency crew whose duty it is to respond to such calls. Emergency trucks should be equipped with gas sampling apparatus and the personnel should be instructed in the proper collection of the air samples. There are a number of cases in the New York Medical Examiner's records in which complications regarding the diagnosis later developed because a sample of the atmosphere was not a part of the evidence.

Collection of Air Samples. The easiest method of collecting samples of the atmosphere is by means of gas collecting tubes of the Shepard type (1) shown in Figure 42-1. These tubes, from 250 ml. to 1 liter capacity, are equipped with vacuum-tight stopcocks at both ends. They are prepared for use by connecting one end to a laboratory vacuum pump and pumping down to a fraction of a millimeter pressure. When evacuated the tubes may be stored with safety for several days in a carrying case. When the cock at one end is opened at the scene, the air rushes into the evacuated tube and reaches atmospheric pressure in a fraction of a second. The advantage of this type of collecting tube is that the operator can hold his breath during the short time necessary to run into the enclosed space, open and close the cock, and return.

When time is not a factor or when it is necessary to collect samples from such places as the bottom of a vat or the hold of a ship, larger quantities of the atmosphere may be collected by lowering two aspirator bottles connected together as shown in Figure 42-2 by means of a rope attached to each bottle. One of the bottles is filled to overflowing with water or calcium chloride solution, specific gravity 1.40 (1). The calcium chloride solution is preferable because gases are less soluble in it than in water. Carbon dioxide is only one sixteenth as soluble in the calcium chloride solution as in water. Mercury can be substituted for the aqueous solution, but smaller aspirator bottles are then needed because of the high density of the liquid mercury. When gas samples are collected over mercury, the solubility of the gases in the collecting medium becomes negligible and the presence of a sulfide is indicated by a darkening of the surface.

955

To collect the gas sample, the pinch clamps at the outlets of both bottles are opened with the bottle containing the liquid held at a level above the empty bottle. As the liquid runs from the filled bottle, the surrounding atmosphere is drawn in. When the liquid has all been transferred, the bottles are withdrawn from the sampling area and the pinch clamps closed. Loss of gas while the sample bottles are being

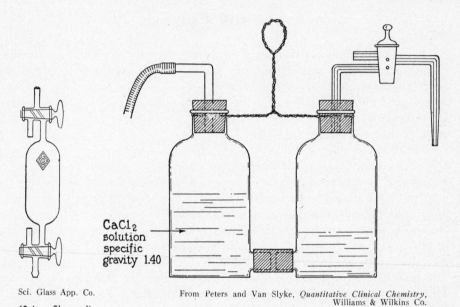

CaCl₂ solution specific gravity 1.40

Sci. Glass App. Co.

Fig. 42-1. Shepard's Pipet for Gas Collecting.

From Peters and Van Slyke, *Quantitative Clinical Chemistry*, Williams & Wilkins Co.

Fig. 42-2. Apparatus for Collection of Gas Samples To Be Analyzed for Carbon Dioxide.

The aspirator bottles are of 250 or 500 ml. capacity. The displacement liquid is a calcium chloride solution of 1.40 specific gravity in which carbon dioxide is only one-sixteenth as soluble as in water.

withdrawn is negligible because of the slow rate of diffusion between air and sample through the capillary inlet tubing. If the apparatus is transported intact to the laboratory, the analyst need only repeat the process in transferring the sample into his gas analysis apparatus.

Carbon Monoxide. Carbon monoxide (CO) is the most common gaseous poison. The chemical analysis is frequently important in determining whether the death was accidental, suicidal or homicidal. Suicidal or homicidal deaths are usually from illuminating gas; accidental deaths occur from large coal gas or charcoal stoves or from defective gas refrigerators burning in closed rooms. Both accidental and suicidal deaths have occurred from the inhalation of fumes from engine exhausts. Since carbon monoxide is an accumulative poison, low concentrations of it in the surrounding atmosphere do not eliminate it as the toxic agent.

When air containing carbon monoxide is drawn into the lungs, the carbon monoxide combines with the hemoglobin of the blood to form cherry red carboxyhemoglobin. The affinity of hemoglobin for carbon monoxide is approximately 200 times as great as for oxygen. Carboxyhemoglobin is a very stable compound; carbon monoxide can be demonstrated in the blood after marked decomposition, as well as in embalmed bodies.

The pathologic report usually furnishes the analyst with definite evidences of carbon monoxide poisoning. The pink tinge of the body and congestion of the brain, heart, lungs and muscle with the characteristic cherry red coloration are in distinct contrast to the reddish purple due to oxyhemoglobin or the dusky violet of reduced hemoglobin.

Quantitative analysis of the blood, collected preferably from the cavity of the heart, is necessary to establish a chemical diagnosis of carbon monoxide poisoning. Analysis of the atmosphere may be helpful in reconstructing the circumstances leading to the death.

ANALYSIS OF BLOOD FOR CARBON MONOXIDE. 1. Alkali Dilution Test. A quick probing test that will indicate a concentration of more than 10 per cent carboxyhemoglobin in the blood consists of placing a few drops of autopsy blood and an equal amount of normal blood in separate test tubes and diluting each with water to a volume of 15 ml. Five drops of 10 per cent sodium hydroxide are added to each tube and mixed. If the autopsy blood contains carboxyhemoglobin it is unaffected by the alkali and the solution retains a pink tinge for some time. The normal blood turns a greenish-brown color due to the formation of alkaline hematin by the action of the alkali. This test is likely to be misleading if performed on normal blood from a human fetus or a recently born infant. Helpern and Strassmann (2) have shown that the formation of alkaline hematin is delayed in infants' blood and the reaction of such blood to the alkali is similar to that of blood containing carboxyhemoglobin. A positive test indicates further analysis of the blood by a quantitative method.

2. Quantitative Estimation of Carbon Monoxide in Blood by Reduction of Palladium Chloride to Palladium. This is a simple and rapid method of analysis (3) and, although the precision is not comparable to that obtainable with the Van Slyke manometric procedure, it is adequate for interpretation in carbon monoxide deaths. A minor objection to the method is that the hemoglobin content of the unknown blood must be determined at the same time. The method depends on the fact that carbon monoxide liberated from the carboxyhemoglobin of the blood by potassium ferricyanide and aerated through palladium chloride reduces the palladium chloride to black metallic palladium according to the equation:

$$CO + PdCl_2 + H_2O \rightarrow Pd + CO_2 + HCl$$

Putrefaction of the blood or the presence of embalming fluid does not interfere in this method.

Reagents.
    (a) 0.5 gm. $PdCl_2$ + 0.5 ml. concentrated HCl diluted to 50 ml.
    (b) 3.2 gm. $K_3Fe(CN)_6$ + 0.8 gm. saponin dissolved in 100 ml. H_2O
    (c) 0.8 ml. lactic acid, specific gravity 1.20, per 100 ml. H_2O
    (d) 10 gm. $Pb(C_2H_3O_2)_2 \cdot 3H_2O$ per 100 ml. H_2O
    (e) caprylic alcohol

Procedure. The apparatus is shown in Figure 42-3. It consists of three 6 inch by ¾ inch potato tubes, a glass flange of 1 cm. internal diameter and a 2 liter Mariotte flask.

Charge tube A with 5 ml. of $PdCl_2$ solution; this serves to remove any CO from the air. Tube B contains 2 ml. of the blood to be analyzed, with 4 ml. of ferricyanide solution and 2 drops of caprylic alcohol. Charge tube C with a 1½ inch layer of glass beads and 5 ml. of $Pb(C_2H_3O_2)_2 \cdot 3H_2O$ solution. It acts to remove any H_2S present in the blood due to putrefaction. Cut a circular paper disk of approximately the same size as the outside diameter of flange D from Whatman #3 filter paper. Treat the disk with a few drops of the $PdCl_2$ solution; remove the excess liquid by pressing between two blotting papers, and then carefully insert the disk between the two sections of the flange, holding it tightly in place by means of two rubber bands, one on each of the sets of hooks on the flange sections. The flange sections must be drawn tightly together around the circumference of the disk in order to prevent air leakage around the paper.

Start the aeration by opening the screw clamp at the outlet of the Mariotte bottle until the rate of flow of water from the bottle is about 400 ml. in 15 minutes. Stop aeration after 15 minutes. Remove the paper disk from the flange and wash it thoroughly in distilled water to remove the unreduced $PdCl_2$. The black stain on the paper disk is then compared with a series of standard stains prepared from blood of known and varying carbon monoxide content.

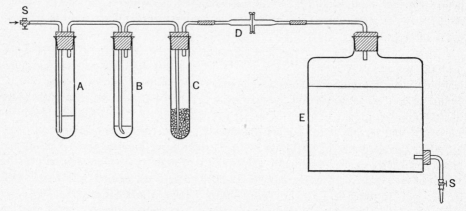

Fig. 42-3. Assembly for the Determination of Carbon Monoxide.

Preparation of the Standard Stains. Saturate 10 ml. of oxalated blood from approximately 50 ml. of a pooled sample having a normal hemoglobin content with CO gas by bubbling it through the blood for about 15 minutes. This treatment produces 100 per cent saturation of the hemoglobin present. Prepare 6 samples of blood containing CO in concentrations of from 10 to 60 per cent saturation by making appropriate dilutions of the 100 per cent saturated sample with CO-free blood. Seven stains on paper disks, prepared by aerating the 6 standards and a control sample of blood, are permanently mounted between glass plates for comparison with the unknown stain.

Estimations to within $\pm$ 4 per cent of the hemoglobin saturation can be made by visual comparison when the hemoglobin content of the unknown blood is the same as that of the blood used in preparing the standard stains. When the hemoglobin content of the unknown blood deviates appreciably from normal (90 per cent hemoglobin), a correction factor must be introduced. For example, if the unknown blood contains only 60 per cent hemoglobin and its stain matches a 30 per cent carbon monoxide saturation standard, the correct percentage of saturation is $\frac{90}{60} \times 30 = 45$ per cent. A slight error is introduced in the method due to the fact that a small amount of the carbon monoxide passes through the palladium paper without reducing the palladium chloride. This is partially compensated for by the equivalent loss that occurs in preparing the standard stains.

The problem of matching the unknown against the standard stains can be simplified by treating the paper disks as colored solutions. The optical density of the standards is easily read in a Stufo photometer with the instrument set at 100 per cent using the grade 3 filter paper. If the optical density is plotted against percentage of carbon monoxide saturation, the curve will serve as the standards. The optical densities of unknown stains are thereafter read on the photometer, the percentage of carbon monoxide saturation obtained from the curve, and the corrections made for variations in hemoglobin content. This procedure is described in detail on page 990 under the determination of arsenic by the Gutzeit method.

3. Van Slyke Manometric Method. This is the most accurate method for the determination of carbon monoxide in blood. Values reported by this procedure are seldom contested in court cases since the method has been thoroughly tested by a large number of investigators and the correction factors verified. There is no excuse for using any other procedure for carbon monoxide in blood when the toxicologic laboratory is located near a chemical laboratory that keeps a Van Slyke apparatus conditioned by constant use. In the toxicologic laboratory where the machine is not used often, the labor used in cleaning, relubricating, testing for leaks and running controls furnishes justification for analysis by the less precise palladium method. The Van Slyke manometric apparatus is standard equipment in most clinical laboratories and, because the procedure is described in detail in texts on clinical chemistry, it will not be repeated (4, 5).

Results should be reported as percentage of carbon monoxide saturation rather than as percentage of carbon monoxide by volume as is frequently done in clinical chemical analyses for gases. Two analyses are run on the autopsy blood. In one, a sample of the blood is saturated with carbon monoxide by passing the gas through it for 15 minutes. Analysis of this sample gives the carbon monoxide capacity or the percentage by volume when the hemoglobin has been completely changed to carboxyhemoglobin. The percentage of saturation is obtained from the ratio

$$\frac{\text{volume } \% \text{ CO content}}{\text{volume } \% \text{ CO capacity}}$$

An alternate procedure is to determine the hemoglobin and to calculate the carbon monoxide capacity. Since 1 gm. of hemoglobin combines with 1.34 ml. of carbon monoxide, the percentage of carbon monoxide saturation equals

$$\frac{\text{volume } \% \text{ CO content}}{\text{gm. hemoglobin per 100 ml. blood} \times 1.34}$$

Interpretation. Gettler and Freimuth (6) have reported values in 65 fatal carbon monoxide asphyxiations. Twenty-three had carbon monoxide saturations below 60 per cent and nine were below 50 per cent. The two lowest values in cases in which death was undoubtedly due to carbon monoxide were 31 per cent and 33 per cent saturation, respectively. Freimuth has made a complete and comprehensive study of the carbon monoxide content of the blood under various conditions of exposure and asphyxia.

ANALYSIS OF AIR FOR CARBON MONOXIDE. Table 42-1, which has been compiled from the files of the New York City Board of Health (G. Lacerre, Oct. 10, 1948), shows the possible effects of exposure to low concentrations of carbon monoxide in the atmosphere.

The standard Van Slyke method should not be used to analyze air containing low carbon monoxide concentrations because of the small capacity of the gas absorption chamber. Standard gas analysis apparatus such as the Orsat or Burrell type of equipment also should not be used because it is not sufficiently sensitive. Commercial carbon monoxide testers, such as the Mine Safety Appliance CO tester, which employ hopcalite * as the catalyst to oxidize the carbon monoxide to carbon dioxide are sufficiently accurate and are convenient to transport. They are specific for carbon monoxide and do not eliminate the need for collecting a repre-

---

* Hopcalite consists of manganese dioxide 50 per cent, cupric oxide 30 per cent, cobalt oxide 15 per cent, and silver oxide 5 per cent.

Table 42-1. Gas Poisoning. Carbon Monoxide Chart

CONCENTRATION OF CO IN AIR, PER CENT BY VOLUME	CONCENTRATION OF CO IN BLOOD AT EQUILIBRIUM, PER CENT BY VOLUME	TIME REQUIRED FOR EQUILIBRIUM, HOURS	SYMPTOMS AT VARIOUS CONCENTRATIONS OF CO IN BLOOD
less than 0.02	less than		0-10%: no symptoms 10-20%: tightness across forehead, slight headache
0.02-0.03	23-30	5-6	20-30%: headache, throbbing in temple
0.04-0.06	36-44	4-5	30-40%: severe headache, weakness, dizziness, dimness of vision, nausea, vomiting, collapse
0.07-0.10	47-53	3-4	40-50%: same as 30-40% plus tendency to collapse and syncope; increased respiration and pulse
0.11-0.15	55-60	1½-3	50-60%: syncope, increased respiration and pulse, coma with intermittent convulsions
0.16-0.20	61-64	1-1½	60-70%: coma with intermittent convulsions, depressed heart action and respiration, possible death
0.20-0.30	68-73	60-90 minutes	
0.50-1.00	73-76	1-2 minutes	70-80%: weak pulse and slowed respiration, respiratory failure and death

sentative sample of the atmosphere in order to rule out the possibility of other toxic gases.

The palladium chloride reduction method is adequate for the analysis of air samples for low concentrations of carbon monoxide. The gas collection apparatus of Figure 42-1 is connected in place of tube B in Figure 42-3 and a volume of gas is run through the palladium chloride paper to give an optimum stain. The displaced water is a measure of the volume of gas analyzed and, on reading the optical density of the stain, the percentage of carbon monoxide by volume is calculated.

Carbon Dioxide. Carbon dioxide (CO_2) is the end product in the combustion of organic materials. Normal air contains 0.03 per cent by volume of carbon dioxide, 21 per cent by volume of oxygen, 78 per cent by volume of nitrogen, and 0.9 per cent by volume of inert gases. In a poorly ventilated room the carbon dioxide concentration may be as high as one volume per hundred. Concentrations of 0.1 to 1 per cent by volume produce languor and headache. In an atmosphere of 8 to 10 per cent by volume, death may occur from asphyxia due to lack of oxygen. In higher concentrations the action is more that of a toxic gas and postmortem examination shows a more drastic picture with hemorrhages in the pericardium, pleura and the galea of the scalp. Death has occurred from exposure to an atmosphere in which dry ice was used as a refrigerant and from exploded carbon dioxide tanks.

It is not possible to demonstrate death from carbon dioxide by chemical tests performed on the blood or the body fluids. Chemical diagnosis is limited to establishing the fact that air samples collected from the area in which the body was found contain carbon dioxide in dangerous quantities (from 1 to 10 per cent or more).

ANALYSIS OF AIR FOR CARBON DIOXIDE. Any one of the conventional gas analysis apparatuses of the Orsat type or other types is adequate for analysis for carbon dioxide in air. The procedure is standard in all texts on gas analysis (7).

A method that does not require specialized equipment is the bubbling of a known volume of the collected sample through a 10 per cent barium hydroxide solution. The following reaction takes place:

$$Ba(OH)_2 + CO_2 \rightarrow BaCO_3 + H_2O$$

The precipitated barium carbonate may be filtered through a sintered glass crucible and weighed, or else it may be calculated after first titrating the excess barium hydroxide with standard acid to a colorless end point with phenolphthalein.

Hydrogen Sulfide. In low concentrations, hydrogen sulfide (H_2S) has an intense odor and is easily recognized. However, as the concentration of the gas in the atmosphere increases, its odor becomes less apparent because the olfactory nerves become paralyzed (8). For this reason, failure of the history to mention a foul odor is not ample evidence to rule out hydrogen sulfide in cases of asphyxia.

In addition to being a by-product in industries utilizing sulfur-containing chemicals, hydrogen sulfide is generated in the decomposition of organic matter by putrefactive microorganisms which are found particularly under anaerobic conditions in sewers and cesspools. Freireich (9) reports two cases, one with fatal outcome, of hydrogen sulfide poisoning incurred in cleaning out a cesspool. According to the data of Haggard (8), 0.01 to 0.015 per cent by volume of hydrogen sulfide in the air will cause symptoms of local irritation after many hours of exposure. Death may be caused in one hour by 0.09 per cent by volume and in 15 to 30 minutes by 0.15 per cent by volume. Almost immediate death from respiratory paralysis will be caused by 0.18 per cent by volume or more. Postmortem findings of greenish-blue cyanosis similar to that seen in advanced decomposition, with a strong odor of hydrogen sulfide gas in the lungs and muscle, are significant.

Hydrogen sulfide can be demonstrated in the blood, lungs and muscle tissue in acute fatal poisonings when postmortem decomposition of the body has not occurred. If putrefaction occurs, hydrogen sulfide is a normal component of tissue degradation.

ANALYSIS OF BLOOD AND TISSUE FOR HYDROGEN SULFIDE. Absorption spectrum methods on blood are unreliable. In the cases reported by Freireich, characteristic bands of neither sulfmethemoglobin nor methemoglobin were observed.

1. Qualitative Analysis. If moistened lead acetate paper is suspended over a cut section of the lungs or muscle tissue contained in a sealed jar, the paper darkens within a few minutes due to the formation of lead sulfide if hydrogen sulfide is present.

2. Quantitative Analysis. Aerate a 10 gm. sample of blood or minced organs into 2 per cent cadmium sulfate dissolved in 0.3 normal hydrochloric acid. The apparatus assembly is similar to that described for carbon monoxide by the palladium chloride reduction method. Tube A contains a 10 per cent basic lead acetate solution. Tube B contains the organs and tube C the 2 per cent acid solution of cadmium sulfate. After 30 minutes aeration, heat the cadmium sulfate solution to coagulate the yellow cadmium sulfide. Weigh the precipitate after filtering it through a microsintered glass filter stick (10).

ANALYSIS OF AIR FOR HYDROGEN SULFIDE. The same procedure is applicable to air analysis by substituting the gas collection bottles in the assembly for tube B.

Sulfur Dioxide. Sulfur dioxide (SO_2) is the product formed in the combustion of sulfur. It is a common constituent, in low concentrations, of the air in industrial centers where coal is burned, particularly in localities containing ore smelting industries. It is used as a refrigerant in some older types of refrigerators, and the burning of sulfur candles and of liquid sulfur dioxide is much used in household fumigation. Medical examiners' cases involving sulfur dioxide are most likely to arise from these domestic uses.

There is little danger of sulfur dioxide poisoning since the fumes are very irritating and give warning of its presence. The odor is detectable in air in concentrations of 5 parts per million, and 20 parts per million cause irritation of the eyes. Exposure to 500 parts of the gas per million parts of air for one hour may cause death by asphyxiation (11). Toxic symptoms are the result of the corrosive action of the sulfurous acid formed when sulfur dioxide dissolves in the moisture of the respiratory tract. Postmortem examination in acute cases shows an inflamed respiratory tract and edema of the lungs. The blood is very dark due to formation of acid hematin. Chemical diagnosis must be made indirectly by analysis of the air.

ANALYSIS OF AIR FOR SULFUR DIOXIDE. 1. Qualitative Analysis. Sulfur dioxide is very soluble in water due to the formation of sulfurous acid:

$$SO_2 + H_2O \rightarrow H_2SO_3$$

Sulfurous acid is a strong reducing agent and readily decolorizes iodine solutions. The presence of the gas in air may be indicated by bubbling a sample of the air through a dilute acid solution of iodine in potassium iodide:

$$SO_3^= + I_3^- + H_2O \rightarrow 2H^+ + 3I^- + SO_4^=$$

2. Quantitative Analysis. Procedure. Connect the gas sampling tube to a glass tubing fitted into a 2 hole rubber stopper fitted to a 6 inch test tube, with the glass tubing submerged in about 20 ml. of a 10 per cent $Ba(OH)_2$ solution. Bubble a measured volume of the gas sample through the solution. CO_2 and SO_2 will be precipitated as insoluble $BaCO_3$ and $BaSO_3$ respectively. Make the $Ba(OH)_2$ solution acid to methyl red indicator with 6N HCl and heat it to just below boiling until the vapors fail to darken lead acetate paper. Then add 0.3 ml. of 30 per cent H_2O_2 dropwise with stirring and boil the solution for 10 minutes. Add an additional 3 ml. of 6N HCl and 2 ml. of 30 per cent H_2O_2 and continue boiling for 15 minutes. Any sulfides present will be volatilized and the $BaCO_3$ dissolved by the acid. H_2O_2 oxidizes the sulfite to insoluble $BaSO_4$. Filter the solution through a weighed sintered glass weighing microfilter, wash it with dilute HCl and then with alcohol, and reweigh it.

Nitrous Oxide. Nitrous oxide (N_2O) is used as an anesthetic in dentistry and in minor operations. The gas is nonpoisonous; the very few deaths that have occurred during its use have been attributed to asphyxia or other causes. It cannot be demonstrated in body fluids, and analysis of the atmosphere in cases of death during anesthesia would be meaningless. Requests for toxicologic analysis have been restricted to the examination of the contents of the gas tank in order to safeguard the doctor against criticism in the use of that particular sample.

Nitric Oxide. Nitric oxide (NO) is of no significance in toxicology since it is not found free in nature and is immediately converted to nitrogen dioxide on exposure to the air.

$$2 NO + O_2 \rightarrow 2 NO_2$$

Nitrogen Dioxide. Fumes of nitrogen dioxide (NO_2) are found only in chemical laboratories and in those industries in which nitric acid is used. It is of little interest to the medicolegal toxicologist. The vapor is heavier than air and brown in color, and has a strong and irritating odor. Accidental deaths from nitrogen dioxide should be indicated from the history and the chemical diagnosis made indirectly by analysis of the atmosphere.

Nitrogen dioxide dissolves in aqueous solutions to form nitrous and nitric acids. Absorption by the blood following inhalation results in the formation of nitrite and nitrate salts which change hemoglobin to methemoglobin. In acute cases, alarming symptoms develop within a few hours after exposure. Postmortem findings show intense congestion of the air passages, marked edema of the lungs and dark colored tar-like blood.

ANALYSIS OF AIR FOR NITROGEN DIOXIDE. 1. Qualitative Analysis. The presence of oxides of nitrogen in the air is indicated by the intense blue color formed when a sample of the gas is passed through a solution of diphenylamine in concentrated sulfuric acid or by the formation of a blue starch-iodine color when it is passed through a mineral acid solution of potassium iodide to which a little soluble starch has been added.

2. Quantitative Analysis (12). Pass a sample of the air through an absorbing solution consisting of 15 ml. of 5 per cent NaOH and 5 ml. of 3 per cent H_2O_2. Oxides of nitrogen will be oxidized to nitrate. Then analyze the absorbing solution for nitrate by observing its action on phenoldisulfonic acid, forming colored nitrophenoldisulfonic acid.

Phenoldisulfonic Acid Reagent. Heat 6 gm. of phenol with 37 gm. of concentrated H_2SO_4 on a steam bath, cool and add 3 ml. of water.

Evaporate the absorbing solution through which the air sample has been passed to dryness on a hot plate. Add 1 ml. of phenoldisulfonic acid reagent and, after mixing, add 1 ml. of water made acid with 4 drops of concentrated H_2SO_4. Heat the solution on a steam bath for 5 minutes, cool, and add an excess of NH_3 and then 25 ml. of water. If the solution is cloudy, add 1 ml. of alumina cream with shaking, filter the suspension with suction into a 50 ml. Nessler tube and dilute to the mark with water. The color is matched against standard $NaNO_3$ solutions containing 0.1 to 1.0 mg. of the salt treated in the same way as the unknown.

Phosgene. Phosgene ($COCl_2$) is a very toxic gas which was used extensively in World War I. One part per 30,000 parts of air is dangerous and one part per 6,000 may cause lung injury after a two minute exposure (13). Its only interest to the toxicologist arises from the fact that chlorinated hydrocarbons such as carbon tetrachloride (CCl_4), chloroform ($CHCl_3$) and trichlorethylene ($CHClCCl_2$) form phosgene by pyrolysis when the vapors come in contact with a flame or a hot surface. Phosgene needs to be eliminated as the toxic agent in deaths under circumstances in which pyrene-type fire extinguishers have been used in an enclosed space.

ANALYSIS OF AIR FOR PHOSGENE. The gas can be demonstrated only in the air. It may be detected when present in a concentration of one part per million parts of air by passing the air sample through a paper disk impregnated with p-dimethylamino-benzaldehyde (14). The disk, held in a flange of the type described under the palladium chloride method for determining the presence of carbon monoxide, develops a yellow to orange stain in proportion to the concentration of phosgene.

A sensitive quantitative method depends on the reaction which takes place when phosgene is absorbed from an air solution by an aqueous aniline solution (15, 16).

$$COCl_2 + 4C_6H_5NH_2 \rightarrow CO(NHC_6H_5)_2 + 2C_6H_5NH_2 \cdot HCl$$

The amount of phosgene present is calculated from the weight of the precipitated s-diphenylurea.

Hydrogen Cyanide. Hydrogen cyanide (HCN) is considered with the gaseous poisons because, during investigations of death from cyanide, the possibility of accidental inhalation frequently arises. Hydrogen cyanide is a highly toxic substance which acts directly on the central nervous system. The liquid has a low boiling point (26° C.). It is used extensively as a fumigant by commercial exterminators to rid warehouses, ships and large evacuated buildings of rodents and vermin. A mixture of sodium cyanide and oxalic acid is a homemade preparation used to polish brass. One part of hydrogen cyanide in 10,000 parts of air is dangerous if inhaled for one hour, and one part in 500 is fatal (17).

Cyanide may be demonstrated in the organs and body fluids of the deceased. In a "general unknown," it first appears when the distillate from the brain is tested for volatile poisons. A positive cyanide reaction in the brain distillate immediately calls for a steam distillation of the stomach contents. Failure to find cyanide in the stomach contents leaves inhalation as a possibility. Chemical diagnosis is made on the basis of quantitative analysis for the cyanide content of the lungs and organs. In inhalation deaths the lungs show a higher cyanide content than the brain and other organs. Moreover, the cyanide content of all organs is much less in inhalation deaths than in cases of suicide by cyanide ingestion.

In the two deaths from cyanide inhalation that were investigated in the New York City Medical Examiner's Laboratory, the distillate from the brain showed only a suspicious reaction. With subsequent concentration of the distillate, the test became clearly positive for cyanide. The distillate from the lungs was positive beyond question but required concentration for accurate quantitative analysis. The stomach contents were negative for cyanide even after extensive concentrating procedures on the distillate. Methods for the analysis are described in the discussion of the volatile poisons (page 1051).

ANALYSIS OF AIR FOR HYDROGEN CYANIDE. The gas may be detected in the air in concentrations greater than 20 μg. per liter by the benzidine-copper acetate test (18).

Reagents (19).
    (a) 3 gm. Cu(Ac)$_2$ • H$_2$O dissolved in 100 ml. H$_2$O
    (b) 1 per cent benzidine acetate solution prepared by heating 2 gm. of benzidine acetate in 100 ml. of H$_2$O at 80° C. for 15 minutes and filtering with suction when cold

Procedure. Prepare a filter disk similar to that used for the detection of carbon monoxide by the palladium chloride reaction by immersing it in a freshly prepared solution consisting of 25 ml. of the benzidine acetate solution and 2 ml. of the copper acetate solution. Insert the paper disk into a glass flange as described for the detection of carbon monoxide and connect the flange directly to the gas-sampling bottle assembly. Force the air sample through the moist reagent paper by elevating the leveling bottle and adjusting the rate of liquid flow into the gas-sampling bottle by means of a pinch clamp on the rubber connecting tube, so that approximately 1 ml. of air sample is displaced per minute. In the presence of cyanide the moist paper turns a blue color. The intensity of the stain may be compared with standard stains or the optical density may be read in a Stufo photometer and the cyanide content determined from a standard cyanide curve, as described under the determination for arsenic (page 990).

Exclusion of Toxic Gases Encountered as Industrial Hazards.

There are many gaseous poisons liberated as products of certain industrial processes that are potential hazards as air contaminants. They include carbon bisulfide (CS$_2$), sulfur monochloride (S$_2$Cl$_2$), sulfuryl chloride (SO$_2$Cl$_2$), carbon oxysulfide (COS), ammonia (NH$_3$), arsine (AsH$_3$), stibine (SbH$_3$), phosphine (PH$_3$), halogen gases (Cl$_2$, Br$_2$) and halogen acids (HCl, HBr, HF). There are also low boiling organic solvents such as the alcohols, ethers, esters and the chlorinated hydrocarbons (methyl chloride (CH$_3$Cl), methylene chloride (CH$_2$Cl$_2$), chloroform (CHCl$_3$), carbon tetrachloride (CCl$_4$), ethyl chloride (C$_2$H$_5$Cl), ethylene dichloride (ClCH$_2$CH$_2$Cl), dichlorethylene (ClCH=CHCl) and trichlorethylene (ClCH=CCl$_2$). Combustible gases containing methane, ethane, propane and unsaturated hydrocarbons of low molecular weight are asphyxiants, and saturated and aromatic hydrocarbons of higher molecular weight in gases and gasoline vapors are irritants and convulsants.

In cases in which a high concentration of carbon monoxide is found in the blood it is frequently necessary to trace the source of the carbon monoxide in order to establish the circumstances leading to the fatality. Whether the death is accidental, suicidal or homicidal will have a great effect on the settlement of insurance claims and civil suits for damages.

Since carbon monoxide may be a component of many gaseous mixtures, as well as a product of incomplete combustion, the question of possible sources for carbon monoxide is always raised during the investigation into the circumstances of the death. In order to be sure of the factors responsible for the death, the possibility of the presence of gases other than carbon monoxide must be eliminated by an analysis of the atmosphere. For example, in the accidental death by asphyxiation of three persons in a closed apartment in New York City, a gas refrigerator was found to be defective. In addition, a slight leak was found around one of the valves of the gas stove. The carbon monoxide content of the air in the room was 0.28 per cent as determined by the Mine Safety Appliance CO analyzer.

Table 42-2. Composition of Some Combustible Gases

COMPONENTS	GAS IN SEWAGE DIGESTION TANKS (23) PER CENT BY VOLUME	GAS IN SEPTIC TANKS (23c) PER CENT BY VOLUME	NATURAL GAS (20) PER CENT BY VOLUME	ILLUMINAT- ING GAS (21) PER CENT BY VOLUME	GAS IN MANHOLES (22) PER CENT BY VOLUME
Methane	63.0-84.2	72.5-78.0	84.7		
Ethane			9.4	14.1	0.1-25.4
Propane			3.0		
Unsaturated hydrocarbons			1.5	10.2	0-2.5
Carbon monoxide			.4	26.1	0-2.4
Carbon dioxide	3.3-29.4	13.6-17.0		4.0	0-8.3
Hydrogen	0-8.2		.3	26.4	0-44.1
Oxygen	0-1.2			1.0	3.7-20.9
Nitrogen	2.9-23.3		.7	18.3	19.5-85.6
Hydrogen sulfide	0-0.1				

New York City illuminating gas (Table 42-2) contains carbon monoxide 26.1 per cent by volume, hydrogen 26.4 per cent by volume, methane and saturated hydrocarbons 14.1 per cent by volume and unsaturated hydrocarbons 10.2 per cent by volume. The ratio of combustibles to carbon monoxide in illuminating gas is approximately 2:1. Analysis of a sample of air in the above-mentioned case for combustible materials other than carbon monoxide showed less than 0.01 per cent. The low combustible value for the atmosphere compared with the carbon monoxide content indicated that the refrigerator was the source of the toxic gas. On further examination the nature of the defect was revealed.

The causes of deaths due to the type of poison classified as an industrial hazard are almost always clearly established from the history; the primary problem is the prevention of a recurrence in the industry. However, in contested court cases, the opposition may attempt to discredit the interpretations drawn from the chemical analysis as to the cause of death by introducing evidence of exposure to one of these poisons prior to the death. Although the problem is of more legal than toxicologic importance, the medical examiner's findings may be jeopardized by failure to consider all the possibilities.

Individual tests for all of the possible compounds cannot be justified on the basis of incidence of death from these poisons. However, a general procedure that is sensitive enough to detect significant amounts of almost all of this group in the air is available to the toxicologist and may be applied in order to exclude them from further consideration. If the findings by this procedure are not negative, and if there is no other lead, the sample should be referred to a laboratory equipped with the specialized apparatus necessary for differential gas analysis.

METHODS FOR THE DETECTION OF COMBUSTIBLE HYDROCARBONS, HALOGENATED HYDRO-CARBONS AND SULFUR-CONTAINING GASES IN AIR. 1. Analysis for Combustible Hydrocarbons. The combustion assembly for microanalysis for carbon and hydrogen should be standard equipment in the toxicologic laboratory. The detailed procedures for the determination of the carbon-hydrogen content of organic microsamples are given in standard texts on organic microanalysis (24, 25). Air samples may be analyzed for traces of combustible organic gases by mixing a sample with oxygen and passing the mixture through the combustion tube charged with the simple band or combination band filling (26). CO_2 and water, the final products of combustion, are absorbed on ascarite and anhydrone respectively and the amount of combustible material is calculated from the increase in weight of the absorption tubes in the combustion of a given volume of gas.

The CO_2 and water vapor present in the sample must be removed before carrying out the combustion. CO, if present, will be absorbed as CO_2. In the analysis of samples connected with CO deaths, in which it is necessary to rule out combustibles as contributing to the asphyxia, it is better to remove the relatively large amount of CO prior to the combustion rather than to correct for it by difference by a separate CO determination.

If the air sampling container is of the vacuum type, connect one end to a mercury leveling bottle so that the gas may be displaced from the air sample container, as described for the apparatus of Figure 42-2. Connect a T tube to the gas outlet end with one outlet connected to a capillary water manometer and the other to the purification train of four absorption tubes. Fill the first tube with loosely packed cotton to serve as a dust filter, the second with desiccant grade silica gel to remove water vapor (27) and the third with hopcalite I to absorb CO. The fourth tube in the train is the same type of combination bubble counter and U tube used in the carbon-hydrogen assembly (28). The bubble counter serves to measure the flow of gas from the sample bottle, and the U tube, packed with ascarite and anhydrone, absorbs the CO_2 and any water vapor from the bubble counter. Connect the end of the U tube to the carbon-hydrogen apparatus by means of a T tube inserted between the oxygen bubble counter and the inlet end of the combustion tube.

To carry out the combustion, the oxygen and air samples are forced through the combustion tube simultaneously by adjusting the pressures on the gas sampling bottle so that the rate of flow, as measured by the bubble counter, is the same as that of the oxygen. The water manometer in the system serves as an indicator in order to keep the pressure of the air sample at approximately the same level as that indicated by the oxygen pressure regulator.

An alternate procedure is to mix one volume of air sample freed of dust, CO, CO_2 and water vapor with four volumes of oxygen and to pass the mixture through the carbon-hydrogen apparatus. More manipulation is required with this procedure and there is the added disadvantage that the carbon-hydrogen apparatus has to be modified and reassembled with each determination.

The volume of air sample necessary for an accurate quantitative analysis is established by a trial determination. The combustion of 1 liter of sample containing 0.01 volume per cent of methane (CH_4) would result in an increase of 200 μg. in the ascarite tube.

All of the precautions required for an accurate carbon and hydrogen determination are not necessary for air analysis, since the primary purpose of the method is to eliminate combustibles as the cause of or as contributing to the asphyxia. In deaths by asphyxiation from this type of substance, the concentration in the atmosphere will be high enough for analysis by any of the standard procedures for gas analysis.

2. Analysis of Air for Halogenated Hydrocarbons (29, 30). When halogenated hydrocarbons are present in air samples in significant amounts, the maximum possible concentration is indicated by elevated values for the combustibles. Differentiation between halogen substituted

hydrocarbons and other combustible substances may be made by application of the dry combustion method for microanalysis of organic compounds. The auxiliary equipment and manipulative procedure are similar to that for the carbon and hydrogen determinations.

Subject the sample to combustion in a stream of oxygen; the decomposition products pass over heated platinum contacts contained in a special combustion tube. The halogen gas, CO_2 and water that are formed pass into an absorbing solution consisting of sodium carbonate and $NaHSO_3$ where the halogen is reduced to halide. On making the absorbing reagent acid with NHO_3 and adding $AgNO_3$, insoluble silver halide is precipitated. The halogenated hydrocarbon is calculated from the weight of the silver halide precipitate.

Since CO, CO_2, water vapor and other gaseous constituents do not interfere with the method, the gaseous sample needs only to be diluted with about four volumes of oxygen and the resulting gaseous mixture passed through the combustion system.

3. Analysis for Sulfur-Containing Gases. The apparatus and combustion tube assembly are identical with that for halogenated hydrocarbons. Pregl (31) determined halogens and sulfur simultaneously by omitting the $NaHSO_3$ in the absorption solution. To determine sulfur, oxidize to sulfates by perhydrol of the sulfur acids absorbed by the sodium carbonate solution. Make the solution acid with NHO_3, precipitate the sulfates with $BaCl_2$ and weigh them. Halogens are then determined in the filtrate by the reduction of higher halogen acids to halide and precipitation with $AgNO_3$. The detailed procedures for sulfur-containing compounds are given on page 138 in Pregl and on page 188 in Niederl and Niederl.

The only precaution necessary in the analysis of air samples for sulfur-containing poisons is in the method of collecting the samples. All of these substances have a foul odor and their presence will probably be suspected. Some are very corrosive and are readily hydrolyzed by water. The sample should therefore be collected over mercury or in an evacuated type of gas sample bottle.

REFERENCES

1. Peters, J. P., and Van Slyke, D. D. Quantitative Clinical Chemistry, Baltimore, Williams & Wilkins Co., 1932, Vol. II.
2. Helpern, M., and Strassmann, G. Differentiation of fetal and adult human hemoglobin, Arch. Path., 35:776, 1943.
3. Gettler, A. O., and Friemuth, H. C. Carbon monoxide in blood; simple and rapid estimation, Am. J. Clin. Path., Sect. 7:79, 1943.
4. Peters, J. P., and Van Slyke, D. D. Quantitative Clinical Chemistry, Baltimore, Williams & Wilkins Co., 1932, Vol. II.
5. Hawk, P. B., Oser, B. L., and Summerson, W. H. Practical Physiological Chemistry, 12th ed., New York, Blakiston Co., 1947.
6. Gettler, A. O., and Freimuth, H. The carbon monoxide content of the blood under various conditions, Am. J. Clin. Path., 11:603, 1940.
7. Fieldner, A. C., Jones, G. W., and Holbrook, W. F. The Bureau of Mines Orsat Apparatus for Gas Analysis, U. S. Bureau of Mines Technical Paper #320, 1925.
8. Haggard, H. W. Toxicology of hydrogen sulfide, J. Indust. Hyg. & Toxicol., 7:113, 1925.
9. Freireich, A. W. Hydrogen sulfide poisoning; report of 2 cases, Am. J. Path., 22:147, 1946.
10. Gettler, A. O., Neiderl, J. B., and Benedetti-Pichler, A. A. The isolation, identification and quantitative determination of ethyl alcohol normally present in human tissues, Mikrochemie, 11:167, 1932.
11. Katz, S. H., and Porter, H. C. Effect of Low Temperature Oxidation on the Hydrogen and the Change of Weight of Coal on Drying, U. S. Bureau of Mines Technical Paper #98, p. 172, 1917.
12. Nelson, G. H., Levine, M., and Buchanan, J. H. Elimination of corrections for nitrites in nitrate determinations, Indust. & Engin. Chem., Anal. Ed., 4:56, 1932.
13. Dept. of Scientific and Industrial Research. Methods for the detection of toxic gases in industry; phosgene, Analyst, 65:290, 1940.
14. Patty, F. A. Rapid methods for the determination of gases in the air, Am. J. Pub. Health, 30:1191, 1940.
15. Olsen, J. C., Ferguson, G. E., Sabetta, V. J., and Scheflau, L. Quantitative determination of phosgene, Indust. & Engin. Chem., Anal. Ed., 3:189, 1931.
16. Yant, W. P., Olsen, J. C., Storch, H. H., Littlefield, J. B., and Scheflau, L. Determination of phosgene, Indust. & Engin. Chem., Anal. Ed., 8:20, 1936
17. Dept. of Scientific and Industrial Research, Great Britain. Methods for the detection of toxic gases in industry, hydrogen cyanide vapor, Leaflet #2, 1938.
18. Sherrod, G. C. Practical Applications of Two Qualitative Tests for HCN in Ship Fumigation, U.S. P. H. S., Reprint #1224, 1928.

19. Dept. of Scientific and Industrial Research. Methods for the detection of toxic gases in industry, II. Hydrogen cyanide vapor, Analyst, 63:658, 1938.

20. Fieldner, A. C. Gases Commonly Used in the Industries and the Home and Their Hazards, U. S. Bureau of Mines Information Circular #6009, 1926.

21. Consolidated Edison Gas Company, New York City. Personal communication.

22. Jones, G. W., Campbell, J., and Goodwin, F. M. Investigations During 1932 of Combustibles in Manholes in Boston, Mass., U. S. Bureau of Mines Report of Investigations, #3213, p. 17, 1933.

23a. Sayers, R. R. Gas hazards in sewers and sewage-treatment plants, Pub. Health Rep., 49:145, 1934.

  b. News Report. Engineering News, 71:760, 1914.

  c. Buswell, A. M., and Strickhouser, S. I. Some observations on sewage tank gases, Indust. & Engin. Chem., 18:407, 1926.

24. Pregl, F. Quantitative Organic Microanalysis, 2nd ed., New York, Blakiston Co., 1930, p. 19.

25. Niederl, J. B., and Niederl, V. Micromethods of Quantitative Organic Analysis, 2nd ed., New York, John Wiley and Sons, Inc., 1942, p. 101.

26. Roth, H., and Daw, E. B. The Quantitative Organic Microanalysis of Fritz Pregl, New York, Blakiston Co., 1937, pp. 15-68.

27. Frevert, H. W., and Francis, E. H. Improved analyzer for carbon monoxide in air, Indust. & Engin. Chem., Anal. Ed., 6:226, 1934.

28. Niederl, J. B., and Niederl, V. Micromethods of Quantitative Organic Analysis, 2nd ed., New York, John Wiley and Sons, Inc., 1942, p. 104.

29. —— and Niederl, V. Micromethods of Quantitative Organic Analysis, 2nd ed., New York, John Wiley and Sons, Inc., 1942, p. 160.

30. Pregl, F. Quantitative Organic Microanalysis, translated by E. Fyleman, 2nd English ed., New York, Blakiston Co., 1930, p. 118.

31. —— Quantitative Organic Microanalysis, translated by E. Fyleman, 2nd English ed., New York, Blakiston Co., 1930, p. 119.

43

Inorganic Metallic Poisons

Inorganic substances are divided into metals and nonmetals on the basis of their physical and chemical properties. The analytic toxicologist further classifies inorganic poisons into four groups depending on the type of analysis which is employed to separate the toxic substance from the organs. The outstanding characteristic of inorganic poisons is that they can be isolated by destruction of the organic matrix; they are elemental in nature and more stable than the surrounding body tissues. Unlike organic poisons they are not altered appreciably by chemical reactions in the body nor by chemical treatment in the isolation process and, therefore, present little difficulty in the interpretation of findings. In some instances, however, it may be more convenient to isolate certain inorganic poisons by solvent extraction, dialysis or aeration.

Four principal methods are employed for the isolation of inorganic poisons from the biologic sample: (1) Ashing of the organs directly in a muffle furnace at 450° C. with neutral tissue or alkalinized tissue; (2) wet digestion with concentrated sulfuric acid, and a mixture of one part concentrated nitric acid and two parts perchloric acid, or a mixture of concentrated mineral acid and a strong oxidizing agent such as potassium permanganate or potassium chlorate; (3) aeration or distillation of the finely ground tissue; and (4) dialysis through permeable membranes.

The inorganic poisons as a class are similar to the gaseous poisons in that there usually is a history which indicates that tests for a particular poison should be carried out. Many give characteristic pathologic findings; therefore, in the absence of any such findings, certain members of the group are eliminated as possibilities. The methods used in the analysis of tissue residues for inorganic substances fall into two categories. Metals are first identified by qualitative analysis for the group, and if a toxic metal is present a quantitative determination is then made by a special procedure on a separate portion of the material. In contrast to the metals, inorganic nonmetals require specific tests for each substance and usually include quantitative estimation as a part of the identification procedure.

The classic sulfide scheme of analysis for metals with its systematic separation and specific identifying reactions for each member is the ultimate in qualitative analysis. Unfortunately, the perfection of which the scheme is capable depends on a reasonable distribution ratio of metals in the unknown sample. When the ratio of two components is of the order of 1000:1, the minor constituent will invariably be lost by occlusion and coprecipitation of the major component. This situation also exists in the toxicologic analysis for metals.

Iron, magnesium, calcium, sodium, potassium, phosphate and silica are present in high concentrations in tissue residues. Moreover, most requests for toxicologic examination for heavy metals are initiated by a history of exposure some months before death, and the amount in the organs at death will be relatively small. Under these conditions the systematic scheme is not adequate to identify a trace of toxic metal contained in a complex inorganic mixture. In a general unknown case, the presence of such metals as cadmium, thallium, barium, beryllium, silver and gold in the organs can never be excluded with certainty with this procedure. In suicides and homicides from the ingestion of metal-containing substances, a high concentration of a single metal is found in the stomach contents, and the systematic scheme is seldom needed for the identification of the metal. It remains as a potential tool of the analytic toxicologist but its inclusion in a text on the subject is merely repetition of general qualitative inorganic analysis.

At present, spectrographic analysis is the only technic that is adequate for the detection of toxic metals in tissue residue, particularly in the general unknown type of case. Individual chemical tests for each element are prohibitive because of the time and labor involved and the limited samples available. The sensitivity of spectrographic analysis is sufficient to detect significant amounts of all the metals except mercury, arsenic and antimony; by this method all of the detectable members of the metal group can be surveyed in one operation. (It is a potential quantitative procedure, but the limited concentration range and restrictions due to possible interfering lines give preference to chemical methods of quantitative analysis in all but a few cases.)

Spectrographic analysis is a valuable screening mechanism capable of semiquantitative interpretation which may indicate that a quantitative chemical analysis for a particular toxic metal should be performed on the organic material or that certain metallic poisons can be eliminated as not significant. Mercury, arsenic and antimony do not give a detectable spectrum unless present in high concentrations because they distill out of the crater of the spectrographic arc at a temperature below that required for activation. Toxic amounts are easily detected by the Reinsch test and this with a spectrographic analysis furnishes a complete examination for toxic metals. The kidney and the liver are the best organs for analysis in metal poisonings. Lung tissue, lymph nodes, spleen and stomach contents are desirable in special cases.

Nonvolatile Metals. Nonvolatile metals are those that are not volatilized in appreciable amounts when tissue or body fluids are ashed in a muffle furnace. Silver, aluminum, bismuth, cerium, chromium, copper, iron, magnesium, manganese, molybdenum, nickel, platinum, radium, silicon, thorium, titanium, vanadium and tungsten are not lost when tissue is subjected to temperatures slightly above red heat. The loss of beryllium, cadmium, lead, tin and zinc at a muffle furnace temperature of 450° C. is not great enough to influence the analysis when toxic doses are present.

Ashing Procedure. Dehydrate 25 gm. of ground organs, 20 ml. of blood or 100 ml. of urine, at 110° C. in a drying oven. Place the dried sample in a muffle furnace maintained at 450° C. and leave for 3 to 5 hours until all the volatile matter has been removed and a soft black ash remains. Inspect the sample in the oven from time to time during the first hour. Keep the thick crust that is baked over the top broken by means of a spatula until gases no longer escape from the sample. Unless the sample is punctured during the initial heating stage, it will swell up to overflowing.

The ashing process is complete when the ground residue fails to burn when heated to glowing with a bunsen burner. It should grind to a light powder with a spatula. When overheated, the residue is gritty and requires a mortar and pestle to grind. Soft ash burns much better than gritty residue in the arc of the spectrograph, with the result that the intensity of the spectral lines is proportionately greater per unit weight of metal contained in the carbon matrix. The soft ash is less desirable for leaching with acids because of the brown color extracted by the aqueous solution. The ash is removed quantitatively from the dish and weighed.

Volatile Metals. Mercury, arsenic and antimony are the only volatile metals in the sense that losses during the ashing process are so great that lethal amounts might not be detected by analysis of the residue. Quantitative analysis and the detection of very small amounts of these metals require a wet digestion for the destruction of the organic material without appreciable loss of metal.

The fact that the results of a Reinsch test are positive when it is applied directly to ground tissue containing toxic concentrations of a volatile metal, and the fact that significant amounts may not be found in a tissue digest by routine spectrographic analysis, would appear to eliminate the need for the laborious wet digestion of the tissue in a qualitative examination for metals. However, there are a number of advantages in performing a spectrographic analysis for many of the nonvolatile metals on a concentrate from a wet digestion. In particular, when the pathology or history is indicative of metal toxicity, using a wet digestion from the beginning will usually reduce the over-all labor involved in the metal analysis. Furthermore, more information is obtainable from a spectrographic examination when both a tissue ash and tissue digest are run on the same sample. The unused portion of the digest remains available for quantitative analysis by chemical or other methods.

The limiting concentration for detecting all metals in tissue by spectrographic analysis is improved when the analysis is performed on the concentrate from a wet digestion. This digestion of a tissue sample leaves a residue of considerably less bulk than the carbonized ash from the same weight of sample. The optical density of the spectral lines for each metal in the sample increases with the number of atoms contained in the core of the electrode. Since the capacity of the electrode is fixed at 0.1 ml., there are more atoms available for excitation per unit volume of wet digestion concentrate.

However, reducing the bulk by digestion to, say, one-tenth that of the bulk of an equal weight of ash sample will only increase the sensitivity by a factor of approximately two, despite the tenfold increase in actual gram atom content. The degree of excitation varies with the nature of the sample and the ratio of the concentrations of the extraneous ions. The presence of the highly conducting carbon in the ash produces a higher degree of activation per atom for all of the inorganic components. Consequently, the increased sensitivity obtained with the wet digest is relative and semiquantitative interpretations based on the density of characteristic lines must be made on spectra from comparable controls.

The losses that occur in ashing tissue containing beryllium, cadmium, lead, tin or zinc are quite small, but the amount may be significant when the metal concentration in the tissue is as low as it is in those cases in which most of the toxic metal is excreted before the time of death. In suspected metal toxicities in individuals who have been under treatment, particularly when compensation is involved, the purpose of the analysis is usually to furnish evidence on the possible extent of the metal damage prior to death. If a careful qualitative analysis for metals is warranted, negative findings for beryllium, cadmium, lead, tin and zinc should not be inferred without a spectrographic examination on the tissue digest. The possible significance of low concentrations combined with the questionable losses in ashing justifies including these metals with the volatiles, as well as the nonvolatiles.

A wet digestion is the better method for preparing almost all of the metals for quantitative analyses and, with the eight metals included in the volatile group, it is the only safe procedure. Only a part of the residue need be used for spectrographic confirmation. If aliquots of the digest are taken, a single wet digestion will serve for all purposes.

In a choice between ashing and wet digestion, the advantages of the latter are great enough to justify the added labor involved. At the same time, the little effort required to prepare a tissue ash is ample argument for a spectrographic examination of both.

Procedure for the Wet Digestion of Tissue and Body Fluids. Evaporate to dryness in a drying oven 50 to 100 gm. of minced tissue, 100 to 1,000 ml. of urine or 20 to 100 ml. of blood. Place the dehydrated sample in a 300 to 500 ml. Kjeldahl flask. Add 5 ml. of concentrated H_2SO_4 for a 50 gm. sample of tissue, 3 ml. for 100 ml. of urine, or 2 ml. for 20 ml. of blood. Larger samples do not require proportionately larger amounts of H_2SO_4. If the tissue sample is increased to 100 gm. or the blood to 100 ml., 7 ml. of concentrated H_2SO_4 will be sufficient. For 1 liter of urine, 12 ml. of acid is adequate. It is important to use the minimal amount of H_2SO_4 in a digestion that is to be analyzed spectrographically because the excess acid is converted to ammonium sulfate. The less acid that has to be neutralized, the less will be the dilution of the tissue residue with the salt.

Cover the sample with a layer of concentrated HNO_3 and allow it to stand overnight at the back of the hot plate so that the mixture remains warm. The HNO_3 digests the sample to a homogeneous solution, except for the fat which floats on the surface of the liquid. Remove the fat by filtration through glass wool.

Add several glass beads to the filtrate and heat the solution to slow boiling in the fume hood. If the boiling is continued without further addition of acid, the solution becomes darker in color as the oxides of nitrogen distill off until it suddenly changes from a dark brown to a black charred suspension. To prevent the charring stage from being reached, add dropwise a mixture of 2 volumes of $HClO_4$ and 1 volume of HNO_3 as the solution shows a tendency to darken. The digestion is complete when an amber color remains that does not become darker on further removal of excess HNO_3. Continue boiling at low heat, removing all of the excess HNO_3 and $HClO_4$, until SO_3 fumes appear. Cool the solution and transfer the contents of the flask quantitatively with water washing into a weighed beaker. Evaporate the wash water by heating on a hot plate and set the beaker under a bell jar with another beaker of NH_3. The NH_3 fumes neutralize the H_2SO_4 with the formation of ammonium sulfate. Bake the residue to dryness at 150° C., weigh and store it in a desiccator. Aliquot weights may then be taken for the analyses.

Modification for Embalmed Tissue. Formaldehyde-fixed tissue froths violently with loss of the sample when the HNO_3 mixture is warmed. With embalmed tissue the HNO_3 to cover the sample must be added slowly over about 8 hours while the sample is kept cooled.

Wet Digestion for Mercury. Mercury is the only metal that is likely to be volatilized by the HNO_3-$HClO_4$ digestion. A cold finger condenser in the neck of the Kjeldahl flask will reduce the losses, but will lengthen the time for the digestion. A safer method of digestion for small amounts of mercury is to omit the $HClO_4$ and employ a cold finger condenser for the final removal of the HNO_3. Losses will not be as great if care is taken to maintain an oxidizing medium at all times. If the solution is allowed to char, the carbonized material reduces the metal to the more volatile lower valence state.

Fortunately, the loss of mercury in the digestion of general unknowns is not too important. The Reinsch test is sufficiently sensitive for mercury to indicate that it is present in tissue and that the special digestion, without $HClO_4$, should be used. Digestion with oxidizing salts such as $KMnO_4$ and $KClO_3$ has been employed (1, 2). Large amounts of nonvolatile solid are introduced into the sample by these procedures. The dilution of the residue as a result of the increased bulk, as well as the addition of extraneous ions, defeats the purpose of the digestion for spectrographic examinations.

THE REINSCH TEST. The Reinsch test is a valuable probing type of reaction, and in the general unknown type of case it should be the first procedure carried out in the examination for metals. The test is applied directly to the ground biologic sample. Stomach contents, kidney or liver tissue are used.

Procedure. Add approximately 25 gm. of finely ground tissue or 5 to 10 gm. of stomach contents to a six inch potato tube and mix with enough water to make a slurry. Next, add 5 ml. of concentrated HCl. Make a copper coil by winding 12 to 14 turns of #20 wire around a lead pencil, leaving about six inches of wire for a handle. Clean the wire by quickly immersing it in HNO_3 and washing with distilled water until the copper shows a bright surface finish. Submerge the coil in the tissue mixture and heat the tube in a boiling water bath for 45 minutes to one hour. Remove the coil, wash in running water to remove any adhering tissue particles, rinse in distilled water and observe it for any discoloration on the surface of the copper.

In performing the test on a general unknown, it is advantageous to add two copper coils or else, when there is ample sample, to run two simultaneous determinations. It is important to detect mercury at this point in order to determine whether or not the special digestion procedure is necessary. The wire must remain in the tissue mixture for a long time when small amounts of metals are present, and the extra wire is then available for the other tests.

Mercury, bismuth, silver, arsenic and antimony and large amounts of selenium, tellurium and sulfide deposit on the surface of the copper under the conditions of the test. Relatively large amounts of mercury produce a silvery deposit which polishes to a high gloss when the wire is rubbed with a piece of lens paper. Small amounts which may not be apparent by visual or microscopic examination of the wire are detected by the cuprous iodide reaction.

CUPROUS IODIDE REACTION FOR METALLIC MERCURY (3). *Reagent.* Dissolve 5 gm. $CuSO_4 + 3$ gm. of anhydrous $FeSO_4$ in 10 ml. of water. Then add 7 gm. of KI in 50 ml. of water with stirring. Filter the precipitated Cu_2I_2, wash with water and then make into a slurry with water. Store in a brown bottle in the form of a suspension.

Procedure. Place a small filter paper on a watch glass and add two drops of the suspension at the center of the paper. Place the copper spiral on the Cu_2I_2 spot, cover it with a watch glass, and allow it to stand about 12 hours. In the presence of as much as 20 μg. of mercury, a salmon pink color develops, due to the formation of cuprous mercuric iodide.

The remaining elements give a black deposit. The easiest method of testing the deposit is with the aid of a spectrograph, using a high voltage condensed spark source. In the direct current arc, mercury, arsenic and antimony are lost unless present in relatively high concentrations. If a high voltage exciting source is not available, an alternate procedure is to volatilize the arsenic and antimony and test for bismuth and silver in the spectrograph.

VOLATILIZATION PROCEDURE FOR MERCURY, ARSENIC AND ANTIMONY. Place the coil in a small reduction tube 3 cm. long and 1 cm. in diameter. Cover the mouth of the tube with the flat surface of a hollow ground slide, and then cover the hollowed surface of the slide with ice. Suspend the tube in a hole in an asbestos board and heat gently 1 to 3 minutes with the oxidizing flame of a microburner. Mercury forms minute globules, arsenic minute octahedral crystals and antimony an amorphous deposit. The deposits are subjected to microchemical tests for the metals.

CONFIRMATORY TEST FOR ARSENIC AND ANTIMONY. With small amounts of arsenic and antimony, it is easier to subject another wire to special tests for the two metals than to carry out a microchemical examination of a sublimate. An arsenic deposit may be separated from antimony by just submerging the wire in a 10 per cent solution of KCN and shaking intermittently for 5 minutes. The arsenic dissolves, as do selenium, tellurium and sulfide, leaving the antimony deposit unaffected. The KCN solution is analyzed for arsenic and the coil for antimony by the modified Gutzeit method described under the respective metals.

Gettler and Kaye (3) described chemical tests for all the metals (except silver) deposited on the copper coils in the Reinsch test. Sulfide deposits are a source of annoyance. They are likely to be obtained when putrefaction has set in, or in the presence of relatively large amounts of sulfa drugs. Sodium formaldehyde sulfoxylate and BAL, used in the treatment of mercury and arsenic poisoning, produce a black sulfide deposit on the wire. If the black deposit dissolves in 10 per cent KCN, the solution should be tested for the sulfide ion. The sensitivity of the Reinsch test for the detection of metals is reduced when sulfide is present, and a more detailed search by other methods must be made before they can be eliminated.

SPECTROGRAPHIC ANALYSIS FOR METALS

The two important constants in the performance of a spectrograph are resolving power and speed. The greater the resolving power, the greater the purity of the spectrum and the better the separation of individual lines. The greater the speed, the greater is the intensity of the spectral lines or the more sensitive the instrument for the detection of low concentrations of metal. In the design of an instrument one of these constants can be increased only at the expense of the other. The minimum requirements for the spectrographic examination of tissue residue are found in the large Littrow type of prism spectrograph which has a linear dispersion of approximately 30 inches and both quartz and glass optics.

The lower resolution of the medium-sized prism instrument with a 10-inch dispersion renders it inadequate for interpretation of spectra for the complex tissue residue. In the past, grating instruments have not been suitable because of their low speed. Recent developments in the manufacturing of ruled gratings have made it possible to construct grating spectrographs with higher speeds and resolution than the Littrow type of prism instrument. If a grating instrument has eliminated interference due to overlapping of higher order spectra, is free of "ghosts" and has resolution and speed equal to or better than the Littrow type of instrument, it has the advantage over prism instruments because there is a linear separation of the spectral lines.

Preparation of the Sample. Grind the tissue ash to a fine powder in a mortar. If it has a greasy consistency with a tendency to lump on grinding, the sample has not been ashed sufficiently. If it is hard and sandy, the ash has been overheated.

Core a one-fourth inch by one inch graphite electrode by drilling a 5 mm. cavity in one end, preferably with a coring machine,* so that the side walls of the core are very thin. Thin walls burn away faster, with the result that poorly conducting samples are made to burn better in the arc. For qualitative analysis fill the core of the electrode with ash by gently tamping the electrode in the sample. When a semiquantitative interpretation is to be made from the line intensities, introduce a 50 mg. weighed sample into the electrode core with the aid of a special electrode funnel.

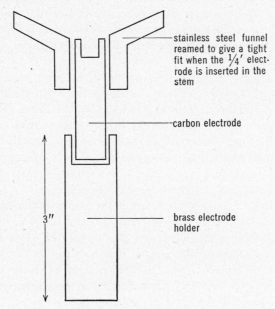

stainless steel funnel reamed to give a tight fit when the $\frac{1}{4}'$ electrode is inserted in the stem

carbon electrode

3"

brass electrode holder

Fig. 43-1. Electrode Assembly with the Loading Funnel.

Grind a three-sixteenths inch by one inch graphite electrode to a point in the shaping attachment for the coring machine or in a pencil sharpener reserved for that purpose and set in a brass holder. The electrodes are mounted in the arc stand of the spectrograph with the bottom sample electrode made the anode and the three-sixteenths inch top electrode the cathode. Residues for tissue digests are mounted in the same way.

The procedure for setting up, aligning and checking the instrument and the details for carrying out the analysis are described in standard texts on spectrographic analysis (4, 5, 6).

Choice of Exciting Source. There are three standard methods for activating the sample, and each has an advantage for the special problems involved in the spectrographic examination in general unknowns. The direct current arc, using 220 volts and 8 to 10 amperes, results in greater sensitivity for tissue ash and digestion residues. The arc wanders considerably during the exposure so that semiquantitative analysis from line intensity comparisons with reference plates is subject to considerable error. The alternating current arc which employs 2,500 to 6,000 volts gives

* Such as the Jaco carbon electrode driller, made by the Jarrell-Ash Co., Boston, Mass.

a more steady source, resulting in more nearly quantitative interpretations. There is less background on the plate and densitometer readings are more easily recorded. The high voltage condensed spark, employing 15,000 to 80,000 volts and a current of a few milliamperes, is not suitable for producing spectra from tissue ash and digestion residues, because the sample burns only on top with very little penetration. Air bands and second order spectral lines complicate the pattern. The spark is essential for analysis of Reinsch wires when spectrographic differentiation between arsenic and antimony is to be made. It is an ideal source for examining single metal particles removed at autopsy and is the only source for use in the special analysis of unashed tissue sections.

Preparation of the Qualitative Plate. The first trial is usually made with the quartz optics of the spectrograph set to cover the region between 3400 and 2380 Å. Practically all of the metals have prominent lines falling within this range, and after an inspection of this region, the other instrument settings for the suspected metal will be indicated.

First, make a qualitative plate, employing the direct current arc with 10 amperes and a 20 micron slit. If a wet digestion was made, load four electrodes comprising two ashed samples and two digestion residues. At the same time, prepare two electrodes, one containing a normal sample of ash and the other a normal sample of digestion residue of the type of material under examination. If only one type of sample, the ashed material or the digestion residue, is to be examined, load only two electrodes with the sample and load a third with a control sample of the same tissue as the test specimen but free of extraneous toxic metals.

Make six exposures through the aperture of the Hartman diaphragm for one type of sample, for example, the tissue ash. Arc the residue from the normal tissue through the #1 aperture of the diaphragm for 30 seconds. Move the #2 aperture in alignment with the slit and then arc the unknown for 30 seconds. Mount pure iron electrodes in the arc and make a three second exposure through the #3 aperture of the diaphragm with the current reduced to three amperes.

The pure iron spectrum serves as the scale on the instrument. The positions of the iron lines are the reference points from which the wavelengths of lines in the unknown sample are determined. The normal tissue spectrum is used for comparison with the unknown to spot quickly those lines in the unknown produced by other than the normally occurring metals and thereby to eliminate the labor of a complete analysis of the unknown spectrum.

The plate holder is racked down so that the position of the #1 aperture of the diaphragm is in juxtaposition with the #3 spectra for the above plate setting. Make three additional exposures of the remaining unknown sample through the Hartman diaphragm apertures without interrupting the arc—a 15 second exposure through the #1 aperture, 60 seconds through the #2, and the #3 is exposed until the sample has been completely burned.

The varying exposures on the same sample give information concerning the nature of the metals in the residue that is not apparent from a single exposure. As the sample burns, the more volatile metals disappear first and their lines are recorded in the earlier stage of the arcing process. By the time the second 60 second exposure has been completed, most of the more volatile metals will have been removed from the sample, and the third exposure will record only the metals with very high melting points. This results in a partial separation similar to that in a fractional distillation. Where there is possible interference of prominent lines of two or more metals, comparison of intensity ratios in the three spectra will aid in the interpretation.

The same set of procedures is repeated with the digestion residue, making a total of 12 exposures for the plate.

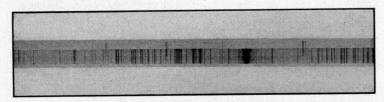

Fig. 43-2. Qualitative Spectrographic Plate.

1. Pure thallium.
2. Kidney ash from a case.
3. Normal kidney ash.

A typical qualitative plate is shown in Figure 43-2.

Examination of the Qualitative Plate. An ordinary hand lens or plate viewing box is not adequate for analyzing the complex spectra of tissue from general unknowns. A plate comparator of the Judd Lewis type *, capable of bringing spectra from two different plates into juxtaposition in an eyepiece, should be a part of the spectrographic equipment. When used as a simple viewing apparatus, the permanent plate mount, with eyepiece mounted on the optical bench carriage, allows the spectra to be scanned without distracting the attention of the observer. The adequately magnified spectrum is always in alignment with the eyepiece, thus greatly reducing eyestrain.

In the spectra, as photographed by the instrument, the top aperture of the diaphragm is represented by the bottom photograph and the bottom aperture is represented by the top photograph. However, if the plate is mounted in the comparator, turned upside down with the emulsion side toward the observer, the wavelengths from left to right will be increasing in order and the position of the spectrum will correspond to the data sheet. The unknown spectrum is first scanned for the purpose of spotting any outstanding abnormal lines in the normal spectral pattern. Certain metals have strong lines appearing in the neighborhood of typical normal spectral lines and, if the normal tissue spectrum is well known, these will be apparent immediately. All lines seen by the operator which are not ordinarily present in the control spectrum should be marked by placing a small black ink dot above the line with a fine pointed pen.

Determination of the Approximate Wavelengths of Abnormal Lines. The pure iron spectrum in juxtaposition to the unknown serves as the scale for determining the approximate wavelength of unknown lines. Obviously, in order to use the iron spectrum as a scale, the wavelengths of all of the iron lines must be known. In this laboratory, the iron lines are identified from a master plate containing pure iron lines with pure copper and tin lines in juxtaposition to those of iron. The iron spectrum is divided into sections of three-fourths inch and one and one-fourth inch between easily identified copper and tin lines. Within each section, 10 to 20 characteristic iron lines or iron pairs are marked by ink dots and numbered in groups of five. A densitometer tracing covering each iron section and an enlarged photograph of the same magnification as the tracing are mounted on a cardboard. The wave-

* Manufactured by Adam Hilger Ltd., London, N.W. 1, England.

lengths of the iron lines are recorded on the tracing, along with the corresponding line number of the master plate.

In determining the wavelength of the unknown line, the master iron plate is placed in the bottom section of the comparator and the iron spectra of the master and unknown plates are brought into alignment in the eyepiece. The two iron lines nearest to the unknown line on either side of it on the unknown plate are noted. These iron lines are then located in the master iron plate and their position with respect to numbered iron lines is determined. The numbered lines are then located on the densitometer tracing and the wavelengths of the iron lines in question are established from the position and intensity ratios within the numbered iron patterns.

By means of the master plate and the densitometer tracing, the wavelengths of all of the iron lines can be determined very quickly. The wavelength of the unknown line is now calculated by noting its position with respect to the two known iron lines. Visual inspection will show the position of the unknown line with respect to the two known iron lines with sufficient precision to allow an estimation of the wavelength to within one Å in the middle ultraviolet region of the spectrum. Within this narrow range it may be assumed that the dispersion is linear with the wavelength. Thus, if an unknown line is halfway between the two known iron lines, its wavelength is half the difference between the wavelengths of the iron lines added to the wavelength of the shorter iron line.

After the wavelength of the unknown has been determined, a table of wavelengths(7) is consulted which lists wavelengths in increasing order with the possible metals. Assuming more than one metal is a possibility, the wavelengths of each metal are examined. Since all metals have a number of strong lines, once one of the lines is identified, the others can be predicted from the table. By reversing the above identification procedure and looking in other portions of the spectrum for predicted lines for a certain metal, the identification can be confirmed. At least three strong lines should be identified for qualitative identification of a metal. Approximately two minutes are required for determining the wavelengths of unknown lines by this procedure.

In certain isolated portions of the spectrum the iron lines are too widely separated for a visual determination of line positions. When this condition exists, the linear distance between the known iron lines and the unknown must be measured with a microscope-micrometer(8) and the wavelength calculated by linear interpretation from the equation:

$$\lambda = \lambda_1 + \frac{\lambda_2 - \lambda_1}{d_2 - d_1}(d - d_1)$$

λ_1 and λ_2 are the wavelengths, and d_1 and d_2 the micrometer readings, for two reference iron lines located on either side of the unknown; λ and d are the same values for the unknown.

In exceptional cases it may be necessary to eliminate the possibility of interference by another element which has a prominent line very close to that of the suspected metal. In those cases subject to review by independent examiners, it is necessary to establish the precision of the wavelength measurement. When the positions of the two possible lines are close to the limits of resolution of the instrument, the wavelengths should be calculated from the Hartman dispersion formula:

$$\lambda = A + \frac{B}{D - d}$$

A, B and D are constants for the instrument calculated from measurements between three known iron lines located on either side of the unknown and within a range of 100 Å of it, and d is the linear distance between the λ_0 iron line (the arbitrary zero point—the shortest of the three iron lines) and the unknown (9). A calculating machine is essential for solving the equations because the B constant must be carried to seven significant figures and the other values to six figures.

Once the identification of an abnormal metal in the unknown spectrum has been established from at least three prominent lines, its spectral pattern can be located quickly by the use of metal reference plates. The procedure for the comparison is the same as that described for the master iron plate. The metal reference plate is substituted for the iron plate in the comparator and the iron spectra of the unknown and metal reference plates are brought into alignment in the eyepiece. Metal lines in the unknown spectrum will then line up with corresponding lines in the reference plate. They are marked with red ink dots to differentiate them from the black dotted abnormal spectral lines in the unknown. The spectral pattern is thus simplified by inspection and the labor of wavelength measurements is reduced proportionately. The process is then repeated for any remaining abnormal lines in the simple spectra.

Metal Reference Plates. The spectrographic laboratory should have a complete series of reference plates on file, including all of the metals and covering the complete spectral range. Six plates are required for each metal; three of these are for ashed samples and three for tissue digests. The three plates on the two samples cover the spectral range of the instrument. Two are taken in the ultraviolet region with quartz optics at instrument wavelength settings of 4100 Å to 2620 Å and 3100 Å to 2300 Å. The third is taken with glass optics at wavelength settings of 6000 to 4000 Å.

Six spectra are photographed on each reference plate through the three apertures of the Hartman diaphragm, thus making two rack settings for the plate. A pure iron spectrum is photographed through the #1 aperture, and the pure metal in the form of oxide, carbonate or sulfate is photographed through the #2 aperture using a current and exposure time to give an optimum optical density for the predominant metal lines. A 30 second exposure with a normal liver or kidney ash or a normal liver or kidney digest is then made through the #3 aperture, using 10 amperes and a 20 micron slit. The plate is racked down so that the #1 aperture of the Hartman diaphragm is in juxtaposition to the #3 photograph and a second set of exposures is made. Pure iron is again photographed through the #1 aperture and the normal tissue through the #3 aperture as in the first setting above. The photograph through the #2 aperture is the important one in that it is the reference spectrum for the plate. The sample is prepared by adding a predetermined weight of pure metal to a known negative tissue sample and carrying out the ashing or digestion process as previously described. The amount of metal is usually tabulated in milligrams per 100 gm. of wet tissue. The actual amount to be added is governed by the sensitivity of spectrographic analysis for the detection of the particular metal. The weight of added metal should be such that the optical density of the strongest lines falls on the linear portion of the plate, under the controlled conditions of excitation and exposure. This optimum concentration is most easily determined by running a series of exposures by diluting a prepared metal sample with the same ash or digest in steps of 1 to 10. Once the proper concentration of metal is known it is a good idea to prepare a large enough sample to have it available for direct comparisons with unknown samples.

The metal-containing sample is photographed through the #2 aperture with a current of 10 amperes for 30 seconds, using a 20 micron slit. This spectrum serves to show not only the positions of persistent metal lines in normal tissue spectra but also the possible interferences and the relation between line intensity and concentration of the metal in the normal tissue matrix. A typical reference plate is shown in Figure 43-3.

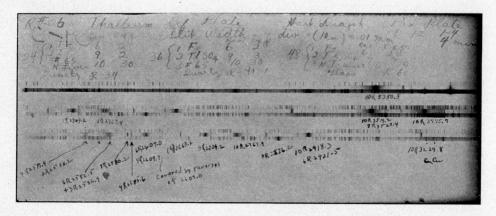

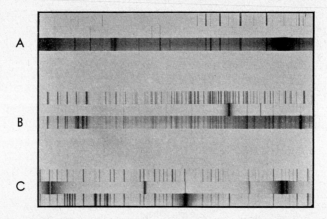

Fig. 43-3. Reference Plate for Thallium (Insert Magnification 1.6).

A, glass optics (4000-6000 Å.)
{ 1. Pure iron.
  2. Pure thallium.
  3. Normal tissue.

B, near ultraviolet (2620-4100 Å.)
{ 1. Pure iron.
  2. Pure thallium.
  3. Normal tissue.

C, ultraviolet (2300-3100 Å.)
{ 1. Pure iron.
  2. Pure thallium.
  3. Normal tissue.

Semiquantitative Interpretations. The qualitative plate is for the purpose of detecting abnormal quantities of metals other than those normally present in the spectrum. If significance were attached to all lines in the spectrum, the analyst would include most of the periodic table in his report. The conditions for obtaining the spectrum are set up for maximum sensitivity, and the presence of common elements such as lead, zinc, tin, manganese, aluminum and chromium in a tissue spectrum is not indicative of poisoning by the metal. Negative findings eliminate the metal from further consideration. Positive findings, however, merely serve to establish the need for a further quantitative examination. In general, quantitative analyses by chemical methods are less troublesome and more accurate than by the spectrographic method. When line intensities in the unknown are intense by comparison with the sample spectrum of the metal reference plate, the analyst can proceed directly to quantitative chemical analysis. In borderline cases with the less toxic metals, labor will be saved by making a semiquantitative plate using the alternating current arc as the exciting source before making a decision as to a chemical analysis.

Alternating Current Arc Spectra. Load a carbon electrode with a 25 to 50 mg. sample of the ash or digest, and add the same weight of control metal sample used in preparing the reference plate to a second electrode. Tissue digests are preferable to tissue ash for this purpose, since the digestion process leaves a residue that is more constant in composition for comparison with the control sample. First, photograph pure iron through the #1 aperture of the Hartman diaphragm, using a three second exposure with 220 volts direct current and three amperes. Then mount the unknown electrodes in the arc stand, and burn them two minutes with the alternating current arc, making the exposure through the #2 aperture of the diaphragm. In this laboratory the alternating current power supply is 6,000 volts open current with a three ampere electrode current. Then arc the control metal sample under the same conditions as the unknown through the #3 aperture of the diaphragm.

Analyze the plate in a densitometer and determine the relation between the line intensities of metal in the unknown and control samples. In addition, examine the spectra of both unknown and control samples to determine the ratios of the intensities of the metal lines to those of the normal tissue metals. The comparison will indicate the order of magnitude of the metal in the unknown and, if it is present in toxic concentrations, an exact quantitative analysis is indicated. Since less than 30 minutes are required for this analysis, the effort involved will be more than compensated for by eliminating chemical analysis in a series of cases requiring metal analysis.

Spectrographic Analysis of Dithizone Extracts. In poison cases involving the very toxic metals such as cadmium or thallium, the metal content in the sample residue may be so low that the wavelength of only one prominent line can be identified with certainty. Interference is always a possibility when less than three prominent lines are apparent. In order to establish the identification, it is necessary to concentrate the metal so that the amount contained in the core of the electrode is sufficient to give a clear-cut spectrum. The increase in line intensity in the sample after concentration not only serves to establish the identity of the metal but is a measure of the original concentration in the sample. Faint lines for the very toxic metals cannot be considered in the same light as those for the less toxic ones such as lead, zinc or tin. These may be normal components in certain cases due to ingestion with food or exposure to low concentrations over a long period of time, and their presence in the spectrum is of no significance in establishing the cause of death. The lowest detectable concentration of the very toxic metals, however, may be significant and their identity must be established with certainty.

A second type of case in which it is essential to determine low concentrations of any one of the metals is in suspected chronic poisonings in which considerable time has elapsed between the exposure and the death. When elimination of the metal by excretion in the urine has reduced the concentration to low levels, the histologic diagnosis may hinge on the detection of small amounts. The best method for concentrating metals in order to obtain electrode samples which give spectra of ample intensity is by the evaporation of a dithizone extract of a sample digest.

A chloroform solution of dithizone, when shaken in a separatory funnel with an aqueous solution containing metal ions, forms dithizonates with many of the metals which are readily soluble in the chloroform but insoluble in water. The dithizone in chloroform is a deep green color, while the dithizonates are yellow-orange, red or violet. If an unknown aqueous solution is shaken out with small volumes of green chloroform-dithizone solution, the formation of a dithizonate will be apparent by the change in color of the chloroform layer, and, if the extraction process is continued stepwise, the removal of the metal ion will be complete when the chloroform layer retains its green color after the shaking. Gold, platinum, palladium, silver, mercury, stannous tin, copper, bismuth, zinc, cobalt, nickel, lead, thallium and cadmium form chloroform-soluble dithizonates. Quantitative methods by dithizone titration have been described for all of them in which controlled pH and the addition of competitive complex forming salts reduce co-extraction to a minimum.

Gold, silver, mercury, stannous tin, bismuth and copper are extracted from mineral acid solutions at a pH of 1 to 4 with the optimum pH for each metal increasing in the order named. Zinc, cobalt, nickel and lead are extracted from neutral or faintly ammoniacal solutions. When the aqueous solution has a pH between 8 and 12, the optimum value for the extraction of the metal increases in this order: stannous tin $<$bismuth $<$zinc $<$thallium $<$lead $<$cadmium (10).* In ammoniacal solutions containing cyanide only stannous tin, bismuth, thallium and lead react with dithizone.

By employing a stepwise dithizone extraction of an aqueous solution of a sample digest and by carrying the titration through the pH ranges 1 to 4 and 8 to 12, all of the above metals are separated quantitatively from the normally occurring tissue metals. Spectrographic analysis of the chloroform evaporate produces a special pattern with line intensities increased in proportion to the degree to which the electrode sample was concentrated. The influence of extraneous ions on the activation in the arc is minimal and, with the resolution of the Littrow model spectrograph, interference due to overlapping with any combination that might be encountered from a biologic sample is of no consequence. An appropriate internal standard may be added to the evaporated dithizonate for precise quantitative analysis.

Procedure. A dithizone solution containing 25 mg. of diphenylthiocarbazone per liter of $CHCl_3$ is used for the extraction. Dissolve the wet digest from 50 gm. of sample in about 100 ml. of water, and adjust the pH to approximately 1.0 by the dropwise addition of NH_3, preferably with a glass electrode. If a residue from a wet digestion was prepared for spectrographic examination an aliquot may be weighed, moistened with a little concentrated H_2SO_4 and diluted to 100 ml. with water.†

Place the aqueous solution in a 250 ml. separatory funnel, add 5 ml. of dithizone solution and shake the mixture. If the green dithizone changes to a yellow or orange

---

* Stannous tin and bismuth have optimum pH values in both acid and alkaline solution, while zinc and lead may be extracted from neutral or strongly ammoniacal solutions.
† It is not necessary to filter off the insoluble silicate precipitate from the digest solution.

color, draw off the 5 ml. and add a second 5 ml. portion. Continue the titration until the dithizone retains its green color after shaking. Then readjust the pH to approximately 4.0, and continue the stepwise dithizone addition until the green dithizone no longer shows a color change. Next, add 10 ml. of 10 per cent citric acid to the solution * and adjust the pH to approximately 8.5 by the addition of NH_3. Again continue the stepwise addition as long as the 5 ml. portion of dithizone changes in color to a red or violet tinge. Repeat the titration process at pH values of 10 and 12, and then evaporate the combined $CHCl_3$ solution of dithizonate to a volume of approximately 5 ml.

If a particular metal is suspected from the examination of the qualitative plate, an appropriate internal standard may be added to the $CHCl_3$ solution at this point. Next, stir 50 mg. of powdered carbon from a spectrographically pure carbon electrode into the $CHCl_3$ solution, and continue the evaporation to dryness. Mix the carbon-dithizonate residue thoroughly by means of a rubber policeman, remove it quantitatively from the beaker to a glazed paper with a camel's hair brush, and pack it into the core of the electrode. Carry out the spectrographic analysis in the 6,000 volt open current alternating current arc at three amperes using a 20 micron slit and an exposure time long enough to burn the electrode sample to completion.

Quantitative Spectrographic Analysis. For precise quantitative spectrographic analysis, internal standards must be used. Line intensity measurements or the logarithmic sector method cannot be relied upon because of variations in the percentage composition of the normally occurring metals in a tissue ash or digestion residue. Extraneous ions in an electrode sample change the sensitivity of spectrum lines (11-14). The varying sodium content of urine ash or digest makes quantitative analysis particularly troublesome. The effect may be either positive or negative for only one or a number of metals in a sample. Because of these possible variations in spectral sensitivity, interpretations from standard quantitative working curves are limited to comparable samples. In general, quantitative chemical methods are preferable for a quantitative analysis, with quantitative spectrographic analysis reserved for those special cases in which sensitivity or interfering ions create a chemical problem. Internal standard methods have been published for most of the metals in biologic samples. Papers by Cholak and his associates (15-19) and the publications of Gerlach and Schweitzer (20) are particularly recommended.

Spectrographic Analysis of Reinsch Wires. Mercury, arsenic and antimony may be detected by spectrographic analysis of a Reinsch wire using an alternating current condensed spark as the exciting source. The 15,000 to 50,000 volts with the milliampere current produce a high degree of activation without creating a high electrode temperature. Bismuth and silver also give a good spark spectrum. Selenium, tellurium and sulfide do not have sensitive spectral lines. The more complicated spectral pattern produced by the spark source does not make interpretation difficult because the number of metals that may be present is limited. The sensitivity for the detection of mercury is considerably less than that by the cuprous iodide method, so that there is no reason for using a spectrographic method to detect mercury. The only advantage of a spectral analysis in a positive mercury finding is to eliminate the possibility of a second metal. Arsenic and antimony show about the same spectral sensitivity as obtainable by chemical tests, while bismuth and silver may be detected in considerably smaller concentrations spectrographically. Spectro-

* Citrates and tartrates prevent the precipitation of the hydroxides or phosphates of the metals in alkaline solutions.

graphic analysis is especially good for differentiating between a sulfide and a metal deposit in the Reinsch test.

With the alternating or direct current arc, the electrode temperatures are so high that the volatile metals distill off without undergoing activation. The arc spectra of bismuth and silver may be photographed without interference from any of the other Reinsch metals that may be present.

CONDENSED SPARK ANALYSIS. Make an electrode holder for the copper coil by drilling a small hole in the top of a three-eighths inch brass rod. Drill and tap the side for a small set screw. Clamp the copper coil in the brass holder and mount it in the bottom arm of the arc stand with a one-eighth inch carbon electrode on top. Spark the sample for 15 and then 30 seconds through the #1 and #3 apertures of the Hartman diaphragm with the spectrograph set to cover the middle portion of the ultraviolet region. Then spark a sample Reinsch coil from the same wire for 15 seconds through the #2 aperture of the diaphragm.

ALTERNATING CURRENT ARC ANALYSIS FOR BISMUTH AND SILVER. Place the Reinsch coil in the core of a three-eighths inch carbon electrode, mounted with a pointed one-fourth inch top electrode in the arc stand, and arc it, with an open circuit voltage between 2,500 and 3,000 and a current of 1 ampere, for 30 seconds through the #2 aperture of the diaphragm. Arc a control wire through the #1 aperture and the carbon electrodes through the #3 aperture under the same conditions as the unknown.

QUALITATIVE AND QUANTITATIVE ANALYSIS FOR SPECIFIC METALS

Mercury. Positive mercury findings are not proof of poisoning by mercury. Enough calomel may be present in the stomach contents to give a strong positive reaction for mercury, with detectable amounts present in the organs. The ingestion of diuretics such as mercuhydrin sodium solution and mercupurin (mercuzanthin) may lead to positive mercury tests for urine or blood. After treatment with organic mercurial antisyphilitics, organs give positive Reinsch tests; the use of organic mercurial antiseptics as preservatives in transfusion blood has been responsible for a mistaken diagnosis of mercury poisoning.

If mercury compounds are the cause of a death, the mercury content of the organs will be high and the kidney sections will show definite pathologic lesions. A negative mercury finding by the Reinsch test justifies elimination of acute mercury poisoning as the cause of death, whereas a positive test demands a quantitative analysis of the organs. The diagnosis hinges on the histologic findings supported by the quantitative chemical results.

ANALYSIS FOR MERCURY. 1. Indications for Mercury: the Reinsch test.

2. Spectrographic Analysis. A mercury spectrum can be obtained only with very high mercury concentrations as sometimes found in the stomach contents, or it can be obtained with condensed spark analysis of the Reinsch wire (see above). The indicating spectral line is 5460.7 Å (glass optics). The confirming spectral lines are 4358.3 and 4046.6 (glass optics) and 2536.5 Å.

3. Microchemical Tests for Mercury on a Reinsch Wire. Mercuric Iodide Test. If the Reinsch wire is treated by the volatilization procedure described under the Reinsch test on page 974, the resulting mercury globules, if examined under the microscope with oblique illumination, show the typical mirror-like reflection. If a small crystal of iodine is placed near the deposit and covered with an inverted watch

glass, the mirror-like particles will turn orange-red due to the formation of a coating of mercuric iodide.

Formation of Aluminum Amalgam. A very sensitive and specific method for the detection of mercury depends on the formation of an aluminum amalgam(21) which, in the presence of moist air, is quickly converted to aluminum oxide. The mercury thus liberated can amalgamate with fresh aluminum and the process of oxide formation is repeated. The liberated aluminum is detected with sodium alizarin sulfonate.

Reagent. 0.2 gm. sodium alizarin sulfonate per 100 ml. water plus 0.5 ml. glacial acetic acid.

Procedure. Volatilize the mercury from a Reinsch coil as described on page 000, using a polished aluminum plate instead of the microscope slide as the collector. After allowing to stand 15 minutes in a moist atmosphere, add a drop of alizarin reagent and let stand 3 minutes. Wash off the excess reagent with water and dry with blotting paper. Repeat the process, rinsing thoroughly with water before blotting. In the presence of mercury, red spots of the aluminum alizarin lake stick to the plate after the washing process.

4. Quantitative Determination of Mercury by the Dithizone Titration (22). Carry out a wet digestion on 50 gm. of tissue or 100 ml. of urine evaporate in a 500 ml. Kjeldahl flask by the procedure described on page 972, with the omission of the $HClO_4$ as described on page 972. When the digestion process has been carried out to the appearance of SO_3 fumes, cool the flask and wash down the cold finger condenser and flask neck with about 50 ml. of water. Add 1 gm. of hydroxylamine sulfate to reduce traces of HNO_2 that may remain in the solution. Rinse the contents of the flask into a 250 ml. separatory funnel with water, making a total volume of not more than 100 ml. Adjust the pH of the solution to approximately 2.0 by partial neutralization with ammonia and re-acidification with 6N H_2SO_4 to a red with Benzo yellow indicator.

Reagent. The dithizone solution is made up of 25 mg. diphenylthiocarbazone per liter of chloroform.

Standardization of the Dithizone. Make a standard mercury solution by dissolving 0.5 gm. of metallic mercury in concentrated HNO_3 and making the volume to 500 ml. with water. Dilute 10 ml. of this solution plus 10 ml. of concentrated HNO_3 to one liter with water. One ml. contains 10 μg. of mercury. Add 10 ml. of this standard mercury solution to a 250 ml. separatory funnel, dilute to approximately 100 ml. with water, and adjust the pH to approximately 2.0 as described previously. Add the dithizone solution contained in a 50 ml. buret in steps of 5 ml., 3 ml., 2 ml. and finally in 0.2 ml. portions from the buret. After each addition, shake the contents and draw off the chloroform after the two layers have separated completely. The mercury dithizone complex is an orange color in the chloroform layer. As the mercury is extracted from the aqueous solution, the chloroform layer becomes lighter in color and finally assumes a green off-color at the end point. The total volume of dithizone solution is read from the buret, and the mercury equivalent to 1 ml. is calculated. Approximately 1 ml. of the dithizone solution is equivalent to 1 μg. of mercury. The titration may be made more precise by back titrating the off-color dithizone portions with standard mercury solution (23, 24).

The dithizone solution deteriorates slowly and must be standardized after standing longer than 24 hours.

Analysis of the Unknown Solution. The titration procedure is carried out in the same manner as in the standardization process. In certain digests the green off-color persists over a greater volume range than will the standard solutions, probably due to complex formation of the mercury in the aqueous phase. When the end point is not sharp, the off-color chloroform solutions are combined and back titrated with standard mercury solution to an orange color in the chloroform layer.

Arsenic. Arsenic is the most common metallic poison. Arsenic trioxide, a frequent component of rat poison, is the arsenic compound most often encountered in toxicology. Lead arsenate is used extensively as an insecticide and is readily obtainable. There are a number of complex organic arsenicals, such as sodium cacodylate, neosalvarsan, arsphenamine and mapharsen, that are used in the treatment of syphilis and other spirillum infections, psoriasis, chronic myeloid leukemia and secondary anemia. Inorganic arsenic is used as a medicinal. Before penicillin was available, the dosage of inorganic arsenic given by intravenous injection in the treatment of syphilis was just below the level producing acute toxic symptoms. This drastic treatment is still used in exceptional cases of syphilis.

ANALYSIS FOR ARSENIC. 1. Indications for Arsenic: the Reinsch test.

2. Spectrographic Analysis. The spectral sensitivity for arsenic is greater than for mercury, and arsenic has been detected in the organs but only in rare cases. The indicating spectral line is 2780.2 Å. The confirming spectral lines are 2745.0 and 2860.5 Å.

3. Microchemical Test for Arsenic on a Reinsch Wire. The Reinsch test is very sensitive for the detection of arsenic; however, positive findings in the organs may be due to arsenic therapy or to the ingestion of food contaminated with arsenic-containing insecticides. Diagnosis of arsenic poisoning is made from quantitative analysis of the organs and from pathologic findings.

(a) The Bettendorff Test. Arsenic when volatilized from the Reinsch wire by the procedure described on page 974 is deposited as arsenous oxide. Traces can be detected by the Bettendorff test.

Reagent. Concentrated HCl saturated with stannous chloride.

Procedure. A drop of the reagent is placed on the deposit from the volatilization of the Reinsch wire. If arsenic is present a brownish black precipitate forms immediately:

$$2 \ As^{+++} + 3 \ Sn^{++} \rightarrow As_2 + 3 \ Sn^{++++}$$

Mercury interferes; if mercury is present the deposited arsenic should be converted to the heat resistant $Mg_2As_2O_7$ before applying the test (25). Antimony deposits do not react with the reagent.

The nature of the arsenic compound in the stomach contents may indicate whether the death was accidental or suicidal. The presence of large amounts of inorganic arsenic is consistent with suicide, whereas organic-bound arsenic may be present from accidental ingestion.

4. Detection of the Presence of Arsenic Trioxide. Arsenic trioxide is easily sublimed from dehydrated stomach contents. Dry 5 gm. of stomach contents at 110° C. in a drying oven. Grind the dehydrated material in a mortar, place it in the sublimation tube described on page 1153 and heat the tube at 250° C. under reduced pressure. The sublimed oxide deposits on the collector of the sublimation tube. The presence of large amounts of lead in the stomach should lead to an examination for lead arsenate.

5. Isolation of Organic Arsenic Compounds. With the exception of the caco-dylates, most of the organic arsenic compounds are soluble in 95 per cent alcohol. Dehydrate 10 to 50 gm. of the stomach contents and grind to a powder in a mortar. Disperse the sample in 95 per cent ethyl alcohol and add enough HCl to give a strong acid reaction. After thorough mixing, preferably in a blender, allow the solid matter to settle out and decant the supernatant alcohol through filter paper. Repeat the process three times in order to extract all of the alcohol soluble components. Then evaporate the combined alcohol solutions to dryness on the steam bath. Run a Reinsch test on the residue and on the alcohol evaporate. A higher arsenic content in the alcohol evaporate than in the residue is an indication of the presence of organic arsenic compounds. The evaporate is further examined by conventional organic methods. A number of these arsenic compounds have amine groups which give a positive alkaline diazo reaction (page 1216). When the concentration is relatively large, the dye formed in the coupling reaction can be salted out with NaCl and the precipitate tested for arsenic.

6. The Marsh Test. The Marsh test is the best all around method for the detection and estimation of arsenic. Analysis is performed on the H_2SO_4 solution remaining after the wet digestion of 10 to 50 gm. of organs as described on page 972. The test depends on the formation of arsine (AsH_3) by the action of hydrogen produced by the zinc and H_2SO_4. The arsine gas is passed through a heated tube where it is decomposed with the deposition of arsenic in the form of a mirror-like coating in the cool portion of the tube. The length of the mirror is proportional to the concentration of arsenic in the sample.

Antimony also gives a mirror. Selenium gives a yellow-red or brownish-red deposit, and H_2S from the reduction of the sulfuric acid breaks down in the hot tube with the deposition of sulfur. Organic substances such as alcohol, if present in the solution, may produce a carbon mirror; however, all organic material will have been removed if the test is performed on the wet digest.

Procedure. The apparatus (26) consists of a 500 ml. Florence flask equipped with a thistle tube and right angle glass tubing in a two hole rubber stopper. The glass tubing is connected to a $CaCl_2$ drying tube by means of a rubber hose connection, and the outlet of the drying tube is connected to a pyrex tube of 7 mm. internal diameter pulled out to form a capillary of 6 inch length and 1 mm. bore. Wire gauze is wrapped around the 7 mm. bore just back of the capillary constriction. The Florence flask is wrapped with a heavy towel to prevent flying glass in the event the generating flask explodes.

Introduce 10 to 15 gm. of arsenic-free mossy zinc into the Florence flask, and insert the stopper into the thistle tube tightly to prevent any air leaks. Introduce enough 12 per cent H_2SO_4 to cover the zinc and to submerge the bottom end of the thistle tube. To catalyze the reduction, add 0.5 ml. of 1 per cent $CuSO_4$. The hydrogen gas is allowed to generate for half an hour in order to remove any air from the apparatus. A rubber hose, connected to the end of the combustion tube is led under water to prevent back diffusion of air.

Wash the H_2SO_4 solution of the tissue digest from the Kjeldahl flask and dilute it with water to make the solution 12 to 15 per cent with respect to the H_2SO_4. Place a Bunsen burner under the wire gauze of the capillary combustion tube and heat the wire to redness. Then introduce the diluted digestion solution into the flask through the thistle tube in 10 ml. portions until a pronounced mirror forms in the capillary of the combustion tube. Allow the hydrogen to generate at a slow rate for about one hour after the addition of the diluted digest.

7. Microchemical Tests for Arsenic on the Marsh Mirror. Cut the capillary at a point about 1 cm. beyond the mirror produced in the Marsh test. Using the mirrored section as a pipet, draw up a microdrop of concentrated HNO_3 through the capillary end until it comes in contact with the end position of the mirror. Arsenic and antimony dissolve readily in the acid. Deposit the acid drop on a hollow ground glass microslide and allow the drop to evaporate to dryness. Prepare several slides in this manner.

Action of H_2S. Allow H_2S gas to pass over the deposit on the slide. With arsenic yellow As_2S_3 is formed.

Bettendorff Test. Add a drop of $SnCl_2$-HCl reagent (page 986). Black metallic arsenic is deposited if the metal is present.

Action of Silver Nitrate Solution. Add a drop of aqueous $AgNO_3$. A precipitate of red Ag_3AsO_4 forms if arsenic is present.

Quantitative Estimation from the Marsh Mirror. The estimation from the Marsh mirror is less accurate than in the Gutzeit method, but the precision is adequate for poison cases and has the advantage that the metal is isolated and its identity confirmed by microchemical tests. The length of the mirror in the capillary is compared with standard mirrors made from solutions of known arsenic content, and the arsenic is calculated from the total volume of the solution digest and the aliquots used to produce the mirror.

8. Quantitative Determination of Arsenic by the Gutzeit Test. The Gutzeit test is more sensitive, more quantitative, less laborious and less specific than the Marsh test. A choice between it and the Marsh test is usually decided on the basis of the results from the Reinsch test. If identification from the Reinsch test is certain, quantitative analysis by the Gutzeit method will save time and give more precise values. When there is a possibility of the presence of metals other than arsenic and when there is sulfide interference in the Reinsch test, the Marsh test is preferable. Arsine is generated as in the Marsh test. The gas reacts with a paper disk impregnated with mercuric bromide, forming a yellow to brown mixture of $As(HgBr)_3$ and As_2Hg_3 (27).

A modified apparatus and procedure designed (28) to eliminate variations in the stain due to changes in the rate of hydrogen liberation when a strip of impregnated paper is inserted in the top tube as in the conventional method, follows: A glass flange with paper disk is substituted for the paper strip. Thus, all of the arsine gas has to pass through the impregnated paper. Changes in the rate of hydrogen generation produce variations in the intensity of the stain at the surface of the paper when comparison with standards is made with reflected light. This error is reduced by reading the optical density with transmitted light as done in solution colorimetry. The modified Gutzeit apparatus is shown in Figure 43-4. It consists of a 50 ml. capacity generating flask with a side arm inlet for admitting the solution. The generating flask is connected to a condensing column by means of a ground glass joint, and a glass flange connected to the top of the column with an interchangeable ground glass joint. The impregnated paper disk is tightly held between the ground surfaces of the flange by means of rubber bands. The apparatus is designed to accommodate flanges 8, 12 and 15 mm. in diameter. The 12 mm. flange is normally used in arsenic determinations in which a positive Reinsch is obtained, and in treatment cases in which the arsenic content lies between 0.5 and 10 gamma. The 8 and 15 mm. flanges are substituted when exceptionally low or high values are expected.

Reagents. Lead acetate impregnated glass wool; solid $NaHSO_3$; 40 per cent $SnCl_2$ in concentrated HCl; 10 per cent $CuSO_4$; and 5 per cent $HgBr_2$ in absolute methyl alcohol.

$HgBr_2$ paper is prepared as follows: A stock supply of impregnated paper may be made at one time and stored in an airtight amber container. Whatman #1 or #2 paper is used. Immerse the filter paper sheets for about 5 minutes in the 5

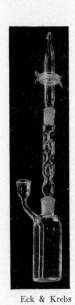

Eck & Krebs

Fig. 43-4. Modified Gutzeit Apparatus.

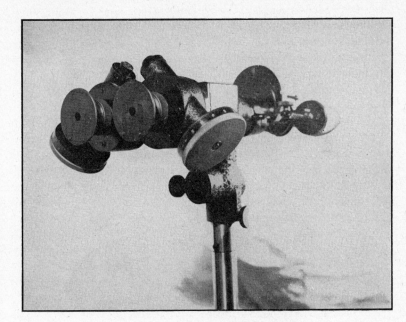

Fig. 43-5. Zeiss Stufo Photometer.

per cent $HgBr_2$ solution of absolute methyl alcohol contained in a petri dish. Remove the paper and suspend it in air to dry. During drying an excess of the $HgBr_2$ diffuses to the outer rim of the filter paper. In order to insure an even impregnation of the disk, cut off and discard a strip about 1 inch from the edge. Cut round disks from the remaining section with a cork borer of a diameter approximately $\frac{1}{16}$ inch less than the outer diameter of the flanges.

Procedure. Reheat the sulfuric acid solution of the wet digest from 50 ml. of urine, 10 ml. of blood or 10 to 25 gm. of tissue to SO_3 fumes for 5 minutes to insure complete removal of the $HClO_4$. Cool the acid, dilute with approximately 2 volumes of water and add 0.1 gm. of solid $NaHSO_3$. Wash down the sides of the flask with water after the addition of the $NaHSO_3$ and boil the solution until all SO_2 is driven off. Transfer the solution to a graduate, washing the flask with small portions of water. Adjust the volume by the addition of water so that the acidity of the solution to be analyzed is 10 per cent by volume with respect to the sulfuric acid. If the wet digestion is made especially for the Gutzeit arsenic determination, 4 ml. of concentrated H_2SO_4 is the desirable quantity to use in order to have the proper acidity in the final volume which does not exceed 40 ml. of solution.

Approximately half fill the condensing column of the apparatus with loosely packed lead acetate impregnated glass wool. Place a plug of absorbent cotton on either side of the glass wool. The apparatus should be conditioned by running a 20 gamma sample of arsenic by the described procedure before analyzing the unknown solution with a new charge of the glass wool. The lead acetate removes any H_2S which may be formed by reduction of the H_2SO_4, particularly if the temperature of the solution is elevated during the reduction process. Add 5 gm. of mossy zinc and 0.5 ml. of 10 per cent $CuSO_4$ to the Gutzeit generating flask, and assemble the charged condenser and appropriate flange containing the $HgBr_2$ impregnated paper. Add three drops of 40 per cent $SnCl_2$ to the 40 ml. of digest containing 10 per cent by volume of the sulfuric acid. Then carefully add the solution through the side arm inlet tube. Allow the reduction to continue for one hour, after which the paper disk is removed and examined.

A quantitative estimation may be made by visual comparison of the unknown with a series of stains made from arsenic concentrations ranging from 0.5 to 10 gamma of As^{++}. Unless care is taken to maintain a constant rate of hydrogen formation, variations in the intensity of the stain at the surface of the paper will occur. Since visual comparison is usually made by reflected light, an error may be made in the matching process. When matched visually by light transmitted through the paper, the higher arsenic concentrations cannot be read. Moreover, the standard stains fade during storage and dilute standard arsenic solutions change with age, due to absorption by the glass container. By preparing a curve from fresh standard, using optical density measurements from photometer readings, the need for standard stains or the alternate procedure of running known solutions along with the unknown may be eliminated. The accuracy with which the density of the stain can be read is considerably greater and the curve constitutes a permanent record for the method.

Photoelectric colorimeters may be adapted for transmission readings of the paper disk in which the instrument is set at 100 per cent with a control disk and the transmission then determined on the stained disk. However, the light source in most machines, after reduction in intensity by the monochromatic filters, does not furnish enough energy for transmission readings with the paper system. Moreover, the surface effects on the matted paper limit their application for this purpose. A Zeiss Stufo photometer, equipped with the low density filters and special adapters for holding the paper disks, is ideal for this type of measurement. The apparatus is shown in Figure 43-5.

In order to adapt the photometer for transmission readings through paper, a special adaptor for holding the paper disks was made to replace the housing in which the absorption cells are normally held. The adaptor consists of two parts. One is a reproduction of the threaded adaptor of the Stufo cell holder with the cell housing removed; the other is the face plate 5 cm. in diameter with a centered collar turned to fit snugly over the one end of the sleeve of the thread. Face plates of 8 and 12 mm. diameter are available for the 8 and 12 mm. flanges respectively. The 15 mm. flange size may be read through the 12 mm. face plate. When the aperture of the Stufo photometer is set at 100 per cent transmission, the diameter of the diaphragm is 12 mm. so that scale readings on the 12 mm. and 15 mm. paper are the same as for solutions. When measurements are made on the 8 mm. flange the aperture corresponding to maximum transmission is 44.4 per cent. Readings with the smaller flange are then calculated on a 100 per cent basis for plotting the curve. The procedure for aligning the instrument and making the readings is described in operating instructions published by Zeiss for the instrument. The L-1 red filter is used for reading the arsenic stains. Arsenic curves for the 8 and 12 mm. flanges are shown in Figure 43-6.

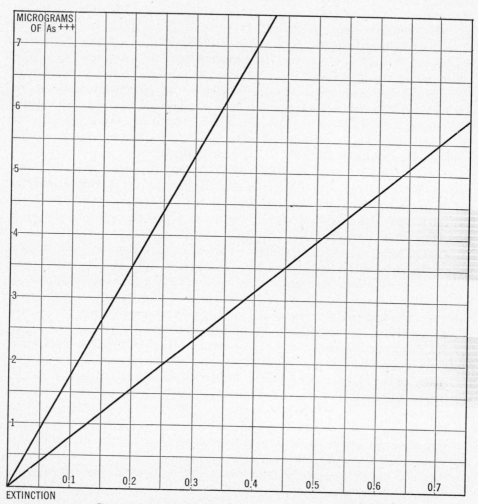

Fig. 43-6. Extinction Values for 8 and 12 mm. Arsenic Disks.

Antimony. Antimony is seldom encountered in toxicologic analysis. Its chief interest to the analyst is due to its similarity to arsenic in chemical behavior. Since it behaves like arsenic in the Reinsch, Marsh and Gutzeit tests it must be excluded in considering quantitative values for arsenic. Organic antimony compounds have limited use in medicine. Tartar emetic, antimony sodium thioglycollate, diramin and similar substances are used as protozoal parasiticides, particularly in certain tropical diseases.

ANALYSIS FOR ANTIMONY. 1. Indications for Antimony: the Reinsch test.

2. Spectrographic Analysis. The spectral sensitivity for antimony is considerably greater than for mercury and arsenic, and it is frequently detected spectrographically in the organs although the major lines are weak and can be easily overlooked. The indicating spectral line is 2770.0 Å. The confirming spectral lines are 2877.9 and 2598.1 Å.

3. Microchemical Tests for Antimony on a Reinsch Wire. The sublimate from volatilization of antimony from a Reinsch wire done by the procedure described on page 974 is amorphous in contrast to the crystalline deposit from the volatilization of arsenic.

Bettendorff Test (page 986). Negative.

Hydrogen Reduction Test. Soluble and insoluble Sb^{+++} and Sb^{++++} compounds are reduced to brown metallic antimony by nascent hydrogen. Tin compounds are also reduced but, if the reduction is carried out in the presence of platinum, tin will deposit as a gray-colored plate on the platinum and also on the zinc added as the source of hydrogen. It is easily distinguished from the brown granular antimony deposit. When the Bettendorff test, applied to a white deposit from the volatilization of a Reinsch wire, is negative for arsenic, the hydrogen reduction test may be continued in the $SnCl_2$-HCl reagent added for the Bettendorff test.

Procedure. Force a piece of mossy zinc the size of a large grain of sand into the loop of a platinum wire, with the wire squeezed so that the zinc is firmly held. Place the loop containing the zinc in the drop of $SnCl_2$-concentrated HCl from the Bettendorff test and observe it after five minutes. In the presence of antimony a dark brown color develops.

4. The Marsh Test. Stibine (SbH_3) is formed in the Marsh test when the procedure described for arsenic (page 987) is followed. Stibine is less stable than arsine and consequently the mirror of antimony usually deposits on both sides of the flame in the combustion tube. Quantitative estimation cannot be made from the length of the mirror as in the case of arsenic. The antimony mirror may be dissolved and determined nephelometrically as the sulfide.

5. Microchemical Tests for Antimony on the Marsh Mirror. The antimony is dissolved in small portions with nitric acid as described for arsenic on page 988.

Action of H_2S. If antimony is present, orange Sb_2S_3 is formed.

Bettendorff Test. Negative. The nascent hydrogen reduction test is positive (see above).

Rhodamine B Test. *Reagent.* 0.01 gm. of rhodamine B per 100 ml. water.

Procedure. Evaporate the nitric acid solution to dryness in the depression of a porcelain spot plate. Add one drop of concentrated HCl and a microcrystal of $NaNO_2$. Add 5 to 10 drops of the rhodamine B reagent. In the presence of antimony the light red dye solution changes to violet.

6. Quantitative Determination of Antimony by the Gutzeit Test. The procedure is the same as for arsenic (page 988). The stain from antimony on the $HgBr_2$ paper is completely decolorized by exposing the paper to HCl fumes whereas the color due to arsenic will persist(29). Five per cent $AgNO_3$ solution has been recommended as superior to $HgBr_2$ impregnated paper for the quantitative determination of antimony(30). Black silver antimonide (Ag_3Sb) is formed.

Bismuth. Bismuth is a relatively toxic metal once it is absorbed from the intestines. Most of the bismuth taken by mouth reaches the intestines where it forms insoluble salts that are not easily absorbed. Bismuth salts are used in medicine as antisyphilitics, frequently in combination with arsenic. The bismuth content of organs in cases in which the metal has been used therapeutically is not large, since absorbed bismuth is eliminated in the saliva, urine, bile and feces. In poison cases large amounts are present in the urine, liver, kidney and spleen, as well as in the bones.

ANALYSIS FOR BISMUTH. 1. Indications for Bismuth: spectrographic analysis of ash and the Reinsch test.

2. Spectrographic Analysis. The indicating spectral line is 3067.7 Å. The confirming spectral lines are 2898.0 and 2938.3 Å.

The most persistent bismuth line occurs at 3067.7 Å. This line is free from interference by the normal constituents of tissue ash, but because of its location in the normal tissue spectrum it is easily overlooked. It is the only line that appears with very low bismuth concentrations. Traces are indicated by an increase in the relative intensity when a digestion residue is arced or in an arc spectrum from a dithizone extraction. The 3067.7 Å bismuth line is located visually in a spectrum from the first strong iron line (3067.3 Å) of the four symmetrical iron lines preceding the triplet. Confirming bismuth lines at 2898.0 and 2938.3 Å are looked for when the iron line at 3067.3 Å appears as a doublet. These lines and the two at 2993.3 Å and 3024.6 Å are not interfered with when bismuth is the only abnormal metal present. In acute bismuth poisonings, the metal content is large and all of the above spectral lines are apparent.

High bismuth concentration is indicated by the appearance in the spectrum of the bismuth line at 2780.5 Å which falls between the second and third lines of the magnesium quintuplet. The appearance of this line is an indication for quantitative chemical analysis by the bismuth iodide method.

In the spark spectra of tissue, a double band occurs at 3068 Å and the 3067.7 Å line can only be identified by the reinforcement that occurs at one part of the band. The spark spectrum of a Reinsch wire gives a clear-cut spectral pattern for bismuth.

3. Microchemical Test for Bismuth on a Reinsch Wire. The combination of arsenic and bismuth as used in antisyphilitics can be demonstrated by carrying out the volatilization procedure on a Reinsch wire. The arsenic is sublimed, leaving nonvolatile bismuth remaining on the wire. The bismuth may then be demonstrated by spectrographic analysis (page 984) or by chemical tests.

Reagent. 1 gm. cinchonine per 100 ml. water made acid with $HNO_3 + .2$ gm. KI.

Procedure. Place the copper spiral in a solution containing 0.5 ml. of 5 per cent $Na_2SO_3 + 0.5$ ml. of 1:7 HNO_3 and allow it to remain 5 to 10 minutes with frequent agitation(30). Impregnate a filter paper with the reagent and add several drops of the acid test solution to the center of the paper. In the presence of bismuth, an orange-red ring of bismuth cinchonine double iodide forms. The Na_2SO_3 prevents the liberation of iodine by any dissolved copper. If the sulfite-nitric acid solution stands too long before testing, oxidation of the SO_3 to SO_4 may occur. Any cupric ion will then react with the KI of the reagent, liberating brown I_2. When this occurs the orange bismuth complex is usually apparent at the center due to diffusion of the I_2 through the fibers of the paper. The orange spot may be made more apparent by adding water dropwise to the paper so that the I_2 further diffuses toward the outer edge of the filter paper(31).

4. Quantitative Determination of Bismuth. Bismuth is a nonvolatile metal and tissue containing it is destroyed by ashing (page 970) or by wet digestion (page 972).

For chemical analysis on acid leaches of ash, the ashing process should be carried to the stage at which the black residue is granular and has a sandy consistency. A brown solution will be obtained if the soft ash prepared for spectrographic analysis is extracted with acids. This brown coloration may be cleared with superoxol but it is preferable to reheat the spectrographic ash or else subject a new sample to longer heating at 450° to 500° C.

Procedure for Extraction of Bismuth from Ash. Cover a weighed sample of the powdered ash with concentrated HNO_3 and warm it on the steam bath for 10 minutes. Then add an equal volume of water and continue the warming with stirring for 10 minutes. Allow the mixture to stand until the solid settles to the bottom; carefully decant the supernatant liquid through a sintered glass filter with suction. Repeat the leaching process with water, twice with 1:2 HCl. Transfer the residue to the filter with 1:2 HCl and wash with water. The filtrate is evaporated almost to dryness on the hot plate.

The method(32) depends on the formation of a yellow bismuth iodide complex in acid solution containing a reducing agent.

Reagents. (a) 1 gm. $NaSO_3$ dissolved in water containing 0.8 ml. concentrated H_2SO_4 and diluted to 200 ml., prepared fresh; (b) 17 gm. KI per liter; (c) 280 ml. concentrated H_2SO_4 per liter.

A standard bismuth solution is made to contain 2.0 mg. of bismuth per 100 ml. of a solution comprising 50 ml. of (c), 16.8 ml. of (b) and 13.4 ml. of (a).

Procedure. The residue from a wet digestion should contain about 7 ml. of concentrated H_2SO_4. If the evaporate from the acid treatment of the ash is to be used, add 7 ml. of concentrated H_2SO_4, heat the solution to SO_3 fumes and add 30 per cent H_2O_2 dropwise to clear up any brown color and to remove all the HNO_3. Allow the flask to cool, add 10 ml. of water and again heat the solution to SO_3 fumes to remove all the H_2O_2. Rinse the contents into a 50 ml. volumetric flask with not more than 25 ml. of water. After cooling, add 6.7 ml. of reagent (1) and 8.4 ml. of reagent (2), and dilute the solution to 50 ml. Centrifuge the solution if it is not clear.

The transmission is measured in a photoelectric colorimeter through a 1 cm. cell depth, using a blue filter with the instrument set at 100 per cent transmission with water. The Lambert-Beer law is obeyed for concentrations of bismuth up to 2 mg. per 100 ml. of solution. The bismuth content is determined from a curve made with various dilutions comparable to the standard bismuth solution.

Silver. Instances of death involving silver as the result of mistakes in pharmaceutical prescriptions have been noted by the New York City Medical Examiner's Office. Silver is not a toxic metal(33) and, when death occurs after the administration of a silver compound, it has usually resulted from the anion or another substance in the silver-containing preparation.

Requests for silver analysis in the toxicologic laboratory are normally confined to analysis of biopsy material to confirm the diagnosis of argyria. A positive Reinsch test is obtained on the stomach contents when silver salts have been ingested but, due to the slow rate of absorption through the intestinal walls and the ready reduction to the metal by the body, silver deposition is not visible when the Reinsch test is carried out on organs and tissue.

ANALYSIS FOR SILVER. 1. Indications for Silver: spectrographic analysis of ash and the Reinsch test.

2. Spectrographic Analysis. The indicating spectral line is 3280.7 Å. The confirming spectral lines are 3382.9 and 4055.3 Å. The spectrographic method is the only reliable procedure for identifying and estimating the silver content of tissue. The 3280.7 Å line is free of interference from normally occurring metals, and quantitative estimation can be made with titanium as the internal standard, using the 3372.8 Å titanium line for comparison. Confirmation is made from the 3382.9 Å line. Two weak iron lines, 3383.7 and 3384.0 Å, are not resolved from the 3382.9

Å silver line with the Littrow spectrograph. However, the presence of the 3382.9 Å line will be apparent from a comparison of the intensity ratios with neighboring iron lines in this region. Final confirmation is made with the 4055.3 Å silver line after preparing a second spectrogram using glass optics.

Silver may be detected spectrographically on a Reinsch wire when the silver plate is not sufficient to be observed visually or detected by chemical tests. The 3280.7 and 3383.9 Å silver lines are sufficient for the identification. They are not interfered with by any copper lines and are immediately apparent when the control wire is arced in juxtaposition to the unknown.

Lead. Lead presents a special problem to the analytic toxicologist in that there are relatively few lead poisonings in comparison to the number of requests for lead analyses. Moreover, the types of cases involving lead determinations fall into three distinct classes: possible chronic lead poisoning, acute lead poisoning and general unknowns. Each requires special consideration for an interpretation.

ANALYSIS FOR LEAD. 1. Indications for Lead: spectrographic analysis of tissue ash or digest and the dithizone determination.

2. Spectrographic Analysis. The indicating spectral line is 2802.0 Å. The confirming spectral lines are 2873.3, 2577.3 and 3220.5 Å.

Possible Chronic Lead Poisoning. In this type of case, there is a previous history of exposure to lead and of an illness extending over some time. The purpose of the analysis is to determine whether or not the symptoms may be attributed to lead. Considerable lead will have been eliminated in the feces and urine during the illness and, in the absense of typical symptoms, the lead content of the organs will not be elevated far beyond the upper limits for normal cases. Dithizone values for normal liver and kidney usually lie between 80 and 150 μg. per 100 gm. of tissue, but in exceptional cases values up to 400 μg. have been observed in accidental deaths with no previous illness. The pathologist makes the diagnosis from the values of the quantitative analysis and the histologic findings in relation to the time of exposure prior to death. The validity of claims for compensation or insurance for death resulting from an industrial occupation is usually concerned.

A spectrographic examination is of little value in this type of case since lead lines are always found in a tissue spectrum. The most that can be accomplished from a semiquantitative interpretation of a spectrogram is to rule out significant amounts of lead. Regardless of the intensity of the spectral lines, the history of illness and exposure to lead makes it imperative to obtain exact quantitative values in order to avoid controversy in settling a claim. Consequently, the analyst will save time by proceeding directly to a quantitative analysis by the dithizone method. Bone should be analyzed as well as samples of liver and kidney. In chronic poisonings estimation of lead deposits in the bone and comparison of bone values with the lead content of the liver or kidney are necessary to differentiate chronic lead poisoning from the exceptionally high normal values.

Acute Lead Poisoning. Death probably does not occur from acute lead poisoning before one or more of the typical symptoms such as basophilic stippling, wrist drop, pain in the extremities, constipation, receding gums or blue gum lines have been observed. The lead content of the liver and kidney is high, ranging between 1 and 10 mg. per 100 gm. of tissue.

Acute poisoning may be immediately recognized from the spectrum of the tissue ash. The intensity of the normally occurring lead lines will be greatly elevated above the normal, with many of the weak lines standing out prominently. The lead chromate method is preferable to the dithizone procedure for quantitative analysis. The sensitivity of the dithizone procedure makes it necessary to use very small aliquots of a digest, thus introducing relatively large dilution errors.

General Unknowns. Lead as well as the other metals must be eliminated in evaluating the spectrum from cases of the "general unknown" type. As mentioned previously, a lead content of 1 mg. or more per 100 gm. of tissue will be apparent by the appearance of weak lines along with the increased intensity of the normally occurring lead lines. When the lead content is within the range for average normals, lead can be eliminated from further consideration by an evaluation of the intensity ratios of the normal lines. Differentiation between an undiagnosed chronic poisoning, a high normal lead content which is without pathologic significance, and pseudosensitivity of lead in the arc spectrum requires a special study.

The spectrum in these conditions shows intensities for the normal lead lines considerably elevated above those for the average normals without the appearance of comparable weak lead lines. Isolated weak lines may show up but the intensity pattern is not complete and is reversed from its normal order. When this type of lead spectrum appears, a quantitative chemical analysis by the dithizone method is necessary before the apparent positive findings can be accepted.

Pseudosensitivity in the spectrum of lead in tissue ash is particularly pronounced. It is this frequent phenomenon that causes lead poisoning to be suspected in many normal cases. The intensity of the normally occurring lead lines is markedly influenced by extraneous ions in the ash and by changes in conditions of excitation in the arc. Fortunately the effect is always positive so that the worst that can occur is to suspect elevated lead values. Comparison of the spectrum of the ash with that of a wet digest of the same sample will usually reveal this phenomenon. The relatively high alkali metals content of digestion residues tends to reduce extraneous ion effects. If the intensity ratios in the spectrum of the digest are not elevated in proportion to those in the ash, a chemical determination can be dispensed with.

Usually the chemical values are not outside the normal range, so that spectrographic examinations for lead tend to increase the number of chemical determinations rather than save labor as they do with the other metals. Spectrographic analysis will avoid overlooking those few chronic cases that were not treated prior to death. When dithizone values actually show a lead content at or above the high normal range, a sample of bone should be analyzed chemically for comparison with the organs. Lead values for bone below those for organs indicate that the elevated lead content, although due to previous exposure to the metal, was not pathologic.

Interpretation of the Spectrum. In the ultraviolet region between 3100 and 2380 Å, lead lines from bone and organs which are located at 2614.2, 2663.2, 2802.0, 2873.3 and 2833.1 Å appear as strong lines. These are the normal lead lines that are due to ingestion of small amounts of lead during life. The 2663.2 and 2833.1 Å lines are invariably too intense to allow any semiquantitative interpretations from line intensities. The others vary in intensity from spectrum to spectrum in normal cases in about the same proportion from very weak lines up to line intensities that stand out prominently. The lead line at 2577.3 Å seldom appears in normal tissue and then only faintly, while lines at 2446.2, 2476.4 and 3220.5 Å do not appear in the spectrum except when the lead content is elevated. Interpretation is based on the relative intensities of the normal lines coupled with the appearance of the weak lead lines in the spectrum.

The 2802 Å lead line is used as the indicating line because of the ease with which it is located. It is next to the strong magnesium line at 2802.7 Å and is clearly resolved under a low power objective. When the lead content is abnormally high, it stands out as a strong dark line with an optical density of one or more; the 2873.3 Å line shows approximately the same intensity and the weaker line at 2577.3 Å is clearly perceptible. The appearance of the 2577.3 Å line with elevated intensities at 2802 and 2873 Å is an indication that a chemical analysis by the dithizone procedure should be performed in order to differentiate between possible chronic poisoning, an abnormally high nonpathologic lead content, and pseudosensitivity of the lead spectrum. A bone analysis should be started at the same time to differentiate between pathologic and nonpathologic elevated lead contents.

As the lead content in the ash increases, the weak lines 2476.4, 2446.3 and 3220.5 Å appear in that order. The appearance of the 3220.5 Å line is indicative of the presence of relatively large amounts of lead. When these weak lines appear in the spectrum, all of the normal lead lines show spreading with the 2802 Å line overlapping the 2802.7 Å magnesium line.

The normal lead spectrum of bone ash shows a slightly greater lead intensity pattern than that of the organs. The 2577.3 Å line usually appears with the other normal lines found in tissue ash. Urine, however, presents a different picture. The high alkali metal content of the ash markedly decreases the spectral sensitivity for lead and the appearance of a clearly perceptible 2802 Å lead line is indicative of abnormal lead excretion.

3. Quantitative Determination of Lead as Lead Chromate(34). This method requires considerable labor and is much less sensitive than the dithizone method. It is specific for lead, and its decreased sensitivity serves to make the method more reliable than any other procedure for interpretations involving lead poisonings. A perceptible precipitate of lead sulfate is obtained when the lead content of the solution is of the order of 60 μg., and inspection of the precipitate at this point furnishes an index of the degree of lead intoxication. The method is not recommended for urine.

Procedure. Treat the ash or digest from 50 gm. of bone, tissue or blood with two 25 ml. portions of 1:2 HCl, heating each portion to boiling and decanting through a filter with suction. Wash the residue onto the filter paper with boiling water, and continue the washing until there are approximately 100 ml. of filtrate. Neutralize the filtrate by dropwise addition of 50 per cent NaOH to the first appearance of a permanent phosphate precipitate. Then add a few drops of concentrated HCl with shaking until the phosphate precipitate is just dissolved. Heat the solution to boiling and pass in H_2S for about 15 minutes. Allow the solution to stand overnight, and then filter it. Wash the precipitate with water saturated with H_2S and dissolve by pouring 10 ml. of hot 1:2 HNO_3 over the paper. Wash the paper with water until it is free of acid. Add 3 ml. of concentrated H_2SO_4, and evaporate the filtrate until white SO_3 fumes appear. Then add 50 ml. of water and 50 ml. of 95 per cent ethyl alcohol, and allow the solution to stand overnight. The appearance of a white precipitate of $PbSO_4$ on the bottom of the beaker is indicative of significant amounts of lead.

Decant the supernatant liquid through a filter paper, and wash the beaker containing the precipitate with 1:2 alcohol-water solution, filtering the washings through the paper. Only a small amount of the $PbSO_4$ precipitate is transferred to the paper in the washing process, the largest portion remaining on the bottom of the beaker. Pour 10 ml. of hot 25 per cent ammonium acetate over the filter paper, and collect the ammonium acetate filtrate in the beaker containing the $PbSO_4$ residue. Wash the paper with three successive 5 ml. portions of hot water and warm the resulting filtrate until all of the $PbSO_4$ has dissolved. Make the solution distinctly acid to litmus by the dropwise addition of glacial acetic acid, then add 1 ml. of saturated K_2CrO_4 to the warm solution. Allow it to stand for two hours; then filter the precipitated $PbCrO_4$ through a #4 sintered glass crucible. The lead may be determined by weighing the lead chromate or else it may be dissolved and analyzed iodometrically. In the iodometric determination the lead chromate is dissolved in 10 ml. of cold 1:2 HCl. Two ml. of 1 per cent KI is added and the liberated iodine is titrated with standard $Na_2S_2O_3$ to a starch end point. One ml. of .005N $Na_2S_2O_3$ is equivalent to .3452 mg. of lead.

4. Quantitative Determination of Lead by the Dithizone Method. This method is best suited for urine analysis and for organs and body fluids when the lead content is not greater than 0.5 mg. per 100 gm. of material. A wet digest is used for the analysis. In the presence of cyanide a cherry red dithizonate is formed in the chloroform layer when an aqueous solution containing lead, bismuth, stannous tin or thallium is shaken out with dithizone solution. The spectrographic analysis will detect the presence of interfering metals. Stannous tin is converted to the stannic state by the oxidizing agents used in the wet digestion and therefore is not a source of interference. Bismuth may be removed by a preliminary extraction of the digest to a pH of 2 to 3. Thallium is a potential source of interference, but fortunately its presence in biologic material is rare.

Dithizone Reagent. Fifteen mg. of diphenyl thiocarbazone per liter of $CHCl_3$.

Procedure. To the digest prepared from 25 to 50 gm. of organs, 15 to 25 ml. of whole blood or 50 to 100 ml. of urine, add 5 ml. of distilled water and 5 ml. of saturated NaCl in 5 per cent HCl for each 2 ml. of concentrated H_2SO_4 used in the digestion process. The NaCl-HCl solution dissolves any insoluble $PbSO_4$. Filter off any insoluble precipitate, washing the filter paper with 5 ml. of distilled water. Add 2 drops of phenol red indicator and make the solution alkaline with ammonia. Add 5 ml. of 10 per cent citric acid. The citric acid dissolves the precipitated phosphates and prevents their reprecipitation when the pH is adjusted. Readjust the pH to 7.6 with ammonia and add 2 ml. of 10 per cent KCN. Transfer the solution to a 250 ml. separatory funnel. Shake out the aqueous solution with small measured portions of dithizone solution, as described under the dithizone titration procedure for mercury (page 985). The end point is obtained when a permanent green color remains in the chloroform layer. One ml. of dithizone solution is equivalent to 3 to 5 μg. of lead. The error is approximately 5 per cent for 20 to 150 μg. of lead per 15 ml. of blood. The reagent should be stored in the refrigerator and restandardized against a standard lead solution after standing for two days.

If the digestion process is not complete, or if all of the oxidizing agents are not removed from the digest, and high concentrations of ferric iron are present, the dithizone end point is not sharp. The color slowly changes from an off-color red to violet and finally to blue green. When this occurs, it is preferable to continue the titration until an excess of dithizone has been added and to determine the lead by photometric measurement of the red color after stripping the uncombined dithizone from the chloroform solution.

Colorimetric Measurement of Lead-Dithizone Complex. *Stripping Reagent.* Five ml. of concentrated NH_4OH + 10 ml. of 10 per cent KCN per 100 ml. of water.

Procedure. At the completion of the titration, draw off the chloroform layer into another 250 ml. separatory funnel, and wash it by shaking with two 10 ml. portions of water, discarding the washings. Then shake out the dithizone solution with 20 ml. of stripping reagent and again wash with two 10 ml. portions of water. Run the chloroform-dithizone solution into a 50 ml. volumetric flask and make up to volume with chloroform. The transmission of the chloroform solution containing red lead-dithizone complex is measured in a photoelectric colorimeter against chloroform, at a wave length of approximately 510 mμ and the lead content is determined from a curve prepared from standard lead solutions treated by the above procedure. The extinction is linear up to 50 μg. with a 5 cm. cell depth (35-40).

Thallium. Thallium is not a normal component of tissue. Therefore, the detection of even very small amounts in postmortem tissue should initiate an investigation to determine the source of the poison.

Thallium sulfate is on the market in the form of a paste for use as an insecticide and rodenticide, and thallium coated grain is available for use against rodents and other pests. Thallium salts are no longer used as therapeutic agents, and the sale of thallium-containing ointments and depilatory creams is not permitted. Accidental deaths have occurred from the ingestion by small children of food coated with thallium rodenticide. Suicidal and homicidal deaths from thallium poisoning are not common, but many accidental poisonings have been reported. In chronic poisonings, thallium is readily eliminated in the urine and after eight weeks is apparently removed from the body. Recovery in all known chronic cases has been complete after two to six months. No fatal cases of poisoning from industrial contact have been reported.

ANALYSIS FOR THALLIUM. 1. Indications for Thallium: spectrographic analysis of ash or digest.

2. Spectrographic Analysis. The indicating spectral line is 2767.9 Å. The confirming spectral lines are 2918.3, 2580.2 and 3229.8 Å.

Thallium is easily detected by spectrographic methods. The metal is very sensitive to excitation by the arc or spark source and produces a simple spectrum containing a number of strong lines free of interference by normal metals in tissue ash. The indicating line at 2767.9 Å is located in the tissue spectrum to the long side of and just resolved from the second strong iron line below the magnesium quintuplet. Thallium is not appreciably volatile at temperatures of 400° to 450° C. and can be detected spectrographically in tissue ash. However, the spreading of the strong thallium lines on the carbon background of the ash spectrum produces more or less diffuse lines. Spectrographic analysis of a digestion residue gives a more sensitive and sharper thallium spectrum. More thallium is deposited in the kidney than in any other organ, although large amounts also deposit in the liver, spleen, pancreas, muscle and bone. The thallium content in fatal subacute and acute poisonings is reported to range from 0.5 to 10 mg. per 100 gm. of tissue(41).

3. Confirming Test for Thallium. Confirmation of thallium as the agent in poison cases is readily made by separating the thallium from the other ions in a tissue digest, and demonstrating the increased intensity of the spectral lines when the thallium-containing precipitate is arced in the spectrograph.

Isolation of Thallium from a Tissue Digest. Transfer the digestion residue from 50 to 100 gm. of tissue or 1,000 ml. of urine to a 50 ml. centrifuge cone and dilute to a volume of approximately 25 ml. Bubble SO_2 through the solution until it is saturated with gas. Add 0.5 ml. of concentrated hydriodic acid dropwise, with the SO_2 bubbled through the solution during the addition and for five minutes thereafter. A turbidity or precipitate develops in the solution. Allow the tube to stand overnight and then centrifuge it and carefully decant the supernatant solution. Dry the precipitate by placing the tube in an oven at 110° C. for ½ hour. Then add enough spectrographically pure carbon powder to give a total bulk sufficient to half fill the core of the carbon electrode. Mix the carbon with the precipitate by grinding with an applicator stick. Transfer the mixture to the core of the electrode and arc for 15 seconds at 8 amperes.

If thallium is present, pale yellow thallous iodide is precipitated, but a yellow precipitate is not proof of thallium. Copper or mercury, if present, or colloidal sulfur from the reduction of SO_2 by the HI will also give a yellow precipitate.

4. Quantitative Determination of Thallium(42). Thallium may be determined quantitatively by the dithizone method described for lead. Results by this method are always open to question, however, because lead is a normal component of tissue and body fluids.

The iodometric titration in which thallium is oxidized to the thallic state with bromine is recommended. The excess bromine is removed with phenol, KI added and iodine is liberated according to the equation:

$$TlCl_3 + 2\ KI \rightarrow TlCl + 2\ KCl + I_2$$

The iodine so liberated is titrated with standard $Na_2S_2O_3$.

Reagents. (a) 5 per cent phenol: 5 gm. of white phenol crystals per 100 ml. of water.

(b) Bromine water. A layer of liquid bromine washed three times with distilled water and stored in a brown bottle layered over with about 10 volumes of distilled water.

(c) Starch-KI-phenol indicator. 0.5 gm. starch mixed with 5 ml. distilled water and added with stirring to 50 ml. of boiling water. 0.5 gm. KI is then added, and when the solution has cooled, 2.5 ml. of 5 per cent phenol solution is added in order to prevent mold formation. The indicator keeps for months.

(d) Standard thallous sulfate. O.3087 gm. of dry Tl_2SO_4 dissolved in 250 ml. of distilled water. 1 ml. of this solution is the equivalent of 1 mg. thallium.

(e) Standard 0.01N $Na_2S_2O_3$. 2.5 gm. pure $Na_2S_2O_3 \cdot 5H_2O$ dissolved in previously boiled distilled water, 1 ml. of 0.1N NaOH added and the solution diluted to 1 liter. The NaOH adjusts the pH to between 9 and 10 and prevents bacterial decomposition of the $Na_2S_2O_3$. The solution keeps several years when stored in the dark.

Titration of Tissue Digests. Dilute the clear colorless digest to about 150 ml. with water, and add 10 gm. of Na_2PHO_4. $12H_2O$ and 20 ml. of 85 per cent H_3PO_4 to buffer the solution and to eliminate any interference due to iron. Add bromine water dropwise until the solution assumes a persistent yellow color. After the solution stands 5 minutes, add 2 ml. of phenol solution to remove the excess bromine. Five minutes later add 0.5 gm. KI. Mix the contents, and allow the solution to stand again for 10 minutes. Add 2 ml. of starch-KI-phenol indicator, and titrate the liberated iodine with the standard $Na_2S_2O_3$ solution using a 10 ml. microburet.

Calculation. 1 ml. of the $Na_2S_2O_3$ is equivalent to 1.06 mg. of thallium. The average of the blanks on 50 gm. of thallium-free tissue is found to be 0.11 ± 0.03 ml. of $Na_2S_2O_3$ solution by this method. The thallium loss during the wet digestion is approximately 10 per cent. Therefore: the number of milligrams of thallium in the weighed sample equals

$$(\text{ml. Na}_2\text{S}_2\text{O}_3 \text{ solution} - 0.11) \times \frac{1.06}{0.9}$$

Interfering Cations. Bismuth, copper and chromium give positive titers with this method. Their presence in the tissue will have been indicated in the spectrographic examination. In the absence of a spectrogram, an aliquot of the digestion solution may be tested by microchemical methods in order to eliminate the possibility of interference. In the presence of one of these ions, the gravimetric TlBr method of Gettler and Weiss(42) is preferable.

Barium. Barium compounds are easily available, and accidental and suicidal barium poisonings occur. Insoluble barium sulfate is given orally in roentgenographic and fluoroscopic studies of the gastrointestinal tract. The other salts of barium are soluble in gastric fluid and, if taken internally, barium ion is readily absorbed through the intestinal wall; 1 gm. or less of a soluble salt may prove fatal. Deaths have occurred from mistakes in which a soluble barium salt instead of insoluble barium sulfate was ingested for roentgenographic purposes. The carbonate and hydrates are used in rat poison, frequently in combination with strychnine, and the fluorosilicate is an agricultural poison. Barium sulfide is used as a depilatory, and the chloride and nitrate are used extensively in industry.

In acute barium poisoning, death may occur in 1 to 12 hours. The absorbed barium is deposited in the organs and bones. In nonfatal cases, it remains in the bones for a long time, but is removed from the circulatory system within a few days as a result of bone deposition and excretion, primarily by the large bowel. The ratio of the concentration in the organs to that in the bones can be determined by the time death was delayed after ingestion of the poison. In most of the cases of barium poisoning seen in this laboratory, big doses of the salt were taken so that large amounts remained in the stomach contents after death. The organs, however, never contain high concentrations of barium. The presence of the other insoluble components of a tissue ash or digest therefore makes the identification of barium in the organs by chemical methods a difficult procedure. It is questionable whether a case of acute barium poisoning can be detected in a routine chemical examination of organs unless the stomach contents or the history first directed suspicion toward such a diagnosis. In the "general unknown" case, nonvolatile metal poisoning is usually ruled out after an examination of the organs, and spectrographic analysis is the only reliable procedure for detecting an unsuspected barium poisoning.

ANALYSIS FOR BARIUM. 1. Indications for Barium: spectrographic analysis of tissue ash.

2. Spectrographic Analysis. The indicating spectral line is 3071.6 Å. The confirming spectral lines are 4554.0, 4934.1 and 5535.5 Å obtained on a second spectrogram with glass optics.

Barium does not show a sensitive spectrum in the ultraviolet region. Only one line, 3071.6 Å, appears in the spectra from liver or kidney ash. Although this line is only of medium sensitivity, it is apparent in tissue from cases of acute barium poisoning. Fortunately, it is free of interference by the normally occurring elements in a tissue spectrum. It is located at 3067.3 and 3075.7 Å midway between the first and second of the four symmetric iron lines preceding the iron triplet. It can be readily observed as an abnormal line upon visual inspection, but a line appearing in this position must first be differentiated from the zinc line at 3072.1 Å before proceeding with the confirming test. The presence of barium must be confirmed spectrographically by taking a second spectrogram with glass optics set at 4000 to 6000 Å. In the visible region of the spectrum the very strong lines at 4554.0, 4934.1 and 5535.5 Å will be very dark in comparison to the ultra-violet line at 3071.6 Å. The sensitivity for the detection of barium spectrographically increases markedly with increased current densities. One finds that 12 to 15 amperes for 30 seconds at 220-volts of direct current gives much darker barium lines than the 10 ampere current normally used. The residue from a tissue digest gives a much stronger spectrum than does the ash. In the digestion process the barium is precipitated as insoluble barium sulfate and much greater sensitivity can be obtained by evaporating off the excess sulfuric acid and arcing the residue after mixing with an equal bulk of powdered spectrographically pure carbon.

In suicidal barium poisoning, large amounts are usually present in the stomach contents and demonstration of soluble barium after finding barium in the organs may be considered evidence of barium poisoning. Therefore, identification of the 3071.6 Å line in a tissue spectrum should be followed by an examination of the stomach contents before confirming by a second spectral examination in the visible region of the spectrum. The presence of water soluble barium is indicated by the appearance of a green flame from a simple platinum wire flame test on an evaporate of the stomach fluid.

Barium, like thallium, is never found as a normal component of tissue and detection of even traces should initiate further investigation into the circumstances of the case. However, the presence of traces of barium in the tissue is not necessarily indicative of barium poisoning, unless the possibility of barium absorption from roentgenographic or fluoroscopic examination has been eliminated. In this connection, five cases of particular interest have been noted in this laboratory. The possibility of barium poisoning was not suspected until the 3071.6 Å line was observed during a routine examination of the liver ash in three of them. On re-arcing the samples with glass optics in the visible region of the spectrum, the 4554.0, 4934.1 and 5535.5 Å lines were quite intense in each of the three cases. An evaluation of these spectrograms indicated barium poisoning. When the histories were examined, it was found that the three cases were infants, all of whom had received barium sulfate for roentgenographic studies not more than 48 hours prior to death. It was then suspected that a soluble barium salt had been accidentally substituted for the barium sulfate or that the barium sulfate was contaminated with soluble barium. However, only the insoluble barium sulfate was found in the stomach contents and the barium sulfate obtained from the original source in each case proved to be chemically pure.

This raised the question of the possibility of insoluble barium sulfate being absorbed through the intestinal walls, and two other cases in which barium sulfate had been administered for roentgenographic analysis before death occurred were subsequently examined. One was an elderly woman who had received barium sulfate a number of times and who had died of malignant melanoma with extensive metastases to the liver. Significant amounts of barium were found in the ash of both the normal and melanomatous liver tissue. In the other case, death, from a hemorrhage following an operation, occurred 48 hours after the administration of barium sulfate. In this case, spectrographic examination of the tissue did not disclose any barium nor did a review of previous cases with a history of having received barium sulfate for diagnostic studies.

In contrast to these cases, there are a number on record in our laboratories of actual barium poisonings such as a suicide from a barium carbonate-strychnine mixture and one in which barium sulfide was mistakenly compounded for barium sulfate for roentgenographic analysis. These cases showed very intense barium lines in the spectra of all the organs. In the cases of the three infants and the elderly woman, the liver ash was leached with 1:2 hydrochloric acid, as in the isolation process on this page, evaporated to dryness and the residue arced in the spectrograph. Barium lines were barely detectable for two of the infants and were not observed for the other two cases. However, when the ash in each case was fused with sodium carbonate, spectrographic examination showed significant amounts of barium. In all the known cases of barium poisoning, strong barium lines are seen in the spectra for the leaches of the ash without fusion.

It is difficult to explain how insoluble barium sulfate can be carried through the intestinal wall and this problem will require more study before the significance of these findings can be justly appraised.

3. Isolation of Barium from Tissue. It is easier to isolate barium for chemical analysis from ashed samples than from digests. The barium sulfate in a digestion residue is mixed with insoluble silicates and sulfates, and the separation following a fusion is quite troublesome. On ashing, a part of the barium is converted to the carbonate which is readily leached out with acid. Some of it is converted to the insoluble sulfate and, for quantitative recovery, the residue remaining after acid leaching must be fused as with the digestion residue.

Procedure. Continue the ashing process at low heat until a white carbon-free ash remains. Leach with hot 1:2 HCl and wash twice with distilled water. Dry the residue and fuse with Na_2CO_3. Leach the fusion mixture with hot water until the washings are sulfate free. Dissolve the residue in dilute HCl and treat according to the procedure for barytes analysis to remove silica and other interfering ions. For a quantitative analysis, combine the two barium fractions, and precipitate and weigh as the insoluble sulfate.

4. Sodium Rhodizonate Test. The acid leach of the ash in acute barium poisonings contains enough barium to be detected by microchemical methods, if relatively large samples are taken for the analysis. For the test with sodium rhodizonate(43), evaporate the aqueous acid solution just to dryness and redissolve in the minimal volume of water. Place two drops of the slightly acid aqueous solution on a filter paper, followed by a drop of 5 per cent aqueous sodium rhodizonate. The formation of a red-brown stain indicates the presence of barium.

Cadmium. Cadmium is a metallic poison analogous in its toxicity to arsenic, antimony and mercury. It is semivolatile, melting at 320.9° C. and boiling at 772° C.; consequently losses occur when tissue samples are ashed. Unlike arsenic, antimony or mercury, cadmium is difficult to detect chemically in the low concentrations that are present in the organs in poison cases.

Industry is finding increased uses for cadmium metal, particularly as a substitute for zinc, tin and nickel in the plating of metal parts for rust prevention. Cadmium plate takes a high polish, and many articles, especially automobile and marine hardware parts, are now supplied with cadmium plated surfaces. Insoluble cadmium salts are used in paints, and cadmium selenide is a substitute for vermilion as a red pigment. The selenide was formerly used in some of the more expensive lipsticks, but the use of cadmium in any oral preparation is now prohibited by law. Cadmium plate on articles for food handling is not permitted, since appreciable amounts of the metal will dissolve in solutions containing the equivalent of 0.5 to 2.5 per cent acetic acid(44).

Cadmium is principally an industrial hazard; cadmium-containing dusts may be inhaled in electroplating and other manufacturing processes. In most of the cases reported, assimilation of the poison has been through the respiratory tract. Cadmium poisoning is not frequently encountered in medical examiners' cases. In this laboratory, examinations have been made in two cases that occurred during World War II from inhalation of cadmium oxide fumes while cutting cadmium plated metal with an acetylene cutting torch. The use of an acetylene flame on a cadmium plated surface is dangerous. The metal is readily burned to a very light finely divided oxide which is blown in colloidal suspension from the hot metal surface by the blast from the burner and envelops the operator in a white cloud.

Cadmium is present in the kidney and liver in poison cases. Prodan(45) reported the highest concentration of the metal in the lungs of cadmium-fed cats, with the liver next, followed by the kidney. Acute cadmium poisoning can be detected by spectrographic analysis but, as in lead poisoning, the question of establishing cadmium poisoning from a routine examination of a spectrogram from a "general unknown" presents a special problem.

ANALYSIS FOR CADMIUM. 1. Indications for Cadmium: spectrographic analysis of liver (not kidney) digest.

2. Spectrographic Analysis. The indicating spectral line is 3261.1 Å. The confirming spectral lines are 3403.7, 3612.9, 3466.2 and 3467.7 Å. Unlike the other metals, final confirmation of cadmium should be made only on a dithizone extract of a liver digest.

The sensitivity of spectrographic analysis for the identification of cadmium in biologic materials is less than that for any of the other metals except mercury, arsenic and antimony. Moreover, in a routine examination, the qualitative plate is exposed in the ultraviolet region which does not include any of the strong cadmium lines except the indicating line at 3261.1 Å. A decision to make a further search for cadmium or to rule out the possibility of cadmium poisoning must depend on an evaluation of the intensity of the 3261.1 Å line. In acute poisoning by inhalation, with a cadmium concentration high enough to produce respiratory symptoms and with autopsy findings that include inflammation of the respiratory tract and congestion of the organs, the 3261.1 Å line will be pronounced in the spectra for kidney or liver ash. A second spectrogram taken with the prism set between 4100 and 2600 Å will show the confirming cadmium lines. The spectrum from a tissue digest will show a more intense spectral pattern and is preferable to the ash spectrum for photographing the confirming lines. However, the increased sensitivity is not in proportion to the degree to which the cadmium was concentrated by the digestion process because the extraneous sulfate residue markedly decreases the spectral response of the cadmium. Improved digest spectra are obtained by arcing a mixture of the digestion residue with an equal bulk of spectrographically pure carbon powder.

Identification of the confirming lines should be followed by a third spectrogram on lung tissue in the near ultraviolet. If the cadmium in the organs came from inhalation, the lung spectrum will show a much greater content of the metal with the appearance of some of the weaker lines in the spectrum below 3261.1 Å, particularly the 2980.6 Å line. Cadmium poisoning is seldom suspected at autopsy. Furthermore, lung tissue is not always submitted for analysis and by the time the organ analysis has been completed, it is no longer available. In such cases, the poisoning must be established from the analysis of the organs.

The confirming lines in the near ultraviolet are in the region of medium resolution that includes many strong iron and other normally occurring metal lines. Although they are free of interference, identification of the confirming lines is complicated by the cyanogen bands and excessive carbon background. The confirming lines are not nearly as persistent as the indicating cadmium line at 3261.1 Å and, since they are in a region of the spectrum in which interpretation is more difficult, the presence of cadmium in toxic amounts is not assured even with a pronounced indicating line. The findings must be confirmed by examination of the spectrum, free of interference, that is obtained from the evaporated chloroform solution of a dithizone extraction or the H_2S precipitate of the digest.

Spectrographic Analysis of a Dithizone Extract. The general procedure is described on page 985. Cadmium is extracted with dithizone by the procedure described on page 1011 for zinc. Evaporate the chloroform-cadmium dithizonate contaminated with zinc and other dithizone extractable metals to dryness after mixing in enough spectrographically pure carbon powder to cover the bottom of the beaker. Rub the walls of the beaker with the carbonaceous residue in order to pick up any adhering particles of the evaporate. Pack the solid in the core of a one-quarter inch carbon electrode and heat by flaming with the bunsen burner to a temperature below red heat in order to pyrolize the organic dithizone. Arc the sample with the spectrograph set at 4100 to 2600 Å for 30 seconds at 10 amperes and 200 volts of direct current. If the cadmium content of the organs is significant, the spectrum will show dark, clear-cut, prominent lines with many of the weaker lines clearly perceptible.

Spectrographic Analysis of the Hydrogen Sulfide Precipitate of a Wet Digest. Isolation of cadmium as the sulfide from a wet digest is not as sensitive as the dithizone method but requires less labor. The extraneous sulfides and the free sulfur that are precipitated along with any cadmium act as entrainer and collector for the cadmium sulfide and do not influence the cadmium spectrum. Make the sulfuric acid digestion solution just acid enough to prevent the precipitation of the phosphates. Add sodium citrate to aid in keeping the phosphates in solution. Dilute the digestion solution from 100 gm. of tissue to about 25 ml. with water, add 2 drops of methyl orange indicator and neutralize the excess H_2SO_4 with ammonia until the indicator just changes from red to yellow. Add 2 gm. of sodium citrate and dilute to approximately 50 ml. with water. Saturate the solution with H_2S by bubbling a stream through it for 15 minutes. Stopper the flask and let stand overnight. Filter through a Schwinger filter tube using an inverted siphon with suction to transfer the solution onto the 10 mm. filter paper disk(46). When all of the solution has been filtered, wash the paper once with water to remove occluded soluble salts. Allow the paper disk containing the precipitate to dry, then fold it over and roll into a ball small enough to fit into the cavity of a one-quarter inch cored electrode. Flame the electrode in the bunsen burner until the paper is charred to a carbon ash. Sprinkle a thin layler of spectrographically pure carbon powder over the charred paper and pack the sample into the electrode by tamping with the back end of a microspatula. Make two exposures on the sample; arc the first one for 30 seconds and follow with a second 60 second exposure, using 10 amperes at 220 volts of direct current with the spectrograph set between 4100 and 2600 Å. The spectrogram will show strong magnesium lines, silica, a small amount of iron and traces of the other normally occurring heavy metals, but the cadmium spectrum will be free of interference.

Interpretation of a Spectrogram for Cadmium. The problem of ruling out the possibility of cadmium poisoning in a routine examination of a spectrogram from kidney or liver tissue is complicated by the peculiar behavior of the indicating cadmium line at 3261.1 Å in a normal tissue spectrum. This is the strongest and most persistent of the cadmium lines. As the cadmium content of tissue ash or digest is decreased, it shows prominently in the tissue spectrum long after the other lines have disappeared. Except for a very weak lead line at 3261.0 Å, there is no other recorded line in the spectrum of normally occurring metals that is not clearly resolved by the Littrow spectrograph. We have not as yet been able to determine whether this line is actually due to normal cadmium or is an unrecorded weak line of one of the metals that is made abnormally intense by an extraneous ion effect. In the absence of proof of possible interference, it must be assumed that cadmium is a potential normal component of tissue.

The 3261.1 Å line is located midway between the two strong copper lines at 3247.0 and 3274.0 Å and is readily found by visual inspection. It shows up as a strong line in many routine spectra with an intensity high enough to suggest an abnormal cadmium content. It is observed frequently in spectra from kidney tissue and less frequently in liver and lung tissue. The appearance of a strong line at 3261.1 Å must be followed by a second spectrogram with the instrument set in the near ultraviolet in order to pick up the confirming lines. The spectral sensitivity of these lines in a tissue matrix is very low compared with the 3261.1 Å line. This and the fact that their evaluation is difficult in the presence of the carbon background sometimes makes it difficult to rule out the possibility of exposure to abnormal amounts of cadmium. In such cases, the final analysis must be based on the spectrum from a dithizone extract or a H_2S precipitate from a tissue digest. The 3261.1 Å line may be absent or appear quite strong but the confirming lines of the cadmium spectrum will be absent if the tissue is normal with respect to its cadmium content.

3. Quantitative Determination of Cadmium. Cadmium may be determined by comparison of the yellow color of the colloidal sulfide in concentrations down to 0.1 mg. per 50 ml. of solution. The sensitivity is increased to 0.01 mg. per 50 ml. if the comparison with standards is made under the quartz mercury vapor lamp(47). It may be determined by the dithizone procedure for zinc if first isolated from the tissue digest by H_2S precipitation with the acidity adjusted to prevent co-precipitation of zinc.

4. Quantitative Spectrographic Analysis. A quantitative analysis using the 3403.7 Å line, with tin as an internal standard may be made directly on a tissue digest when the cadmium concentration is high enough to give a pronounced 3403.7 Å line. Attempts to evaluate the possible cadmium content of normal tissue by comparison of the 3261.1 Å line with the titanium line at 3242.0 Å have not been successful.

Chromium. Some chromium salts such as carbonate or phosphate do not produce harmful effects when fed to animals in large doses. Derivatives of chromic acid however are quite toxic due to their strong oxidizing ability. Chromates and dichromates are used in electroplating, as mordants in dyeing, in the manufacturing of paper, dyes, oils and fats and in paint pigments. A number of industrial poisonings and accidental and suicidal deaths from the ingestion of salts of chromic acid have been reported. The postmortem findings are those of an irritant poison, and since the toxic dose is relatively high, poisonings are readily detected in a routine examination for heavy metals.

ANALYSIS FOR CHROMIUM. 1. Indications for Chromium: spectrographic analysis of ash.

2. Spectrographic Analysis. The indicating spectral line is 2780.7 Å. The confirming spectral lines are 3053.8, 3005.1 and $\begin{cases} 3578.7 \\ 3593.5 \text{ Å} \\ 3605.3 \end{cases}$

Chromium is very sensitive spectrographically. It produces a complex spectrum analogous to that of iron except for a wider variation in the intensity ratios of the lines. The spectrum shows many prominent lines free of interference by the inorganic components of tissue. Comparison of an unknown spectrum with a chromium reference plate in any region of the spectrum will verify the presence of the metal. The indicating and confirming lines are chosen for the ease with which they are located visually, rather than for specificity or sensitivity. The indicating line at 2780.7 Å is located between the third and fourth magnesium lines of the magnesium quintuplet. The arsenic line at 2780.2 Å is not present in tissue ash and the bismuth line at 2780.5 Å does not appear except with high bismuth contents. Both of these are resolved from the chromium line with the optics of the comparator.

Chromium is nonvolatile and samples can be ashed carbon free without loss of metal. A second exposure of an arced sample gives a stronger spectrum than the first exposure except at the higher current densities.

Chromium is not present normally in tissue and the appearance of the 2780.7 Å line in the spectrum is indicative of an abnormal chromium content. Care must be taken to exclude the possibility of contamination when fixed tissue shows chromium, since Zenker's solution which contains potassium bichromate is a common fixative in the pathologic laboratory.

3. Quantitative Determination of Chromium. Chromium may be determined quantitatively by oxidizing to the chromate by sodium peroxide fusion of the ash and comparing the violet color produced with diphenylcarbazide in acid solution with standard chromate solutions. The ashed sample used for the analysis must be carbon free or some reduction may occur when the fusion mixture is acidified.

Reagent. 0.1 gm. of diphenylcarbazide reagent is dissolved in 10 ml. of glacial acetic acid and diluted to 100 ml. with 95 per cent ethyl alcohol.

Procedure. Heat the sample in the muffle furnace at a temperature not above 500° C. to a white carbon-free ash. Transfer the ash to a spun iron crucible of 50 ml. capacity and add 2 gm. of solid Na_2O_2. Heat the crucible in a bunsen burner with a rotary motion, not allowing the temperature to go much above red heat. Fusion is complete when the melt becomes a homogeneous liquid. Cool while continuing the rotation of the crucible so that the melt solidifies in a thin layer around the sides and in the bottom of the crucible. When cold, add about 25 ml. of water, slowly heat to boiling and continue the boiling for 10 minutes in order to destroy the excess Na_2O_2. Allow the solution to partially cool, add 10 ml. of cold water and sprinkle in, with stirring, 2 gm. of powdered ammonium carbonate. As soon as the ammonium carbonate * dissolves, filter with suction and wash the crucible and filter paper twice with hot water. Carefully neutralize the solution by dropwise addition of concentrated HCl and add an excess equivalent to 5 ml. of concentrated

---

* The ammonium carbonate partially neutralizes the NaOH. It must not be added without destroying the Na_2O_2 by boiling or else some ammonium nitrate will be formed and give abnormally high results.

acid per 100 ml. of solution. Aliquots of the solution are then treated with 1 ml. of diphenyl carbazide reagent and the intensity of the violet color is compared with that of standard chromate solutions.

Manganese. Although manganese is present in small amounts in all plant and animal tissue, an elevated manganese content in the body results in toxic symptoms. The neuromuscular system is affected, resulting in muscular stiffness and incoordination which progresses until disability occurs. Poisoning has occurred from long exposure to dust from ore-crushing which was high in manganese content. Chronic manganese poisoning does not cause fatal results. Except for complications from the crippling disability, longevity is not apparently affected. Acute poisoning from ingestion of manganese salts is not common.

Permanganates are stronger oxidizers than chromates and ingestion of large doses of permanganate salts would be expected to produce death from the corrosive action of the oxidant, if not from the toxicity of the ion. In this laboratory we have examined the stomach washings in several cases of attempted suicide by ingestion of potassium permanganate tablets and have found large quantities of manganese in the washings. All of these cases recovered after hospital treatment. A major proportion, if not all, of the manganese in the stomach was in the form of insoluble manganese dioxide. It is probable that the reduction which takes place in the low acidity of the stomach renders the permanganate relatively inactive physiologically by the formation of the insoluble manganese dioxide.

In a death in which potassium permanganate was used as a douche following a mechanical abortion with rupture of the uterus, an exceptionally high concentration of manganese was found in the blood, liver and kidneys. The pathologic and bacteriologic examination did not indicate that complications from the abortion were the direct cause of death. In this case, permanganate ion was absorbed directly into the blood by way of a neutral and highly buffered system. At a pH of 7 the oxidation potential of permanganate ion is low and one would predict that reduction by the tissue fluids would be much less than reduction occurring in the acid environment of the stomach. The permanganate ion may be quite toxic if it is absorbed as such into the blood. Failure to produce death in the attempted suicides was possibly due to the fact that the manganese that reached the blood stream from the permanganate ingestion was in the reduced state. The question of permanganate toxicity needs more experimental work before definite conclusions can be drawn.

ANALYSIS FOR MANGANESE. 1. Indications for Manganese: spectrographic analysis of ash.

2. Spectrographic Analysis. The indicating spectral lines are $\begin{cases} 2794.8 \\ 2798.3 \\ 2801.1 \end{cases}$ Å. The

confirming spectral lines are $\begin{cases} 2933.1 \\ 2939.3 \\ 2949.2 \end{cases}$ and 2572.8, 2595.8, and 2584.3 Å.

Manganese is nonvolatile and, if tissue samples are ashed carbon free, the effective manganese content of the residue and the sensitivity for detection are increased. As with chromium the second exposure of an arced sample of manganese shows a more intense spectrum. Even though the manganese is not lost when heated to high temperatures, the ashing process should not be conducted at temperatures above 500° C. At high temperatures in the muffle furnace, the ash is fused to a sintered mass and the powdered electrode sample is made much less conductive to the electric current in the arc of the spectrograph. The sensitivity for the detection of manganese is particularly influenced by the physical nature of the ash.

Manganese produces a complex spectrum containing many weak lines with only a few sensitive lines that are free of interference and are easily located. The three lines at 2794.8, 2798.3 and 2801.1 Å are always present in normal tissue spectra. They are of equal density and do not show a wide variation in intensity in normal liver and kidney ash. With elevated manganese concentrations, their intensity is markedly increased; the unusually high density serves to indicate abnormal manganese concentrations in the sample. With exceptionally high manganese concentrations, as found in the previously mentioned abortion case, the lines show up in the spectrum as reversals. The entire tissue spectrum appears exceptionally complex, because of the appearance of many of the manganese lines.

The indicating lines at 2733.1, 2939.3 and 2949.2 Å, as well as those at 2572.8, 2584.3 and 2595.8 Å, do not appear in the spectra of normal tissue. They are all of about equal sensitivity and, if one is present, the others should also be apparent. In examining a spectrogram from a tissue unknown, the observation of abnormal densities for the indicating lines should be followed by a search for the confirming lines; if they are present, a quantitative chemical analysis is indicated. Several exceptional cases have been observed in which spectrographic analysis showed an elevated manganese content of the organs. The abnormal manganese concentration was confirmed by chemical analysis, yet there were no symptoms of manganese poisoning and the cause of death was clearly established at autopsy. One of these deaths was a suicide from an overdose of mercuric chloride. Apparently, the manganese content of the organs can become unusually high under certain conditions. Caution must therefore be exercised in attributing an elevated manganese concentration to manganese exposure.

3. Quantitative Determination of Manganese. Manganese is determined chemically by oxidation to permanganate and comparison of the color with standard permanganate solutions. All organic matter and chlorides must be removed, since they are readily oxidized by the hot permanganic acid. The tissue may be prepared by wet digestion or ashing. Ashed samples must be burned until carbon free and then treated with sulfuric acid to remove chlorides.

Procedure(48). To ashed samples in a silica dish add enough 1:2 H_2SO_4 to give a suspension of material in the acid solution, and about 1 ml. of concentrated HNO_3. Heat to slow boiling and evaporate to SO_3 fumes on a hot plate. Continue the heating on a sand bath until most of the H_2SO_4 has been removed. Care must be taken to prevent spattering in the final stages of the evaporation process. The treatment removes chlorides and oxidizes iron to the ferric state.

Chlorides are removed from digests during the digestion and the metals are in the oxidized state. Transfer the H_2SO_4 residue from a digest with water to a beaker and evaporate almost to dryness, as with the ash, in order to permit adjustment of the acidity. Add 2.5 ml. of 1:2 H_2SO_4 and dilute with 10 to 50 ml. of water depending on the bulk of the evaporate. Heat to boiling with stirring and filter through a sintered glass filter with suction, using hot water to make the quantitative transfer and to wash the precipitate. Evaporate the filtrate to approximately 10 ml., thus giving a solution of approximately 6 per cent with respect to H_2SO_4. Add several glass beads and sprinkle in 0.5 gm. of potassium periodate. Gently heat to boiling and immerse in a boiling water bath for 30 minutes. Cool and transfer to a volumetric flask of a capacity to give a readable pink color after dilution to the mark. Match the color against standard permanganate solutions of comparable intensity.

Copper. Copper is one of the trace metals necessary for human metabolism and small amounts are present in all tissues of the body. Abnormal concentrations of copper in the organs are harmful and produce anemia, nausea, vomiting, colic and diarrhea. The copper content of the liver is greatly elevated in hemochromatosis (49). Normal levels for copper in the liver vary between 0.1 mg. and 1.0 mg. per 100 gm. of tissue. Gerlach(50, 51) reported the experimental production of cirrhosis of the liver from copper in food.

Copper poisoning is rare in spite of the extensive use of the metal. Suicides and homicides from copper salts have been reported. The copper content of the organs is high in arsenic poisonings from Paris green. The organic cuprous compound cupraline® (sodium benzoate n-allyl cuprothiocarbamide) which contains 19 per cent copper has been used as a source of copper in the treatment of arthritis. The copper content of the organs reaches levels far above normal with the administration of this drug.

ANALYSIS FOR COPPER. 1. Indications for Copper: spectrographic analysis of ash.

2. Spectrographic Analysis. The indicating spectral line is 2618.4 Å. The confirming spectral lines are 2766.4 and 2829.4 Å. The copper spectrum contains two very sensitive copper lines at 3267.6 and 3274.0 Å. These lines always appear in a spectrogram of biologic or plant material and because of their extreme sensitivity are of no value in determining copper levels in a routine analysis. The lines at 2618.4, 2766.4 and 2824.4 Å are sometimes very faintly visible in a normal tissue spectrum; they become quite pronounced when the copper level is above the upper limits for normal. They are greatly increased in intensity when the sample is ashed carbon free, as recommended for the spectrographic determination of chromium or manganese. For this reason, an evaluation of the plate for copper should always be made on the carbonized soft ash described on page 970. Spectrographic analysis of skin for copper is frequently of importance in reconstructing the circumstances of or in establishing the cause in deaths by accidental electrocution.

3. Quantitative Determination of Copper. The analysis is done with sodium diethyldithiocarbamate (a modification of the method of McFarlane(52)). Ash the sample at 400° to 450° C. to a carbon-free ash. Add 5 ml. of 1:2 H_2SO_4 solution and 1.0 ml. of concentrated HNO_3 and evaporate almost to dryness on a sand bath. Cool, add approximately 30 ml. of water, bring the solution to a boil, and continue the heating, breaking up any undisintegrated particles with a glass stirring rod. Filter the hot solution with suction through a DeWitt filter into a 125 ml. Ehrlenmeyer flask and wash with hot water. If the total volume exceeds 50 ml., evaporate down to approximately this volume. Add concentrated NH_4OH dropwise until the solution is distinctly alkaline; then add 50 per cent sodium citrate with shaking until the phosphate precipitate is redissolved. Add 2 ml. of 1 per cent sodium diethyldithiocarbamate, shake and let stand 10 minutes. Transfer the solution to a 125 ml. separatory funnel and shake out with 10 ml. of amyl alcohol. Separate the layers and read the transmission of the amyl alcohol solution in a photoelectric colorimeter at 465 mμ, with the instrument set at 100 per cent against amyl alcohol. Determine the copper content from a curve prepared by treating standard copper solutions the same way as the unknown.

Zinc. Zinc, like copper, is a normal component of plant and animal tissue(53).

The average excretion per day has been reported to be 10.7 mg.(54) so that the zinc intake from food ingestion and the use of zinc coated utensils is appreciable. Gettler and Bastian(55) found the average normal zinc content of liver and kidney tissue to be of the order of 5 mg. per 100 gm. of tissue. Noncaustic zinc compounds are relatively nontoxic, and ingestion of moderate amounts of the salts does not produce any ill effects. The inhalation of high concentrations of zinc oxide fumes may produce symptoms similar to those caused by other finely divided metals and oxides, characterized as metal fume fever(56).

Zinc ion is a weak base, and salts with strong acids are corrosives and irritants. Ingestion of other than neutral salts produces symptoms of poisoning. In one case 6 gm. of zinc chloride caused death several weeks after ingestion of the salt. Zinc sulfate is less toxic, its action being more irritating than corrosive. Recovery has occurred after ingestion of one ounce of the sulfate(57). Suicides involving zinc are almost always from the ingestion of soldering fluid which is made by allowing concentrated hydrochloric acid to react with an excess of zinc metal until all action ceases. In acute poisoning with toxic zinc salts the metal content of the organs is very high and no difficulty is encountered in differentiating between a possible high nontoxic zinc level and a poisoning.

ANALYSIS FOR ZINC. 1. Indications for Zinc: spectrographic analysis of digest.

2. Spectrographic Analysis. The indicating spectral line is 3072.1 Å. The confirming spectral lines are 2770.9, 2771.1 and 3282.3 Å

Zinc is a semivolatile metal and losses occur when tissue samples are prepared for analysis by ashing at 450° C. The normal zinc content of organs is relatively high, but if the strong lines of the zinc spectrum appear at all in the spectrogram of ashed samples of the normal tissue, their intensity is very low due to the loss in the ashing process. The wet digest of normal liver and particularly that of lung tissue may show a pronounced zinc spectrum. In cases of chronic or acute zinc poisoning, the zinc content of the tissue is so much greater than the high normal zinc levels that losses due to ashing are of no significance in detecting abnormal zinc concentrations. The spectrum of the ashed sample in cases of poisoning shows strong zinc lines and, since normal zinc is almost entirely lost in the ashing process, the appearance of zinc in the spectrum from ash is indicative of toxic concentrations of the metal.

The indicating line at 3072.1 Å must not be mistaken for the barium line at 3071.6 Å. The confirming lines at 2770.9 and 2771.1 Å are free of interference, but the line at 3282.3 Å must not be confused with the 3280.7 Å silver line.

3. Quantitative Determination of Zinc(58). The method depends on the fact that only cadmium and cobalt are extracted with zinc by dithizone from an aqueous solution with a pH of 5.5 and containing sodium potassium tartrate, sodium thiosulfate, potassium cyanide and sodium acetate. Cobalt is not likely to occur with zinc in human organs, and any cadmium may be removed by hydrogen sulfide precipitation.

Reagents. (a) Dithizone solution: 0.04 gm. per liter of $CHCl_3$.

(b) Standard zinc solution: 63.5 mg. zinc metal dissolved in 1:2 HNO_3. 5 ml. of concentrated H_2SO_4 is added, the solution heated to SO_3 fumes, and diluted to 500 ml. with water. 1 ml. is equivalent to 0.127 mg. of zinc.

(c) Buffer solution: 55 gm. $Na_2S_2O_3 \cdot 5H_2O$, 1.0 gm. KCN, and 9 gm. NaC_2-$H_3O_2 \cdot 3H_2O$ are dissolved in 100 ml. H_2O. 1:4 acetic acid is added until the pH is 5.5 and the solution is then diluted to 200 ml.

(d) Sodium potassium tartrate solution: 20 gm. dissolved in 80 ml. of water.

(e) Acid metacresol purple indicator, 1 per cent.

(f) Methyl red indicator, 1 per cent.

Procedure. Dilute the wet digest from 25 to 50 gm. of tissue or 200 ml. of urine to approximately 30 ml., filter and make up to a volume of 50 ml. in a volumetric flask. A 10 ml. aliquot is adequate for the analysis. If the spectrum shows cadmium, make the aliquot sample alkaline to acid metacresol purple with concentrated ammonia, dilute to 50 ml. and then make slightly acid with concentrated HCl. Heat to 70° C, pass H_2S in for 5 minutes, and then allow it to stand about one hour. Filter any precipitate, wash with small portions of water, adding the washings to the filtrate, and boil the filtrate to reduce the volume to about 10 ml.

In the absence of cadmium, the H_2S precipitation is omitted and a 10 ml. aliquot of the digest is treated by the following procedure: add 2.0 ml. of 20 per cent sodium potassium tartrate, and add concentrated NH_4OH dropwise until the solution is alkaline to acid metacresol purple. Add two drops of methyl red indicator, introduce a small piece of litmus paper, and add 1:5 ammonium hydroxide dropwise until the solution is alkaline to methyl red, but acid to litmus. Then add 50 ml. of buffer solution, and transfer the solution to a 250 ml. separatory funnel with water washing to bring the volume to about 75 ml. The solution will have a pH of 5.5 ± 0.2. Carry out an extractive titration with dithizone as described on page 998 for lead, using 5 ml. portions of dithizone near the end point. Smaller portions of dithizone are not necessary because the error involved in this volume is not more than 10 μg. of zinc.

4. Confirmatory Test for the Presence of Zinc. In order to avoid the possibility of any interference in the titration and to confirm the presence of large amounts of zinc in the sample, the combined chloroform solution containing the dithizonate may be evaporated to dryness and analyzed spectrographically as described on page 1005 for cadmium. As an alternative the zinc may be isolated from the chloroform solution by aqueous acid extraction. Wash the chloroform dithizonate with 10 ml. of buffer solution, 10 ml. of water, and then shake it out with 10 ml. of 1:2 HCl. Wash the aqueous solution with three successive 10 ml. portions of $CHCl_3$ and evaporate to about 5 ml. Make it alkaline with ammonia and then just acid with acetic acid. White ZnS will be precipitated on bubbling H_2S through the solution.

Tin. The salts of tin are not highly toxic but rarely may cause a fatal poisoning (see page 768). Some salts of tin when ingested act as gastrointestinal irritants. Salant(59) fed 20 mg. per liter doses of the tartrate and chloride daily to cats for three months without harmful effect. The metal is used extensively as a rust preventative for food containers; it is important in toxicologic analysis principally because of the frequency with which it is encountered in the examination of organs and tissue for heavy metals.

Although tin melts at 231.9° C. it is relatively nonvolatile. The boiling point is 2,270° C. and losses in ashing at temperatures below red heat are negligible. It burns at high temperatures to the nonvolatile stannic oxide (SnO_2). The oxide is a light, soft microcrystalline powder which is readily dispersed as a colloidal dust by air drafts.

Inhalation of dust by workers in plants processing nonferrous metals and alloys may result in exceptionally high tin concentrations in the organs. Postmortem examination of an apparently normal lung of a worker who had cast tin ingots showed an uncommonly high tin content. Death occurred as a result of injuries sustained in an accident, and there was no pathologic evidence of metal damage.

The metal is quite sensitive spectrographically, giving a simple spectrum with a number of strong and prominent lines. Since spectrographic analysis of tissue ash or digest usually shows some tin, the metal may be considered a normal component of tissue. The concentration found in the organs in different cases is quite variable and ranges from a trace to amounts suggestive of tin exposure. This variability is probably due to differences in assimilation with food from tin cans. Spectrographic analysis of lung tissue shows particularly variable concentrations of tin with unusually high amounts in some exceptional cases. Several deaths have been noted in which there were extensive granulomatous changes of the lungs. In these cases, the lungs contained peculiar birefringent bodies which were found to have abnormal amounts of tin. It has not yet been established whether or not the tin is significant in these undiagnosed cases.

ANALYSIS FOR TIN. 1. Indications for Tin: spectrographic analysis of ash or digest.

2. Spectrographic Analysis. The indicating spectral line is 3262.3 Å. The confirming spectral lines are 3330.6 and 2661.3 Å.

The indicating line at 3262.3 Å is almost always present in a tissue spectrum. It is located just to the long side of the midpoint between the two strong copper lines. With elevated tin concentrations the density of the indicating line is greatly increased. The confirming lines at 3330.6 and 2661.3 Å were selected because they are weaker spectral lines that are not normally present in a tissue spectrum. Strong tin lines at 3175.1, 3034.1, 3009.1 and 2840 Å are free of interference, but are normally occurring spectral lines.

3. Quantitative Determination of Tin. Tin is determined by reduction to $SnCl_2$ and titration with standard iodine solution. Stannic ion is reduced to the stannous state in acid solution by means of iron, antimony metal or sheet nickel. The analysis may be performed on tissue digest or ash. An alkali fusion of the ash is made in order to insure the complete solution of the tin. The nitric acid treatment in the wet digestion of the tissue may form some insoluble metastannic acid (H_2SnO_3) and, for this reason, the diluted digest is not filtered prior to the reduction. Moreover, any insoluble inorganic salts do not interfere with the iodine titration. The large amounts of copper that interfere with the titration are not encountered in tissue.

Reagents. (a) Standard 0.01 N iodine solution. Dissolve approximately 0.65 gm. of iodine in 500 ml. of cold solution containing 1.2 gm. of KI. Standardize against 0.01 N $Na_2S_2O_3$.

(b) 1 per cent starch solution.

Procedure for Tissue Ash. Ash 50 to 100 gm. of tissue in a nickel crucible at 400° C. to a soft carbonaceous ash. When cool, mix an equal bulk of powdered NaOH with the ash and heat gently with a Meker burner to avoid spattering; gradually increase the heat until a melt is obtained. Continue the heating at the maximum burner temperature for 10 minutes or until no further action is seen. Cool, add water and bring to a boil to partially dissolve the cake. Transfer the contents of the crucible with hot water washing to a beaker. Cool and add concentrated H_2SO_4 dropwise until the solution is distinctly acid. Add four iron nail rods three to four inches long, cover the beaker with a watch glass and warm gently for

30 minutes to effect a free evolution of hydrogen. Set the beaker in a dish of ice water until the solution is cold. Add 1 ml. of 1 per cent starch solution and titrate to a blue end point with the standard iodine solution.* One ml. of 0.01 N iodine solution is equivalent to 0.6 mg. tin.

Procedure for Tissue Digest. Transfer the digest quantitatively to a beaker and dilute with water to give an acid concentration approximately 1 to 25. Continue with the procedure described for tissue ash.

REFERENCES

1. Gettler, A. O., and Lehman, R. A. Simplified procedure for determination of mercury in urine, Am. J. Clin. Path., Tech. Supp., 2:161, 1938.
2. Schumacher, and Jung, W. L. Eine einfache und zuverlässige Methode zur quantitativen Bestimmung des Quecksilbers im Harn, Ztschr. f. anal. Chem., 39:12, 1900.
3. Gettler, A. O., and Kaye, S. Simple and rapid analytical method for Hg, Bi, Sb, and As in biologic material, J. Lab. & Clin. Med., 35:146, 1950.
4. Brode, W. R. Chemical Spectroscopy, New York, John Wiley and Sons, Inc., 1939.
5. Harrison, G. R., Lord, R. C., and Loofbourow, J. R. Practical Spectroscopy, New York, Prentice-Hall, Inc., 1948.
6. Gerlach, W., and Schweitzer, E. Foundations and Methods of Chemical Analysis by the Emission Spectrum, London, Adam Hilger, Ltd., 1929.
7. Harrison, G. R., Ed. New Wave Length Tables (M. I. T.) 100,000 Principal Spectrum Lines, New York, John Wiley and Sons, Inc., 1939.
8. —— Lord, R. C., and Loofbourow, J. R. Practical Spectroscopy, New York, Prentice-Hall, Inc., 1948, p. 209.
9. Sawyer, R. A. Experimental Spectroscopy, New York, Prentice-Hall, Inc., 1944, p. 229.
10. Wickmann, H. J. Isolation and determination of traces of metals, Indust. & Engin. Chem., Anal. Ed., 11:66, 1939.
11. Negresco, T. Technique de l'analyse spectrale, J. de chim. phys., 25:216, 1928.
12. van Someren, E. H. S. Spectrographic analysis of some alloys of aluminum, J. Inst. Metals, 55:409, 1934.
13. Duffenbach, O. S., Wolfe, R. A., and Smith, R. W. Quantitative analysis by spectroscopic methods, Indust. & Engin. Chem., Anal. Ed., 5:226, 1933.
14. Twyman, F., and Hitchen, C. S. Determination of metals in solution by means of their spark spectra, Proc. Roy. Soc., London, s.A., 133:72, 1931.
15. Cholak, J., and Bambach, K. Determination of lead in biological material, Indust. & Engin., Anal. Ed., 13:583, 1941.
16. —— Hubbard, D. M., and Story, R. V. Determination of aluminum in biological material, Indust. & Engin. Chem., Anal. Ed., 15:57, 1943.
17. —— and Hubbard, D. M. Determination of cadmium in biological material, Indust. & Engin. Chem., Anal. Ed., 16:333, 1944.
18. —— Hubbard, D. M., and Burkey, R. E. Determination of zinc in biological material, Indust. & Engin. Chem., Anal. Ed., 15:754, 1943.
19. —— and Hubbard, D. M. Microdetermination of antimony in biological material; spectrographic method, J. Indust. Hyg. & Toxicol., 28:121, 1946.
20. Gerlach, W., and Schweitzer, E. Foundations and Methods of Chemical Analysis by the Emission Spectrum, London, Adam Hilger, Ltd., 1929.
21. Cucuel, F. Detection and determination of small quantities of mercury, Mikrochemie, 13:321, 1933.
22. Gettler, A. O., and Lehman, R. Simplified procedure for determination of mercury in urine, Am. J. Clin. Path., Tech. Supp., 2:161, 1938.
23. Winkler, W. O. Determination of small quantities of mercury in leafy vegetables by means of diphenylthiocarbazone (dithizone), Journal of Association of Official Agricultural Chemists, 18:638, 1935.
24. —— Report on the determination of mercury in foods, Journal of Association of Official Agricultural Chemists, 19:233, 1936.
25. Feigl, F. Spot Tests, New York, Elsevier-Nordeman, 1939, p. 50.
26. Autenrieth, W. Laboratory Manual for the Detection of Poisons and Powerful Drugs, 6th ed., New York, Blakiston Co., 1928, p. 200.

* Filtration is not necessary since carbon particles or insoluble silicates do not interfere. The presence of carbon in the mixture aids in the fusion reaction.

References 1015

27. Treadwell, F. P., and Hall, W. T. Analytical Chemistry, 7th ed., New York, John Wiley and Sons, Inc., 1929, p. 254.
28. Umberger, C. J., and Goldbaum, L. Unpublished data. Laboratory of the Chief Medical Examiner, City of New York.
29. Kaye, S. Simple procedure for detection of arsenic in body fluid, Am. J. Clin. Path., Tech. Supp., 8:36, 1944.
30. Gettler, A. O., and Kaye, S. Simple and rapid analytical method for Hg, Bi, Sb, and As in biologic material, J. Lab. & Clin. Med., 35:146, 1950.
31. Feigl, F. Spot Tests, New York, Elsevier-Nodeman, 1939, p. 33.
32. Sproull, R. C., and Gettler, A. O. Application of a photoelectric colorimeter, Indust. & Engin. Chem., Anal. Ed., 13:462, 1941.
33. Gettler, A. O., Rhoads, C. P., and Weiss, S. Contribution to pathology of generalized argyria with discussion of fate of silver in human body, Am. J. Path., 3:631, 1927.
34. ———— Unpublished data.
35. Methods of Analysis (Official and Tentative). Association of Official Agricultural Chemists, 4th ed., Washington, D. C., 1935, pp. 375-385.
36. Tompsett, S. L., and Anderson, A. B. The lead content of human tissues and excreta, Biochem. J., 29:1851, 1935.
37. Lynch, G. R., Slater, R. H., and Osler, T. G. The determination of traces of lead in biological materials, with special reference to bones, Analyst, 59:787, 1934.
38. Cholak, J. Quantitative spectrographic determination of lead in biological material, Indust. Engin. Chem., Anal. Ed., 7:287, 1935.
39. Ross, J. R., and Lucas, C. C. A new method for the determination of minute amounts of lead in urine, J. Biol. Chem., 111:285, 1935.
40. Horwitt, M. K., and Cowgill, G. R. A titrimetric method for the quantitative estimation of lead in biological materials, J. Biol. Chem., 119:533, 1937.
41. Gettler, A. O., and Weiss, L. Thallium poisoning; clinical toxicology of thallium, Am. J. Clin. Path., 13:422, 1943.
42. ———— and Weiss, L. Thallium poisoning; quantitative determination of thallium in biologic material, Am. J. Clin. Path., 13:368, 1943.
43. Feigl, F. Spot Tests, New York, Elsevier-Nordeman, 1939, p. 137.
44. Gronover, A., and Wohnlich, E. Cadmium als Ueberzugsmetall für Gebrauchsgegenstände, Ztschr. f. Untersuch. d. Lebensmitt., 53:392, 1927.
45. Prodan, L. Cadmium poisoning; experimental cadmium poisoning, J. Indust. Hyg., 14:174, 1932.
46. Emich, F. Microchemical Laboratory Manual, translated by F. Schneider, New York, John Wiley and Sons, Inc., 1932.
47. Jacobs, M. B. Analytical Chemistry of Industrial Poisons, Hazards and Solvents, New York, Interscience Publishers, Inc., 1946, p. 213.
48. Willard, H. H., and Greathouse, L. H. The colorimetric determination of manganese by oxidation with periodate, J. Am. Chem. Soc., 39:2366, 1917.
49. Funk, E. H., and St. Claire, H. Hemochromatosis: report of a case, with studies of the copper content of the liver, Arch. Int. Med., 45:37, 1930.
50. Gerlach, W. The copper content of human and animal organs, Virchows Arch. f. path. Anat., 294:171, 1934.
51. ———— The copper content of human organs in special cases, Virchows Arch. f. path. Anat., 295:394, 1935.
52. McFarlane, W. D. Application of the sodium diethyl-dithiocarbamate reaction to the micro-colorimetric determination of copper in organic substances, Biochem. J., 26:1022, 1932.
53. Lutz, R. E. Normal occurrence of Zn in biologic materials: a review of the literature and a study of the distribution of zinc in the rat, cat and man, J. Indust. Hyg., 8:177, 1926.
54. Drinker, K. R., Fehnel, J. W., and Marsh, M. Normal excretion of zinc in urine and feces of man, J. Biol. Chem., 72:375, 1927.
55. Gettler, A. O., and Bastian, R. Zinc in human tissues, detection and determination by dithizone, Am. J. Clin. Path., 17:244, 1947.
56. Koelsch, F. Metal-fume fever, J. Indust. Hyg., 5:87, 1923.
57. McNally, W. Toxicology, Chicago, Industrial Medicine, 1937, p. 298.
58. Gettler, A. O., and Bastian, R. Zinc in human tissues; detection and determination by dithizone, Am. J. Clin. Path., 17:244, 1947.
59. Salant, W. Pharmacology of heavy metals, J. Indust. Hyg., 2:72, 1920.

44

Inorganic Nonmetallic Poisons

The inorganic nonmetallic poisons are characterized by the fact that, with the exception of a few special members, they cannot be determined from the analysis of the organs, tissues or body fluids. Because the elements are normal constituents of tissue, they can be identified only by examination of the stomach contents. Almost all the compounds are extremely reactive as they are acids, bases, oxidizers or reducers. Once absorption takes place through the intestinal wall, the reactive properties of the molecule are nullified as a result of their action on the tissue and, after distribution throughout the body, any increase in the elemental content of the tissue will not exceed possible normal variations. When ingested, these poisons are taken invariably in large dosages, particularly when the intent is suicidal. Being corrosive substances, their possible presence will be indicated from the postmortem examination of the mouth, esophagus and stomach lining. Since they are difficult to ingest and produce violent pain before death, there is usually some of the original material to be found at the scene, either from the container or dispersed in the vomitus. Isolation of the soluble compounds is made by dialysis of the fluid from the stomach contents. Fluorides, phosphorous and borates are determinable from analysis of the organs as well as the stomach contents. The chemistry for the detection and quantitative analysis of this type of poison requires no special treatment other than conventional inorganic macro analysis. The limited number of these poisons, coupled with autopsy findings which indicate or exclude specific substances, permits the use of individual tests for each compound without employing any particular analytic scheme.

EXAMINATION OF THE STOMACH CONTENTS

A *physical examination* of the stomach contents will frequently reveal undissolved inorganic particles. These should be separated mechanically or by flotation in a nonpolar liquid. The particles of food and any other solid structures in the contents should be separated for possible future examination in case the question of poison in the food should arise.

Examination of Insoluble Inorganic Material. 1. Combustion Test. A sample of any unusual material should be tested for combustibility by igniting to red heat on a platinum crucible lid to rule out organic compounds.

2. Solubility Test. The solubility of the isolated substance should be determined in water and in N/10 HCl. A water soluble substance may have been ingested in sufficient quantity to exceed its solubility in the aqueous phase of the stomach contents. Some toxic salts, such as barium carbonate, which are insoluble in neutral or alkaline solution are rendered sufficiently soluble by the action of the normal stomach acid to produce death.

3. Spectrographic Examination. The noncombustible residue from the combustion test should be subjected to a spectrographic examination to determine its metal content. A sample of about 25 mg. is treated by the procedure for the

spectrographic examination of tissue ash (page 975), using 10 amperes and a 30 second exposure with a 20 μ slit. At the same time, a sample of the original solid should be run on the same plate under the same conditions. The volatile metals such as mercury, arsenic and antimony, which may be lost on ignition, may be detected spectrographically because, if present, they will be in relatively high concentrations. Ingested permanganate may be completely reduced to insoluble manganese dioxide or chromates may be reduced to a slightly soluble chromous state by the action of the organic compounds of the stomach contents and the tissue of the stomach lining.

4. Digestion with 3 Normal Sodium Carbonate Solution. The identification of the anion of a soluble salt taken in excess or of a salt which is only soluble in acid solution (see 2. Solubility Test above) is necessary in establishing the identity of an ingested preparation even though it is nontoxic. Identification of extraneous insoluble inorganic matter which could not have had an effect on the cause of death may furnish the key to the legal question of suicide or accidental death and the nature of the anion may then become of prime importance.

If a soluble salt is treated with sodium carbonate solution, all of the metals except sodium, potassium, lithium and NH_4^+ are precipitated as the insoluble carbonates, leaving the anions in solution as the soluble sodium salts. If an insoluble salt is digested with sodium carbonate solution, the same change occurs at a slower rate by metathesis. Filtration of the insoluble metal carbonates then leaves a solution of all the anions except in the case of the few salts not attacked by boiling sodium carbonate. Many metal sulfides are not decomposed and the halides of silver are not affected. All the insoluble metal phosphates and barium sulfate are acted on only slightly. Metals which are both acidic and basic, such as manganese, chromium and arsenic, may be in solution as the anions. The few metals like aluminum, chromium, antimony and tin which form amphoteric hydroxides may also be rendered soluble. The only possible change in the composition of the anions by the carbonate treatment occurs when reducing constituents such as sulfide, sulfite, arsenite, lead, antimony, stannous tin and ferrous iron are present in a mixture with an oxidizing anion. Hypochlorite can be decomposed to chloride and chlorate, ferricyanide to the ferro state, MnO_4^- to MnO_2, and $CrO_4^=$ to the chromous state. Chlorate, nitrate, nitrite, sulfide and sulfite are not affected by other components in the boiling sodium carbonate solution.

Reagent. 3 normal sodium carbonate.

Procedure (1). A 0.1 to 0.3 gm. sample of the inorganic substance is placed in a crucible and boiled gently for 10 minutes with about 5 to 10 ml. of 3 N sodium carbonate solution, replacing the water as it evaporates. The solution is filtered, the precipitate washed with water and the solution examined by the procedures for the stomach filtrate and diffusate (pages 1017 to 1023).

Examination of the Fluid Fraction. If the stomach contents are not sufficiently fluid for filtration, enough distilled water is introduced to form a filterable slurry. The water and contents are measured in order to permit corrections for the dilution in subsequent tests. The contents are thoroughly mixed, filtered through fluted filter paper and the insoluble portion and paper washed with water.

1. Hydrogen Ion Concentration. A small aliquot of the filtrate is tested for acidity or basicity with indicators or the hydrogen ion concentration measured with a pH meter. The normal gastric residuum in the stomach varies between 50 and 150 ml. and contains, at most, 0.3 per cent total hydrochloric acid. The maxi-

mum acidity expected is, therefore, of the order of 0.09 normal for the original fluid of the stomach and it will have been reduced in proportion to the dilution for the filtration. Any acidity above this in the filtered solution is suggestive, therefore, of an ingested acid substance.

2. Titration for Total Acid. When the hydrogen ion concentration is elevated, the total acidity should be determined by titration of an aliquot of the filtrate with 0.1 N alkali (2) and the acid calculated as HCl after correction for the dilution prior to filtration.

3. Chlorides. The total chloride content is seldom above 500 mg. per 100 ml. except during digestion, when it may reach 600 mg. per 100 ml. (3). If the acidity is found to be only moderately in excess of the upper limits for normal, the total chloride content should be determined by any of the standard procedures for chlorides in gastric contents (2). If it is not elevated in proportion to the acidity, an acid salt may be present.

4. Titration for Total Alkali. The gastric residuum is never on the alkaline side and pH findings above 7.0 are suggestive of the presence of bases or salts of weak acids and strong bases. The total alkali should be determined by titrating an aliquot of the filtrate with 0.1 N HCl to a methyl red end point, following the methods in step 2 for the total acid.

(a) Test for Carbonate. The stomach is usually washed with sodium bicarbonate when patients showing signs of poisoning are admitted to a hospital. This information is seldom available at the time of autopsy so that an alkaline stomach filtrate should be examined for carbonates before drawing conclusions from the findings for alkali.

Procedure. Two milliliters of filtrate are placed in a 3 inch test tube fitted with a one-hole cork containing a 4 mm. piece of glass tubing extending down to several centimeters above the surface of the liquid. The lower end of the glass tubing is charged with a drop of strong $Ba(OH)_2$ solution so that the end of the tube is sealed by the solution. Several drops of concentrated hydrochloric acid are introduced into the filtrate and the tube is quickly closed with the cork containing the glass tube and the $Ba(OH)_2$ solution. If carbonates are present, the solution shows effervescence and the CO_2 produced clouds the barium hydroxide solution in the glass tube as a result of the formation of insoluble barium carbonate.

If carbonates are found, the possibility of sodium or other soluble carbonates must still be excluded. The pH of sodium bicarbonate is about 8.5 regardless of the concentration while sodium carbonate has a pH of 9.0 to 10.0. Carbonates other than those of potassium and lithium are insoluble in neutral or basic solution.*

5. Detection of Oxidants. Colorless inorganic oxidizers such as nitrate, nitrite, chlorate, hypochlorite, bromate, hypobromite, iodate, persulfate, peroxides, perborates, arsenates are readily detected with diphenylamine reagent (page 1055). A drop of reagent added to a small portion of filtrate gives an immediate intense blue coloration. A slight blue color may be produced as a result of the action of the reagent on organic matter but the intensity and speed of color formation is slight in contrast to the immediate intense reaction with oxidants.† Chromates, ferricyanide and permanganates which react with the reagent are indicated by their reddish or

---

* After ingestion of an insoluble carbonate such as barium carbonate, there will be some soluble barium ion and dissolved carbon dioxide from the action of the stomach acid on the carbonate.

† Some organic oxidants such as nitroglycerine also give an immediate reaction.

yellow colored solutions, providing all of the oxidant has not been reduced by the organic content of the stomach.

6. Examination for Ferri- and Ferrocyanide and Thiocyanate with Ferric and Ferrous Ion. Ferric and ferrocyanide is slightly decomposed during the steam distillation for the volatiles (page 1046) and, with weak positive findings for cyanide in the distillate, the stomach contents should be examined for these ions. In acid solution, ferrocyanide reacts with Fe^{+++} to form insoluble Prussian blue, while ferricyanide produces only a brown coloration. Ferrous ion, on the other hand, reacts with ferricyanide to form Turnbull's blue. Thiocyanate reacts with ferric ion to form blood red ferric thiocyanate.

Reagents. (a) 5 per cent aqueous $FeCl_3$; (b) 5 per cent aqueous $FeSO_4$.

Procedure. A drop of the 5 per cent ferric chloride solution is added to 1 ml. of filtrate, slightly acidified with HCl if it is not already acid. A blue precipitate indicates ferrocyanide and a red color indicates thiocyanate. If there is no reaction, a drop of 5 per cent ferrous sulfate is introduced. A blue color indicates ferricyanide.*

Isolation of Soluble Inorganic Chemicals by Dialysis. Dialysis is normally used for removing soluble ions from colloids or soluble substances of high molecular weight. The solution or colloidal suspension is placed inside the membrane compartment and the membrane bathed in water or other solvent until all diffusible substances have passed through the membrane. Since the solution containing the diffusible substances is not wanted, large volumes of solvent are usually circulated over the membrane surface in order to hasten the diffusion process.

Since it is the diffusible ions that are sought in the dialysis of stomach contents, the standard procedure should be modified to permit use of the minimum volume of bathing solution. Electrodialysis is not a safe procedure because of possible electrochemical changes in the diffusate. Factors other than permeability and surface of the membrane affect the rate at which diffusion occurs. A layer of pure solvent continuously circulated over the surface of the dialylic membrane (4) and elevated temperature of the dialysate (5) hastens the process.

The apparatus most suitable for toxicologic work is a modification of the Star dialyzer of Zsigmondy and Heyer (6). The cell consists of a hard rubber ring provided with a groove at the bottom, in which the membrane is held by means of a cord or rubber band. The ring fits into a bottom compartment the size of a petri dish. The dish contains baffles running parallel, spaced 1 cm. apart and opened at alternate ends, so that a channel of about 0.5 cm. is at each end of the baffle. The baffles are about half the height of the dish and are ground flat so that they act as a support for the membrane when the ring assembly is placed inside the dish. Two short pieces of 5 mm. bore glass tubing are sealed into opposite sides of the dish at points perpendicular to the baffles to serve as inlet and outlet for the bathing solution. The inlet tube is located at a level in the side wall below the top level of the baffles, while the outlet tube is located just above the baffles. The inlet tube is connected to a Mariotte flask through a rubber tubing equipped with pinch clamp to serve as the reservoir for the bathing solution. The assembled apparatus is located on a stand so that the outlet tube empties into a beaker which serves as collector for the bathing solution after it bathes the membrane while flowing through the channels of the dish.

---

* Ferric or ferrous solutions may contain both ferrous and ferric ion so that the differentiation between the ferro- and ferri- ion is not conclusive.

PREPARATION OF THE MEMBRANES. Highly permeable membranes are desirable for recovery of all the diffusible ions. The permeability of different membranes made from the same source material varies with the nature of the solvent, the concentration of membrane substance in the solvent, the time of drying, the amount of swelling of the film and its thickness (7). The method for the preparation of a highly permeable membrane is taken from the process of Brown for the preparation of graded membranes (8, 9).

An 8 per cent solution of Celloidin * in a mixture of equal volumes of absolute ethyl alcohol and ethyl ether is prepared. A glass plate larger than the diameter of the rubber ring of the dialysis apparatus is dipped in the Celloidin solution and allowed to drain while suspended over it for 5 minutes. The plate is exposed to air for one minute, following which it is plunged into water at 20° C. for one minute and the films removed from the plate. The films are thoroughly dried out by exposure to air overnight. The dry membrane is soaked in 95 per cent ethyl alcohol for 24 hours at a temperature of 20° C. and then thoroughly washed in distilled water for 24 hours, after which it is ready for use. The prepared films may be stored under water at a temperature not exceeding 20° C.

Procedure. The membrane is carefully fitted over the rubber ring and tied securely to it by means of a string or rubber band at the groove of the ring. The ring is then placed inside the dish with the membrane supported by the baffles. Fifty to 100 ml. of filtrate from the stomach contents is introduced into the rubber ring compartment and about 500 ml. of distilled water into the Mariotte flask. The dialysis cell and Mariotte flask are placed on a ring stand with the Mariotte flask elevated slightly above the level of the dialysis dish. The pinch clamp is regulated so that water flows through the dish and out of the outlet tube at the rate of a few drops per minute. The discharge, which is collected in a beaker, is returned to the Mariotte flask before the latter is completely emptied. In this manner, a continuous flow of solution is maintained across the membrane for six to eight hours. The stomach filtrate is maintained at a temperature of 70 to 90° C. during that time by partially submerging a 30 watt pilot light bulb into the solution. The use of a small laboratory reciprocating pump to return the solution from the beaker to the Mariotte flask and moderate mechanical agitation of the filtrate inside the cell compartment makes the process automatic. At the end of the dialysis, the aqueous solution is carefully evaporated to a small volume on a hot plate.

Examination of the Diffusate. 1. Evaporation of the Solution. The relative hydrogen ion concentration of the small volume of solution remaining after the evaporation is determined with indicator paper or indicator solutions. If it is decidedly acid, about half the solution is neutralized with ammonia and carefully evaporated to dryness on a hot plate. The acid solution is used to identify the acid constituent and the neutralized residue is used for the anions (pages 1021-1022). If the solution is neutral or alkaline all of it may be evaporated to dryness.

2. Tests for the Anions in the Dialysis Residue. (a) Anions Forming Insoluble Barium and Calcium Salts in Acetic Acid Solution. Sulfates, sulfites and chromates react with barium to form salts that are insoluble in dilute acetic acid solution while fluorides and oxalates form insoluble calcium salts under the same conditions. Barium sulfate is insoluble in concentrated mineral acid solution and calcium fluoride, a gelatinous precipitate which is difficult to filter, is insoluble in con-

---

* Product of Schering.

centrated acetic acid solution. The insolubility of the other barium and calcium salts depends on the limited hydrogen ion concentration of the buffered solution. With the exception of sulfates, they are very toxic anions. They are excluded as a group when a mixture of barium and calcium ions, added under controlled conditions, fails to give an insoluble precipitate.

Reagents. 6 normal acetic acid; 1 normal barium chloride; 1 normal calcium chloride (sulfate free); 50 per cent sodium acetate.

Procedure (10). About 50 mg. of residue from the dialysis is dissolved in 1 ml. of water and the solution, if alkaline, neutralized to litmus with acetic acid. Three-tenths milliliter of 50 per cent sodium acetate, 1.0 ml. of 6 normal acetic acid, 1.0 ml. of normal barium chloride and 3.0 ml. of normal calcium chloride solutions are added, the solution heated to near boiling and allowed to stand at least 10 minutes. Any precipitate is allowed to settle and is filtered and examined by tests for the individual anions (pages 1021, 1023, 1032, 1039).

(b) Reducing Substances. Sulfide, sulfite, meta bisulfite, nitrite, iodide, arsenite and ferrocyanide ions have sufficiently high reducing potentials to reduce ferricyanide to ferrocyanide in weakly acid solution. Ferricyanide reacts with ferrous iron but not with ferric iron, while ferrocyanide reacts with ferric iron to form Prussian blue (page 1051). The formation of a green or blue coloration or a blue precipitate when a solution of ferricyanide and ferric ion is added to an acid solution is, therefore, indicative of reducing substances. The test is given by many organic compounds. It is one of the procedures recommended for differentiation between morphine and heroin (11).

Positive findings will not be obtained on the residue from the dialysis of stomach contents except where an abnormal substance is present and, on elimination of organic interference by mild ignition (page 1016), the test is indicative of one of the inorganic reducing anions. Strong reducers such as sulfite act partly by reducing the ferric ion to ferrous which then reacts with the ferric cyanide to form Turnbull's blue. Care must be taken to use pure reagents and to run a control at the same time since the presence of any ferrous ion in the ferric reagent or ferrocyanide contamination of the ferricyanide reagent will give a false positive reaction.

Reagents. 2 normal HCl; normal $Fe(NO_3)_3$ free of ferrous ion; normal $K_3Fe(CN)_6$ free of ferrocyanide ion.

The ferric nitrate and potassium ferricyanide should be prepared fresh.

Procedure (12). Dissolve about 50 mg. of residue in 1 ml. of water and carefully neutralize with the appropriate strength HCl selected to avoid excessive dilution of the sample.* Measure the final volume and then add the calculated volume of 2 normal HCl to make the solution $\frac{1}{2}$ normal with respect to HCl. Add one drop of normal $Fe(NO_3)_3$ and one drop of normal $K_3Fe(CN)_6$. Let stand two to three minutes to observe the color.

(c) Anions Forming Insoluble Silver Salts in Dilute Nitric Acid Solution. Insoluble salts are formed when silver ion is added to a dilute nitric acid solution containing chloride, bromide, iodide, cyanide, thiocyanate, ferro- and ferricyanide or sulfide ion. $AgCl$, $Ag_2(CN)_2$, $AgSCN$ and $Ag_4Fe(CN)_6$ are white while $AgBr$ is light yellow, AgI dark yellow, $Ag_3Fe(CN)_6$ brown and AsS black. A little chloride will always be present so that, in a test on the dialyzed residue from a natural death, a white precipitate is to be expected. Cyanides will have been found in the volatile

---

* The concentration of HCl to select is determined by the alkalinity of the sample.

poisons (page 1051) and the absence of soluble thiocyanates or ferrocyanide would have been shown by the failure of ferric ion to give a red or blue color in the tests on the stomach filtrate (page 1019).

The value of the test with silver ion is limited then to the detection of bromides, iodides and sulfides with positive findings indicated by a colored precipitate.* If the test is put on a semiquantitative basis it may be used to indicate chlorate and hypochlorite ion which may be present if the diphenylamine-sulfuric acid test was positive (page 1018). These ions are readily reduced to chloride in nitric acid solution by sodium nitrite. The procedure, modified to include chlorate and hypochlorite, consists of dissolving the sample in water, dividing the solution into equal portions and treating both solutions by the procedure which follows, with the addition of three drops of 3 normal $NaNO_2$ to one portion before adding the silver nitrate solution. A large white precipitate of silver chloride in the tube containing the sodium nitrite is indicative of chlorate or hypochlorite.

Reagents. normal $AgNO_3$; 6 normal HNO_3; 3 normal $NaNO_2$.

Procedure (13). About 50 mg. of residue is dissolved in 6 ml. of water and neutralized with nitric acid solution, if alkaline. One milliliter of 6 N HNO_3 and 1 ml. of normal $AgNO_3$ are then introduced. A colored precipitate indicates a positive reaction.

(d) Iodine-Sodium Azide Reaction for Sulfur-Containing Anions. The iodine-sodium azide reaction is described for the detection of sulfur-containing molecules in the volatile distillate (page 1062). The decolorization of the iodine by sodium azide is catalyzed by sulfur-containing organic compounds such as CS_2, mercaptans, thioketones and inorganic sulfur compounds such as sulfides, thiocyanates and the poly sulfur anions such as thiosulfate and meta bisulfite. The reaction is not affected by free sulfur, sulfite or sulfate. The procedure is described on page 1053.

3. Tests for Metals in the Residue. (a) Flame Spectra. A flame spectral examination of the residue may eliminate chemical testing. If an abnormal metal is present, there will usually be relatively large amounts in the evaporate. Moreover, it is rare that more than one metal is present. A normal diffusate shows only a yellow sodium flame and any other coloration is indicative of an abnormal metal.

A yellow-green flame is an indication for an examination for barium as the most probable substance giving this coloration with thallium as the next choice. These metals are in use in rat and roach powders and are commonly found in suicides. Borates give a green color in acid solution and phosphates also do so in the presence of sulfuric acid. The copper halides and tellurium also color the flame green. Red flames are indicative of lithium, strontium or calcium and light blue of selenium, arsenic or lead. The potassium flame can be seen in the presence of the normal sodium without the aid of a cobalt glass filter or pocket spectroscope.†

Procedure. A loop about 2 mm. in diameter is made in the end of a platinum wire previously cleaned by repeatedly moistening with concentrated hydrochloric acid and heating to red heat in the bunsen burner until the flame fails to show any yellow color. A portion of the residue is taken up on the end of the platinum loop. A small drop of concentrated hydrochloric acid is placed on the wire in back of the

---

* Silver bromide does not always settle out as a yellow colored precipitate. If the conditions are not proper, it may have a dirty gray appearance and be mistaken for chlorides contaminated with foreign material. Also, the color difference between $Ag_3Fe(CN)_6$ and AgI is not always distinctive and the ferricyanide can be mistaken for iodides.

† Rubidium and caesium give the same flame spectra as potassium.

sample and allowed to run down the wire to the loop. The middle portion of the wire is inserted into the lower edge of the flame of a microburner and held until the heat transferred along the wire to the loop evaporates the excess acid, leaving the hydrochloride of the metal. The glowing wire is then slowly moved through the edge of the flame until the loop reaches the oxidizing cone. Sodium interference is lessened and flashes of color are better observed by this technic than by inserting the sample directly into the flame.

(b) Spectrographic Examination. A 25 mg. sample of the residue is treated in the arc of the spectrograph in the same manner as a tissue ash (pages 974 to 976). It is preferable to take two exposures on the one sample, using 10 and 30 seconds at 8 amperes with a 20 μ slit. A comparison of the intensities of the lines of the spectrographically sensitive metals in the two exposures furnishes a better semi-quantitative measure of their concentrations. For example, potassium will always be present but when the amounts are excessive, the potassium lines in the 10 second exposure will be almost as intense as at the 30 second exposure. Metals which may be missed in the spectrographic examination of the tissue such as mercury, antimony, arsenic, selenium and tellurium may be present in concentrations high enough to give a clearcut spectrum.

DIFFERENTIAL AND SPECIFIC TESTS FOR INDIVIDUAL SUBSTANCES

CORROSIVE ACIDS AND THEIR SALTS

Sulfuric Acid. 1. Test for Strong Sulfuric Acid Solution. If the acid is present in high concentration it will give a color reaction with a number of organic compounds (pages 1203 to 1206), particularly the alkaloid veratrine. A drop of stomach contents containing strong sulfuric acid on a crystal of veratrine gives a play of colors ending with a crimson red.

2. Identification of barium sulfate.* Insoluble barium sulfate is formed by the action of Ba^{++} (section 2(a), under Examination of the Diffusate, page 1020) even from concentrated mineral acid solution. The barium sulfate is confirmed by adding several drops of concentrated sulfuric acid to the precipitate in a test tube and heating to SO_3 fumes. The barium sulfate dissolves in the hot acid but on the addition of a microdrop of water it reprecipitates immediately.

Halogens. 1. Detection of High Concentrations of Hydrochloric Acid. The concentration of free hydrochloric acid in the stomach contents may be well above 0.3 per cent in cases with gastric ulcers. It will not be elevated to a concentration high enough to convert red brown silver chromate to colorless silver chloride when a solution of the stomach filtrate is brought to boiling with a silver chromate paper suspended over the vapors unless the free acid solution was ingested. Suicides have occurred from the ingestion of the free acid and also of "killed spirit" (the soldering flux made by dissolving zinc in concentrated hydrochloric acid (14)).

Procedure. A silver chromate impregnated paper is prepared by dipping the paper into 10 per cent potassium dichromate, allowing it to partially dry and then quickly immersing in a dilute silver nitrate solution. The paper is thoroughly washed in water to remove any silver nitrate and is air dried. A section of the paper is placed over a test tube containing a few milliliters of the stomach filtrate and the solution brought to the boiling point. HCl vapors immediately decolorize the paper on coming

---

* This is a confirmation test for $BaSO_4$ in the group test (page 1020) and for the detection of $BaSO_4$ in the water-insoluble matter of the stomach contents after gastrointestinal x-ray studies.

in contact with it and, on washing out the displaced chromate, a clear spot of white silver chloride is obtained.*

2. **Differentiation Between Silver Halides and Other Silver Salts Insoluble in Nitric Acid Solution.** Establishing a silver salt insoluble in dilute nitric acid as a halide may be made by the process of elimination because all the other anions have characteristic distinguishing tests. However, the question of the identity of the silver precipitate from the stomach contents may arise when it is contaminated with occluded foreign matter. In addition, there may be the problem of distinguishing between a normal and abnormal chloride content. Hot potassium dichromate and sulfuric acid oxidize the silver halide with the formation of chlorine and bromine. One of the most sensitive tests for chlorine and bromine is the displacement of I^- from KI with the formation of I_2. Iodine is detectable in minute concentrations by the reaction with starch. The formation of a blue color when moist starch-KI paper is suspended over a tube containing the silver salt in the hot oxidizing mixture shows that the silver salt was a chloride or bromide. Iodine is not liberated from the solution, probably because it is converted into iodate. When silver iodide is heated in a few drops of a mixture of equal volumes of phosphoric and perchloric acids, iodine is liberated and colors starch paper blue in the absence of potassium iodide.

Procedure. A sample of the washed silver precipitate is placed in a microtest tube, several crystals of potassium dichromate introduced, one drop of water and 3 drops of concentrated sulfuric acid added. The mouth of the tube is covered with filter paper which has been dipped into a 10 per cent solution of KI containing 1 per cent starch solution and allowed to drain until moist. The acid is heated just to the boiling point in a microburner. A blue color on the starch-KI paper shows the presence of halides.‡

3. **Differentiation Between Silver Chloride and Silver Bromide.** Since some silver chloride usually will be found in a silver precipitate from stomach contents, bromides and iodides must be detected in the presence of chlorides. Bromine reacts with acid fuchsin (reagent on page 1048) to form a violet brominated dyestuff (15). The test is not given by chlorine or iodine and, therefore, serves to detect silver bromide in a silver precipitate.

Procedure (16). The silver bromide is oxidized to bromine as described in 2 above, in a microtest tube which is equipped with a rubber stopper containing a small medicine dropper. A drop of the acid fuchsin, held in the constricted end of the dropper, absorbs the liberated bromine and gives an intense violet color.†

4. **Differentiation Between Silver Bromide and Silver Iodide.** When silver bromide fails to settle out of solution as a light yellow precipitate, it is usually grayish, resembling silver chloride, but under different conditions it can precipitate with a decided yellow color indistinguishable from silver iodide. The iodide can be distinguished from the bromide by the action of gold chloride on the precipitated halide. Gold ion displaces silver from silver iodide, forming dark brown gold iodide while silver bromide and silver chloride are not affected by the reagent. Consequently, a darkening of the halide precipitate on the addition of a 5 per cent gold chloride solution shows that silver iodide is present.

---

* Hydrobromic and hydriodic acids will react like hydrochloric acid. CN^- in acid solution will also decolorize silver chromate but the concentration will be high enough to be recognized from its odor.

‡ Iodine, even if formed in the chromate oxidation, would not be volatilized in sufficient quantity to react with the starch, under the mild heating conditions.

† This test is more sensitive than the bromine reaction with fluorescein.

Procedure. A small portion of the precipitate produced in section 2(c) under Examination of the Diffusate (page 1021) is moistened with a drop of 5 per cent gold chloride solution. An immediate darkening to brown or black is indicative of silver iodide. If the test is carried out on a microscope slide and viewed under low power as the reagent is added, the silver iodide can be detected in the presence of other insoluble silver salts.

5. Detection of Iodides. Iodides are more readily detected in the original sample material. Iodide is oxidized to iodine in acid solution by nitrite and may be detected by the blue color with starch solution. Organic compounds, particularly phenols, proteins and cyanides interfere with the iodine-starch reaction (17), so that the test is best carried out on the diffusate after dialysis.

Procedure. A few milliliters of solution are made acid with HCl and boiled to remove cyanides, if they are present. When 3 drops of 3 N potassium nitrate and 3 drops of 1 per cent starch solution are added, the blue iodine-starch color develops if iodides are present.

6. Free Halogens. Chlorine is a heavy yellow green gas, bromine a dark reddish brown liquid of low vapor pressure and iodine a crystalline dark purplish solid. Chlorine is used as a bleaching agent and disinfectant. Although a number of commercial preparations are available which are alkaline and liberate chlorine on acidification of the solution, it is questionable whether the toxicologist would have occasion to test for free chlorine. When inhaled, the gas is converted into hypochlorous acid which would be indicated by its strong oxidizing properties (pages 1018 and 1032). On ingestion of a quantity of an alkaline bleaching solution in excess of that required to neutralize the available stomach acid, chlorine will remain in the stomach contents. It would be recognized from the characteristic odor of the gas liberated in the test for carbonates (page 1018) and confirmed by the displacement of iodine from starch-KI paper (page 1024). Bromine is used primarily as a chemical reagent. It is extremely pungent and corrosive and deaths other than accidental ones from the free halogen are unlikely. Unlike chlorine, bromine dissolves in water without undergoing a reaction with it. Bromine water may contain up to 3.6 parts bromine per 100 parts water and the solution is stable in the dark. On long standing it slowly decomposes with formation of hydrobromic acid and oxygen. Bromine water is a strong oxidizing solution. When alkali is added, bromide and bromate are formed. Free bromine is detectable by volatilization of the element into acid fuchsin (reagent on page 1048) or on fluorescein-impregnated filter paper (18). Iodine solution is a common household antiseptic and suicides with it are common. It is recognized at autopsy by the permanent staining around the mouth and oral cavity. Iodine on the skin can be confirmed by the blue color produced by swabbing the brown area with a cotton applicator stick moistened with a normal potassium iodide solution containing 1 per cent starch.

Nitrogen Acids. Free nitric acid not only combines readily with proteins but also acts as a digestive agent on the tissue. Therefore, it would not remain as such in the stomach unless the ingested solution was dilute (19). Nitrate salts are oxidants in the presence of the acid in the stomach so that nitrite can always be expected when nitrates are taken internally. Nitrates and nitrites are used as meat preservatives. The legal limit is 200 parts per million of either or both, and very small amounts in the stomach contents may not be significant. Accidental deaths have occurred from the ingestion of meat treated with excess nitrite (14). The analytic problem involves the detection of nitrates in the presence of nitrites and the determination of an excessive nitrate and/or nitrite content. Nitrites in high concentrations will have been indicated by the yellow coloration produced in the test for chloral hydrate on the steam distillate (page 1052). Both are indicated in the diphenylamine test for oxidants (page 1018); nitrite also gives the test for reducers (page 1021) and forms a blue color by liberating iodine in starch-KI paper.

1. Quantitative Estimation of Nitrites. The Griess diazo reaction (20) which is specific for nitrites may be made quantitative by carrying out the test in sufficiently dilute solution and comparing the color with that of a standard potassium nitrite solution.

Reagents. (a) 0.5 gm. sulfanilic acid dissolved in 150 ml. of 2 normal acetic acid.

(b) 0.2 gm. of solid alpha-naphthylamine is boiled with 20 ml. of water. The supernatant solution, which should be colorless,* is decanted from the undissolved residue and diluted to 150 ml. with 2 N acetic acid.

(c) The separate solutions are stored in the dark and the reagent is prepared before use by mixing equal volumes of (a) and (b).

(d) Standard sodium nitrite solution: 0.5 gm. of pure sodium nitrite is dissolved in 1 liter of water. Ten milliliters of this is again diluted to 1 liter. One milliliter of the standard solution contains 0.005 mg. sodium nitrite.

Procedure (21). One-half milliliter of filtrate or a very small measured amount of diffusate is diluted to 50 ml. in a volumetric flask. The solution should be neutral or only slightly acid. One milliliter of the sample solution and 1 ml. of standard sodium nitrite solution are diluted with 9 ml. of water and 1 ml. of mixed reagent (c) introduced. An immediate red color develops if nitrites are present. If the color in the sample is more intense than in the standard, the procedure should be repeated, using an appropriate dilution to obtain a sample color with an intensity of the order of the standard or less. The nitrite content is estimated from optical density comparison of the standard with the sample.

2. Detection of Nitrates. When a significant nitrate concentration is found in the stomach it is probable that the nitrate alone was ingested, since the amount to be expected as an impurity in a commercial nitrite or from a meat preservative would be reduced in the stomach and escape detection. Practically all tests for nitrate are interfered with by nitrite. Nitrite, however, is broken down in dilute acid solution with the formation of nitrogen by the action of ammonium sulfamate. Since nitrates are not affected by sulfamate, the removal of nitrite with this compound makes tests such as that with brucine in concentrated sulfuric acid nearly specific for nitrate.†

Reagents. (a) Solid ammonium sulfamate; (b) 0.2 per cent brucine alkaloid dissolved in concentrated sulfuric acid, freshly prepared.

Procedure. A very small portion of diffusate dissolved in water, or a few milliliters of stomach filtrate, is acidified with 6 N acetic acid until the solution is distinctly acid. Ammonium sulfamate is introduced, a few crystals at a time, until all effervescence ceases and starch-potassium iodide paper fails to show a coloration. The solution is boiled to remove dissolved gases, cooled and the brucine-sulfuric

---

* If the supernatant solution is not colorless the alpha-naphthylamine is impure and must be recrystallized since the colored reagent may give a color with the sulfanilic acid alone.

† Chlorates in significant concentrations interfere but their presence along with nitrites is highly improbable.

acid reagent carefully layered under the aqueous solution. In the presence of nitrates, an intense red ring is formed at the interface.

3. Confirmatory Test for Nitrate. Nitrate may be confirmed after removal of nitrite with the phenoldisulfonic acid method described for organic nitro compounds on page 1055. A quantitative estimation can be made by both the brucine-sulfuric acid and phenoldisulfonic acid tests (22).

Phosphoric Acid. Poisoning with phosphoric acid solution has not been reported. It is improbable that the acid would be detected as such from the stomach contents in a routine chemical examination. A careful quantitative analysis of the diffusate would be necessary in order to draw the distinction between free phosphoric acid and phosphates ingested as salts in an acid solution.

1. Detection of Phosphates. Small amounts of phosphates are normally present in the stomach contents. Findings for large amounts would logically lead to a search for a cation in comparable concentration. Only its absence would lead the analyst to suspect the presence of the acid. Phosphates are readily detected by precipitation as phosphomolybdic acid. Arsenates and silicates react like phosphates. Arsenic will have been detected by the Reinsch test (page 973). It can be removed by hydrogen sulfide precipitation from 0.3 N hydrochloric acid solution and the phosphate precipitated after boiling to remove dissolved sulfides. Silicates are unlikely components of stomach contents but can be removed by evaporation to dryness of a solution strongly acidified with perchloric acid (23) (sodium silicate, page 1032). Oxalates and fluorides in high concentrations interfere by the formation of stable molybdate complexes, but will be indicated in the barium and calcium ion acid precipitation test (page 1020).

Reagents. (a) 3 normal nitric acid; (b) ammonium molybdate reagent: 9 gm. ammonium molybdate $((NH_4)_6Mo_7O_{24} \cdot 4H_2O)$ is dissolved in 10 ml. of 6 normal ammonium hydroxide. Twenty-four grams of ammonium nitrate is added and the solution is diluted to 100 ml. with water.

Procedure. The test is carried out on a sample of the diffusate, or the original stomach contents are made just alkaline, evaporated to dryness and ashed carbonfree in a muffle furnace at a temperature below 500° C. The sample is dissolved in 5 to 10 ml. of water and an equal volume of 3 normal nitric acid and half the volume of ammonium molybdate reagent is added. The solution is heated nearly to boiling and allowed to stand 5 to 10 minutes. A fine yellow precipitate is indicative of phosphate.

2. Confirmation Test for Phosphates. White to pale yellow molybdic oxide sometimes precipitates from the strongly acid solution due to extraneous ion interference or too intense heating. When the quantity of precipitate is small or its composition is questionable, the complex molybdate can be confirmed by its oxidizing action on benzidine in acetic acid solution.

Reagent. 0.10 gm. benzidine dissolved in 100 ml. of 10 per cent acetic acid.

Procedure. A portion of the precipitate is spread on a filter paper, moistened with several drops of benzidine reagent and the paper allowed to air dry. When the spot is held over concentrated ammonia solution, an intense blue color develops with the molybdate complex.

Acetic Acid. Vinegar contains 3.5 to 6 per cent acetic acid and, as the end product of fermentation, it is present in undistilled beverages which have gone sour. Acute poisonings have occurred from the ingestion of the concentrated acid.

Dilute solutions are administered as an antidote in the treatment of poisonings with corrosive basic substances. A quantitative determination is necessary in order to draw a distinction between acetate which is incidental and a toxic amount. Qualitative tests are not sensitive and are subject to interference by many compounds. Both qualitative and quantitative analysis are best made after distillation of the stomach contents.

1. Qualitative Tests for Acetate. (a) Cacodyl Reaction. The stomach filtrate or the distillate, if acidic, is made alkaline by the addition of 10 per cent sodium carbonate and evaporated to dryness on a hot plate. An equal bulk of arsenic trioxide is mixed with dry residue and the mixture gradually heated up by flaming with a bunsen burner. In the presence of acetates, the cacodyl oxide which is formed is recognized by its garlic-like odor.

$$4 NaC_2H_3O_2 + As_2O_3 \rightarrow 2 Na_2CO_3 + CO_2 + [(CH_3)_2As]_2O$$

Aliphatic organic acids which give a similar reaction are not found in the distillate.

(b) Lanthanum Nitrate-Iodine Test (24).

Reagents. (a) 5 per cent lanthanum nitrate solution; (b) 0.02 normal iodine in alcohol; (c) Normal ammonium hydroxide.

Procedure. An equal volume of lanthanum nitrate is added to a small volume of unevaporated acidic diffusate (page 1020) or distillate. Half the volume of iodine solution is added and the solution neutralized by dropwise addition of the ammonium hydroxide. In the presence of acetate ion a blue color resembling that of starch-iodine appears. The color is intensified on heating to boiling.*

Oxalic Acid. Oxalic acid is strong enough in its acid properties to be corrosive. In addition, oxalates are quite toxic and are readily absorbed through the intestinal walls. Absorbed oxalates are precipitated in the tissue as calcium oxalate, particularly in the tubules of the kidney. The free acid is solvent-soluble and, if present as such, will be extracted from the tissue in the isolation of the non-volatile organic fraction (page 1142). However, except in acute cases in which a large amount was ingested, all of it may be in the tissue as a salt, in which form it is alcohol insoluble (page 1146). The kidney is the best organ from which to isolate oxalates. The pathologist will see the crystals during the histologic examination of the kidney and in most acute cases the oxalate crystals can be removed mechanically.

Free oxalic acid can be extracted directly from the stomach contents with organic solvents but sodium oxalate or other salts are alcohol- and organic-solvent-insoluble. The distinction between oxalic acid or sodium oxalate poisoning can be made on the basis of solvent solubility or in an examination of the diffusate. In oxalate poisoning, large quantities of the typical calcium oxalate crystals are seen in the microscopic examination of the urine sediment or centrifugate but a distinction must be made between those from an oxalate toxicity and the relatively large calcium oxalate urinary content from oxalate-containing foods such as rhubarb.

1. Confirmatory Test for Oxalates. A few milligrams of solid sample placed on a microscope slide are covered with an equal bulk of resorcinol. The slide is gently warmed until the resorcinol melts. After cooling, a drop of concentrated sulfuric acid is added and the slide warmed up by flaming over a microburner until SO_3 fumes are produced. A variety of colors, with dark blue predominating, is

---

* Sulfite, phosphate, fluoride, oxalate and cations precipitated by ammonia interfere and propionate gives the same reaction.

characteristic of oxalates. Many other organic substances give colorations other than blue.

Citric Acid. Citrates are not toxic. Salts, particularly magnesium citrate, are used as cathartics and citrates are common constituents of fruit juices and other foods. Free citric acid, however, in high concentrations is sufficiently acidic to produce the clinical signs of a corrosive acid. The acid is soluble in water and alcohol but only slightly soluble in organic solvents.* It may be identified from the fluorescence of the ammoniacal solution after conversion into citrazinic acid with thionyl chloride (26).

Procedure. A few crystals of the solid or residue from the evaporated solution in a microtest tube are covered with a few drops of thionyl chloride and gently heated to fuming. An excess of concentrated ammonia is added and the mixture boiled to near dryness. Six to 10 drops of concentrated sulfuric acid are added after cooling and the contents reheated to SO_3 fumes. About 0.5 ml. of water is added and the solution made ammoniacal by the dropwise addition of concentrated ammonium hydroxide. If citrates are present, an examination of the solution in ultraviolet light, using a Wood's filter, will show an intense blue fluorescence.†

Tartaric Acid. Tartaric acid has about the same acidic properties as citric. Although no cases of poisoning from the ingestion of the acid are known it is a potential corrosive. Tartrates are present in foods and may be isolated in small amounts in the dialysis of the stomach contents. They are of interest in a toxicologic examination when antimony is found (page 991). Tartar emetic (potassium antimony tartrate) at one time was used as an emetic, administered in doses of 0.03 gm., and is still used in dosages of 3 to 6 mg. for the treatment of some tropical diseases. A suicidal death from the ingestion of a large quantity of tartar emetic has occurred (14). When the antimony content is relatively small, the question arises as to whether its presence resulted from the medicinal use of tartar emetic or from an antimony poisoning with elimination of most of the antimony prior to death. The tartrate content of the stomach may aid in settling the question.

Tartaric acid is soluble in water and alcohol but is insoluble in ether and other organic solvents. It is added to the stomach contents or tissue in the isolation process for the organic volatiles (page 1046) and care must be taken that a portion of the sample prepared for this purpose is not used in the chemical examination for the inorganic anions.

1. Detection of Tartrates. The acid and its salts char, giving off an odor of burnt sugar when heated with a few drops of concentrated sulfuric acid to SO_3 fumes.* Tartrates may be detected by the reaction with ferrous ion and hydrogen peroxide (27).

Reagents. (a) Freshly prepared 10 per cent solution of ferrous ammonium sulfate; (b) 3 per cent hydrogen peroxide; (c) 50 per cent sodium hydroxide.

Procedure. Several milligrams of tartaric acid or the soluble salt are dissolved in 0.5 ml. of water. One drop of ferrous ammonium sulfate reagent and two drops of hydrogen peroxide are added and the solution is shaken for a few minutes; then one drop of sodium hydroxide is introduced. A control is run at the same time with

---

* The Molisch-type reaction for citric, tartaric and malic acids, as described in Mulliken (25) is neither sensitive nor specific since it is given by other nonhydroxylated acids and is entirely negative when carried out by the slide technic (page 1244).

† The test is reported to be specific for citrates and citrazinic acid.

0.5 ml. distilled water. In the presence of tartrates, a violet color resembling that with salicylates and ferric ion is formed.*

ALKALINE CORROSIVES

Detection of Strong Alkali. Although soda ash and other alkaline salts are strongly basic, their aqueous solutions do not reach a pH of 14. A 1 per cent solution of 1,3,5 trinitrophenol in 95 per cent alcohol acts as an indicator for strongly alkaline solution, changing from colorless to deep red at pH 14. The color change when a drop of the indicator solution is placed on the skin or added to the stomach contents may be used, therefore, to differentiate between basic salts and free alkali. Strong ammonia and the strong aliphatic amines react positively.

Ammonium Hydroxide. Ammonia can be recognized usually at autopsy from its odor. The odor, however, may be misleading since it is a product of tissue degradation (page 1047) and may be quite pronounced, particularly under conditions of putrefaction. In addition, ammonia salts used as an inhalant is sometimes used to treat individuals with prostration. Ammonia is not distinguishable from some aliphatic amines by the odor. It may be detected by the yellow to orange color produced with Nessler's reagent or by the formation of hexamethylenetetramine-tetraiodide (page 1077).

1. Nessler Test for Ammonia. *Reagent.* For the method of preparation consult Hawk, Oser and Summerson (28).

Procedure. A drop of reagent, placed on a piece of filter paper, is suspended above the alkaline sample for several minutes. A deep yellow to orange stain is indicative of ammonia. Volatile aliphatic amines may react, with the formation of a white precipitate, but if any coloration is produced it is no more than a pale yellow.

Sodium Hydroxide. Indications of the presence of strong alkali, with ammonia absent, should initiate an examination for large amounts of sodium. Commercial sodium hydroxide contains significant amounts of carbonate and is a mixture of the hydroxide and carbonate. The persistent flame spectra and the intense sodium lines in the spectrographic examination are usually sufficient to establish the presence of the metal. If a quantitative determination is required, the sodium may be determined with zinc uranyl acetate after fusing about 0.5 gm. of ashed sample in a platinum crucible with a mixture of one part ammonium chloride and 8 parts calcium carbonate (29). By this process, the alkali metals and some calcium are converted into their water soluble chlorides while the remaining metals form the water insoluble oxide or carbonate. After leaching with water, the calcium is removed by precipitation with ammonium carbonate and the sodium determined on an aliquot of the solution (30). If the nature of the ingested sample is important, the ratio of carbonate to free alkali is determined by titration (page 1031).

Potassium Hydroxide. Potassium hydroxide is not likely to be encountered in deaths but potassium salts are quite common and significant concentrations in

---

* The test is not sensitive enough to detect traces of tartrate and the conditions must be carefully controlled. On adding hydrogen peroxide to the control, the solution turns light yellow, due to the oxidation of ferrous to ferric ion, while, if sufficient tartrate is present in the test sample, the yellow which first forms disappears, leaving a colorless solution. If the tartrate content is not high enough to discharge the yellow coloration, ferric hydroxide separates as a dark black to brown precipitate. In the absence of tartrate, the ferric hydroxide precipitate has a yellow brown color. If the hydrogen peroxide had aged so that there was not enough oxidant to convert ferrous to ferric ion, greenish ferrous hydroxide is precipitated on the addition of the alkali.

the stomach contents indicate that a substance other than food was ingested. Although potassium is present in food preparations, the normal potassium intake is small in comparison with sodium. A normal potassium concentration in the stomach will not be detectable by flame spectra in the presence of the normal sodium, and the potassium lines of the spectrogram will be only slightly more intense than those from tissue. The easiest procedure for distinguishing between normal and significant potassium concentrations in the stomach contents is by precipitation as the perchlorate from the filtrate obtained for the determination of sodium by the J. Lawrence Smith method for the fusion of the ash.

Procedure (31). The method depends on the insolubility of potassium perchlorate and the solubility of sodium and other perchlorates in ethyl alcohol. An aliquot of the neutral filtrate is treated with one-quarter the volume of perchloric acid and evaporated on a hot plate until all the hydrochloric acid is expelled and the heavy white fumes of perchloric acid are given off. About 20 ml. of 95 per cent ethyl alcohol are added to the solution after it has cooled and the crystals are separated by filtration through a washed sintered glass filter, using alcohol to make the transfer and to wash the crystals. The crucible is dried at 130° C. and weighed. The weight of potassium perchlorate multiplied by 0.283 equals the weight of potassium.

Detection of Alkali Hydroxide or Alkali Bicarbonate in the Presence of Alkali Carbonate. With alkaline stomach contents when a significant carbonate content is found (page 1018), it may be necessary to differentiate between bicarbonate taken as a home remedy or acid antidote and corrosive carbonate with or without hydroxide.

When a solution of alkali hydroxide is titrated with N/10 hydrochloric acid, the reaction is practically complete at pH 11, while in the titration of sodium carbonate the carbonate is changed into bicarbonate at pH 10. If the titration is carried to pH 4, bicarbonate is completely changed to chloride. Phenolphthalein shows a color change after all hydroxide has been neutralized and after carbonate has been converted into bicarbonate while methyl orange shows an acid reaction after conversion of bicarbonate to chloride. Since bicarbonate cannot exist in the presence of free alkali, alkaline solutions will contain only the carbonate and bicarbonate ions or carbonate and hydroxide ions and the ratio of the titration values with phenolphthalein and methyl orange determines the nature of the alkaline solution and the ionic concentration.

Procedure (32). A one to 5 ml. portion of stomach filtrate is diluted to 10 ml., chilled in the icebox and 2 drops of phenolphthalein indicator added. The solution is slowly titrated with N/10 hydrochloric acid to the rose color indicative of the change at the pK value for phenolphthalein. A second portion is then titrated with N/10 hydrochloric acid until methyl orange shows a change from yellow to pink. With a solution containing only sodium carbonate, the methyl orange titration will be just twice that for the phenolphthalein titration. If the acid used in the methyl orange titration is over twice that used in the phenolphthalein titration the solution is a mixture of carbonate and bicarbonate. If the acid used in the phenolphthalein titration is over one-half as large as that used in the methyl orange titration, the solution contains carbonate and hydroxide.

Alkali Cyanide. Cyanides of sodium and potassium, being salts of a strong base and a very weak acid, are quite alkaline and, if ingested in moderate amounts, will produce alkaline corrosion. In corrosive amounts the cyanide will probably be present in high enough concentrations to be recognized from the odor, and a strong copper-benzidine reaction will be obtained by suspending a filter paper impregnated with the reagent over the stomach contents (page 964).

Sodium Silicate. Aqueous sodium silicate is an alkaline solution known as water glass, and is used as a preservative. Accidental poisoning has been reported (33). When the solution is made acid, insoluble silicic acid precipitates. The normal silica content in the ash of stomach contents is of the same order as that in tissue and larger amounts are readily detected from the increased intensity of the silica lines in the lower wavelength region of the spectrum. Silicate may be determined quantitatively as the silicomolybdate (34).

OXIDANTS

Permanganates. Ingested permanganate may be completely reduced to manganese dioxide by the organic matter and tissue of the stomach. The black particles of dioxide are readily seen clinging to the stomach walls and dispersed in the solution. The reaction of the dry solid with diphenylamine reagent is delayed but an aqueous suspension gives an immediate reaction. The manganese will be detected in the spectrum (page 1008) or it can be converted to permanganate after ashing a portion of the stomach contents by the periodate oxidation (35) (page 1009).

Chromates. Like permanganates, chromates may be reduced in the stomach but not as completely. There is usually free chromate ion remaining, particularly when a neutral salt was taken. Chromates may be confirmed in the acidified filtrate with diphenylcarbazide, as described in the last part of the procedure for the quantitative determination of chromium in tissue (page 1007).

Differentiation Between Chlorates and Hypochlorites. Although chlorates have been used in suicidal deaths, hypochlorites, which are present in household bleaching solutions, are far more likely to be encountered. Both are immediately reduced to chloride by nitrous acid. They may be detected in the presence of chloride by the addition of an excess of silver nitrate to a nitric acid solution (page 1021) and the removal of the insoluble silver chloride by filtration. On the addition of a few drops of sodium nitrite to the nitric acid solution, chloride from the reduction of the oxidizing ions is precipitated (page 1022). Hypochlorites are converted into chloride and chlorate by boiling with sodium bicarbonate. Hypochlorite, in solutions made acid with acetic acid, is reduced to chloride by the addition of normal sodium arsenite solution. In the presence of silver ion, the chloride from the reduction is precipitated and, if removed by filtration, the addition of sodium nitrite reduces chlorate, so that preferential chloride precipitation can be used to detect the three ions in the presence of each other.

Hypochlorites in neutral or alkaline solution liberate iodine from potassium iodide, while chlorates do not react unless the solution is acid. Weakly acid solutions oxidize a solution containing 2 per cent benzidine in 10 per cent acetic acid to benzidine blue (36). Other oxidants such as hypobromite, persulfate, ferricyanide, chromate, permanganate and metal peroxides like PbO_2 also give a blue color with the reagent, but alkali peroxides, 3 per cent hydrogen peroxide, perborates, chlorates, bromates, iodates, nitrates and perchlorates do not react in the weakly acid solution.

Peroxides. Alkali peroxide is not likely to be encountered as a poison but hydrogen peroxide is a common household antiseptic and hair bleach. Hydrogen peroxide decomposes on standing, particularly at elevated temperatures. Peroxide may be detected by the reaction with titanium trichloride. A small volume of stomach filtrate is overlayed with an equal volume of ethyl ether and, unless already acidic, made acid to litmus by the dropwise addition of dilute sulfuric acid. One drop of 15 per cent titanium trichloride is added and the mixture shaken. A yellow to deep orange coloration in the aqueous layer, due to the formation of $H_2I_2O_4$ is indicative of peroxides.

REDUCERS

Reducers. Inorganic ions that have reducing properties will have been detected by one of the tests already described. If the test for reducing substances (page 1021) is strongly positive and the inorganic reducers were not found, the reaction is due most likely to an organic substance and the analytic process should be directed toward extraction with organic solvents by one of the processes described in Chapter 47.

INORGANIC SALTS

Differentiation Between Ferro- and Ferricyanide. A blue color with ferric and/or ferrous ion (page 1019) may not be conclusive in distinguishing between ferro- and ferricyanide because of the possible interferences and both may be present. Ferricyanide may be confirmed by the formation of the brown silver salt (page 1021). Ferrocyanide can be separated from ferricyanide by precipitation as lead ferrocyanide by the addition of lead acetate to a dilute nitric acid solution of the ions. White silver ferrocyanide can be distinguished from the other colorless insoluble silver salts by conversion to brown silver ferricyanide on the addition of a drop of concentrated nitric acid to the solid.

Prussian blue is used as a pigment and has been found, along with metals, in cases of small children who died after eating paint or window putty. Insoluble ferro- and ferricyanides are converted into the soluble sodium salts on boiling with caustic alkali solution from which the insoluble metal hydroxide is separated by filtration and the ions detected after acidification of the solution. All complex soluble and insoluble cyanides are converted into mercuric cyanide when boiled with a suspension of yellow mercuric oxide. Tests for cyanide can then be made on the solution after filtering off the insoluble metal oxides and hydroxides.

Arsenate and Arsenite. When arsenic is found in the examination for the metals and the question of suicide or accidental poisoning arises, it may be important to establish the nature of the arsenic compound. Trivalent arsenic is more commonly used. The trioxide is a common constituent of rodenticides. The use of relatively large doses to build up a high arsenic level in the treatment of luetics has been largely replaced by the use of the antibiotics (page 986). Both trivalent and pentavalent arsenic are present in the organic arsenic compounds used in the treatment of spirochetal and protozoal diseases and small amounts of arsenate and arsenite are used in medicinal preparations. Arsenate is used extensively in spray material as the lead or calcium salt. Copper biarsenite, known as Scheele's green, was formerly used as a pigment, and copper acetoarsenite (Schweinfürter or Paris green) is an insecticide used principally on potato and tobacco plants.

The following tests may be used to differentiate between arsenate and arsenite:

1. Formation of Arsine. Although arsenate and arsenite are reduced to arsine in acid solution, only arsenite is reduced by aluminum turnings in 10 per cent sodium hydroxide solution. If the stomach filtrate is treated by the Gutzeit procedure

(page 988), replacing the zinc-hydrochloric acid solution with alkali and aluminum, a yellow coloration on the silver impregnated paper disk indicates that arsenite is present.

2. Precipitation of Arsenate as Magnesium Ammonium Arsenate. Arsenate and phosphate are precipitated in weakly ammoniacal solution with magnesium ion. The solution, if basic, is first neutralized with nitric acid. Ammonia is added dropwise until the mixture turns red litmus paper blue.* Any precipitate is filtered off and one-half the volume of normal magnesium nitrate solution added. The mixture is allowed to stand for at least 10 minutes. Crystals of $MgNH_4AsO_4$ form slowly and crystallization is sometimes aided by scratching the sides of the tube with a stirring rod. The solution is filtered and the precipitate washed with normal ammonium hydroxide.†

3. Confirmatory Test for Arsenate. The precipitate on the filter paper is treated with a small volume of normal silver nitrate solution made faintly acid with acetic acid. A brownish red color, due to the formation of silver arsenate, occurs if the precipitate is magnesium ammonium arsenate.‡

4. Action of Arsenate on Iodide. In strong acid solution, arsenate oxidizes iodide to iodine. If the precipitate from 2 is dissolved in a small amount of 6 N hydrochloric acid and a small volume of normal potassium iodide containing 1 per cent starch is introduced, the blue color of the iodine-starch absorption complex forms if arsenate is present.

Alum. Alum is a hydrated double sulfate with the structural formula Al_2-$(SO_4)_3 \cdot M_2SO_4 \cdot 24H_2O$ where M is usually potassium or ammonia although other metal salts are known. Sodium alum is very water-soluble and difficult to prepare. The term alum normally implies the potassium salt. It is an acid type salt used as an astringent and styptic. It is used extensively as a chemical in industry and is the acidic component in some baking powders. Alum is not a poison, having been used as an emetic and an antidote in acute lead poisoning. It has been taken by mistake, producing toxic symptoms as a result of the gastrointestinal irritation from the acid solution. The salt will probably not be encountered except in stomach washings from a living patient. Aluminum absorbed through the intestinal walls is indicated by the elevated intensity of the normal aluminum lines in the spectra of the blood ash. Sodium bicarbonate, used as a gastric lavage, precipitates aluminum as the hydroxide.

Magnesium Sulfate. Magnesium sulfate is marketed as Epsom salts for use as a purgative. Absorption occurs with repeated doses and may cause symptoms of poisoning. Absorption is greater with ingestion of the dry salt than with a dilute aqueous solution. Magnesium has a high spectral sensitivity and the normal magnesium content of food or biologic material makes the strong magnesium lines in a spectrogram of an ash about as intense as the silver in the plate emulsion will permit. Elevated magnesium in the stomach contents or tissue may be easily overlooked by spectrographic analysis unless recognized from the very weak lines that do not appear normally. Qualitative tests for magnesium are futile since it is always present in detectable amounts. It may be determined quantitatively by precipitation

---

* If the concentration of ammonia is too high, $Mg(AsO_3)_2$ will precipitate when large amounts are present.

† Arsenite forms an immediate precipitate when hydrogen sulfide is passed into the filtrate, after it is made acid to litmus paper with hydrochloric acid.

‡ Silver phosphate and silver arsenite, if present, would react but would give a yellow color readily distinguishable from the dark colored arsenate.

from ammoniacal solution with 8-hydroxyquinoline after removal of the interfering metals by precipitation of the sulfides from a solution made basic with ammonia. Metals of the alkaline earth and alkali groups do not interfere.

Reagent. 1 gm. of 8-hydroxyquinoline is dissolved in 3 ml. of glacial acetic acid and 5 ml. of water, then diluted to 50 ml.

Procedure (37). The sample to be analyzed is ashed carbon-free in a muffle furnace, the ash dissolved in a small volume of nitric acid and diluted to 50 ml. Ammonia is then added to a 25 ml. aliquot until a pronounced ammoniacal odor persists. Hydrogen sulfide is passed through the solution until all precipitation has ceased and the solution is saturated with sulfide. The precipitate is allowed to flocculate and the solution filtered, using 1 per cent ammonia as a wash solution. The filtrate is acidified with hydrochloric acid, boiled to remove hydrogen sulfide, diluted to 50 ml. with water and 2 ml. of concentrated ammonium hydroxide added. The reagent of 8-hydroxyquinoline is introduced dropwise, with stirring, until the solution retains a permanent yellow color. The solution is digested at low heat on a hot plate without boiling, until the precipitate coagulates. It should maintain a decided ammoniacal odor during the digestion; if necessary, add ammonia in small portions during the heating process. When the precipitate has coagulated, the solution should have a yellow color about as intense as that of the reagent. If considerably less, add more reagent and continue the digestion. Remove from the hot plate, cool, filter through a weighed sintered glass crucible and wash the precipitate with 1 per cent ammonia.* Weight of precipitate multiplied by 0.116 equals magnesium, as magnesium oxide.†

BORATES, PHOSPHORUS AND FLUORIDES

Unlike other inorganic nonmetallic poisons, borates, phosphorus and fluorides are detectable in the organs and body fluids. They are distinctive because their presence is not readily indicated in the course of a general screening procedure and special tests must be performed for each one. In sufficiently high concentration, phosphorus may have been indicated by the phosphorescence during the distillation for the volatiles (page 1048). Boron is only moderately sensitive spectrographically and has very few strong lines. Borate is suspected when the line pair at 2496.8 Å and 2497.7 Å are found in the ash. Irritation from the alkali in high concentrations of fluorides may be found at autopsy.

Borates. Boric acid is used as an antiseptic lotion in eye, nasal, oral and aural washes and as a dusting powder in abrasions of the skin. Boric acid and borax have been used as food preservatives and borax is a common household cleaner. Boric acid is somewhat volatile with steam and may be present in the distillate prepared for the analysis of the volatiles (page 1046). Borates are best detected in the residue from a sample ashed at low heat. Boric acid is not lost on ashing the dried sample as it is converted into boron trioxide at elevated temperatures. The oxide, however, is difficult to leach out and the ashing process is best carried out after making the sample alkaline with sodium hydroxide or, preferably, with a mixture of sodium carbonate and sodium nitrate.

---

* Magnesium 8-hydroxyquinoline has a tendency to adhere to the sides of the beaker. The addition of a small amount of sodium taurocholate to the hot solution just before filtering greatly reduces this tendency.

† More accurate results are obtained in this method with a relatively small magnesium concentration. Values are invariably low when the magnesium ion exceeds 20 mg./50 ml. of solution.

1. Formation of Boric Acid Methyl Ester. A sample of the ash contained in a porcelain crucible is moistened with a small volume of 10 per cent sodium hydroxide and evaporated to dryness. About 2 ml. of absolute methyl alcohol and 0.5 ml. of concentrated sulfuric acid * are introduced and the supernatant alcohol is ignited by flaming with a burner. If the alcohol burns with a green flame, borate is present.

2. Detection in the Ash—Reaction of Boric Acid with Turmeric.† A portion of the ash is digested with water made decidedly acid with hydrochloric acid and filtered. The acid filtrate is evaporated to dryness ‡ in a porcelain crucible and dissolved in a small amount of dilute acetic acid. Three to 5 drops of a saturated solution of turmeric powder in 95 per cent ethyl alcohol are added and the solution is re-evaporated to dryness. The residue is stained reddish brown and, on moistening with alkali, the color becomes bluish black if as little as 2 μg of boric acid are present §.

3. Detection in the Stomach Diffusate. Borate isolated as a solid can be detected by the green color of the flame spectra. A small particle is placed in the loop of a platinum wire, moistened with a drop of hydrofluoric acid and heated in the edge of the bunsen flame (page 1022). The volatile boron fluoride formed burns with a green flame.||

Boric acid in the stomach contents may be distinguished from borax by its solubility in ethyl alcohol.

Phosphorus. Phosphorus differs from other poisons in that the tests for its detection are made directly on the tissue, body fluid or stomach contents without preliminary treatment of the sample material. Only the white form of the element is toxic. White phosphorus melts at 44.1° C. and boils at 287° C. It is practically insoluble in water but dissolves in organic solvents such as benzene and turpentine and is quite soluble in carbon bisulfide. It oxidizes spontaneously in air at room temperature to the pentoxide, giving off a greenish glow or phosphorescence. At slightly elevated temperatures it ignites spontaneously on exposure to dry air. In the absence of oxygen, under the influence of light or slightly elevated temperature, it slowly changes into the more stable red form which is nontoxic and odorless and does not ignite in air until heated to about 240° C. It is used in matches and in rat poisons, the most common being J O Paste. In suicides, it is often recognized at autopsy from the odor and, in the laboratory, from the phosphorescence in the condenser during the steam distillation for the volatiles (page 1048).

1. Silver Nitrate Flange Test. Phosphorus vapor reacts with some heavy metal salts to form the metal phosphide. At the same time, some of the metal ion is reduced to the metal. The reaction with silver nitrate is particularly sensitive and is the basis for its detection. The mechanism for the test, first described by Scheuer (38), is thought to involve the reaction of phosphorus with water ¶ as the first step (39).

$$P_4 + 6\,H_2O \rightarrow 3\,H_3PO_2 + PH_3$$

* The test may be carried out directly on the sulfuric acid solution from the wet tissue digest. Boric acid may be lost entirely during the evaporation, however.

† Fluoride interferes, due to the formation of fluoboric acid.

‡ Any oxidizers that would affect the color of the turmeric are removed.

§ Molybdic, titanic and zirconic acids also react with turmeric to form a red brown color.

|| Barium and copper interfere.

¶ This mechanism is not in line with the observation that dry silver nitrate paper gives a darker spot for the same phosphorus content. On the basis of the reaction given, moist paper should be more sensitive.

Both phosphine and hypophosphorus acid then react with the silver nitrate, producing brown to black silver phosphide and silver.

$$H_3PO_2 + 2 H_2O + 4 AgNO_3 \rightarrow 4 HNO_3 + H_3PO_4 + 4 Ag$$
$$\text{and } PH_3 + 3 AgNO_3 \rightarrow 3 HNO_3 + Ag_3P$$

The apparatus shown in Figure 44-1 consists of a bubble counter (A) to control the flow of nitrogen used to aerate the sample, a 100 ml. potato tube (B) containing the sample and suspended in a boiling water bath (C), a calcium chloride drying tube (D) packed with glass wool impregnated with lead acetate, and a flange (E) to hold the filter paper disk impregnated with silver nitrate. The

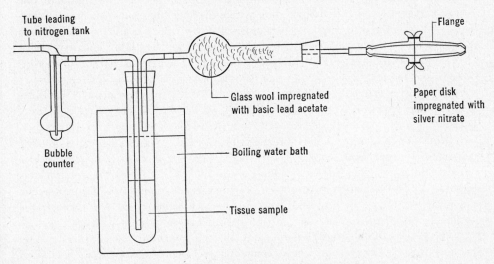

Fig. 44-1. Assembly for the Determination of Phosphorus.

flange has a 1 cm. internal diameter and accommodates a paper disk 1 inch in diameter.

Preparation of the Silver Nitrate Reagent Paper. A sheet of Whatman #2 filter paper is steeped in a methyl alcohol solution saturated with silver nitrate. The paper is allowed to dry while suspended in air. About 1 inch is cut from the outer edge and discarded.* Paper disks are prepared from the central portion by cutting on a rubber mat with a 1 inch cork borer.

Procedure (40). An equal quantity of water is added to 10 to 20 gm. of finely ground tissue, urine or stomach contents, the sample made distinctly acid with dilute sulfuric acid and placed in the potato tube. The silver nitrate impregnated paper is fitted between the faces of the flange and held secure by means of rubber bands wound around the glass connecting hooks. The apparatus is assembled as shown in Figure 44-1, and the nitrogen pressure is adjusted to pass about one bubble per second through the counter. The water bath is heated to boiling with a Meker burner and heating is continued for about 30 minutes while maintaining a steady flow of nitrogen through the system. The paper disk is stained brown to black, depending on the phosphorus content. Excess silver nitrate is removed by washing in water.† The paper is dried and viewed by transmitted light (Fig. 43-5,

---

* The reagent concentrates unevenly in the outer portion of the paper.
† The paper will darken on exposure to light unless the silver ion is removed.

page 989). Compounds other than phosphorus stain silver nitrate paper. Arsine, stibine, volatile aldehydes, particularly formaldehyde, formic acid and reactive ketones reduce silver nitrate. Hydrogen sulfide is removed by the glass wool impregnated with lead acetate but some organic sulfur-containing compounds interfere.

Although there is an invariable darkening of the silver nitrate under conditions of even moderate putrefaction, there is little change of interference with fresh tissue. Arsenic from urine was found to give a positive test (41) but it is readily detected in the examination for the metals. Confirmation is made by converting the phosphide in the paper to phosphate.

2. Confirmatory Test for Phosphorus. The dry disk is cut in half and one section is placed on a microscope slide. About 20 mg. of solid bleaching powder are spread over the darkened area and pressed down with a spatula to form a thin layer of solid covering the spot.* The slide is placed in a humidity chamber (page 1258) and allowed to remain 5 to 10 minutes during which the darkened area, as viewed from the under side of the slide, should be completely decolorized.

The excess calcium hypochlorite is washed from the paper disk by carefully adding water dropwise with the slide held at an inclined angle.† Water droplets surrounding the paper disk are removed from the slide by blotting with filter paper. Two drops of ammonium molybdate reagent (page 1027) are added after making the reagent 2 normal with respect to nitric acid. The slide is allowed to stand several minutes and is then placed on a heating block at 100° C. until the solution has evaporated from the paper. A drop of 0.05 per cent benzidine in 10 per cent acetic acid is added and the disk is held over concentrated ammonium hydroxide. If the blackening of the silver was due to phosphorus, an intense blue color develops from the action of the phosphomolybdate on the benzidine. Since silicates and arsenates are the only other complex molybdates giving the reaction, arsenic is the only possible interference.‡

Fluorides. Fluorides are more likely to be missed in a routine toxicologic analysis than any other inorganic poison. Soluble fluorides and fluorosilicates are very toxic for all living organisms, yet fluoride is a normal component of human tissue and body fluids. Large amounts of insoluble fluorides are present in rock and clay formations and all soil contains a small amount of soluble fluoride. It is present in food in amounts varying between 0.059 and 13.87 mg. per 100 gm. of dried sample (43). Water may contain significant amounts. In Arizona, as much as 7.15 mg. of fluorine per liter was found and the high incidence of mottled enamel of the teeth in certain western areas has been reported to be due to the elevated fluorine intake (44). There is evidence that an optimum fluorine intake is beneficial

---

* Many oxidants convert the phosphide to phosphate. Calcium hypochlorite was found to be preferable because, in employing the solid and allowing it to wet by deliquescence, a relatively low acidity is maintained and the oxidized phosphate is fixed in the paper because it is precipitated as insoluble calcium phosphate. In this manner the phosphate ion does not become soluble during the conversion process and spread throughout the paper by diffusion in the solution. The final blue color is made more intense, since it is confined to the area of the paper exposed to the phosphorus vapors.

† If the excess calcium hypochlorite is not removed, a transient blue color will form with the benzidrine. For this reason, Schwartz and Posnick (page 1037) prefer reduction to molybdenum blue with 0.25 per cent 1-amino-4-naphthol sulfonic acid in a mixture of 20 per cent sodium sulfite and 15 per cent sodium bisulfite solutions.

‡ According to Feigl (42), arsenate interference is eliminated in the molybdate-benzidine reaction by the addition of 15 gm. of tartaric acid to 100 ml. of the ammonium molybdate-nitric acid reagent.

in preventing dental caries (45, 46). The normal daily excretion by man has been estimated at 0.3 to 0.5 mg. per day (47). The fluorine present in the body is probably deposited as the calcium salt. The fluorine content of teeth and bone is between 0.01 and 0.03 per cent, while the organs do not normally contain more than 80 μg per 100 gm. of dried tissue.

Fluorides and fluorosilicates are easily obtained. They are used in wood and other preservatives and in insecticides. Fluoride is the most common component of roach powders. Almost all commercial preparations for this purpose are now colored with a dye, but many accidental deaths have occurred through use of the roach powder in place of ingredients common to the household. Death occurs after ingestion of a lethal dose in from 45 minutes to 24 hours. Characteristic symptoms include severe vomiting and intense burning pain over the whole abdomen. When death occurs within a few hours, large amounts of fluorides will be found in the stomach despite the severe vomiting. When death is delayed, the fluoride may be entirely absorbed from the stomach. The organs never reach a high fluoride content. In acute poisoning and in experimental poisoning in dogs, the fluoride was between 0.14 and 1.6 mg. per 100 gm. of tissue for both fluoride and fluorosilicate. In experimental chronic poisonings of dogs in which death occurred after two weeks, the fluorine content was between 20 and 50 μg per 100 gm. of dried tissue, indicating that there is little tendency for the accumulation of fluorine in the internal organs (48). Since fluorine is rapidly excreted by way of the kidneys, urine is the first choice as sample material for the detection of absorbed fluoride. There is little preference between kidney, liver, lung and spleen as sample material. Blood values are more variable than the organs and depend on the period of absorption.

1. Detection of Fluorides. Large amounts of fluorides in the stomach are indicated by the gelatinous precipitate with barium and calcium ions (page 1020). The precipitate is almost impossible to filter because of its slimy consistency. The precipitation should be repeated, adding potassium sulfate to the solution. The barium sulfate which is formed simultaneously with the calcium fluoride makes the precipitate filterable (49). After washing, it may be confirmed as fluoride by the formation of sodium fluorosilicate crystals.

(a) Qualitative Detection of Fluoride by the Formation of Sodium Fluorosilicate. This test depends on the conversion of fluoride into volatile silicon tetrafluoride by reaction with silica in sulfuric acid solution.

$$2 \, CaF_2 + 2 \, H_2SO_4 + SiO_2 \rightarrow 2 \, CaSO_4 + SiF_4 \uparrow + 2 \, H_2O$$

The silicon tetrafluoride is collected in a drop of water and reacts to form silicic acid and hydrofluorosilicic acid.

$$3 \, SiF_4 + 4 \, H_2O \rightarrow 2 \, H_2SiF_6 + H_4SiO_4$$

On addition of sodium chloride to the solution, typical crystals of sodium fluorosilicate are deposited.

This test is subject to the variations characteristic of all tests depending on crystal habit. With the proper concentration of fluoride ion for the reagents used, the crystalline form is typical and reproducible. When the fluoride is too low, crystal growth is not normal and typical crystals, if formed, may be occluded by sodium chloride crystallization. If the fluoride content is too high, precipitation without the characteristic crystalline form can occur. However, in this case the cloudiness (due to the precipitation of the larger amount of silicic acid) is suspicious for silicon tetrafluoride and indicates that the test should be repeated on a smaller sample. In the presence of large amounts of chlorides, hydrochloric acid may be volatilized during the heating with sulfuric acid and influence the crystalline form. Good crystalline formation is obtained with 50 μg of fluorine, although 10 μg can be detected. In acute poisonings, the fluoride is between 0.14 and 1.6 mg. per 100 gm. of tissue, so that 10 gm. of tissue sample furnishes about the proper fluoride content for the test in these cases. Five to 10 ml. of urine are usually adequate and, in some cases, fluoride can be detected in as little as 2 drops. Twenty gram samples of normal tissue or body fluid always give negative results in this test so that positive findings on 10 gm. or less are indicative of abnormal amounts of fluoride.

Preparation of the Sample. Twenty grams of finely ground tissue are mixed in a silica dish with 0.4 gm. of sodium carbonate plus 0.2 gm. of powdered silicic acid,* and enough water is added to make a thick slurry. The mixture is evaporated to dryness on the steam bath and ashed carbon-free at about 450° C. in the muffle furnace. The dish is then heated in the free flame of a bunsen burner until a fusion melt is obtained, cooled and leached by boiling with about 80 ml. of water. The insoluble portion is removed by filtration and washed with 20 ml. of boiling water added in small portions. The filtrate is evaporated to dryness on a hot plate and the residue is divided into equal portions to make the equivalent of 10 gm. of original sample.

Procedure (48). The residue is mixed with an equal bulk of powdered glass † and transferred to a micro test tube about 2½ inches high with a 1 cm. internal diameter. The mixture is moistened with a few drops of concentrated sulfuric acid and quickly covered with a cover slip with a drop of water suspended from the under surface as a hanging drop. The tube is placed in a heating block maintained at a temperature of approximately 150° C. After three to five minutes, the cover slip is removed and a small crystal of sodium chloride is pushed into the edge of the drop with a capillary stirring rod. When the cover slip is observed under the microscope, using the high-dry magnification, the presence of six-pointed stars or hexagonal crystals showing pink pleochroism is indicative of sodium fluorosilicate.

(b) Isolation of Fluoride by Distillation. When the findings with the sodium fluorosilicate method are questionable and in cases where it is known that death was delayed more than 24 hours after the onset of symptoms, fluoride is more easily determined after separation from the extraneous ions in the ash by perchloric acid distillation. The sensitivity is increased by volatilizing the fluorine as SiF_4, collecting it in water and determining the silicate by the silicomolybdate benzidine reaction (page 1041). Phosphates, sulfates and chlorides are not distilled with the fluoride and a portion of the distillate may be used for quantitative analysis. When the sodium fluorosilicate test is inconclusive and the hanging drop is not cloudy, a larger sample should be analyzed.

Procedure. About 50 gm. of tissue are ashed by the same procedure described under the sodium fluorosilicate test (page 1039), increasing the quantities of sodium

---

* Silicic acid is prepared by the addition of dilute hydrochloric acid to a sodium silicate solution. The precipitate is then filtered and air dried.

In the presence of silica, any calcium fluoride is converted into calcium fluorosilicate which, unlike calcium fluoride, is readily converted into sodium fluoride by the sodium carbonate during the fusion.

† Different forms of silica are attacked differently by H_2F_2. Freshly precipitated and ignited SiO_2 reacts immediately with evolution of heat while the rate of reaction with quartz is relatively slow. Powdered glass is attacked almost as readily as precipitated SiO_2.

carbonate and silicic acid in proportion to the increase in tissue sample. Instead of leaching the ash with water, it is dissolved in 10 ml. of 60 per cent perchloric acid and transferred to a 150 ml. distilling flask with about 20 ml. of water. Twenty milliliters of 60 per cent perchloric acid, enough water to make the total volume about 80 ml.* and several small glass beads are introduced. Ten per cent potassium carbonate is added dropwise until a small crystalline precipitate of $KClO_3$ forms † and about 0.1 gm. of silver sulfate is mixed into the solution.‡

The distilling flask is fitted with a two-hole rubber stopper containing a 150° C. thermometer and a dropping funnel, with the lower end of the stem pulled into a capillary of about 1 mm. bore, which extends to within a few millimeters of the bottom of the distilling flask. The flask, fitted with a water cooled condenser, is mounted on an asbestos mat over an opening of about 1 inch cut from the center and the unit is clamped with the neck of the distilling flask inclined at an angle of about 50° with the horizontal.§ The condenser is fitted with an adaptor which extends into 2 ml. of 10 per cent sodium hydroxide solution in a 500 ml. receiving flask. The flask is heated with a low flame from a bunsen burner and the distillation is carried out until the boiling point rises to 140° C. It is then maintained at 135 to 140° C. by the gradual introduction of water from the dropping funnel while 250 ml. of distillate is collected. The distillate, which should still be alkaline, is evaporated on a hot plate to a volume of about 5 ml., quantitatively transferred to a 10 ml. volumetric flask and diluted to the mark. For qualitative analysis by the molybdate method, 5 ml. may be withdrawn, evaporated to near dryness, transferred to a microtest tube with $\frac{3}{8}$ inch bore and $2\frac{1}{2}$ inch length and evaporated to dryness. The remaining 5 ml. may be used for quantitative analysis.

(c) Silicomolybdate-Benzidine Test for Detection of Fluoride. The residue in the microtest tube is mixed with an equal bulk of powdered glass and moistened with a few drops of concentrated sulfuric acid. The mouth of the test tube is quickly capped with a moist paper disk cut with a ½ inch cork borer and a microscope slide is placed over the paper.‖ The test tube is then heated in a heating block, maintained at a temperature of 150° C., for 5 minutes. The slide with the damp paper disk adhering to it is then removed, a drop of 6 normal ammonium hydroxide added ¶ and the slide is heated on a heating block at 100° C. until the paper disk has about half dried.

Two drops of ammonium molybdate reagent which has been made 2 normal with respect to nitric acid (page 1027, procedure for phosphate) are added to the paper. The slide is placed on a heating block maintained at 100° C. and allowed to heat until the solution has just evaporated from the paper.** A drop of 0.1 per cent

---

* At this dilution the solution should boil at about 110° C.

† $KClO_3$ crystals serve as nuclei for the formation of bubbles of steam and prevent bumping.

‡ This prevents the distillation of chloride as HCl.

§ In case of bumping, liquid is not thrown up the neck of the flask and into the condenser.

‖ The sensitivity may be increased by using a ½ inch paper disk with an outer paraffin ring to prevent diffusion of the solution and to maintain the reactants in the central portion. The disk is prepared by clamping it in a C-clamp between two $\frac{5}{16}$ inch rods faced on a lathe and cut to a length to fit the clamp. The end of the clamp containing the rods and paper disk is then dipped into a molten paraffin bath.

¶ Ammonia acts on the fluorosilicic acid to form fluoride and silicic acid.

** Elevated temperature favors the formation of the silicomolybdate complex. The block should be at 100° C. and the slide placed on it immediately so that the solution is evaporated by heating, not spontaneous evaporation during the time the block is reaching the maximum temperature.

benzidine in 10 per cent acetic acid is added and the paper disk held over concentrated ammonium hydroxide. A blue color is indicative of silicic acid volatilized as silicon tetrafluoride.

2. Quantitative Determination of Fluoride (48). The method depends on the fact that, in titrating fluoride ion with thorium in the presence of sodium alizarinsulfonate, the end point is indicated by the formation of a thorium alizarinsulfonate lake when all the fluoride has been precipitated as insoluble thorium fluoride. The titration, made on the concentrated distillate (page 1041), is in itself a qualitative test for fluoride, since all interfering ions have been removed by the distillation. The advantage of carrying out the qualitative test before the quantitative determination is that an estimate of the fluoride content is obtained and the appropriate strength thorium nitrate titrating solution can be selected.

Reagents. (a) 95 per cent ethyl alcohol.

(b) 50% ethyl alcohol.

(c) 0.05% aqueous sodium alizarinsulfonate.

(d) dilute (1:50) hydrochloric acid.

(e) sodium hydroxide-chloracetic acid buffer prepared by dissolving 1.0 gm. of sodium hydroxide and 4.72 gm. of chloracetic acid in 100 ml. of solution.

(f) stock 0.01 normal thorium nitrate.

(g) standard 0.001 normal thorium nitrate prepared by a 1:10 dilution of (f).

(h) blank reference standard prepared by adding 0.03 ml. of sodium alizarinsulfonate solution and 1 ml. of buffer to 20 ml. of 50 per cent ethyl alcohol and titrating with 0.001 normal thorium nitrate until a faint pink color appears. This determines the amount of thorium nitrate necessary to produce the end color with the indicator. This value is the blank to be subtracted from the titration for the distillate before calculating the fluoride content.

Procedure. To the distillate remaining from the silicomolybdate qualitative test (page 1041) or an aliquot, add 10 ml. of 95 per cent ethyl alcohol, 0.03 ml. of sodium alizarinsulfonate solution, dilute hydrochloric acid dropwise until the yellow acid color of the indicator appears and 1.0 ml. of buffer solution. The solution is then titrated with 0.01 or 0.001 normal thorium nitrate solution (depending on the amount of fluoride predicted from the qualitative test) from a microburet until a faint orange color develops. The titration is then continued, adding a microdrop per minute until the solution assumes a permanent pink color of the same intensity as the blank reference standard.

One milliliter of 0.001 normal thorium nitrate is equivalent to 19 μg of fluorine. The fluoride content of the tissue in milligrams per cent is:

$$\frac{(\text{ml. for the titration} - \text{ml. for the blank}) \times 0.019 \,* \times 10}{\text{grams of tissue distilled} \times \text{volume of aliquot}}$$

REFERENCES

1. Noyes, A. A. Qualitative Chemical Analysis, 9th ed., New York, The Macmillan Co., 1937, p. 136.
2. Hawk, P. B., Oser, B. L., and Summerson, W. H. Practical Physiological Chemistry, 12th ed., New York, The Blakiston Co., 1947, pp. 343-353.
3. Kolmer, J. A. Clinical Diagnosis by Laboratory Examinations, 2nd ed., New York, Appleton-Century-Crofts, Inc., 1949, p. 243.
4. Neidle, M. Temperature effect in dialysis and a simple dialyzer, J. Am. Chem. Soc., 38:1270, 1916.

* Obviously, the factor becomes 0.19 if 0.01 normal thorium nitrate is used.

5. Neidle, M., and Barab, J. Studies in dialysis. II. Hot dialysis of the chlorides of ferric iron, chromium and aluminum, and the rapid preparation of their colloidal hydrous oxides, J. Am. Chem. Soc., 39:71, 1917.

6. Zsigmondy, R., and Heyer, R. Purification of colloids by dialysis, Z. anorg. Chem., 68:169, 1910.

7. Thomas, A. H. Colloid Chemistry, 1st ed., New York, McGraw-Hill Co., Inc., 1934, p. 74.

8. Brown, W. The preparation of collodion membranes of differential permeability, Biochem. J., 9:591, 1915.

9. ——— Further contributions to the technic of preparing membranes for dialysis, Biochem. J., 11:40, 1917.

10. Noyes, A. A. Qualitative Chemical Analysis, 9th ed., New York, The Macmillan Co., 1937, p. 141.

11. Autenrieth, W. Laboratory Manual for the Detection of Poisons and Powerful Drugs, 6th American ed., translated by Warren, W. H., New York, The Blakiston Co., 1928, p. 406.

12. Noyes, A. A. Qualitative Chemical Analysis, 9th ed., New York, The Macmillan Co., 1937, p. 142.

13. ibid., p. 140.

14. Office of the Chief Medical Examiner of the City of New York.

15. Wieland, H., and Scheuing, G. Fuchsin-sulfurous acid and its color reaction with aldehydes, Ber. d. deut. chem. Ges., 54B:2527, 1921.

16. Feigl, F. Spot Tests, 2nd ed., translated by Matthews, J., New York, Elsevier-Nordeman Publishing Co., 1939, p. 163.

17. ibid., p. 166.

18. ibid., p. 162.

19. Partington, J. R. A Text-book of Inorganic Chemistry, 3rd ed., London, Macmillan & Co., Ltd., 1930, p. 569.

20. Treadwell, F. P., and Hall, W. T. Analytical Chemistry, Vol. I. Qualitative Analysis, 7th English ed., John Wiley and Sons, Inc., 1929, p. 352.

21. ibid.

22. Snell, F. D., and Snell, C. T. Colorimetric Methods of Analysis, Vol. I. Inorganic, 2nd ed., New York, D. Van Nostrand Co., Inc., 1936.

23. Fish, F. H., and Taylor, F. M. Effect of the presence of perchloric acid in the proximate analysis of limestone, J. Chem. Ed., 10:246, 1933.

24. Engelder, C. J., Dunkelberger, T. H., and Schiller, W. J. Semi-micro Qualitative Analysis, New York, John Wiley and Sons, Inc., 1936, p. 216.

25. Mulliken, S. P. A Method for the Identification of Pure Organic Compounds, Vol. I, 1st ed., New York, John Wiley and Sons, Inc., 1904, p. 83.

26. Feigl, F. Spot Tests, 2nd ed., translated by Matthews, J., New York, Elsevier-Nordeman Publishing Co., Inc., 1939, p. 340.

27. Mulliken, S. P. A Method for the Identification of Pure Organic Compounds, Vol. I, 1st ed., New York, John Wiley and Sons, Inc., 1904, p. 48.

28. Hawk, P. B., Oser, B. L., and Summerson, W. H. Practical Physiological Chemistry, 12th ed., New York, The Blakiston Co., 1947, p. 1229.

29. Low, A. H. Technical Methods of Ore Analysis, 10th ed., New York, John Wiley and Sons, Inc., 1927, J. Lawrence Smith method, p. 189.

30. Cumming, A. C., and Kay, S. A. Quantitative Chemical Analysis, 7th ed., revised by Guthrie, F. C., and Nance, J. T., New York, D. Van Nostrand Co., Inc., 1939, p. 335.

31. Scott, W. W. Chemical Methods for the Analysis of Metallurgical Products, 2nd ed., New York, D. Van Nostrand Co., Inc., 1927, p. 469.

32. Treadwell, F. P., and Hall, W. T. Analytical Chemistry, Vol. II. Quantitative Analysis, 8th ed., New York, John Wiley and Sons, Inc., 1935, p. 512.

33. Eichhorst, H. Ueber Vergiftung mit Wasserglas, Schweiz. med. Wchnschr., 1:1081, 1920.

34. Gettler, A. O., and Umberger, C. J. A colorimetric method for the determination of silica in human tissues, Am. J. Clin. Path., 15:1, 1945.

35. Official and Tentative Methods of Analysis of the Association of Official Agricultural Chemists, 3rd ed., Washington, D.C., Association of Official Agricultural Chemists (A.O.A.C.), 1930, p. 267.

36. Feigl, F. Spot Tests, 2nd ed., translated by Matthews, J., New York, Elsevier-Nordeman Publishing Co., 1939, p. 208.

37. Research Laboratory Staff. Organic Reagents for Metals, 3rd ed., London, Hopkins and Williams, 1938, p. 65.

38. Scheuer. Ann. Chem. Phys., 112:214, 1859.

39. Treadwell, F. P., and Hall, W. T. Analytical Chemistry, Vol I. Qualitative Analysis, 7th English ed., John Wiley and Sons, Inc., 1929, p. 408.

40. Schwartz, H., and Posnick, D. Laboratory of the Chief Medical Examiner of the City of New York, unpublished.

41. Hoffman, H. Laboratory of the Chief Medical Examiner of the City of New York.

42. Feigl, F. Spot Tests, 2nd ed., translated by Matthews, J., New York, Elsevier-Nordeman Publishing Co., Inc., 1939, p. 218.

43. Gautier, A. Sur le rôle du fluor chez les animaux, Compt. rend. Soc. de biol., 76:107, 1914.

44. Smith, M. C., Lantz, E. M., and Smith, H. V. The cause of mottled enamel, Science, 74:244, 1931.

45. Ast, D. B., Finn, S. B., and McCaffrey, I. Newburgh-Kingston caries fluorine study; dental findings after 3 years of water fluoridation, Am. J. Pub. Health, 40:716, 1950.

46. ——— Finn, S. B., and Chase, H. C. Newburgh-Kingston caries fluorine study; further analysis of dental findings including permanent and deciduous dentitions after 4 years of water fluoridation, Am. Dent. A., 42:188, 1951.

47. Gautier, A., and Clausmann, P. Fluorine in animal organisms, Compt. rend., 157:94, 1913.

48. Gettler, A. O., and Ellerbrook, L. Toxicology of fluorides, Am. J. M. Sc., 197:625, 1939.

49. Woodman, A. G., and Talbot, H. P. The etching test for small amounts of fluorides, J. Am. Chem. Soc., 28:1437, 1906.

45

Inorganic and Organic Poisons Volatile with Steam

Poisonous substances classified as volatiles are those compounds which volatilize with steam from a weakly acid solution. Isolation from tissue and body fluids is accomplished by a steam distillation of the biologic material and the collection of the distillate in a weakly basic solution. The distillate is tested directly for the few reactive members of this group, using reactions that are sensitive for small amounts of the compounds in the aqueous solution. The distillate may then be concentrated by fractionation and the less reactive members of this class isolated by rectification and identified by their physical properties.

Distillation serves a purpose other than isolation of the volatiles. During the heating process, proteins are coagulated and a part of the lipid fraction is split into less complex molecules. The filtrate from the tissue after distillation contains many of the heat stable, water soluble poisons. By using this aqueous filtrate in analyzing for the nonvolatile organic poisons, the residue containing the isolated poison is contaminated with less of the normally occurring tissue extractives than are tissue residues obtained by any other isolation procedure.

Analysis for the volatiles is a logical first step in attacking a general unknown. Establishing the presence or absence of ethyl alcohol is usually the first consideration. Many other members of this group are common poisons. Moreover, the volatiles are more readily lost when the tissue stands around pending the analysis. Since the filtrate has been made available as a result of the analysis for the volatiles, it is logical to subject it to analysis for the nonvolatiles even though the comprehensive isolation by direct extraction of the tissue must be carried out later on. If a poisonous substance is detected in the residue from the filtrate, the amount may be sufficient to warrant eliminating the labor of the exhaustive tissue extraction. The fewer compounds detectable in the filtrate is an advantage in their detection, and the saving in sample material and manipulative labor justifies the practice of conducting an analysis for the nonvolatile organics on the filtrate after distillation prior to direct extraction of tissue.

In the test procedures which are described in this section, the quantities of distillate utilized in a single determination are maximal for concentrations of unknown that will be recovered when the substance is present in the tissue in amounts that warrant consideration in establishing the cause of death. If all of the procedures are followed as written, there will not be enough distillate from the 500 gm. sample to complete the examination. These specifications were set up for the routine toxicology laboratory where a number of cases are being processed at one time and where the analyst does not have time to give each test special consideration. In examinations that are not routine, smaller quantities of distillate with proportionately smaller quantities of reagents will give comparable results.

The order of performing the tests is determined by the early chemical findings, the history or the pathologic report. For example, if an oil is observed in the distil-late, one might better proceed directly to the extraction of the distillate and the examination of the extracted residue or, if an ethereal or hydrocarbon-like odor is evident, the isolation procedure is indicated as the first step in the analysis. With the exception of ethyl alcohol, more than one unrelated volatile poison is seldom encountered in a toxicologic examination. Consequently, in order to conserve the sample, the first positive chemical findings should initiate a search for a member of the type of compound indicated by the test, before proceeding with tests for other poisons.

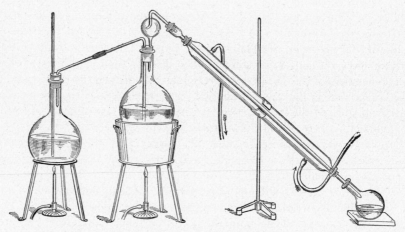

From Peterson, Haines and Webster, *Legal Medicine and Toxicology*, W. B. Saunders Co., 1923.

Fig. 45-1. Steam Distillation Apparatus.

Steam Distillation Procedure. Mince 500 gm. of chilled tissue or one third of the stomach contents in a meat grinder and add the material to the 2-liter Claissen distilling flask of the distillation apparatus shown in Figure 45-1. Submerge the tip of the condenser adapter in 5 ml. of approximately 0.01 N NaOH contained in the 250 ml. receiver flask. Cover the ground tissue with 600 ml. of distilled water to which 3 ml. of saturated tartaric acid are added. The water bath and steam generator are brought to boiling. Permit steam to generate until 100 ml. of distillate are col-lected. Then replace the receiver flask by a second one and continue the distillation until the second portion of distillate is 150 ml. This second portion of distillate is seldom utilized in the qualitative examination. It is collected to insure recovery of those substances that are not readily volatile with steam. It is held in reserve for aliquoting with the first 100 ml. portion for certain quantitative analyses or for further qualitative examination when the findings on the first portion warrant such an investigation. Chill the distillates in the ice box before testing for the volatile components. Transfer the hot tissue and aqueous solution remaining in the Claissen flask immediately to 20 cm. filter containing a fluted filter paper and set aside to filter overnight. The filtrate is treated by the procedure described in Chapter 47.

Alternate Alkaline Distillation. In isolated cases in which the history indicates the possibility of a basic poison which is volatile with steam, it may be advisable to continue the steam distillation after making the tissue slurry basic with magnesium oxide. Coniine, nicotine, aniline, primary and secondary aliphatic amines, *d*-desoxy-

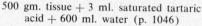

Outline for the Detection of the Volatile Poisons

Steam Distillation

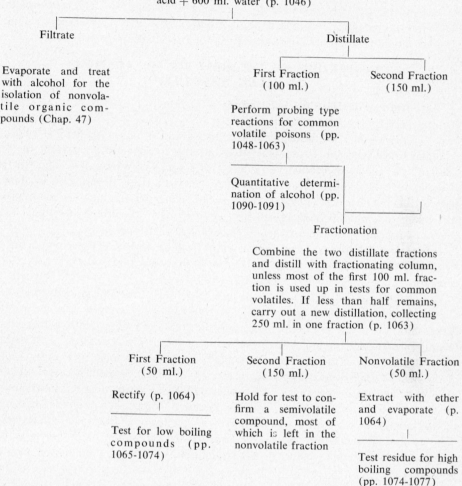

500 gm. tissue + 3 ml. saturated tartaric acid + 600 ml. water (p. 1046)

Filtrate

Evaporate and treat with alcohol for the isolation of nonvolatile organic compounds (Chap. 47)

Distillate

First Fraction (100 ml.)

Second Fraction (150 ml.)

Perform probing type reactions for common volatile poisons (pp. 1048-1063)

Quantitative determination of alcohol (pp. 1090-1091)

Fractionation

Combine the two distillate fractions and distill with fractionating column, unless most of the first 100 ml. fraction is used up in tests for common volatiles. If less than half remains, carry out a new distillation, collecting 250 ml. in one fraction (p. 1063)

First Fraction (50 ml.)

Second Fraction (150 ml.)

Nonvolatile Fraction (50 ml.)

Rectify (p. 1064)

Test for low boiling compounds (pp. 1065-1074)

Hold for test to confirm a semivolatile compound, most of which is left in the nonvolatile fraction

Extract with ether and evaporate (p. 1064)

Test residue for high boiling compounds (pp. 1074-1077)

ephedrine, ephedrine and amphetamine may be isolated from tissue by this procedure. Varying amounts of ammonia will be collected in this distillate from degradation of the normal tissue components by the steam. The degradation of putrefied material produces other bases and is so extensive that the basic steam distillation is impractical. Subjecting the filtrate to analysis for non-volatile organics after the basic distillation is optional, but this procedure is less desirable because the residue will contain a greater proportion of tissue impurities.

Procedure. Disconnect the steam generator and set the Claissen flask containing the tissue slurry in the ice box until cool. Add solid MgO in small portions with shaking until the aqueous solution is distinctly basic. Reconnect the steam generator and steam distill with the condenser tip submerged in 5 ml. of N/10 HCl until 250 ml. of distillate has been collected.

See page 1077.

Phosphorus. At the start of the distillation, the condenser should be examined for any phosphorescence. The room is darkened by drawing the shades and the upper end of the condenser is screened by encircling it with a black cloth. The condenser is examined as soon as the distillate starts to collect at the point where steam condenses in the condenser by observing it through the fold in the cloth. Phosphorescence indicates large amounts of phosphorus; if it is observed a sample of tissue should be analyzed quantitatively by the procedure on page 1036.

EXAMINATION OF THE FIRST 100 ML. PORTION OF STEAM DISTILLATE

Detection of Oxidizable Substances (7). *Reagent.* 0.05 N $K_2Cr_2O_7$ in 50 per cent H_2SO_4.

Procedure. Add 1 ml. of distillate to 5 ml. of reagent in a test tube and heat in a boiling water bath for 10 minutes. If oxidizable compounds are present in the distillate, the yellow dichromate is reduced to a green chromic color. The test is meaningless with distillates from putrefied tissue, since tissue degradation products are reducing substances. A negative reaction eliminates the necessity for conducting tests for the common alcohols, aldehydes, unsaturated hydrocarbons, terpenes, and many commercial preparations such as flavoring extracts and elixirs.

Aldehydes. SCHIFF'S TEST, FOLLOWING COPPER OXIDE OXIDATION. *Schiff's Reagent.* Dissolve 50 mg. of basic fuchsin in 20 ml. water and add H_2SO_3 solution containing the equivalent of 0.1 gm. SO_2.

Procedure. Add 20 ml. of distillate to a 6 inch test tube and plunge a red hot nitric acid-cleaned copper spiral, made by winding # 14 copper wire around a pencil until a ½ inch coil is obtained, into the solution 8 times while holding the test tube under cold running water. Add 5 ml. of the oxidized distillate to a 3 inch test tube and 5 ml. of the unoxidized distillate to another test tube; then add 0.5 ml. of the Schiff's reagent to each. Observe after 15 minutes. A reddish color in both tubes indicates aldehydes,* whereas a reddish color in only the oxidized tube shows the presence of alcohol (probably ethyl or methyl). Comparison of the intensity of the red color with standard solutions of ethyl or methyl alcohol shows the approximate alcohol concentration. With experience, visual estimation of the intensity of the color will determine whether or not a quantitative alcohol determination should be made.

The copper spiral should be observed while carrying out the oxidation process. If the wire has a bright luster after it is plunged into the solution, the presence of some component, oxidizable by hot copper oxide, is indicated. With a normal distillate, the surface remains a dull brown.

With putrefied tissue, a positive test for aldehydes will invariably be obtained, but large amounts of alcohol should be suspected when the test on the oxidized portion of the distillate shows a much deeper red than the unoxidized one. An exception is the analysis of liver for alcohol in cases of submersion in which body decomposition is extensive. Liver distillates in such instances invariably give indications of large amounts of alcohol. Confirmation must be made in the quantitative analysis with a procedure that removes interfering substances. When death has occurred under ether anesthesia, a weak positive reaction is obtained, due to hydrolysis of the ether by the hot copper. A methyl chloride poisoning will show a

---

* Benzaldehyde does not give an immediate color with Schiff's reagent (see page 1049). If benzaldehyde is present it is probably from oil of bitter almonds (see page 1051 for cyanide).

positive methyl alcohol test. Urotropin will give a positive aldehyde reaction, as it readily hydrolyzes on steam distillation with the formation of formaldehyde. About 25 per cent of the alcohol sedative methylparafynol comes over during steam distillation and gives a positive Schiff's reaction.

Methyl and Ethyl Alcohols. PHENYLHYDRAZINE-SODIUM NITROPRUSSIDE TEST. *Reagents.* (a) saturated aqueous phenylhydrazine solution; (b) saturated aqueous sodium nitroprusside solution.

Procedure. If the Schiff test is positive for the presence of alcohol, add 10 ml. of the oxidized distillate to a 6 inch test tube, followed by 1.5 ml. of saturated phenylhydrazine solution and 2 drops of saturated aqueous sodium nitroprusside. Mix the contents and add 5 drops of 10 per cent NaOH by allowing the drops to run down the sides of the inclined tube. Observe the drops as they pass through the solution. Ethyl alcohol gives a red color, whereas the color from methyl alcohol is blue. In the presence of both methyl and ethyl alcohol, blue streamers will radiate from the descending drop while the solution takes on a reddish color. In the presence of benzaldehyde, there is an immediate heavy white precipitate of the hydrazone.*

Formaldehyde. CHROMOTROPIC ACID TEST. Methyl alcohol is confirmed by a positive formaldehyde reaction on the oxidized distillate. When the Schiff test is positive on both the oxidized and the unoxidized distillates, the unoxidized portion should be examined for formaldehyde. Add 5 drops of distillate to 2 ml. of 1 to 2.5 (72 per cent) H_2SO_4 and sprinkle in a few crystals of chromotropic acid. Warm the tube in a water bath at 60° C. for 10 minutes. A violet color is produced in the presence of formaldehyde. Acetaldehyde and higher aliphatic aldehydes do not interfere. Furfural gives a red color in high concentrations.

MILK TEST. This test is specific and, being less sensitive, is more conclusive than the chromotropic acid test for significant amounts of formaldehyde. Mix 3 ml. of whole milk with 3 ml. of distillate and add a drop of 5 per cent $FeCl_3$. Add 5 ml. of concentrated H_2SO_4 slowly, with stirring, and place the mixture in a boiling water bath. A violet color indicates the presence of appreciable amounts of formaldehyde. Filter the solution and observe the precipitate. With small amounts of formaldehyde, the curdled milk on the filter paper shows a pink coloration.

Brain tissue from persons who have died in diabetic coma may give a positive test for methyl alcohol. When the test shows only small or moderate amounts of methyl alcohol, the urine and blood should be examined for ketone bodies and sugar. If the examination indicates ketosis at the time of death, the possibility of methyl alcohol from this condition must be ruled out (9).

Acetaldehyde. SODIUM NITROPRUSSIDE-PIPERIDINE TEST. A positive Schiff's reaction for the unoxidized distillate from unputrefied tissue, with a negative chromotropic acid reaction, points to the probable presence of acetaldehyde in the distillate.

Reagents. (a) piperidine; (b) freshly prepared saturated sodium nitroprusside solution.

Procedure. Add two drops of freshly prepared sodium nitroprusside solution to

---

* The method for detection of methyl alcohol by oxidation to formaldehyde according to Merley and Bueding (8), in which they use 3 drops of 5 per cent $KMnO_4$ and 4 drops of 10 per cent H_3PO_4 for 5 ml. of distillate, is more sensitive and less troublesome than the copper oxide oxidation. We have not found it reliable as a method for ethyl alcohol, and it fails almost entirely with the higher alcohols. Moreover, we are not able to vary the procedure by using stronger acid and heat to permit the detection of the higher alcohols and the alcohol sedative methylparafynol.

2 ml. of unoxidized distillate to give a pale yellow color to the solution. Then allow one drop of piperidine to run down the side of the inclined tube. In the presence of acetaldehyde a green to deep blue color is obtained. On the addition of glacial acetic acid, the color changes to deep green and then fades. Acetone gives a red color with piperidine and a mixture of acetone and formaldehyde gives a violet color. On the addition of glacial acetic acid, in the presence of acetone, the red color deepens to magenta and then slowly fades (see test for acetone on this page). Formaldehyde does not react in this test.*

Paraldehyde. The odor of the tissue at autopsy will indicate the presence of significant amounts of paraldehyde. It is hydrolyzed during the steam distillation and appears in the distillate as acetaldehyde.

Isopropyl Alcohol. Acetone is produced in the copper oxide oxidation of a distillate containing isopropyl alcohol.

Acetone. SODIUM NITROPRUSSIDE-SODIUM HYDROXIDE TEST.† *Reagents.* (a) freshly prepared aqueous saturated sodium nitroprusside solution; (b) 10 per cent sodium hydroxide.

Procedure. To 1 ml. portions of oxidized and unoxidized distillate in 3 inch test tubes, add 2 drops of freshly prepared sodium nitroprusside solution and 1 drop of 10 per cent sodium hydroxide. With acetone and ketones containing the

$$CH_3C\overset{\displaystyle O}{\overset{\|}{}}-$$ group, a red color which changes to a deep magenta appears which becomes, on standing, a violet color when the solution is acidified with glacial acetic acid. Acetaldehyde gives a red color but, on the addition of acetic acid, the color decreases in intensity and fades to a light yellow.

Removal of Interfering Aldehydes from the Distillate. When aldehydes interfere with the tests for alcohols or ketones, they may be separated by moist silver oxide oxidation to the acids and distilled from a basic solution.

Reagents. (a) freshly prepared silver oxide; (b) sodium bicarbonate.

Procedure. Add approximately 2 gm. of the silver oxide to 10 ml. of distillate. Tightly stopper the tube and allow it to stand for 2 days with intermittent shaking. Filter the solution, make it alkaline with $NaHCO_3$, and distill it in a microdistillation apparatus. Collect 5 ml. of distillate and subject it to the tests described previously, using smaller aliquots of solution and reagents.

---

* The *p*-hydroxydiphenyl procedure for acetaldehyde is more sensitive than the sodium nitroprusside-piperidine reaction. Sensitivity is not needed for acetaldehyde since it is sometimes present in small concentrations as a normal component and, when acetaldehyde or ethyl alcohol is significant in the case, the concentration is quite high. For this reason, we prefer the less sensitive sodium nitroprusside-piperidine reaction as an indicating test. The *p*-hydroxydiphenyl procedure for acetaldehyde is carried out by adding copper sulfate solution and concentrated sulfuric acid to the distillate, cooling, and then adding *p*-hydroxydiphenyl. A reddish or blue violet color develops in the presence of acetaldehyde (8, 10).

For ethyl alcohol, the oxidation to acetaldehyde is carried out by Merley and Bueding by the addition of 3 drops of 5 per cent potassium permanganate and 4 drops of 10 per cent phosphoric acid to 5 ml. of distillate and decolorizing with oxalic acid.

† Another test for acetone uses furfural, sodium hydroxide and hydrochloric acid.

Reagents. (a) 3 gm. potassium permanganate + 15 gm. 85 per cent phosphoric acid made up to 100 ml. with water; (b) 5 per cent furfural solution in water; (c) 10 per cent sodium hydroxide; (d) concentrated hydrochloric acid.

Procedure. Add 2 ml. of (a) to 1 ml. of distillate. Bring to a boil and allow to stand 5 minutes, add 0.5 ml. of (b) and 0.5 ml. of (c). Bring to a boil, cool, filter off the excess MnO_2, and layer over with concentrated HCl. A red color indicates the presence of acetone. Use unoxidized and oxidized portions of distillate (11).

Cyanide. PRUSSIAN BLUE TEST. *Reagents.* (a) 50 per cent sodium hydroxide; (b) freshly prepared 10 per cent ferrous sulfate solution; (c) 5 per cent ferric chloride solution; (d) concentrated hydrochloric acid.

Procedure. Treat 5 ml. of distillate with 1 ml. of (a), 3 drops of the freshly prepared (b), and 3 drops of the (c) solution, and heat almost to boiling. Cool the solution and add (d) dropwise until the brown $Fe(OH)_3$ precipitate is dissolved. A blue color due to colloidal ferric ferrocyanide indicates the presence of cyanides. With significant amounts of cyanide, a blue precipitate separates on standing.

The test is specific and sensitive enough to indicate cyanide in deaths from ingestion of the poison, but at best, it will only give a suspicious reaction in deaths due to inhalation of hydrocyanic acid which is sometimes used in fumigation. If a green color is produced in the Prussian blue test, allow the solution to stand for 2 hours and then filter. If there is a bluish deposit on the filter paper, a sample of lung tissue should be steam distilled. Concentrate the distillate by fractionation and test the concentrated solution for cyanide by the more sensitive sulfocyanate test. The Prussian blue test for cyanide has been made much more sensitive by the procedure described by Gettler and Goldbaum (12).

Cyanide may or may not be present in oil of bitter almonds. If it is present, the concentration will be high enough to give a positive Prussian blue reaction. However, if the cyanide comes from oil of bitter almonds, benzaldehyde will also be present (see test on page 1049).

SULFOCYANATE TEST FOR CYANIDE IN INHALATION DEATHS. *Reagents.* (a) ammonium polysulfide; (b) 5 per cent hydrochloric acid; (c) 10 per cent ferric chloride; (d) 5 per cent sodium hydroxide.

Procedure. When the circumstances suggest cyanide inhalation or in cases of accidental death in which the CN^- concentration in the organs is low, steam distill a fresh 500 gm. sample of tissue, collecting 250 ml. of distillate in 5 ml. of 5 per cent NaOH. Make the distillate acid and fractionate it in three steps, collecting 90, 30 and 10 ml. of distillate in alkaline solution. Add 1 ml. of ammonium polysulfide to the 10 ml. of distillate in an evaporating dish and evaporate the solution to dryness on the water bath. Add 5 ml. of 5 per cent HCl to the dry residue, warm the solution with stirring to dissolve the salts, allow it to stand 2 hours and then filter it with suction. If cyanide is present, the solution turns blood red on the addition of 5 drops of 10 per cent $FeCl_3$, due to the formation of ferric thiocyanate.

Death by inhalation is proved by the absence of CN^- in the stomach and by a higher CN^- content in the lung tissue than in the other organs.

QUANTITATIVE DETERMINATION OF CYANIDE (13). Cyanide is produced in small amounts during putrefaction of tissue. Gettler and Baine found 0.01 to 0.03 mg. per 100 gm. of tissue when organs in sealed containers were allowed to stand at room temperature for 1 to 5 days. Even larger amounts of cyanide may be produced as a result of tissue degradation with marked putrefaction. When brain tissue is stored from 5 to 8 days in an icebox above freezing temperature, the tissue distillate may give a positive Prussian blue reaction, even though the odors of putrefaction are not apparent. A quantitative determination is necessary, therefore, for the interpretation of results from tissue that has been stored prior to the analysis.

Reagents. (a) concentrated NH_4OH; (b) 10 per cent potassium iodide solution; (c) 0.005 N silver nitrate.

Procedure. For the volumetric silver nitrate titration for cyanide, add 10 to 25 ml. of alkaline absorbed distillate to a 50 ml. Erlenmeyer flask. For 25 ml. of distillate add 2 ml. of (a) and 1 ml. of (b). Titrate the cyanide with (c). The end point is denoted by the formation of a bluish white opalescent cloud of AgI. The sharp end point is best observed against a black background. Each milliliter of (c) is equivalent to 0.266 mg. of HCN.

Halogenated Aliphatic Compounds. The most common halogenated compounds encountered in toxicology are chloroform and chloral hydrate. These and the chlorinated solvents such as carbon tetrachloride, ethylene dichloride, trichlorethylene, perchlorethylene, tetrachlorethylene, and pentachlorethylene are detected by the Fugiwara reaction. Other common halogenated compounds giving a positive, although less sensitive Fugiwara reaction are bromoform, iodoform, tetrachlorethane, methyl bromide, ethyl bromide, methylene chloride, the local anesthetic chlorobutanol, and the rectal anesthetic tribromoethanol.

PYRIDINE-SODIUM HYDROXIDE REACTION (FUGIWARA). *Reagents:* (a) pyridine; (b) 10 per cent sodium hydroxide.

Procedure. Treat 5 ml. of distillate with 2 ml. of pyridine and 2 ml. of sodium hydroxide. Heat the solution in a boiling water bath until the temperature reaches approximately 90° C. A pink to deep red color in the pyridine layer indicates halogenated aliphatic compounds. The pyridine must be pure or false positive results will be obtained. A blank test should be run simultaneously with the test on the unknown.

Chloral Hydrate. Chloral hydrate readily decomposes in the organs after death unless the organs have been preserved in a deep freeze. For this reason the compound may be missed when the organs have been held without proper storage for some time before the analysis.

RESORCIN TEST. *Reagents.* (a) saturated resorcinol solution; (b) saturated sodium carbonate solution.

Procedure. Add 6 drops of (a) and 1 ml. of (b) to 3 ml. of distillate. After allowing it to stand for 1 hour, dilute the solution with 10 ml. of water and observe it under the quartz ultraviolet lamp. A green fluorescence indicates the presence of chloral hydrate.

Chloroform and other chlorinated compounds do not react to this test. Nitrites give a strong yellow color with resorcinol and sodium carbonate. A yellow color from the organ distillate should, therefore, initiate a search for nitrites in the stomach contents. Distillates from the stomach contents in a case of nitrite intoxication are a deep orange color without fluorescence in this test.

CORROBORATING TEST FOR HALOGENATED HYDROCARBONS (14). *Reagents.* (a) 2 per cent phloroglucinol in cyclopentanol; (b) concentrated sulfuric acid; (c) solid sodium hydroxide.

Procedure. Shake the distillate and add a 5 ml. portion to a test tube containing one quarter of a pellet of (c). Add 1 ml. of (a), shake the contents and warm the mixture to approximately 80° C. Let stand until two layers separate and note the color in the bottom layer. Allow 2 drops of (b) to run down the side of the tube, shake, let stand until the two layers separate, and again note the color in the bottom layer. The top layer is yellow or colorless.

This test confirms the positive findings by the Fugiwara reaction and further differentiates between chloroform, carbon tetrachloride, chloral hydrate and the other halogenated solvents. The colors in the bottom layers before and after acid treatment are recorded in Table 45-1.

Table 45-1. Color Reactions in Phloroglucinol-Cyclopentanol Test

HALOGENATED COMPOUND	BOTTOM LAYER	
	Before Acid	After Acid
Chloroform	blue → orange	bright yellow
Carbon tetrachloride	blue → dark brown	yellow brown
Chloral hydrate	brown → orange	bright yellow
Other halogenated solvents	blue → violet	colorless

If the halogen compound is a halogenated solvent, it must be isolated from the distillate (pages 1063-1065).

Odor of the Distillate and Putrefaction and Test for Thio Compounds. Distillates from fresh tissue have only a faint characteristic tissue odor. The offensiveness of the odor increases with the degree of putrefaction. In distillates from fresh tissue, an unusual odor indicates abnormal components. Unfortunately, the analyst cannot always differentiate odors from decomposition of tissue that may appear fresh by gross examination from those of volatile chemicals in the distillate.

Sulfides and thio compounds produced during putrefaction are partially responsible for the disagreeable odor of distillates. Their presence in a distillate can be detected by the sensitive sodium azide-iodine reaction. Therefore, when a distillate has a pronounced odor and gives a negative azide-iodine reaction, the conclusion can be drawn that the distillate comes from tissue that has not undergone decomposition and that the odor is indicative of the presence of a chemical compound. The analyst should then proceed to isolate the compound by the method described on pages 1063 and 1074. Conversely, a distillate with a strong odor that gives a positive azide-iodine reaction is either from tissue that has undergone degradation during the distillation process or else from tissue containing a poisonous thio compound recovered in the distillate. The sulfur-containing compounds from tissue degradation are held back when the distillate is redistilled in the presence of mercuric chloride, whereas sulfur-containing compounds like carbon disulfide and most volatile thio compounds pass over into the distillate.*

SODIUM AZIDE-IODINE REACTION (17). *Reagent.* 1 gm. sodium azide and 1 gm. sodium iodide dissolved in 3 ml. of water. Powdered iodine crystals are sprinkled in, with stirring, until the solution is amber colored.

Procedure. Add 2 drops of the reagent to 1 ml. of distillate. The immediate disappearance of the brown color, accompanied by effervescence, indicates that there was tissue breakdown during distillation or that there are thio compounds in the distillate. A negative test, indicated by the continued presence of a yellow brown color, shows that the tissue components were not broken down during the distillation process. Any pronounced odor in the distillate is due, therefore, to an odorous volatile chemical.

TEST FOR VOLATILE THIO COMPOUNDS CONTAINING ACTIVE —SH OR C=S GROUPS. The odor of the distillate from tissue that has undergone putrefaction is more or less characteristic and distinctive from that of sulfur-containing chemicals so that, in the light of the other finding, the following procedure is rarely necessary. It should be performed when the presence of carbon disulfide is a possibility and when aliphatic or aromatic hydrocarbon mixtures are found. Petroleum or tar hydrocarbon fractions may contain thio compounds as impurities; also they are

---

* Low molecular weight aliphatic mercaptans form insoluble mercaptides of mercury (15, 16).

sometimes added to toxic solvents to give them an odor. Mustard oils are used in commercial preparations, and commercial mixtures of the relatively nonvolatile thiocyano esters, which are active ingredients with DDT in some fly sprays, usually contain steam-volatile thio impurities.

Procedure. Add 1 gm. of $HgCl_2$ to 5 ml. of distillate in a micro distilling flask and distill until approximately 2.5 ml. of distillate have been collected. Place 1 ml. of the original distillate and 1 ml. of the distillate collected from the $HgCl_2$ into separate test tubes and add the azide-iodine reagent, a drop at a time, to each distillate, holding the tubes side by side to compare the rate of decolorization. If the decolorization in the first test with azide-iodine reagent was due to the presence of putrefaction, the $HgCl_2$ distillate will retain the yellow color from the reagent after the second drop. Immediate decolorization in both tubes after 2 to 4 drops of reagent should initiate a search for active thio compounds in the distillate. A portion of the distillate should be fractionated or extracted and examined further by reagents to determine the nature of the sulfur linkage (18, 19, 20. See also sodium fusion on page 1250 and Grote's reagent on page 1222).

Phenolic Compounds. MILLON'S TEST. *Reagent.* Dissolve metallic mercury in an equal weight of concentrated HNO_3, warming gently to start the reaction. Dilute with an equal volume of distilled water, let stand 24 hours and decant the clear liquid.

Procedure. Add 1 ml. of Millon's reagent to 3 ml. of distillate, heat to boiling, and boil for 2 minutes. A yellow, brownish or red color, with or without a precipitate, indicates the presence of a phenolic compound.

Phenols other than carbolic acid and cresol are seldom encountered and the primary purpose of Millon's test is to detect these substances. Since normal distillates do not give a color with the reagent, the development of any color change in the test solution indicates the presence of an abnormal volatile compound. Results for the more common reactive volatiles are shown in Table 45-2.

Table 45-2.   Reactions with Millon's Reagent

COMPOUND	COLOR DEVELOPED IN COLD	COLOR DEVELOPED ON HEATING
Phenol (carbolic acid)	reddish yellow	wine red
o-Cresol	yellow	red
m-Cresol	orange	orange red
p-Cresol	orange	wine red
Creosote	reddish yellow	reddish brown
Eugenol	wine red	darker wine red
Guaiacol	reddish yellow	brown
Resorcinol	yellow precipitate	wine red
Pyrocatechol	brown red	black
alpha-Naphthol	yellow	yellow + precipitate
beta-Naphthol	yellow	orange
Salicylic acid	negative	red + brown precipitate
Hydroquinone	negative	reddish → brown → black → brown precipitate
Pyrogallol	negative	yellow + yellow precipitate
Thymol	negative	yellow
Eucalyptol	negative	yellow

Dinitro-o-cresol (elgetol), menthol and camphor do not react with Millon's reagent. When salicylic acid is present in the sample material, only a small part will be carried over into the distillate. Its presence in the volatile fraction is, therefore, indicative of a high concentration as, for example, in the stomach contents in cases of suicides from salicylates. Large amounts will be isolated from the tissue with the nonvolatile organics. If any color change is noted in the Millon test, the distillate should then be extracted with organic solvents as described on page 1056 and further examined for phenolic substances (pages 1056-1057).

Oxidizing Compounds. Oxidizing compounds which are readily broken up in the body cannot be detected except in distillates from the stomach contents.

DIPHENYLAMINE TEST. *Reagent.* Enough diphenylamine to cling to the tip of a microspatula is added to 1 ml. of concentrated sulfuric acid and stirred with a glass rod to dissolve the crystals. Prepare fresh.

Procedure. Carefully layer about 1 ml. of the reagent under about 2 ml. of distillate. A blue ring at the interface indicates the presence of oxidizing compounds. The compounds most probably present if a positive reaction occurs are the inorganic nitrites, isoamyl nitrite or nitroglycerine. If a positive test is obtained, a sample from the stomach should first be examined for inorganic nitrites. If these are excluded, a portion of the unground sample should be taken immediately, slightly acidified with sulfuric acid, and treated with about 6 times its volume of a mixture of 2 volumes of methyl alcohol to 1 volume of acetone, allowing the mixture to stand 24 hours with intermittent stirring. The mixture is then filtered and the filtrate distilled to remove most of the alcohol-acetone solution. The undistilled liquid is extracted with ether and the ether evaporate examined for organic oxidants such as nitroso compounds, aliphatic nitro compounds, and esters of nitrous and nitric acid (21, 22, 23).

CONFIRMATION TEST FOR ESTERS OF NITROUS AND NITRIC ACID. Esters and a few aliphatic nitro compounds hydrolyze with alkali to nitrate and nitrite. The nitrate and the nitrite, after oxidation, will react with the phenoldisulfonic acid reagent (24). The diphenylamine-sulfuric acid reagent reacts positively with all types of oxidants, whereas the yellow color formed by the nitration of phenol-disulfonic acid is specific for nitrate. Inorganic nitrates are nonvolatile and positive findings are, therefore, indicative of the presence of easily hydrolyzable aliphatic nitrites or nitro esters, the most probable of the pharmaceuticals being nitro-glycerine.*

Reagent. Dissolve 2.5 gm. of phenol in 15 ml. concentrated sulfuric acid + 7.5 ml. fuming (13 to 15 per cent SO_3) sulfuric acid and heat in a boiling water bath for 2 hours.

Procedure. Redissolve the residue in a 3-part methyl alcohol, 1-part acetone mixture and add to an aliquot of this solution in a test tube about one-quarter the volume of 5N aqueous potassium hydroxide. Evaporate to dryness in a water bath and allow the dried residue to bake for about 1 hour. Add 0.1 ml. of phenoldisul-fonic acid reagent, mixing the residue and reagent by grinding with a glass rod. Dilute with 5 ml. of water, add 3 to 4 drops of 3 per cent hydrogen peroxide and heat almost to boiling. Cool and add concentrated NH_4OH dropwise until the solution is distinctly ammoniacal. A clear yellow color in the solution shows that nitrate was present in the residue.

ETHER EXTRACTION OF THE DISTILLATE

Many poisons volatile with steam are more soluble in organic solvents than in water and can be separated from the distillate by extraction with ether. This extraction isolates high-boiling liquids and solids which may not boil without decom-

* Ethylene glycol dinitrate, used widely in explosives, reacts like nitroglycerine.

position at atmospheric pressure but which have a vapor pressure low enough to permit them to be steam distilled. Solids which are mechanically carried over by the steam are also isolated. In addition, liquids with moderate vapor pressures, such as the alcohols above propyl, ketone, aldehyde and ester solvents and some acids are extractable with ether. Because this type of compound is better isolated by the fractionation procedure, the tests for their detection are described under fractionation (pages 1065-1070) although it may be desirable to test for them at this point if evaporation of the ether leaves an oily residue, particularly one with a marked odor. Higher alcohols which might influence the tests for low-boiling alcohols (such as ethyl alcohol) by the copper oxide oxidation, if present in significant amounts, will be isolated by ether extraction in amounts sufficient to give the positive generic test for alcohols (page 1076). Negative findings for alcohols in the residue from the ether extract confirm the significance of positive findings for low-boiling alcohols on the unextracted distillate (page 1048).

Procedure. Extract the remaining distillate from the first 100 ml. fraction (of which at least 40 ml. should remain *) with two 50 ml. portions of ether. Wash the combined ether extracts with two 20 ml. portions of water and dehydrate the ether by shaking with about 5 gm. of anhydrous sodium sulfate. Filter the ether through paper and evaporate to a volume of approximately 2 ml. on the steam bath. Allow the remaining ether to evaporate spontaneously at room temperature.† Note the odor after the ether has disappeared and the color and nature of the residue.

Tests on the Residue. NITROSYLSULFURIC ACID. Nitrosylsulfuric acid ($HNOSO_4$), like concentrated sulfuric acid, dissolves many organic compounds and, being a strong oxidizer, produces colors with many of them. With most phenols, nitrosamines are formed which may condense with excess phenol to form a dye stuff. The acid is analogous to Liebermann's reagent but is more drastic in its action and consequently reacts with a larger number of compounds. It gives positive results for all substances that react in the Liebermann reaction or the Eijkman modification. The reagent is not specific for phenols. Secondary aliphatic and aromatic linkages react to form nitroso compounds and, when water is present, the liberation of nitrous acid may result in diazotization of an aromatic amino group.

Some relatively high molecular weight alcohols and esters give colorations, probably as a result of dehydration with addition to the unsaturated linkage. The nitrosylsulfuric acid reaction differentiates a number of the volatile phenols which give a positive Millon's test and also indicates several of the nonphenolic volatiles.

Procedure. Place a microcrystal or drop of the residue on a microscope slide and cover it with a very small drop of nitrosylsulfuric acid, added by use of a stirring rod drawn at the end to a diameter of about 1 mm. Note any color changes. After 5 minutes, add a small drop of distilled water and observe the reaction. After effervescence has subsided, add a drop of concentrated NH_4OH from a 1 ml. serologic pipet beside the reaction mixture and observe any color changes as the ammonia flows into the acid solution. Color changes are tabulated in Table 45-3.

VANILLIN-SULFURIC ACID REACTION. When aldehydes in concentrated sulfuric acid condense with phenols, as well as other of the aromatic structures, the complex molecule that is formed is usually colored. Formaldehyde, *para*-dimethylamino-

---

* Compounds only moderately volatile with steam will be present in significant amounts in the second 150 ml. portion of distillate. All of these are relatively water insoluble and ether soluble, and may be recovered by extraction.

† When ether evaporates to dryness on a steam bath, the odor due to slight ether decomposition may mask that of another organic substance.

Table 45-3. Color Reactions with Nitrosylsulfuric Acid Reagent

Compound	Reaction with Concentrated Reagent	Reaction after Addition of Water	Color Change on Addition of Concentrated NH_4OH
Phenol	black tarry residue	brown red color	blue green
Creosote	black tarry residue	brown red color	blue green
m-Cresol *	black tarry residue	brown red color	blue green
o-Cresol *	black tarry residue	blood red color	blue green
p-Cresol *	black tarry residue	yellow precipitate + dark oil	yellow brown
Pyrogallol	black tarry residue	light yellow color	dark brown
Phloroglucinol	black tarry residue	light yellow color	dark brown
Resorcinol	tarry residue with green cast	light yellow color + black precipitate	blue (colloidal) particles
Catechol	tarry residue with green cast	yellow color	brownish
Eugenol	tarry residue with blue green cast	brown color	dark brown
Guaiacol	blue→black tarry residue	deep blue + blue precipitate	green
Hydroquinone	black precipitate with violet cast	brown precipitate	dark brown colloidal suspension
Eucalyptol	dark brown color	yellow precipitate	no change
Thymol	yellow brown color	white precipitate + brown oil	greenish yellow
Camphor	canary yellow color	light yellow precipitate	white precipitate
alpha-Naphthol	blue green color	light yellow color	canary yellow
beta-Naphthol	dark green color	light yellow color	no change
Menthol	violet + pale green precipitate	yellow color	white precipitate

* The behavior with nitrosylsulfuric acid serves to distinguish between o, m, and p-cresols when the compounds are pure.

benzaldehyde, vanillin and other aldehydes in concentrated sulfuric acid have been used as reagents for performing color tests (25, 26, 27). With most phenols the reaction takes place in the cold, whereas less reactive compounds require heat before condensation takes place. The vanillin-sulfuric acid reagent has some minor advantages over the other aldehyde-sulfuric acid reagents in the examination of the volatiles. The vanillin-acid mixture is more stable, as well as being more selective with regard to certain organic structures with which it will react. Concomitant with the nitrosylsulfuric acid reaction, it serves as a rapid color test to further differentiate the volatiles.

Reagent (1 per cent). 0.266 gm. vanillin dissolved in 15 ml. concentrated sulfuric acid.

Procedure. Add a microquantity of residue to a microscope slide and cover with a small drop of vanillin-sulfuric acid reagent. If no color develops in the cold or if the color is very faint, warm the slide just to SO_3 fumes. Allow the drop to cool, add a drop of water and note any color change. If a pronounced color develops in the cold, omit the warming. After allowing the slide to stand approximately 2 minutes, add a drop of water. The possible results after each of the three steps of the test are shown in Table 45-4.

The cresols show a much greater reactivity than phenol with the reagent. The differences are more apparent when a control phenol and cresol test is run simultaneously with the unknown. *Alpha* and *beta* naphthol also show differences which permit distinguishing between the two compounds. Menthol in the cold shows color

Table 45-4. Color Reactions with Vanillin-Sulfuric Acid Reagent

COMPOUND	COLOR IN THE COLD	COLOR ON HEATING TO SO_3 FUMES	COLOR AFTER ADDITION OF DISTILLED WATER
Phenol	orange	orange red	colorless
Creosote	dark red → magenta	—	magenta precipitate which fades
m-Cresol	dark red → magenta	—	magenta precipitate which fades
o-Cresol	dark red → magenta	—	magenta precipitate which fades
p-Cresol	dark red → magenta	—	magenta precipitate which fades
Guaiacol	red → maroon	—	magenta precipitate which fades
Eugenol	red black	—	maroon precipitate
Eucalyptol	dark brown with violet cast	—	magenta → violet → colorless
Thymol	deep orange	—	magenta → colorless
Menthol	orange → cherry red → wine red	—	maroon
alpha-Naphthol	magenta → maroon	—	blue → colorless
beta-Naphthol	violet increasing in intensity	—	colorless
Pyrogallol	orange red	—	colorless
Catechol	rose	no increase in color intensity	colorless
Terpin hydrate *	brown	red → red violet	intense violet (stable)
Camphor	negative	orange red	violet precipitate → colorless
Resorcinol	orange	orange red	colorless
Phloroglucinol	yellow	orange red	colorless
Hydroquinone	negative	negative	—
Dinitro-o-cresol	negative	negative	—

* Terpin hydrate is only slightly volatile with steam, about 5 per cent being carried over into the first 100 ml. fraction; more will be present in the second 150 ml. fraction. An indication of its presence in the volatiles should initiate a search in the original sample.

changes that are exceptional, and the increased intensity of the color with terpin hydrate after addition of water is characteristic. Thymol and camphor show pronounced color changes in contrast to the relatively insignificant reaction with nitrosylsulfuric acid.

DIFFERENTIATION BETWEEN PHENOL AND CRESOLS. 1. Separation. Separation depends on the fact that phenol is only sparingly soluble in petroleum ether whereas the cresols are quite soluble. Also, only phenol is sufficiently acidic to form a water soluble ammonium salt when a nonaqueous solution of phenol is shaken out with concentrated NH_4OH (28).

Add petroleum ether to the residue from the ether extract of the distillate and allow the solution to stand without agitation for about 10 minutes. Remove the liquid phase carefully with a capillary syphon and repeat the petroleum ether washing twice more. Shake out the combined petroleum ether washings in a separatory funnel with about one-tenth the volume of concentrated NH_4OH and, after separation, wash the nonaqueous phase twice with water. Cresol and other petroleum ether-soluble phenolic compounds remain as oily residues on evaporation of the petroleum ether.

Make the NH$_4$OH solution acid with HCl, extract with ether, and evaporate the ether in the container from which the original petroleum ether extraction was made.

2. Confirmation Tests. (a) Tetranitromethane * Reaction. A drop of tetranitromethane shows only a light yellow color when added to a droplet of phenol, whereas a deep orange to brown coloration develops with minute droplets of the cresols. Eugenol and guaiacol, which have creosote-like odors, react like the cresols. Thymol and *alpha*-naphthol crystalline residues stain deep orange but no coloration is imparted to the liquid.

(b) Brominated Derivatives. Add 2 ml. of warm water (60° C.) to the suspected phenol or cresol residue and stir the aqueous solution with a glass rod to form a suspension of residue in the aqueous phase. Decant into a centrifuge cone and add saturated bromine water dropwise until the solution retains a permanent yellow color. Centrifuge the precipitate and decant the liquid. Cover the precipitate with water, add 1 drop of sulfurous acid or acid sodium sulfite solution,† break up the precipitate with a stirring rod, and warm the suspension to 40° C. Recentrifuge the precipitate, decant the supernatant, and then wash the precipitate twice with cold water. Dissolve the precipitate in boiling 40 per cent ethyl alcohol and allow the solution to stand until crystals separate out. Centrifuge, decant and allow the crystals to air dry. Phenol forms 2,4,6-tribromphenol which has a melting point of 92.5 to 93.5° C. Tribromphenol is also formed when salicylic acid is treated with bromine water. The tribromcresols and other brominated phenolic compounds melt at much higher temperatures.

DIFFERENTIAL TESTS FOR OTHER VOLATILES. 1. Ferric Chloride Reaction for Phenols. Ferric chloride shows differences between individual compounds whose possible presence has already been indicated by the more sensitive but less specific reactions previously described. The behavior in aqueous and alcoholic ferric chloride solution is quite different with the different phenolic compounds and comparison in the two solvents serves to further distinguish between some of the closely related members. Of the two reactions, that in alcoholic solution is more significant since those compounds that give positive reactions only in aqueous solution will probably have been identified by other tests. The deep blue color developed by eugenol in alcohol differentiates it from the cresols and guaiacol which react similarly with tetranitromethane. Salicylic acid and methyl salicylate give violet colors in both aqueous and alcoholic solution.

Reagent. 5 per cent ferric chloride in 1 N hydrochloric acid.

Procedure. In one of two microtest tubes place 2 drops of aqueous solution or suspension, and in the other tube place 2 drops of an alcoholic solution of the unknown. Layer a drop of the reagent over the contents of each of the tubes and observe the color as the reagent diffuses down through the solutions. The color reactions are listed in Table 45-5.

2. Tollen's Reagent (page 1079). *Procedure.* Add a drop of freshly prepared reagent to a small portion of residue on a microscope slide and place a second drop near the first as a control. A positive reaction is indicated by reduction to black Ag^0 within 30 seconds.

---

* Obtainable from Nitroform Company, Newark, New Jersey.
† Excess Br$_2$ precipitates C$_6$H$_2$Br$_4$O (melting point 131° C.) with phenol and it is converted to C$_6$H$_2$Br$_3$OH by the acid sulfite.

Table 45-5.   Color Changes with Ferric Chloride in Aqueous and Alcoholic Solutions

Compound	Aqueous Solution	95 per cent Ethyl Alcohol Solution
Salicylic acid	deep violet	deep violet
Methyl salicylate	deep violet	deep violet
Salol (phenyl salicylate)	—	violet
Eugenol	white precipitate	deep blue
Guaiacol	dark brown	grass green
Creosote (Merck)*	brown turbidity	blue green
o-Cresol	blue violet	—
m-Cresol	blue violet	—
p-Cresol	blue violet	—
Phenol	violet	—
Resorcinol	light blue	—
Pyrogallol	dark brown	green
Pyrocatechol	blue green	green
alpha-Naphthol	—	yellow green
Thymol	—	light green
Hydroquinone	decolorizes $FeCl_3$ with a precipitate of green black quinhydrone	—

* Coloration with commercial creosote or lysol® depends on the other impurities. Mixtures of pure *o, m,* and *p*-cresol give a color in alcohol that is only a slightly darker yellow green than the control.

Catechol, pyrogallol, hydroquinone, and quinone show immediate reduction. Crystals of phlorglucinol and *alpha*-naphthol darken immediately but require about 30 seconds for the reduced Ag^0 particles to appear in the solution. Positive but slightly delayed reduction is distinguished from decomposition of the reagent by the appearance of a blue halo around the residue prior to the blackening.

3. Chloroform-Potassium Hydroxide Test (29). *Reagents.* (a) solid potassium hydroxide; (b) chloroform.

Procedure. Dissolve a small portion of the unknown in 3 to 4 drops of chloroform in a microtest tube and add about one eighth of a pellet of solid potassium hydroxide. Heat the chloroform solution to boiling. A positive reaction is indicated by a pronounced color in the chloroform solution.

With guaiacol, thymol, creosote and *o*-cresol, a deep maroon color develops. Salol produces a pink coloration with a significant concentration. *Alpha*-naphthol gives blue and *beta*-naphthol gives green. *Alpha* and *beta*-naphthol stain the potassium hydroxide particle a deep blue, while catechol colors it dark green and pyrogallol brown with the chloroform remaining colorless. Phenol, phloroglucinol, resorcinol and *m*-cresol stain the potassium hydroxide rose to red without color in the solution.

DISTINGUISHING TEST FOR THYMOL. Thymol in concentrated sulfuric acid is a sensitive reagent for titanium (30). Also, the yellow brown color develops with small amounts of thymol when $TiCl_3$ in concentrated sulfuric acid is used as a reagent. Other phenols react with the $TiCl_3$-H_2SO_4 reagent (31) but these will have been indicated by other phenolic reagents which do not react with thymol.

Reagent. Titanous chloride-sulfuric acid reagent is made by adding a 15 per cent $TiCl_3$ solution dropwise to about 1 ml. of concentrated sulfuric acid until a faint blue color persists. Make up fresh each time.

Procedure. Add a drop of reagent to the residue from the ether extraction of the distillate or to its glacial acetic acid or acetone solution. In the presence of thymol, a deep yellow to brown color develops.

DETECTION OF NITRO COMPOUNDS. Nitrobenzene, present in most shoe polishes and in a few soap preparations, is the most common of the nitro compounds encountered in toxicologic analysis. The odor strongly resembles that of oil of bitter almonds, and, if the concentration in the distillate is high enough to form a visible oily layer on the surface, its presence will be suspected by the odor.

Dinitro-o-cresol is used extensively as a dormant spray material under the trade name of elgetol®. It is a yellow solid only slightly volatile with steam, about 10 per cent being carried over into both the first and second fractions, producing light yellow colored distillates. The undistilled aqueous phase remains yellow after the distillation is completed. Solutions of dinitro-o-cresol stain the skin and cloth fibers yellow, in a manner similar to that of dilute solutions of picric acid. It is closely related to picric acid in structure and the chemical properties of the two compounds are so similar that the cresol can very easily be mistaken for picric acid.

Reagents. (a) magnesium powder; (b) furfural-acetic acid reagent (page 1079).

Procedure. Place a small drop of liquid or solid residue from the ether extraction of the distillate on a watch glass and sprinkle a thin layer of powdered magnesium on top of the unknown. Add the furfural-acetic acid reagent dropwise in minute droplets from a capillary to the top of the magnesium powder until effervescence ceases. After about 10 minutes, observe the magnesium acetate formed by the action of the acetic acid on the metal. In the presence of nitro compounds the white magnesium acetate is stained dark red.

This test (36) depends on the reduction of NO_2^- to NH_2 by the magnesium and the acetic acid in the furfural reagent. The furfural then condenses with the amine to give the colored dye which is absorbed by the magnesium acetate residue (page 1079).

The procedure works equally well as a paper spot test. Impregnate filter paper with the unknown and sprinkle a layer of powdered magnesium over the surface. Add the furfural reagent a little distance from the unknown so that it diffuses to the magnesium powder. The red stain is visible on the reverse side of the paper.

The color with dinitro-o-cresol has a brownish cast and the positive reaction is not immediately apparent as in the case of nitrobenzene and other mono nitro compounds.

1. Differential Test for Mono and Polyaromatic Nitro Compounds. The presence of two or more nitro groups in the benzene nucleus makes the nitro compounds more reactive toward alkali. A few polynitro compounds give colors with aqueous and alcoholic alkali alone and still others with alkali in solutions of different ketones (32-35). The reactivity of some polynitro compounds toward alkali is enhanced by treatment of the aqueous or alcoholic solutions with $TiCl_3$ before the addition of the alkali (36).

Reagents. (a) 15 to 16 per cent $TiCl_3$ solution; (b) concentrated NH_4OH.

Procedure. Dissolve enough residue in two drops of 95 per cent ethyl alcohol to give the alcohol a faint yellow color. Heat to boiling and add 1 drop of $TiCl_3$ solution to the hot alcohol solution. Cool and add a drop of concentrated NH_4OH.

With dinitro-o-cresol and picric acid a dark red colored crystalline precipitate is formed with high concentrations and a reddish solution with smaller amounts of the compounds. The red precipitate is more soluble in water, giving a red solution. It dissolves in excess ethyl alcohol to give a less intense yellow-red coloration.*

2. Distinguishing Tests for Dinitro-*o*-cresol and Picric Acid.§ Dinitro-*o*-cresol is much less soluble in water and readily crystallizes out of a hot saturated solution in long yellow needles which melt at about 86° C. Picric acid melts at 122 to 123° C. Both dinitro-*o*-cresol and picric acid are insoluble in petroleum ether and give reddish colors when the aqueous solution is boiled with dilute potassium cyanide solutions.† Both give reddish colors in the so-called picramic acid test in which a solution to which lactose has been added is made alkaline with sodium carbonate and heated.

The ability of aqueous solutions of picric acid to precipitate alkaloids and complex basic substances serves to distinguish the two compounds. Dinitro-*o*-cresol does not form insoluble complexes with this type of molecule. Nitron is a very sensitive precipitant for picric acid.

Reagent. 10 per cent solution of nitron in 1 N sulfuric acid.

Procedure. A drop of reagent is added to several drops of aqueous unknown heated almost to boiling. Picric acid gives an immediate dense yellow crystalline precipitate whereas dinitro-*o*-cresol does not react.‡

DETECTION OF ORGANIC THIOCYANATES. The presence of significant amounts of hydrocarbons in the sample material may be apparent to the analyst by the odor of the oil droplets on the surface of the distillate. If kerosene is present, it may have been the carrier for a fly spray preparation. Many fly sprays contain lethane® mixtures with or without DDT. Lethane ‖ is composed of a number of organic thiocyanates and their presence in the distillate, along with hydrocarbons, is indicative of fly spray material. About a fourth of a commercial lethane® preparation distills over during the steam distillation process and can be recovered by ether extraction of the distillate. The evaporate is a clear, colorless liquid with a pronounced odor. Ether extraction of the undistilled solution removes the remaining fraction of the preparation as a brown viscous oil with an odor similar to that of the volatile fraction. Undistilled lethane® gives a strong sodium azide reaction (page 1053) but the reaction is negative or only weakly positive on the steam volatile fraction. The test for organic thiocyanates depends on the formation of the typical blood red color of ferric thiocyanate on addition of the Fe^{+++} ion to the solution after alkaline hydrolysis.

Reagents. (a) solid Na_2S; (b) absolute methyl alcohol; (c) 1:2 hydrochloric acid; (d) 5 per cent ferric chloride.

Procedure. Evaporate an aliquot of ether extract of the distillate in a 3 inch test tube to remove all of the ether. The residue should be about 0.1 ml. in volume.

---

* 3,5-Dinitrobenzoic acid forms a light rose colored precipitate when similarly treated. This behavior was observed in an attempt to reduce the NO_2 to NH_2 with $TiCl_3$. No amine is formed under the conditions of the test. The formation of this red precipitate resembles the behavior described for 1,3,5-trinitrobenzene in methyl alcohol with KOH in which the red compound $[(C_6H_3NO_2)_3CH_3OK]_2 \cdot H_2O$ is precipitated (37).

§ Picric acid is not volatile with steam but could be mechanically carried over into the distillate.

† Trinitrocresol reacts even more readily with potassium cyanide solution and would be expected to give the other tests described for picric acid and dinitro-*o*-cresol. The less commonly used spray material 2,4-dinitro-6-cyclohexylphenol would also be expected to react similarly.

‡ Inorganic ions such as Br^-, I^-, NO_2^-, $CrO_4^=$, ClO_3^-, ClO_4^-, $Fe(CN)_6\equiv$, $Fe(CN)_6\equiv$, and thiosulfate all precipitate nitron but will not extract with ether.

‖ Lethane is the Rohm and Haas trade name for *beta*-butoxy-*beta*-thiocyanodiethyl ester and *beta*-thiocyanoethyl esters of aliphatic acids.

Introduce approximately 20 mg. of reagent (a), followed by a volume of reagent (b) equal to that of the unknown. Clamp the tube upright with the bottom suspended over a hot plate at a distance sufficient to make the solution reflux. Continue refluxing for 15 to 20 minutes with the addition of methyl alcohol to maintain nearly constant volume. Cool the solution, acidify it to Congo red paper by the dropwise addition of reagent (c) and add a drop of reagent (d). A red color in the solution due to $Fe(CNS)_3$ indicates the presence of organic thiocyanates.

FRACTIONATION OF THE DISTILLATE

Detection of Low-Boiling Volatiles. Alcohols other than methyl and ethyl, particularly the fusel oils, aromatic hydrocarbons such as benzene, toluene and xylene, aliphatic hydrocarbons and their mixtures such as kerosene, gasoline and naphtha, ester and ketone solvents, especially those used in lacquer solvents, halogenated solvents, turpentine and special compounds such as ethyl ether are relatively inert chemically and cannot be identified by the type of reactions already described. Nevertheless, during the examination, the analyst may become aware of the presence of the relatively inert component in the distillate, and may, in addition, obtain some idea of its volatility. With significant amounts, he should recognize its presence during the distillation process, from the odor, the separation of oily droplets or the Schlieren effect inside the condenser or in the distillate as it collects in the receiver. At the first indication of the presence of this type of chemical substance, the analytic approach should be altered to include detection of these compounds.

A fractional distillation of the collected distillate is essential in order to concentrate these lower boiling, less reactive compounds and to separate them from the bulk of the aqueous phase. The very volatile inert members must be further concentrated by rectification before adequate tests can be applied. Fractional distillation prior to carrying out any extensive chemical examination not only serves to indicate the volatility of any of the low boiling substances, but conserves ample material in view of the fact that any of the tests already described become even more sensitive when applied to the fractions.

In the general unknown type of examination, theoretically the logical starting point is the elimination of the inert volatiles before examining for the more reactive compounds. However, the sequence in the discussion of the tests has followed a pattern applicable to the general run of toxicologic examination rather than to the exceptional case. Since there is usually some history or other evidence involving inert volatile chemicals associated with such deaths, it is the common practice first to eliminate the most probable types of the volatile poisons.

If a fractional distillation has to be made after using up a significant amount of the original distillate, a new sample of the biologic specimen must be steam distilled in order to insure isolation of an adequate quantity of these less reactive poisons. In general, the final sample will not exceed a few tenths of a milliliter in volume and methods of testing for this class are limited to the determination of physical properties or, at best, reactions of low sensitivity.

Fractional Distillation of the Steam Distillate. Because of the relatively small amount of material compared with the total volume of distillate, the conventional fractionation in which fractions are selected on the basis of change in boiling point cannot be used. In the usual case, the best that can be accomplished is a separation into three groups: compounds with boiling points below and up to

100° C., most of the water making up the distillate plus any compounds boiling close to 100° C., and the undistilled portion containing compounds boiling above 100° C. In order to effect the separation, a fractionating column of the Hempel or Widmer type (38) is utilized. The only restriction on the type of column used is that the design must permit it to be readily washed with solvents after the distillation is completed.

Procedure. Place the total distillate (250 ml.) collected during the steam distillation of the sample in a flask connected with the packed fractionating column and thermometer. The condenser is equipped with a condenser adaptor which extends to the bottom of the receiver flask kept submerged in a salt-ice bath.* Carry out the distillation with a low flame protected from drafts by a chimney, and allow it to proceed until about 50 ml. of distillate has been collected.† Observe the temperature as the condensate starts to collect in the receiver and note any changes between this point and 100° C. Change the receiver and continue the distillation without attention at a slow rate until all but about 50 ml. of undistilled solution remains in the distilling flask.

Disconnect the apparatus and wash out the fractionating column by pouring a 25 to 50 ml. portion of ether through several times. Saturate the undistilled portion with powdered sodium chloride ‡ and extract it first with ether, including the portion used to wash out the fractionating column, and then with chloroform. Evaporate the ether and chloroform in separate containers and examine the residues as described on page 1075.

The analyst must use his judgment regarding extraction of the second fraction of the distillate. Almost all of the possible water soluble volatiles will appear in the first fraction and, unless the second fraction is turbid or contains some insoluble oil, it may be ignored. The first fraction must be further concentrated by rectification for analysis.

Isolation of the Low-Boiling Volatiles by Rectification. Gettler, Niederl and Benedetti-Pichler have described the rectification procedure in their study of ethyl alcohol normally present in human and animal tissue (42). Gettler and Siegel applied the principle to the isolation of ethyl alcohol from tissue of alcoholics (43, 44) using a modified rectification flask. Their apparatus is suitable for the isolation of any of the volatiles although a flask of smaller capacity is adequate.§

Procedure. Cool the first fraction of distillate in an ice bath and saturate it with anhydrous sodium fluoride by addition of small portions of the salt to the solution with stirring. Introduce the solution into the rectification flask through the safety tube and add about 1 gm. of granulated zinc to prevent bumping. Keep the receiver, which is a graduated 3 inch by 10 mm. test tube, submerged in a cooling bath of dry ice and acetone. The best source of heat is a hot plate with a variable resistance to control the current through the heaters. The flask should be protected from cross drafts by wrapping the bulb with asbestos cloth. The use of a magnetic stirrer gives more even heating and helps prevent bumping. Apply heat

---

* The distillation apparatus used in the New York City Medical Examiner's Laboratory was specially designed for distillation of the very volatile liquids. The condenser is a new type constructed to maintain a state of equilibrium between liquid and vapor and to avoid dead spaces or losses of vapor at the tip (39).

† This assumes that the thermometer has reached 100° C. before the 50 ml. have been collected.

‡ Adapted from the Allen-Marquardt method for amyl alcohols (40, 41).

§ Eck and Krebs catalogue item # 3540, Long Island City, New York.

to the flask so that the liquid just comes to boiling temperature. A ring of steam condensate develops in the neck of the flask and slowly rises toward the bulb. The temperature is then regulated through the variable resistance to maintain the steam condensate below the bulb in the neck for 20 to 30 minutes.

During this time, the upper portion of the neck of the flask acts as a fractionating column, allowing the more volatile vapors to rise above the less volatile ones and to finally condense in the receiver. The uniform controlled heating permits a state of equilibrium to exist between liquid and vapor phase in the neck of the flask so that an efficient separation from the water vapor is obtained. The heating temperature is then increased to drive the ring of steam condensate up the neck of the flask at the rate of about 0.5 cm. per minute. When the steam finally passes the bend of the tube leading into the receiver, the distillation is completed.* The delivery tube is removed and the volume of liquid above the solidified water vapor in the receiver is recorded.

If the receiver does not have a liquid layer when it is removed from the dry ice-acetone bath, volatiles are not present in significant amounts. A microboiling point (45) should first be done on the liquid layer to determine the precautions necessary for handling the sample in subsequent tests, as well as to indicate the presence of a common substance. A boiling point of 34° to 35° C. indicates the presence of ethyl ether. When ethyl chloride is present in conjunction with ethyl ether it will lower the boiling point below 34° C. (45). Methylene chloride boils at 40° to 41° C. If the microboiling point corresponds to that of another pure substance it can be verified by a refractive index measurement. However, microboiling points do not indicate mixtures, as in macroboiling point determinations, and this constant alone is not proof of the identity of a substance.

If the isolated product is not ethyl ether from anesthesia it is very likely to be a mixture. Kerosene, gasoline and halogenated solvents are commonly encountered and preliminary tests to determine the type of product isolated should be made before proceeding with an analysis on the assumption that the odor, boiling point or other physical characteristic designates the class of compound.

Reactions for the Distillate Isolated by Rectification. FORMALDEHYDE-SULFURIC ACID TEST FOR AROMATIC COMPOUNDS (46).

Reagent. 0.1 ml. of 40 per cent formaldehyde in 2 ml. concentrated sulfuric acid.

Procedure. Add a drop of reagent in the cavity of a hollow ground microscope slide. Immerse a clean glass stirring rod pulled out at the end to a diameter of about 1 mm. into the sample so that the surface of the rod at the tip is wet with a film of the unknown. Dip the end of the rod into the reagent while viewing the slide against a white background. This reagent reacts with aromatic hydrocarbons and some unsaturated aliphatics to give orange to dark brown colorations. The reaction is very sensitive and serves as an exclusion test for this type of sample material. A positive reaction should be followed by the test for benzene and closely related compounds (page 1073).

BROMINE-CARBON TETRACHLORIDE TEST FOR UNSATURATED COMPOUNDS (47). Bromine in carbon tetrachloride adds to olefinic or acetylenic linkages to form bromine addition compounds. Decolorization of the brown carbon tetrachloride

---

* If heating is too rapid, the water vapor will be condensed with the formation of ice in the base of the delivery tube. This will be apparent by the back pressure developing in the safety tube of the flask. The delivery tube can be cleared by removing it from the receiver and warming with the hand.

without effervescence with an anhydrous unknown is therefore indicative of aliphatic unsaturations. To discharge the color completely, the unknown must be in amounts equivalent to or in excess of the bromine-carbon tetrachloride reagent. In mixtures in which unsaturated compounds are the minor components, the color may only be reduced in intensity and on a microscale the interpretation is difficult. However, if the test is carried out in a capillary with a bore of 0.5 to 1.0 mm. so that the reagent is layered over the unknown without mixing with it, the reaction can be observed at the interface and rendered more sensitive and specific.

Other compounds such as phenols, aromatic amines, aldehydes, ketones, and molecules with active methylene groups discharge the color by reaction with substitution of bromine into the molecule and the liberation of hydrobromic acid. Hydrobromic acid is insoluble in carbon tetrachloride and, when the reaction is one of substitution rather than addition, the discharge of color is accompanied by effervescence. The only exceptions are additions to tertiary bases such as pyridine which form perbromides and substitutions in a few isolated aromatic bases such as aniline in which the first mole of hydrobromic acid adds to the base to form a salt.

Reagent. 5 per cent liquid bromine in carbon tetrachloride.

Procedure. Warm to body temperature by holding in the hand a 0.5 to 1.0 mm. capillary melting point tube sealed at one end. Quickly dip the open end into the unknown and allow a small drop of liquid to rise in the tube by the contraction of the air inside it. Centrifuge the sample to the bottom of the tube and introduce a drop of the bromine-carbon tetrachloride reagent in the same manner. Drop the capillary down through a 3 foot piece of 7 mm. glass tubing with the end resting on a soft wooden block, in the manner of loading a capillary for a melting point determination. The impact forces the reagent down the tube, overlayering the unknown. Decolorization proceeds from the interface upward. If gaseous hydrobromic acid is formed the drops move forward in the capillary.

Other chemical evidence may eliminate the need for this test which is used to corroborate the aromatic hydrocarbon test with formaldehyde-sulfuric acid. If the bromine-carbon tetrachloride test is negative, the possibility of interference from aliphatic hydrocarbons in the formaldehyde-sulfuric acid test is ruled out and the analysis is directed toward the identification of aromatic ring compounds (page 1070).

HYDROXAMIC ACID TEST FOR ESTERS (48, 49). Volatile esters are seldom encountered as a single compound in a toxicologic analysis, but are common components of solvent mixtures, particularly in lacquer solvents. They are easily overlooked in a mixture containing other types of solvents. They may be identified in a mixture by conversion to hydroxamic acids which give a red to violet color on the addition of Fe^{+++} ion. Many complex drugs give positive reactions with this test (50) but none of these will be isolated in this fraction.

Reagents. (a) saturated solution of potassium hydroxide in ethyl alcohol; (b) saturated solution of hydroxylamine hydrochloride in ethyl alcohol; (c) 1 percent ferric chloride in ethyl alcohol; (d) acid methyl alcohol (10 ml. concentrated hydrochloric acid plus absolute methyl alcohol to make 100 ml.).

Procedure (50). Add two small drops of alcoholic potassium hydroxide from a capillary pipet to a 2 by 50 mm. microtest tube and introduce a microdrop of unknown.* Add one drop of hydroxylamine hydrochloride solution † and seal

---

* Adequate unknown can be transferred to the test solution by means of a 1 mm. glass fiber, fire polished on the end to form a small glass bead, since the film of liquid which collects on the end of the rod when it is dipped into the unknown is approximately equal to a microdrop from a capillary pipet.

the open end of the microtest tube by heating in an open flame. Mix the contents of the closed tube by tapping with the finger, and heat for five minutes by laying the tube lengthwise on a hot plate with a surface temperature of approximately 100° C. After cooling, force the solution to the bottom of the tube by centrifugation in a hand centrifuge. Reopen the end, add one drop of ferric chloride and mix with the contents.†

Then layer several drops of acid alcohol solution over the alkaline test solution. Neutralization takes place at the surface and continues as the acid diffuses down through the solution. A positive reaction is indicated when a red to violet color develops after acidification.

DETECTION OF ALCOHOLS. Low-boiling alcohols such as methyl, ethyl and isopropyl will have been detected in the original distillate (page 1048). A portion of the alcohols with intermediate boiling points will be removed in the rectified distillate, along with the low-boiling ones. A reliable qualitative generic test for the detection of microquantities of the alcohols has not been available. The conventional reactions in organic analysis with metallic sodium or acyl halides for indicating an alcoholic hydroxy group requires macroquantities of purified sample and, consequently, cannot be readily adapted for microsamples. On the other hand, the detection of very small quantities of aldehydes by Schiff's reagent is a practical test in organic analysis when proper precautions are taken to exclude interferences (page 1068).

Oxidation of alcohols to aldehydes and the subsequent detection of the aldehyde appeared to be a practical solution to the problem of detecting alcohols. Oxidants such as potassium permanganate, potassium dichromate, iodic acid and hydrogen peroxide oxidize alcohols to aldehydes but, with many of the individual compounds, the oxidation proceeds further, with the formation of the acid. The conditions required for controlling the oxidation so that the principal product is aldehyde are so variable with the different alcohols, that these reagents cannot be used to set up standard conditions applicable to alcohols as a class.

In a study of the effect of various oxidizing agents on alcohols, it was found that benzoyl peroxide, with nitrobenzene as a solvent, produced some aldehyde with all of the alcohols studied (36). Aliphatic alcohols were more readily oxidized than some of the aromatic ones but sufficient aldehyde was formed under the conditions of the test to give a good positive Schiff's reaction. This reagent was found to be a mild oxidant, capable of satisfying the conditions necessary for the detection of primary alcohols as a class by oxidation to their respective aldehydes and furnishes a new generic alcohol test for organic analysis as well as toxicology. Since the recovery of the higher boiling alcohols is not complete in the rectified fraction and the largest proportion is found in the unrectified distillate, this procedure for their detection is described under Analysis of the Undistilled Portion of the Fractionated Distillate (pages 1074-1077).

DETECTION OF KETONES WITH 3,5-DINITROBENZOIC ACID. Ketone solvents are finding more extensive use in industry primarily because of their solvent power for the synthetic resins, particularly the vinylite and cellulose ester and ether types. Commercial solvents containing mixtures of ketones and esters are common and

† Care must be taken in introducing the microdrop of reagent to have the bores of the capillary pipets used nearly the same. The volumes of the reagents added should be in the ratio 2:1:1 in the order listed.

identification of the components of these complex mixtures on a limited sample is difficult. A prerequisite to a successful analysis on such small samples is the detection of the ester and keto groups. The hydroxamic acid reaction is a generic test for the esters. Detection of ketones has depended on the formation of insoluble oximes or hydrazones. Unfortunately, the formation of these derivatives is quite variable with different types of ketones and does not serve as an infallible generic test. A modification of the Janovsky reaction (32) has been developed in the New York City Medical Examiner's Laboratory and serves as an indicating test for compounds containing active carbonyl groups in solvent mixtures (51).*

Reagents. (a) 20 per cent alcoholic sodium hydroxide; (b) 10 per cent alcoholic 3,5-dinitrobenzoic acid.

Procedure. Add three drops of each of the above reagents and one drop of unknown introduced by means of a glass stirring rod to a small test tube (see footnote, page 1066). An immediate red to violet color in the cold indicates the presence of ketones.

The Janovsky reaction and its modifications (52) utilize *m*-dinitrobenzene, 3,5-dinitrobenzoyl chloride and 2,4-dinitrochlorobenzene; and probably numerous other dinitro compounds give colorations with ketones. 3,5-dinitrobenzoic acid appears to be a little more sensitive for a larger number of ketones. The reaction is not entirely specific for the carbonyl group in the ketone structure. Acetaldehyde, phenyl acetyl chloride and acetamide give a positive test. All aliphatic primary amines tested reacted positively, although the coloration was deep red in contrast to the violet cast for the ketones. None of the ethers, esters or alcohols tested gave a reaction except for ethylene glycol monoethyl ether which acted like the ketones. Under the conditions of the test, amines and most other interfering substances are excluded, so that the positive findings should be followed by the procedure (page 1069) for the preparation of a derivative.

FUCHSIN TEST FOR ALDEHYDES. Aldehydes other than formaldehyde, acetaldehyde and benzaldehyde are rarely found in the analysis of biologic samples and will have been detected in the preliminary tests on the distillate. There are relatively few volatile aldehydes of commercial use and any of them, if present, give the fuchsin reaction when applied directly to the distillate. Application of the fuchsin test at this point is warranted only when the reaction was positive on the distillate and the presence of the aldehydes noted above was not confirmed by more specific tests.

The violet color depends on the liberation of basic fuchsin from the fuchsin-sulfite addition compound and any substance that has a greater affinity for sulfurous acid than for the basic fuchsin will, therefore, give the reaction. Since salts such as sodium bicarbonate, some digestion products of tissue, particularly those from putrefied material, and some reactive ketones give positive reactions, the question of the significance of findings, when they are positive for the distillate (page 1048), must depend on the isolation of the product and identification from its derivatives. A positive test on this low-boiling fraction excludes aldehydes resulting from tissue degradation or hydroxyl ion interference. If the test is negative, an examination of the undistilled fraction (page 1064) for aldehydes is indicated (page 1075).

Reagent. Schiff's reagent (page 1048).

Procedure. Add a microdrop of sample (see footnote, page 1066) to approximately 0.1 ml. of acid-fuchsin reagent in a 10 mm. test tube. An immediate red to violet coloration indicates the presence of aldehydes or reactive ketones.

---

* Umberger, C. J., and Eagleson, D. A. Unpublished.

ISOLATION OF ALDEHYDES AND KETONES AS THE 2,4-DINITROPHENYL-HYDRAZINES. *Reagent.* A saturated solution (approximately 1 per cent) of 2,4-dinitrophenylhydrazine in 95 per cent alcohol containing 1 per cent hydrochloric acid.

Procedure. Add a drop of unknown to 2 drops of reagent in a 1 ml. centrifuge cone and mix by stirring with a glass fiber. If a precipitate does not separate immediately, allow the tube to stand several hours at room temperature. If crystallization does not occur, warm the tube gently in a bath, cork it and allow it to stand overnight. If a reaction is still not apparent, introduce a trace of concentrated hydrochloric acid by stirring with a glass fiber which has been dipped into concentrated hydrochloric acid. Cork the solution tightly (as in Mulliken, 53) and heat just below boiling temperature for 5 minutes and again allow to stand (54, 55). When crystals separate from the solution separate them from the liquid by centrifugation, wash with cold 95 per cent ethyl alcohol, and recrystallize them from hot chloroform or ethyl acetate. The melting point (56) of the 2,4-dinitrophenylhydrazine is determined on a Kofler hot stage.

FERROX TEST FOR OXYGEN-CONTAINING NEUTRALS. Davidson (57) introduced the ferrox test as a procedure in qualitative organic analysis to supplant the concentrated sulfuric acid solubility test of Kamm and the auxiliary solubility test of Shriner and Fuson with 85 per cent phosphoric acid for oxygen containing compounds. Davidson's test depends on the fact that ferric thiocyanate (correct name: ferric hexathiocyanatocyanate) is insoluble in saturated and unsaturated aliphatic and aromatic hydrocarbons and their halides but is readily soluble in liquid compounds containing neutral oxygen, particularly alcohols and ethers. It also becomes soluble in a saturated hydrocarbon after a liquid or solid oxygen-containing neutral has been dissolved in it. Only a trace of ferric thiocyanate is required to impart a deep red color to the solution and, in the absence of structures containing nitrogen and sulfur linkages,* the appearance of a red color after the addition of a small particle of the solid to an anhydrous organic solution is indicative of alcohols, ethers, aldehydes, ketones or esters. In Davidson's procedure, filter paper is impregnated with ferric thiocyanate, cut into 3 mm. squares, and a square of paper is immersed in a drop of unknown. In conjunction with the hydroxamic acid test for esters (page 1066) and the 3,5-dinitrobenzoic acid test for ketones (page 1067), the ferrox test may be used to rule out the possibility of the presence of ethers and inert esters and ketones in the rectified distillate.

Preparation of the Ferrox Paper. Dissolve 1 gm. ferric chloride and 1 gm. KCNS in 10 ml. of absolute methyl alcohol and filter off the precipitate of potassium chloride. Drench the paper with the solution and quickly air dry. Repeat until the paper assumes a greenish tinge. Cut into 3 mm. squares and store in a dark bottle containing sodium sulfate decahydrate as a humidifying agent.

Procedure. Dehydrate the sample by adding several milligrams of calcium oxide to a drop of unknown contained in a microcentrifuge cone and allow it to stand until anhydrous. Insert a square of the reagent paper into the drop and note any coloration imparted to the unknown. The reagent is very sensitive to ethyl ether.

PHLOROGLUCINOL-CYCLOPENTANOL TEST FOR HALOGENATED HYDROCARBONS. The presence of chloroform, chloral hydrate and carbon tetrachloride will have been established from tests performed directly on the distillate (pages 1052 to 1053). If the presence of one of the other halogenated solvents is indicated, this test will

---

* Amides and a number of thio compounds react positively.

confirm the findings and will establish the halogenated solvent as being one of the more volatile members.

Procedure. The test works only when applied to an aqueous suspension of the compound. Add a drop of unknown to a test tube containing one fourth of a pellet of solid sodium hydroxide overlayed with 2 ml. of water. Carry out the procedure as described on page 1052.

IDENTIFICATION OF ALIPHATIC HYDROCARBONS. Aliphatic compounds are characterized by their nonreactivity and will be indicated only when the findings in the tests for the other types of molecules are negative. The odor may be suggestive, but the presence of tissue or natural impurities may mask the hydrocarbon odor. Aliphatic hydrocarbons are invariably encountered in toxicology as complex mixtures in commercial preparations. Fortunately, deaths in which this type of preparation is involved are usually accompanied by a history suggestive of the lethal agent. If the mixture is isolated in a general unknown, the true identity of the preparation can seldom be established. Cyano esters with a hydrocarbon are indicative of fly sprays (see pages 1053, 1062). A high percentage of unsaturated hydrocarbons (see page 1065 for test), with or without an objectionable odor and traces of sulfur compounds (see page 1053 for test), indicates a cheap grade of naphtha (gas naphtha). A positive reaction for aromatic hydrocarbons (pages 1065, 1073), with a high percentage of high-boiling aliphatic hydrocarbons (see pages 1071-1072), would be indicative of a fuel oil from coal tar. Almost all of the aliphatic hydrocarbon mixtures for industrial use are obtained from the destructive distillation and cracking of petroleum (58). Petroleum ether (benzin) is a purified aliphatic hydrocarbon fraction boiling between 30° and 60° C.,* used principally as a fat solvent. Petroleum benzine is a higher fraction boiling between 40° and 90° C. Naphtha is a more complex mixture from either a petroleum or tar distillate of varying grades of purity; it is used extensively in dry cleaning and dewaxing and has a boiling range which is approximately between 60° and 120° C. Ligroin is a commercial solvent which boils between 90° and 102° C., and benzine or benzine-naphtha is a solvent fraction boiling between 110° and 150° C.

Gasoline is a mixture of hydrocarbons having a variable and wide range for the boiling temperature of the components. Approximately 10 per cent boils below 65° C. and practically all is volatile below 200° C. It is rich in octane, with saturated hydrocarbons from pentane up, depending on the grade and blend. Kerosene is a higher boiling fraction than the others and is used principally as a low boiling fuel or cheap solvent. It is of variable purity † depending on the source. The major components are aliphatic hydrocarbons, but significant amounts of unsaturated compounds and small amounts of aromatic compounds may be present. The boiling range may be from 150° to 300° C. with the major fraction boiling above 200° C. Small amounts of volatiles may come over well below 150° C. Since the mixture is predominantly decanes and larger molecules, the major portion will appear in the undistilled fraction of the distillate (pages 1064, 1071). Although commercial fuel oil contains a much higher percentage of high-boiling components than kerosene, a small amount of volatile hydrocarbons may be isolated from it in the rectified fraction. The source may be either petroleum or tar and,

---

* Microboiling points by the capillary method (page 1065) are of no value for mixtures, since the indicated boiling temperature is only that of the low-boiling component.

† The term purity as used here refers to the absence of unsaturated or aromatic hydrocarbons as well as other structures.

from either source, the mixture might be composed of saturated aliphatic hydro-carbons alone or aliphatics with varying amounts of unsaturated components and aromatics. The purity of kerosene and fuel oil depends on the efficiency of the concentrated sulfuric acid treatment and, with the modern tendency to isolate all possible by-products, these commercial mixtures are likely to be practically free of all but the saturated aliphatic series.

1. Dimethylsulfate Test. A negative test for alcohols on the distillate (pages 1048-1050) and negative findings for compounds with reactive functional groups (pages 1065-1070) are indicative of the presence of aliphatic hydrocarbons. However, positive findings do not rule out the presence of saturated aliphatic compounds, since these sensitive methods will detect reactive compounds in a hydrocarbon mixture. The solubility test with dimethyl sulfate may be used to indicate saturated hydrocarbons in a complex mixture (59, 60).

Procedure. Layer a small drop of dimethyl sulfate over an equal volume of unknown in a melting point capillary by the technic described on page 1066 for the determination of unsaturations. Quickly observe the capillary under a low power objective on a microscope with a micrometer eyepiece, and measure the lengths of the two liquid layers. Then seal the open end of the capillary and mix the contents by centrifugation with inversion of the capillary tube. Again measure the two layers with the micrometer eyepiece and compare the ratios of the lengths before and after centrifugation. Aromatic hydrocarbons, in general, dissolve in all proportions, probably due to the formation of addition products between the ester and aromatic nucleus. The solubility of the alkyl halides is significant and variable, depending on the structure of the halogen derivative.

Examination of the Hydrocarbon Mixtures by Infrared Absorption. Determination of the infrared absorption is the only reliable procedure for evaluating mixtures of inert compounds in which the quantity is not sufficient or in which the mixture is too complex to permit separation of the components. It is particularly suitable for hydrocarbons since absorption curves for practically all of the members of the various series are available in the literature pertaining to petroleum and allied products. In a mixture, the absorption characteristics of the components are additive, so that considerable information can be obtained from the curves of very complex solutions. The absorption spectra of the aliphatic hydrocarbons are quite simple compared with those for molecules containing reactive functional groups and, even though the identity of any of the separate components may not be apparent, the presence of significant concentrations of other substances in the mixture may be ruled out. The sensitivity for the detection of compounds by infrared analysis is considerably less than by other analytic methods. With this particular type of sample, the lack of sensitivity is an advantage because small concentrations of impurities in the sample material or from tissue breakdown will not interfere with the pattern for the major components.

Recent developments in infrared instrumentation have removed many of the technical difficulties associated with infrared analysis. Introduction of the double beam compensated and recording infrared spectrophotometer has changed infrared analysis from a technic restricted to research to an analytic tool for the chemist. The compensating and recording features are indispensable for the usual type of medicolegal problem requiring infrared for solution. However, application to the analysis of the volatiles is an exception, because the liquid samples do not require solution in a solvent. Since the need for compensation is eliminated, the apparatus is used as a single beam instrument. A cell depth of 0.1 mm. or less is adequate. Two or three drops of sample are sufficient to fill the cavity of the macrocell. The only restriction is that the sample material be anhydrous and that methyl alcohol and other reactive chemicals which corrode the sodium chloride cell windows be absent. The rectified samples may be rendered sufficiently free of moisture by cooling in the dry ice-acetone bath to a temperature low enough to cause any dissolved water to solidify.

Additional information may be obtained by determining the absorption spectrum of several dilutions of the sample using chloroform as the solvent (61). In this case the compensating feature of the spectrophotometer is used with pure chloroform as the reference. By analyzing a series of dilutions in steps such as 1:2, 1:4, 1:8, 1:16, and so on, the absorption spectrum of the major component of the mixture will be the last to disappear.*

In those cases in which a history is available or, better still, when a sample of the suspected poison has been submitted as evidence, the analyst will save time and material by proceeding directly to infrared analysis after isolation of the sample by rectification. This applies to any type of volatile compound or mixture discussed under the heading of volatiles. By running an absorption curve on the isolated sample, using the spectrophotometer as a single beam instrument and comparing its curve with that of the known sample similarly treated, the identity of the unknown will be apparent from the absorption spectra. Moreover, if both samples are run using the compensation system with either sample as the reference, the similarity in composition will be shown by the absence of absorption bands in the spectrum, due to the compensation in the absorption of the solution in the sample beam by the one in the reference beam of the spectrophotometer.

Confirmatory Tests for Special Low Boiling Volatiles. Iso-Amyl Nitrite. The use of iso-amyl nitrite in medicine is now rare, and the probability of encountering this compound in a toxicologic analysis is remote. Its presence in insignificant concentrations in the distillate would be indicated by a positive diphenylamine reaction (page 1055). Because of its volatility, it is very likely to be lost during the procedure for isolating the organic oxidants (page 1056). Failure to recover an oxidizing substance and the absence of inorganic nitrites should lead to the application of the diphenylamine-sulfuric acid reaction on the rectified distillate. If the results of that test are positive, the test for iso-amyl nitrite should be performed.

Eijkman's Reaction (62). Wet the end of a stirring rod with the unknown and dip it into about 0.1 ml. of approximately 1 per cent phenol in 95 per cent ethyl alcohol. Carefully layer 3 to 4 drops of concentrated sulfuric acid underneath the alcohol solution. A red ring at the interface is indicative of the presence of nitrite.

Ethyl Ether. Since ethyl ether is usually encountered in cases in which death occurred under ether anesthesia, the presence of the compound is known from the circumstances and the problem is only to determine the level at the time of death. If the case should be a general unknown, the microboiling point (page 1065) plus the odor should be an indication. Confirmation may be made by conversion of the ether to ethyl iodide, using the apparatus described on page 1093 for the quanti-

---

* This is analogous to the dilution method in spectrographic analysis in which the concentration is determined by the dilution at which a persistent line starts to disappear. It assumes that the mixture is composed of components which have comparable molecular extinction coefficients, as occurs in a homologous series. Obviously, the presence of a lower concentration of a highly absorbing compound would lead to an erroneous interpretation, particularly if the other structures were the hydrocarbons with relatively weak absorption.

tative ethoxy determination of small quantities of ethyl and methyl alcohol, substituting an empty receiver flask submerged in dry ice and acetone for the flask containing the absorbing solution. A quantitative analysis can be made by the same procedure for alcohol.

$$\text{mg. ethyl ether} = \text{ml. sodium thiosulfate} \times \text{normality of the sodium thiosulfate} \times 6.15$$

Siegel (63) has developed a quantitative method for ether based on the dichromate oxidation.

BENZENE: QUANTITATIVE DETERMINATION. Indications of the presence of aromatic hydrocarbons from positive findings with the formaldehyde-sulfuric acid reaction (page 1065), after the elimination of reactive unsaturated hydrocarbon interference by means of the bromine-unsaturation test (page 1065), justify a quantitative analysis for benzene. A quantitative determination is essential whether the aromatic compound is the only substance present or is one component in a mixture. At the same time, the quantitative analysis serves as a qualitative test to further confirm the presence of benzene or closely related substances.

The method of Yant, Schrenk, and Mantz (64, 65) for the determination of benzene in biologic material and air may be applied to the isolated volatile fraction, to the aqueous distillate, or directly to the frozen tissue with equal success. In the case of an unknown, the rectified sample will be available and is therefore the most logical source of sample material. Although the precision will be less than that for a determination made directly on the tissue, any added error due to recovery losses will be more than compensated for by the information concerning the ratio of the aromatics to the other volatile components when the sample is a mixture. The method is an application of the Janovsky reaction for ketones with *meta*-dinitrobenzene (pages 1068, 1228).

Reagents. (a) Nitrating mixture: equal volumes of fuming nitric acid and concentrated sulfuric acid.

(b) 10 N sodium hydroxide: 40 gm. sodium hydroxide per 100 ml.

(c) Sodium nitrate-sodium sulfate solution: 1.32 gm. $NaNO_3 + 0.67$ gm. sodium sulfate per 100 ml.

(d) Commercial methyl ethyl ketone.

(e) Standard *meta*-dinitrobenzene solution: 53.8 mg. *meta*-dinitrobenzene per 5 ml. of nitrating mixture (1 ml. is equivalent to 5 mg. of benzene).

Procedure. Introduce 1 ml. of nitrating mixture into a 50 ml. pyrex® NPN test tube and let stand in the icebox until cool. Pipet off 0.05 ml. of the rectified distillate with a blood counting pipet for leukocytes, wiping off the tip of the pipet with cotton. Slowly add the distillate to the nitrating mixture by placing the pipet into the test tube and carefully pinching the rubber connecting tube of the pipet so that the displaced air forces the liquid sample into the cooled reagent. Mix by shaking and allow the tube to stand at room temperature for half an hour. Dilute the acid mixture with 2 ml. of distilled water, cool to 0° to 10° C. in an ice-salt bath and make the acid mixture neutral to litmus by a dropwise addition of 10 N sodium hydroxide from a buret. Then add 0.1 ml. excess of alkali. Warm the solution to slightly above room temperature (30° C.), add 10 ml. of methyl ethyl ketone, stopper the tube, and shake occasionally over a period of 10 minutes. Centrifuge, or let stand, until the layers separate. Pipet 5 ml. of the methyl ethyl ketone layer into a separate tube, add 0.75 ml. of 10 N sodium hydroxide, shake vigorously several minutes and then occasionally for more than one hour to allow the red color to develop fully. One ml. of standard *meta*-dinitrobenzene nitrating mixture containing the equivalent of 5 mg. of benzene is run simultaneously with the unknown.

The method as worked out for benzene in air is for much lower concentrations (0.01 to 0.06 mg.) than will be encountered in 0.05 ml. of rectified distillate in a case of benzene poisoning. Both the unknown and the standard will show color intensities that are too intense for quantitative comparisons and appropriate dilutions will be necessary before the transmission can be read in a colorimeter.*

According to the authors, it is necessary to maintain a constant salt concentration in the methyl ethyl ketone aliquot prepared from the standard and unknown solution for quantitative comparison.† In making appropriate dilutions for optimal color intensity, an aliquot of the solution is diluted with methyl ethyl ketone to a measured volume, shaken out with sodium nitrate-sodium sulfate solution in the proportion of 0.1 ml. of salt solution per milliliter of pure methyl ethyl ketone, and 10 N sodium hydroxide is added. The reagents are added in amounts to maintain the same conditions as in the original solution. For example, if the dilution is 1:10 with the addition of 9.0 ml. of methyl ethyl ketone to 1.0 ml. of the original, then 9 ml. of sodium nitrate-sodium sulfate solution and 1.5 ml. of 10 N sodium hydroxide are used.

ANALYSIS OF THE UNDISTILLED PORTION OF THE FRACTIONATED DISTILLATE

The major portion of the higher boiling volatiles will be held back by the fractionating column in the fractional distillation (page 1063). Significant amounts of any compounds with boiling points close to and slightly above 100° C. may pass over with the water in the second fraction of distillate; however the possibilities are few, and since all such compounds are water insoluble, their presence in this fraction will be indicated by a turbidity or oil dispersed in the distillate. If there is any indication of the presence of a compound in the second fraction, it is saturated with sodium chloride, extracted with ether and chloroform, and the residue is subjected to the tests to be described for the residue for the undistilled portion.

These residues will contain the higher boiling compounds of any mixture and, in those cases in which more than one compound was present in the rectified fraction, it is highly probable that a greater proportion of the mixture will be found in one or more of the residues from the extraction. All organic structures discussed under the examination of the rectified distillate are possible, with the exception of special compounds such as benzene and ethyl ether which can be eliminated because of their low volatility. Most of the components of kerosene, gasoline, naphtha and coal tar solvent mixtures are higher boiling compounds. Halogenated compounds, commercially used aldehydes, ketones, esters and ethers of higher molecular weight are possibilities that may be detected by repeating the tests described

---

* The best color intensity for photometric measurements is at transmissions of approximately 38 per cent.

† The color intensity is a function of the solubility of the NaOH in the methyl ethyl ketone solution and the salts present from neutralization of the nitrating mixture reduce the NaOH solubility in the methyl ethyl ketone.

for the rectified fraction. Oxidants (other than iso-amyl nitrite), the fusel oils, turpentine and thiocyano esters will not appear in the rectified fraction and tests for their detection are added. In addition, a few nitrogen- and sulfur-containing neutrals would be isolated in the residues from the extraction and, therefore, provision is made to exclude such compounds as possibilities.

Tests Described Under the Examination of the Rectified Fraction of the Distillate. 1. Formaldehyde-sulfuric acid reaction for aromatic ring compounds (page 1065).

2. Bromine-carbon tetrachloride addition reaction for aliphatic unsaturated compounds (page 1065).

3. Hydroxamic acid test for esters (page 1066).

4. 3,5-dinitrobenzoic acid test for ketones (page 1067).

5. Fuchsin test for aldehydes (page 1068).

6. Ferrox test for ethers (page 1069).

7. Dimethyl sulfate solubility test for saturated aliphatic compounds (page 1071).

8. Infrared spectrophotometric examination (page 1071).

Tests for the Detection of Organic Structures Not Indicated by the Reactions Previously Described. OXIDIZING COMPOUNDS (page 1055). Wet the end of a stirring rod with the unknown and mix with a drop of diphenylamine reagent (page 1055) on a glass slide. A deep blue color indicates the presence of an oxidizing compound.

THIOCYANO ESTERS. If kerosene is found, the test for thiocyano esters (page 1062) should be repeated at this point even if it is negative on the residue from the solvent extraction of the distillate (page 1055). Because of the relatively poor recovery by steam distillation, the concentration of thiocyano esters isolated by direct extraction of the distillate may be below the sensitivity of the method. If they are present, their concentration will be maximum in this portion of the original steam distillate.

Higher Molecular Weight Alcohols and Turpentine. VANILLIN-SULFURIC ACID REACTION. Alcohols from propyl up react with complex aldehydes in concentrated sulfuric acid on heating to give colors.* The reaction with alcohols and vanillin-sulfuric acid is less sensitive than that for phenols (pages 1056-1058) although a few of them, particularly those of higher molecular weight, give colorations in the cold. Normal-amyl alcohol gives an intense violet color which changes to indigo on standing. This differentiates it from iso-amyl alcohol which only gives a light green, increasing in intensity on standing. Iso-butyl alcohol is the lowest molecular weight member that gives a definite color without heat. The alkyne alcohol sedative, methylparafynol, gives an intense maroon color in the cold, while benzyl alcohol gives a flesh colored precipitate. Turpentine gives an immediate deep orange-brown coloration which distinguishes it from the mineral spirits used in painting as a turpentine substitute. Because of the variety of substances giving a positive reaction, this test serves only as an exclusion reaction in which negative findings eliminate the positive reacting substance as possibilities. Some positive-reacting compounds that will not have been indicated by previous tests are tabulated in Table 45-6.

---

* Dimethylaminobenzaldehyde, salicylaldehyde and furfural in concentrated sulfuric acid have also been used as reagents for the alcohols.

Table 45-6.   Color Reactions in Vanillin-Sulfuric Acid Test for Alcohols *

COMPOUND	COLOR DEVELOPED IN COLD	COLOR ON WARMING TO SO_3 FUMES
n-Amyl Alcohol	violet → indigo	blue violet → blue
iso-Butyl alcohol	reddish → maroon	blue violet → blue
Methylparafynol	maroon	maroon
Octyl alcohol	light green → blue green	violet
Benzyl alcohol	flesh colored precipitate	green
Turpentine	orange brown	maroon
iso-Amyl alcohol	light green → darker green	maroon
n-Propyl alcohol	negative	reddish violet
n-Butyl alcohol	negative	reddish violet
Mineral spirits †	negative	rose → blue
Mineral oil ‡	negative	negative

* See page 1057 for reagent.

† Mineral spirits is a mineral oil distillate with kerosene-like odor containing fewer of the high boiling hydrocarbons. The coloration is apparently due to impurities in the mixture.

‡ Mineral oil or higher boiling alcohols, when used as antifoam agents, may be mechanically carried over and recovered in the residue. Mineral oil may be detected by its insolubility in 95 per cent ethyl alcohol.

GENERIC TEST FOR ALCOHOLS (36). *Reagents.* (a) solid benzoyl peroxide; (b) nitrobenzene; (c) acid fuchsin-Schiff's reagent (page 1048).

Procedure. Add 3 drops of nitrobenzene and 1 drop of unknown to 20 to 30 mg. of benzoyl peroxide in a 3 inch test tube. Tightly stopper (as in Mulliken, 53). Heat in a boiling water bath for 5 minutes. Cool and add 4 drops of Schiff's reagent and mix by shaking. Observe the color after the two layers separate and again after standing 30 minutes. The formation of the sulfite addition compound is relatively slow with some of the high molecular weight aldehydes, but a strong violet color develops in all of them within half an hour. The control remains yellow.*

Table 45-7.   Color Development in Benzoyl Peroxide-Nitrobenzene Test for Alcohols *

COMPOUND	COLOR DEVELOPMENT AFTER 30 MINUTES
Methyl alcohol	2 +
Ethyl alcohol	3 +
n-Propyl alcohol	4 +
iso-Propyl alcohol	0
n-Butyl alcohol	4 +
iso-Butyl alcohol	4 +
n-Amyl alcohol	4 +
iso-Amyl alcohol	4 +
Octyl alcohol	3 +
Benzyl alcohol	1 +
Methylparafynol †	4 +
Turpentine ‡	2 +
Commercial mineral spirits	1 +
Fusel oil	4 +

* The relative intensities are based on the maximum color development, scaled from one plus to four plus.

† Methylparafynol can be differentiated from the other compounds by its immediate strong (4 +) reaction in the cold.

‡ Oil of turpentine contains the alcohol terpineol as well as other hydroxy compounds.

CONFIRMATORY TEST FOR METHYLPARAFYNOL.† *Reagent.* Ammoniacal silver nitrate: concentrated NH_4OH added dropwise, with shaking, to 10 per cent silver nitrate until the precipitate of silver oxide is just dissolved.

* After 1 to 2 hours, the control test will begin to show a slight pink to violet coloration.

† This test is characteristic of the alkyne linkage which may be partially or entirely reduced by the detoxification process in the body.

Procedure. Add a drop of ammoniacal silver nitrate to a drop of methylparafynol on a microscope slide. An immediate heavy white precipitate is formed.

Differentiation of Turpentine.† Concentrated sulfuric acid distinguishes turpentine from all of the alcohols except methylparafynol. The addition of a drop of the acid produces an intense brown coloration which develops a red cast on standing. Mineral spirits does not produce a color with sulfuric acid.

1. Distinction Between Turpentine and Methylparafynol. A drop of tetranitromethane added to a drop of turpentine produces an intense orange color whereas methylparafynol does not react with this reagent. Mineral spirits gives a yellow color much less intense than that with turpentine.

2. Differentiation Between Turpentine and Pine Oil (68). Some grades of pine oil have a turpentine-like odor and react chemically like oil of turpentine. In addition, commercial turpentine sometimes contains pine oil as a diluent. Pine oil differs from oil of turpentine by the presence of reducing substances which are capable of converting ferricyanide to ferrocyanide.

Reagents. (a) 0.4 per cent ferric chloride, prepared fresh; (b) 0.2 per cent potassium ferricyanide, prepared fresh.

Mix equal volumes of (a) and (b).

Procedure. Add 2 drops of oil to 0.5 ml. of a mixture of equal volumes of the reagents and shake thoroughly. The formation of a precipitate of Prussian blue indicates the presence of reducing substances in the oil.

ANALYSIS OF THE ALKALINE STEAM DISTILLATE FOR VOLATILE BASES

Detection of Ammonia. (1). The presence of ammonia in suicide cases is indicated at autopsy by its odor and by the corrosion of the esophagus. It is best detected in the original stomach contents. Ammonia is formed in small amounts during the alkaline steam distillation of fresh tissue and in larger amounts in the presence of moderate to extensive putrefaction. Its presence in the distillate may complicate the detection of strong organic bases and for this reason its relative concentration in the distillates should be known. Comparison of the first 100 ml. fraction of the steam distillate with the second 150 ml. portion will differentiate ingested ammonia from that formed by tissue degradation. When the ammonia is from tissue breakdown, the second fraction will contain as much ammonia as the first fraction, or more.

Procedure. Dilute 4 ml. of distillate with water until the basic odor is barely detectable, recording the amount of dilution. Add 12 drops of 40 per cent formaldehyde to 4 ml. of solution. If a precipitate forms, remove it by filtration. Heat the clear solution nearly to boiling, let stand one minute, cool to room temperature and add 10 drops of a solution containing 12.5 gm. of I_2 and 16.5 gm. of KI per 100 ml. of solution. Shake and let stand 5 minutes. Hexamethylenetetramine tetraiodide ($C_6H_{12}N_4I_4$) is formed. It starts to darken at 115° C., and melts with decomposition at 200° to 204° C. One mg. of NH_3 per 4 ml. of solution will give a detectable precipitate which settles on standing for 4 to 10 minutes.

Confirmatory Test for Ammonia. Evaporate a portion of the distillate to dryness in a 6 inch test tube after making it acid to Congo red paper with N/10 HCl. Heat the residue gently by flaming the bottom of the tube with a bunsen burner. NH_4Cl sublimes at room temperature without melting or decomposition. The hydro-

---

† The color tests described for turpentine are only manifestations of the reactions of turpentine with sulfuric acid alone (66, 67).

chlorides of low molecular weight amines melt and darken in the free flame of the burner.

Examination of the Distillate for Organic Bases. The presence of basic organic poisons, volatile with steam, is detected by means of the indicator reactions described on page 1151. A small portion of the distillate is tested or an ether extract of a small portion is evaporated in a test tube and the test performed on the residue. Evaporation of the last portion of ether should be allowed to proceed spontaneously to avoid overlooking volatile aliphatic bases.

Procedure for Isolation. Make the distillate basic with NaOH, transfer to a 500 ml. separatory funnel and shake out with 250 ml. portions of ether. Evaporate about 10 ml. of the ether by dropwise addition to a watch glass placed on a hot plate at 60° C. Observe the odor during evaporation and check the alkalinity of the residue. A very basic liquid suggests the presence of aliphatic amines. To the remaining ether solution, add 2 drops of N/10 hydrochloric acid * and set on the steam bath until all but about 1 ml. of the ether has evaporated. Remove the beaker and allow final evaporation to take place at room temperature.

TEST FOR PRIMARY AND SECONDARY ALIPHATIC AMINES. Volatile primary and secondary aliphatic amines can be identified more readily after isolation by steam distillation than in the residue after extraction for the nonvolatile poisons. The free aliphatic bases react readily with carbon disulfide to form dithiocarbamates which break down, with the formation of sulfide ion, on treatment with a nitric acid solution of silver nitrate (2).

A portion of the residue is re-extracted with ether from a NaOH solution. The ether is evaporated at below boiling temperature in a round bottom microbeaker. A strip of filter paper the size of a piece of litmus paper is dipped in the ether while it is evaporating. The amine remains on the filter paper after evaporation of the ether. Add 3 drops of a solution containing equal volumes of carbon disulfide-ethyl alcohol to one end of the paper and allow it to diffuse along the paper strip. After the paper has completely air dried, add 1 drop of the silver nitrate-nitric acid reagent as used in the test for chloride ion. Blackening due to AgS, with effervescence from the liberation of nitrogen, indicates that the basic compound is aliphatic.

TEST FOR PRIMARY ARYLAMINES BY THE CARBYLAMINE REACTION. Primary amines, except those of high molecular weight, react with chloroform, in the presence of strong alkali, to give isocyanides recognized by their nauseating and penetrating odors.

$$RNH_2 + HCCl_3 + 3\ KOH \rightarrow RNC + 3\ KCl + 3\ H_2O$$

Aniline is the most probable low molecular weight aromatic amine.

Procedure. Transfer a small portion of the residue from the ether extract of the distillate (see above) to a microtest tube and add 0.25 ml. of an ethyl alcohol solution prepared by dissolving a pellet of KOH in 1 ml. of 95 per cent ethyl alcohol. Add 2 drops of chloroform and warm gently until the solution comes to a boil. Note the odor and, if a carbylamine is not detected, wait for 2 minutes and again heat to boiling. Aniline gives an immediate reaction. Secondary and tertiary amines do not react.

Detection of Aniline. Dissolve a portion of the ether residue from the extract of the distillate in about 0.5 ml. water in a centrifuge tube and add saturated bromine

---

* Many acetate salts of organic bases are volatile.

water dropwise until a permanent yellow color persists. Centrifuge the precipitate, wash by suspending in water, recentrifuge, and transfer to a porous tile to dry. Aniline reacts with bromine water, forming the tribromaniline which melts at 118° C.

CONFIRMATORY TEST FOR AROMATIC AMINES (FURFURAL-ACETIC ACID REAGENT) (3). Furfural in an alcohol-glacial acetic acid solution condenses with primary arylamino groups that are distinctly basic in character, producing deep red colors. Aniline, the toluidines, *para*-phenylendiamine, *para*-aminophenol and the aminobenzoic acids are equally sensitive toward the reagent. Secondary and tertiary arylamines and tertiary cyclic amines like pyridine and piperidine, as well as all aliphatic amines do not give colors with the reagent. As a generic test, the furfural reaction is almost as specific as the carbylamine reaction and the ease with which it is performed makes it preferable in some respects as first choice for the arylamine-indicating reaction. In the few anomalies that have been observed, colors other than red developed or precipitates were formed.

Reagent. 0.25 ml. furfural added to a mixture of 2.25 ml. of 95 per cent ethyl alcohol and 7.5 ml. glacial acetic acid.

Procedure. Add a drop of reagent to a crystal of the hydrochloride residue from the ether extract of the distillate (page 1078). A deep red to maroon coloration indicates the presence of an arylamine.

TESTS FOR CYCLIC BASES AND TERTIARY ALIPHATIC AMINES. 1. Precipitation with 10 Per Cent Alcoholic Picric Acid. Add a microdrop of 10 per cent picric acid in 95 per cent ethyl alcohol to a drop of base isolated from the distillate by ether extraction. Volatile compounds with pyridine, piperidine, pyrrole, pyrroline, pyrrolidine, quinoline and isoquinoline structures give an immediate white or yellow precipitate. Pyridine is not precipitated by aqueous picric acid.

2. Formation of Iodomethylates with Methyl Iodide. Tertiary aliphatic amines and cyclic nitrogen bases form addition products with methyl iodide. A few aliphatic secondary amines and an occasional primary amine will react but these will have been excluded by the test described on page 1078.

Procedure. Add methyl iodide to the base contained in a capillary test tube in the ratio of 1 drop of base to 2 drops of CH_3I. Reactive bases such as piperidine form an immediate precipitate with fuming and the development of heat. If a precipitate does not form, seal the open end of the test tube with a burner and submerge the tube in a hot water bath maintained at a little below boiling temperature for about 30 minutes. Remove the test tube and cool under the cold water tap. A precipitate on the walls of the tube is indicative of the formation of an iodomethylate (4).

REDUCTION TEST WITH TOLLEN'S REAGENT (5). Tollen's reagent is reduced by many nitrogen-containing organics of the most diverse type. However, there are no reducing basic drugs that are volatile with steam and a positive reducing test indicates the presence of a commercial preparation for industrial use, such as an intermediate dyestuff, rather than a pharmaceutical preparation. The literature covering basic substances encountered as industrial hazards should be consulted if the test is not negative (6).

Reagents. (a) 10 per cent $AgNO_3$ in 1 volume concentrated NH_4OH + 1 volume of water; (b) 10 per cent aqueous NaOH.

Add equal volumes of (a) and (b) just before using.

Procedure. Place a small portion of the residue from the ether extract of the distillate on a microscope slide and add 1 drop of Tollen's reagent. Let stand in the cold (the reagent gives a black precipitate if warmed) and observe after 5 minutes. A positive test is indicated by a black grayish or brownish black precipitate or a silver mirror.

Tests for the other volatile bases are described in Chapter 47.

REFERENCES

1. Mulliken, S. P.   A Method for the Identification of Pure Organic Compounds, New York, John Wiley and Sons, Inc., 1916, Vol. II, p. 20.
2. Feigl, F.   Spot Tests, New York, Elsevier-Nordeman Co., 1939, p. 304.
3. Frehden, O., and Goldschmidt, L.   The use of spot tests for the testing of drugs. II. New tests for amines with particular attention to p-phenylenediamine, Mikrochim. Acta, 1:338, 1937.
4. Feigl, F.   Spot Tests, New York, Elsevier-Nordeman Co., 1939, p. 326.
5. Mulliken, S. P.   A Method for the Identification of Pure Organic Compounds, New York, John Wiley and Sons, Inc., 1904, Vol. I, p. 22.
6. Jacobs, M. B.   Analytical Chemistry of Industrial Poisons, Hazards and Solvents, New York, Interscience Publishers, Inc., 1941.
7. Feldstein, M.   Personal communication, May, 1952.
8. Merley, R. W., and Bueding, E.   Systematic qualitative analysis of biological materials for common steam volatile organic poisons, J. Lab. & Clin. Med., 33:371, 1948.
9. Siegel, H., and Schwartz, H.   Positive methyl alcohol reactions in the tissues of a young person dying in diabetic coma, J.A.M.A., 141:194, 1949.
10. Feigl, F.   Spot Tests, New York, Elsevier-Nordeman Co., 1939, pp. 33-34.
11. Goldbaum, L.   Personal communication, May, 1952.
12. Gettler, A. O., and Goldbaum, L.   Detection and estimation of microquantities of cyanide, Anal. Chem., 19:270, 1947.
13. ———— and Baine, J. O.   The toxicology of cyanide, Am. J. M. Sc., 195:182, 1938.
14. Weber, H. N.   Methods for the analysis of technical solvents. IV. Color tests for trichloroethylene, carbon tetrachloride and other chlorinated hydrocarbons of the aliphatic series, Chem. Ztg., 57:836, 1933.
15. Kamm, O.   Qualitative Organic Analysis, New York, John Wiley and Sons, Inc., 1922, p. 76.
16. Hickinbottom, W. J.   Reactions of Organic Compounds, New York, Longmans Green and Co., 1938, p. 106.
17. Feigl, F.   Spot Tests, New York, Elsevier-Nordeman Co., 1939, p. 195.
18. ———— Spot Tests, New York, Elsevier-Nordeman Co., 1939, p. 294.
19. Hickinbottom, W. J.   Reactions of Organic Compounds, New York, Longmans Green and Co., 1938, p. 106-108.
20. Hawk, P. B., Oser, B. L., and Summerson, W. H.   Practical Physiological Chemistry, 12th ed., New York, Blakiston Co., 1947, p. 129.
21. Jacobs, M. B.   Analytical Chemistry of Industrial Poisons, Hazards and Solvents, New York, Interscience Publishers, Inc., 1946, pp. 521-522.
22. Mulliken, S. P.   A Method for the Identification of Pure Organic Compounds, New York, John Wiley and Sons, Inc., 1916, Vol. II, pp. 23-50.
23. Hickinbottom, W. J.   Reaction of Organic Compounds, New York, Longmans Green and Co., 1938, pp. 311-333.
24. Methods of Analysis (Official and Tentative) of the Association of Official Agricultural Chemists, 3rd. ed., Washington, D. C., 1930, p. 405.
25. Pougnet, J.   A general reagent for phenols, Bull. sci. pharmacolog., 16:142, 1909.
26. van Urk, H. W.   p-dimethylaminobenzaldehyde as a reagent for organic drugs, Pharm. Weekblad., 66:101, 1929.
27. Carletti, O.   A borneol reaction, Boll. chim, farm., 75:299, 303, 1936.
28. Read.   Test for Differentiating Phenol and Creosote, cited by The Merck Index, 5th ed., Rahway, N. J., Merck and Co. Inc., 1940, p. 874.
29. The Merck Index.   Test #1620, 5th ed., Rahway, N. J., Merck & Co., 1940.
30. Griel, J. V., and Robinson, R. J.   Spectrophotometric characteristics for the determination of titanium with thymol, Anal. Chem., 23:1871, 1951.
31. Lehner, V., and Crawford, W. G.   A new colorimetric method for titanium, J. Am. Chem. Soc., 35:138, 1913.
32. Janovsky, J. V., and Erb, L.   Zur Kenntniss der directen Brom- und Nitrosubstitutions producte der Azokörper, Ber. d. deutsch. chem. Gesellsch., 19:2155, 1886.

33. Janovsky, J. V. Ueber eine Reaction der Dinitrokörper, Ber. d. deutsch. chem. Gesellsch., 24:971, 1891.
34. Bittó, von B. Ueber eine Reaction der Aldehyde und Ketone mit arom. Nitroverbindungen, Liebig's Annalen der Chemie, 269:377, 1892.
35. Reitzenstein, F., and Stamm, G. Janovsky's reaction for dinitro compounds and Bittó's reaction for aldehydes and ketones with aromatic compounds, J. prakt. Chem., 81:167, 1910.
36. Umberger, C. J. Unpublished data, Laboratory of the Chief Medical Examiner, City of New York.
37. Lobry de Bruyn, C. A. Le sodium et les alcalis caustistiques par rapport à quelques substances polynitrées, Rec. d. trav. chim. d. Pays-Bas, 14:89, 1895.
38. Smith, M. E., and Adkins, H. The relative reactivity of amines in the aminolysis of amides, J. Am. Chem. Soc., 60:657, 1938.
39. Umberger, C. J. Alcohol Normally Present in Blood, Ph.D. Thesis, New York University, 1940.
40. Allen and Chattaway, cited by Jacobs, M. B. Analytical Chemistry of Industrial Poisons, Hazards and Solvents, New York, Interscience Publishers, Inc., 1941.
41. Marquardt, L. Quantitative Bestimmung des Fuselöls im Branntwein, Ber. d. deutsch. chem. Gesellsch., 15:1370, 1882.
42. Gettler, A. O., Niederl, J. B., and Benedetti-Pichler, A. A. The isolation, identification, and quantitative determination of ethyl alcohol normally present in human tissues, Mikrochemie, 11:167, 1932.
43. ——— and Siegel, H. Isolation of ether from human tissues, Arch. Path., 17:510, 1934.
44. ——— and Siegel, H. Quantitative isolation of ethyl alcohol from tissues of alcoholics, J. Clin. Path., 7:85, 1937.
45. ——— and Siegel, H. Isolation of ether from human tissues, Arch. Path., 17:510, 1934.
46. Great Britain Scientific and Industrial Research Dept. Methods for the Detection of Toxic Gases in Industry. Benzene Vapor, Leaflet #4, London, H. M. Stationery Office, 1939.
47. Shriner, R. L., and Fuson, R. C. The Systematic Identification of Organic Compounds, 2nd ed., New York, John Wiley and Sons, Inc., 1940, p. 36.
48. Feigl, F. Spot Tests, New York, Elsevier-Nordeman Co., 1939, p. 295.
49. Schmall, M., Houghton, R. E., and Wollish, E. G. Applications of the reaction of hydroxylamine with esters of p-hydroxy benzoic acid, presented at the meeting of the Northern New Jersey Section of the American Chemical Society, January 28, 1952, Newark, New Jersey.
50. Umberger, C. J., and Stolman, A. A systematic approach to the identification of toxic organic compounds isolated from tissues and fluids. IV. Specific group tests, Ann. West. Med. & Surg., 6:232, 1952.
51. ——— and Eagleson, D. A. Unpublished data from the Laboratory of the Chief Medical Examiner, New York City, 1952.
52. Zimmerman, W. Eine Farbreaktion der Sexualhormone und ihre Anwendung zur Quantitativen colorimetrischen Bestimmung, Ztschr. f. physiol. Chem., 233:257, 1935.
53. Mulliken, S. P. A Method for the Identification of Pure Organic Compounds, New York, John Wiley and Sons, Inc., 1904, Vol. I, p. 112.
54. Allen, C. F. H. The identification of carbonyl compounds by use of 2,4-dinitrophenyl-hydrazine, J. Am. Chem. Soc., 52:2957, 1930.
55. Brady, O. L. The use of 2:4-dinitrophenylhydrazine as a reagent for carbonyl compounds, Journal of the Chemical Society, London, part 1:756, 1931.
56. Shriner, R. L., and Fuson, R. C. The Systematic Identification of Organic Compounds, 2nd ed., New York, John Wiley and Sons, Inc., 1940, pp. 221-224.
57. Davidson, D. A qualitative test for oxygen in organic compounds, Indust. Engin. Chem., Anal. Ed., 12:40, 1940.
58. Rogers, A. A Manual of Industrial Chemistry, 3rd ed., New York, D. Van Nostrand Co., Inc., 1919, p. 588.
59. Die chemische Industrie Rufslands. Ueber die Schädliche Einwirkung von Schwefelsäure dimethylester auf die Athmungsorgane, Chemische Industrie, 23:559, 1900.
60. Kamm, O. Qualitative Organic Analysis, 2nd ed., New York, John Wiley and Sons, Inc., 1938, p. 44.
61. Umberger, C. J., and Adams, G. Identification of malonyl urea derivatives, Anal. Chem., 24:1309, 1952.
62. Eijkman, J. F. Eine empfindliche Phenolreaction, Ztschr. f. anal. Chem., 22:576, 1883.
63. Siegel, H. Unpublished data, Laboratory of the Chief Medical Examiner, City of New York.
64. Yant, W. P., Schrenk, H. H., and Mantz, P. H. A Microcolorimetric Method for the Determination of Benzene, U. S. Bureau of Mines, Circular R. I. 3287, October, 1935.

65. Yant, W. P., Schrenk, H. H., and Mantz, P. H.   A Procedure for the Removal and Determination of Small Amounts of Benzene in Biological Material, U. S. Bureau of Mines, Circular R. I. 3282, August, 1935.

66. Dragendorff.   Reactions for Volatile Oils, cited by The Merck Index, 5th ed., Rahway, N. J., Merck & Co., Inc., 1940, p. 698.

67. Reichard.   Reaction for Terpineol, cited by The Merck Index, 5th ed., Rahway, N. J., Merck and Co. Inc., 1940, p. 876.

68. Wolff, H.   Pine oils (Kienöle), Farben Ztg., 17:1709, 1912.

46

Ethyl Alcohol

The fact that ethyl alcohol warrants a separate discussion under the heading of volatile poisons indicates its importance in the field of toxicology. Whether or not the vast amount of experimental work that has been done on this one substance is justified, in contrast to the relatively few investigations on other toxic substances, is a debatable question. Almost everyone concerned with the chemical aspects of analytic toxicology has done work on the alcohol problem at one time or another, and, from the volume of published literature, it might appear to one not familiar with the science that the field is concerned primarily with ethyl alcohol and its relation to alcoholic intoxication.

More methods have been recommended for the quantitative analysis of ethyl alcohol than for any entire class of the pharmaceuticals (1), yet all of them together comprise only five different analytic principles (2). The number of the published methods is evidence in itself that the interpretations from the analytic findings are not always undisputed.

Quantitative analysis of organs or body fluids for alcohol is primarily for the purpose of furnishing evidence about an individual's probable behavior and extent of responsibility at the time of sampling. Almost all of the experimental work, however, has been concerned with methods, rate of absorption, rate of oxidation, tolerance, distribution, and the ratio of the alcohol concentration in the different organs and body fluids. Unfortunately, no reliable test has been developed which will permit a quantitative measure of the physiologic response of an individual in relation to the alcohol level in the organs and fluids of the body (3, 4, 5, 6, 7). Most of the correlation between the degree of intoxication and *brain* alcohol levels has been based on the histories furnished to the investigator by the police or by witnesses after accidental or homicidal deaths.

A great deal has been written about the relative merits of one chemical method of analysis in comparison with others. In the process of developing any procedure for quantitative chemical analysis, the nature of the sample material, the number of determinations that must be made in a given time, the manipulative labor required for a single determination, the purpose for which the method is to be applied, and the precision * required for an interpretation, all influence the choice of a method. The aim, however, in any chemical procedure is for maximum precision with minimum time and manipulative labor irrespective of the significance which is to be placed on the final results. Conversely, interpretations of the final results from a quantitative chemical procedure have the same limitations regarding significance of the values as in any other type of precision measurement.

In any text which includes a discussion of errors and precision (8), the subject matter is developed starting with the fundamental rule that the precision of the final result can be no greater than that of the least precise factor entering into the com-

---

* Precision is defined as the narrowness of the limits within which true values may be assumed to lie with respect to the measured value.

putation. The purpose of a quantitative alcohol analysis is to permit evaluation of the degree of intoxication, but the physiologic response to varying alcohol concentrations in the organs cannot even be expressed in terms of values that have significance. Until a physiologic procedure is developed in which measurable values have a significance comparable to those in the chemical determinations, the values for the alcohol levels, regardless of their chemical accuracy,* are analogous in their physiologic significance to retail listings of items priced with the values used by the wholesaler in the cost accounting for bulk quantities. For example, a tenth of a cent may represent a large profit or loss to the wholesaler on bulk quantities but the retail purchaser cannot pay in tenths of a cent for a single item and listing a price in such terms has no meaning for him. Similarly, a tenth of a per cent error in the method is the ideal from a chemical standpoint, but unless the physiologic response to alcohol can be measured to this same precision, alcohol findings, listed within their chemical precision, cannot have the physiologic meaning that they imply.

From the point of view of the physiologic interpretation, the subject of alcohol methodology has been overemphasized, and, in this sense, the least desirable of the chemical methods for alcohol is adequate if it is without interference and follows the laws of stoicheiometry. For the same reason, the controversies on whether brain, blood, spinal fluid, saliva or urine is the most reliable criterion of intoxication are futile (9-21).

The questions of the precision of the degree of intoxication established from the chemical values and the precision of the analytic procedure used to determine those values are, therefore, two entirely different problems. From the chemical point of view, methodology in the analysis of ethyl alcohol is as important as in any other type of analysis, for the primary responsibility of the analyst is to the values reported. Before the question of interpretation can even be discussed, it must be shown that the findings are significant for alcohol only and that the values have been determined within the limits of accuracy that are accepted chemical practice. Particularly in contested cases, the analytic toxicologist, as a chemist, must be prepared to defend his findings. In the practice of analytic chemistry where certain procedures and technics, being less subject to error and criticism than others, take precedence, the final selection of a method for ethyl alcohol becomes more than a mere matter of choice. From the chemical standpoint, the toxicologist cannot permit the significance of the analytic values to be of the low order set by the limitations on predicting physiologic response to varying alcohol levels. In this difference of the two responsibilities of the analyst, namely, reliability of his values and the physiologic interpretation, lies the dilemma which produces the scientific arguments and contrasting opinions that are part of the subject of the toxicology of ethyl alcohol.

Survey of Analytic Methods. There are five analytic principles on which the published alcohol methods depend:

1. Oxidation to acetic acid.
2. Mild oxidation to acetaldehyde.
3. Conversion of ethyl alcohol to ethyl iodide.
4. Conversion of ethyl alcohol to ethyl nitrite.
5. Determination of the physical properties of the distillate.

---

* Accuracy is defined as the concurrence between the measured value and the true value.

Of these, only two meet the requirements for analysis of biologic materials. Almost all of the accepted alcohol procedures rely on oxidation of the alcohol to acetic acid and determination of the amount of acid produced or the amount of oxidizing agent consumed. All oxidation methods are open to the criticism that they are not specific for ethyl alcohol. The procedure assumes that all other possible reducing substances have been removed from the solution by purification steps or have been proven absent by a qualitative examination prior to the quantitative determination. The advantages of oxidation methods over others are the simplicity of the procedure and the relatively small amount of manipulative labor required for a series of analyses. It is the only type of method applicable for routine work in a medical examiner's laboratory where a series of determinations must be made each day.

Lack of specificity is only a minor objection when the analyses are performed by an experienced and competent analyst. With fresh tissue or body fluids, blank values from normally occurring volatile oxidizable components are negligible (22). The probability of the presence of another volatile reducing substance in blood in amounts comparable to ethyl alcohol without accompanying signs or symptoms of a toxic poison is remote. Ketone bodies produced in diabetic coma are eliminated if the method includes purification as a part of the procedure. Moreover, interference from ketone bodies does not produce values calculated as alcohol that would lead to an interpretation of intoxication. Methyl alcohol, isopropyl alcohol, paraldehyde and other interfering compounds have been eliminated by the qualitative examination. Quantitative alcohol values on putrefied or embalmed samples are not reliable (pages 1111, 1115) and are of no value in predicting the behavior that might be associated with such values determined for fresh tissue. The reliability of the alcohol values from oxidation methods narrows down to the reliability of the person who performs the analysis.

Quantitative alcohol methods which depend on the conversion of ethyl alcohol into ethyl iodide have the advantage of specificity and sensitivity. Extremely small samples of material may be analyzed. Methyl alcohol and ethyl ether are the only common interferences. Formaldehyde from embalmed tissue or ketone bodies in diabetic cases do not influence the results. Values obtained from putrefied tissue that did not contain alcohol are only moderately elevated above those for fresh tissue. A modified procedure permits the simultaneous determination of methyl and ethyl alcohol with a precision adequate for toxicologic interpretations. The disadvantage of this type of method is its complexity. The technics and apparatus are complicated and the operations should be performed only by a trained chemist. The methods are applicable to special samples where oxidation procedures cannot be used and as reference procedures in contested cases.

Evaluation of Oxidation Methods for Ethyl Alcohol. There are a number of reliable oxidation procedures, each of which has been developed with a particular purpose in mind. In the method of Gettler and Tiber (2) and the application of Gettler and Freireich (23) of the same procedure to blood and spinal fluid, relatively large sample weights are taken for the analysis. Errors which are likely to occur in small samples, such as evaporation or surface losses on the apparatus, and magnified error in calculating on a percentage basis are reduced to a minimum. The calculation is based on the titration of the acetic acid produced in the oxidation and, consequently, there are fewer grounds for criticism regarding possible interferences than in those procedures in which the alcohol is estimated from the excess of oxidant remaining after the oxidation process is completed. Considerably more labor and time are required than in methods using smaller samples and there is always the danger of carrying over small amounts of SO_3 fumes with the acetic acid, due to bumping or superheating of the dichromate-sulfuric acid solution. However, the use of a magnetic stirrer and a hot plate with proper shielding is an adequate safeguard against errors due to SO_3 fumes. Besides, this possible source of error can always be excluded by testing the final distillate for $SO_4^=$ with Ba^{++} ion.

The work of Gorr and Wagner (24) showed that aldehydes and ketones can be removed completely from an alcohol solution by refluxing the mixture for 2 to 5 hours with mercuric chloride in 1 or 2 normal sodium hydroxide and then distilling the alcohol. Friedemann and Klaas (25) utilized mercury salts to remove interfering substances in their method for the determination of alcohol in 0.2 to 10 ml. of blood, urine, and saliva. The alcohol is isolated by distillation after dilution of the sample with water to a volume of 50 to 60 ml. and addition of 5 ml. of 10 per cent sodium tungstate, 5 ml. of 10 per cent mercuric sulfate acidified with 10 per cent sulfuric acid, and a small amount of powdered talc as an inert antifrothing agent. Thirty to 35 ml. of distillate is collected. The reagents precipitate the proteins and remove most of the aldehyde and ketone impurities. When exceptionally large amounts of impurities are present in the distillate, a second distillation is carried out after the addition of 5 ml. of 10 per cent mercuric sulfate and sufficient calcium hydroxide to render the solution alkaline. The alcohol is determined by oxidation to oxalic acid with permanganate and the calculation of the alcohol concentration is made from an iodometric back titration of the excess permanganate after acidification of the solution. However, the conditions for the alkaline oxidation of alcohol are critical and this phase of the procedure offers no advantage over acid oxidation with dichromate.

Kozelka and Hine (26) have simplified the purification process by employing a closed apparatus in which the isolation of the alcohol by steam distillation and the distillation from alkaline mercuric oxide solution are carried out in one operation. Interfering substances are reported to be removed quantitatively when the steam distillate from 1 to 2 ml. of blood or urine, which has been treated with 5 ml. of 10 per cent sodium tungstate and 5 ml. of 1N sulfuric acid, is passed through a solution containing 10 ml. of saturated mercuric chloride and 10 ml. of saturated sodium hydroxide. The 25 to 30 ml. of distillate which is collected in the digestion flask is oxidized with 10 ml. N/10 $K_2Cr_2O_7$ and 5 ml. concentrated sulfuric acid, heated in a water bath for 20 minutes, and diluted with water. Then 0.2 gm. of potassium iodide is added and the liberated I_2 titrated with N/10 $Na_2S_2O_3$ to a starch end point.

The primary feature in the method of Newman (27) for alcohol in 1 ml. samples of body fluids consists of the distillation of the sample under reduced pressure. Equal volumes of N/10 dichromate and concentrated sulfuric acid are used as the oxidizing mixture with iodometric determination of the excess dichromate. There is no advantage to the use of reduced pressure and an objection to its use is that frothing is enhanced.

The micro method of Nicloux (28) for 0.2 to 5.0 gm. of blood or tissue was one of the first of the reliable alcohol procedures. The distillation is carried out in a special apparatus and the distillate is oxidized with dichromate and sulfuric acid. The excess dichromate is back titrated past the end point with standard ferrous ammonium sulfate and the end point established by titration of the excess ferrous ammonium sulfate with standard permanganate. The use of iodometry or other indicators has eliminated the need for the additional back titration. McNally and Coleman (29) described essentially the same method with a higher concentration of $K_2Cr_2O_7$ in order to extend the range to 0.88 per cent ethyl alcohol in 1 ml. samples of blood. Titration of the excess $K_2Cr_2O_7$ is made with potassium iodide and $Na_2S_2O_3$.

Harger's method (30) for the distillates containing 0.02 to 0.5 mg. of alcohol employs an improved direct titration of the excess dichromate remaining after oxidation of the distillate. The oxidizing solution, consisting of 1 ml. of 0.21 per cent $K_2Cr_2O_7$ and 1 ml. concentrated sulfuric acid is titrated directly with a reducing solution made of ferrous sulfate and methyl orange. The ferrous sulfate performs about 80 per cent of the reduction while the methyl orange, which is decolorized by the minute concentration of acid dichromate, acts both as a reducer and indicator.* A major advantage of this procedure over iodometric and other back titration methods is that the titration can be made directly on the concentrated sulfuric acid-dichromate solution without dilution.

Chaikelis and Floersheim (31) aerate the diluted gastric fluid into a maximum of 10 ml. of 0.43 per cent $K_2Cr_2O_7 + 10$ ml. concentrated sulfuric acid and employ ferrous sulfate and Congo red to titrate the unreduced dichromate remaining in the oxidizing solution. Johnston and Gibson (32) distill 1 ml. specimens from 20 ml. of picric acid solution into dichromate-sulfuric acid and carry out the titration with Harger's titrating solution.

The official U.S. Army method (33, 34) employs the Scott-Wilson reagent (page 1091) for removing interfering substances (pages 1089, 1091). This method uses the aeration of 4 ml. samples of blood or urine to which 2.0 to 4.0 ml. of Scott-Wilson reagent and sufficient water to make the final volume 10 ml. are added. The sample tube is connected to a receiver tube containing 9 ml. of Anstie's dichromate-sulfuric acid oxidizing mixture † and the tube is heated in a boiling water bath for 15 minutes with air drawn through the solution by means of an aspirator pump connected to the receiver tube. The oxidizing solution is made up to a volume of 10 ml. by the addition of water and the alcohol is determined by visual comparison of the yellow-green color with a series of nine dichromate standards. The standards are prepared by the addition of 1 ml. solutions of standard alcohol to the dichromate solution. The alcohol standards are made by diluting 2 per cent absolute ethyl alcohol to prepare a series of alcohol solutions differing by 0.5 mg./ml. to a maximum alcohol concentration of 4 mg./ml. (page 1089).

Haggard and Greenberg (16) developed a method for alcohol in air, blood and urine based on the procedure for carbon monoxide and ethyl ether in which the alcohol is oxidized to carbon dioxide by I_2O_5. Calculation is made from titrations of the I_2 and hydriotic acid liberated in the oxidation. Although the method eliminates steam distillation, it is complicated and requires considerable manipulative labor. Since iodine pentoxide is a more drastic oxidant than dichromate-sulfuric

---

* Harger's titrating solution: (a) 0.1 per cent methyl orange prepared by dissolving 1 gm. of methyl orange in 1 liter of approximately N/4 sodium hydroxide and filtering. (b) 20 per cent $FeSO_4$ made by dissolving 50 gm. $FeSO_4 \cdot 7H_2O$ in 150 ml. water + 30 ml. concentrated sulfuric acid and diluting to 250 ml. The titrating solution is prepared by adding 15 ml. of (a) and 1 ml. of (b) to 35 ml. of 62 per cent sulfuric acid in a flask, shaking during the addition. Keeps 3 to 4 days.

† Anstie's reagent: 3.7 gm. $K_2Cr_2O_7$/150 ml. water + 280 ml. concentrated sulfuric acid + water to make 500 ml.

acid, any volatile organic substance other than alcohol is a potential source of interference in the method.

Of all the procedures described for the quantitative analysis of alcohol, the chemical principles in the classic micromethod of Widmark (35) for 100 mg. samples of blood more closely meet the theoretical requirements for a quantitative chemical analysis. In addition, the principles can be defended more readily in contested cases than those of some of the other methods because the procedure automatically compensates for most of the possible errors. This method, which was developed for the purpose of analyzing the small blood samples obtained by finger puncture, utilized the principle of desiccation of water and alcohol by concentrated sulfuric acid. The desiccant was a dichromate-sulfuric acid solution contained in a special flask with a cup holding the sample suspended over the oxidizing solution. Widmark pointed out that although the theoretical oxidation of alcohol proceeds according to one of three equations, all three stages occur with the products of oxidation formed in varying proportions which depend on the conditions under which the oxidation is carried out.

$$3\ C_2H_5OH + K_2Cr_2O_7 + 4\ H_2SO_4 \rightarrow 3\ CH_3CHOH +$$

$$K_2SO_4 + Cr_2(SO_4)_3 + 7\ H_2O$$

$$3\ C_2H_5OH + 2\ K_2Cr_2O_7 + 8\ H_2SO_4 \rightarrow 3\ CH_3COOH +$$

$$2\ K_2SO_4 + 2\ Cr_2(SO_4)_3 + 11\ H_2O$$

$$C_2H_5OH + 2\ K_2Cr_2O_7 + 8\ H_2SO_4 \rightarrow 2\ CO_2 + 2\ K_2SO_4 + 2\ Cr_2(SO_4)_3 + 11\ H_2O$$

Under controlled conditions, the difference between the amount of dichromate remaining in a control and in a test flask is proportional to the amount of alcohol regardless of the products of oxidation. An empirical relation between alcohol and reduced dichromate is obtained experimentally by carrying out a series of determinations with known alcohol solutions of varying concentrations. The dichromate in the control and test solutions is determined iodometrically with sodium thiosulfate and the alcohol constant related to the difference in the volumes of sodium thiosulfate needed in the two titrations. Micrograms of alcohol in the sample are calculated from the equation:

$$\text{micrograms of alcohol} = 113\ (b\text{-}a)$$

where b = ml. of 0.01 N $Na_2S_2O_3$ used to titrate the control and a = ml. of 0.01 N $Na_2S_2O_3$ used to titrate the test solution. The amount of alcohol is thereby related through the constant 113 to the easily standardized sodium thiosulfate and is independent of small amounts of reducing materials in the reagents and slight variations in the concentration of the dichromate-sulfuric acid solution.

A number of variations of the Widmark method have been described. In Abels' (36) modification of the methods of Widmark and Heise (35, 22), the blood sample is absorbed on filter paper and suspended over the oxidizing solution. Sheftel (37) absorbed blood and urine samples on filter paper suspended over the oxidizing solution but determined the reduced dichromate colorimetrically with a blue filter. A correction for the absorption of light by the $Cr_2(SO_4)_3$ formed in the test sample was made by employing a slightly different dilution ratio of the standard and test dichromate solutions. Levine and Bodansky (38) used Widmark's method with the filter paper technic for desiccating the sample and Harger's (30) titrating solution for determining the dichromate in the control and test solutions. Cavett (39) employed distillation with the oxidation technic of Widmark and titration with Harger's solution. Shupe and Dubowski (40) have published a photometric method for analyzing the dichromate-sulfuric acid solution.

Quantitative Determination of Alcohol in the Toxicologic Analysis of Organs for Poisons. Most of the quantitative methods for ethyl alcohol have been developed for the purpose of establishing the alcohol level in living persons. In medical examiner's cases where organs and tissue must be examined for other substances, a steam distillation is a prerequisite in the isolation and separation of the volatile poisons. Since the alcohol will have been quantitatively recovered in this distillate, analysis of a separate sample of material is not warranted. A quantitative analysis of the distillate is made only when the qualitative tests for ethanol (page 1048) indicate that it is present in significant concentration. Samples of 500 gm. of brain and sometimes the less desirable liver tissue (page 1111) are used for the distillation in order to isolate an ample quantity of an unknown substance. The quantitative method for the alcohol in the 100 ml., or at most 250 ml., of distillate (page 1046) must be applicable to considerably higher alcohol concentrations than in those methods for the body fluids of living patients.

Regardless of the limitations in predicting physiologic response to different alcohol concentrations (page 1101), in selecting a procedure for the quantitative determination of ethyl alcohol for medicolegal purposes, certain quantitative procedures take precedence over others and, since the method of Widmark has the soundest chemical basis, it is our method of choice. To avoid any question regarding the quantitative recovery, the alcohol should be separated from the sample by distillation and the analysis performed on the distillate since aeration and desiccation procedures are potentially open to criticism, no matter how reliable the values are to the analyst. Although the use of the Scott-Wilson reagent or other mercury-containing solutions to remove aldehyde and ketone interference makes oxidation methods quite selective for alcohol even those continuous distillation-oxidation procedures which incorporate a purification step put the burden of proof on the analyst to show the absence of all possible interfering substances. Therefore, to avoid any controversy in cases which come to court, a preliminary examination of a distillate should be made to exclude interferences in the oxidation procedure. There is little justification for performing an analysis on very small samples of tissue or body fluids in medicolegal cases. Even in the case of blood from living patients, the sample should be taken by a competent person only and a large quantity taken by vena puncture is as easy to obtain as a small sample from a finger puncture.

In our opinion, adaptations which incorporate colorimetric analysis of dichromate-sulfuric acid solutions are not as practical as titration since the partially reduced oxidant comprises a two component yellow-green system. Moreover, a titration can be performed in about the same time as that required to prepare the solution for photometric measurement. The possibility for large errors to occur is considerably greater than in titration procedures, particularly when the technician is not familiar with the shortcomings of the method. Iodine-sodium thiosulfate solutions give good end points for the back titration of the dichromate-sulfuric acid solution and are easier to prepare and standardize but Harger's titrating solution (page 1087) would appear to be equally good.

METHOD FOR THE QUANTITATIVE DETERMINATION (41).* The Widmark method for the analysis of a distillate was developed to cover the range of alcohol concentrations to be expected in 2 gm. of sample material when the ratio of the volume of distillate collected to the weight of sample distilled is not more than 1 ml. of distillate per gram of sample. The maximum alcohol content is rarely in excess of 5 mg. per gram and the optimum value expected in acute intoxications is of the order of 3 mg. per gram. The dichromate concentration was selected to make the control titration slightly less than 10 ml. with $N/10$ $Na_2S_2O_3$. The potassium dichromate equivalent to 10 ml. of $N/10$ $Na_2S_2O_3$ is 0.049 gm. which in turn is equivalent to 11.119 mg. of ethyl alcohol, assuming the oxidation is stoichiometric with the formation of acetic acid. This dichromate concentration then permits the analysis of 2 ml. of distillate from a sample with a distillate to sample ratio of 1:1, titrating with $N/10$ $Na_2S_2O_3$ from a 10 ml. buret.

Some unreduced dichromate should always remain after completion of the analysis and, in those exceptional cases where the alcohol content is nearly equal to or in excess of the dichromate,† the analysis can be repeated with a 1 ml. sample without fear of exceeding the maximum possible alcohol content to be found in biologic material. $K_2Cr_2O_7$ is not too soluble in strong sulfuric acid solution and, in order to prepare a stable oxidizing solution, the 0.049 gm. $K_2Cr_2O_7$ requires 2 ml. water + concentrated sulfuric acid to make 3 ml. This restriction automatically sets the minimum volume of reagent at 3 ml. for 2 ml. of sample. Although concentrated sulfuric acid is diluted with 4 volumes of water, making the solution far below the acid concentration used by Widmark, values obtained by other procedures which use still greater acid dilution ‡ have shown that oxidation readily proceeds beyond the aldehyde stage.

Reagents. (a) Dichromate-sulfuric acid oxidizing solution: dissolve 4.85 gm. of $K_2Cr_2O_7$ in 200 ml. of distilled water and add concentrated sulfuric acid to 300 ml., with cooling.

(b) $N/10$ sodium thiosulfate solution: dissolve 25 gm. of $Na_2S_2O_3 \cdot 5H_2O$ in 900 ml. water, add 1 ml. of 0.1N sodium hydroxide and dilute to 1 liter.

(c) Standard $KH(IO_3)_2$ solution: carefully weigh approximately 0.155 gm. $KH(IO_3)_2$ and let stand, with intermittent shaking, in a 250 ml. volumetric flask nearly filled with distilled water until dissolved. Then dilute to the mark.

(d) 1 per cent starch solution: add 1 gm. potato starch to a 100 ml. volumetric flask containing 60 ml. hot water and continue warming until dissolved. Dilute nearly to the mark, cool and adjust volume to 100 ml. The starch solution should be prepared fresh each day.

(e) Solid potassium iodide.

(f) 0.5 per cent ethyl alcohol solutions: pipet 6.33 ml. of absolute ethyl alcohol into a 1 liter volumetric flask containing distilled water, dilute to the mark, and mix.

(g) Standard alcohol solutions: a series of standards are prepared by diluting the 0.5 per cent solution with water according to Table 46-1.

To standardize the $Na_2S_2O_3$ solution, pipet 50 ml. of standard $KH(IO_3)_2$ solution into a 125 ml. Erlenmyer flask, add 25 ml. water, 2 drops of concentrated sulfuric acid, and 1.5 gm. of solid potassium iodide. After standing 15 minutes,

* Umberger, C. J., and Ames, A. Unpublished.
† This is indicated when the sample titration approaches or equals the control.
‡ In the Harger method (page 1087) the final dilution is 1 volume acid to 6 volumes water.

Table 46-1.

STANDARD	VOLUME 0.5% ETHYL ALCOHOL TO VOLUMES WATER	DILUTION RATIO	MG. ETHYL ALCOHOL PER ML.
#1	1 + 4	1:5	1
#2	2 + 3	2:5	2
#3	3 + 2	3:5	3
#4	4 + 1	4:5	4
#5	5 + 0	5:5	5

titrate to a pale yellow iodine color with the $Na_2S_2O_3$ solution, add 1 ml. of starch solution and continue the titration to a colorless end point.

$$\text{Normality of } Na_2S_2O_3 = \frac{0.03077 \times \text{mg. } KH(IO_3)_2/50 \text{ ml.}}{\text{ml. } Na_2S_2O_3 \text{ solution}}$$

Procedure. The distillate from the 500 gm. of tissue (page 1046) remaining after completion of the qualitative examination (pages 1048-1055) will have been 100 or 250 ml. in volume. All but a negligible amount of alcohol will be recovered in the first 100 ml. portion of distillate and recovery will be complete even at high tissue alcohol levels with the collection of 250 ml. of distillate (2). In order to make the distillate volume to sample ratio of 1:1, the 100 ml. portion collected is diluted fivefold, the 250 ml. portion is diluted 1 to 2. If separate 100 and 150 ml. portions were collected, aliquots of both may be recombined in their proper proportion and diluted twofold. Three ml. of dichromate-sulfuric acid solution are pipeted into each of two 125 ml. Erlenmeyer flasks equipped with ground glass stoppers, labelled "control" and "sample." Two ml. of distilled water are added to the control and 2 ml. of distillate are added to the sample. The flasks are placed in a drying oven set at 70° C. and heated for 5 minutes. They are then cooled to room temperature, diluted with 50 ml. water and 1.5 gm. of solid potassium iodide is added. The liberated I_2 is titrated with the N/10 $Na_2S_2O_3$ to a straw color. One ml. of starch solution is introduced and the titration continued to a colorless end point.

Milligrams of ethyl alcohol in the sample = 1.25 (ml. N/10 $Na_2S_2O_3$ to titrate the control − ml. N/10 $Na_2S_2O_3$ to titrate the sample). The 1.25 is the average value found in this laboratory for the Widmark factor from analysis of 2 ml. of the standard alcohol solutions, Table 46-1.

Estimation of Ethyl Alcohol in Distillates from Partially Putrefied Tissue. (See Interpretations of Alcohol Values, pages 1101-1116.) The offensive odor of both the tissue and distillate will indicate even moderate putrefaction. In questionable cases, the appearance of a red color after the addition of the nitroprusside to the unoxidized portion of the distillate in the tests for formaldehyde and acetaldehyde (pages 1048-1050) or a positive finding in the iodine-sodium azide test for thio compounds (page 1053) will indicate tissue degradation which interferes with the oxidation test for ethyl alcohol. With fresh tissue, positive findings in the qualitative examination for acetone or other volatile oxidizable substances make it necessary to introduce a purification step before the quantitative analysis. A second distillation with the reagents of Friedemann and Klaas (page 1086), Kozelka and Hine (page 1086) or the Scott-Wilson reagent (see below) removes all but negligible amounts of thiol, aldol and keto interferences. Scott-Wilson's reagent has some minor advantages, particularly the removal of a greater variety of possible interfering substances, which make it the preferred reagent.

Scott-Wilson Reagent (34). Five grams of $Hg(CN)_2$ per 300 ml. of water and 1.45 gm. $AgNO_3$ dissolved in 200 ml. water is added to a solution of 70 gm. NaOH per 300 ml. Any precipitate which settles out after mixing is filtered off. The solution keeps for 6 months.

Procedure. Add 5 ml. of the Scott-Wilson reagent to 5 ml. of distillate * in a 25 ml. microdistillation apparatus, using a 25 ml. flask as the receiver. Mount the distillation flask on a hot plate with asbestos shielding and distill until approximately 5 ml. of distillate has been collected.† Dilute to the 25 ml. mark, so that 1 ml. of distillate will represent 1 gm. of tissue and analyze a 2 ml. aliquot by the procedure on page 1090.

Determination of Alcohol in Blood, Urine or Small Amounts of Tissue. In the steam distillation of small samples, it is necessary to collect proportionately larger volumes of the steam distillate for complete recovery of the alcohol. Recovery in the collection of 100 ml. of distillate from 500 gm. of brain is quite different from that in 1 ml. of distillate from 5 gm. of brain because of the lag in the heat transfer of flask and sample and surface losses in the apparatus. Using a macro-distillation, Gettler and Freireich (23) isolated most of the alcohol from 10 ml. of blood in the first 30 ml. of a steam distillation and all but traces at very high alcohol concentrations were recovered after collection of 50 ml. of distillate. The recovery is considerably improved by employing microdistillation technics with adequate shielding and controlled heating of the sample flask.

Procedure. Two to 10 ml. of blood or urine is added to a distillation flask or, in the case of tissue, 10 to 25 gm. is minced in a Waring Blendor after the addition of enough water to give a thick slurry and washed into a distillation flask with water. One ml. of saturated tartaric acid is added and the sample is steam distilled, collecting 5 ml. of distillate per gram of sample. Five ml. of distillate, representing 1 gm. of sample, may be analyzed by the procedure on page 1090 or the distillate may be redistilled with addition of the Scott-Wilson reagent as described on this page.‡ When the second distillation is made, only one-half the volume of the original distillate is collected so that the final distillate represents 2 grams of tissue per 5 ml. of distillate. Analysis of the more dilute distillate (1 gm. is equivalent to 5 ml. distillate) limits the range of the method and decreases the precision somewhat at low alcohol concentrations.

Ethoxy Method for Ethyl Alcohol (42). In this method, Pregl's application of the Zeisel reaction for the determination of alkoxyl groups was adapted to the

---

* The use of 5 ml. of distillate is based on the assumption that the original was a 100 ml. portion, collected from 500 gm. of tissue (page 1046).

† From the data of Nicloux and Bandner, *Ztschr. f. anal. Chem.*, 38:258, 1899, all of the alcohol is recovered from 0.01 and 0.03 per cent ethyl alcohol solutions when one quarter of the volume is distilled. Straetar, *Ztschr. f. physiol. Chem.*, 50:24, 1906, reported complete recovery of the alcohol from a 1.5 per cent solution when two fifths of the volume was distilled. Donitz, in *Spiritus Fabrikation Maerker-Delbuseck*, page 694, 1908, shows complete recovery from a 2.5 per cent solution with distillation of one fifth of the volume.

‡ When alcohol only is to be determined on small samples of tissue, blood or urine, distillation may be made with addition of the Scott-Wilson reagent directly to the sample. However, a still larger volume of distillate per unit sample weight needs to be collected for complete recovery of the alcohol and it is then necessary to carry out a second distillation in order to have an alcohol content sufficient to give an adequate sample titration. Because the alcohol is determined by titration difference, titration and dilution errors are magnified when a dilute alcohol solution is analyzed with the relatively concentrated dichromate reagent and the calculation then made on a percentage basis. Since the maximum precision in the method is attained at that alcohol content which reduces approximately 70 per cent of the dichromate, in applying the procedure to small samples with a single distillation, the dichromate concentration should be halved and the titration made with 0.05 N $Na_2S_2O_3$.

determination of small amounts of alcohol. It depends on the conversion of ethyl alcohol into ethyl iodide by interaction with constant boiling hydriodic acid.

$$C_2H_5OH + HI \rightarrow C_2H_5I + H_2O$$

The ethyl iodide is absorbed in a potassium acetate, glacial acetic acid and liquid bromine solution where IBr is formed according to the reaction:

$$C_2H_5I + Br_2 \rightarrow C_2H_5Br + IBr$$

On the addition of water, the excess Br_2 oxidizes the IBr to iodate:

$$IBr + 3\,H_2O + 2\,Br_2 \rightarrow HIO_3 + 5\,HBr$$

After removal of the excess bromine, addition of KI liberates 3 molecules of I_2 for each molecule of iodate and, hence, each molecule of ethyl iodide, thereby increasing the sensitivity of the reaction 6 fold (43):

$$2\,HIO_3 + 10\,KI + 10\,HAc \rightarrow 10\,KAc + 6\,H_2O + 6\,I_2$$

The liberated iodine is titrated with standard sodium thiosulfate and the ethyl alcohol is calculated from the thiosulfate used in the titration.

The apparatus * is a modified Pregl alkoxy apparatus equipped with a side arm test tube for the sample and an enlarged wash chamber. The chamber is charged with a suspension of lead thiosulfate and basic lead carbonate to remove any vaporized iodine or HI from the hydriodic acid or sulfides from the sample material. While the sample tube is immersed in a boiling water bath and the bulb containing the HI in a constant temperature oil bath, a steam of CO_2 aerates the alcohol from the sample into the HI. The ethyl iodide that is formed is carried over into the receiver flask by the stream of CO_2.

The method, as described, was developed for the determination of the very small concentration of alcohol in normal blood but it is equally applicable to the determination of alcohol in blood, tissue, urine or in distillates in cases involving questionable intoxication. Samples from 0.1 to 1 gm. may be analyzed by addition of the minced tissue, blood or urine to the side arm test tube after acidifying with tartaric acid. Titration is made with $0.1N\ Na_2S_2O_3$ rather than the $0.01N\ Na_2S_2O_3$ used for the nonalcoholic sample material. One ml. of $0.1N\ Na_2S_2O_3$ is equivalent to 0.86 mg. ethyl alcohol.

Although the method is less subject to interference than other alcohol procedures, any compound volatile at $100°$ C. that will react with HI to form a volatile alkyl iodide will interfere with the alcohol determination. Methyl alcohol and normal and isopropyl alcohols give quantitative values. Secondary and tertiary butyl alcohol give positive titrations but the values are not quantitative. Ethyl ether may be determined quantitatively on brain tissue in deaths from anesthesia (44). Normal and isopropyl ether and ethyl acetate react in this method but have not been studied quantitatively.

Since formalin and other volatile aldehydes do not interfere, this method can be applied to the determination of alcohol in embalmed tissue. Methyl and ethyl alcohol may be estimated simultaneously by replacing the absorbing solution with an alcoholic solution of trimethylamine as described by Küster and Maag (45) for the determination of methoxyl and ethoxyl groups in organic compounds. Methyl iodide reacts to form insoluble tetramethyl ammonium iodide while ethyl iodide

* Made by Eck and Krebs, Long Island City, New York, catalogue item #3000A.

forms trimethylethyl ammonium iodide which is readily soluble in the alcoholic absorbing solution. The ethoxy method is particularly valuable in detecting alcohol in distillates from putrefied tissue when the findings by an oxidation method are questionable. Even with extensive putrefaction of nonalcoholic tissue, the values do not exceed 0.1 per cent which is below the limit for significant findings. Alcohol values on normal tissue with moderate putrefaction are usually of the order of 0.05 per cent.

This method is too complicated and time consuming for routine laboratory examinations. It is only recommended for confirmation in contested cases and for those special determinations where the quantity of sample material is quite small or where oxidation procedures are not applicable due to interference. The original article should be consulted for the detailed procedure.

SURVEY OF THE EXPERIMENTAL WORK ON THE MEDICOLEGAL ASPECTS OF INTOXICATION

When alcohol is introduced into the stomach, within 2 to 10 minutes (46) some of it passes through the intestinal wall and appears in the blood. The rate of absorption is quite rapid and, if sufficient quantities are present in the stomach, the alcohol passes into the blood stream at a much greater rate than can be utilized, or eliminated, by the body. Therefore, there is a piling up of alcohol in the blood, the surplus depending on the amount consumed. The excess alcohol is deposited in all parts of the body, particularly in the brain, and the nervous system. According to Miles (47) the fatty substances in the nerve cells and tracts have a particular affinity for alcohol, and its presence at the cell junction interferes with the passage of nerve impulses along the regular routes. Numerous experiments (48-50) have shown that alcohol, even in concentrations below that which causes intoxication, markedly decreases the efficiency of the individual to perform tasks that require thinking and reasoning. In excessive doses, besides the loss of equilibrium and the production of mental instability, alcohol causes various emotional reactions, ranging from friendliness to a state of irritation or anger, which may lead to acts of violence (51). The prevalence of alcoholics among sex offenders is well known. Alcohol may be a contributary cause of many accidents. In a study of the alcohol content of the blood of persons involved in 661 automobile accidents Koller (52) found that appreciable amounts were present in 79.3 per cent of the cases. Because of the diminished mental responsibility of persons under the influence of alcohol in accident cases and fatalities, it is important in medicolegal work to show the presence of appreciable amounts of alcohol. Of all the issues in forensic medicine, none is of greater concern than the problem of establishing the degree of intoxication.

Alcohol in the Organs and Body Fluids. Gréhant, in 1885, was one of the first chemists to attack the problem of alcoholic intoxication. In numerous experiments (53-60) he demonstrated the presence of alcohol in all the organs after its introduction into the stomach and showed that when a large part of the alcohol has been taken up from the stomach by the blood there is a point reached where the blood content remains stationary. At this high level, "Gréhant's plateau," he believed that the alcohol content of the blood and organs were in equilibrium. Nicloux (46) studied the distribution of alcohol in dogs and guinea pigs and showed that it was present in the body fluids, urine, bile, lymph, saliva, pancreatic juice, spinal fluid and mother's milk.

Abel (61), in a report on the physiologic aspects of the liquor problem, demonstrated that it is not the quantity of alcohol in the stomach but that which is in contact with the nervous system which produces the effects of intoxication.

Mellanby (62), after an extensive study of the alcohol content of the blood of dogs dosed with varying amounts and concentrations, arrived at the following conclusions: (a) intoxication is related to the amount of alcohol in the blood, (b) dilute solutions are less intoxicating than strong solutions containing the same amount of alcohol, (c) the presence of food in the stomach inhibits intoxication, (d) water taken after the absorption of alcohol intensifies intoxication, from which recovery appears to be more rapid than normal.

Carpenter (63), upon investigating the relation between the alcohol content of the blood and that of the organs, reported that the content of the brain, lungs, kidney, spleen, muscle and skin is usually less than that of the blood.

In 1927 Gettler and Tiber (64) reported their analyses on the organs of 6,000 alcoholic cadavers in which, in many cases, complete histories were available. From their data they concluded that the alcohol concentration of the brain furnishes the best index for the degree of intoxication. They graded the various stages of intoxication into five classifications as shown in Table 46-2.

Table 46-2.

CLASSIFICATION	PERCENTAGE OF ALCOHOL IN THE BRAIN	PHYSIOLOGIC EFFECTS
1. Trace	0.005 to 0.02	normal
2. +	0.02 to 0.10	normal
3. ++	0.10 to 0.25	less sense of care
4. +++	0.25 to 0.40	less sense of equilibrium
5. ++++	0.40 to 0.60	unbalance, intoxication

In a study of 500 cases involving alcoholic intoxication, Bogen (65) set up five classifications based on the alcohol concentration of the urine (Table 46-3).

Table 46-3.

GROUP	MG. ETHYL ALCOHOL/ML. URINE	PHYSIOLOGIC SYMPTOMS *
I	0 to 1	insufficient for diagnosis of intoxication
II	1 to 2	borderline
III	2 to 3	slight intoxication
IV	3 to 4	unmistakable intoxication
V	4 to 5	dead drunk

* The physiologic heading is the writer's abbreviated interpretation of Bogen's discussion of the different groups.

His comparison of urine values with blood, spinal fluid and alveolar air showed comparable values in some cases. However, some overlapping occurred to either side of the urine group in other cases.

In the Laboratory Manual of the United States Army (34) interpretations of the degree of intoxication are based on values for the alcohol in the blood (Table 46-4).

It is noted that urine alcohol values may be higher or lower depending on the state of absorption or elimination.

In the report of the Committee of the American Medical Association to Study Problems of Motor Vehicle Accidents (66), it is recorded that the concentration of alcohol in the blood is one of the best criteria of intoxication because blood alcohol concentrations closely parallel detrimental effects noted in carefully con-

Table 46-4.

MG. ETHYL ALCOHOL/ML. BLOOD	REMARKS
0.5	May have been drinking but values may also be due to interference from reducing substances other than alcohol.
1 to 1.5	Under the influence of liquor but definitely not intoxicated.
2 to 2.5	Definitely intoxicated.
3 to 3.5	Seriously intoxicated.
4 to 4.0 +	Close to dead drunk.

ducted experimental tests. Although this relationship is not mathematically exact because of slight variations resulting from inherent differences in human beings, it is sufficiently accurate for practical purposes. The relationship between the concentration of alcohol in blood, urine, saliva and breath has been shown to be sufficiently definite so that chemical tests on any of these body fluids can furnish a reliable measure of the degree of alcoholic influence. For medicolegal purposes, the Committee recommended the following interpretation of chemical tests for alcohol:

"1. Although there is no minimal figure which can be set at which there will be absolutely no effect from alcohol, persons with concentrations of less than 0.05 per cent in blood or its equivalent in urine, saliva or the breath should not be prosecuted for driving while under the influence of liquor.

"2. All persons show a definite loss of that clearness of intellect and control of themselves which they would ordinarily possess when the concentrations are above 0.15 per cent in blood or its equivalent in other body fluids and should therefore be considered as under the influence.

"3. When the alcohol concentrations are between 0.05 and 0.15 per cent in blood, a great many persons will be under the influence of alcohol but the committee recommends prosecution only when the circumstances and results of physical examination give definite confirmation of such influence" (66).

The recommendations of the Committee of the American Medical Association to Study Problems of Motor Vehicle Accidents is apparently based on the report of the Committee on Tests for Intoxication of the National Safety Council (67). From the study of published information and the experience of the members, the National Safety Council Committee concluded that all persons having a level of alcohol in the blood above 0.15 per cent by weight are sufficiently impaired to be unsafe automobile drivers and recommended that a finding of 0.15 per cent should be considered as conclusive evidence that the person is under the influence of alcohol from the standpoint of car operation. They further recommended that in every case all available evidence of abnormal actions or conditions should be obtained to permit presentation of a more convincing case. This appears to be at variance with the recommendation concerning acceptance of the chemical analysis as conclusive evidence.

The Committee suggested that in those few cases where the blood concentration is greater than 0.15 per cent and there is no evidence of driving error, abnormal actions or other physical symptoms of intoxication, that it will be better not to prosecute for an intoxication charge unless chemical tests are used exclusively in the locality, are accepted by the courts and are fairly well known to the average person who is to serve on the juries. This suggestion is hardly in line with the previous recommendations of the Committee. If 0.15 per cent alcohol is the critical limit for intoxication and the value is based on scientific evidence that is conclusive, no exceptions should be permitted. If the evidence is uncertain enough to permit exceptions, recommendations with such a sharp distinction are not warranted.

The Committee pointed out that many persons with blood alcohol concentrations below 0.15 per cent are sufficiently impaired to be unsafe automobile drivers. In such cases it recommended that abnormal actions and the unusual external symptoms of intoxication should be considered in determining whether to prosecute. When the blood level is below 0.07 per cent, prosecution is generally not warranted. It is reported that a urine alcohol concentration of 0.2 per cent can be accepted as equivalent to a 0.15 per cent blood alcohol and 0.10 per cent as equivalent to 0.07 per cent.

The data presented in the report to substantiate the selection of 0.15 per cent blood alcohol as the limiting value for intoxication are from the work of Holcomb, Heise, Whitney, Bavis, Friedemann and others, Harger and others, and experiments on automobile drivers at Dresden, Germany (68, 69, 70, 71, 72, 73, 21, 67). In a statistical analysis of the data of Holcomb by the Committee it was determined that the chance of being involved in an auto accident increased from 14.5 to 1 at a blood level from 0.11 to 0.14 per cent, to 55 to 1 at a level of 0.15 per cent and above.

Stages of intoxication in terms of concentrations of alcohol in blood and urine, as determined by C. W. Muehlberger, are tabulated in the Committee's report (Table 46-5).

Table 46-5. Stages of Intoxication

Prepared by Dr. C. W. Muehlberger (74).

ALCOHOL CONCENTRATIONS

STAGE	PER CENT IN BLOOD	IN URINE	PARTS PER THOUSAND IN BLOOD	IN URINE	CLINICAL
Subclinical	0.01 to 0.12	0.01 to 0.16	0.1 to 1.2	0.1 to 1.6	Normal by ordinary observation. Slight change by special tests.
Stimulation	0.09 to 0.21	0.13 to 0.29	0.9 to 2.1	1.3 to 2.9	Decreased inhibitions. Emotional instability. Slight incoordination. Slowing of stimuli response.
Confusion	0.18 to 0.30	0.26 to 0.42	1.8 to 3.0	2.6 to 4.2	Disturbance of sensation. Decreased pain sense. Staggering gait. Slurred speech.
Stupor	0.27 to 0.39	0.38 to 0.54	2.7 to 3.9	3.8 to 5.4	Marked stimuli decrease. Approaching paralysis.
Coma	0.36 to 0.48	0.51 to 0.67	3.6 to 4.8	5.1 to 6.7	Complete unconsciousness. Depressed reflexes. Subnormal temperature Anesthesia. Impairment of circulation. Stertorous breathing. Possible death.

Overlapping stages of intoxication are shown to take into account the variation to be expected in the relationship between blood alcohol concentrations and the physical and mental impairment of different individuals.

Other investigators who have attempted to correlate the degree of intoxication with the alcohol concentration of the blood report higher values for the limiting blood alcohol concentration. Turner and Loew (75) believed the subject to be intoxicated if the alcohol concentration in the blood exceeded 0.25 per cent while later Turner (76) set the limit for the blood alcohol concentration of intoxicated persons between 0.2 and 0.5 per cent. Andresen (77) concluded that two hours after alcohol had been consumed, a blood alcohol concentration of over 0.24 per cent indicated intoxication. If the values were under 0.08 per cent, no symptoms were noticeable. Between these values he suggests that chemical analyses be used in conjunction with clinical and psychical symptoms for a correct interpretation.

Widmark (78) states that when blood levels are above 200 mg. per cent, individuals are almost without exception intoxicated; with a value of over 160 mg. per cent and less than 200 mg. per cent, the probability of intoxication is very great. Ladd and others (79) report that on the basis of European investigations 200 mg. per cent in blood has been recognized in Sweden and Germany as a state of intoxication. Widmark and Jungmichel (80) believe that blood alcohol may be used to determine the degree of intoxication, providing equilibrium conditions have been established in the body. Widmark has made an extensive study (81) of the relation between the alcohol concentration of the blood and its distribution in and the rate of removal from the body. He expressed these relations in the mathematic equation:

$$A = PR\ (C_t + \beta_t)$$

where A = total number of grams of alcohol consumed; P = body weight in kilograms; R = ratio of the average concentrations of alcohol in the entire body to the concentration in the blood; C_t = alcohol concentration in milligrams per milliliter of alcohol in the blood at the time, t; β = rate of disappearance of alcohol from the blood in per cent per minute; t = time in minutes following the ingestion of alcohol.

From this equation, it should be possible to estimate the concentration of alcohol in the blood at any particular time following ingestion of alcohol and also to estimate the quantity of alcohol consumed. The validity of the equation necessitates constant values for R and B in different individuals. Widmark obtained close agreement between the calculated and observed values on individual animals, but as shown by Meyer (82) and Le Breton (83), the constants not only vary widely between different animals but are affected by variables such as habitation and temperature in a particular animal. Kozelka (84) also believes that the best chemical criterion of the degree of alcoholic intoxication is furnished by analysis of blood. In general, the data on the relation of the alcohol content of the different organs and body fluids by different authors is not in agreement (85-87, 12, 63).

Establishing intoxication from the analysis of postmortem material involves the same problems as those of living persons with the exception that the sample material is limited to body fluids. Gettler and Freireich (23), following the work of Gettler and Tiber (64) in which the quantity of alcohol found in the brain determined the degree to which an individual is affected by alcohol, presented evidence showing that spinal fluid more closely parallels the alcohol content of the brain and, hence, serves as a better index of the degree of intoxication than other body fluids. In dogs, the blood-brain ratios varied over a wide range and they concluded that blood alcohol does not give reliable information concerning the state of persons under the influence of alcohol. Their findings are supported by Tuovinen (88) who found that the same quantity of alcohol consumed by human subjects under closely controlled conditions gave quite different blood alcohol values at the end of definite time intervals. Mehrtens and Newman (89), and Fleming and Stotz (90) found a lag in the lumbar spinal fluid alcohol as compared with the blood following small doses of alcohol in human beings and for this reason Mehrtens and Newman contend that spinal fluid is less satisfactory than blood for predicting the brain alcohol content. On the other hand, Harger, Hulpieu and Lamb (12) show a nearly constant value not only for blood-brain ratios but between the brain and other organs as well.

Renaux (14) and Naville (15) claim that the alcohol content of the urine may be used to establish the degree of intoxication. Haggard and Greenberg (17), and Bornstein and Budelman (19) report a constant ratio between blood and urine alcohol. Abels (20) has proposed the use of saliva while Harger (21) suggests expired air will serve as a measure of intoxication. Mozes and Katonak (91), in discussing the operation of motor vehicles by intoxicated persons, state that expired air furnishes a far more reliable index of the degree of alcoholic influence than the most carefully detailed clinical study.

Factors Affecting Intoxication. In contrast to the limited experimental work in which attempts were made to evaluate quantitatively the degree of intoxication at different alcohol levels in the body, many careful and detailed studies have been made concerning the factors other than the quantity of alcohol consumed that have an influence on the degree of intoxication. Most of these studies were initiated in an attempt to explain why some persons can consume larger amounts of alcohol than others and yet show fewer clinical signs of intoxication.

Strong alcohol solutions were found to be more intoxicating than dilute solutions containing the same quantity of alcohol and that water, taken after the absorption of alcohol, intensifies intoxication (62). The fact that recovery appears more rapid than normal was thought to be due to the diuretic effect of the water. It has been demonstrated (62, 92, 93) that the rate of absorption through the intestinal walls depends not only on the quantity but the nature of the material already in the stomach. Widmark (94) has suggested that the lowered rate of absorption of alcohol in the presence of foods rich in protein, compared to that of foods rich in carbohydrates, is the result of a combination of alcohol with the amino acids. Le Breton (95) believes that this lowered rate is due to an increase in the rate of oxidation of the alcohol, in the presence of the amino acids which have been absorbed by the blood stream.

Nicloux (96) has shown that higher temperatures hasten the removal of alcohol from tissues. In experiments on frogs he noted that the rate of oxidation was almost doubled for each 10° rise in temperature. Nyman and Palmlöv (97) found that the alcohol content of the sweat of persons in a heated room was about 80 per cent of that in the blood. That the physical state of the individual has some bearing on intoxication is indicated by experiments on rats (98) in which their ability to utilize alcohol was decreased from 20 to 40 per cent when starved to 10 to 20 per cent of their normal body weight.

The most important factor relating to the degree of intoxication is the phenomenon of tolerance. It has long been recognized that there is not only a wide range of natural susceptibility to alcohol in different persons, but those who use it habitually acquire a tolerance for (or a resistance against) it. Folger (99) showed that the ability of the tadpole to withstand higher alcohol concentrations was greatly increased after having lived in 1 per cent solutions of alcohol for a few weeks.

Gettler and Freireich (100) converted dogs into habitual alcohol drinkers by giving alcohol in water for periods ranging from six months to two years. At the end of these periods they gave the alcoholic dogs and control animals of equal weight the same quantity of alcohol and compared the physiologic effects. The alcoholic dogs were much less affected than the control animals.

The cause of tolerance is a much debated question. The following four possibilities have been suggested as an explanation: (1) increased elimination, (2) delay in the absorption, (3) more rapid destruction by oxidation, (4) an acquired resistance of the tissue.

1. *Increased Elimination*. A number of investigations have revealed that increased elimination is not a contributing factor. Pringsheim (86) found that the excretion of alcohol in abstainers and alcoholics was about the same. The work of Cushny (101) and Bödlander (102) who claim that only small amounts of the absorbed alcohol is excreted through the lungs is in agreement with that of Atwater and Benedict (103) who found that between 1 and 2 per cent of the ingested alcohol was excreted through the lungs, kidneys and skin. Miles (104) reported that only 1.5 per cent of the ingested alcohol was excreted in the urine during the first two hours, while only 0.3 per cent was excreted during the following six hours.

2. *Delayed Absorption*. Absorption processes have likewise been shown to have no bearing on tolerance. The data of Gettler and Freireich (100) showed the absorption of alcohol from the gastrointestinal tract of alcoholic dogs was somewhat more complete than that of the control animals. Bernhard and Goldberg (105) found that the maximum in the blood curve was reached at an earlier time in chronic drinkers than in abstainers. Fleming and Stotz (90) obtained similar results working on blood and spinal fluid alcohol. Their blood alcohol values rose more rapidly in heavy drinkers than in abstainers.

3. *More Rapid Destruction by Oxidation*. Numerous investigations indicate that the tissues of habitual drinkers acquire the ability to oxidize alcohol more rapidly than those of abstainers. Rosenfeld (106) expressed this belief as early as 1901. Pringsheim (86) claims that rats and rabbits habituated to alcohol destroy it in about two-thirds the time of normal animals. He also states that normal animals reach a 66 per cent higher alcoholic content in the blood. The results of Schweisheimer (107) who investigated the alcohol content of normal and of alcohol-accustomed persons, also showed a higher maximum alcohol content in normal persons. This maximum was reached in one and a half to two hours in normal persons, remaining at this level for about five hours, then gradually diminishing; in alcoholic persons the maxima were reached much more quickly, and remained for about two hours, before subsiding very rapidly. He states that he could find no indication of increased resistance of the tissues, and in a later paper (108) points out that in people who have been chronic alcoholics for about 10 years or more the tissues may lose their previously acquired oxidizing power.

Gettler and Freireich (100) have presented very conclusive evidence of the increased oxidizing ability of alcoholic individuals. When the dogs which had been converted into alcoholics were killed simultaneously with control animals of the same weight, and the organs analyzed in 12 separate experiments, the alcohol content of the organs, blood and spinal fluid of the alcoholics was much lower than that of the control animals, without exception. These results are in agreement with those of Turner (76). Jungmichel (109) however, believes that the difference in combustion power of alcoholics and abstainers exists only when there is a pronounced addiction to one particular beverage. These results are supported by the work of Barach (110) who found that the oxygen treatment of intoxicated persons increases the intelligence and improves the sensory functions.

Additional evidence in favor of increased oxidation in alcoholics is furnished by respiratory quotient (R.Q.) experiments. Le Breton (111), working with pigeons on a sugar diet, obtained R.Q. of 1.03 to 1.08; when alcohol was given the R.Q. dropped to 0.77 to 0.96, which approaches the theoretical value of 0.667. From the change in R.Q. the approximate rate of oxidation of alcohol was calculated. These values corroborate those of Fleischmann (112) on isolated frog muscle. He obtained a value of 1.06 for the R.Q. during the period of recovery, while with the muscle provided with alcohol, the R.Q. was 0.86. Canzanelli and others (113) concluded from R.Q. measurements on dogs that alcohol is oxidized in the body but that it is not utilized as a source of energy.

Aggazzotti (114, 115), who studied the rate of combustion of alcohol at increased pressures, claims that although the respiration increases at higher pressures, the R.Q. remains unchanged.

4. *Acquired Tissue Resistance*. There is no direct evidence in favor of an acquired resistance or tissue tolerance. Because Newman and Cutting (116, 117) found no significant change in the alcohol metabolism of their normal and alcoholic animals, they concluded that if tolerance exists in dogs, it is due to a tissue tolerance and not to an increased oxidation. Their results are based on determinations with only three dogs, and it is possible that the negative results are due to the comparatively short period of habituation. Lévy (118) also contends that the rate of oxidation in those accustomed to alcohol is comparable with abstainers.

Evaluation of the Experimental Work on Alcohol in Relation to Establishing the Degree of Alcoholic Intoxication. In view of the number of known variables which have an influence on the physiologic response to absorption, utilization and elimination of alcohol by the body, it is not surprising that the physiologists have not yet found a quantitative method for establishing the state of intoxication. Many of the conclusions which have been reached regarding intoxication in living persons are based on data obtained in animal experiments under carefully controlled conditions. In many of the experiments the studies were confined to the post-absorptive state during a limited period when it was believed that an equilibrium had been established in the body. Unfortunately, the analyst cannot control the conditions dealing with living persons. Although values given for the rate of oxidation or removal of alcohol from the system are in fair agreement (62, 16, 17, 18, 119, 120, 105, 121) and the rate of absorption through the intestinal walls into the blood stream is reasonably uniform in different individuals (105, 85, 122, 123, 124, 125, 87), the time and conditions under which the alcohol was consumed can seldom be established. Therefore, information regarding the period of absorption and state of equilibrium is seldom available in a medicolegal case. However, in spite of all the variables and factors which introduce an element of uncertainty in chemical analyses for alcohol and the lack of a quantitative method for measuring the disturbances of alcoholic behavior known as intoxication, some definite conclusions can be reached from the chemical values for the concentration of alcohol in the organs and body fluids. The quantitative determination of alcohol must remain, therefore, as one of, if not the primary chemical procedure in toxicologic analysis.

The major criticism in a discussion of interpretation of the chemical values lies in the failure of investigators in general to recognize and accept the existing limitations. The following section is a discussion of the limitations on the interpretations of chemical findings for alcohol. That it is a controversial question can be seen from the subject matter already presented.

After consulting the literature pertaining to ethyl alcohol in relation to intoxication, one is impressed by the fact that the values reported by the various workers are in reasonably close agreement, considering the many variables that enter into the problem. The differences are far more pronounced in the conclusions by the authors than in the data. The explanation for the difference in the opinions expressed by various investigators narrows down to the failure of many to recognize that it is an individual who is under consideration in a medicolegal problem involving intoxication.

In almost all alcohol studies, the data have been collected from a large number of individuals and, invariably, the values on which interpretations have been made were the statistical averages for a group. Fine distinctions have been drawn relating to the degree of intoxication from alcohol concentrations in different organs or body fluids which unquestionably represent a true picture for any group large enough to permit a statistical evaluation. However, because of the many variables that affect the state of intoxication, the alcohol range which includes the physiologic response for the members within the group is much wider than the average. Thus, when this average is applied to an individual, as in a medicolegal case, the interpretation may be in error if he is not this statistically "average" person.

Although the tables (pages 1095, 1096, 1097) relating alcohol concentrations to the degree of intoxication have a range of alcohol values for each physiologic state, the available data show that there are many exceptions, particularly at the lower alcohol range in which the so-called borderline cases fall. The tables fail to establish limits that are wide enough to include all individuals. The overlapping of the values for the different stages in the data of Muehlberger (page 1097) adds another physiologic state without extending the range of values within a particular stage. From the discussion of the experimental work on which the different tables were based, it appears that the range of alcohol concentrations within a stage were optimum values from studies of a group. The uncertainty of the physiologic interpretation is apparently responsible for the failure to include in the evaluation those exceptional cases in which wide deviations occur. In fact, most of the conflicting opinions regarding the question of establishing the degree of intoxication equivalent to the chemical value result from the uncertainty of the physiologic interpretation.

In most of the data expressing the physiologic state in terms of the alcoholic concentration there is a nearly constant difference in the alcohol values in passing from one stage to the next. For example, the mean values with their mean deviations in parts per 1000 from the data in Table 46-5 for the successive stages of intoxication are: stage I, 0.65 ± 0.55; stage II, 1.5 ± 0.6; stage III, 2.4 ± 0.6; stage IV, 3.3 ± 0.6; stage V, 4.2 ± 0.6. A plot of the mean value against the number corresponding to that stage gives a straight line, implying a linear physiologic response to varying alcohol concentrations. Regardless of the physiologic aspect, it would be more illuminating if the data were tabulated as a mean value with its deviation from the mean to represent the physical state.

Those not familiar with the significance of alcohol data are likely to interpret the physiologic response, as tabulated in the conventional manner, as falling strictly within the alcohol range specified by the tables. In this sense, a sharp line is drawn between one physiologic stage and another. Although it may appear captious to criticize the manner in which data are recorded, the primary purpose of most investigations concerning the state of intoxication is to aid in the solution of legal problems and the practice of recording the mean value with the mean deviation would stress the existing variations in the biologic response that are not made apparent to the untrained in the conventional tables.

Up to the present, little experimental work has been done to establish the limiting value for a state of intoxication which pertains to all persons. There is certainly an upper limit for the alcohol concentration of tissue or body fluids at or above which a comatose condition is produced and beyond which toxic symptoms and death may occur. An exact value for this upper limit has not, as yet, been unanimously accepted. From the published literature, as well as the records of this office, there has not been a case reported in which, with an alcohol concentration of 0.46 per cent or greater, there was evidence that the subject was able to walk and coordinate well enough to commit any acts other than damage to himself through falling.* This value, then, would appear to be close to the upper limit at or beyond which the term "dead drunk" would apply to all individuals. It would appear to be independent of all factors that affect intoxication. For practical purposes, it is independent of the organs or tissues used for the analysis, with the possible exception of alveolar air. Another possible, but improbable, exception is the value for the blood alcohol in the very early absorptive state after ingestion of a large amount of alcohol (Table 46-8; and 126-129, 64, 65, 34). On this basis, all limits for the various stages of intoxication then fall above 0 and below 0.46 per cent.

When one attempts to establish some optimum lower limit, below which no individual will show sufficient depression of the sensory system so that alcohol, although present, could be held responsible for any abnormal behavior, the problem appears much more complicated. One of the most careful and complete studies on the relation of alcohol concentration to the physiologic response is the work of Bjerver and Goldberg on the effect of alcohol on driving ability (7). One can find little fault with the methods used and the observations recorded. Their findings indicate that an alcohol concentration of 0.035 to 0.04 per cent in the blood is near the threshhold of impairment of driving ability in expert drivers accustomed to consume moderate amounts of alcohol. They conclude that the role played by alcohol in causing traffic accidents is probably considerably greater than appears from official statistics.

According to their findings there was a 3.3 per cent to 71.8 per cent impairment in driving ability on separate tests, averaging 27.9 per cent, with a blood level between 0.04 and 0.05 per cent. If one takes the individual whose function is 71.8 per cent impaired at a level of 0.05 per cent and projects this impairment to a blood level of 0.15 per cent, assuming the implied linear relationship between alcohol concentration and physiologic response, a 215.4 per cent impairment in driving ability results. In the case of a 3.3 per cent impairment of driving ability with the 0.05 per cent blood alcohol, the blood level would have to reach 1.09 per cent in order to give him the 71.8 per cent impairment of the first individual. This represents more than twice the blood alcohol level of 0.46 per cent which is indicative of a condition corresponding to "dead drunk" while in the first case, the driver is not merely 100 per cent incapable of operating a car but is a little over twice incapable.

---

* This implies that, if even one exception should be proven to this upper limit, the value must be raised accordingly.

Obviously something is wrong in the physiologic interpretations as they pertain to the individual and analogy with other biologic phenomena would lead one to believe that the relation between alcohol concentration and physiologic response must follow a curve more complex than a straight line over the entire alcohol range.

On the basis of Bjerver and Goldberg's findings of only 27.9 per cent as an average for the impairment at an alcohol level up to 0.05 per cent, with a 71.8 per cent maximum impairment, an alcohol level of 0.05 per cent is obviously too low for the boundary line separating possible borderline intoxication and impairment of function from a nonintoxicated state. Projecting the impairment of the single individual to 100 per cent impairment on the basis of a linear response would lead to an alcohol value of 0.07 per cent. Accepted values for the lower limit start at 0.1 per cent. There are more people in the class that responds to lower concentrations of alcohol than are in the group that can tolerate larger amounts. Therefore, to include those individuals who are sensitive to alcohol, the accepted lower limit should be reduced. The more rapid increase in the symptoms in comparison with the alcohol concentration in the phase of increasing intoxication, described by Alha (page 1100), also favors a reduced lower limit. Although the National Safety Council considers values as low as 0.05 per cent as indicative of possible mild intoxication, consideration of the available literature indicates that 0.07 per cent is a more probable value for the lowest limit bordering on intoxication.

A definite impairment of function obviously occurs for all individuals at an alcohol concentration above which all persons could be said legally and morally to be in a state of intoxication. This value constitutes the lower limit for the intoxicated state. The National Safety Council and the American Medical Association Committee to Study Problems of Motor Vehicle Accidents concluded that a blood alcohol concentration of greater than 0.15 per cent is conclusive evidence of intoxication and practically identical interpretations have been incorporated into the laws of several states. Gettler and Tiber (64) analyzed brains in cases of accidental death which were accompained by histories and concluded from their study that when the alcohol content is 0.25 per cent or above, the person is in a condition generally known as intoxication. Turner and Loew (75) set the limit at 0.25 per cent for blood and Andresen (77) at 0.24 per cent. Widmark (78) reports that almost without exception a blood level above 0.2 per cent corresponds to intoxication. Turner (76) later reduced his limit to 0.2 per cent. Although many cases of well defined intoxication have been reported at blood alcohol values below 0.15 per cent, other cases are on record where clinical signs were absent at values well above 0.15 per cent. These cases become fewer in number as the alcohol value approaches 0.21 per cent and no living cases have been cited with values up to 0.25 per cent. In the criticism by Gettler and Freireich (10) of the National Safety Council's limiting value of 0.15 per cent, the fallacy of applying average values to specific cases was pointed out. A survey of the available data indicates that the 0.15 per cent is an optimum rather than the average value for a large group but it is apparent that it is not high enough to include all cases. A mean value which would be characteristic for the larger number of persons who do not have a particular tolerance for alcohol appears to be of the order of 0.12 per cent. On this basis, the borderline range of intoxication becomes 0.12 per cent $^{+\ 0.09\ \text{per cent}}_{-\ 0.05\ \text{per cent}}$ with the probability being greater that intoxication will occur in the average normal person at a value much closer to 0.12 per cent than 0.21 per cent. The data on which these values are based were primarily from blood alcohol analyses and, admittedly, the mean value is dependent on the source.

Mozes and Katonak (91) state that as far as operation of a motor vehicle is concerned, the alcohol concentration of various body fluids and expired air furnishes a far more reliable index of the degree of alcohol influence than the most careful and detailed clinical study. Intoxication is a clinical state defined in clinical terms. The word implies a behavior pattern with dimensions that are based on observation. By definition, then, a person is not intoxicated until he shows the clinical signs which define the term. The Committee on Tests for Intoxication of the National Safety Council (67) stated that when the blood level is between 0.07 per cent and 0.15 per cent the symptoms observed in the medical and physical examination should be considered. This statement should be made to apply to all examinations for intoxication because, in lieu of a physiologic test, the nature of the supporting evidence must determine the significance of the chemical findings. In almost all of the discussions by investigators in the field of alcoholic intoxication, the emphasis has been placed on the chemical findings and, when it has been recommended that a clinical evaluation be made, the clinical findings are supposed to substantiate the stage of intoxication as indicated by the chemical findings. If the problem is to establish the clinical state of the individual, then the clinical findings should take priority, with the chemical values reinforcing the clinical picture.

If the behavior in any of the alcohol ranges for a particular stage of intoxication cannot be predicted, it is illogical to explain actions in retrospect on the basis of chemical analyses. The degree of coordination in living persons should be evaluated by the clinical signs between 0.21 per cent and 0.46 per cent as well as in the lower range and their inclusion in the examination makes it ambiguous to subdivide intoxication into so many stages. In fatal cases in which intoxication is a problem and supporting evidence is not available, the chemical values can provide information on the probable degree of inebriation only.

It does not require a physician to determine well defined intoxication and no cases have been observed in which there was a question in the clinical interpretation with alcohol values of the order of 0.3 per cent. The alcohol range covering the stage designated as definite intoxication then becomes 0.3 per cent $\begin{array}{l} + \ 0.16 \text{ per cent.} \\ - \ 0.09 \text{ per cent.*} \end{array}$

This analysis of the chemical values in terms of the limits for interpreting the stimulation effect is summarized in Table 46-6.

Table 46-6.

CLINICAL STAGE	PER CENT ALCOHOL	OBJECTIVE SIGNS
Subclinical	0.04 $\begin{array}{l}+\ 0.03 \\ -\ 0.03\end{array}$	nonintoxication
Borderline intoxication	0.12 $\begin{array}{l}+\ 0.09 \\ -\ 0.05\end{array}$	nonintoxication to decreased sensitory response
Intoxication	0.3 $\begin{array}{l}+\ 0.16 \\ -\ 0.09\end{array}$	unmistakable intoxication

If clinical signs are a necessary part of an examination for inebriation, the question might be raised concerning the value of any chemical determination. In

---

* The question of the significance of values which express physiologic response (above 0.21 per cent) ceases to be a part of the problem because all persons reaching this level show a definite decrease in sensory response. However, if attempts are made to grade the sensory response within the range of definite intoxication, the physiologic response must be in terms of significant measurements, as in the stage of borderline intoxication.

the first place, from a medicolegal point of view it must be determined that the clinical signs are due to alcohol and not to some other cause. Also, under many circumstances it is important merely to show that alcohol was consumed. In accident cases, as a result of traumatic injury or mental shock, the clinical signs may be entirely misleading when the alcohol values are definitely in the subclinical stage and the determination makes it obvious that other factors are involved. On the other hand, the person involved in the accident may be in such a state of intoxication that clinical signs cannot be evaluated. In other words, from the alcohol analysis, there is no question about the subclinical and unmistakable stages of intoxication. As pointed out by many investigators, the questioned stage is the region designated as the borderline of intoxication. As more supporting evidence becomes available, the chemical value becomes more than probable and the limits within which the chemical values can be said to conform to the physiologic stages as designated in the tables of Muehlberger, Gettler and the others are narrowed (pages 1095, 1096, 1097).

For example, in a hypothetical vehicular homicide in which the deceased is found to have an alcohol value of 0.12 per cent and a witness testifies to his unsteady gait prior to the accident, a conclusion of inebriation is warranted. If, on examination of the driver, a blood alcohol of 0.12 per cent is also found and evidence is shown that the car was being driven in a reckless or careless manner, a verdict of intoxication is also justified. In each case there is evidence to support the fact that both are normal in their response to alcohol. Inconclusive clinical findings for the driver at this alcohol level should not outweigh the testimony of witnesses for, as pointed out by Ladd, Mason and Gibson (79), shock or a feeling of apprehension tend to produce a sobering effect during the examination. In the absence of any supporting evidence, the most that can be said for the chemical values is that both driver and victim were probably in a state of intoxication, as the majority of individuals who react to this alcohol level are intoxicated. It can be said with certainty that both are more liable for the damage done or were more irresponsible for their actions than they would have been without the alcohol, as the experimental evidence is conclusive that alcohol does decrease the physiologic response of the sensory nervous system.

In this discussion of the alcohol values, little has been said about the choice of organs or body fluids. The values from which interpretations regarding living patients have been made were blood alcohol values. Spinal fluid, urine, saliva and alveolar air have been proposed and there has been considerable controversy over the use of spinal fluid values versus blood values as the index of the brain alcohol concentration in living persons (9, 10). A spinal tap is out of the question even if it were the most accurate because it is a procedure incurring some danger. Urinary values obtained in this laboratory (page 1113) have shown much greater variation than blood in comparison with the other tissues. Available data on alveolar air values show it to be less reliable than other materials. The values for saliva are likewise questionable and, considering the ease with which a blood sample can be obtained at the time of a physiologic examination, there is little justification for using any other sample material from living patients.

In the work of Gettler and Tiber (64) the brain was suggested as the true index on which to base the degree of intoxication. Most investigators have been in agreement with this postulation and considerable work has been done in determining the ratio of brain alcohol values to the blood and other organs (11, 12). The brain does control the central nervous system and alcohol is included in pharmacologic texts (130) in the discussion of the central nervous system depressants along with ethyl ether and chloroform, but to postulate that brain alcohol values determine the state of intoxication, although a logical assumption, is nevertheless based on logic for which there is no scientific proof. If one determines the particular concentration of ethyl ether that just produces sleep, the ether level becomes a definite value in terms of the physiologic response. That level is the anesthetizing concentration and, if one repeats the experiment using one-half the anesthetizing concentration of ether and uses the accepted linear interpretation of the ethyl alcohol response to predict the ether effect, then the conclusion would be that the subject is half asleep. This is a fine expression figuratively but literally is of no scientific value. The effect of ethyl alcohol on the brain may not necessarily follow what would appear to be the logical sequence and one could argue just as logically that, because the blood feeds the brain, its level controls the state of intoxication.

There is evidence that the brain does not function as an independent organ in the body and, consequently, interpretations of physiologic response in terms of concentrations of a reactive substance would also be expected to depend on the other factors which control brain function.

In cretinism, the success of therapy depends largely on how early it is instituted, with normal development in every respect resulting if an adequate dosage of U.S.P. thyroid is given in the first few months (131) and this and the fact that disturbances in the cortical architecture of the brain are found in cretins dying at an early age has suggested that the thyroid hormone is not only necessary for proper morphologic development of the central nervous system but also for continuation of its normal function (132).

In Addison's disease in which there are manifestations of a neurologic disorder, the disease is accompanied by focal electroencephalographic changes (133) and both the personality abnormalities and the abnormally slowed electroencephalograms are corrected by administration of either adrenocorticotrophic hormone or cortisone (134, 135). The delirium tremens of acute alcoholism and Addisonian crisis are biochemically and clinically quite similar and adrenocortical extract and ACTH have been found to be one of the most effective treatments of acute alcoholic intoxication (136).

ACTH, cortisone and thyroid extract have been shown to have a marked effect in inducing hypermetabolism (137). This suggests that the rate of oxidation of alcohol is influenced by the function of the endocrine system and, in view of the rapid response of the hormones in producing hypermetabolism, it is to be expected that any factor which sets off the "alarm reaction" should have a rapid and noticeable influence on the state of intoxication. Ingle (138) has stated that he does not know of "any metabolic process which is exclusively the function of any single organ" and, since the physiologic response to alcohol must be related to its metabolism, the manner in which the brain reflects various alcohol levels would not necessarily be expected to follow the same pattern for different individuals at the same alcohol level. Idiosyncrasies and variations in response to drugs are well known. For example, persons with myxedema react with marked narcosis to small doses of morphine whereas hyperthyroid patients tolerate morphine well (139). In discussing the mechanism of anesthetic requirements, Guedel (139a) states "the employment of a routine dose of morphine (for preoperative sedation) is folly." He shows the curve of the normal metabolic rate for individuals from infancy to

80 years of age and discusses the influences on the metabolic rate of endocrine imbalance, fever, pain and emotional excitement. The anesthetic requirements are determined by the condition of the patient. There is no reason to believe that alcohol would show a behavior different from other drugs.

An evaluation, based on studies done in this laboratory (41),* of postmortem cases in which there were discrepancies among the alcohol values of the different organs and which were at variance with the histories could lead to the conclusion that the alcohol content of striated muscle is the best index of the physiologic state when conditions are other than at equilibrium. This proves only that the problem is far from settled, in spite of all the work that has been done, since accurate histories are very difficult to obtain and the number of comparisons of muscle with other tissue in alcohol cases has not been done in enough laboratories to be statistically significant.

Our own animal experiments (41, 126) * † indicate that, at a condition of equilibrium, the difference between the alcohol concentration in the blood, spinal fluid, brain and other organs is negligible in comparison with the limitations for interpreting physiologic response. Values are shown in Table 46-7 for the alcohol concentration which had reached a condition of equilibrium as determined by the percentage of ingested alcohol found in the stomach after the animals were sacrificed. The time interval for absorption was from 50 minutes to 2¼ hours. The data represents selected experiments in which the percentage of ingested alcohol not absorbed from the stomach was not greater than 8.0 per cent or less than 2.3 per cent.

Table 46-7. Per Cent Ethyl Alcohol in Fluids and Tissues of Animals at the Absorption Stage Corresponding to a Condition of Equilibrium

BRAIN	BLOOD	SPINAL FLUID	LIVER	KIDNEY	SPLEEN	MUSCLE	URINE
0.31	0.36	0.35	0.28	0.30	0.30	0.29	0.36
0.24	0.25	0.27	0.23	0.29	0.20	0.22	0.24
0.20	0.23	0.25	0.17	0.22	0.23	0.18	0.30
0.18	0.22	0.20	0.17	0.19	0.17	0.15	0.26
0.16	0.19	0.18	0.14	0.18	0.13	0.11	0.23
0.12	0.13	0.17	0.10	0.11	0.14	0.10	0.18

The findings are in agreement with the conclusions of Harger, Hulpieu and Lamb (12) in their study of the stage of absorption corresponding to a condition of equilibrium.

When the conditions deviate from equilibrium, values of the different biologic samples vary accordingly and, in view of the fact that in a practical case one cannot establish the particular stage in the absorption process, then the controversy over drawing fine distinctions with regard to the selection of the sample material has little meaning. An exception to this is in the absorptive state as equilibrium is being approached. With ingestion of a relatively large amount of alcohol, the blood alcohol concentration may reach a level far in excess of that of the other organs and fluids without clinical signs that are at all close to those that might be predicted from the blood alcohol concentration. Values in the absorptive state of animals given varying quantities of alcohol in a 25 per cent solution are shown in Table 46-8 (126).†

In an extreme case in which a large amount of alcohol was consumed on a bet and in which death occurred within one-half hour, the brain value was 0.72 per

---

* Umberger, C. J., and Ames, A. Unpublished.
† Siegel, H., and Umberger, C. J. Unpublished.

Table 46-8. Per Cent Ethyl Alcohol in Dogs in the Absorptive Stage of Intoxication

WEIGHT IN KG.	GM. ALCOHOL PER KG.	TIME BEFORE DEATH (MIN.)	ALCOHOL INGESTED (GM.)	ALCOHOL REMAIN-ING IN STOMACH (PER CENT)	BRAIN ALCOHOL (PER CENT)	BLOOD ALCOHOL (PER CENT)	SPINAL FLUID ALCOHOL (PER CENT)	URINE ALCOHOL (PER CENT)
11.5	12	37	175	21	0.241	0.756	0.344	0.426
17.0	6	24	125	38	0.211	0.310	0.230	0.277
7.0	9	9	75	28	0.203	0.608	0.218	0.232
8.0	6	17	75	24	0.188	0.401	0.196	0.180
10.0	3	12	50	26	0.141	0.251	0.146	0.145
7.0	6	42	75	12	0.403	0.435	0.422	0.415

cent with a blood alcohol of 0.95 per cent and a urine value of 0.65 per cent (140). In a similar case reported by Ellerbrook (11), the brain concentration was found to be 0.62 per cent with a blood alcohol of 0.94 per cent, a spinal fluid alcohol of 0.98 per cent and a urine alcohol of 0.55 per cent.

From data in Table 46-7, at equilibrium alcohol values for urine are of a similar order of magnitude as the blood and other sample material, while, as seen in Table 46-8, during the absorptive state the urine values are well below those of the blood. Heise has shown the relation between blood and urine alcohol during the absorptive and postabsorptive states (141).

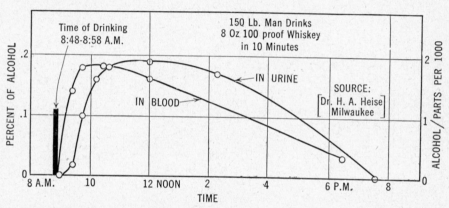

Fig. 46-1. Comparison between Concentrations of Alcohol in Blood and Urine for One Subject at Different Times.

It is improbable that an official examination for intoxication would be made while the subject is in the absorptive state. Nevertheless, findings in which the urinary values are much less than the blood are indicative of the absorptive state. In a case in which both blood and urine are analyzed and the urine concentration is close to or greater than that of the blood, it cannot be maintained that the blood alcohol level was elevated out of proportion to the physiologic response merely because the subject was still absorbing alcohol. In a medicolegal case involving intoxication, the analytic determination should include the analysis of urine as well as blood in order to eliminate any questions concerning the absorptive state. It has even been recommended by the Blood Alcohol Committee in Finland (142) that at least two blood alcohol determinations be done at half hour intervals in order to differentiate between the so-called phases of decreasing and increasing intoxication but a urine analysis would appear to be just as reliable a guide to the condition in which absorption is occurring and intoxication is progressing.

Soon after between 90 and 98 per cent of the ingested alcohol has been absorbed from the intestinal tract into the blood stream and the distribution process by which the various organs and body fluids receive the alcohol is completed, the subject is in the postabsorptive state. The concentration of alcohol starts to decrease from this point on in all the organs and fluids of the body as a result of the oxidation and elimination processes. The rate of oxidation and elimination of alcohol is dependent on such variables as tolerance, physical condition, activity and temperature; consequently, it is not even a constant for the same individual at different times, much less for different individuals (143-146).

This variability in response is clearly demonstrated in the recent comprehensive study of alcohol and its relation to intoxication by Alha in Finland (147). He has shown that, in the postabsorptive stage during the period of decreasing drunkenness, a phase is reached in which the rate of recovery of the sensory system as determined by the clinical signs of intoxication is considerably greater than the rate at which the alcohol concentration of the blood decreases. His graphs showing the blood alcohol concentrations and objective findings for intoxication at different time intervals after ingestion of varying quantities of alcohol are reproduced in Figure 46-2.

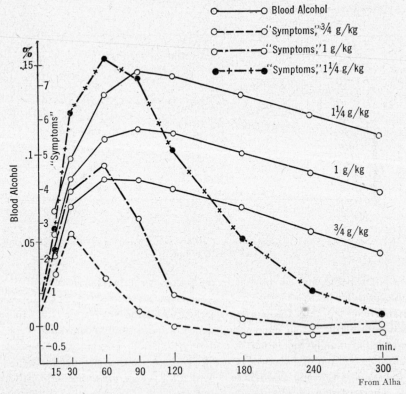

Fig. 46-2. The Average Curves of the Sum of the Clinical Symptoms and of the Blood Alcohol Concentrations on Different Amounts of Alcohol.

The curves show that in a practical examination, the conclusions concerning the degree of intoxication from the blood alcohol level at 90 minutes, for example, are out of proportion to the clinical state that would be predicted from the blood alcohol concentration after 300 minutes, even if physiologic response to alcohol could be measured quantitatively. Since there is no way of estimating the particular phase in the postabsorptive stage, other than in controlled experimentation, the evidence is convincing that a physiologic, as well as a chemical, examination should be a part of any investigation of intoxication.

In spite of the experimental indications that at equilibrium the choice of the biologic sample is immaterial and, even if one is willing to admit that the brain or the blood level is not necessarily the true index of the intoxicated state, there are still definite reasons why the brain should be used rather than other materials in postmortem analyses for alcohol. These are not based on theoretical considerations or on animal experiments but are the result of evaluating a number of analyses of postmortem cases that showed indications of intoxication.* In attempting to determine a constant relating the ratios of the alcohol concentration in the different organs, it was observed in certain cases that marked deviations occurred. Check analyses involving redistillation with duplicate determinations confirmed the fact that these variations were real and not the result of experimental error in the isolation or analytic determination. The only feasible conclusion was that the time interval was far enough removed from any condition which might correspond to equilibrium and that, in the metabolism of alcohol in the body, the rate in the later stages varied with the different organs.

If variations among the different organs occur, while at the same time there is a more consistent relationship between one organ and the fluids which supply the organs, then it is more logical to select that sample material, namely brain, which shows a more constant behavior (Table 46-9). Moreover, in a problem in which there are so many variables to begin with, there should be standard acceptance of the sample material so that there is a uniform basis of comparison of the results of different laboratories. When brain is not available, there is evidence that muscle tissue is the next choice rather than liver, kidney or spleen (Table 46-9).

Another factor in favor of the use of brain is the possibility of early putrefaction. Tissue degradation sets in after death and proceeds more rapidly after the sample material is exposed to the air. In most of the organs, particularly liver, volatile oxidizable products are developed to a greater extent than in brain. Thus, the chance of interference in the determination is less with brain and less extensive purification treatment is needed.

Alcohol findings cannot be used to draw conclusions concerning the probable degree of intoxication under conditions of definite putrefaction. In many cases of suicide and homicide, the body is not discovered until putrefaction has set in and, although the degree of intoxication cannot be established, it is important to determine the presence of significant amounts of alcohol from which it can be inferred that alcohol was consumed prior to death, and depending on the magnitude of the values, that some state of intoxication existed.

Little experimental work has been done on the alcohol values for nonalcoholic tissue that has undergone putrefaction. Wagner (148) reported variable results on the alcohol content of cadaver blood in nonsterilely stored bottles. Nicloux (149-151), on examination of the specially purified distillates of blood and tissue from five cadavers examined at intervals from 12 to 25 days, found alcohol values varying between 0.04 and 0.13 per cent. Experimental work in this laboratory indicates that although oxidizable material is produced somewhat in proportion to the degree of putrefaction, the values reach a maximum which does not exceed the lower range

* Umberger, C. J., and Ames, A. Unpublished.

Table 46-9. Per Cent Ethyl Alcohol in the Postmortem Tissue of Random

Brain	Spinal Fluid	Brain Spinal Fluid	Blood	Brain Blood	Liver	Brain Liver	Kidney
0.28	0.36	0.78	0.32	0.88	0.20	1.40	0.19
0.20	0.24	0.83	0.21	0.95	0.18	1.11	0.15
0.17	0.21	0.81	0.16	1.05	0.11	1.54	0.19
0.38	0.47	0.80	0.41	0.93	0.25	1.52	0.31
0.11	0.15	0.73	0.13	0.85	0.13	0.85	0.12
0.13	0.17	0.76	0.15	0.87	0.07	1.86	0.13
0.27	0.35	0.77	0.30	0.90	0.20	1.35	0.29
0.18	0.22	0.82	0.19	0.95	0.15	1.20	0.22
0.07	0.11	0.64	0.08	0.88	0.09	0.78	0.10
0.10	0.14	0.72	0.09	1.10	0.06	1.67	0.07

in the borderline stage of intoxication. Oxidation values (see page 1090 for oxidation method) for brain, blood and liver from medical examiner's cases in which there was no evidence of ingestion of alcohol prior to death and in which putrefaction had occurred are shown in Table 46-10 (41).*

Table 46-10. Per Cent Alcohol in Nonalcoholic Putrefied Human Tissue

Brain	Blood	Liver	Apparent Putrefaction
0.024	0.033	0.042	slight
0.015	0.037	0.029	slight
0.033	0.043	0.056	moderate
0.043	0.061	0.068	moderate
0.084	0.052	0.107	moderate
0.110	0.143	0.165	advanced
0.093	0.072	0.122	advanced
0.070	0.111	0.145	advanced

Alcohol values determined by the ethoxy method (page 1092) give consistently lower values for nonalcoholic tissue as shown in Table 46-11 (41).*

Table 46-11. Per Cent Alcohol in Nonalcoholic Putrefied Human Tissue by the Ethoxy and Oxidation Methods

Brain		Liver	
Ethoxy	Oxidation	Ethoxy	Oxidation
0.016	0.024	0.019	0.040
0.013	0.027	0.021	0.035
0.081	0.110	0.107	0.145
0.060	0.092	0.077	0.140
0.102	0.125	0.113	0.161
0.008	0.036	0.013	0.077

The lower values by the more specific ethoxy method indicate that oxidizable materials other than alcohol are produced during putrefaction which are not entirely removed by purification of the distillate with the Scott-Wilson reagent.

Experimental work on the so-called normal alcohol (152) demonstrated that the ethyl alcohol isolated from normal tissue by Gettler, Niederl and Benedetti-Pichler (153) was produced in the tissue distillation process. The fact that the normal alcohol increased with the increase in the ammonia liberated during the distillation led to the postulation that the alcohol was formed by hydrolysis of compounds containing the amino linkage. The same phenomenon was found to be more pronounced under conditions of mild putrefaction and the isolation of significant

* Umberger, C. J., and Ames, A. Unpublished.

Cases Examined in the New York City Medical Examiner's Office

BRAIN KIDNEY	SPLEEN	BRAIN SPLEEN	MUSCLE	BRAIN MUSCLE	URINE	BRAIN URINE	BLOOD URINE
1.47	0.22	1.27	0.23	1.22	0.32	0.88	1.00
1.33	0.13	1.54	0.18	1.11	0.25	0.80	0.84
0.89	0.13	1.31	0.13	1.31	0.27	0.63	0.59
1.22	0.40	0.95	0.33	1.15	0.43	0.88	0.93
0.92	0.10	1.10	0.12	0.92	0.15	0.74	0.87
1.00	0.12	1.08	0.13	1.00	0.23	0.57	0.65
0.93	0.31	0.87	0.25	1.08	0.41	0.62	0.73
0.82	0.21	0.86	0.14	1.29	0.29	0.62	0.66
0.70	0.13	0.54	0.09	0.78	0.18	0.39	0.43
1.43	0.11	0.91	0.08	1.25	0.15	0.67	0.60

amounts of ethyl alcohol from these purified distillates points to the fact that it is ethyl alcohol that is primarily responsible for the increased oxidation.

Under conditions of normal refrigeration, the formation of oxidizable substances during putrefaction is not significant. Values for nonalcoholic blood stored in uncorked bottles in the icebox are shown in Table 46-12.* A pronounced odor developed after three days and putrefaction was extensive on the final day of the test.

**Table 46-12. Per Cent Alcohol in Nonalcoholic Human Blood
Stored Under Normal Refrigeration**

TIME (DAYS)	PER CENT ETHYL ALCOHOL
0	0.001
7	0.004
35	0.015
47	0.040

In submersion cases in which putrefaction has progressed to the floater stage, alcohol findings are at a level comparable to that of intoxication. Values for the brain are usually elevated above those in nonsubmersion cases of comparable decomposition while findings for the liver may indicate extensive intoxication. For this reason, liver tissue should not be used for alcohol analysis in drowning cases. It is probable that anaerobic bacterial fermentation processes occur under water that are not pronounced in the absence of submersion. Some brain and liver values in drowning cases with extended submersion are shown in Table 46-13 (41).*

Table 46-13. Per Cent Alcohol in Tissue from Submersion Cases

BRAIN	LIVER
0.21	0.43
0.15	0.35
0.08	0.28
0.12	0.37

Although histories are seldom available in these cases, the consistently high alcohol findings are out of proportion to the probable percentage of intoxication in such cases and positive findings should be evaluated accordingly.

Very little study has been done on the fate of ethyl alcohol in alcohol-containing tissue undergoing putrefaction. Weinig (154) found that a difference in the blood alcohol values appeared from the second day after death and Nicloux (155) showed that some of the alcohol added to blood was lost during putrefaction. When Nicloux

* Umberger, C. J., and Ames, A. Unpublished.

(156) dosed mice with alcohol, killed and stored them under various conditions at a temperature of 20° to 22° C., he found that most of the added alcohol disappeared at the end of 26 days. Control animals stored under the same conditions were found to contain about 0.1 per cent alcohol. Whether the added alcohol was lost as a result of some bacterial action or by simple diffusion and evaporation was not established.

Alcohol losses in blood and brain during putrefaction under conditions of normal refrigeration are not enough to influence the interpretation of the values, as shown in Table 46-14 (41).*

Table 46-14. Per Cent of Alcohol in Alcohol-Containing Tissue under Normal Refrigeration

TISSUE	TIME AFTER DEATH	PER CENT ETHYL ALCOHOL
Brain	5 hours	0.46
	7 days	0.36
	35 days	0.31
	47 days	0.30
Blood	3 hours	0.35
	22 days	0.30
	84 days	0.34
Blood	8 hours	0.25
	11 days	0.23
Blood	4 hours	0.33
	14 days	0.34

When alcohol-containing tissue undergoes putrefaction at room temperature, the picture is quite different. There usually is a rapid initial decrease in the alcohol content which levels off as putrefaction progresses. Values for different portions of the same sample material are quite variable when carried out under the same conditions, indicating that the putrefaction process does not progress in a constant or uniform manner in different samples. Losses during putrefaction in material from medical examiner's cases found to contain alcohol after storage in closed containers at room temperature are shown in Table 46-15 (41).*

Table 46-15. Per Cent Alcohol in Alcohol-Containing Human Tissue Stored at Room Temperature

		PER CENT ALCOHOL	
TISSUE	HOURS STORED AT ROOM TEMPERATURE	OXIDATION METHOD	ETHOXY METHOD
Brain #1	0.0	0.29	0.31
	9	0.16	0.12
	28	0.13	0.09
	62	0.15	0.08
Brain #2	0.0	0.41	0.39
	14	0.27	0.18
	71	0.19	0.10
Brain #3	0.0	0.41	0.39
	14	0.32	0.29
	71	0.28	0.25
Blood #1	0.0	0.36	0.34
	18	0.23	0.18
	96	0.25	0.21
Blood #2	0.0	0.22	0.24
	18	0.15	0.12
	96	0.11	0.07

* Umberger, C. J., and Ames, A. Unpublished.

The evidence is convincing that ingested alcohol is lost during putrefaction and the few in vitro studies that have been made indicate that the values approach the range of the borderline intoxication as a limit. No in vivo experiments have been performed to determine whether changes in the ingested alcohol content of tissue occurring in the body during ordinary putrefaction are comparable to in vitro findings but available evidence suggests that, when changes occur, the ingested alcohol concentration will always decrease in value. On the other hand, as putrefaction progresses in nonalcoholic tissue, alcohol is produced somewhat in proportion to the extent of putrefaction, also reaching a borderline value as a limit.

In an examination of tissue for alcohol from cases that have undergone putrefaction under conditions other than water submersion, positive alcohol findings with values in the intoxicated range are not only indicative of ingested alcohol, but also furnish evidence that the deceased was in an intoxicated state at the time of death to a degree equal to or greater than that indicated by the alcohol values.

Unfortunately, no data are available on the changes that occur during putrefaction of tissue containing borderline concentrations of alcohol but the consistent loss of higher concentrations and the failure of nonalcoholic tissue to exceed the lower range of borderline values suggests that there would be no increase in the alcohol values which might result in an unjust interpretation.

Alcohol in the Organs of Embalmed Cases. Infrequently, investigations of the cause of death are not initiated until after the body has been embalmed, and requests are sometimes made for the determination of the ethyl alcohol content of the organs in these cases. Whether the analysis is worth the effort depends on the circumstances, for the most that can be said with certainty from the findings is that ethyl alcohol is absent. Almost all embalming fluid contains some methyl alcohol as an impurity in the commercial formalin, and some embalming fluids may contain significant amounts of ethyl alcohol as well as many other volatile oxidizing components. Any method of analysis is therefore troublesome and subject to indeterminate errors. A method has been described (157) for the estimation of ethyl alcohol in the presence of embalming fluid, which depends upon the oxidation of methyl alcohol and formaldehyde to carbon dioxide and water, and the simultaneous oxidation of the ethyl alcohol to acetic acid, which is then distilled off and titrated. The success of this procedure depends upon rigidly controlled conditions for the oxidation process, and the absence of titratable compounds in the oxidized sample other than acetic acid. Failure to oxidize all of the methyl alcohol and formalin to carbon dioxide results in a high positive error, while excessive oxidation can cause low results, due to breakdown of the acetic acid to carbon dioxide.

The ethoxy method (page 1092) offers the best possible procedure for determining ethyl alcohol in embalmed cases. Although methyl alcohol reacts, a simultaneous ethyl and methyl analysis can be made (page 1093), or the methyl alcohol content can be corrected for, if a sample of the embalming fluid is available. Analysis of a few commercial embalming fluids by the ethoxy method are shown in Table 46-16.

Table 46-16. Alcohol Content of Commercial Embalming Fluids by the Ethoxy Method

SAMPLE	PER CENT ETHYL ALCOHOL
A₁	0.96
A₂	0.87
B	1.34
C	0.58
D	0.72

Analyses of the distillate of brain tissue of some embalmed cases in which death occurred more than 24 hours after hospital admission are shown in Table 46-17.

Table 46-17. Analysis of Embalmed Normal Brain Tissue for Alcohol

CASE	PER CENT ALCOHOL
1	0.027
2	0.015
3	0.032
4	0.064
5	0.045
6	0.038

With the better grades of embalming fluid, the methyl alcohol and other impurities are apparently not present in the distillates in amounts which cause significant interference in the determination, and negative findings in any case rule out alcohol as a factor in establishing the cause of death.

Legal Aspects of the Alcohol Problem. One cannot study the literature and experimental work and read the legal reports on alcoholic cases without forming an opinion about the scope of the medicolegal problem regarding alcoholism in living persons. Any recommendations would be inconsistent with the previous discussion if they did not provide that a person suspected of alcoholic intoxication should have a physical examination and a quantitative chemical analysis of some biologic sample to determine if a charge of intoxication is warranted. In any case, the chemical examination is a necessary step in indicating the possible level of intoxication (as discussed on page 1106) but, within the level of borderline intoxication, a consideration of the circumstances and the results of the physical examination should take priority over the chemical findings in evaluating the condition of the suspect. Thus, the problem becomes one of securing a workable procedure for accomplishing this objective.

Regardless of the reliability of alveolar air for quantitative analysis, it offers an easily performed qualitative test which excludes the presence of alcohol when it is negative and can distinguish between traces and significant amounts when it is positive. Its use has been criticized because occasionally the results may be abnormally high or may give a false positive reaction. Such errors or slight inaccuracies would become apparent when the suspect is given a further clinical and quantitative chemical examination. Since interpretations of the results of quantitative determinations on alveolar air, saliva or urine alone may be questionable or sometimes erroneous, blood remains the only body fluid which meets the requirements of a quantitative scientific analysis as far as the determination of alcoholism in the living patient is concerned. At the time the blood sample is taken, a sample of urine should be collected, if possible, as an aid in evaluating the stage of the absorption process.

For a workable method, the law should provide for a complete physical and chemical examination. Positive findings from the alveolar air test could then serve more properly as justification for such examinations rather than as a measure of intoxication. This, of course, creates the problem of examining a suspect and performing necessary chemical tests without violating the legal rights of the individual but, unless the clinical examination and the procurement of a sample for chemical analysis are made compulsory, on the basis of positive findings and objective observations, the use of alveolar air as a qualitative test would not be practical. If the suspect refuses to be examined, his objections would be difficult to surmount under the present law and his failure to cooperate makes evaluation of the clinical signs difficult. The law could be altered to make examination mandatory over the objections of the suspect, although many people do not regard this as a desirable solution of the problem. However, positive qualitative findings in the alveolar air test have the effect of placing the suspect on the defensive and, if he is familiar with the legality of the procedure, his failure to cooperate only increases the suspicion of his intoxication. A nonintoxicated person has little difficulty in convincing an examiner of his sobriety, if he so desires, whereas the same person, in a state of intoxication, only adds further evidence of his alcoholic state in his effort to appear sober.

If this problem of intoxication is sufficiently important to require legislation, it is just as important to provide the machinery for fair, competent and impartial investigation. A trained police officer can easily carry out the simple test on alveolar air when it is used only as a qualitative procedure. However, specially trained personnel are necessary to carry out the examinations which have been outlined above. Such a staff should be organized after the pattern of a medical examiner's office and be independent of the police and district attorney.

The alcohol problem has been settled in Sweden in a drastic fashion, where the law governing intoxication sets the limits for the concentration of alcohol in the blood at which a vehicle can be operated, without regard to a specific stage of intoxication. For discussion about the situation in the United States, see page 183.

REFERENCES

1. Dubowski, K. M.   An Evaluation of Methods for the Determination of Ethyl Alcohol in Biological Materials, Ph.D. Thesis, Abstracts of Doctoral Dissertations, No. 61, Ohio State University Press, 1951.
2. Gettler, A. O., and Tiber, A.   The quantitative determination of ethyl alcohol in human tissues, Arch. Path. Lab. Med., 3:75, 1927.
3. Fleming, R., and Goldman, N.   Experimental studies in alcoholism. III. The effect of alcohol on a complex reaction time, J. Gen. Psychol., 14:392, 1936.
4. Hansen, K.   Ein exakteres Mass. f.d. Alkoholizierungsgrad des Organimus, usw. Arch. internat. de pharmacodyn. et de thérap., 30:355, 1925.
5. Graf, O.   Über den Zusammenhang zwischen Alkoholblut konzentration und psychischer Alkoholwirkung, Arbeitsphysiol., 6:169, 1932.
6. Fleming, R.   A psychiatric concept of acute alcoholism intoxication, Am. J. Psychiat., 92:89, 1935.
7. Bjerver, K., and Goldberg, L.   The effect of alcohol ingestion on driving ability, Quart. J. Stud. on Alcohol, 11:1, 1950.
8. Fales, H. A.   Inorganic Quantitative Analysis, 1st ed., New York City, The Century Co., 1925, pp. 9 and 58.
9. Heise, H. A., Harger, R. N., Muehlberger, C. W., and Jetter, W. W.   Comments by members of Committee on Tests for Intoxication of National Safety Council on blood alcohol and intoxication: its value in borderline cases, Am. J. Clin. Path., 15:613, 1945.
10. Gettler, A. O., and Freireich, A. W.   Answers to comments by members of the Committee on Tests for Intoxication, Am. J. Clin. Path., 15:618, 1945.
11. Ellerbrook, L. D., and Van Gaasbeek, C. B.   The reliability of chemical tests for alcoholic intoxication, J.A.M.A., 122:996, 1943.
12. Harger, R. N., Hulpieu, H. R., and Lamb, E. B.   The speed with which various parts of the body reach equilibrium in the storage of ethyl alcohol, J. Biol. Chem., 120:689, 1937.
13. Newman, H. W., and Mehrtens, H. G.   Reliability of spinal fluid analysis in the diagnosis of drunkenness, Proc. Soc. Exper. Biol. & Med., 30:725, 1933.
14. Renaux, E.   Determination of alcohol in the blood and urine, J. Pharm. Belg., 12:639, 1930.

15. Naville, F. Chemical proof of drunkenness and the chemical measurement of its intensity, Rev. méd. de la Suisse Rom., No. 13:849, 1928; Schweiz. Apoth. Ztg., 67:246, 1929.

16. Haggard, H. W., and Greenberg, L. A. The absorption, distribution and elimination of ethyl alcohol. I. The determination of ethyl alcohol in air, blood and urine by means of iodine pentoxide, J. Pharmacol., 52:137, 1934.

17. ———— II. The excretion of alcohol in urine and expired air and the distribution of alcohol between air and water, blood and urine, J. Pharmacol., 52:150, 1934.

18. ———— III. Rate of oxidation of alcohol in the body, J. Pharmacol., 52:167, 1934.

19. Bornstein, A., and Budelman, G. Excretion of alcohol and ether through the kidneys, Arch. f. exper. Path. u. Pharmakol., 150:47, 1930.

20. Abels, J. C. Determination of ethyl alcohol in saliva, Proc. Soc. Exper. Biol. & Med., 34:504, 1936.

21. Harger, R. N., Lamb, E. B., and Hulpieu, H. R. A rapid chemical test for intoxication employing breath, J.A.M.A., 110:779, 1938.

22. Heise, H. A. The specificity of the test for alcohol in body fluids, Am. J. Clin. Path., 4:182, 1934.

23. Gettler, A. O., and Freireich, A. W. Determination of alcoholic intoxication during life by spinal fluid analysis, J. Biol. Chem., 92:199, 1931.

24. Gorr, G., and Wagner, J. A new method for the separation of ethyl alcohol from acetaldehyde and acetone, Biochem. Ztschr., 161:488, 1925.

25. Friedemann, T. E., and Klaas, R. The determination of ethyl alcohol, J. Biol. Chem., 115:47, 1936.

26. Kozelka, F. L., and Hine, C. H. Method for the determination of ethyl alcohol for medicolegal purposes, Indust. & Engin. Chem. (Anal. Ed.), 13:905, 1941.

27. Newman, H. W. The determination of ethyl alcohol in body fluids, J. Pharmacol. & Exper. Therap., 56:278, 1936.

28. Nicloux, M. Simplification de la méthode de dosage de l'alcool dans le sang et dans les tissus, Compt. rend. Soc. de biol., 60:1034, 1906.

29. McNally, W. D., and Coleman, H. M. A micro method for the determination of ethyl alcohol in blood, J. Lab. & Clin. Med., 29:429, 1944.

30. Harger, R. N. A simple micromethod for the determination of alcohol in biologic material, J. Lab. & Clin. Med., 20:746, 1935.

31. Chaikelis, A. S., and Floersheim, R. D. A micro method for the quantitative estimation of alcohol in gastric or intestinal contents, Am. J. Clin. Path., 10:180, 1946.

32. Johnston, G. W., and Gibson, R. B. A distilling apparatus and a procedure for the determination of alcohol in blood and urine, J. Lab. & Clin. Med., 26:399, 1940.

33. United States War Department, Technical Manual 8-227, Methods for Laboratory Technicians, Washington, D. C., Government Printing Office, 1941, p. 132.

34. Simmons, J. S., and Gentzkow, C. J. Laboratory Methods of the United States Army, 5th ed., Philadelphia, Lea and Febiger, 1944, p. 342.

35. Widmark, E. M. P. A micromethod for the estimation of alcohol in blood, Biochem. Ztschr., 131:473, 1922.

36. Abels, J. C. A simple method for the determination of ethyl alcohol in blood, Proc. Soc. Exper. Biol. & Med., 34:346, 1936.

37. Sheftel, A. G. A simple colorimetric method for the determination of the alcohol concentration in urine and blood, J. Lab. & Clin. Med., 23:534, 1938.

38. Levine, H., and Bodansky, M. A simple accurate method for the determination of alcohol in body fluids, Am. J. Clin. Path., Tech. Suppl., 4:103, 1940.

39. Cavett, J. W. The determination of alcohol in blood and other body fluids, J. Lab. & Clin. Med., 23:543, 1938.

40. Shupe, L. M., and Dubowski, K. M. Ethyl alcohol in blood and urine. A simple photometric method for its forensic determination, Am. J. Clin. Path., 22:901, 1952.

41. Umberger, C. J., and Ames, A. Unpublished data, Laboratory of the Chief Medical Examiner of New York City.

42. Gettler, A. O., and Umberger, C. J. A quantitative method for ethyl alcohol normally present in blood, J. Biol. Chem., 143:633, 1942.

43. Vieböck, F., and Brecher, C. New method for the volumetric determination of methoxy- and ethoxy- groups. II. Microanalysis. Ber. chem. Ges. 63B:3207, 1930.

44. Umberger, C. J., and Ellerbrook, L. D. Unpublished data, Laboratory of the Chief Medical Examiner of New York City.

45. Küster, W., and Maag, W. The microdetermination of methyl and ethyl groups in the presence of each other., Ztschr. f. physiol. Chem., 127:190, 1923.

46. Nicloux, M. Recherches Expérimentales sur l'Élimination de l'Alcool dans l'Organisme. Détermination d'un "Alcoolisme Congénital," Paris, O. Doin, 8°, no. 523, 1900.

47. Miles, W. R. Alcohol and Human Efficiency—Experiments with Moderate Quantities and Dilute Solutions of Ethyl Alcohol on Human Subjects, Washington, D. C., Carnegie Institute Publ. #333, 1924.

48. Vernon, H. M. The Influence of Alcohol on Normal Work and Neuro-muscular Co-ordination, London, H. M. Stationery Office, 1919.

49. Hollingworth, H. L. The influence of alcohol. I., II., J. Abnorm. & Social Psychol., 18:204, 1924.

50. Meyer, F., and Atzler, E. Strenuous work by a heavy drinker as influenced by alcohol, Arbeitsphysiol., 4:410, 1931.

51. Koren, J. Alcohol and Society, New York, Henry Holt and Co., 1916.

52. Koller, J. Methods and results of our blood alcohol investigations, Deutsche Ztschr. f. d. ges. gerichtl. Med., 26:234, 1936.

53. Gréhant, N. Injection d'alcool éthylique dans le sang veineux, Compt. rend. Acad. d. sc., 120:1154, 1895.

54. ―――― Dosage de l' alcool éthylique dans le sang après l'injection dirècte dans les veins ou après l' introduction des vapeurs alcooliques dans les poumons, Compt. rend. Acad. d. sc., 123:192, 1896.

55. ―――― Dosage de l'alcool dans le sang recueilli d' heure en heure après l' injection intra-veineuse d' une certaine dose d' alcool éthylique, Compt. rend. Soc. de biol., 48 (10. s. iii):839, 1896.

56. ―――― Toxicité de l' alcool éthylique, Compt. rend. Soc. de biol, 55:225, 1903.

57. ―――― Démonstration du passage dans l' estomac contenant de l' eau et de l' alcool éthylique injecté dan le sang, Compt. rend. Soc. de biol., 55:376, 1903.

58. ―――― Influence de l' exercice musculaire sur l' élimination de l' alcool éthylique introduit dans le sang, Compt. rend. Soc. de biol., 55:802, 1903.

59. ―――― Dosage de l'alcool dans le sang après l' ingestion dans l' estomac d'un volume mesuré de ce liquide; courbe complète, Compt. rend. Soc. de biol., 55:1264, 1903.

60. ―――― Chimie physiologique; recherches sur l' alcool éthylique injecté dans le sang ou dans l' estomac et sur ce qu'il devient dans l' organisme, J. de physiol. et de path. gén., 9:978, 1907.

61. Abel, J. J. The Physiological Aspects of the Liquor Problem, 2nd ed., Boston and New York, 1903, pp. 1-167.

62. Mellanby, E. Alcohol: Its Absorption into and Disappearance from the Blood under Different Conditions, Great Britain M. Res. Comm., 1919.

63. Carpenter, T. M. Ethyl alcohol in fowls after exposure to alcohol vapor, J. Pharmacol., 37:217, 1929.

64. Gettler, A. O., and Tiber, A. The alcoholic content of the human brain, Arch. Path. Lab. Med., 3:218, 1927.

65. Bogen, E. Drunkenness: a quantitative study of acute alcohol intoxication, Am. J. M. Sc., 176:153, 1928.

66. Heise, H. A., Shurly, B. R., McGoldrick, T. A., and Roberts, C. W. Report of the Committee to Study Problems of Motor Vehicle Accidents, J.A.M.A., 112:2164, 1939.

67. Report of the Committee on Tests for Intoxication, National Safety Council, Chicago, 1938.

68. Holcomb, R. H. Alcohol in relation to traffic accidents, J.A.M.A., 111:1076, 1938.

69. Heise, H. A., and Halporn, B. Medicolegal aspects of drunkenness, Pennsylvania M. J., 36:190, 1932.

70. Whitney, C. F. Comparison Between Urine Alcohol Concentrations and Degree of Intoxication, Report of the Committee on Tests for Intoxication, National Safety Council, Chicago, 1938, p. 31.

71. Bavis, D. F. Correlation Between Amount of Alcohol in Blood and Urine, Report of the Committee on Tests for Intoxication, National Safety Council, Chicago, 1938, p. 32.

72. ―――― Comparison Between Urine Alcohol Concentrations and Degree of Intoxication, Report of the Committee on Tests for Intoxication, National Safety Council, Chicago, 1938, p. 32.

73 Friedemann, T. E., Motel. W. G., and Necheles, H. The excretion of ingested ethyl alcohol in saliva, J. Lab. & Clin. Med., 23:1007, 1938.

74. Muehlberger, C. W. Report of the Committee on Tests for Intoxication. National Safety Council, Chicago, 1938, pp. 12-13.

75. Turner, R. G., and Loew, E. R. Blood alcohol and its relation to intoxication, J. Pharmacol., 44: 305, 1932.

76. ―――― Blood alcohol and its relation to intoxication in man, Proc. Soc. Exper. Biol. & Med., 32:1548, 1935.

77. Andresen, P. H. Estimation of alcohol in blood for medico-legal purposes, Medico-Legal Criminol. Review, 1:223, 1933.

78. Widmark, E. M. P. Die theoretischen Grundlagen und die praktische Verwendbarkeit der gerichtlich-medizinischen Alkoholbestimmung, Berlin, Urban and Schwarzenberg, 1932.

79. Ladd, Mason, and Gibson. Iowa Law Review, XXIV, #12: 1939.

80. Jungmichel, G. The importance of alcohol estimation in blood in forensic and clinical medicine, München. med. Wchnschr., 82:365, 1935.

81. Widmark, E. M. P. Distribution and transformation of ethyl alcohol in the organism of the dog, Biochem. Ztschr., 267:128, 1933.

82. Meyer, H. H. Relation between the Widmark factors β and γ in rabbits and the action of alcohol on its own oxidation in the organism, together with a comparison of the blood-alcohol and blood-sugar curves, Biochem. Ztschr., 276:174, 1935.

83. Le Breton, E. Relation of the concentration of ethanol in the blood to its rate of oxidation in the organism, Compt. rend. Soc. de biol., 117:707, 1934.

84. Kozelka, F. L. Medicolegal aspects of alcoholism, Wisconsin M. J., 34:816, 1935.

85. Le Breton, E. Speed of diffusion of ethanol in the organism in relation to the method of administration, Compt. rend. Soc. de biol., 117:704, 1934.

86. Pringsheim, J. Chemical investigation of the nature of the tolerance of alcohol, Biochem. Ztschr., 12:143, 1908.

87. Harger, R. N., and Hulpieu, H. R. Extent of absorption of alcohol at various intervals after oral administration, Proc. Soc. Exper. Biol. & Med., 32:1247, 1935.

88. Tuovinen, P. Alcohol content of the blood under different conditions (Über den Alkoholgehalt des Blutes), Skandinav. Arch. Physiol., 60:1, 1930.

89. Mehrtens, H. G., and Newman, H. W. Alcohol injected intravenously. Its penetration into the cerebrospinal fluid in man, Arch. Neurol. & Psychiat., 30:1092, 1933.

90. Fleming, R., and Stotz, E. Experimental studies in alcoholism. I. The alcohol content of the blood and cerebrospinal fluid following oral administration in chronic alcoholism and the psychoses, Arch. Neurol. & Psychiat., 33:492, 1935.

91. Mozes, E. B., and Katonak, L. J. One hundred drunken drivers, Ohio State M. J., 37:21, 1941.

92. Southgate, H. W. Effect of alcohol under varying conditions of diet on man and animals with some observations of the fate of alcohol in the body, Biochem. J., 19:737, 1925.

93. Elbel, H., and Lieck, G. Alcohol resorption after eating, Deutsche Ztschr. f. d. ges. gerichtl. Med., 26:270, 1936.

94. Widmark, E. M. P. Effect of the composition of food on the alcohol content of the blood, Biochem. Ztschr., 267:135, 1933.

95. Le Breton, E. Influence of the nature of the food oxidized on the rate of oxidation of ethanol in the animals. Case of proteins, Compt. rend. Soc. de biol., 117:709, 1934.

96. Nicloux, M. Combustion of alcohol in a cold blooded animal. Value of the temperature coefficient, Compt. rend., 193:364, 1931.

97. Nyman E., and Palmlöv, A. Elimination of ethyl alcohol in sweat, Skandinav. Arch. Physiol., 74:155, 1936.

98. Le Breton, E. Effect of fasting on the rate of oxidation of ethyl alcohol in the white rat, Compt. rend. Soc. de biol., 122:330, 1936.

99. Folger, H. T. Acclimatization of Bufo tadpoles to ethyl and methyl alcohols, Science, 66:18, 1927.

100. Gettler, A. O., and Freireich, A. W. The nature of alcohol tolerance, Am. J. Surg., 27:328, 1935.

101. Cushny, A. R. On the exhalation of drugs by the lungs, J. Physiol., 40:17, 1910.

102. Bödlander, G. Die Ausscheidung aufgenommenen Weingeistes aus dem Körper, Arch. f. d. ges. Physiol., 32:398, 1883.

103. Atwater and Benedict, cited by Emerson, Alcohol and Man, New York, The Macmillan Co., 1932, p. 8.

104. Miles, W. R. Comparative concentrations of alcohol in human blood and urine at intervals after ingestion, J. Pharmacol. & Exper. Therap., 20:265, 1922.

105. Bernhard, C. G., and Goldberg, L. Absorption and oxidation of alcohol in alcoholics, Acta med. Scandinav., 86:152, 1935.

106. Rosenfeld, G. Der Einfluss des Alkohols auf den Organismus, Wiesbaden, J. F. Bergmann, 1901.

107. Schweisheimer, L. Der Alkoholgehalt des Blutes unter verschiedenen Bedingungen, Deutsches Arch. f. klin. Med., 109:271, 1913.

108. ———— Behavior of alcohol in the human body, Schweiz. Chem. Ztg., 524, 1920.

109. Jungmichel, G.   The physiology of alcohol oxidation after beer and meals, Deutsche Ztschr. f. d. ges. gerichtl. Med., 22:153, 1933.
110. Barach, A. L.   The action of oxygen in counteracting alcoholic intoxication. Am. J. Physiol., 107:610, 1934.
111. Le Breton, E.   Untilization of variations in the respiratory quotient for determining the part played by the oxidation of alcohol. Case of carbohydrate diet, Compt. rend. Soc. de biol., 119:1014, 1935.
112. Fleischmann, W.   The utilization of the oxidation energy of alcohol in muscle work, Biochem. Ztschr., 219:7, 1930.
113. Canzanelli, A., Guild, R., and Rapport, D.   The use of ethyl alcohol as a fuel in muscular exercise, Am. J. Physiol., 110:416, 1934.
114. Aggazzotti, A.   Action of compressed air on animals. XVII. Combustion of ethyl alcohol injected in rats, Boll. Soc. ital. biol. sper., 10:782, 1935.
115. ———— Action of compressed air on animals. XXVIII. Combustion of ethyl alcohol injected in increasing doses, Boll. Soc. ital. biol. sper., 10:784, 1935.
116. Newman, H. W., and Cutting, W. C.   Alcohol injected intravenously. Effect of habituation on rate of metabolism, J. Pharmacol., 55:82, 1935.
117. ———— and Cutting, W. C.   Alcohol injected intravenously. The effect of habituation on rate of metabolism, J. Pharmacol., 57:388, 1936.
118. Lévy, J.   Experimental alcoholism. Mechanism of alcohol tolerance, Compt. rend., 199:973, 1934.
119. Le Breton, E.   Influence of the concentration of alcohol in the tissues on the rate of oxidation in vivo, Compt. rend. Soc. de biol., 119:572, 1935.
120. Nicloux, M.   The combustion of alcohol in vivo. Its measurement: apparatus and technic, Compt. rend. Soc. de biol., 107:529, 1931.
121. Newman, H. W., and Cutting, W. C.   Alcohol injected intravenously. Rate of disappearance from the blood stream in man., J. Pharmacol., 54:371, 1935.
122. Goldhahn, R.   Determination of blood alcohol in cases of accident, Medico-legal Criminol. Review 2: Pt. 1, 80; Klin. Wchnschr., 1834-6, 1932.
123. Cori, C. F., Villiaume, E. L., and Cori, G. T.   Intestinal absorption. II. The absorption of ethyl alcohol, J. Biol. Chem., 87:19, 1930.
124. Delhougne, F.   Experimental studies on absorption in the stomach, Arch. f. exper. Path. u. Pharmakol., 159:128, 1930.
125. Vahlmering.   Zentralbl. biochem. biophys., 14:520, 1912.
126. Siegel, H., and C. J. Umberger.   Unpublished data, Laboratory of the Chief Medical Examiner of the City of New York, 1935-1936.
127. Fry, A.   Private communication.
128. Jetter, W. W.   Studies in Alcohol. I. Diagnosis of acute alcoholic intoxication by a correlation of clinical and chemical findings, Am. J. M. Sc., 196:475, 1938.
129. ———— Studies in alcohol. II. Experimental feeding of alcohol to non-alcoholic individuals, Am. J. M. Sc., 196:487, 1938.
130. Edmunds, C. W., and Gunn, J. A.   Cushny's Pharmacology and Therapeutics, Philadelphia, Lea & Febiger, 1940, p. 289.
131. Duncan, G. G.   Diseases of Metabolism, Philadelphia, W. B. Saunders Co., 1942, p. 239.
132. Grinker, R. R.   Neurology, 2nd ed., Springfield, Ill., Charles C Thomas Co., 1937, p. 305.
133. Thorn, G. W., Forsham, P. H., Prunty, F. T. G., Bergner, G. E., and Hills, A. G.   Clinical studies in Addison's disease, Ann. New York Acad. Sc., 50:646, 1949.
134. ———— Forsham, P. H., Bennett, L. L., Roche, M., Reiss, R. S., Slessor, A., Flink, E. B., and Somerville, W.   Clinical and metabolic changes in Addison's disease following the administration of compound E acetate, Tr. A. Am. Physicians, 62:233, 1949.
135. Hoefer, P. F. A., and Glaser, G. H.   Electroencephalographic and Neuropsychiatric Changes in Patients Treated with Adrenocorticotrophic Hormone (ACTH), Proceedings of the First Clinical ACTH Conference, New York, The Blakiston Co., 1950, pp. 536-543.
136. Smith, J. J.   The Role of the Adrenal Gland in Alcoholism, Proceedings of the First Clinical ACTH Conference, New York, The Blakiston Co., 1950, p. 566.
137. Werner, S. C., Hamilton, H., and Frantz, V. K.   Some Effects of ACTH in Chronic Thyroiditis and Myxedema, Proceedings of the Second Clinical ACTH Conference, New York, The Blakiston Co., 1951, Vol. II. Therapeutics, pp. 521-528.
138. Ingle, D. J.   Some studies on the role of the adrenal cortex in organic metabolism, Ann. New York Acad. Sc., 50:592, 1949.
139. Goodman, L., and Gilman, A.   The Pharmacological Basis of Therapeutics, New York, The Macmillan Co., 1941, p. 204.
139a. Guedel, A. E.   Inhalation Anesthesia, New York, The Macmillan Co., 1937, Chap. 5, p. 61.

140. Laboratory of the Chief Medical Examiner of the City of New York.
141. Heise, H. A. Report of the Committee on Tests for Intoxication, National Safety Council, Chicago, 1938.
142. cited by Alha, A. R. Blood alcohol and clinical inebriation in Finnish men. A medico-legal study., Ann. Acad. Scient. Fennicae V. Medica-Anthropologica 26, 1951.
143. Mayer, R. M. Intermittent alcohol resorption, saliva-alcohol curve and alcohol effect, Deutsche Ztschr. f. d. ges. gerichtl. Med., 26:250, 1936.
144. Newman, H. W. J. Clin. Psychopath., 8:83, 1943.
145. ———— and Fletcher, E. The effect of alcohol on driving skill, J.A.M.A., 115:1600, 1940.
146. ———— Fletcher, E., and Abramson, M. Alcohol and driving, Quart, J. Stud. on Alcohol, 3:15, 1942.
147. Alha, A. R. Blood alcohol and clinical inebriation in Finnish men. A medico-legal study., Ann. Acad. Scient. Fennicae V. Medica-Anthropologica 26, 1951.
148. Wagner, K. Variability of the alcohol content of cadaver blood in non-sterilely stored blood samples, Deutsche Ztschr. f. d. ges. gerichtl. Med., 26:276, 1936.
149. Nicloux, M. Neoformation of alcohol in human cadavers during putrefaction, Compt. rend. Soc. de biol., 121:975, 1936.
150. ———— Alcohol in putrefied blood and in cadavers. Microdetermination. Chemical study. Neoformation., Bull. soc. chim. biol., 18:318, 1936.
151. ———— Determination of alcohol in putrefied blood and tissues, Compt. rend. Soc. de biol., 120:1301, 1935.
152. Umberger, C. J. A study of the ethyl alcohol normally present in the tissue and body fluids, Ph.D. thesis, New York University, 1940.
153. Gettler, A. O., Niederl, J. B., and Benedetti-Pichler, A. A. The isolation, identification and quantitative determination of ethyl alcohol normally present in human and animal tissues, Mikrochemie, 11:167, 1932.
154. Weinig, E. The alcohol level in cadaver blood, Deutsche Ztschr. f. d. ges. gerichtl. Med., 26:293, 1936.
155. Nicloux, M. Fate of alcohol in blood allowed to putrefy in vitro, Compt. rend. Soc. de biol., 120:1304, 1935.
156. ———— The fate of alcohol in the dead body of a mammal given alcohol. Neoformation of alcohol in the dead bodies of animals not given alcohol, Compt. rend. Soc. de. biol., 120:1306, 1935.
157. Abernethy, R. J., Russell, E. R., and Thienes, C. H. The estimation of alcohol in the brain, J. Lab. & Clin. Med., 19:1014, 1934.

47

The Nonvolatile Organic Poisons

Analysis of organs and body fluids for the nonvolatile organic poisons is by far the most difficult of the toxicologic procedures. When the toxicologist receives organs from a case in which the history, autopsy report or both suggest the presence of a particular substance, he need only look up the drug in some text and select the best isolation procedure and qualitative and quantitative methods described. However, he will find no procedure described for those cases of the general unknown type in which reports of the circumstances of death and of the autopsy findings fail to indicate a cause of death. Toxicologists usually develop or adapt their own general methods, patterned after the classic Stas-Otto extraction procedure for alkaloids (1, 2, 3), for isolating drugs. Unfortunately, so little of this work has been published that there has been little agreement concerning a standardized working procedure for the isolation and purification processes in the analysis. Any information pertaining to losses during the recovery of different substances is usually limited to the experience of the individual applying his own methods. The problems are understood by most of the analysts and, in scientific meetings (4), they have discussed the shortcomings of the processes of isolation, recovery and identification of materials from tissues. Simple solubility data, except for the common solvents, are rarely available unless listed by the manufacturer in his advertising literature, so that the development of a process generally applicable to the isolation of unknown drugs meets with many obstacles. Furthermore, conventional organic qualitative methods of identification such as those developed by Kamm (5), Shriner and Fuson (6) and Mulliken (7), with Beilstein (8) as the reference, are not adaptable to toxicologic analysis.

In a death from poisoning, the causative agent is more likely to be one of the common drugs. In a general unknown case, even if it is a newly developed drug rather than a standard proprietary, at least a detectable quantity *may* be recoverable by application of any one of a number of isolation technics to the tissue sample. The problem of its identification is quite different from a case in which there is some evidence to suggest a particular poison. The analyst may determine the physical and chemical properties of the isolated substance but, because no references are available which catalogue drugs according to their properties, he must make a page by page comparison with known compounds in an attempt to find properties corresponding to those of the unknown substance. Methods for the isolation, chemical testing and quantitative determination of most drugs, along with their medicinal use, pharmacologic activity and dosage, are described in the literature and in toxicologic textbooks but all these references tabulate the chemical and physical properties under the name of the particular substance. As a result, the existing process for the identification of unknown drugs has been little more than a guessing game in which success has depended on the analyst's experience to permit him to select the right series of reagents or to apply the correct physical test in seeking a positive result suggestive of a particular substance. The process has been one of random testing and, if it has failed to indicate a substance known to the analyst, the sample material has soon been exhausted, followed by the logical report that nothing toxic could be found.

The use of the term toxic substance is inappropriate as far as the chemical analysis is concerned, for it cannot be determined that a substance isolated from tissue is toxic until it has been identified. Outside of drug sensitivities, most pharmaceutical compounds are toxic only when taken in excess of the prescribed dose. Any compound taken in large enough amounts is a potential poison. For the analyst, the nontoxic drugs with properties which permit them to be isolated from tissue are as important as any of the physiologically more potent drugs for, once the qualitative examination begins, any unidentified substance isolated in abnormal amounts is a potential poison. Cholesterol, some amino and fatty acids, benzoic acid, para-aminobenzoic acid, hippuric acid, saccharin, the chemically reactive vitamins, phenolphthalein, and all organic solvent-soluble drugs prescribed in large doses should be included in the subject matter covering the chemical phase of toxicology. Positive identification of an isolated substance is imperative, for the term unknown poison has no place in a pathologic report, regardless of the circumstances.

The rapid advances in the pharmaceutic field have resulted in a continuous flow to the market of new and more reactive synthetic drugs whose properties have not been compiled in the reference literature. In toxicologic laboratories where attempts are made to keep active files for qualitative analysis, there is seldom time or personnel to study new drugs in order to place them in their proper analytic category. It is not uncommon for the laboratory handling medical examiner's cases routinely to isolate a substance giving positive results in any number of chemical reactions; although melting points and molecular weights may be known, the identification of the substance can rarely be made unless it has been studied and its properties tabulated in the laboratory file. If the case remains under investigation long enough, the substance may be recognized eventually by its resemblance to a known compound studied at a later time in the laboratory. For this reason, the usual practice of setting time limits for processing medicolegal cases which involve the identification of organic compounds should be discouraged because chemical findings that are not negative are indeterminable only when the sample material is no longer available.

The obvious solution to the problem of the general unknown in analytic toxicology is the development of a systematic scheme of analysis, in which the drugs and related compounds are tabulated according to their reactivity with reagents into groups and subgroups. Starting with a general type of reaction and following with more specific testing would be expected to lead to identification of the substance, as long as it is included in the scheme. Toxicologic analysis, however, is complicated by factors not encountered in other analytic fields. Because the analyst has only a limited amount of sample material at his disposal, he can expect to isolate only micro quantities of the chemical substance, at most. Once the isolated material is exhausted, no other source of supply is available and the failure is permanent. The analyst is compelled, therefore, to use only those tests which give maximum information and the preliminary testing must be limited to sensitive nonspecific reactions that are positive for a large number of compounds.

The purity of the isolated compound is of major importance, for in any of the conventional processes of isolation of the drugs from tissue and body fluids, varying amounts of normally occurring tissue extractives are always removed simultaneously with the drugs. Each purification step is also attended by loss of the unknown compound. Since a purification method presupposes a knowledge of the unknown sought, the general nature of the unknown compound must be ascertained before the final purification can be made with safety. This factor limits the type of identifying reactions to those which are possible in the presence of the naturally occurring tissue impurities.

These complications which circumscribe the use of conventional organic micromethods, coupled with the vast scope of the field and the diversified nature of the pharmaceutics encountered, make it unlikely that a successful systematic toxicologic scheme of analysis can be devised. On the other hand, chemical analysis that is not systematic does not meet the requirements for a scientific process. The basic principles to be followed in this section for the analysis of general unknown have been termed a systematic approach (9) which differs from a systematic scheme in that the course of the analysis is more or less open to the analyst, depending on his experience and whatever information is obtained from the clinical symptoms and pathologic report (10). A systematic scheme rigidly followed in toxicologic analysis is not only impractical, but dangerous, since a mistake in any one step in the scheme misleads the analyst in all succeeding steps.

The major difference between a toxicologic analysis of organs and tissues and any other analytic chemical problem is that the analyst first has to separate the chemical from the tissue matrix before he can begin his analysis. Once the isolation and purification phases have been completed, the limiting factors for identification of the unknown are the quantity of sample available, and the state of purity of the isolated product. In the identification process, reactions must be selected for their sensitivity and specificity on the basis of available sample weight. The smaller the sample of unknown available for analysis, the more conservative must be the analytic approach, with the chances for success reduced proportionately. Isolation is, then, the primary factor for determining the success or failure of the analysis.

The sensitivity for the detection of an unknown substance by color or precipitation reactions is a function of the concentrations of the normally occurring tissue extractives in the residue. A single microcrystal of a pure compound will show a far more sensitive and clear-cut reaction than the extracted substance of many times its weight contaminated with the lipid-like material that is always extracted from the tissue along with the organic compound. Purity of the isolated product, therefore, controls the sensitivity of the reaction for detection of the poison.

In attempting to develop a general scheme for the isolation of all types of drugs, with maximum recovery from the tissue and maximum purity of the isolated product, two opposing factors are encountered. All available isolation methods for the non-volatile organics utilize extraction with organic solvents. The more exhaustive the extraction, the better the recovery of the drug; but at the same time the greater will be the contamination of the isolated product. The more contaminated the product, the more involved the purification process must become, and the introduction of each additional purification step entails a loss of the unknown compound. Consequently, if the extraction process is carried beyond the stage for optimum removal of the drugs, the further extraction only serves to add more impurities to the residue, with increased losses of drug when the final separation of the normal tissue components is made.

The process for isolation of drugs for qualitative examination must be a compromise procedure, therefore, with an adequate recovery in a tissue extraction residue that can be purified to yield detectable amounts of the different substances if taken in quantities corresponding to their lethal dosages. The minimum tissue sample from which a sufficient quantity of isolated compound can be extracted in an adequate state of purity for its detection as an unknown is of the order of 500 gm. for the more toxic drugs (page 1190). In cases where the cause of death is not indicated, it is futile for the pathologist to submit small samples of tissue with a request for an analysis for poisons. Disposal is the least difficult of the toxicologic processes and the pathologist would do better to submit too much rather than too little of the autopsy material.

Since the qualitative isolation and purification processes are compromises, with only adequate recovery in order to gain maximum purity of the final product, the yield is not necessarily quantitative. The amount recovered from the tissue must not only be sufficient for performing a series of qualitative tests, but also a separate tissue sample must be available after the substance has been identified for a special isolation process which may be modified to give a quantitative recovery for the quantitative determinations.

The opinion of practising toxicologists is not unanimous regarding the use of one relatively large sample in order to isolate enough compound to carry out the variety of tests necessary for the detection of all possible drugs. The opposite school recommends the use of very small tissue samples, with a separate isolation procedure as a part of each test. Usually, reliance is placed on sensitive physical methods to indicate the substance. The basic argument for this approach is based on the fact that the more commonly used drugs are more likely to be encountered, and chance is in favor of a solution during the course of testing for the more probable poisons. In addition, savings in time and labor, with more quantitative recovery requiring less purification, are claimed.

In cases where enough information is available to suggest a particular substance, this testing process has advantages over the involved procedure utilizing large tissue samples. The laboratory following this practice for all cases, however, can only hope for successful solution of its analytic problems on a percentage basis, for the growing number of available pharmaceutics that are toxic when taken in excess makes it increasingly difficult to predict the agent in a death from poison.

As sample material for starting the analysis for the detection of the nonvolatile organics, the stomach contents are the first choice, when available. If the dose of ingested drug was large enough to produce death before absorption through the intestinal walls was complete, then larger recoveries in a purer state are possible from stomach contents than from any organ or body fluid. Metabolites or detoxification products of the compound are not isolated as in extracts from organs, and the reactions are more comparable to the control tests. Analysis of an organ must still be made to prove absorption, but identification is usually much easier on extracts from the viscera, particularly with the substances of low lethal dosage. Furthermore, once identification is made, shortcuts in the procedure can be devised for the organs.

Brain tissue is the best organ for the analysis. Solvent extraction residues from brain contain smaller amounts of the extractable normal tissue components, and most organic substances may be recovered from it with better yields.

More recent distribution studies in animals indicate that lung tissue is potentially good sample material for the isolation of organic compounds. Purification of lung extracts incurs more difficulty than that of brain, and it has been used very little in toxicologic analysis.

Urine is the best source material in cases where death was delayed. If enough time has elapsed to permit concentration of the drug in the urine, the extra yields will more than pay for the labor involved in the special purification to remove pigments and chromogens.

Extracts from blood are relatively pure except for cholesterol, which interferes with some color reactions carried out in sulfuric acid. Blood is the only source material for compounds like the sulfa drugs, but it is seldom available in quantity sufficient to isolate detectable amounts of the more toxic substances.

Deposition of the unmetabolized ingested drugs has been shown to occur extensively in fatty tissue, but the lack of a suitable purification procedure for fatty extracts makes it an impractical source material.

Liver is the source material most frequently used when brain is not available, but purification of liver extracts is far more difficult than purification of brain, and the final product is never as free of interferences. Reactions on brain extracts invariably show much greater sensitivity than on the liver in the same case. Infrared absorption studies of fresh liver extracts still show significant absorption after extensive purification, while extracts from brain show little or no absorption with only moderate purification.

The purification problem increases with the age of the sample material, and if putrefaction has set in, contamination of the extracts with tissue degradation products will require such extensive purification that many of the toxic substances will be completely lost before removal of the interferences is completed. Brain that has been stored in the refrigerator overnight will contain a larger percentage of tissue impurities than the same sample removed and immediately placed in alcohol. A brain that stands for three hours at the autopsy table in a hot room will not give as pure an extraction residue as it will when analyzed immediately. To avoid deterioration, a deep freeze should be standard equipment in the autopsy room, as well as in the laboratory, and samples removed for analysis should be stored at low temperatures as quickly as possible.

The chances for the successful isolation of an adequate quantity of drug from embalmed tissue are even less than from putrefied tissue. Putrefaction is not a problem, provided the compound can be extracted. The fixing action on the tissue occludes intracellular substances so that they are not readily extractable from the homogenized sample. The solvent action of the formalin with postmortem diffusion also acts to reduce the yield.

In the preceding discussion, the terms isolation and purification have been used both together and separately. An isolation procedure includes partial purification as an integral part of the extraction process. In the subject material which follows, the term purification is reserved for the special processes by which the small amounts of normal tissue components are separated from the organic poison in the residue after the isolation process has been completed.

ISOLATION AND EXTRACTION

ISOLATION

A. Water- and Alcohol-Soluble, Nonvolatile, Organic Compounds from the Steam Distillation Filtrate.

A. Water- and Alcohol-Soluble, Nonvolatile, Organic Compounds from the Steam Distillation Filtrate. Steam distillation of a sample of brain tissue (see Chapter 45) is the logical first step in toxicologic analysis. Many of the nonvolatile poisons are water-soluble and heat stable up to the temperature of 100° C. and during the distillation process will be extracted from the tissue suspension and remain dissolved in the undistilled aqueous phase which can be separated from the tissue residue by filtration. Since the brain sample has to be sacrificed for the volatile analysis and the distillation filtrate may contain the substance sought, an examination of this aqueous filtrate is the logical starting point for the nonvolatile organics. During the steam distillation the heat coagulates the tissue; and as a result of the cooking process the normal tissue extractables are rendered more insoluble than by any other treatment. The final residue therefore is obtained in a state of greater purity than by any other isolation process. Less time is required to process the filtrate than in any other procedure, and the water-soluble compound that is recovered in the more readily purified residue will respond to the tests for its detection with the maximum sensitivity for the reaction. If, after identification, the quantities recovered are comparable to a lethal dose, there is no need for the more involved isolation process. If nothing is found, or the concentration recovered leaves doubt as to the cause of death, the analysis has served to indicate a further and more complete extraction.

There are three possible sources of error when this procedure is used in the general unknown type of case:

1. Certain organic poisons are not stable at 100° C. and are lost as a result of hydrolysis.

2. Coagulation of the proteins in the distillation process produces a densely packed insoluble mass in which appreciable quantities of water-soluble substances are found by occlusion. With some types of organic structure, absorption is extensive and the occlusion and absorption phenomena may result in very low recoveries.

3. Water-insoluble drugs will not be recovered in this extraction process.

In the laboratory where routine toxicologic analysis is being done the advantages of beginning the analysis on the aqueous filtrate far outweigh the objections. The biggest percentage of the common drugs are sufficiently soluble in water to permit their detection from analysis of this residue.

On a yearly basis, the added labor in carrying out both isolation procedures on those special cases where the more involved extraction has to be made will result in an over-all saving of time and labor for all cases processed, because in approximately 80 per cent of those cases in which nonvolatile organics are present, the identification can be made from the extract of the distillation filtrate alone.

Procedure. The steam distillation is carried out on 500 gm. of ground tissue to which about 600 ml. of water and 3 ml. of 50 per cent tartaric acid are added. The final volume of tissue suspension is approximately 1,500 ml. Filter while still hot through 38 cm. fluted filter paper, collect about one liter * and begin evaporation. Allow to drain overnight and add to original filtrate. Open paper and allow the residue to air dry. Hold it for extraction with alcohol (page 1130), in the event that it becomes necessary to make an examination for water-insoluble, alcohol-soluble substances. Transfer the filtrate to a round bottomed evaporating dish, set in the open steam bath, and evaporate to a thick syrup. About eight hours are required for the evaporation. Overnight in the bath will give nearly the proper consistency, but the residue must not be allowed to evaporate to near dryness. Add slowly with stirring 600 ml. of 95 per cent ethyl alcohol. Let stand with intermittent stirring for at least one hour and preferably overnight. Protein material is precipitated by the alcohol, and if it is added too rapidly, the immediate precipitation will occlude some of the drug. Filter off the precipitate through a

* The aqueous suspension should be distinctly acid to litmus. If not, add tartaric acid dropwise until acidic.

cotton plug, and reevaporate the alcohol solution on the steam bath until the consistency is that of a thick syrup and the odor of alcohol is absent. Take up the residue in approximately 80 ml. of cold water, mixing with a rubber-tipped stirring rod. Filter through a cotton plug and then through paper into a 300 ml. separatory funnel. The aqueous solution is then extracted by the procedure on pages 1138, 1139 (Table 47-1).

Table 47-1. Isolation of Water- and Alcohol-Soluble Compounds

Aqueous Tissue Suspension from Steam Distillation (page 1128)

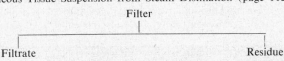

Filter

Filtrate	Residue
Check acidity and evaporate to a syrup on the steam bath. Slowly take up in approximately 600 ml. 95% ethyl alcohol. Let stand one hour or more	Hold for possible extraction of water-insoluble compounds (page 1130)

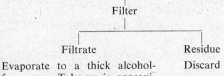

Filter

Filtrate	Residue
Evaporate to a thick alcohol-free syrup. Take up in approximately 80 ml. water	Discard

Filter

Filtrate	Residue
Extract with organic solvents (pp. 1138, 1139)	Discard

This process is designed for speed and simplicity. Under conditions of mild to severe putrefaction, better purification is attainable by repeating the alcohol and water extractions alternately.

B. Water-Insoluble, Alcohol-Soluble, Heat-Stable Compounds from the Steam Distillation Filtrate.*

B. Water-Insoluble, Alcohol-Soluble, Heat-Stable Compounds from the Steam Distillation Filtrate.* Ingestion of the insoluble type of poisons produces pathologic signs that furnish a clue to their presence. At least partial solubility is a prerequisite for absorption of ingested material through the intestinal walls; and, in the manufacturing process for the synthetic drugs, the purification steps depend on solubility with but few exceptions. Consequently, practically all the nonvolatile organics that can produce death without pathologic findings are either water- or alcohol-soluble, or both. Heat-stable, water-insoluble drugs and occluded water-soluble compounds remaining in the residue from the steam distillation filtrate can be recovered by extraction with alcohol. The water-insoluble, alcohol-soluble members are comparatively few in number and the procedure for processing this residue is quite laborious in comparison with the filtrate. Only under unusual circumstances will it be needed; for, in those cases where findings from the filtrates indicate a more complete extraction, the continuous extraction procedure on uncooked tissue (page 1139), is the only plausible choice.

Although the final extract contains somewhat smaller proportions of fatty material than with uncooked tissue, the interference is great enough to require final purification of the extracted residue. There is a tendency for hydrolytic products to produce anomalies in the chemical reactions; and considering the possibility of changes occurring in the structure of the drugs, there is considerably more to gain by analysis of a residue from uncooked tissue.

* The procedure as described includes the complete isolation from uncooked tissue as well as the residue from the distillation.

This procedure, which is only a modification of the original Stas-Otto method for alkaloids, is more likely to find use where there is a shortage of sample material and extensive occlusion and absorption of the water-soluble compounds are suspected. Although recoveries are not nearly as good, it can be applied to uncooked tissue when the apparatus for continuous extraction is not available. Its main use in toxicologic analysis is for the extraction of the stomach contents or residues from the evaporation of urine samples.

Procedure. 1. Approximately 500 gm. of cooked or uncooked tissue, nearly half of the stomach contents or the residue from the evaporation of a urine sample is mixed with about 4 volumes of 95 per cent ethyl alcohol, and enough 50 per cent tartaric acid

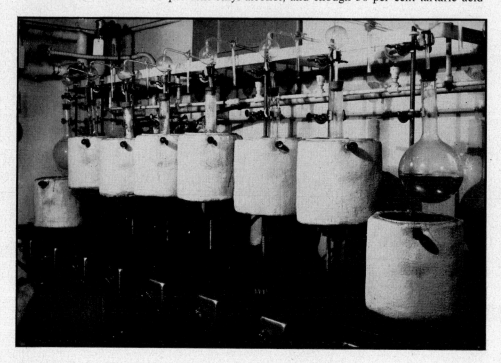

Fig. 47-1. Vacuum Evaporators.

added to make the mixture distinctly acidic. If heavy solid material immediately settles out on stirring, homogenize the mixture in a Waring Blendor to give a fine suspension of solid dispersed in the alcohol. Digest the mixture with intermittent stirring, at a temperature which should not exceed 60° C. for the uncooked tissue, for at least two hours. Following this, filter the mixture through cheesecloth, then through cotton, and wash the residue with 95 per cent alcohol.

2. Again extract the residue with 95 per cent alcohol as in step 1. Combine the filtrates and evaporate them to a syrupy consistency. With uncooked tissue, in order to avoid decomposition of some heat-labile compounds, carry out the evaporation preferably in a vacuum evaporator at a temperature not exceeding 60° C. (Fig. 47-1). Cooked tissue may be evaporated at the temperature of the steam bath, but in either case in the interest of economy a condensing system should be used to recover the alcohol. During the evaporation, rotate the container occasionally to prevent overheating on the sides, and thus obviate the formation of a brown water-insoluble pigment which is difficult to remove during the subsequent purification steps.

The tissue residue from the extraction in steps 1 and 2 is reserved for extraction with water (step 7).

3. To the syrupy liquid from the evaporation of the combined filtrates from step 2, add an equal volume of absolute ethyl alcohol and stir and reevaporate the mixture. Continue the evaporation process until the odor of alcohol has disappeared, taking the

same precautions as in step 2. The evaporate should be of free-flowing syrupy consistency, but not viscous.

If there is a relatively large bulk of undissolved suspension or the alcohol solution is quite turbid, the addition of absolute alcohol and evaporation should be repeated. The alcohol treatment further denaturizes any protein material and dehydrates lipids and glycolipids, rendering them less colloidal.

4. Take up the syrupy liquid from step 3 in about 3 volumes of water made acid with tartaric acid; add one-half the volume of acetone. Allow the mixture to stand several hours to let the suspended matter settle out, then filter it first through a cotton plug and then through filter paper with suction. A DeWitt type of filter with platinum cone speeds up the filtration. Reserve the residue for step 6. The acetone treatment precipitates lecithin type lipids.

5. Again evaporate the filtrate, taking precautions as in step 3. Take up the syrupy liquid in 50 to 100 ml. of water, filter it through paper with suction, and hold the filtrate for extraction with organic solvents (page 1137).

6. Air-dry the cotton plug and filter papers containing the residues from steps 4 and 5 and store them in a desiccator. When dehydration is complete extract them with about 100 ml. of ethyl alcohol or other nonaqueous solvent, filter through paper, and hold the filtrate for examination of substances insoluble in water, such as croton and ricin oils, cantharadin or nonvolatile esters and ethers.

7. Mix the tissue residue from the alcohol extractions in steps 1 and 2 with an equal volume of water, made acidic to Congo red paper with mineral acid and heated on the steam bath to near boiling. Allow the mixture to cool and filter it through a combination of cotton cloth and fluted filter paper. The cotton cloth contains the filter paper and residue, and is used to squeeze out the absorbed water without the residue breaking through the paper. Evaporate the aqueous filtrate to a voulme of about 100 ml., refilter through paper, and reserve the filtrate to test for alcohol-insoluble, water-soluble substances, such as toxalbumins and salts of acids stronger than tartaric, such as sodium oxalate.

8. Dehydrate the tissue residue in a vacuum desiccator, immerse it in a nonpolar organic solvent, and store it in a closed container.

The only toxic substances not removed up to this point are the very few water-insoluble, alcohol-insoluble, special solvent-soluble materials, such as the rat poison alphanaphthylthiourea (ANTU). The residue is relatively free of fats and fatty acids, and proteins have been made insoluble by denaturization. Some lipids, like cephalin and cerebrocide-like material, still remain. If the residue is allowed to dry in air, particularly with brain tissue, it darkens, becomes tough and leathery in consistency, and is impermeable to the special solvents which may be required for the extraction.

9. The aqueous solution remaining from the solvent extraction in the separation of the acidic and basic compounds may contain water- and alcohol-soluble, solvent-insoluble compounds (pages 1138, 1141, 1144) (Table 47-2).

The experienced operator may make any number of shortcuts in this method, depending on the nature and the condition of the original sample material. On the other hand, more extensive treatment may be required, particularly with putrefied tissue. Additional alcohol treatment (step 3), or alternate alcohol and water treatment (steps 4 and 5), may be necessary when the syrupy residue is unusually large and readily dissolves on addition of the solvent with formation of highly colloidal solutions. Where the history points to the absence of heat sensitive poisons, preliminary heat treatment, using a cooking process analogous to that in the steam distillation, will yield a final aqueous filtrate of greater purity.

The biggest objection to this procedure is that experience is a necessary part of the process. To obtain a final residue that is clear with adequate recovery, the operator must be able to recognize the necessity for changes in the method, from the way in which the precipitation occurs, and its size, color, and consistency.

C. Continuous Extraction.

C. Continuous Extraction. There has long been a need for a standardized isolation procedure in which the experience of the analyst was not the controlling factor in determining purity and yield of the isolated product.

Table 47-2. Isolation of the Nonvolatile Compounds *

Ground Brain or Other Residue from a Steam Distillation, Urine Evaporate, Uncooked Organs or Stomach Contents

|

Add 95% ethyl alcohol made acid with tartaric (step 1)

|

Filter through gauze, then cotton

1st Alcoholic Filtrate — **Residue**

Repeat 95% alcohol extraction (step 2)

Filter

2nd Alcoholic Filtrate — **Residue**

Extract with equal volume H₂O (acid to Congo red paper) (step 7)

Filter

Combine

Evaporate to a syrupy consistency and take up in 100 ml. absolute alcohol (step 3)

Filter

Filtrate — **Residue**

Re-evaporate to a syrup and take up again in 100 ml. absolute alcohol — Discard †

Filtrate — **Residue**

Evaporate and examine for alcohol-insoluble, water-soluble compounds | Dehydrate and extract with nonpolar solvents (step 8)

Filter

Filter

Filtrate — **Residue**

Re-evaporate to a syrup. Take up residue in 3 volumes H₂O and add ½ the volume of acetone (step 4) — Discard †

Filtrate — **Residue**

Evaporate and examine for alcohol-insoluble, water-insoluble compounds — Discard †

Filter through cotton, then gauze

Filtrate — **Residue**

Evaporate to remove acetone and take up in acid water (step 5)

Filter

Filtrate — **Residue**

Extract with organic solvents by the procedure on page 1137.

Combine

Dry and extract with alcohol or other nonaqueous solvent (step 6)

Filter

Solvent layer — **Aqueous layer**

Examine for water-, alcohol- and solvent-soluble compounds | Examine for water- and alcohol-soluble, solvent-insoluble compounds (step 9)

Filtrate — **Residue**

Examine for water-insoluble, alcohol-soluble compounds — Discard †

* This is the flow sheet for the complete isolation from any type of biologic material. Steps 1, 2, 3, 4, 5 are essentially the same as Table 47-1, except that they include isolation of the alcohol-soluble, as well as water-soluble compounds.

† The term discard means that the residue, wash water, etc. are set aside and are not used further in the extraction process. They are not thrown away until the analysis is completed.

More complete extraction is possible from fresh untreated tissue, and use of an apparatus for continuous extraction was expected to be an improvement over manual extractions. Several years ago attempts to adapt various types of continuous extractors to tissue analysis were so discouraging that the project was abandoned. Best results were obtained using a glass extraction thimble with a bottom made from a sintered glass filter disk (10). The homogenized tissue dispersed in alcohol was put in the glass extraction thimble which was placed inside a standard ether-water type continuous extractor. Although extraction proceeded in the usual manner, heavy tissue particles finally settled out on the bottom, plugging up the filter plate; and all attempts to prevent it from plugging by mechanical or air agitation failed. Glass filter plates with coarser grain allowed considerable solid matter to pass through before they, too, finally blocked up. Recoveries were variable and the operation was too troublesome to be practical.

The recent increase in drug addiction, along with deaths from apparent drug sensitivity and the advent of infrared spectrophotometry, which requires much larger samples for the analysis, created the immediate need for improved recoveries of drugs from tissue. Processes for continuous extraction were therefore reexamined. In order to improve recoveries, occlusion and absorption had to be at a minimum, and consequently extractions of the tissue had to be more exhaustive. The more exhaustive extraction, with greater removal of the normal tissue extractables, made improvements in the purification of the extract necessary. It was obvious that simplicity in the design of the apparatus and brevity of operating time in the procedure had to be sacrificed in the interest of efficient recovery. The difficulties in the early attempts at continuous extractions were overcome after the proper design for the extraction apparatus had been determined, by adding the alcoholic tissue suspension to a paper thimble placed inside the glass extraction thimble. The apparatus shown in Figure 47-2 was made to specifications by E. Machlett and Son.* It consists of a 1 liter receiver flask mounted on a 1,200 watt hot plate, and connected to the extraction chamber through a side arm by means of a #24/40 interchangeable glass joint. Two such flasks should be available so that the alcohol can be quickly replaced with a fresh solution by interchanging the receiver flasks. The extraction chamber has a capacity of approximately 1 liter up to the side arm tube; the distance from the bottom of the chamber to the side arm outlet is 25 cm. The internal diameter (I.D.) of the extraction chamber is 7 cm. The total height from the bottom to the #71/60 ground glass joint is 51 cm. A reducing adapter with #60/71 and #40/50 joints connects the extraction chamber with a 35 cm. bulb condenser. A glass extraction thimble, 50 cm. high with a 57 mm. I.D. with an extra coarse sintered glass plate fits into the extraction chamber, which is mounted on an 800 watt hot plate.

The dimensions of the inner paper thimble are such that it fits snugly against the walls of the glass extraction thimble. The pores of the paper thimble are small enough to prevent tissue particles from passing through, and the glass thimble reinforces the walls so that the tissue mixture does not break through the paper. Agitation is necessary to prevent packing of the tissue in the thimble assembly. Better mixing is accomplished by passing in gas under pressure through a 7 mm. I.D. glass tube resting on the bottom of the paper thimble. This glass tube, bent to form a small U at the bottom, passes up through the condenser and is connected through a rubber hose with a pressure regulator on a compressed nitrogen tank. The sintered glass disk of the thimble assembly serves to set up a static pressure head, rather than act as a filter. The alcohol level rises in the thimble about one-half the height of the column above the side arm of the extraction chamber as a result of the back pressure created when the apparatus is in operation.

Paper thimbles can be obtained from the Carl Schleisher and Schmell Co.† It has been found that thimbles constructed from 23 by 23 inch Whatman filter paper #2 are equally good. The sheet of filter paper is rolled to a diameter that will fit into the glass thimble. A fold is made from one-half to three quarters of an inch from the loose open edge of the paper. Under this fold the entire cylinder is creased down and clipped flat through all thicknesses of the paper by standard sized staples spaced 1 inch apart. The stapled edge is folded over to make a seam with the smooth side of the staples inside toward the cylinder and pressed flat. The bottom of the cylinder is turned up about 1 inch and clipped with 4 staples, 2 horizontal ones on each end and 2 vertical on either side of the seam.

Time has long been recognized as one of the best reagents for the separation of

* E. Machlett and Son, 220 East 23rd Street, New York, N. Y.
† Carl Schleisher and Schmell Co., 116-118 West 14th Street, New York 11, N. Y.

tissue extractives from the drugs. Once the initial extraction is made, the longer the solutions stand around, the less trouble there is in making the separations. Alcohol has a denaturizing effect, as shown by the fact that the more extensive the alcohol treatment, the less is the solubility of the tissue components. Dehydration also decreases the solubility of the tissue extractives, and the longer the dried residues stand in air, the

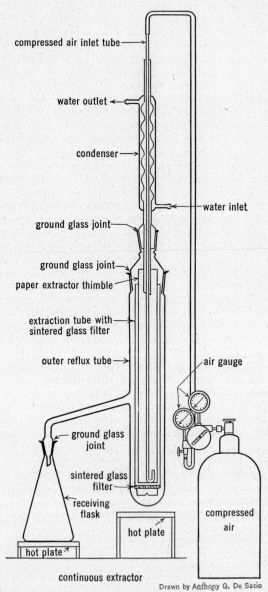

compressed air inlet tube

water outlet

condenser

water inlet

ground glass joint

ground glass joint
paper extractor thimble

extraction tube with
sintered glass filter

outer reflux tube

air gauge

ground glass
joint

sintered glass
filter

receiving
flask

compressed
air

hot plate

hot plate

continuous extractor

Drawn by Anthony G. De Sario

Fig. 47-2. Continuous Extractor.

less soluble they become. Strangely enough, spontaneous drying at room temperature gives the most insoluble tissue residues.

Experience, as well as theoretical considerations, has shown that the ultimate in separating the tissue components from the drugs would involve crystallization, rather than precipitation of the tissue impurities from the alcohol, and efforts to obtain purer drug residues were directed toward maximum crystallization with a minimum precipitation in an optimum operating time.

An analogy can be drawn between the crystallization of tissue impurities and the precipitation of aluminum ion as the hydroxide with the formation of a crystalline precipitate. If ammonia is added to an aqueous solution of aluminum ion containing small amounts of other ions, the white flocculant precipitate of $Al(OH)_3$ will contain large amounts of the other ions that were in the solution. It is common practice in microchemistry to add an ion called a carrier to a solution which, when precipitated, will occlude or adsorb small amounts of another ion which in itself cannot be precipitated. Willard and Tang (11) published a method in which $Al(OH)_3$ was precipitated by the addition of urea. In aqueous solution urea slowly breaks down with the formation of ammonia. The slow production of ammonium ion resulted in such a slow formation of $Al(OH)_3$ that the precipitate came down crystalline without the removal of other ions from the solution.

A variety of procedures were tried in an effort to favor crystallization. Quick cooling by dry ice, low temperature refrigeration, the addition of flocculating agents, and salting effects were not found to aid the recovery process. As a result of a study of optimum conditions of temperature, volume of solution, and time of standing, on the rate of precipitation of impurities from alcohol, a standardized method of processing was worked out which gives precipitates of tissue extractives with much larger particle size and a more crystalline structure than previously obtainable. Filtration is possible through a Buchner filter with an asbestos mat. A considerably greater volume of alcohol is used, so that a process for reclaiming alcohol is essential. Adherence to detail is important. Some of the steps are hard to justify theoretically, but experience has shown that the conditions are critical.

Extraction Procedure (10). 500 gm. samples of tissue homogenized in alcohol are extracted. Because the capacity of the Waring Blendor is not sufficient to macerate the entire sample, it is divided into two 250 gm. portions for emulsification with alcohol in the Blendor.

Grind 500 gm. of tissue in a meat grinder and divide into two 250 gm. portions. Place 250 gm. in the quart size container of the Blendor, and add 500 ml. of 95 per cent ethyl alcohol containing 5 ml. of saturated tartaric acid. After the mixture is homogenized transfer it to a 3 liter beaker. Then homogenize the second 250 gm. portion and add it to the first in the 3 liter beaker. Wash out the Blendor with 500 ml. of the 95 per cent ethyl alcohol-tartaric acid solution. Set the beaker on the back edge of the steam bath overnight, and then heat it the next morning over the open steam vent to a temperature of 50° C.

Add approximately 250 ml. of 95 per cent ethyl alcohol to the absorption chamber containing the glass-paper extraction assembly. The extraction apparatus is mounted on the stand with the bottom resting on the 800 watt hot plate. When the alcohol has heated to a temperature of approximately 60° C., carefully pour the warm tissue homogenate in small portions through a long stem funnel into the paper thimble. Wash out the 3 liter beaker with approximately 250 ml. of warm alcohol. A 4 liter beaker, placed at the outlet of the side arm, catches the alcohol which overflows during the charging process. Set this overflow sample aside as the first portion in the extraction process. Place about 300 ml. of 95 per cent alcohol containing 3 ml. of saturated tartaric acid in the collection flask with several glass beads to prevent bumping, then connect it to the side arm of the extraction chamber. Clamp the apparatus securely in place, with the collection flask resting on the 1,200 watt hot plate, and the extraction chamber on the 800 watt hot plate. Care must be taken to keep the alcohol in the extraction apparatus hot after the addition of the tissue, or the sintered glass plate will clog.

Insert the 7 mm. I.D. glass tube for nitrogen agitation through the bottom of the bulb condenser and connect it to the pressure regulator. Adjust the valve to give approximately #8 pressure on the gauge and connect the condenser to the apparatus through the adapter joint while holding the glass tubing above the liquid in the extractor. Then slowly lower the tube, using a rotating motion to give mechanical mixing with the U end of the tubing while it passes through the tissue layer which has settled on the bottom. When the tube rests on the bottom of the paper thimble, the nitrogen should rise through the liquid at the rate of about one bubble per second.

The extraction should continue for five hours. Usually three changes of alcohol in the receiver flask are required during this time. Interchange the receiver flask with one containing fresh alcohol-tartaric acid when foam starts to rise to the side arm of the extractor, and when the solution in the receiver flask starts to bump or gets cloudy. The alcohol develops a green color soon after the extraction starts. If after five hours the alcohol in the receiver and extraction flasks is not clear and colorless, continue the extraction process. When the extraction is completed, decant the alcohol in the extraction chamber into the 4 liter beaker. The residual tissue may be held for examination for alcohol-insoluble compounds, as in steps 7 and 8, page 1131.

Processing Method. Lipids start to settle out of the alcohol as a fine granular precipitate as soon as the extract reaches room temperature, and the beaker is set in the refrigerator overnight to allow further crystallization. Carry out the filtration the next morning through a Gooch filter with an asbestos mat. The solubility of the lipid fraction is appreciable at room temperature, and care must be taken to keep the alcohol solution cold during the filtration. After the asbestos mat is prepared, wash it with alcohol, and set the filtering apparatus in the refrigerator until cold. Make the filtration with suction, and wash out the precipitate with about 200 ml. of cold alcohol. In order to recover the alcohol in concentrating the extract, transfer the filtrate to a 4 liter distilling flask and distill it under reduced pressure until the volume remaining is 450 ml. Then transfer the solution to a 1 liter beaker, and wash the distilling flask with about 50 ml. of hot alcohol. Cool the alcohol solution to room temperature, and slowly add, with stirring, 300 ml. of distilled water. This is the most important step in the procedure, since the addition of water at this point precipitates the fats and oils from the solution.

A flocculent precipitate, well dispersed throughout the solution, should form after the water addition. If a heavy gelatinous precipitate immediately settles on the bottom, the proportion of water to alcohol was too great. Add additional alcohol with stirring to give a dispersed precipitate. A better corrective measure is to evaporate the solution under vacuum to a thick syrup, take it up in alcohol, and reprecipitate with water. When a precipitate of the proper consistency has been obtained, set the solution in the refrigerator overnight and filter it cold through asbestos as before. Then evaporate the filtrate under vacuum to a syrup, and take it up by the slow addition of 300 ml. of absolute alcohol, with stirring. If the absolute alcohol is not added in small portions, a heavy muck will precipitate out. The precipitate should be flocculent and granular. Let the solution stand about two hours, and filter. Evaporate under vacuum and repeat the absolute alcohol treatment a second and third time if a large precipitate forms.

Evaporate the last alcoholic filtrate under vacuum to a thick syrup, and then add 100 ml. of water. Heat the aqueous solution to 50° C. on the steam bath, with stirring; allow it to cool to room temperature; and filter it through paper, using a DeWitt suction filter. Transfer the contents of the flask quantitatively to the paper with water washings. Allow the precipitate to air dry, and then it may be examined for water insoluble, alcohol soluble organics, as in step 6, page 1131. Extract the filtrate, which should still be acid to Congo paper, with solvents to separate the organic acids and neutrals from the bases (page 1137).

Recoveries are better than previously obtainable by other extraction procedures, although sufficient quantitative data have not yet been accumulated for a quantitative evaluation of the recovery process. Morphine, one of the most difficult drugs to isolate from tissue, can be recovered in yields of 45 to 55 per cent when 1 mg. is added to 500 gm. of homogenized brain tissue. Seventy per cent of a 0.5 mg. sample of pentobarbital was recovered from 500 gm. samples; and when 2 mg. of meperidine, codeine, or heroin was added, the yield of compound was ample for colorimetric and crystallographic examination.

Prior to the use of continuous extraction, heroin and morphine were rarely detected in organs from known addicts. Good positive reactions can now be obtained by the continuous extraction process in many of the addict cases. In two cases that died during operation after receiving thiopental as a preoperative anesthetic, positive identification of the drug was made in residue from the brain extract. Without continuous extraction, negative findings were obtained in attempts to detect thiopental in deaths under similar circumstances.

Examination of the residue which results when an alcoholic extraction is made of uncooked tissue from the brain reveals fats, fatty acids, some protein, phospholipids, cerebrosides, purines and small amounts of other complex molecules. This residue, commonly labelled muck, is fatty in appearance, but does not have the physical properties of true lipids. Cerebrosides, which are only moderately alcohol-soluble, constitute a big proportion of this residue from brain tissue. The solubility of each specific residue in 95 per cent alcohol is variable, but if any sample of residue is re-extracted with alcohol, only a part of the evaporate will redissolve. Moreover, the alcohol solution shows a very intense Tyndall effect. On standing for some time, a cloudy solution develops, a precipitate then settles out and continues to grow in proportion to the time the solution stands. A large amount, if not the major portion, of the muck is colloidal and probably dispersed in the liquid phase by tissue dispersing agents in a manner analogous to the dispersion of protein and fats in blood serum.

The simplest purification method for any residue from an alcohol extraction of tissue consists of a series of extractions with water and immiscible solvent, changing the acidity of the water so that the compound alternately passes from aqueous to solvent phase and back again. Each extraction gives better purification, but with loss of compound. The organic compounds that are readily isolatable * fall into one of five categories depending on their acidity and basicity. Acids are those compounds which have ionization constants greater than carbonic acid and therefore form water-soluble, solvent-insoluble sodium salts on the addition of sodium bicarbonate to the aqueous solution. Phenols or intermediate acids are compounds with ionization constants less than carbonic acid but whose pK values are still on the acid side. They form water-soluble, solvent-insoluble alkali salts on the addition of alkali to the aqueous solution. Neutral organics are neither acidic nor basic and, because they do not form salts and are, with few exceptions, more soluble in solvents than in water, they always pass into the solvent layer in the extraction. The organic bases are compounds which form water-soluble, solvent-insoluble salts with mineral acid. There are two classes: bases and amphoteric bases. In addition to the basic group in the molecule, the amphoteric bases have some functional group which acts as an acid in forming a water-soluble, solvent-insoluble salt in an aqueous solution which is strongly basic. The organics that are entirely basic are made insoluble when an aqueous solution of the acid salt is made alkaline.

There are, therefore, two possible methods for extracting the aqueous solution containing the muck.

1. The acidified solution may be extracted with organic solvents to remove the acid, phenolic and neutral compounds together, then made alkaline with ammonia and again extracted to remove bases and amphoteric bases at the same time. Acid and base extraction should include both ether and chloroform,† since almost all organics are soluble in one or the other, if not both.

2. The acidified solution may be extracted as in 1 and the acids, phenolics and neutrals separated by the three-component extraction (page 1139). The original aqueous solution is then made decidedly alkaline and extracted to remove bases, then neutralized with acid, made faintly ammoniacal and extracted to remove the amphoterics. Only ether is used for the basic extraction and chloroform for the amphoteric group in contrast to the use of both solvents independently for the separation of the acidic compounds. Consequently, any basic drug that is ether-insoluble will be separated out in the amphoteric group, despite the fact that it is a true base.

In the first process, the isolated organics are divided into two main acid and basic groups, while in the second process, five classifications are obtained. Certain considerations favor the first extraction process as the starting point when the toxicologic analyses are daily routines.

The major decision is to establish whether extraneous organic matter is present in the extract in sufficient quantity to be of possible significance. In this connection it

---

* Alcohol- and water-soluble drugs.

† A number of the salts of the organic bases are somewhat soluble in chloroform and, on chloroform extraction, some salt will appear in the acid fraction. Fulton pointed out (176) that those salts which are chloroform-soluble are carbon tetrachloride-insoluble. Consequently, carbon tetrachloride should be substituted for chloroform as the solvent for removing those acidic or neutral compounds that are only slightly soluble in ether. This change is practical in all cases studied but, because the data in the tables were based on a chloroform extraction, this change has not been made in the text.

should be pointed out that, with few exceptions, acute deaths do not occur from minute traces of poisons and, in suicides or homicides in which the causative agent is an isolatable toxic substance, enough will have been isolated to be apparent. The major exceptions are delayed deaths in which the poison is the indirect cause and extensive elimination has taken place or in drug sensitivities in which death occurred soon after the administration of a small amount of the poison. Regardless of the implications of the history, one can only do an analysis when there is something to analyze and, if it can be determined at the start that the isolated residue is that of a normal extract of tissue, it is futile to proceed further with chemical testing.

The indicator reactions are invaluable as probing tests on all of the five solubility classes of tissue residues.* Only neutral compounds will not be detected but their chemical nature makes them less toxic and the larger lethal dose will result in the recovery of quantities that can be seen on microscopic examination. Indicator tests for bases should only be done on ammoniacal extracts in order to avoid the possibility of inorganic base being mechanically carried into the nonaqueous phase and interfering with the test on the residue. Tests on the dried residues of the acid extracts should be made after extraction with hydrochloric acid acidification for the same reason.

Once there are positive indications that an organic substance has been isolated, a further purification is invariably required regardless of the isolation process and extraction procedure that were used. Both partial purification and a separation will be attained by making the initial extraction by the first extraction procedure (see below) and following with the second procedure (page 1139) which gives the five group separation. Comparison of the factors and the over-all labor involved for a series of cases with the usual spread of positive and negative findings is in favor of this, with a preliminary examination of the acidic and basic residues before carrying out the second extraction. The saving in the labor from the negative cases will compensate for the additional work in the two series of extractions in the positive cases.

First Extraction Procedure—Extraction Separation into Two Main Acid and Basic Groups.

1. Acids. Acidify the aqueous solution obtained from one of the isolation procedures (pages 1128-1136) with hydrochloric acid to Congo red paper and place it in a 300 ml. Squibb separatory funnel. Make two extractions with approximately 50 ml. portions of ethyl ether and one extraction with about 50 ml. of chloroform.† ‡ Allow the funnel to stand, after shaking, until separation of the layers is complete. Wash each organic extract once with water and filter the final nonaqueous solution through paper.§ Evaporate the ether and chloroform extracts to almost complete dryness on the steam bath, with rotation of the container.¶ Dehydrate the residues preferably by storing overnight in a H_2SO_4 or vacuum desiccator.

2. Bases. Add ammonia dropwise to the aqueous solution remaining from the acid extraction until a faint ammoniacal odor persists after shaking. Shake it out twice with ether and once with chloroform containing 10 per cent butanol.‖ The nonaqueous extracts may be combined or evaporated in separate beakers.

Reserve the aqueous layer for examination to exclude the very few water- and alcohol-soluble, organic solvent-insoluble drugs that have not been removed by the ether or chloroform in the acid and basic extractions. Highly hydroxylated compounds,

* 1. Water-, alcohol- and solvent-soluble compounds, page 1142.
  2. Water- and alcohol-soluble, solvent-insoluble compounds, page 1144.
  3. Water-insoluble, alcohol-soluble compounds, page 1145.
  4. Water-soluble, alcohol-insoluble compounds, page 1146.
  5. Water and alcohol-insoluble, special solvent-soluble, page 1146.

† Chloroform has a greater tendency to form emulsions than ether and may require longer standing for complete separation. Any emulsion may be broken by mixing with more $CHCl_3$ with gentle agitation or, in exceptional cases, transferring the contents of the separatory funnel to a beaker and warming on the steam bath.

‡ Some neutral compounds such as diphenylhydantoin are removed only in small amounts by ether and, if the $CHCl_3$ is eliminated, they will appear in the fraction with the amphoteric bases. See footnote, page 1137.

§ The organic solvent is filtered through paper to absorb occluded water.

¶ A round bottomed microbeaker of about 25 ml. capacity is preferable to a flat bottomed beaker because distribution of the residue over the surface of the container is lessened.

‖ Ten per cent ethyl alcohol in chloroform increases the solubility of the opium alkaloids. Butyl alcohol is a little better solvent, although it has an objectionable odor on evaporation.

glucosides, some lower molecular weight acids, low concentrations of sulfa drugs and choline derivatives may be present.* † If the probing tests (pages 1150-1152) show any indications of a base, while the methyl orange test indicates that only small amounts are present, examine this aqueous solution and the fraction containing the water-insoluble, alcohol-soluble drugs (page 1145) for bases.

In contrast to the acid group, evaporation of the bases requires the close attention of the analyst, as well as judgment in determining how far the process can proceed. Isolation of the free base is essential for the indicator reactions and all the color tests should be performed on the base rather than one of its salts. On the other hand, some of the bases such as amphetamine and coniine are volatile and, if not immediately lost by over-evaporation, will disappear on standing overnight. The bases cannot be dehydrated over H_2SO_4 as with the acids.‡ However, evaporation should be carried far enough to remove any trace of ammonia mechanically carried over and not removed by the water washing. The presence of volatile bases must be detected, therefore, before evaporation is complete and their loss prevented by the addition of a few drops of hydrochloric acid § just before the last trace of solvent has volatilized. The acetate salt can then be dehydrated by desiccation but the indicator reactions cannot be made on the residue.

Any volatile bases are ether soluble and the safest plan is to evaporate the ether and chloroform solutions separately. First carefully evaporate about one quarter of the volume of ether extract and note the odor and physical appearance at the point of near dryness.¶ Make indicator tests and other preliminary tests (page 1150) immediately on this partially dried residue and, if volatile bases are indicated, add a few drops of acetic acid before evaporation of the remaining ether. The chloroform extract may be handled like the acids. With positive indications for volatile bases, initiate an isolation by steam distillation from an alkaline solution (page 1046). At this point it may be advisable to carry out the preliminary examination of the residues by the procedures on pages 1147 to 1152, or to proceed directly with the second extraction procedure.

Second Extraction Procedure—Five Group Extraction Separation of the Residue.

If the history suggests a particular preparation, it may be advisable to proceed directly with this procedure in order to make a separation before any preliminary testing with indicators or probing reactions.‖ In this case, make the acid extraction on the aqueous extract (pages 1128-1136) exactly as in the procedure described on page 1138, and follow it up to evaporation of the solvents. The three component separation starts with the ether, chloroform ** or a mixture of both solvents. Also, if there is an indication of a mixture at any time during the preliminary testing, time will usually be saved by proceeding directly to this group separation. The flow sheet for the entire separation is shown in Table 47-3. The first steps in the flow sheet include the first extraction procedure (page 1138).

1. Three Component Separation of the Acid Group. Extract the ether and/or chloroform solutions discussed on this page or, if the extraction on page 1138 was made, dissolve the residues in about 50 ml. of the more appropriate solvent as determined by the solubility of the unknown during the extraction.

Shake out the nonaqueous solution in a 300 ml. Squibb separatory funnel with an equal volume of 4 per cent $NaHCO_3$ solution.†† After separation, draw off the aqueous

* Vitamin B_1 produces an intense yellow-colored solution which does not decrease in intensity on extraction with solvents.
† The water-soluble, solvent-insoluble drugs are more readily detected from analysis of the blood.
‡ $CaCl_2$, $Mg(ClO_4)_2$ or anhydrous Na_2SO_4 can be used as desiccants.
§ Morgan, C. E., has shown (177) that the acetates of several volatile bases are almost as volatile as the free base.
¶ Addition of ethyl chloride in the last stage of the evaporation hastens it and reduces the loss of volatile base.
‖ If the first extraction procedure (page 1138) is omitted, the aqueous layer remaining from the amphoteric extraction is reserved to examine it for water and alcohol-soluble, solvent-insoluble drugs, as described on page 1144.
** See footnote, page 1137.
†† The sodium bicarbonate solution should not be an old reagent, as it changes on standing with an increase in pH due to the formation of carbonate which will extract the weak and intermediate acids as well as the strongly acidic compounds.

Table 47-3. Five-Group Separation of Water- and Alcohol-Soluble Drugs

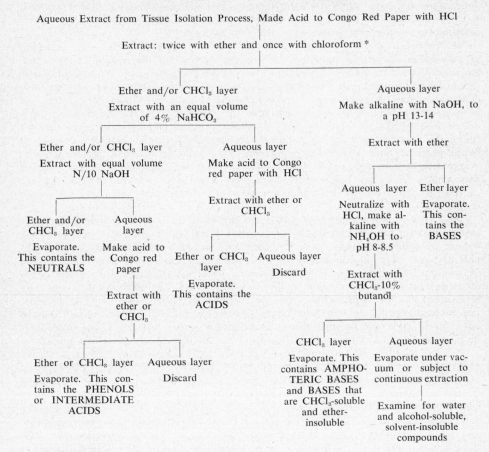

Aqueous Extract from Tissue Isolation Process, Made Acid to Congo Red Paper with HCl

Extract: twice with ether and once with chloroform *

Ether and/or CHCl₃ layer
Extract with an equal volume of 4% NaHCO₃

Aqueous layer
Make alkaline with NaOH, to a pH 13-14

Ether and/or CHCl₃ layer
Extract with equal volume N/10 NaOH

Aqueous layer
Make acid to Congo red paper with HCl

Extract with ether

Ether and/or CHCl₃ layer
Evaporate. This contains the NEUTRALS

Aqueous layer
Make acid to Congo red paper

Extract with ether or CHCl₃

Aqueous layer
Neutralize with HCl, make alkaline with NH₄OH to pH 8-8.5

Ether layer
Evaporate. This contains the BASES

Extract with ether or CHCl₃

Ether or CHCl₃ layer
Evaporate. This contains the ACIDS

Aqueous layer
Discard

Extract with CHCl₃-10% butanol

Ether or CHCl₃ layer
Evaporate. This contains the PHENOLS or INTERMEDIATE ACIDS

Aqueous layer
Discard

CHCl₃ layer
Evaporate. This contains AMPHOTERIC BASES and BASES that are CHCl₃-soluble and ether-insoluble

Aqueous layer
Evaporate under vacuum or subject to continuous extraction

Examine for water and alcohol-soluble, solvent-insoluble compounds

* See footnote, page 1137.

layer, acidify it to Congo red paper with HCl and re-extract it with the solvent. The residue, on evaporation, contains compounds acidic enough to form sodium salts in aqueous solution at pH 8.5 or below.

Then shake out the nonaqueous layer with an equal volume of N/10 NaOH. After separation of the layers, neutralize the aqueous solution, then make it acid to Congo red paper and shake it out with the solvent. The residue, on evaporation, contains phenols or intermediate acids whose acidity is great enough to form alkaline salts in strongly alkaline solutions but not in solutions of pH 8.5 or less.

Wash the nonaqueous layer twice with acidified water and, on evaporation, it will contain the neutral organics. The residues are then examined by the indicator tests and probing reactions (pages 1147 and 1148).

2. Separation of Bases from Amphoteric Bases. In the event that the extraction (page 1138) was omitted, neutralize the aqueous solution from the acid separation with sodium hydroxide, then make it decidedly alkaline to pH 13-14 and extract it twice with ether, washing each extract twice with water. The residue, on evaporation, contains the bases.

The aqueous solution is just neutralized with HCl, then made faintly alkaline with ammonia (pH 8.0) and extracted with chloroform containing 10 per cent ethyl or n-butyl alcohol. Evaporation of the solvent gives a residue consisting of those amphoteric type bases that have a functional group acidic enough to form a water-soluble, solvent-insoluble sodium salt at pH 13-14, and the nonamphoteric, chloroform-soluble, ether-insoluble bases.

If the extraction (page 1138) was made, and a separate ether and chloroform evaporate was obtained, the ether extract is dissolved in ether, while the chloroform extract is washed with ether.* Combine the two ether solutions and make an extraction with an equal volume of water made alkaline with sodium hydroxide to pH 13-14. Evaporation of the ether gives the bases.† The aqueous solution is just neutralized with HCl and made faintly basic with ammonia and extracted with chloroform containing 10 per cent ethyl alcohol or normal butyl alcohol as described above. The evaporate contains only the amphoteric bases.

Any undissolved base from the extracted ether-washed, chloroform residue is an ether-insoluble, chloroform-soluble one which may or may not be amphoteric and the above process serves as a separation and purification for it. Preliminary tests are made on these residues the same as for the others.

The aqueous solution may be discarded only if the five group extraction separation was preceded by the acid-base extraction (footnote, page 1139).

The classification of the drugs according to their separation in the extraction with immiscible solvents is shown in Table 47-4.

The efficiency for the separation by extraction is determined by the deviation of the physical properties of the compounds from those of the ideal organic. A clear-cut separation is obtained with a mixture of salicylic acid, phenobarbital, acetophenetidin, scopolamine and morphine, each of which is typical of acids, phenolics, neutrals, bases and amphoterics, respectively. Salts of these compounds are water-soluble, solvent-insoluble while in the free state they are nearly water-insoluble, solvent-soluble. In the extraction they pass almost completely from one phase to the other, depending on the hydrogen ion concentration of the aqueous solution. As the water solubility of a solvent-insoluble compound in the free state increases, the partition between organic solvent and the aqueous phase becomes greater and the number of extractions required for the separation is increased proportionately (12). Since the solubility behavior is not known during the extraction stage of the analysis, the best practice is to keep extracting in any one step as long as a significant amount of unknown is being removed.‡

In the extreme case, the compound is water-soluble, solvent-insoluble and a separation by extraction with immiscible solvents is not possible. These solvent-insoluble drugs fall into a separate group listed in Table 47-5 (page 1144).

In the analysis for an unknown drug where all manner of structures and wide variations in solubility behavior exist, more or less overlapping into different groups is to be expected. Overlapping may even be an index to the substance if its behavior has been established. In any case, the fact that all drugs do not fall completely into one category in the extraction process does not detract from the value of this procedure, because more information concerning the general nature of the unknown can be gained from it than from all other physical or chemical testing.

The best possible extraction is attained with acids and phenolics because all of their alkali salts are completely solvent-insoluble. Separation of acids from phenols with sodium bicarbonate is less complete since some intermediate acids have pK_a values on the borderline of that value necessary to form a sodium salt at the pH of the sodium bicarbonate solution. Not many of the drugs are decidedly acid, so that the problem of the incomplete separation of phenols from acids is of minor importance. The most

---

* The ether wash is best made by layering ether over the sample, allowing it to stand and siphoning off the supernatant.

† If indicator reactions are to be made on this residue, the nonaqueous solution must be carefully washed in order to remove all NaOH mechanically carried over with the solvent. NaOH contamination can be detected with phenolphthalein paper but, to insure purity where the indicator reactions are of importance, the residue should be re-extracted from ammoniacal solution.

‡ The usual procedure is to test each abstract by quickly evaporating a few drops on a watch glass. If there is evidence that a substance is being extracted, the entire solvent should be evaporated and examined before proceeding with the next step. The procedure (page 1138) which calls for two extractions with ether and one with chloroform in the separation of the acids, for example, is adequate for removal of the average drug, but if a small residue is obtained from a relatively large bulk of sample, the separation may be incomplete because of low solvent solubility or relatively high water solubility. The extraction should then be made repeatedly as long as a residue of constant composition is being removed.

Table 47-4. Separation of Drugs into Five Groups by Extraction

ACIDIC GROUP DRUGS

Acids

Acetylsalicylic acid	Cinchophen	Ethyl biscoumace- tate	Levulinic acid	Phenylbutazone
p-Aminobenzoic acid	Citric acid	Glutaric acid	Mandelic acid	Saccharin
	Dimenhydrinate	Glycine	Oxalic acid	Salicylic acid
Benzoic acid	(acid extraction product)	Hippuric acid	Phenylacetyl- urea	Sclererythin *
				Sulfisoxazole

Phenols

Amobarbital	Estrone	Phanadorn	Piperidione
Aprobarbital	Hexobarbital	Phenobarbital	Probarbital
Barbital	Meconin	Phenylacetyl- urea	Pyrithyldione
Butabarbital	Mephobarbital		Sandoptal
Chrysazin	Neonal	Phenylbu- tazone	Secobarbital
Cyclopal	Ortal		Thiopental
Diphenylhydantoin	Pentobarbital	Picrotoxin	Vinbarbital

Neutrals

Acetanilid	Chlorobutanol	Emetine	Phenylsalicylate	Theobromine
Acetophenetidin	Cholesterol	Isoamylethyl- acetylurea	Pregnenolone	Theophylline
Antipyrine	Coniine.HCl		Santonin	Tribromo- ethanol
Benzocaine.HCl	Digitoxin	Methylphenyl- ethylhydantoin	Sedormid	Trimethadione
Bromural	Dimenhydrinate	Pavatrine	Sulfonethyl- methane	Urethan
Caffeine	(basic extrac- tion product)	Phenylacetylurea	Sulfonmethane	Xylocaine.HCl
Carbromal				

BASIC GROUP DRUGS

Bases

Aconitine	Codeine	Emetine	Optochin	Quinine
Adiphenine	Coniine	Ephedrine	Pamaquine	Scopolamine
N-Allylnormorphine	Delphinine	Ethylmorphine	Pentamethylene- tetrazol	Solanin
Aminopyrine	d-Desoxyephe- drine	Heroin		Sparteine
Amphetamine		Homatropine	Phenindamine	Strychnine
Amprotropine	Dibucaine	Hyoscyamine	Physostigmine	Tetracaine
Apothesine	Dicyclomine	Larocaine	Piperine	Thenylpyra- mine
Atabrin	Dimenhydrinate	Lobeline	Piperocaine	
Atropine	(basic extrac- tion product)	Meperidine	Prisilidene	Thiazolsulfone
Brucine		Methadon	Procaine	Thonzylamine
Butamin	Diothane	Nicotine	Procaine amide	Trihexyphenidyl
Cinchonidine	Diphenylhydra- mine	Nicotinic alcohol	Pseudopelle- tierine	Veratrine
Cinchonine				Xylocaine
Cocaine	Dromoran	Nikethamide	Pyrilamine	Yohimbine

Amphoterics

N-Allynor- morphine	Digitalin	Dromoran	Morphine	Procaine amide
	Dihydromor- phinone	Eucupin	Narceine	Pyrilamine
Apomorphine		Heroin	Narcotine	Strychnine
Brucine	Dimenhydrinate	Hydrastine	Nicotinic alcohol	Thiamin (decom- position product)
Codeine	(basic extrac- tion product)	Metopon	Pilocarpine	
Curarine				
Digalen				

* Sclererythin from ergot is indicated when the sodium bicarbonate solution turns red in extraction of the other for the separation of the acid.

important application of the acid-phenol separation is in the removal of salicylic acid and acetylsalicylic acid from barbiturates.

In this classification of drugs, the designation of the compound is independent of the chemical structure. Saccharin which is an imide structurally reacts chemically as a strong acid while barbiturates are malonyl ureas with the phenolic properties due to the enolization of a secondary amino group.

Neutrals extract with the acidic compounds in the first separation only because the acid extraction is carried out first. Since they are more organic solvent-soluble, in general, and are neither acidic enough to form salts with bases or basic enough to form salts with acids they always pass more readily from the aqueous to the solvent phase. If, in the extraction process, the aqueous tissue extract is made alkaline at the start, in order to remove the bases first, the neutrals would come out in the basic fraction (footnote, page 1151). The sodium hydroxide separation of phenols from neutrals is of particular importance when the tissue residue shows a positive Koppanyi reaction. Theophylline and acetophenetidin are commonly used along with barbiturate preparations. Theophylline gives the Koppanyi reaction and acetophenetidin in the mixture makes it difficult to identify the particular barbiturate even after partial purification.

Acidic and neutral compounds are generally ether-soluble. Mineral acid salts of the bases are ether-insoluble but there are some notable exceptions. Benzocaine comes out entirely in the acid fraction. Bases like xylocaine® and emetine are removed in significant amounts in the acid extraction and appear in the extraction classification in the neutral fraction as well as in the basic fraction.*

With all of those compounds in which appreciable overlapping occurs, the names are listed in each group of Table 47-4 in which they are removed in significant amounts. Codeine is both a base and an amphoteric because, in the somewhat higher hydroxyl ion concentration than normally used for the bases, partial salt formation occurs with its free hydroxyl group.

An anomaly exists in the amphoteric fraction as a result of the extraction procedure. Some bases are relatively ether insoluble but are chloroform soluble. Because chloroform is used for the amphoterics, it is omitted in the extraction for the bases. Those relatively ether-insoluble compounds, such as narcotine, which are not amphoterics appear in the amphoteric fraction because they are not removed until the chloroform extraction for the amphoteric group. Strychnine is listed as both a base and an amphoteric because it is much more soluble in chloroform and may be only partially extracted with the bases when significant concentrations are present. Phenylbutazone is listed as both an acid and a phenol, although the acidic properties are those of a phenol. It is very soluble in ether but significantly soluble in water. Consequently, some passes into the bicarbonate solution, due to its water solubility. It is then removed as a strong acid on acidification and extraction with ether. Neutrals that are both water- and solvent-soluble may overlap extensively. Phenylacetylurea, which is not very organic solvent-soluble, overlaps into all fractions. Contamination of the bases is more likely to occur with the neutrals. Neutral compounds, such as diphenylhydantoin, which are only partially soluble in ether but significantly soluble in chloroform, will not be removed completely in the extraction for the acidic group if the chloroform extraction is omitted and will appear in the amphoteric fraction. Many neutrals such as caffeine are very weak bases and, although they appear predominantly in the neutral fraction, they will be found also in the basic fraction if incompletely removed in the first extraction of the acidified aqueous solution.

If the solubility and acidic and basic properties of all drugs were ideal, the position of the compound in Table 47-4 could be predicted from the acidity and basicity in Table 47-10 and there would be no need for both tables. The anomalies existing between the classification, based on indicator reactions, and extractability actually aid in the identification process. Deviations in indicator reactivity from the behavior expected on extraction rule out all those compounds that are known to show the proper indicator tests corresponding to the extraction group. Indicator reactions are an aid in detecting overlapping of a single drug and, at the same time, furnish an index to the solubility of the compound. When the unknown is a mixture containing compounds falling into different extraction groups, incomplete separations may be detected and the efficiency of the purification process followed. For example, an acid extraction group that did not give a positive Congo red test could not contain salicylic acid. If the acidity reaction is that of an intermediate acid while the original acid residue (page 1138) indicated a barbiturate, acetylsalicylic acid interference with the barbiturate reaction should be investigated. On the other hand, acetylsalicylic acid that gives an acidity reaction for a strong acid will not give the typical pink color in the Koppanyi reaction.

Barbiturates show indicator reactions for weak acids. When there are positive findings for barbiturates and the phenolic fraction gives an indicator reaction for intermediate acids, there is contamination of the isolated barbiturate and a special purification of the individual member of the extract should be made before attempting to identify

---

* The solubility of the salts of the bases in ether is exceptional behavior and is not to be confused with the variable chloroform solubility of salts of the bases (see footnote, page 1137).

the individual compound.* Conversely, if the phenolic fraction shows the typical weak acid reaction and nothing was isolated in the neutral fraction, the isolated barbiturate is usually pure enough for immediate identification from the micromelting point.

Indicator reactions for intermediate acids in the neutral fraction suggest the few basic compounds such as pavatrine®, xylocaine® or benzocaine that are extracted from acid solution because of solvent solubility of their salts. The xylocaine® hydrochloride that is isolated in the neutral fraction tests as a strong acid while benzocaine hydrochloride shows the acid properties of an intermediate acid. When the acid or phenolic fraction shows indicator reactions for nonacids, the compound can only be a neutral one like phenylacetylurea which is decidedly water-soluble as well as solvent-soluble.

Indicator reactions for bases are of special value in detecting a basic substance in the tissue extract. Since the basic fractions are rarely crystalline, positive findings for a base show that the extract is not merely tissue residue. Most true amphoterics are weak bases and indications for an intermediate base in the amphoteric fraction points to the few amphoterics that are decidedly basic (apomorphine) or suggests a non-amphoteric which appears in this fraction because it is relatively ether-insoluble, chloroform-soluble (procaine amide). The basic indicator reactions serve as an exclusion test for the basic extraction group to differentiate between the members that are intermediate and weak or nonbases. For example, diphenhydramine and amphetamine give similar colorations with Marquis reagent but diphenhydramine is excluded if the indicator fails to show an intermediate base.

A few compounds are hydrolyzed as a result of the alkaline treatment in the acid extraction. Dimenhydrinate may be partially broken down with the formation of a basic component and the action of alkali on thiamin produces an extractable decomposition product which gives indicator and precipitation reactions for a base and is found principally in the amphoteric fraction. Under conditions of partial putrefaction, basic tissue degradation products are a potential source of interference.

Groups Other Than the Water-, Alcohol- and Solvent-Soluble Group.

Organic drugs not water- and alcohol-soluble enough to be isolated by the routine extraction (pages 1128-1136) in quantities sufficient for their detection are few in comparison with the water-, alcohol-, solvent-soluble group and relatively few of these are in common use. Because of their limited number, special procedures may be applied for the individual substances if further examination is indicated after exclusion of the major group.

1. Water- and Alcohol-Soluble, Solvent-Insoluble Compounds. This group, listed in Table 47-5, which appears in step 9 of the isolation process (page 1131) can be

Table 47-5. Acidity and Basicity of Water- and Alcohol-Soluble, Solvent-Insoluble Drugs

ACIDIC GROUP DRUGS

Strong Acids

Ascorbic acid	Maleic acid	Succinic acid	Succinylsulfathiazole	Tartaric acid

Intermediate Acids

Thiamin *

Weak Acids or Non Acids

Acetylcholine bromide	Carbamylcholine chloride	Salicin
Acetylcholine chloride	Choline chloride	Sulfadiazine
Acetyl-β-methylcholine chloride	Digitonin	Sulfanilamide

* Thiamin produces an intense yellow-colored aqueous solution after addition of the alkali in the separation of the bases, and it does not decrease in intensity after extraction with solvents.

recovered by vacuum evaporation of the aqueous solution or it may be subjected to continuous extraction with an immiscible solvent. Tartaric acid will always be present since it is added at the beginning of the analysis. An examination for other acids may

* Increased acidity in the phenol fraction containing barbiturates is usually due to acid products from tissue degradation.

be of value in establishing the nature of the original pharmaceutic preparation. In the absence of a yellow colored aqueous solution, any basic reaction in the amphoteric group of the water-, alcohol- and solvent-soluble group is not due to thiamin (page 1144). A reddish solution may be due to sclererythrin and tests for the ergot alkaloids should then be made on the basic fraction (Table 47-4). Sulfa drugs may be eliminated by direct application of the diazo reaction (13) page 1246 on the aqueous solution but these are more readily detected by analysis of the blood. Glucosides or highly hydroxylated substances not listed may be excluded by the anthrone reaction (14, 15) or the Molisch reaction (16) (pages 1243, 1252). Choline-type drugs are neutral compounds but react with some alkaloidal precipitants. Silicotungstic acid gives an immediate white precipitate while picric acid does not react. There are no important basic organic medicinals that are alcohol-insoluble.

2. Water-Insoluble, Alcohol- and Solvent-Soluble Compounds. Pharmaceutics shown in Table 47-6 and many of the compounds which appear in Tables 47-10 and 47-4 may

Table 47-6. Acidity and Basicity of Water-Insoluble, Alcohol- and Solvent-Soluble Drugs

ACID GROUP DRUGS

Strong Acids

| Pthalylsulfathiazole | Sulfacetimide |

Intermediate Acids

| Croton oil | Dicoumarol | Ethylphenylhydantoin |
| Desoxycholic acid | Diphenylhydantoin | Sulfisoxazole |

Weak Acids or Non Acids

| Antabuse | Cantharidin | Sulfathiazole |

BASIC GROUP DRUGS

Intermediate Bases

Quinidine

be present in this group as a result of occlusion and absorption in the isolation process as well as from relatively low water solubility. The purification problem is quite difficult since the drug must be separated from relatively large amounts of cerebrosides, lipids and fatty material. Special purification procedures are required for a good separation from the tissue extractives (17, 18, 19).

Chromatographic (20, 21) and ionophoretic (22, 23) technics can be applied to the isolation of these compounds (page 1163). These methods are best applied when there is evidence for a particular substance so that the proper conditions and solvent can be selected without the need for trial analyses. Column chromatography is especially useful in checking this class for the incomplete removal of some of the less water-soluble compounds of the major group. The column has the advantage over paper chromatography and ionophoresis in that larger samples can be processed and the compound readily recovered from the adsorbent by alcohol extraction. In addition, the packed column acts partly as a filter for the semicolloidal tissue extractables.

Quinidine (24) is the only important basic drug that may not be isolated in detectable amounts in the water-, alcohol- and solvent-soluble group. The alcohol solution gives a blue fluorescence with ultraviolet irradiation.

Antabuse, although reportedly nontoxic (25), may become significant in deaths involving alcoholics under treatment. A method has been described in which the compound is extracted from blood, plasma and urine with ethylene dichloride and determined by the ultraviolet absorption in the region between 250 and 350 mμ (26). It was readily isolated from stomach contents when ingested in amounts exceeding the medicinal dose but was not obtained in detectable amounts from the brain (27). It has not been isolated from blood or urine in living cases under treatment (26).

Diphenylhydantoin and ethylphenylhydantoin will be present in detectable amounts in the major group of water-, alcohol- and solvent-soluble compounds, but if it is necessary to determine whether the amount ingested was in excess of a medicinal dose, the water-insoluble portion should be determined. Desoxycholic acid is nontoxic and will be of interest only in the analysis of stomach contents when there is some question relating to the ingestion of preparations containing bile salts. Croton oil would be indicated by its purgative action prior to death and cantharidin shows postmortem findings of corrosion and irritation with symptoms of violent pains, particularly in the bladder, kidney and urethra, prior to death. It may be detected by the marked irritation of the skin when a small amount of residue is applied to a noncalloused area. Sulfa drugs may be detected by the application of the sensitive diazo reaction (13) to the alcohol solution after partial dilution with water.

3. Water-Soluble, Alcohol-Insoluble Compounds. The water-soluble, alcohol-insoluble compounds appear in the isolation procedure in step 7, page 1131. The toxic ones listed in Table 47-7 are drastic purgatives and would only be of significance with

Table 47-7. Acidity and Basicity of Water-Soluble, Alcohol-Insoluble Compounds

ACIDIC GROUP DRUGS

Strong Acids

Gluconic acid (from calcium gluconate)	Glutamic acid *	Oxalic acid (from sodium oxalate)

Intermediate Acids

Abrin	Crotin	Jalap	Ricin

* Food seasoning and source of HCl.

pathologic findings that included unusual cathartic action. Some oxalic acid would be present in the major group with ingestion of sodium oxalate as a result of the action of the hydrochloric acid in the stomach. Nontoxic compounds such as gluconic or glutamic acid will be of interest only when it is important to determine the nature of the ingested preparation. Alcohol and solvent solubility decreases with the increase in the number of hydroxyl groups in the molecule. There are a number of protein-like resins, some glucosides and other carbohydrate-containing molecules that have been used at some time in pharmaceutic preparations and would appear in this group but are not listed because they are not in current use.

4. Water- and Alcohol-Insoluble, Special Solvent-Soluble Compounds. Compounds falling into this category are listed in Table 47-8 and appear in step 8, page 1131 of

Table 47-8. Acidity and Basicity of Water- and Alcohol-Insoluble, Special Solvent-Soluble Drugs

ACIDIC GROUP DRUGS

Weak Acids or Non Acids

α-Naphthylthiourea (ANTU)—soluble in dioxane	Phenylbutazone— very soluble in ether	Sulfadiazine—soluble in alkaline H_2O and dilute acid H_2O	Sulfapyridine—soluble in alkaline H_2O and acid H_2O

the extraction procedure. There are relatively few water or alcohol insolubles of interest in toxicologic analysis because some solubility is a prerequisite for absorption through the intestinal walls. Special isolation procedures are better applied directly to the tissue sample, since some of the compound is lost during the extensive extractions on the sample in the course of the isolation. Alpha-naphthylthiourea (ANTU) is probably the only commercial substance of toxicologic importance. It is used as a rat poison and usually comes to the laboratory in connection with the death of domestic animals. It has emetic properties and is not considered toxic to humans or animals that can regurgitate.

Phenylbutazone will be present in detectable amounts in the main extraction group. Relatively large dosages are used in the treatment of gout and the rheumatic diseases but, because of its low alcohol solubility, recovery will only be partial. The relatively insoluble sulfa drugs are not of toxicological importance unless it is necessary to identify the particular compound after analysis of the blood has indicated an abnormally high sulfa drug level.

PRELIMINARY EXAMINATIONS, SPECIAL PURIFICATION METHODS, AND IDENTIFICATION OF SEDATIVES

PRELIMINARY EXAMINATIONS

A. Preliminary Examination of the Residues from the Acid Extraction and/or Three Component Separation (pages 1138 and 1139).

A. Preliminary Examination of the Residues and/or Three Component Separation. 1. Physical Examination of the Residue. If the visual or microscopic examination reveals a crystalline residue, substances other than the normal tissue extractables are present. Acidic and neutral compounds are less toxic, in general, than the bases and, if anything is present, the residue will usually consist of a significant deposit of the sample.

2. Indicator Reactions. Indicator reactions as applied to toxicologic analysis (9) were developed by Davidson (28) for qualitative organic analysis. They are particularly suited to the analysis of tissue residues since they are carried out in nonaqueous media and utilize only minute quantities of sample. The Congo red and sodium alizarinsulfonate tests (9) are supporting tests for the nonaqueous indicator tests.

Reagents. (a) Congo red test paper; (b) Davidson's indicator reagents (29): stock solutions of the indicators in their appropriate solvents and the additional reagents are listed in Table 47-9, along with the volumes required for the preparation of the separate reagents.

Table 47-9.

STOCK SOLUTIONS AND SOLVENTS	INDICATOR REAGENTS (ML.)			
	A1	A2	B1	B2
Methanol	21.25	44.4		46.65
Alizarin yellow R (0.1% in MeOH)	1.25			
Bromothymol blue (0.1% in MeOH)	1.25	1.25		1.25
Bromocresol purple (0.1% in MeOH)		1.85		1.85
Thymol blue (0.1% in 0.05 M KOH in MeOH)		1.25		
Benzeneazodiphenylamine (0.1% in AcOH)			2.5	
Potassium hydroxide (2 M MeOH)	1.25	1.25		
Pyridine	25.00			
Glacial acetic acid			47.25	
Hydrochloric acid (36%)			0.25	0.25

From Davidson (28)

(a) Congo Red Test. The residue should be anhydrous to insure the removal of the last trace of hydrochloric acid which may have been carried over into the solvent layer by incomplete separation of the aqueous and solvent phases. All acids change Congo red paper to blue when the pH of the aqueous solution is 4.1 or lower. A positive Congo red test is an indication, therefore, that an acid is present in the extract which is sufficiently strong to form a sodium salt in sodium bicarbonate solution.

Procedure. Pick up a very small quantity of solid on the end of a microspatula and transfer it to a piece of dry Congo red paper. Then place the indicator test paper on a microscope slide and add a drop of water to one end of the paper. Observe the spot containing the extract after the water diffuses through the paper. A positive test is indicated when a blue halo surrounds the solid.

A positive test is indicative of carboxy or sulfonic acids, a few amides such as saccharin or phenols in which the acidity of the OH$^-$ is enhanced by negative groups in the ring. Positive findings on the acid residue from the first extraction procedure (page 1138) should initiate a three component extraction (page 1139) because phenols and neutrals may also be present and further indicator tests will only respond to the strong acid. If the test is negative, proceed with the Davidson indicator tests to differentiate phenols or intermediate acids from the neutrals.

(b) Davidson's Indicator Test for Acids. *Procedure.* Introduce a microquantity of residue into a capillary tube * about 1 x 15 mm. and add an amount of indicator suffi-cient to observe a color and force it into contact with the drug. With an oily or a resinous-like drug place a small portion inside the bore of the capillary and, on addition of the indicator solution, it is carried into the body of the tube. The color changes are immediate with most compounds but some require as much as 4 to 5 minutes for com-plete color development. Indicator changes for acids are shown in Figure 47-3.

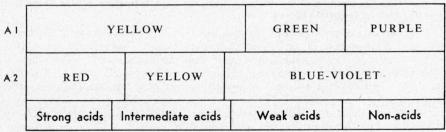

A 1	YELLOW		GREEN	PURPLE
A 2	RED	YELLOW	BLUE-VIOLET	
	Strong acids	Intermediate acids	Weak acids	Non-acids

From Davidson

Fig. 47-3. Indicator Changes for Acids.

After the original work on the application of the indicator method to toxicologic analysis (9), it was found that, with few exceptions, adequate information could be obtained by the use of A2 alone (30). The lack of a sharp distinction between weak and nonacids did not justify the use of sample material for the test with A1 and weak and nonacids were therefore classified in a single group.

Positive findings for an intermediate acid may be due to the presence of phenols or barbiturates. Neutrals may also be present and the three component extraction (page 1139) should be carried out to make the separation, eliminating the first extraction with sodium bicarbonate. Classification of the acidic, with the basic, drugs according to the indicator reactions is shown in Table 47-10.

B. Probing Reactions on the Residues from the Acid Extraction and/or Three Component Separation.

B. Probing Reactions on the Residues from the Acid Extraction and/or Three Component Separation. 1. Ferric Chloride Reaction for Salicylates. Ingested aspirin is always partially hydrolyzed to salicylic acid except in rare cases when isolated from the stomach contents in large amounts. Its detection is an indication for a three com-ponent separation of the residue since it is frequently present with barbiturates.

Reagent. 5 per cent aqueous ferric chloride containing 1.0 ml. N HCl/100 ml. of solution.

Procedure. A drop of reagent is added to a crystal from the residue on a micro-scope slide. An immediate coloration is indicative of salicylic acid.† ‡

2. Alcoholic Ferric Chloride Confirmatory Test for Salicylates.

Reagent. The 5 per cent aqueous $FeCl_3$ is added dropwise to 95 per cent ethyl alcohol to form a brown colored solution.

Procedure. A crystal from the residue is placed in a microtest tube and a drop of reagent introduced. Salicylic acid is the only phenolic substance giving the same shade of color in alcoholic $FeCl_3$ as in water.

3. Koppanyi Reaction for Barbiturates (31). Barbiturates are the most common drugs encountered in suicidal deaths. The Koppanyi reaction is sensitive, although not specific, and, in the absence of salicylates, can be made on residues that are not entirely pure. If salicylates are found the test should be delayed until the separation is made and then performed on the phenolic fraction. There are two procedures, one carried out in $CHCl_3$ solution and the other on filter paper. The filter paper technic is the more

---

* Due to creeping of the nonaqueous solvents used in the indicators listed, the slide method of observing a color change proved inadequate. The color can best be observed in a capillary tube.

† Acetylsalicylic acid (aspirin), if pure, does not react until hydrolyzed.

†† Antipyrine gives a deep red and amidopyrine a violet color. There are other nonvolatile phenolic substances which react positively.

Table 47-10. Acidity and Basicity of Water- and Alcohol-Soluble Drugs

* This requires special isolation procedures because of its extreme toxicity (page 1254). It is only dispensed when colored with a dye.

ACIDIC GROUP DRUGS

Strong Acids

Benzoic acid	Fluoroacetic acid *	Hippuric acid	Mandelic acid	Saccharin
Citric acid	Glutaric acid	Levulinic acid	Oxalic acid	Salicylic acid

Intermediate Acids

Acetylsalicylic acid   Cinchophen   Pavatrine
p-Aminobenzoic acid   Dimenhydrinate   Phenylbutazone
Cholesterol   (acid extraction product)   Sulfisoxazole
Chrysazin   Ethyl biscoumacetate   Xylocaine

Weak Acids or Non Acids

Acetanilid	Chlorobutanol	Hexobarbital	Phenobarbital	Sedormid
Acetophenetidin	Coumarin	Isoamylethyl-	Phenylacetylurea	Sulfonethyl-
Amobarbital	Cyclopal	acetylurea	Phenylsalicylate	methane
Antipyrine	Diallylbarbi-	Meconin	Picrotoxin	Sulfonmethane
Aprobarbital	turic acid	Mephobarbital	Piperidione	Theobromine
Barbital	Digitoxin	Methylphenyl-	Pregnenolone	Theophylline
Benzocaine	Diphenyl-	ethylhydantoin	Probarbital	Thiopental
Bromural	hydantoin	Neonal	Pyrithyldione	Tribromoethanol
Butabarbital	Emetine	Ortal	Sandoptal	Trimethadione
Caffeine	Estrone	Pentobarbital	Santonin	Urethan
Carbromal	Glycine	Phanadorn	Secobarbital	Vinbarbital

BASIC GROUP DRUGS

Intermediate Bases

Aconitine	Butamin	Dicyclomine	Optochin	Quinine
Amprotropine	Cinchonidine	Diphenhydramine	Piperocaine	Tetracaine
Apomorphine	Cinchonine	Homatropine	Prisilidene	Thenylpyramine
Apothesine	Cocaine	Hyoscyamine	Procaine	Thonzylamine
Atropine	Codeine	Lobeline	Procaine amide	Veratrine
Brucine	Dibucaine	Methadon	Pseudopelletierine	Xylocaine

Weak Bases or Non Bases

Adiphenine	Digalen	Eucupin	Nikethamide	Solanin
N-Allylnor-	Digitalin	Heroin	Pamaquine	Sparteine
morphine	Dihydromorphinone	Hydrastine	Pentamethyl-	Strophanthin
Aminopyrine	Dimenhydrinate	Larocaine	enetetrazol	Strychnine
Amphetamine	(basic extrac-	Meperidine	Phenindamine	Thiamin (de-
Atabrin	tion product)	Metopon	Physostigmine	composition
Coniine	Diothane	Morphine	Pilocarpine	product)
Curarine	Emetine	Narceine	Piperine	Thiazolsulfone
Delphinine	Ephedrine	Narcotine	Pyrilamine	Trihexyphenidyl
d-Desoxyephedrine	Ethylmorphine	Nicotinic alcohol	Scopolamine	Yohimbine

sensitive and considerably more specific since it depends on solubility of the compound in the n-butylamine reagent.

Reagents. (a) $Co(Ac)_2$ in absolute methyl alcohol: 1.25 gm. of $Co(Ac)_2$ is dissolved in 100 ml. of absolute methyl alcohol.

(b) 5 per cent normal butylamine reagent: 2 ml. of n-butylamine is added to 35 ml. of absolute methyl alcohol.

(c) Cobalt acetate impregnated paper: #2 Whatman filter paper is dipped into the reagent (a), partially dried and the process repeated several times until the paper has a decided pink cast on drying. The outer edge containing the ring of concentrated $Co(Ac)_2$ is cut away and discarded and the paper is cut into strips the size of litmus paper. It can be stored indefinitely in the dark in a closed container.

Procedure. (a) Reaction on Cobalt Acetate Impregnated Paper. Place a microcrystal of residue on a strip of the cobalt acetate impregnated paper and add a drop of n-butylamine reagent near the crystal so that it diffuses across the paper and wets the crystal. A pink spot in the area of the crystal which is particularly apparent after drying is indicative of barbiturates.

(b) Reaction in Chloroform. Dissolve a crystal of residue contained in a microcentrifuge tube of 1 to 2 ml. capacity in 3 drops of chloroform, add 1 drop of $Co(Ac)_2$ and mix the solution by tapping the tube with the finger. Then carefully layer the n-butylamine reagent over the chloroform solution. A positive reaction is indicated by a violet ring at the interface.

The reaction appears to be related to the acidic character of the compounds in nonaqueous solution (32).

All the barbiturates react positively, while the substituted alkyl ureas such as sedormid® do not. Reaction with succinamide, p-toluenesulfonamide, p-toluenesulfonylaniline and the sedative pyrithyldione are particularly sensitive. Some of the sulfa drugs such as sulfanilamide and sulfathiazole give a red-violet in both tests and sulfadiazine gives a good color in chloroform but a very slight one on the paper. Theophylline and the compound diphenylhydantoin, when pure, give good reactions in chloroform but not on the paper. Dimenhydrinate which contains theophylline gives a positive paper reaction, and a pink color which is not intensified by the added base on addition of the cobalt acetate to a chloroform solution. Benzimidazole gives a decided pink color without addition of the base. Benzoic acid from urine gives a weak reaction in chloroform only, while salicylic acid produces a deep green color which prevents the detection of the barbiturates. Acetylsalicylic acid reacts peculiarly. When crystalline and free of salicylic acid, it gives a strong reaction but if the preparation contains enough free salicylic acid to give a positive chloroform reaction only the green color is obtained. An extract from empirin®,* which is a sticky resin resembling secobarbital in consistency gave a negative reaction even though dissolved in chloroform. On crystallization from alcohol a strong reaction was obtained with the crystalline residue, as previously observed on the original preparation.

Acetylsalicylic acid can be detected by preliminary hydrolysis with mineral acid solution or by simply boiling with water, after which the salicylic acid produces the green color in the test.

The most troublesome interference is a degradation product from normal brain tissue. It has been isolated only in cases which were in the early stage of putrefaction. The brain distillate has a distinct odor and shows a strong azide-iodine reaction without apparent degeneration of the tissue structure. The residue shows a strong Congo red test and, after the three component separation, the positive Koppanyi reaction, in contrast with the barbiturates, is found to be much stronger in the residue from the bicarbonate extraction. Confusion arises from the fact that the other fractions also react, due to the incomplete separation of the fractions and the problem is to determine whether a barbiturate may also be present in the phenol fraction.

The original extract is exceptionally fatty and, on sublimation (page 1153), crystals are obtained in a large amount of oily deposit. All attempts at isolation in pure form have failed because it is considerably more water soluble than solvent soluble and has the physical properties of the other nonreactive fatty tissue compounds.

It may be recognized in the residue from the bicarbonate extraction by the addition of concentrated nitric acid, followed by strong alkali. After spontaneous evaporation of the HNO_3, a yellow deposit similar to the acetophenetidin color is obtained and, on addition of alkali, the typical red color characteristic of dinitro substitution in the benzene ring forms (33). It is not a barbiturate metabolite, as shown by infrared absorption and failure to obtain a substance giving a positive Koppanyi from the liver in the same case.

4. Test with Concentrated Nitric Acid. Acetophenetidin is a common drug frequently present with either salicylates or barbiturates. It is separated from both in the three component separation but their presence does not cause interference in the test.

Procedure. Add a drop of concentrated nitric acid to a crystal from the residue on a microscope slide.

A deep canary yellow coloration is indicative of acetophenetidin. If a large amount of muck is present, it may produce a brown which can mask the yellow coloration.

C. Preliminary Examination of the Residues from the Basic Extractions (pp. 1138, 1140).

C. Preliminary Examination of the Residues from the Basic Extractions. 1. Physical Examination of the Residues. Establishing the presence of a drug in the basic extract requires considerably more care than with the acid fraction. Some bases are very toxic drugs of low lethal dosages and many are noncrystalline. Because of the microquantities mixed with varying but comparatively large amounts of muck in the extracts, visual or

---

* An APC combination of aspirin, phenacetin and caffeine.

microscopic examination will not always reveal their presence so that preliminary chemical testing is essential.

The acidic extraction produces a partial purification for the bases * but, in exceptional cases particularly under conditions of putrefaction, further purification (page 1153)
may be desirable before starting any chemical examination.

2. Indicator Reactions (page 1147). (a) Sodium Alizarinsulfonate Test. This
reagent is especially useful in determining the presence of volatile bases in the final
stage of the evaporation (page 1139).

Reagent. Sodium alizarinsulfonate. A saturated aqueous solution is prepared.

Procedure. Place a small quantity of basic extract on a microscope slide and moisten
it with the sodium alizarinsulfonate reagent. The color change from yellow to red,
which is observed against a white background or microscopically, is indicative of a
substance with decidedly basic properties. A positive reaction should be followed by
the separation of bases from amphoterics (page 1140).†

The sodium alizarinsulfonate reaction is indicative of strong bases and when it is
positive, tests with the Davidson indicators B1 and B2 will always show the reaction
for intermediate bases. Under these conditions this procedure should be delayed and
carried out on the basic and amphoteric fractions after their separation (page 1140).
On the other hand, some bases that are negative with sodium alizarinsulfonate react
as intermediates with B1 and B2 and the reactions serve as a differential test for these
substances.

(b) Davidson's Indicator Tests for Bases. The procedure has been described for
acids on page 1147. Indicator changes are shown in Figure 47-4.

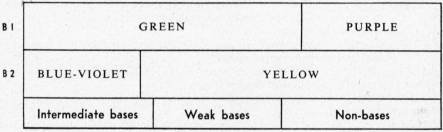

From Davidson

Fig. 47-4. Indicator Changes for Bases.

Classification of the basic, with the acidic, drugs according to the indicator reactions
is shown in Table 47-10.

Further work on the Davidson indicators (30) has pointed to the fact that the
distinction between weak and nonbases is not sufficiently clear-cut to justify their division
into separate groups.

Negative findings are not conclusive for the absence of basic substances since the
toxic ones can be present in concentrations that are below the limits for detecting a
positive reaction.

D. Probing Reactions for the Bases.

D. Probing Reactions for the Bases. 1. Picric Acid Precipitation (page 1260). Picric
acid is the most universal of the basic precipitants and a cloudy solution due to the
separation of an oil or colloidal precipitate, if not a crystalline precipitate, occurs with
most of them with this reagent. At this point, it is useful as a sensitive precipitant to
indicate the presence of bases.

Reagent. 10 per cent aqueous solution.

---

* A few investigators have proposed an extraction in which bases are removed from the aqueous
extract before the acids. The normal tissue components pass into each phase during an extraction
so that the more difficult basic group is in a state of greater purity by removing the acids as the
first step.

† Care must be taken that the positive test was not from ammonia mechanically carried into the
solvent and incompletely removed in the evaporation.

Procedure. Place a small amount of residue on a microscope slide with a micro-spatula * and allow a drop of reagent to flow across it.

Any cloud or crystalline precipitate in the drop is indicative of basic compounds.

2. Marquis Reagent for Morphine. Morphine is one of the few substances that does not react in the methyl orange procedure (see below) and should, therefore, be excluded before proceeding with this test when there are positive indications for a base.

Reagent. Add three drops of 40 per cent formalin to 1.0 ml. of concentrated sulfuric acid, cool the solution and allow it to stand from 10 to 15 minutes. This should be prepared fresh each time.

Procedure. Add a drop of reagent to a small amount of residue placed on a microscope slide.

Morphine gives an immediate red-purple color. The reaction is not specific for morphine. The opium alkaloids and many other substances react (page 1214) so that positive findings do not necessarily eliminate the methyl orange procedure unless a further examination (page 1250) indicates that it is present.

3. Methyl Orange Reaction. The method was developed by Brodie et al. (34) for the determination of bases in pharmacologic studies and applied as a quantitative determination in toxicologic analysis by Gettler and Sunshine (35). It is applied here to the basic residues from the combined or separate ether and chloroform extractions as a qualitative indicating test as well as a semiquantitative reaction, in order to establish whether the concentration of base that was isolated is significant. The semiquantitative estimation determines the use of sample material in carrying out further tests as it permits a selection of reactions on the basis of their sensitivity and specificity.

Reagents. (a) Chloroform, analytical grade.

(b) Methyl orange solution: Add 250 mg. methyl orange to 50 ml. water and heat at 40° C. for 20 minutes. Cool, filter, shake out with chloroform once and refilter.

(c) Boric acid, saturated aqueous solution.

(d) Methyl orange reagent: Prepared just before using by mixing equal volumes of boric acid solution and methyl orange solution.

(e) Phosphate buffer, pH 8.0: Mix 62.5 ml. of 0.2 M KH_2PO_4 and 117.1 ml. of 0.1 M NaOH. Dilute to 250 ml. with distilled water.

(f) Ethyl alcohol, acidified: Add 2 ml. concentrated H_2SO_4 to 100 ml. absolute ethyl alcohol.

Procedure (36). Dissolve the residue to be examined in 10 ml. of chloroform and add a 0.25 ml. aliquot in a 4 inch test tube.† Add 4.75 ml. of chloroform and 0.3 ml. of methyl orange reagent. Stopper the tube with a tin foil-covered cork and shake it 100 times. Transfer the contents to a small separatory funnel and allow them to stand until the layers separate. Draw the chloroform off carefully into a 10 ml. graduate, measure the volume, add 0.1 ml. of the acid ethyl alcohol for each ml. of chloroform solution and mix the contents by shaking. Prepare a reagent blank at the same time by adding 0.3 ml. of methyl orange reagent to 5.0 ml. of chloroform and treat it in the same manner as the unknown. Transfer the solutions to 1 cm. Beckman DU Spectrophotometer Corex cells and read the optical density of the unknown against the reagent blank with the wave length set at 520 mμ. Normal tissue that has not undergone any putrefaction gives optical density readings up to 0.025. Values above 0.05 are indicative of a basic substance present in the residue in abnormal amounts and should initiate a thorough chemical examination of the residue.* Higher values are obtained under conditions of moderate to marked putrefaction. With residues from tissue that is not fresh, the procedure should be modified. Dilute the 0.25 ml. aliquot of the chloroform solution with 4.75 ml. of chloroform and shake it out in a separatory funnel with 5.0 ml. of

---

* The basic residue is not always bulky enough to permit a sample to be removed by a spatula. There are a number of microtechnics for picking up small samples. The bottom of the container may be wiped with a small piece of Whatman #50 filter paper about 1 x 1 mm. and the test done on the paper. A part of the residue may be taken up in a small amount of solvent and placed dropwise on a slide that is warmed near the boiling point of the solvent. Nonaqueous solvents creep on glass and spread the sample rather than concentrate it in a very confined area. One of the best procedures is to take up the solvent in a capillary tube open at both ends and, when enough evaporation takes place at one end, the solid is transferred to a slide with a microscalpel.

† It is best to take duplicate samples of the unknown when performing this test.

phosphate buffer. Draw off the chloroform layer, add 0.3 ml. methyl orange reagent and follow the procedure as described.

SPECIAL PURIFICATION PROCEDURES

A partial purification of the tissue extract was made during the isolation process and, as previously pointed out (page 1127), the term purification is restricted here to mean the special procedures for removing the small amount of normal tissue extractables, commonly labeled tissue muck (page 1137), that remain in the residue after the isolation process has been completed. The proportion of muck to isolated compound determines the extent of special purification needed. Since the sensitivity of all the reactions used in the identifying stage of the analysis is determined by the purity of the test material (page 1125) and since the varying amounts of muck are invariably obtained from different extracts of even the same source material despite the care exercised in the extraction process, the analyst must rely on his judgment in determining the extent of purification needed. Because any purification process results in loss of material, the extent of the purification must be a compromise in order to obtain a final product of sufficient purity to give adequate sensitivity in the tests without incurring losses that prevent carrying out a sufficient number of the test reactions.

Because of the higher lethal dosages of the acidic type substances, the ratio of the isolated test material to tissue extractables will be higher so that, in some cases, no special purification is needed. With the basic drugs, purification is invariably necessary except, perhaps, in extracts of stomach contents. Under conditions of putrefaction (page 1127), it may be necessary to carry out a special purification before attempting the preliminary examination of the extracted residue (page 1147). Under any circumstances, in the first attempts at purification, preference should be given to those procedures that permit reclaiming all of the products in case the process is not successful.

1. Vacuum Sublimation.

1. Vacuum Sublimation. Sublimation under reduced pressures offers one of the best purification methods for tissue extracts. Practically all of the pharmaceutic compounds that are acidic, phenolic or neutral readily sublime while only a small amount of oil from degradation of the normal tissue components undergoes sublimation. Many basic drugs also sublime but considerably higher temperatures are required with the result that tissue breakdown is increased and the smaller amount of sublimed product is contaminated with a greater proportion of oil from the tissue residue. A few basic drugs undergo pyrolysis at or below the sublimation point and, in a general unknown, sublimation of the basic extract should not be attempted without a preliminary trial on a small portion of the sample. A special technic has been developed for the sublimation of tissue residues.

FRACTIONAL SUBLIMATION ON A REMOVABLE TRANSPARENT FILM (37). Many sublimation apparatus and technics have been described (38), in which the sublimate is usually collected on the surface of a glass receiver. In order to perform subsequent chemical or microscopic tests, the crystalline sublimate must be removed either by a scraping process or by dissolution in a suitable solvent. If a scraping procedure is employed, the more or less well formed crystals are likely to be damaged. If two or more components of a mixture have been fractionally separated by a single sublimation, a subsequent dissolution procedure will obviously defeat the original purpose of the sublimation.

To overcome this difficulty, a procedure was devised whereby the sublimed crystals, without further manipulation, may be examined directly on the collecting surface. A sublimation tube consisting of two cylindrical sections connected by a ground-glass joint was designed and constructed as shown in Figure 47-5. The male ground-glass joint is of constant diameter throughout its entire length and has exactly the same diameter as the rest of the tubing to which it is connected. This feature eliminates the dead space at the joint usually found in the standard type of ground-glass joints. The

---

* The method as described is sensitive to 6 mg. and will readily indicate the presence of 0.25 mg. of base in the entire residue.

use of this straight-walled sublimation tube permits the insertion of a transparent cellophane film (which serves as a condensing surface for the sublimate) without the presence of any dead space between the film and inner wall of the tube. When sublimation is complete, the film is removed from the tube without disturbing the crystalline pattern of the sublimate. This procedure results in quantitative deposition of the sublimate on a flat, transparent surface, so that crystalline forms may be easily distinguished microscopically and individual crystals may be readily removed for physical and chemical examination.

Several sublimation devices (39, 40) have been designed for depositing the sublimate on a removable collector. The latter, however, is in one plane, so that the deposit consists of aggregates rather than individual crystals. In the authors' apparatus the removable transparent film is in a vertical position during the sublimation procedure and hence individual crystals deposit in the uppermost part of the sublimate. Fractionation of two or more components is conducted in one uninterrupted sublimation. This cannot be done by methods previously described in the literature.

Mixtures which contain components that sublime at different rates can be fractionally separated during one sublimation step by controlling the temperature and rate of heating. Components that sublime under different conditions may be made to deposit at different levels on the film, and where the separation is not sharp, overlapping bound-

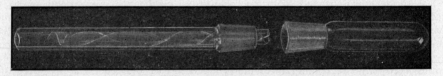

Fig. 47-5. Sublimation Tube With Cellulose Film.

aries may be cut out and resublimed. The characteristic forms of the different crystals in the sublimed mixture can usually be recognized by their optical properties, even in mixtures where complete fractional separation is not attainable (Fig. 47-10). Pure individual crystals to be used for the determination of melting point and other physical, as well as chemical, properties may be picked from the mass by the use of a micromanipulator. Quantities of organic material ranging from 0.05 to 50 mg. can be conveniently sublimed.

Sublimation Apparatus. The sublimation apparatus (Fig. 47-6) may be readily constructed of materials available from any laboratory supply house.

The parts consist of a cylindrical aluminum block, *A,* 6 inches (15 cm.) high and 4.5 inches (11.25 cm.) in diameter, obtainable from the Aluminum Company of America; Cenco mechanical latch electric reset relay, No. 98330, *B;* Cenco de Khotinsky single-pole double-lock bimetallic thermoregulator, No. 90025, *C;* four General Electric 120-watt 115-volt, 3×0.5 inch cartridge heaters, *D;* ten voltmeter-type binding posts, *E;* and a 300° C. thermometer, *F.*

The auxiliary equipment includes a vacuum pump, vacuum gage, freezing trap, and Dewar flask.

The aluminum block and assembly are mounted on a 0.5-inch Transite board with three 1-inch legs. The electric connections for the thermoregulator and relay accompany the apparatus supplied by the manufacturer. The leads for each of the four cartridge heaters connect to a pair of binding posts and a 110-volt direct current supply, and the lines from the regulator and relay are connected to the two remaining binding posts. In this way, any combination of heaters with series or parallel connections can be made with jumpers across the binding posts. No thermal insulation is used on the heating block, as a constant temperature can be maintained with the thermoregulator. When a temperature differential is to be maintained within the block, insulation is unnecessary and is actually detrimental.

Sublimation Tube. The sublimation tube (Fig. 47-5) may be obtained from Eck and Krebs, Long Island City, N. Y., supplied as No. 5600. The outer diameter of the

* Obtainable from Otis Benedict, Jr., 31 Stevenson Street, Lynbrook, New York.

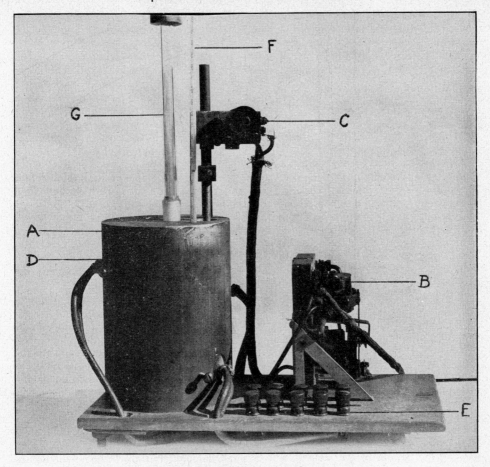

Fig. 47-6. Sublimation Apparatus.

A, aluminum block. B, relay. C, thermoregulator. D, cartridge heaters. E, binding posts. F, thermometer. G, sublimation tube.

lower section is 1.8 cm., and the over-all length is 7.6 cm. including a No. 14/20 female ground-glass joint. The tube fits tightly into the hole, with the bottom edge of the joint at the upper level of the aluminum block. The top section of the sublimation tube is 18.5 cm. in length with constant inner diameter of 8 mm., and the wall thickness is 2 mm. The male joint is made by building up glass on the outside of the thick-walled tube and then grinding a 14/20 taper male joint. In this way the inside of the tube is of uniform diameter throughout its entire length.

Cellulose sausage casing (Visking Corporation, Chicago, Ill.) was found the most suitable lining to function as a condensing surface for the sublimate. This film will not char when the block is heated to 300° C. It is relatively alkali-resistant, insoluble in most organic solvents, and unaffected by cold concentrated hydrochloric or sulfuric acid. A 1.5 × 6 inch strip of the cellulose casing is cut from the roll, washed by dipping in ethyl ether, and dried. The paper is rolled around a glass rod and inserted through the joint end of the upper section of the sublimation tube, about 0.25 inch of the paper projecting from the joint. The rod is then removed and the cellulose film is grasped by the 0.25-inch excess projecting above the joint. The roll of cellulose film is rotated in clockwise direction until it forms a spiral inside the tube, then in a counter-clockwise direction until the coil partially unwinds, causing it to expand and wedge tightly against the internal walls of the sublimation tube. Any excess of cellulose film extending beyond the ground-glass joint is trimmed flush with the end of the joint. Figure 47-5 shows the cellulose film properly inserted in the sublimation tube.

Sublimation Procedure. The following procedure was developed primarily for the investigation of substances extracted from unknown medicinal mixtures and biologic materials by immiscible solvents.

The extracted substance or its solution is placed in the bottom section of the sublimation tube. Any solvent present is evaporated by heating on a hot plate. The upper portion of the tube is connected to a vacuum pump assembly capable of furnishing a pressure of 1 mm. or less. The ground-glass joints are connected while the vacuum is being applied. The rate of heating is controlled by the proper combination of the heating elements at the binding posts. For unknown mixtures the heating elements are connected in parallel with the thermoregulator set at about 150° C., causing the temperature to rise approximately 2° per minute. The cellophane film condensing surface is observed from time to time. When a sublimate begins to appear, the thermoregulator is cut back to maintain that temperature as long as crystals continue to deposit. It is then advanced to a higher level and further observations are made as the sublimation progresses. In this manner components of mixtures are deposited at different levels on the film.

The nature of the deposition levels is an indication of the possible number of components as well as the sublimation conditions that will give the best possible separation of the mixture. A preliminary trial sublimation of an unknown mixture will usually establish the conditions of temperature, rate of heating, and time necessary for the best separation of a component from a mixture. In subsequent sublimations, the thermoregulator can be set accordingly and the operation can proceed with but little attention.

Examination of Sublimate. When sublimation is complete, the tube is disconnected at the joint and the film is removed by hooking it with a dental probe. The film coil is carefully unwound, then fastened by thumbtacks to a cork pad for a few hours, after which time it will remain flat. The sublimate can be examined microscopically on the cork board by reflected light with a vertical illuminator, or the film may be removed from the cork and examined by transmitted light. The crystal area is studied under low magnification to determine the number and relative purity of the crystalline forms present.

If fractional separation of the mixture is evident, the different crystalline deposits are separated by cutting the cellulose film into strips. Sections of the film, approximately 2×3 mm., containing the crystals are removed and then mounted on glass slides by coating the bottom of the sections with a small amount of colorless fingernail polish. These slides are used to obtain photomicrographs of the crystals and measurements of the crystal angles. Well-formed crystals are removed from the film by means of a small dental scalpel mounted as a probe on a micromanipulator for the determination of melting point, examination by polarized light, and determination of refractive indexes. Micromelting points are determined on a Kofler hot stage. Particles of cellulose which may be removed with the crystals in the scraping process do not appreciably affect the melting point, because the cellulose and crystalline melt are mutually insoluble.

The sublimates from tissue extracts are generally contaminated with an oily deposit which is not entirely removed in the preliminary extraction process. In such cases a film section containing the crystals for melting point determination is cut out and washed by allowing petroleum ether or ethyl ether to flow across the film while it is held at an acute angle. Because of the relatively small exposed surface of the sublimed crystals, they can be washed several times without appreciable loss of crystalline material.

Cut film sections are advantageous in the chemical examination of sublimates. The resistance of the film to alkalies and cold concentrated acids permits the direct execution of color reactions and formation of crystalline derivatives on a small section of the film. Interference due to charring of the film occurs only in those color reactions which require hot concentrated sulfuric acid. For such tests, crystals are carefully removed from the film so that there is no contamination by cellulose particles, because any fibers that may dissolve in the hot acid will produce a brown coloration which will alter or mask the color of a particular reaction. Crystals must be removed from the paper for optical studies under polarized light. Although the crystalline forms are clearly defined when the film mounts are observed under crossed Nicols, the paper is birefracting and the optical constants of the crystals are altered accordingly.

In carrying out microprecipitation reactions for the production of characteristic crystals, the reagents may be added directly to cut film sections, inasmuch as the transparent film particles floating in the drop on a microscopic slide do not interfere with the formation or observation of the crystalline precipitate. Because the film is insoluble in most organic solvents, except such cellulose solvents as acetone and ethyl acetate, crystals can be dissolved from the film by immersion in suitable organic solvent.

In the preparation of derivatives where microcondensation-type reactions are to be carried out in nonaqueous solution, cut film sections are of a decided advantage because organic liquids have much less tendency to creep on the film than on a glass surface; consequently, the reaction mixture remains as concentrated droplets on the film surface.

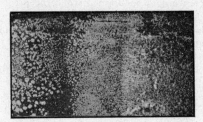

Fig. 47-7. Left to Right, Separation by Sublimation of a Mixture of Phenobarbituric, Acetylsalicylic and Salicylic Acids × 2.5

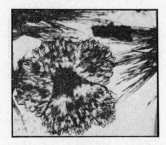

Fig. 47-8. Phenobarbituric Acid Sublimate (Fig. 47-7) × 75

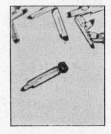

Fig. 47.9 Acetylsalicylic Acid Sublimate (Fig. 47.7) × 70

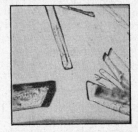

Fig. 47-10. Salicylic Acid Sublimate (Fig. 47-7) × 70

If resublimation is necessary, the sublimate may be transferred to the lower half of the sublimation tube by means of an organic solvent, or the film sections may be used directly. Charring of the film at the higher temperatures inside the heating block will not affect the nature of the sublimate. The fractional sublimation of a few drugs commonly encountered is illustrated in Figures 47-7 and 47-11.

Fig. 47-11. Wider Separation of Phenobarbituric and Salicylic Acids Produced by Higher Sublimation Temperature × 4.5

2. Multiple Extraction with Immiscible Solvents.

2. Multiple Extraction with Immiscible Solvents. As previously pointed out (page 1137), extraction with immiscible solvents offers one of the simplest purification methods for the residues from tissue containing the water and solvent-soluble drugs. Because a large proportion of the normal tissue residue is colloidal in nature, there is a greater tendency for dispersion of the particles in the aqueous than in the solvent phase (page 1137) and each transfer mechanically removes some of the muck in the aqueous phase. In addition, the purity of the more solvent-soluble drugs is increased in the solvent layer

with each extraction as a result of the normal distribution of components of the mixture between solvent and aqueous solutions. The multiple extraction technic has been highly developed under the heading of counter current distribution and applied particularly to the separation of organic substances in biologic mixtures (41). Counter current distribution, as practised, is not yet applicable to tissue residues because the purity of the final product is attained as a result of so many transfers that there is considerable loss of sample material. It can be applied in principle to extracts from tissue however, with the exception that a test be made of the solvent phase after each transfer in order to have a qualitative measure of the recovery of sample after each extraction. The process should be stopped when the purity is adequate for testing rather than continued in attempting a more complete purification. In a toxicologic analysis for poisons it is seldom that more than enough drug will have been isolated than is needed for the identification * (page 1126) so that no purification process should be carried beyond the stage needed for adequate sensitivity in the reactions.

SPECIAL SOLVENTS. (a) Petroleum Ether. Petroleum ether is one of the best fat and lipid solvents while many organic drugs are insoluble or only slightly soluble in this solvent. It may be used to leach out fatty tissue substances from the residue when the solubility of the isolated compound in it is not significant. It is particularly useful in leaching out residues that are oily in consistency and in removing the oily tissue degradation products produced from the breakdown during sublimation. Although a significant number of the synthetic pharmaceutics and organics of lower molecular weight are petroleum ether soluble, nothing is lost by the leaching process since any soluble compounds are recovered on evaporation of the solvent.

In the Haines modification of the Dragendorff process (42) for extraction of drugs from biologic material, petroleum ether is used as one of the solvents in the original extraction of the isolated residue. The disadvantage of this procedure is that the petroleum ether residue is always exceptionally fatty and any soluble compounds are as badly contaminated as before the extraction. Of more importance is the fact that a significant loss of many of the partially soluble substances can occur. The petroleum ether residue contains a higher percentage of low-melting lipids from the tissue extract which obscure any crystalline formation. The sensitivity of the probing tests for drugs in this residue is often less than on the original because of concentration of the low-melting fatty substances. Much of the oily lipid material is removed during the group separation with ether and chloroform and application of petroleum ether as a purification procedure to the separate groups not only achieves the same separation as in the Haines process but also permits an interpretation of the physical action of the petroleum ether on the sample without the danger of losses of test material.

Procedure. Petroleum ether is layered over the dried residue and any solid is put into suspension with a stirring rod. The beaker is allowed to stand in the refrigerator until all solid particles have settled out and the solvent is cold.† The beaker is then carefully removed without disturbing the sediment on the bottom and all but about 0.5 ml. transferred into another container by means of an inverted microsiphon of not more than 1 mm. bore ‡ (Fig. 47-12). The leaching process can be repeated to remove all the extractable components. The petroleum ether extracts and the residue are then evaporated to dryness on the steam bath.

(b) Dioxane. Dioxane is a good fat solvent and some compounds that are petroleum ether soluble are insoluble in this solvent. It may be used as a leaching agent on the residue in the same manner as the petroleum ether but it is more troublesome because of its higher boiling point (105° C.) and odor.

(c) Ethyl Chloride. Ethyl chloride is put up in a special bottle for use in anesthesia. It is stable in the tightly closed container under its high vapor pressure but evaporates almost spontaneously at room temperature and atmospheric pressure (boiling point 12.2° C.). The rapid evaporation lowers the temperature of the solution to near freezing. Many drugs are soluble in ethyl chloride and, because of its special properties, it may

---

* The greater the coefficient for the distribution of drug between aqueous and solvent phase, the greater the number of transfers that can be made without significant loss of sample.

† Solubility of most organics in petroleum ether is significantly less at lower temperatures.

‡ Filtration through paper and solvent extraction of the filter is not advisable because of the comparatively large surface losses incurred.

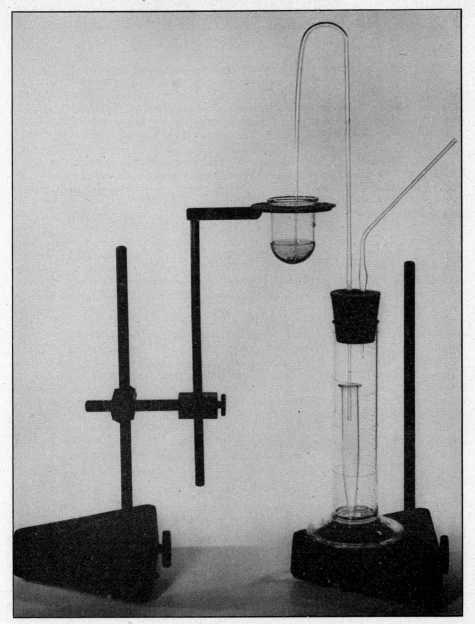

Fig. 47-12. Microsiphon.

be used as a kind of wash solution for purification of crystalline material in the tissue residue.

Procedure. Two to 5 ml. of ethyl chloride are quickly poured over the residue contained in a beaker and the contents mixed by using a rotating motion so that the solvent layer moves over the residue while it is evaporating. If the organic compound is appreciably C_2H_5Cl soluble, relatively pure crystals will be deposited on the sides of the beaker, leaving the bulk of the tissue residue on the bottom.

This solvent is excellent for washing a sublimed deposit on the transparent paper collector of the sublimation apparatus (page 1154). If a few drops are allowed to flow across the deposit on the paper mounted on a cork board, evaporation occurs before the liquid runs off the paper strip. A partial separation, somewhat like the effect obtainable in paper chromatography, is possible with isolatable crystals separated from the bulk of the deposit.

3. Precipitation.

3. Precipitation. (a) *Stannic Chloride-Ethylene Dichloride and Benzene.* In developing the stannic chloride-benzotrichloride color test for drugs (43) it was observed that the stannic chloride precipitates many of them from the ethylene dichloride solution. This suggested the use of stannic chloride as a precipitation reagent for purification from tissue components. The main advantage is that precipitation is from nonaqueous solution and occlusion and adsorption phenomena are minimal.

Procedure (30).* The residue is taken up in a minimal volume of a mixture of 1 part ethylene dichloride and 3 parts benzene.† The solution is transferred to a 10 ml. centrifuge cone and fuming stannic chloride added dropwise as long as precipitation occurs. The precipitate is centrifuged, the solution decanted and the precipitate washed not more than twice with the ethylene dichloride-benzene solution.‡ The precipitate is then dissolved in a small amount of N/10 sodium hydroxide solution, extracted with ether and the ether evaporated to dryness on the steam bath.

Clean precipitates are obtained from muck of residues containing compounds which are precipitated by stannic chloride (Table 47-33). The procedure is not applicable to morphine, heroin and other substances not quantitatively precipitatable by stannic chloride.

(b) *Silicotungstic Acid.* Silicotungstic acid solution is one of the most sensitive precipitants for the bases. The precipitates are granular and generally lack any characteristic crystalline form so that the reagent is not suitable for their identification. Proteins and other high molecular weight compounds are readily precipitated from aqueous solution and these complex silicotungstates are more tightly bound than those of many of the bases. If the water soluble components from an acidified tissue residue are precipitated with silicotungstic acid reagent, the drugs which form weaker complexes can be leached from the precipitate with organic solvents, leaving the tissue components bound by the reagent. Evaporation of the solvent leaves a dry residue in a more purified state. The silicotungstate complexes are insoluble in acid solution but are readily dissolved by dilute alkali from which the base may be recovered by ether or chloroform extraction.

The silicotungstates of the bases are attacked by oxidizing agents and many color tests can be performed directly on the precipitate with greater sensitivity than on the original residue. The binding of the tissue components by the reagent apparently reduces their normal effect of decreasing the sensitivity of the reaction (page 1184).

Reagent. 5 per cent aqueous solution of $SiO_2.12WO_3.26H_2O$

Procedure. The residue is taken up in 1 to 5 ml. of N/10 HCl or N HAc, transferred to a 10 ml. centrifuge cone and the silicotungstic acid reagent added dropwise as long as any precipitation occurs. The tube is allowed to stand until flocculation of the precipitate is complete, then centrifuged and the aqueous solution carefully decanted from the precipitate.§

A few milliliters of a solvent such as methyl alcohol, acetone, ethyl acetate or benzene is then introduced and the precipitate is kept dispersed in the solvent by stirring with a small rod for several minutes. It is then recentrifuged and the solvent decanted and evaporated to dryness on the steam bath. Some solvents are better leaching agents for certain compounds than others. The selection of the solvent is a matter of choice and, if there is only a small residue from one of the solvents in proportion to the bulk of the silicotungstate precipitate, a second leaching with a different solvent is preferable to repeating the process with the original one. Not all of the base will be removed from

---

* Umberger, C. J., and Eagleson, D. A. Unpublished.

† Ethylene dichloride alone is not satisfactory as it does not dissolve the muck. Although the addition of benzene does not completely dissolve the residue, it loosens it and permits a suspension to be obtained. The solution of the unknown is then readily dissolved by the solvent. Precipitation by stannic chloride does not take place in solvents such as alcohol, acetone or ethyl acetate.

‡ If the precipitate is washed further, it may suddenly dissolve in the solvent solution.

§ A small sample of the silicotungstate precipitate should be tested with one of the color reagents for bases (page 1191). A good positive reaction may be obtained on the precipitate and this test is then used to control the purification process.

the precipitate by this procedure.* The primary purpose is to isolate a portion of the compound in a state of purity adequate for a special test or a possible micromelting point. The base remaining in the precipitate after the leaching process is recovered by dissolving the precipitate in about 2 ml. of N/10 NaOH, extracting the alkaline solution with ether or chloroform and evaporating the solvent.

(c) Potassium Bismuthous Iodide (44, 45). Kraut's reagent forms crystalline precipitates with many basic drugs from acid solution. The insoluble complex is decomposed by moderately strong alkali and the base may be recovered by extraction of the alkaline solution with solvents. Some sodium hypoiodite is formed by the action of alkali on the iodide and can react in the alkaline solution with organic compounds having an acetyl group to give iodoform. This side reaction is prevented by the addition of sodium sulfite to the alkaline solution.

Kraut's reagent may be used as a method of purification for bases that form insoluble bismuth iodide complexes (page 1265) when the conditions for the reaction are adjusted to favor a crystalline formation rather than straight precipitation (page 1256). If occlusion and absorption of the tissue components from the acid solution are minimal, the alkaloid can be recovered from the washed crystalline precipitate in a pure state. An objection to the procedure is that, at the concentration of alkali necessary to dissolve the potassium bismuth iodide salt, hydrolysis of some of the unstable drugs may occur.

Reagent (46). 4 gm. of bismuth carbonate are dissolved in 23.5 ml. of nitric acid (sp. gr. 1.18). This solution is added slowly, with constant stirring to a solution containing 13.6 gm. of potassium iodide in 25 ml. H_2O. The orange-red solution is placed in the icebox for 2 hours, after which the potassium nitrate which precipitates is filtered off and the filtrate is diluted to 200 ml. The solution is allowed to stand overnight and the fine black precipitate which settles is removed by centrifugation. The reagent is stable when stored in the dark.

Procedure. The residue is taken up in 0.5 to 5 ml. of 0.5 N H_2SO_4, depending on the quantity of residue. It is added to a 10 ml. centrifuge cone and any insoluble portion is separated by centrifugation. Kraut's reagent is added dropwise, slowly and with constant agitation, and the solution allowed to stand until the crystalline precipitate has settled to the bottom. The tube is centrifuged and the supernatant solution carefully decanted. The precipitate is then washed twice by suspension in 0.5 N sulfuric acid and centrifugation. The precipitate is dissolved in the minimal volume of a 2.5 N sodium hydroxide solution containing 3 gm. anhydrous sodium carbonate and 0.1 gm. sodium sulfite per 10 ml. The alkaline solution is extracted with ether or chloroform and the solvent evaporated to dryness on the steam bath.

(d) Iodine and Potassium Iodide. The precipitates of many of the bases with Wagner's reagent are crystalline and it may be used for precipitation of the tissue residue from the basic extraction in the same manner as Kraut's reagent (page 1265). The tendency for crystallization over precipitation is somewhat less than with Kraut's reagent but the precipitated iodides are dissolved in sodium thiosulfate made only slightly alkaline with sodium hydroxide so that there is little possibility of alkaline hydrolysis of the drug.

Reagent. 5 gm. of iodine are dissolved in 100 ml. of H_2O containing 10 gm. of potassium iodide.

Procedure. The residue is taken up in N/10 hydrochloric acid or normal acetic acid solution and Wagner's reagent added dropwise. The precipitate is separated and washed as described under Kraut's reagent (see above), dissolved in a small volume of N/10 sodium thiosulfate made akaline to phenolphthalein with sodium hydroxide and the base removed by extraction with an organic solvent.

(e) Basic Lead Acetate. Basic lead acetate precipitation is useful for the removal of tissue muck in cases where relatively large amounts are present, as in putrefaction. It is not applicable to bases that are water-soluble in weakly alkaline solution other than some true amphoterics (47) but can be used for water-soluble acidic or neutral compounds where significant amounts of compound have been recovered. The purification

---

* In certain cases, it may be advisable to quantitatively extract the precipitate in a micro Soxhlet extraction apparatus.

depends on precipitation of the soluble tissue components with absorption of the colloidal components of muck from the aqueous solution. There may be appreciable loss of material as a result of occlusion of the water-soluble compounds by the gelatinous precipitate.

Reagent. Lead acetate, 18 gm.; lead monoxide (PbO), 11 gm.; distilled water to make 100 gm.

Dissolve lead acetate in about 80 ml. H_2O with boiling. Add this hot solution to the finely powdered lead oxide and boil for one-half hour with occasional stirring. Cool, filter and add H_2O to make 90 ml.

Procedure. The residue is treated with enough warm water to dissolve or at least to form a colloidal solution with it. The warm solution is transferred to a centrifuge cone and basic lead acetate reagent is added dropwise, with shaking, until no further precipitation occurs. The tube is allowed to stand until aggregation of the flocculant precipitate has occurred, centrifuged and the clear supernatant solution decanted. Excess lead is then precipitated by the addition of dilute sulfuric acid until the solution is acid to Congo red paper. The acid solution containing the insoluble lead sulfate suspension is extracted with ether or chloroform, the separated solvent phase filtered through paper and evaporated to dryness on the steam bath. Insoluble neutrals and bases may be recovered from the basic lead acetate precipitate by suspending it in enough acetic acid to make the mixture distinctly acid and extracting with a solvent.*

(f) Methyl Iodide (48). Methyl iodide is a special reagent which must be used with caution when applied to an unknown sample. When it is applicable, good results are obtained; otherwise sample material may be lost. It is a moderately good solvent for tissue extractables and many drugs are significantly soluble and can be recovered unchanged on evaporation. With tertiary aliphatic amines and nitrogen heterocyclic compounds such as quinoline and piperidine, addition of methyl iodide takes place in a suitable solvent with the formation of quaternary salts (49). The quaternary ammonium type of salts are less solvent-soluble and when addition occurs, precipitation of a solid or oil occurs in the nonaqueous solution. Petroleum ether further reduces the solubility and its addition to the solution induces crystallization of some of the more soluble products of the addition reaction.

Methyl iodide is useful for purification from nonaqueous solution of drugs which form crystalline addition compounds. It is particularly applicable to bases such as diphenhydramine and methadon which are obtained as oils in the extract and are precipitated as crystalline addition compounds with methyl iodide. The formation of a substituted alkyl iodide does not influence the color reactions for a number of the drugs and tests may be made directly on the methyl iodide derivative. Substituted alkyl iodides and their hydroxides are decomposed on heating in an aqueous solution. With some bases, the original compound is recovered while others undergo rearrangement or an alteration in structure is accompanied by liberation of ammonia and an olefin (50). The use of the reagent is therefore limited to heat stable compounds which form crystalline addition products in nonaqueous solution and give the same color tests as the parent substance or which can be recovered unaltered in structure after mild alkaline hydrolysis of the methyl and hydroxyl group from the molecule. Methyl iodide should not be applied to an unknown sample without a preliminary trial on an aliquot to determine whether a reaction occurs and if the chemical properties of the substance will be changed as a result of the addition.

Reagent. Methyl iodide.

Procedure. The basic residue is taken up in 1 to 2 ml. of dry ethyl ether and filtered through an Emich filter stick (51) into a 3 ml. centrifuge cone. Add 0.1 to 0.5 ml. of methyl iodide dropwise with shaking and allow the tube to stand about 30 minutes. If any cloudiness develops the tube is stoppered and placed in the icebox overnight. If a precipitate settles out the tube is centrifuged and the supernatant decanted into a second 3 ml. centrifuge cone. About one-half the volume of petroleum ether is then added to the ether solution with shaking and any precipitate separated from the supernatant by centrifugation.

If there is no evidence of precipitation in the ether-methyl iodide solution after standing 30 minutes, one-half the volume of petroleum ether is added to it and the solution

---

* Some relatively strong water-soluble acids may be precipitated as the insoluble lead salt.

allowed to stand an additional 30 minutes. If a cloudiness then develops, the tube is allowed to stand until flocculation is complete and the precipitate separated from the supernatant as before. The solution is evaporated to dryness on the steam bath and the residue examined for basic substances not precipitatable with methyl iodide. The precipitates are washed twice with petroleum ether, dried and small portions tested with one or more of the color reagents (page 1191).

The precipitate remaining from the chemical examination is heated in a boiling water bath with about 0.5 ml. of a ¼ per cent by volume aqueous solution of methyl alcohol made alkaline to phenolphthalein with potassium hydroxide. The solution is cooled, extracted with ether in a microseparatory funnel and the purified drug recovered on evaporation of the solvent.

4. Chromatography.

4. Chromatography. Chromatographic procedures have been developed almost exclusively for the isolation and separation of small amounts of organic compounds from complex samples (52). Applications to the separation of components in biochemical, pharmaceutic and organic problems are innumerable and it is strange, therefore, that practically no experimental work has been done toward developing chromatographic analysis for the purification of drugs isolated from tissue and contaminated with the normal tissue extractables. The possibilities for applying the various adsorption technics are unlimited, since all of them have been highly developed and used for purification under conditions and with concentrations comparable to those encountered in a residue from a tissue extract. One factor which may have discouraged toxicologic work in this direction is that the principle on which adsorption analysis depends is in opposition to a fundamental rule in microanalysis of working within the smallest possible surface when the sample is an unknown and limited in amount.

Chromatographic analysis depends on adsorption by a solid. Adsorption is a distribution process in which the adsorbed substance is distributed between a fluid and an interfacial phase of extremely large surface area. The purification process, in effect, spreads the sample over a large area from which it must be recovered. Surface area is the bugaboo in microanalysis since sample losses in the course of manipulation and transfer are significant and limiting sensitivity is determined, not by the quantity of material but rather the amount that can be heaped in the smallest possible area (page 1190). The possibility for losses of colorless substances as a result of incomplete zoning or incomplete recovery because of high binding with a reactive adsorbent prevents the indiscriminate use of chromatography for an unknown mixture. In addition, reactive compounds may undergo chemical or physical change when in the adsorbed state. Isomerization occurs when some complex structures such as the vitamins (53, 54) are adsorbed on some highly activated adsorbents. Oxidation (55), hydrolysis (56), aminolysis (57) and decomposition of molecular complexes (58) have been recorded for a variety of structures during the process of adsorption or desorption. Despite the limitations on the general use of chromatography (59) for purification of an unknown residue, the technics have definite application under circumstances in which a preliminary examination has furnished some knowledge concerning the general nature of the isolated product and studies for their application to tissue residues should be pursued.

(a) Column Chromatography (60, 20, 21). Column chromatography appears to be more generally applicable to purification of a tissue residue than the newer chromatographic technics. Larger quantities of sample material can be processed with a good chance for recovery of the sample material when the procedure fails as a purification or separation process. The difficulties involved in carrying out the procedure are mainly mechanical. The adsorbent to be used is packed in a Tswett tube and the sample, dissolved in a nonpolar solvent, allowed to slowly flow down through the packed column by gravity or with the aid of gentle suction or pressure. The adsorbent must be uniformly packed so that the zones will maintain a regular contour as they are developed, while the adsorbent must allow passage of the liquid phase without channelling within the column. Considerable practice is required before uniformity of packing in the column can be attained by mechanically tamping the adsorbent with a dowel. Special methods of filling the columns such as allowing the adsorbent, in the form of a slurry in the solvent, to settle out in the tube (61) or diluting the adsorbent with a filter aid

(62) have been shown to aid in the preparation of an evenly packed column. A wide variety of adsorbents of varying adsorbing ability are available (63, 64) and the choice of adsorbent is usually determined empirically by trial analysis.

Trial adsorption tests are impractical as well as dangerous when applied to tissue residues containing unknown compounds. As a general purification procedure, the medical examiner's laboratory has restricted chromatographic analysis to the use of the less reactive adsorbents such as talc, $CaCO_3$ moderately packed to a depth of about 6 inches in a 1-inch diameter tube and treated with relatively dilute solutions of sample in a nonpolar solvent. The application is not strictly chromatography as the column is not developed to produce the conventional zones. The adsorption is evaluated from an examination of the solution leaving the column as in the Tiselius principle for liquid chromatography (65). The process is part filtration and part adsorption. The tissue extractables that are only partially soluble in the nonpolar solvent and are dispersed in colloidal suspension are removed at the upper end of the column by a filtration process probably analogous to the action of a Berkfeld-type filter. Varying amounts of the tissue extractables are adsorbed as the solution passes through the column, while the organic unknown compound may be completely or partially adsorbed or entirely unadsorbed. An indicating type of test, preferably a color reaction, which was selected from a preliminary examination of the residue (page 1147) is used to locate the unknown. The solvent is first evaporated and the intensity of the reaction on the residue is compared with that on the original. If all or a major portion remained in the column, it is developed with more solvent in the conventional manner except that the additions are stepwise with evaporation of each portion and examination of any residue. The column is then carefully pushed from the tube, air dried and cut into $\frac{1}{2}$ to 1-inch sections. Each section is eluted separately with methyl or ethyl alcohol, the eluent evaporated and the residues examined. Those showing the same general characteristics are combined. If no efficient purification was attained, the entire adsorbent is extracted in a Soxhlet extractor and the separate residues recombined.

Morphine has been separated from codeine and heroin by adsorption from an aqueous solution containing 5 per cent trichloracetic acid to which 25 ml. of 95 per cent ethyl alcohol per 100 ml. of acid solution was added and the pH adjusted to 6-8. Adsorption was on a Florisil * column previously treated with methyl alcohol (66). The methyl alcohol treatment prevented the adsorption of the morphine while the codeine and heroin were completely removed. Morphine was then isolated by adsorption from the same type of solution through Florisil and purified by successive treatment with formic acid, ethyl alcohol and ethyl acetate. Barbiturates, which are not adsorbed by the Florisil from the aqueous solution, were purified by adsorption on coconut shell charcoal from the same solution adjusted to a pH of 5.5 (67).

(b) Paper Chromatography. Paper chromatography is rapidly becoming a standard procedure for the separation of the organic components of a mixture. It can only be used for relatively small amounts of mixture and would appear to be ideal for tissue residues, since the yield of isolated drug is, at most, of milligram quantities. However, the amount of muck in which the drug is dispersed may be considerable and the total sample weight in the tissue extracts will then be too great for the use of paper chromatography as a purification procedure. Basic extracts from the five component separation (page 1140) are more suitable with regard to ratio of drug to tissue extractables. The disadvantages for unknown mixtures lie in the necessity for selecting the solvent systems empirically and the requirement of 18 to 36 hours for completion of the partition. On the other hand, recovery of the original sample is easier from a paper chromatogram than from a column and the chances for surfaces losses and changes in the structure of the compounds are lessened. Although the technic appears to be better suited for separations of purified drug mixtures in the course of the identification process, the possibilities for application as a purification process for tissue extracts are unlimited. Unfortunately, very little experimental work has been done in this direction. Measurement of the R_f values has been used as a means of identifying the different barbiturates (68) and some drugs have been separated on paper strips and identified by spraying the developed chromatogram with color reagents (69-72). The technic of locating the or-

---

* Floridin Co., Inc., Pennsylvania.

ganic compound on the paper by spraying it with a reagent and identifying the compound from its position and color reaction on the paper has been highly developed in related fields and should find more extensive use in the toxicologic analysis of organic drugs (73).

(c) Ionophoresis (Paper Electrophoresis). Electrophoresis on paper is a special application of paper chromatography in which migration on the paper is augmented by a potential applied across the paper strip. The assembly is, in principle, that for the classic measurement of ionic velocities in which the paper containing the sample serves as the bridge between the two half cells. Buffer solution placed in the cells keeps the paper wet by capillarity and serves as the conductor for the current. The 110 to 4,000 volts D.C. which are applied across the electrodes increase the mobility of the polar components in the sample so that the rate of the adsorption distribution is decreased.

Pioneer work in the development of ionophoresis for the separation of amino acids and proteins has been done by Durrum (22, 74-76). He has applied the procedure to the unidimensional, two dimensional and continuous technics of paper chromatography and contributed numerous studies concerning the factors affecting the complex equilibria. Lederer (77) suggests that, for every paper chromatographic separation of ions, an equally sufficient ionophoretic procedure is possible. Although other investigators have applied the method to various inorganic and biologic problems (23, 78-81), Goldbaum, in a study of the purification of morphine and related alkaloids (82), is apparently the only investigator to apply paper electrophoresis to toxicologic analysis.

(d) Ion Exchange. Ion exchange polymers are water-insoluble macromolecular substances which bind ions by an adsorption process which is reversible; the bound ions are readily replaced by others from solution in contact with the exchangers. They may be classified as inorganic and organic exchangers and each group subdivided into anion and cation exchangers. Some are capable of either anion or cation exchange depending on the pH of the solution and the pretreatment of the polymetric substance.

Considerable work has been done in the organic and biologic fields in the use of organic exchange resins for the separation of organic mixtures (83-85). Aside from the study by Feldstein and Klendshoj (86) on the determination of morphine by ion exchange, the procedure apparently has not been used in toxicologic analysis.

Applications in related fields suggest possibilities for the use of ion exchange in the purification of tissue residues in a manner closely related to the basic principle on which the division of drugs in this system depends. Cannan (87), Tiselius and others (88) and Winters and Kunin (89) have devised procedures for the separation of the amino acids into the three basic charge groups—acidic, neutral and basic. Separations based on differences in acidity and basicity have been achieved by choosing the appropriate exchanger that has either the acidity or basicity that is sufficiently strong to neutralize but one ionic species of a mixture. In a mixture of weak and stronger acids, removal of the stronger acids was made by selection of a weakly basic anion exchange resin that was not sufficiently basic to neutralize the weak acids (90). In a similar manner, the separation of weakly basic alkaloids from the more basic ones has been made by utilizing the appropriate cation exchange (89).

Behavior other than ion exchange is shown by exchange polymers because of their large surface area, porosity and chemical nature. Nonexchange adsorption, occlusion, dissolution and chemical reaction can occur, so that ion exchange resins cannot hope to be used indiscriminately on an unknown sample. Nevertheless, the ion exchange phenomenon appears to offer greater possibilities for special purification of tissue residues than the other types of adsorption analysis.

IDENTIFICATION OF SEDATIVES

Before proceeding to apply the general testing procedure for unknown compounds, examination for the common substances whose presence was indicated in the probing tests (page 1147) should be completed. The possible presence of malonylurea derivatives will be apparent from the positive findings in the Koppanyi reaction. In most deaths from sedatives, there will be some history or clinical findings which point to them. In cases of death involving known epileptics and also in deaths following coma, sedatives should be ruled out before proceeding with the more detailed examination. The sedatives which are hydantoins or substituted ureas may not be detected in the probing procedure but are included here with the barbiturates since they are common, frequently combined with barbiturates and may be detected by more specific tests than those used in the general procedure.

A. Barbiturates.

A. Barbiturates. Malonylurea and all its derivatives are intermediate acids and, in the three-component separation (page 1139), they are obtained predominantly in the phenol fraction. The overlapping that does occur is with the less acidic derivatives and small amounts of these may, therefore, appear in the neutral fraction. Barbiturates do not appear in the acid fraction of this extraction procedure and positive findings with the Koppanyi reaction on this fraction are not due to malonylurea derivatives.* When a positive Koppanyi reaction in chloroform or with the more selective paper technic (page 1149) is obtained on the phenol fraction, a number of possible interferences with the reaction are ruled out. Nevertheless, even the test on the phenol fraction can only serve as an indication for barbiturates, since any compound containing the structure

$$-C-NH-C- \quad \overset{O}{\underset{||}{}}$$

as well as other types which are intermediate acids in nonaqueous solution, is potentially reactive until proven otherwise by experimentation.

Both infrared and ultraviolet absorption may be used as confirmatory procedures for barbiturates. Infrared spectrophotometry is more specific but is less sensitive, requiring a much larger quantity of sample material. The decreased sensitivity is an advantage in those cases in which there is sufficient source material to permit isolation of milligram quantities of the unknown. The normal tissue extractables, particularly those from brain, do not show significant infrared absorption and, consequently, unknown residues do not require the degree of purification necessary for ultraviolet measurements. All barbiturates show a characteristic infrared absorption with a similar pattern in the regions between 2.83 and 3.5, 5.65 and 6.7, 6.75 and 7.9 microns (91).

Barbiturates are extremely sensitive to ultraviolet absorption. Significant optical density readings are obtained in alkaline solution with as little as 2 μg. of sample per ml. of solvent. The high sensitivity makes ultraviolet measurements preferable for the quantitative analysis (92, 93, 94). Since tissue impurities have a fairly intense absorption, the isolated material must be relatively pure. Tissue impurities give a "washed out" type of absorption curve and, if not too extensive, may be corrected for by treating a normal sample in the same manner as the unknown and plotting a curve obtained by subtracting the optical densities of the normal tissue from those of the unknown (93). With the exception of the N-methyl and thio-derivatives which give different absorption spectra, the barbiturates, when dissolved in .45 to .5 N sodium hydroxide, show a maximum in the optical density curve at 255 mμ and a minimum at about 235 mμ. In buffered solutions at pH 9.8 to 10.5 a higher maximum occurs at 240 mμ with no minimum. Normal tissue interference can be minimized by the device of plotting a "difference curve" obtained by subtracting the optical density values for the compound in the buffered solution from corresponding readings in the stronger alkaline solution (91). Unless an exceptionally reactive tissue degradation product from putrefaction or drastic chemical treatment of the sample during the isolation procedure is present which also changes in absorption with a change in pH, the usual washed out type of curve for a normal tissue residue is cancelled. The optical density values for the difference curve are greatest at 260 mμ, decreasing through zero at about 250 mμ (the isobestic point for the two curves) to a maximum negative at around 240 or 235 mμ and increasing through zero at the lower wave isobestic point about 227 mμ to positive differences in the lower wave length region.

The N-methyl derivatives (hexobarbital and mephobarbital) show only a washed out, noncharacteristic absorption curve in both buffer at pH 10.5 and in 0.45 N sodium hydroxide. Thiopental, when dissolved in 0.1 N sodium hydroxide, has a maximum at

---

* See last footnote, page 1139.

305 mμ in the absorption curve. In 0.1 N hydrochloric acid, there are two maxima, the smaller one at approximately 240 mμ and the higher maximum at approximately 290 mμ (95).

A positive Koppanyi reaction on the phenol fraction of a tissue extract with characteristic infrared or ultraviolet absorption behavior is adequate proof for the presence of barbituric acid derivatives but, except in those exceptional cases in which the quantitative analysis shows values that are equal to or above the lethal dose of the least active of the barbiturates, the findings are inconclusive for determining the cause of death. The physiologic activity of the 20 odd malonylurea derivatives available for medical use varies over a wide range. Thiopental, used in anesthesia, and the beta-bromallyl members, used in obstetrics, are the most active while barbital has the least physiologic activity. There are five malonylurea derivatives known as the common barbiturates because they are used far more often than the others. These barbiturates, listed in order of decreasing activity are secobarbital > pentobarbital > amobarbital > phenobarbital > barbital. Many outpatients under treatment are prescribed a daily maintenance dose of some barbiturate while other persons, not under the care of a physician, indiscriminately take without thought of harmful effects any barbiturate they are able to obtain. The physiologic activity varies over such a wide range that a level which constitutes a lethal dose for one derivative may be only a medicinal level for another. Goldbaum of the U. S. Army Medical Service Graduate School has made the most extensive study of the content of the various barbiturates in tissue and body fluids. His files, which contain the analyses for barbiturates on over 100 cases from Walter Reed Hospital, include patients on daily maintenance levels, comatose patients and fatal barbiturate deaths. The quantitative values for these cases were obtained by the ultraviolet spectrophotometric method (92). Table 47-11 shows the lowest blood levels (in round figures) found for the different barbiturates from determinations on adult comatose patients.

Table 47-11.

Barbiturate	Blood Level per 100 ml. Blood	Barbiturate	Blood Level per 100 ml. Blood
Barbital	10 mg.	Pentobarbital	2.5 mg.
Phenobarbital	8 mg.	Secobarbital	2 mg.
Amobarbital	4 mg.	Thiopental	1.5 mg.

In this group, barbital and phenobarbital are the longer acting compounds while the others are shorter acting, with increased activity in descending order. The usual blood level found for barbital in comatose patients was closer to 15 mg. per 100 ml. of blood while phenobarbital was around 9 mg. per cent. Patients on phenobarbital with blood levels up to 6 mg. per cent were never comatose and on a daily maintenance dose of 8 grains, levels were consistently around 4.5 mg. per cent. In a number of deaths from phenobarbital, the brain level was not less than 10 mg. per 100 gm. and in deaths from pentobarbital the brain content did not exceed 4 mg. per 100 gm. of tissue.

Animal studies on the different barbiturates (96) showed that there is considerable difference between the blood content and that of the organs for the longer acting and the quick acting barbiturates. With a blood level of about 10 mg. per cent for barbital and 8 mg. per cent for phenobarbital, the brain will contain slightly greater than 12 and 10 mg. per cent respectively for the two barbiturates. The greatest concentration is in the liver which may contain as much as 1.5 times the amount in the blood, although, in general, liver and brain values are closer with the longer acting barbiturates. About 90 per cent of the ingested barbital appears unchanged in the urine while urinary recovery for phenobarbital is about 50 per cent. With the shorter acting barbiturates, the brain level is 1.5 to 2 times that of blood while the liver contains 2 to 3 times as much as the blood. They are stored in the fat which usually contains at least 3 times the blood concentrations of the intermediate members such as pentobarbital. The fat content of thiopental may be as much as 9 times the blood level (95, 97). Barbiturate levels on human patients closely parallel animal values (98). Therefore, if the patient on a maintenance dose of 8 grains of phenobarbital daily, with a blood level of 4.5 mg. per 100 ml., died from natural or accidental causes, analysis of the brain would reveal at least 5.5 mg. per cent of barbiturate. This is well above the brain value found for pentobarbital and secobarbital in deaths from acute barbiturate poisoning. Therefore, to establish barbiturate poisoning, the individual malonylurea derivative must be identified and an evaluation made on the basis of the quantitative analysis of a specific sample. Unless the identification is included, the toxicologic report which merely states "barbituric acid derivative present in large amounts" is little more than meaningless.*

Identification of the Different Barbiturates. The different barbiturates may be identified from the minor differences in the infrared absorption bands within the characteristic absorbing regions (page 1166) of the malonylurea molecule, together with the melting point. However, better purity is required to make the distinctions than is neces-

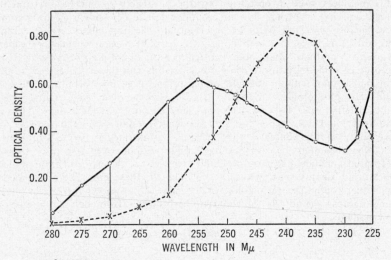

o. In 0.45 N NaOH.
x. In borate buffer, pH 10.5
    Vertical solid lines indicate differences between optical densities in pH 10.5 and in 0.45 N NaOH.

Wavelength, mμ	270	260	252	249	247	240	235	232	228
Differences	+0.22	+0.43	+0.24	+0.05	−0.09	−0.43	−0.46	−0.38	−0.14

From Goldbaum, *Anal. Chem.*, 24:1605, 1952

Fig. 47-13. Ultraviolet Absorption Spectra of Amobarbital.

sary to merely establish the malonylurea structure. The hydantoins and substituted urea sedatives also may be identified from their characteristic spectra which are quite different from those of the barbiturates. Mixtures of barbiturates and substituted ureas are fairly common and are more readily detected by infrared absorption than by any other procedure (91).

The ultraviolet difference curve (see above) may be used to identify a number of the barbiturates. Absorption curves for amobarbital in buffer at pH 10.5 and in .45 N alkali are shown in Figure 47-13. The magnitude of the vertical lines drawn at the different wave lengths represents the difference between the optical densities at each point and these values, plotted with their proper sign against the wave length, give the difference curve. With different barbiturates, significant variations in the relative optical density differences occur at the various wave lengths and these are made more apparent when the differences at a number of wave lengths are compared with the value at 260 mμ. Table 47-12 shows the difference ratios for several representative barbiturates obtained by dividing the optical density difference at the indicated wave length by the value at 260 mμ.

The magnitude of the ratios at a given wave length are independent of the concentration within a limited range and are not influenced by minor concentrations of

* A recent tendency in the pharmaceutic field is toward more complex mixtures of different barbiturates. This really creates a major problem for the analyst because involved methods for separating closely related compounds must be developed.

Table 47-12. Differentiation of Several Representative Barbiturates by Their Difference Ratios (92)

	\multicolumn{9}{c|}{Optical density difference at given wave length}								
	\multicolumn{9}{c|}{Optical density difference at 260 mμ}								
Wave Lengths, mμ	270	260	252	249	247	240	235	232	228
			RATIOS						
Amobarbital	+0.52	1.00	+0.56	+0.12	−0.21	−1.00	−1.09	−0.88	−0.33
Pentobarbital	+0.61	1.00	+0.40	−0.05	−0.38	−1.02	−1.00	−0.80	−0.15
Secobarbital	+0.69	1.00	+0.30	−0.13	−0.39	−1.04	−0.89	−0.63	+0.21
Butallylonal	+0.81	1.00	+0.07	−0.35	−0.63	−1.03	−0.72	+0.20	+0.96
Phenobarbital	+0.59	1.00	+0.36	−0.09	−0.36	−0.96	−0.84	−0.48	+0.43
Cyclopal	+0.80	1.00	+0.11	−0.34	−0.63	−1.10	−0.94	−0.50	+0.71

After Goldbaum, *Anal. Chem.*, 24:1605. 1952.

tissue impurities. The order in which the ratios change with wave length is indicative of the structure. Probarbital, the ethylisopropyl derivative, shows ratios very similar to those of pentobarbital which is an ethylmethylbutyl derivative. However, the former melts at 200 to 203° C. while the latter melts at 127 to 130° C. Barbital, with a melting point of 188 to 191° C., shows a pattern similar to amobarbital with a melting point at 152 to 155° C. Aprobarbital, with a melting point of 140 to 142° C., is very close to secobarbital which does not crystallize for a long time when extracted from tissue.

Although physical methods are safer, furnish a more convincing record and the sample can be recovered, identification of the individual barbiturates usually can be made quickly on a few crystals by means of chemical tests. The best approach for the detection of the barbiturates is through a chemical examination with physical measurements used for confirmation, because mixtures or residues contaminated with excess tissue impurities or detoxification products will not be apparent until the physical testing has failed.

Chemical Testing of the Different Barbiturates (99).* Barbiturates, hydantoins and substituted urea sedatives are best purified by sublimation at reduced pressure as described on pages 1153 to 1158. A few of them form characteristic and distinctive crystalline patterns on the paper collector which point toward their identity. There is a similarity in the crystalline pattern of certain of the other sedatives which permits them to be grouped together on the basis of their sublimation behavior. The paper collector containing the sublimate is mounted on a cork board and is examined by means of the vertical illuminating microscope shown in Figure 47-14. Figures 47-15 through 19 show photomicrographs of the barbiturates which have distinctive crystalline deposits.

Secobarbital gives a noncrystalline, sticky semisolid from which random needle growth develops on long standing. Barbital, probarbital and diphenylhydantoin deposit as long, thin needles which aggregate to form asterisk and starlike forms. Ortal, pentobarbital, neonal®, cyclopal®, butabarbital and sigmodal® deposit as long blades or rectangular rods with a tendency for the aggregate to radiate from a focal point. Butallylonal, sandoptal®, aprobarbital, amobarbital, phenobarbital and nostal® are short, thick prismatic or plate types which aggregate to produce crystalline deposits with random forms. Angles between the faces are usually measurable and end forms are often characteristic.

Several typical crystals should be removed from the collector, mounted on a microscope slide and examined with the polarizing microscope shown in Figure 47-20 under crossed Nicols. Extinction angles should be recorded and face angles should be measured when the crystalline form is well defined.

The identification process depends on the separation of the different barbiturates into groups on the basis of the order of magnitude of the micro melting point of the sublimate. In Table 47-13 the barbiturates are listed in order of their increasing melting points. The micro melting point as determined on the Kofler micro hot stage (Fig. 47-21) requires only a few crystals and differs from the capillary procedure in that impurities do not have as great an influence on the melting temperature. Mixed melting points can be measured only on mixtures that have been fused previously. The

* Umberger, C. J., and Feldstein, M. Unpublished.

melting temperature is not as sharp as in the capillary tube and usually cannot be considered significant to better than ± 4° C. Consequently, a micro melting point alone on even a pure barbiturate is not sufficiently accurate for differentiating between the compounds.

Many crystalline organic compounds undergo one or more transitions as the temperature rises toward the melting point. The changes in crystalline form are characteristic for many substances, and compounds showing similar behavior can often be

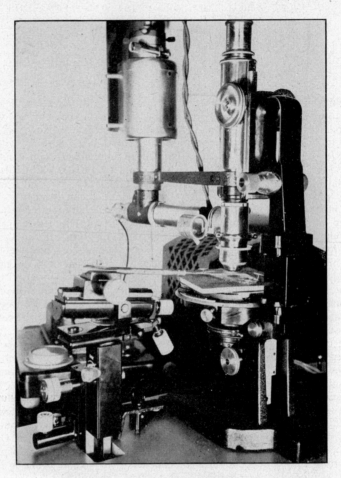

Fig. 47-14. Vertical Illuminating Microscope.

differentiated by measurements of the transition forms under the polarizing microscope. In addition, many compounds sublime at atmospheric pressure before melting, with the formation of characteristic crystals. The outstanding feature of the hot stage technic is that the behavior of the crystals may be observed while the temperature approaches the melting point and any transition or sublimation forms can be removed for microscopic study. In carrying out the procedure, three slides are prepared by placing several crystals on a microscope slide and covering with a cover slip. One preparation is centered on the hot stage with the diaphragm partially closed in order to give a shadow at the outer edge of the field. The other two preparations are placed on either side of the first slide on the stage. As the stage heats up, the temperature at which any changes occur, such as sweating or the beginning of a new crystalline form, is recorded. If a transition occurs with the formation of a new or distinct crystalline form, one of the two slides on the side is removed for optical measurements. If a second form appears, the other preparation on the side is removed. The temperature at which melting starts,

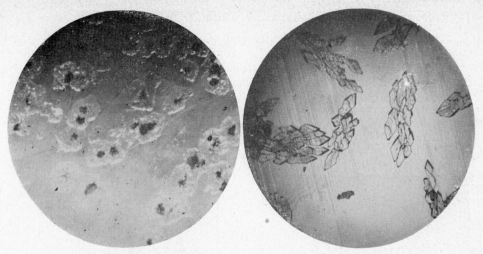

Fig. 47-15. Thiopental Sublimate on Paper.   Fig. 47-16. Diallylbarbituric Acid Sublimate on Paper.

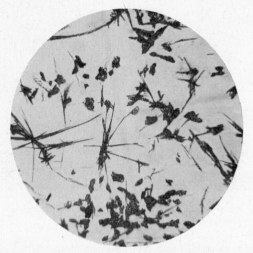

Fig. 47-17. Phanadorn Sublimate on Paper.

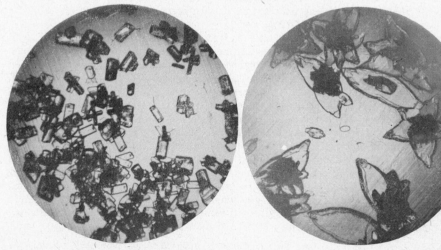

Fig. 47-18. Hexobarbital Sublimate on Paper.   Fig. 47-19. Vinbarbital Sublimate on Paper.

the temperature range over which melting is rapid and the temperature at which the last bit of solid liquefies are recorded.

The relative purity can be estimated from the melting range. Pure compounds do not have more than a 4° temperature differential between the temperature at which melting is rapid and the point of final melting except for a few compounds in which characteristic transition forms remain in the melt over a wide temperature range. The temperature at which the solid phase has just disappeared * is closest to and slightly higher than the capillary value. After completing the melting point study and removing

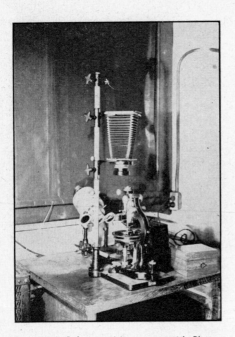

Fig. 47-20. Polarizing Microscope with Photo-micrographic Camera.

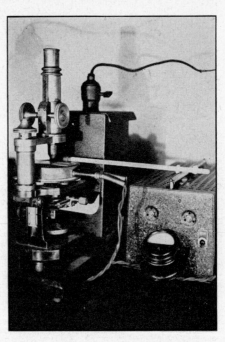

Fig. 47-21. Kofler Micro Hot Stage.

the cover slips to which some of the crystals adhere, six preparations are made available for chemical testing. Figure 47-22 shows the first transition which occurs at around 165° C. with barbital. Characteristic rectangular plates with an acute angle of approximately 60° develop and, as the temperature rises, a second transition occurs with the formation of long prismatic rods (Fig. 47-23).

The melting points of the different barbiturates in Table 47-13, starting with ortal®, increase slowly through butallylonal, then show a significant difference between butallylonal and sandoptal®. From sandoptal® up to amobarbital, the increase between the different sedatives is again small, passing gradually from amobarbital through thiopental to vinbarbital. However, if thiopental, which is a sulfur derivative and easily identified, is ignored, the spread between amobarbital and vinbarbital becomes significant. From vinbarbital on, the increase is gradual. Nostal, a beta-bromallyl derivative, separates mephobarbital from barbital and if it, like thiopental, is ignored, a significant difference in melting points appears between mephobarbital and barbital. Secobarbital is distinct from all the others because it is recovered as a gummy residue which does not crystallize on standing for less than one to two weeks.

If the barbiturates are classified into separate groups, based on the gaps which appear in the melting point table, five groupings result, with one of the five common barbiturates present in each group. Group I contains only secobarbital. The melting point range for Group II, allowing a ± 4° variation for the hot stage method, varies

---

* When viewed by polarized light, this temperature is readily detected. With crossed Nicols, the melting temperature is indicated when the field becomes dark.

between 118° and 137° C. and is designated as the pentobarbital group. Group III, with a melting range of 134° to 159° C., becomes the amobarbital group. The line separating Groups III and IV is drawn after amobarbital because thiopental, separating amobarbital and vinbarbital, is detectable by sensitive tests for the thio group. Group IV, the phenobarbital group which melts between 155° and 181° C., is separated by nostal®, which may be detected readily by determining the presence of the halogen. Nostal is then included in the barbital group which melts above 173° C.

The melting point of any organic compound is always lowered by impurities. Consequently, when the melting point is determined on the sublimate of the unknown compound isolated in the phenol fraction, the unknown, if it is a barbiturate, must be one that lies above the observed melting point in Table 47-13. The melting point in this sense is used as a *designating* reaction rather than a physical property, as it designates the probable group in which the unknown is found. The common barbiturates are the most

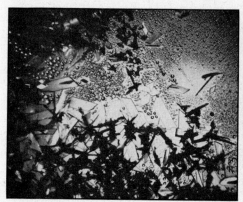 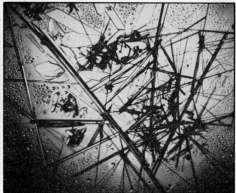

Fig. 47-22. First Transition Phase in Melting of Barbital.   Fig. 47-23. Second Transition Phase in Melting of Barbital.

likely and it is more logical to exclude them before looking for the derivatives used less frequently. The description of the testing procedure, however, is much less complicated if all the possibilities are discussed as a whole. Although secobarbital in Group I is characterized by its noncrystalline, gummy consistency, other barbiturates, particularly when in mixtures with other medicinals, leave a similar extraction residue. On standing for one to two days, crystals develop in the sticky deposit and, when sublimed, the sublimate is always crystalline. Secobarbital does not crystallize in less than one week and the sublimate retains the same gummy consistency. The only difficulty encountered is a mixture of secobarbital with other barbiturates, as in the secobarbital-amobarbital preparation of tuinal®. There is a separation of the sublimate on the paper collector, with deposits of secobarbital but the crystalline member, contaminated with secobarbital, is difficult to identify. Secobarbital gives an oil with the precipitating tests used for the other barbiturates. Crystallization of the oil does not occur except with magnesia mixture in which needles start to radiate from the oil droplets after standing overnight.

In the four remaining groups, certain members can be excluded by the application of *differential* reactions. The physiologically active beta-bromallyl derivatives butallylonal, sigmodal® and nostal® occur in Groups II, IV and V. These are distinguished by means of the Beilstein test for halogens (168, 5, 6). Thiopental in Group IV gives the iodine-sodium azide test for thio compounds when a drop of the reagent (page 1249) is added to a crystal of the sublimate. It also reacts with aquo-ferriate reagent (Table 47-29, page 1223).

In Groups II, III and IV, there are five reactive derivatives which give red colors with vanillin-sulfuric acid reagent (Table 47-36, page 1239).

A drop of reagent is added to a crystal on a microscope slide and observed in the cold for about one minute. The slide is then warmed at 125° C. for 30 seconds by placing the slide on a hot stage maintained at 125° C. Diallylbarbituric acid, vinbarbital, hexobarbital, cyclopal® and phanadorn® all develop a deep red color within this time.

Table 47-13. Malonylurea Sedatives

$$\text{Barbituric Acid Nucleus} = B = CO \begin{array}{c} NH-CO \\ NH-CO \end{array} C \begin{array}{c} R_1 \\ R_2 \end{array} \rightleftarrows HO-C \begin{array}{c} N=C=O \\ N-C=O \\ H \end{array} C \begin{array}{c} R_1 \\ R_2 \end{array}$$

Group	Barbiturate	Chemical Name	Formula	Melting Point
I	Secobarbital	5-Allyl-5-(1-methyl-butyl)barbituric acid	$B \begin{cases} CH_2-CH:CH_2 \\ CH-CH_2-CH_2-CH_3 \\ \quad\vert \\ CH_3 \end{cases}$	96-100° C. Crystals form only on long standing
II	Ortal	5-n-Hexyl-5-ethyl-barbituric acid	$B \begin{cases} C_2H_5 \\ CH(CH_2)_4CH_3 \end{cases}$	122-125° C.
	Neonal	5-n-Butyl-5-ethyl-barbituric acid	$B \begin{cases} C_2H_5 \\ CH(CH_2)_2CH_3 \end{cases}$	127-130° C.
	Pentobarbital	Ethyl (1-methylbutyl) barbituric acid	$B \begin{cases} C_2H_5 \\ CH(CH_2)_2CH_3 \\ \quad\vert \\ CH_3 \end{cases}$	127-130° C.
	Butallylonal	5-sec-Butyl-betabro-mallylbarbituric acid	$B \begin{cases} \quad\quad Br \\ \quad\quad\vert \\ CH_2-C:CH_2 \\ CH-CH_2-CH_3 \\ \vert \\ CH_3 \end{cases}$	130-133° C.
III	Sandoptal	Isobutylallyl-barbituric acid	$B \begin{cases} CH_2-CH \begin{array}{c} CH_3 \\ CH_3 \end{array} \\ CH_2-CH:CH_2 \end{cases}$	138-139° C.
	Aprobarbital	5-Allyl-5-isopropyl-barbituric acid	$B \begin{cases} CH_3 \\ CH-CH_3 \\ CH_2-C:CH_2 \end{cases}$	140-142° C.
	Cyclopal	Cyclopentenylallyl-barbituric acid	$B \begin{cases} CH_2-CH:CH_2 \\ C \begin{array}{c} CH-CH_2 \\ \vert \\ CH_2-CH_2 \end{array} \end{cases}$	140-143° C.
	Hexobarbital	N-Methylcyclo-hexenylmethyl barbituric acid	$B-C \begin{array}{c} CH_3 \\ CH-CH_2 \\ C \begin{array}{c} CH_2 \\ CH_2-CH_2 \end{array} \\ CH_3 \end{array}$	143-145° C.
	Amobarbital	Isoamylethyl-barbituric acid	$B \begin{cases} CH_2-CH_2-CH \begin{array}{c} CH_3 \\ CH_3 \end{array} \\ C_2H_5 \end{cases}$	152-155° C.
IV	Thiopental	5-Ethyl-5-(1-methyl-butyl) thiobarbi-turic acid	$\begin{array}{c} O \\ \parallel \\ C_2H_5 \\ \quad\quad C \\ CH_3(CH_2)_2-CH \\ \quad\quad\vert \\ CH_3 \end{array} \begin{array}{c} C-NH \\ C=S \\ C-NH \\ \parallel \\ O \end{array}$	159-160° C.
	Vinbarbital	5-Ethyl-5-(1-methyl-1-butenyl) barbi-turic acid	$B \begin{cases} C_2H_5 \\ C=CH-CH_2-CH_3 \end{cases}$	162-163° C.

Table 47-13 (cont.). Malonylurea Sedatives

GROUP	BARBITURATE	CHEMICAL NAME	FORMULA	MELTING POINT
	Butabarbital	5-Ethyl-5-*sec*-butyl-barbituric acid	C_2H_5 / $CH-CH_2-CH_3$ / CH_3 (B)	168-170° C.
	Sigmodal	*Sec*-Amyl-betabromallyl barbituric acid	$(CH_2)_4CH_3$ / $CH_2-C=CH_2$ / Br (B)	169-171° C.
	Diallylbarbituric acid	Diallylbarbituric acid	$CH_2-CH=CH_2$ / $CH_2-CH=CH_2$ (B)	171-173° C.
	Phanadorn	Cyclohexenylethyl-barbituric acid	C_2H_5 / C=$CH-CH_2$ CH_2 / CH_2-CH_2 (B)	171-174° C.
	Phenobarbital	Phenylethyl-barbituric acid	C_2H_5 / C_6H_5 (B)	173-174° C.
	Mephobarbital	N-Methylethylphenyl barbituric acid	CH_3 / C_2H_5 / C_6H_5 (B)	175-177° C.
V	Nostal	5-Isopropyl-5-beta-bromallyl barbituric acid	$CH_2-CBr=CH_2$ / CH CH_3 CH_3 (B)	177-179° C.
	Barbital	Diethylbarbituric acid	C_2H_5 / C_2H_5 (B)	188-191° C.
	Probarbital	5-Ethyl-5-isopropyl-barbituric acid	C_2H_5 / CH CH_3 CH_3 (B)	200-203° C.
	Rutonal	Methylphenyl-barbituric acid	CH_3 / C_6H_5 (B)	220-223° C.

The reactivity increases in the order listed. Cyclopal and phanadorn® react in the cold, hexobarbital and vinbarbital react with slight warming and diallylbarbituric acid reacts well below the temperature at which sulfuric acid fumes. On cooling and adding a drop of water, the red color changes to magenta which fades, leaving a greenish precipitate with all but diallylbarbituric acid. Secobarbital, ortal®, pentobarbital, aprobarbital and sigmodal® give a less intense pink to reddish coloration when heated long enough to produce SO_3 fumes and amobarbital, phenobarbital, barbital and butallylonal develop a brownish cast. Since the test is based on the degree of reactivity rather than actual color development, the safest procedure is to run diallylbarbituric acid simultaneously with the unknown as a control. Hexobarbital, cyclopal® and phanadorn® give dark red colors with para-dimethylaminobenzaldehyde-sulfuric acid reagent and orange colors with Mecke's reagent in the cold. Cyclopal and phanadorn® give brown to orange colorations, respectively, with cold concentrated sulfuric acid. Variable color changes occur if the other barbiturates are heated with the color-producing reagents. Mephobarbital is a special case as it produces an emerald green color changing to blue with Mandelin's reagent in the cold while remaining relatively nonreactive with the other color reagents.

Differentiation between the remaining barbiturates is made from the crystalline habit of the compound. Barbiturates obtain their acid properties from the imino nitrogen groups but in alkaline solution they exist as the enol form (see top of Table 47-13) forming salts with metal ions. There are, then, two main crystalline forms possible, depending on whether the crystal is from acid or basic solution. The most characteristic and easily obtained crystals are those formed by acidifying an aqueous solution of the salt.

Procedure. A few crystals of the sublimate on a microscope slide are dissolved by the addition of a small drop of 6 N ammonium hydroxide. A drop of 6 N sulfuric acid is then added. An immediate white cloud should form on neutralization with the acid, indicating that the solution is saturated. If a cloud does not appear, the test should be repeated with a larger quantity of material or a smaller drop of the reagent.

The precipitate with pentobarbital, when viewed under the low-power objective of the microscope, shows an almost solid field consisting of small crystalline forms resembling bundles of wheat tied in the middle (Fig. 47-24). The central portion may be elongated and even consist of a single rod but the ends are always branched. Neonal acts in a similar manner but the branched end forms are much larger and are less symmetrical. Acid amobarbital gives a variety of forms but the only characteristic one is a square plate with a clear-cut notch in one corner. However, these do not always appear even when the test is repeated on the same preparation. Acid phenobarbital is as characteristic as pentobarbital. It first precipitates as an oil which slowly develops into little burrlike growths, followed by an aggregation into the needle masses shown in Figure 47-25. Sandoptal forms square plates somewhat similar to those of amobarbital. Under crossed Nicols the appearance is that of the typical biaxial interference figure but it does not become hyperbolic toward the position of brightness (Fig. 47-26). Butabarbital forms feather-like blades and some random hexagonal prisms with chisel-pointed ends as seen in Figure 47-27. Extinction is slightly oblique. Vinbarbital crystallizes slowly into rosette forms which give the appearance of crystals under polarized light without interference colors (Fig. 47-28).

The second main crystalline form is obtained by allowing the crystals to grow after dissolving some of the sublimate in a drop of 6 N ammonium hydroxide. Precipitation is slower and larger crystal types develop. The drop is viewed under low power at its edge where crystallization starts. The types which develop early are most characteristic. If allowed to stand until crystallization is complete, the aggregate clumps are usually so thick and overlaid that typical forms are masked. With amobarbital, a brushlike needle growth with parallel extinction starts at the edge and small plates shaped like benzene rings develop inside the drop (Fig. 47-29). Benzene ring type structures occur with other barbiturates in basic solution but growth is slower and the ring types are considerably larger. Ortal slowly develops a needle growth with crossed bundle forms and rods with branched ends predominating (Fig. 47-30). The needles show both parallel and oblique extinction. Hexobarbital may be differentiated from cyclopal® by crystallization from ammonia. Cyclopal (Fig. 47-31) is similar to ortal®, while hexobarbital, with a type of square plates with notched corners, is similar to the acid form of amobarbital (Fig. 47-32). With aprobarbital, a variety of needles, rods, parallelograms and elongated benzene rings develop as seen in Figure 47-33.

Crystalline habit is influenced by the pH of the solution and the presence of relatively high concentrations of extraneous inorganic ions. Various modifications of the acid or basic forms crystallize when salt-containing reagents are added to an aqueous solution of the barbiturate. A few crystals of the sublimate, dissolved in a small drop of 6 N ammonium hydroxide, are treated with a drop of the reagent as in the acid precipitation (see above). The following reagents have been found to influence the crystallization habit of one or more of the barbiturates and are an aid in distinguishing between members which melt close together and are not clearly differentiated by their acid or basic forms.

Acidic Reagents: (a) Eder's reagent: Add 1 gm. bromine (0.32 ml.) to 20 ml. of water containing 2 gm. of potassium bromide.

(b) Wormley's reagent: Concentrated hydrobromic acid saturated with bromine.

Basic Reagents: (a) Copper ethylenediamine: Add ethylenediamine dropwise to a 0.5 per cent aqueous copper acetate solution until the precipitate which first forms just dissolves.

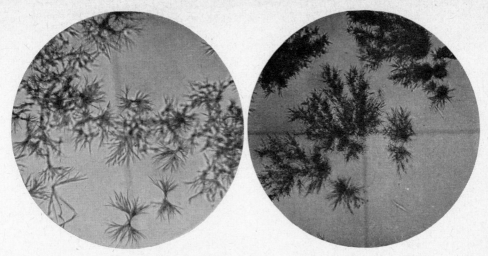

Fig. 47-24. Acid Pentobarbital.   Fig. 47-25. Acid Phenobarbital.

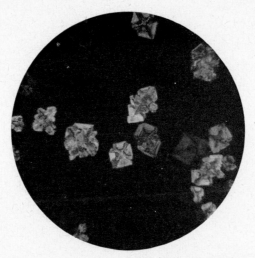

Fig. 47-26. Acid Sandoptal (Polarized Light).

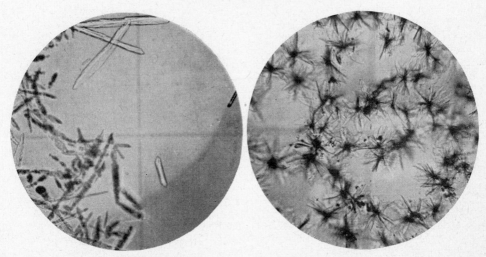

Fig. 47-27. Acid Butabarbital.   Fig. 47-28. Acid Vinbarbital.

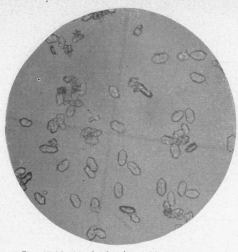

Fig. 47-29. Amobarbital in 6 N Ammonium Hydroxide.

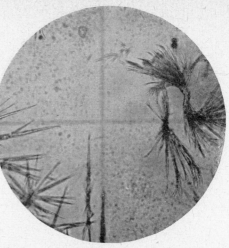

Fig. 47-30. Ortal in 6 N Ammonium Hydroxide.

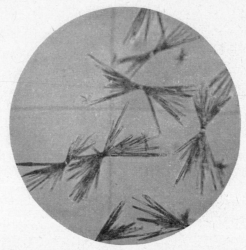

Fig. 47-31. Cyclopal in 6 N Ammonium Hydroxide.

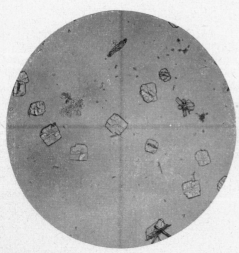

Fig. 47-32. Hexobarbital in 6 N Ammonium Hydroxide.

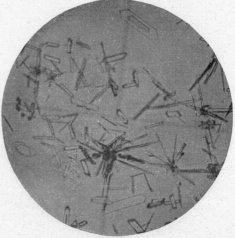

Fig. 47-33. Aprobarbital in 6 N Ammonium Hydroxide.

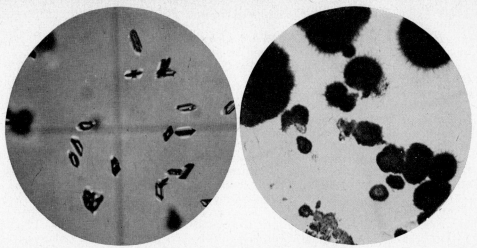

Fig. 47-34. Probarbital with Eder's Reagent.   Fig. 47-35. Aprobarbital with Wormley's Reagent.

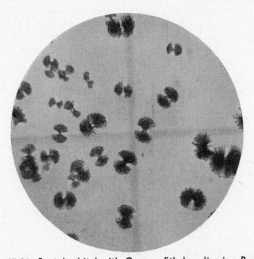

Fig. 47-36. Pentobarbital with Copper Ethylenediamine Reagent.

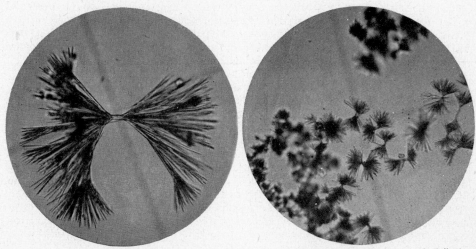

Fig. 47-37. Neonal with Copper Ethylenediamine   Fig. 47-38. Diallylbarbituric Acid with Tollen's
Reagent.   Reagent.

(b) Tollen's reagent: Add concentrated ammonium hydroxide dropwise to a 5 per cent aqueous solution of silver nitrate until the precipitate just dissolves.

(c) Magnesium ammonium nitrate: Dissolve 13 gm. of $Mg(NO_3)_2.6H_2O$ and 24 gm. of NH_4NO_3 in water, add 3.5 ml. of 6 N ammonium hydroxide and dilute the solution to 100 ml. with water.

Eder's reagent is useful in differentiating between barbital and probarbital which gives thick, short hexagonal prisms with beveled ends (Fig. 47-34). Vinbarbital and butabarbital show similar types but they are much larger and not as clearly defined. Barbital forms square and triangular rod forms.

Wormley's reagent produces the same type of formation with phenobarbital as found in the acid precipitation and it reacts characteristically with aprobarbital in forming an oil which changes into bundles of micro needles resembling the first stage in the acid precipitation of phenobarbital. It differs from phenobarbital in not forming the coral-like growth as noted in Figure 47-35. Amobarbital produces benzene ring types which grow into three dimensional hexagonal prisms with beveled ends.

The behavior in copper ethylenediamine differentiates pentobarbital from neonal®. Crystals which are somewhat similar to the acid form quickly develop with pentobarbital but they are smaller and more branched at the ends (Fig. 47-36). Neonal shows the typical pentobarbital acid form but much larger in size. The type is similar to the neonal® acid form but more clearly defined (Fig. 47-37). Other barbiturates give a variety of crystalline types in this reagent.

Tollen's reagent is of little value except in confirming diallylbarbituric acid. It gives amorphous precipitates with most of the other reagents and is reduced to black metallic silver by phanadorn®. Diallylbarbituric acid is exceptional in that an oil separates, followed by crystallization into the typical acid pentobarbital form as seen in Figure 47-38.

Magnesium ammonium nitrate reagent produces crystals with nearly all the barbiturates that are related, in general, to the structures produced with ammonia. Growth is slower and the geometric forms tend to be more clearly defined, particularly with respect to their ends.

Amobarbital is the most troublesome barbiturate to identify. When impure, it is likely to crystallize out in any form, even though the melting point is close to that of the pure compound. When isolated with secobarbital in a case involving ingestion of the commercial preparation of tuinal®, the best indication of its presence is its erratic behavior. It may be confirmed without extensive purification by preparation of a derivative. Aprobarbital, in the preparation allonal®, is troublesome but is suspected from the presence of acetophenetidin with which it is compounded.

Derivatives of the Barbiturates. Derivatives are seldom required since the compounds are isolated in barbiturate deaths in adequate quantity for purification and chemical testing. Their principal value is in cases where contamination is excessive, either from tissue impurities or detoxification products. The decision concerning a derivative usually narrows down to the question of whether it is easier to make the derivative or to further purify the isolated compound. The choice between the xanthydrol and para-nitrobenzylchloride derivative is made on the basis of the melting point spreads of the derivatives of the suspected barbiturates.

(a) Xanthydrol Derivative (100). A ratio of 1 mg. of barbiturate to about 4 mg. of xanthydrol in a 5 ml. centrifuge cone is just moistened with glacial acetic acid and heated in a boiling water bath until the mass dissolves. The tube is removed from the bath and allowed to stand one-half hour. If crystals do not separate, the sides are scratched with a stirring rod to initiate crystallization. Then about 3 ml. of absolute methyl alcohol are added dropwise, with stirring, to complete precipitation. The contents are well mixed, allowed to settle, centrifuged and the alcohol decanted. The methyl alcohol washing is repeated once or twice, depending on the bulk of the precipitate. Xanthone, which may be formed from the xanthydrol, is removed by the methyl alcohol washing.* The washed precipitate is recrystallized from a small amount of hot benzene and the melting point determined. The xanthydrol derivatives contain two molecules of xanthydrol attached to the imino nitrogen groups and all of the high molecular weight

---

* Xanthone, which melts at 170° C., readily sublimes and also may be separated from the derivative by sublimation (page 1153).

derivatives melt at around 200° C. or above. The N-methyl derivatives, hexobarbital and mephobarbital, do not form xanthydrol derivatives. Melting points are observed better at this higher temperature by the conventional capillary technic of organic analysis. Melting points are shown in Table 47-14.

Table 47-14. Melting Points of Xanthyl Derivatives of Barbiturates (101)

	DEGREES C. (UNCORRECTED)			DEGREES C. (UNCORRECTED)	
BARBITURATE	U.S.P. METHOD	BLOCK METHOD	BARBITURATE	U.S.P. METHOD	BLOCK METHOD
Amobarbital	241.5-243.5	250 -251	Pentobarbital	207 -209	219 -222
Aprobarbital	216 -220	225.5-227.5	Phanadorn	229 -232	214 -231*
Barbital	235 -239	248 -249	Phenobarbital	205.5-208	217 -218
Butallylonal	229.5-231.5	257 -259	Probarbital	197.5-199	208.5-210.5
Cyclopal	225.5-226	236 -238	Sandoptai	235.5-237	247 -248
Diallylbarbituric acid	231.5-232.5	242.5-243.5	Secobarbital	175.5-177	180 -184
Neonal	240 -243	249 -251	Sigmodal	188 -191	191 -193.5
Nostal	240 -242.5	265.5-267	Thiopental	156.5-158.5	163.5-165.5
Ortal	197 -198	201 -205	Vinbarbital	218.5-219	224 -226

*Other investigators have reported a melting point of 257° C. for the xanthyl derivative of Phanadorn.

(b) Para-Nitrobenzylchloride Derivatives (100). Weigh 5 mg. of anhydrous sodium carbonate into a 10 ml. pear-shaped micro flask and dissolve in 0.2 ml. of water. Introduce about 1 mg. of the barbiturate into the flask and add 1 ml. of an ethyl alcohol solution of p-nitrobenzylchloride (containing 7.5 mg. of the chloride per ml.). Fit a micro reflux condenser to the flask and reflux the mixture for 1 hour on a hot plate held at a temperature which will maintain gentle boiling of the alcohol. If alcohol evaporates during the heating, add more to maintain the 1 ml. volume. Cool, transfer the contents to a 3 ml. centrifuge cone and wash several times with water to remove the sodium carbonate. Dissolve the precipitate with a minimum volume of chloroform and reprecipitate by the dropwise addition of ethyl alcohol. Centrifuge, decant and dry the precipitate on a porous tile. Determine the melting point by the capillary tube method. Excess p-nitrobenzylchloride is partially converted to the water soluble sodium salt while any that remains is dissolved by the ethyl alcohol. Melting points of the derivatives, according to Goldbaum (100), are shown in Table 47-15.

Table 47-15. Melting Points of the p-Nitrobenzylchloride Derivatives of Barbiturates

BARBITURATE	DEGREES C.	BARBITURATE	DEGREES C.
Amobarbital	188	Mephobarbital	114
Aprobarbital	192	Pentobarbital	142
Barbital	183	Phanadorn	197
Diallylbarbituric acid	192	Phenobarbital	183
		Probarbital	160

B. Hydantoin Sedatives.

B. Hydantoin Sedatives. The hydantoins shown in Table 47-16 should be suspected when the history is suggestive of epilepsy. Diphenylhydantoin is the most common drug in this class. It gives a weak Koppanyi reaction when pure but may not react positively when isolated from tissue after sublimation until extensively purified. It is only slightly soluble in ether and, consequently, will appear predominantly in the chloroform extraction of the acidic group. It is readily identified by the characteristic behavior on the Kofler micro hot stage and its high melting point.

Ethylphenylhydantoin,* formerly used for the treatment of chorea and high blood pressure, has not been imported from Germany since 1938 and has not been studied.

N-Methylphenylethylhydantoin is used infrequently because of the possibility of drug sensitivity with the production of fulminating dermatitis which has occurred with it (102) and the related anticonvulsant trimethadione. It is chemically unreactive, showing only a yellow to orange color with nitrosylsulfuric acid. The Koppanyi and other indicating reactions are entirely negative. In the three-component extraction, it is dis-

* Formerly marketed as Nirvanol by Heyden Chemical Corp., New York City.

Table 47-16. Hydantoin Sedatives

HYDANTOIN	FORMULA	MELTING POINT
Methylphenylethylhydantoin	$\begin{array}{c} CH_3 \\ | \\ NH\!-\!C\!=\!O \quad C_6H_5 \\ | \qquad\qquad C \\ O\!=\!C\!-\!NH \qquad C_2H_5 \end{array}$	135-139° C.
Ethylphenylhydantoin	$\begin{array}{c} NH\!-\!C\!=\!O \quad C_6H_5 \\ \qquad\qquad C \\ O\!=\!C\!-\!NH \qquad C_2H_5 \end{array}$	199-200° C.
Diphenylhydantoin	$\begin{array}{c} NH\!-\!C\!=\!O \quad C_6H_5 \\ \qquad\qquad C \\ O\!=\!C\!-\!NH \qquad C_6H_5 \end{array}$	293-299° C.

tributed in about equal proportions between the phenol and neutral fractions. It shows characteristic crystalline transitions before melting. A needle growth which starts at about 105° C. undergoes a transition with the formation of plates resembling phenobarbital and, at the same time, typical three-dimensional plates with ends shaped like the benzene rings shown in Figures 47-29 and 47-33 for amobarbital and aprobarbital respectively. The transition crystals start to melt at 135° C. and disappear suddenly at 139° C.

C. Substituted Ureas.

C. Substituted Ureas. The substituted ureas (listed in Table 47-17), like the hydantoins, are relatively unreactive chemically. The anticonvulsant, phenylacetylurea, is relatively new on the market. Sedormid is sometimes used in epilepsy and the bromine-containing derivatives are frequently found in mixtures with the barbiturates. Sedormid, carbromal and bromural come out in the acidic extraction and they are separated from

Table 47-17. Substituted Urea Derivatives

* Experimental drug.

SUBSTITUTED UREA	CHEMICAL NAME	FORMULA	MELTING POINT
Carbromal	Bromodiethyl-acetylurea	$\begin{array}{c} C_2H_5 \\ \diagdown \\ CBr\!-\!C\!-\!NH\!-\!C\!-\!NH_2 \\ C_2H_5 \quad\ \| \qquad\ \| \\ O \qquad\ O \end{array}$	116-117° C.
Isoamylethyl-acetylurea *	————	$\begin{array}{c} CH_3 \\ \diagdown \\ CH\!-\!CH_2\!-\!CH_2 \\ CH_3 \qquad\qquad\qquad \diagdown \\ CH\!-\!C\!-\!NH\!-\!C\!-\!NH_2 \\ C_2H_5 \qquad \| \qquad\ \| \\ O \qquad O \end{array}$	130-131° C.
Bromural	alpha-Monobromo-isovalerylurea	$\begin{array}{c} CH_3 \\ \diagdown \\ CH\!-\!CHBr\!-\!C\!-\!NH\!-\!C\!-\!NH_2 \\ CH_3 \qquad\qquad \| \qquad\ \| \\ O \qquad\ O \end{array}$	147-149° C.
Sedormid	Allylisopropyl-acetylurea	$\begin{array}{c} CH_3 \diagdown \quad \diagup CH_3 \\ CH \\ | \\ CH_2\!:\!CH\!-\!CH_2\!-\!CH\!-\!C\!-\!NH\!-\!C\!-\!NH_2 \\ \| \qquad\ \| \\ O \qquad\ O \end{array}$	194° C.
Phenylacetyl-urea	————	$\begin{array}{c} C_6H_5\!-\!CH_2\!-\!C\!-\!NH\!-\!C\!-\!NH_2 \\ \| \qquad\ \| \\ O \qquad\ O \end{array}$	215° C.
Diethylacetyl-urea *	————	$\begin{array}{c} C_2H_5 \\ \diagdown \\ CH\!-\!C\!-\!NH\!-\!C\!-\!NH_2 \\ C_2H_5 \quad \| \qquad \| \\ O \qquad O \end{array}$	217-219° C.

the barbiturates by the three-component separation since they appear in the neutral fraction. Phenylacetylurea is only sparingly soluble in all solvents and is found, therefore, in both the acidic and basic extractions and in all three groups of the three-component separation. Its low solubility furnishes a method for its separation from most of the other drugs. The two bromine-containing members may be differentiated from the others by application of the Beilstein test for halogens (168, 5, 6). When halogen is present and a positive Koppanyi reaction is obtained, the analytical problem is to distinguish between a bromine-containing barbiturate and a barbiturate mixed with a bromine-containing substituted urea. Enough of the substituted urea may carry over into the phenol fraction to give a positive halogen test and a weak positive Koppanyi reaction may be obtained on the neutral fraction but the magnitude of the two reactions on the separate fractions will usually draw the distinction between the two possibilities.

Substituted ureas may be identified by a generic test which is specific for urea or straight chain substituted ureas. It does not react with thiourea derivatives or give the typical coloration with closely related structures. It is one of the few ideal tests for pharmacologic analysis since it designates a specific structure. The method for substituted ureas was adapted from the procedure of Archibald (103) for urea in blood. The procedure (104) depends on the formation of urea by hydrolysis of the substituted ureas with the sulfuric acid-phosphoric acid solution and its reaction with alpha-isonitrosopropiophenone. The rate of hydrolysis is constant for each urea derivative but differs considerably with each compound. Reaction is complete at the end of two hours heating with all those studied. By comparing the color developed at the end of 45 minutes of heating with the color developed at the end of two hours, a ratio is obtained which is a characteristic constant for the substance:

SUBSTITUTED UREA	RATIO	$\dfrac{\text{O.D. 2 hours}}{\text{O.D. 45 minutes}}$
Urea		2
Bromural		3
Carbromal		12
Sedormid		6

Reagents. (a) Alpha-isonitrosopropiophenone, 4 gm., in 100 ml. of 95 per cent ethyl alcohol.

(b) A mixture of 3 parts syrupy (85 per cent) phosphoric acid to one part concentrated sulfuric acid to one part of distilled water.

Procedure. Dissolve the unknown sample, purified by sublimation, in absolute ethyl alcohol to give approximately 1.5 mg./ml. of substituted urea. Add 1 ml. of this solution to each of two 3-5 inch test tubes. Add to each tube 0.7 ml. of alpha-isonitrosopropiophenone reagent, 4.9 ml. of water and 3.5 ml. of the acid-water mixture (water, acid-water and alcoholic reagent are in the ratio of 7:3:1). Set up two reagent blanks at the same time and place all the tubes in a boiling water bath. At the end of 45 minutes, if a red color has developed, remove one test tube with sample and one reagent blank and allow them to stand. The second test tube with the sample remains in the boiling water bath and is removed, with the reagent blank, at the end of two hours (one hour and 15 minutes after the first tube was removed). The tubes are allowed to cool for 15 minutes and then the four tubes are brought back to the original volume with water. Each sample is read against the reagent blank at a wave length of 545 mμ.

IDENTIFICATION PROCESS

At this stage of the analysis, the isolated drug should be sufficiently pure to permit application of chemical tests to determine the general nature of the compound. From the tables which follow, it is possible to devise a systematic method of analysis in which the organic compounds are classified according to color and precipitation reactions. The only prerequisite, other than that adequate material be isolated, is that the compound is one listed in the tables and not a new drug that has not been studied or a substance not considered important enough to include. By following the systematic order of testing as outlined in the flow sheet, almost every compound should become delineated. However, although such a system looks good on paper, it does not follow that it works in practice. As previously pointed out (9), a systematic scheme of analysis for drugs is not only impractical but is also dangerous, since each reaction is an essential part of the scheme and a misinterpretation of one step of the process would probably mislead the analyst in all others. Moreover, if an attempt is made to apply tests in a definite order in such a scheme, the sample is invariably used up before the scheme can be completed.

Because of uncontrollable variables in the analysis of organic substances isolated from tissue, an infallible interpretation cannot be made from any single chemical test. The quantity of sample material available for analysis varies from one case to another and the smaller the quantity of sample, the more conservative must be the analytic testing procedure. The intensity of the individual reaction is a function of the quantity used for the test and, where the reaction depends on color formation, the shade at some optimum concentration may even appear as a different coloration at a lower concentration. The isolated product is never chemically pure, whereas the control reactions must be based on relatively pure substances. The presence of normal tissue extractables can alter both color and precipitation reactions but, even when the results are comparable to the pure compound, the sensitivity is lessened in proportion to the normal tissue contaminants. The composition of the normal tissue extractables varies from case to case and influences the reactions with different compounds differently. Metabolic products formed as a result of the detoxification process in the body may be present in varying amounts and alter the reactions. The term specific test is inappropriate in organic toxicologic analysis; in fact, in any testing procedure, it is the entire process, including separation and purification as well as the reaction itself, which makes a specific test.

Random testing is the only alternative to nonsystematic qualitative analysis and, with the restrictions of limited irreplaceable sample material, the chances for its success are extremely small. Since a systematic scheme is not workable, yet system is necessary for qualitative analysis, the process must be a compromise which is systematic without being schematic. This procedure for attacking the problem has been termed a systematic method of approach (9) and differs from a systematic scheme of analysis in that selection from the number of courses open to the analyst is made on the basis of information already available to him.

The testing process is one of *exclusion* in which the approach is through the use of very sensitive but nonspecific reactions which serve to rule out a large number of compounds from a group. A negative finding, therefore, assumes equal importance with a positive test in a given reaction. Classification is based solely on chemical reactivity without regard to chemical genus, physical or other chemical properties. The compounds are listed under the name of each reaction and fall into two main families, one giving positive and the other negative findings in the test. The reagent, rather than the compound, is then the index to the classification system. Thus, a positive chemical reaction on an unknown compound rules out all drugs known not to react with the reagent and the problem is further narrowed, depending on the degree with which the findings can be interpreted within the positively reacting family. By applying a series of sensitive, nonspecific reactions which overlap in their behavior toward individual drugs, groups of compounds within the positive and negative classification for one reagent are excluded. Chemical and physical behavior, pharmacologic activity, pathologic findings or indications from the history may then point to a single substance or type within the smaller group that remains after elimination of other compounds.

The system depends on all drugs reacting positively in at least one test, for if one were completely nonreactive it would still remain questionable after the testing procedure was exhausted. The selection of the excluding type reactions by the analyst is made after he has evaluated all information concerning the unknown and it follows that the more experience he has, the more readily will he select the proper test. The key to success in the analysis of an unknown organic drug is a knowledge of the type of structure which reacts positively in a given test and the limitations and sensitivity of the test for, if positive results are obtained in a reaction which is understood, the selection of tests for confirmation follows automatically.

Drugs are too diverse structurally to make the conventional type of organic reactions that characterize functional groups of any value, even if they could be made sufficiently sensitive. Although the types of reactions that are applicable vary over a wide range with regard to mechanism, specificity and sensitivity, this variation actually aids in the exclusion process. In developing this approach it was found useful to characterize the reactions in terms of the use to which they are put in the procedure. There can be no clear-cut demarcation between types and any reaction may shift into another category, depending on its use in a particular analysis.

Probing reactions are those used sparingly in random testing for those relatively few substances that are encountered with such frequency that it becomes logical to sacrifice enough sample at the start in order to exclude them. In this sense, any reaction could become a probing reaction but the process then reverts entirely to random testing.

Exclusion reactions must be sensitive and the more nonspecific the better. Their purpose is to divide drugs into two main categories, one being positive, the other negative. They should not be influenced materially by the presence of normal tissue extractables.

Indicating reactions should be equally sensitive but less nonspecific and are used after the exclusion reactions to reduce the number of possibilities within a group. The exclusion reactions have already indicated certain possibilities.

Designating reactions are still more specific, possibly because of the limitations set by the previous reactions, but their purpose is to point toward a type, if not a specific structure.

Differential reactions are any applied toward distinguishing between a small number of possibilities of a particular type. The reactions have attained this specificity as a result of the information obtained from the previous reactions, but they are not necessarily specific themselves.

Confirmatory reactions, by the time they are applied, should have become specific by virtue of the exclusion of all other possibilities through the use of other reactions. These reactions should be confirmatory for the analyst, but are not final; the final identification must rest on the physical properties after the chemical nature of the compound has been established.

Limitations in the Interpretation of Positive Reactions.

Limitations in the Interpretation of Positive Reactions. With reactions having adequate sensitivity, there is usually no question about whether a reaction occurred nor is there usually a question as to whether a false positive is obtained as a result of tissue contamination. The distinction between positive and negative findings is, therefore, rather clearly defined. Since the reactions which are suitable must have sensitivity, the type that is applicable for exclusion and indication tests is limited to color reactions. The interpretation of color changes is far more involved than has been assumed by investigators in dealing with color phenomena. Besides, it is subject to a human element, with the result that interpretation within a positively reacting group cannot be made with the certainty implied in the table for the reaction. Reactions which depend on color changes have certain limitations which must be recognized and the understanding of these limitations requires a fundamental knowledge of the physical phenomenon of color.

Color is a sensation resulting from a stimulation of light of different wave lengths on the retina of the eye. The sensitivity for the detection of different light waves varies over the visible region of the spectrum, the maximum visibility for average normal vision occurring at 555 mμ (105). However, the visibility curve for different individuals varies over a considerable range, with the result that the response to light for different color-producing pigments depends on the observer and the finer distinctions in the colors may not be interpreted in the same way by two different individuals. Moreover, color is a gradation of sensations which the commonly accepted names fail to define. In order to characterize color phenomena, not one but three attributes are required. The attributes, in turn, depend on whether the definition is in terms of the physical properties of the reflected light or the physiologic response to the color sensation that is produced. In the physical sense, the attributes are dominant wave length, brightness and purity (105), while the corresponding physiologic terms are hue, value and chroma (106). The practical theory for the physiologic basis of color as developed by Albert H. Munsell (106), which is the theoretical basis for interior design and decorating, serves equally well in establishing limitations for the interpretation of chemical color reactions.

If a color photograph of a spectrum cast by a prism is coiled to form a cylinder in such a way that the short wave violet end of the spectrum merges with the longest visible waves in the red, a color circle is produced containing all possible hues merging by indistinguishable degrees one into the other. The circle can be divided into 6 or 10 equal segments in such a way that major colorations fall into separate segments. In the Munsell system there are 10 segments with the major or primary colors being designated as the principal *hues*. These are red, yellow, green, blue and purple. With six segments, the primary colors become red, yellow-green, and blue-violet or an indigo. Regardless of the divisions, a line drawn from a primary color segment through the center of the circle extends through the color segment which is the complement of the primary. Of more importance, however, is the fact that a line drawn through two hues that are not complementary shows the coloration resulting from mixing the two colors. The process of forming colors by mixing light waves is called addition and is the opposite of color formation by subtraction in which the color is formed by mixing colored pigments. In subtraction, the color from the mixture is that of the light not absorbed by either of the two pigments. The theory for the color circle is the same, whether the color is produced by addition or subtraction, but in color formation by addition the resultant color from mixing two or more light waves is lighter or more on the white side than either of the original lights. In producing color by subtraction the resultant hue has a darker cast in contrast to those of either of the original pigments.

The coloration of pigments is due to the preferential absorption of certain waves of the spectrum by chromophore groups in the molecule. If absorption is complete, the pigment is black. If there is an absence of absorption, the substance is white. Not only do absorbing pigments have hue but, depending on the magnitude of the over-all absorption, the hue can be on the black or white side and it is for this reason that color cannot be defined in less than three dimensions.

For the three dimensional representation, the color circle circumscribes the center of a pole which is pure white at the top and black at the bottom. The center of the pole, therefore, represents half-white and half-black or neutral gray. All colored pigments may be located within the sphere created by the diameter of the color circle and the neutral pole as axes, in terms of their hue and the degree of whiteness of the hue. A pink, which is a red on the white side, is located in the red segment of the circle but at a level above the neutral gray of the pole while a maroon or red on the dark side of neutral gray is at a lower level in the red segment. This quality of being light or dark constitutes the *value* for the color and, if an arbitrary scale from 1 to 10 is laid out on the pole, the value becomes a number, with 5 representing a neutral coloration.

Some red pigments of the same hue and value are stronger than others as the reflected red light reaching the retina contains more energy in the red. There is no adequate description, except that one pigment is a redder red than another. This quality of being stronger or weaker is called *chroma* and is determined by the proportion of the dominant rays in the reflected light. If the strongest neutral red is placed in the plane of the color sphere perpendicular to the center of the neutral pole and its distance made an arbitrary 10 units from the pole, the chroma also acquires a numeric measurement in terms of the strongest red pigment. The scientific designation for the physiologic response to colors is, then, in terms of the hue and numbers representing value and chroma. Thus, the reddest of the red pigments becomes R 5/10, indicating that it is neutral in value, having a shade comparable to that of spectral red, and maximal in chroma, or spectral red intensity.* Color spheres are available † showing all the varieties of tints and shades in a particular hue and any of the colors observed in a color-producing chemical reaction can be clearly defined in terms of the three attributes by comparison of the observed coloration with the shades in the standard color sphere. Mulliken (107) has approached this precision for recording colorations by using color cards as the reference standards in his procedure for the analysis of commercial dyes.

Data recorded by various investigators for the color changes with different com-

* Since the Munsell scale was devised, newer pigments have been developed which have extended his chroma scale to 14 units.
† The Munsell Color Company, Baltimore, Maryland.

pounds in a given reaction are not only indefinite but are also confusing, if not con-flicting, at times. Terms such as beige, tan, sand, ecru do not mean the same thing to different individuals although each may be a distinct coloration. Many pure com-pounds in adequate concentration give reproducible color in a reaction and the shade may be a distinguishing characteristic. For example, with both compounds run simul-taneously, codeine may be differentiated from morphine by the green cast in the blue produced with Mecke's reagent. In separate tests, the color difference is not sufficiently characteristic to make the distinction. Therefore, the recorded colorations of the pure substance, which serve as the basis for comparison in the examination of an unknown compound, should be put on a more scientific basis and, to be clearly defined, the three attributes for the color must be specified. What is true of the substance in the pure state in adequate concentration and, therefore, free of interference cannot apply to an unknown compound, particularly when isolated from biologic material.

Color sensitivity varies with each reagent and each compound. With limited sample material, the concentration used in a test may be below that necessary for development of maximum color intensity, with the result that there may be, at least, an alteration in shade and even a change in hue. On the other hand, with high concentrations of a substance normally producing a dark coloration, the observed color may be so intense as to appear black. The color shade may even depend on the physical structure of the substance. For example, mephobarbital crystallized from chloroform gives a far more intense color with Mandelin's reagent than the same quantity of mephobarbital crystal-lized from ether. Extraneous impurities that do not give colors themselves can influence the color of a reacting substance, due to the formation of crystalline complexes, solid solutions or even mixed crystals. Normal tissue contaminants decrease the sensitivity for all color reactions and exert varying influences on the shade produced. As it is logical to specify the color of the pure substance in exact terms, it is just as illogical to attempt to interpret color findings in the reaction on an unknown substance in more than general terms. In this respect, the popular names for the various color shades are over descriptive and the problem in the interpretation of a reaction is to decide the possible variations in the color produced by the unknown from that of the suspected pure substance when tested under controlled conditions. This apparent contradiction in which it is proposed that color tables be specified in exact terms while the data can only be interpreted within a wide latitude, is not as inconsistent as might first appear. The unknown *may* be a pure substance tested in adequate concentration without inter-ference and the fine distinction in color shade then becomes significant. The problem, therefore, narrows down to the ability to put an interpretation on the observed colora-tion, and the basic principles on which the physical and physiologic properties of color depend are an aid in establishing the limitations.

Certain basic requirements are necessary in setting up a color system for unknown substances in which all manner of hues and shades are encountered with variable and limited ability for interpretation of the color phenomena. The logical order for tabu-lating the color-producing compounds is that of the spectrum colors. The gradation of color at the lower end of the spectrum containing indigo and violet is gradual and passes into magenta which is a combination of the red with the blue ends of the spectrum. A magenta can, therefore, be misinterpreted for either a deep red or a violet and there is no practical basis for including both violet and magenta as separate colors in a system for tabulating color reactions. The eye is least sensitive to the violet region of the spectrum and, as fine distinctions in violet shades cannot be made, neither can a line of demarcation be drawn in the gradation of violet to magenta without matching against standards. Since magenta is red with a violet cast as well as violet with a red cast and, since red-violets cannot be classified without including magenta in the scheme, magenta takes precedence over violet in a choice between the two colors. As colors corresponding to light waves in the indigo region of the spectrum appear to the eye as deep blues, indigo is not required in designating hues for color reactions.

Brown results when an orange or deep yellow color is darkened. Therefore, it is a shade of yellow to orange, low in value and moderate to low in chroma. Many organic structures undergo some charring in using concentrated sulfuric acid as the solvent for color reactions. A brown can result from the formation of some black carbonized residue by charring of either an impurity or the reacting substance when the products of the reaction are yellow to orange; or the reaction can produce yellow to orange, producing chromophores of value and chroma which give brown. The first case is one of interference whereas in the second, the shade of the color is that developed in the reaction. Although not a color, brown is so frequently encountered and so readily distinguished from the parent yellow or orange that it warrants a place along with the colors. The extremes in color measurement are black and white, although they are not colors in themselves. The formation of black residues in reactions of substances which readily char in the cold may be just as characteristic as color reactions. The formation of black as a color must be differentiated from true color reactions in which the normal low value color is so intense as a result of a high concentration of reactant that very little light reflects from the solution. The distinction between black and true color formation is readily made by diluting the black solution with solvent until some light is transmitted or reflected.

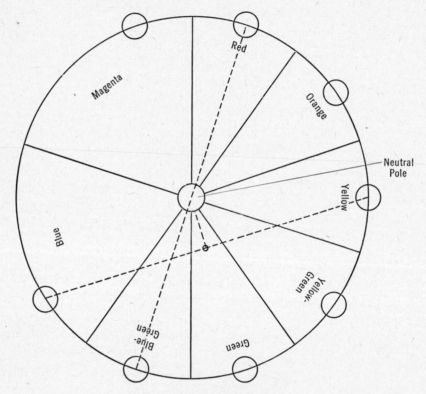

Fig. 47-39. Color Reaction Circle.

The distinction between yellow-green and blue-green and a green or blue is not nearly as sharp as that between orange and red or yellow, magenta and blue or red. Because of the limitations for interpreting yellow or blue-greens, they may just as well be catalogued under the yellows, greens or blues depending on which color predominates, although recorded by their observed intermediate hue in the table. The perceptible colors for interpreting color reactions then are, in their spectral order, red, orange, brown, yellow, green, blue, magenta and black. By analogy with the Munsell system for pigments, the color reaction circle (Fig. 47-39) is divided into eight segments with red, yellow, green, blue as primary hues and intermediate hues of orange, yellow-green, blue-green and magenta. Figure 47-39 would not be a true representation of color by subtraction if it were divided into eight equal sectors which would make red and green and yellow and blue complementary pigments. In the Munsell system the hues were selected so that opposite sectors would be true complements whose admixture would produce a perfectly neutral gray. The color reaction circle described here is merely a device to give a theoretical basis for the prediction of color shades. It also aids in interpreting the possible effects of interference in a color reaction in which the inability of the eye to draw the fine distinctions that are possible when matching pigments in a colorimeter is balanced by a distortion in the color circle of the spectral hues for the short wave region of the visible spectrum.

The circumference of the color reaction circle represents the strongest colorations or those maximal in chroma. The plane of the circle represents a neutral value with the center as neutral gray. The colors represented at or near the circumference may be higher or lower in value, depending on their position in the color sphere, but possess a brilliance comparable to that of the visible light rays dispersed by a prism. Therefore, a term is needed to distinguish the colors which have a luster because they are low in gray from less striking colors. Since the distinction is physiologic, those colors which make a pronounced impression have been designated as "spectral colors." The small circles on the circumference represent the mid-portion of the spectral region comprising the various hues. According to the basic theory of color mixtures, if a line is drawn from any point on the circumference through the center and extended to the opposite side of the circle (dotted line between red and blue-green, Fig. 47-39), it will connect colors which are complementary and a mixture of the two pigments in equal proportions will result in a gray or a combination of black and white. If a chord is drawn between two sectors to form a segment with the circumference of the circle, the intersection of the perpendicular of the chord to the center of the color circle will represent the color obtained with equal amounts of the pigments, with colors represented by the points at which the chord intersects with the circumference, are mixed. This is shown by the dotted line connecting the mid-point in the blue and yellow sectors. The resultant color is a pure green, since it lies along the line connecting the mid-point of the green sector, but, since it is close to the neutral pole, it is low in chroma and has a gray cast which differentiates it from the spectral green of the same value at the circumference.

The most common interference in a color reaction is that from the action of the reagent on the normal tissue extractives. The color produced is a dirty yellow or brown and, for this reason, yellow colors mean very little and browns mean less when obtained on an unknown residue. Normal tissue interference with the color produced in a reaction can be predicted from the color reaction circle. A yellow coloration decreases the strength or chroma of all reaction colors and the greater the brown coloration from the tissue, the more the observed reaction color is on the dark side or the lower is its value. The greatest influence will be exerted in the opposite side of the circle or on the blue or violet colors. Greens and reds will be less affected than blue while orange and yellow-green will only undergo slight changes, except in value. Fortunately, the perception for blue is high and moderate interference will only throw the blue to the green side. Violets will be most affected and, for this reason, a large range of color shades needs to be classified under blue and magenta (see Fig. 47-39). Since tissue interference decreases both the chroma and the value, it follows that, when a spectral color *is* produced in a reaction on an unknown compound, the probability for interference is small and the stronger the observed color, the greater the certainty in the interpretation. The yellow of the reaction of acetophenetidin with concentrated nitric acid, for example, is quite different from the possible yellow of a tissue residue, and the yellow coloration then takes on definite meaning. If the brown or yellow colorations, other than spectral colors, mean very little because of the limitations on their interpretation, the question arises concerning their inclusion in a color reaction table. However, even though the pale yellows which are not usually interpretable are listed, these weak colorations are not without significance. In the absence of any yellow coloration in the reaction on the unknown, those substances which are known to give weak colorations are excluded.

As previously discussed, the color formed by the action of a reagent on a compound is influenced by a number of factors that cannot always be controlled even in the absence of interference. The color results from the chromophore groups in a particular structure, and, naturally, cannot be random. The limits for interpretation in the absence of tissue interference then depend on the possible variations in the color or its shade. When the color of a compound isolated from tissue differs from that of the pure substance in adequate concentration, the shift is *usually* toward the long wave region of the spectrum. Thus, a shift from blue would tend toward green, green toward yellow,

yellow toward orange and orange toward red. Violet will shift toward the long wave region but will pass through magenta to red rather than by way of the blue. The chroma is usually decreased and, if the concentration is below an optimum, the value changes toward the white or high side. The transition also can occur with a shift to the shorter wave region of the spectrum, with normal red developing as orange or magenta. A red, however, will never go as far astray as the yellow or pure violet, and yellow does not develop as green nor green as blue. In searching for an unknown compound from the color table for the reaction, neighboring colors must always be considered, with the greatest possibility for confusion being between violet and magenta or red and orange colors. Color reactions in which blue or green colors develop, therefore, make for more specific reactions with less chance for extraneous interference to influence the color. The exception to the rules is the transition color formation in which the reaction progresses in stages with different structures, each with a definite chromophore group and, consequently, a different color. Veratrine, for example, is oxidized in stages by concentrated sulfuric acid, with the formation of yellow, then orange, then red and finally magenta. However, when changes do occur as a result of minor interference, they are usually with colors at the extreme ends of the spectrum. In this case, the widest latitude occurs between violet and red, and any violet may be shifted over to a magenta or even a red. Yellows frequently crop up as orange and orange colors may develop a red cast but changes in the blue or green are infrequent.

Concentration is the limiting factor in a color reaction when the compound has been isolated in a pure state. When the quantity of material to be tested is decreased below an optimum value, a lighter color or an increase in the color value results. However, it is not concentration per se which determines sensitivity in a reaction between a solid phase and a liquid reagent. The term limiting concentration is exact in solution testing, but the limit of identification for a solid is determined solely by the analytic technic. Working with small samples demands micro technic, but a micro process is only macro chemistry carried out under controlled conditions which maintain the surface area for the reaction within narrow confines. A limited surface area must then be the chief precept of the analytic toxicologist, and his creed must be "avoid spreading, pile up the sample." A 100 μg sample consisting of minute crystals spread over the surface of a microscope slide will not develop the color intensity of a single 5 μg crystal which has depth. As discussed before (pages 1125, 1163), the same crystal mounted upright on the slide can be treated with the reagent in such a way that it will develop a more intense color than when it is lying lengthwise.

In using color reactions in the identification phase, reliance is not placed on the appearance or absence of a color from a single reaction but rather on the continuity in the findings from a number of tests which, taken alone, are of limited interpretability. The greater the number of tests which can be applied to the sample material, the more narrow the limits become until the exclusion process finally points to a few possibilities. Differential and confirmatory reactions then make the distinction, with final identification made on the basis of the physical properties of the parent substance or one of its derivatives. Successful completion of the process depends, therefore, on the careful allocation of the isolated material for the testing process. Purity of the sample is the controlling factor for, if a death resulted from poisoning by a drug, there will be a sufficient amount of test material from 500 gm. of the appropriate tissue. This amount of biologic sample (see page 1126) was selected as the optimum because at least 0.5 mg. of the more toxic drugs can be isolated from this amount of sample when the dosage was lethal.

The exclusion and indicating tests are sensitive to at least 10 μg. of pure compound. With a 500 μg. sample, 25 separate tests are then possible, with 0.25 mg. remaining for final identification from the physical properties, after which the reclaimed sample is available for review in case the findings are contested. Allocation of the isolated residue is more easily made on a volume basis and, if the residue from 500 gm. of sample is dissolved in 2.5 ml. of solvent (assuming 20 drops per ml.), the sample contained in one drop of solvent may be used for each test without fear of uselessly sacrificing test material. Obviously, since tissue impurities reduce the sensitivity, the quantity of sample necessary in each test must be increased in proportion to the contamination.

The tables for the color reactions which follow are an accumulation of data by various investigators in this laboratory over a period of about 11 years. Although minor colorations are of little practical significance, they are included with the more definite color reactions, with the distinction between very faint colors and colorless based solely on the behavior of the material at hand. The inclusion of nonreactants in each test is repetitious, but it serves to show all those substances that have been examined. The observations may be aberrant at times because of the human element, but of greater importance is the fact that the material was obtained from many different sources, some as pure drugs, some purified from pharmaceutic mixtures and others isolated from tissue. Inconsistencies are to be expected, but inconsistency in the reactivity of drugs isolated from tissue is the factor which makes analytic toxicology different from all other branches of analytic chemistry.

COLOR REACTIONS

The manipulative procedure which is to be used for carrying out a color test will depend on the quantity of sample material and its purity. When it is necessary to limit the test sample to very small amounts, the reactions are more readily observed in small capillaries viewed with vertical illumination. A micro manipulative unit is necessary for adding the reagents to the mounted capillaries and considerable labor is required to gain the added sensitivity in the observation. Various compromise technics may be used, such as carrying out the test on acid resistant filter paper or by mounting the sample on the immersion objective of the vertical illumination microscope (Fig. 47-14). In most cases, the quantity of isolated sample will be sufficient to permit the use of the simple microscope slide technic.

Organic solvents creep when placed on a microscope slide and, for this reason, reactions in nonaqueous solution are better performed in capillary test tubes about 2 mm. in diameter and 1 cm. in length. These may be mounted vertically in a clamp and viewed by transmitted light with a low power objective in a manner analogous to nephelometric observations. The slide technic is carried out by merely adding a drop of the reagent to a particle of solid sample on a microscope slide. Tissue residues, even when fairly pure, are often fatty in consistency and tend to adhere to the spatula or stirring rod. In attempting the transfer from the spatula to the slide, the sample is likely to be spread over the surface of the slide, resulting in decreased sensitivity of the test due to the surface area effect (page 1190).

The most efficient procedure consists of using a very small scalpel as a spatula and of transferring the sample from it by scraping the very edge of the slide so that the sample material is piled up on the top edge. The reagent drop is added in back of it but far enough away to prevent it from flowing to the sample while the slide is maintained level. The preparation is placed on the microscope stage under a low power objective with long working distance and the slide is tilted upward at about 45° so that the reagent runs into the sample while it is being viewed under the microscope. In this way, the drop is held at the edge of the slide and, at the same time, it acts as a refracting body for the transmitted light, giving added depth for the color observation. A microscope for observation with reflected light should also be at hand and a comparison of any apparent color change made with both transmitted and reflected light. Intense colors which appear dark in transmitted light are more readily distinguished with reflected rays and some colorations actually differ in the two types of illumination.

The shade of color produced by certain compounds is influenced by their specific structure. In general, the free acids or bases that are isolated in the extraction process give better colorations than their salts. Therefore, salts were not used in carrying out the control color reactions except where indicated. There may be a question concerning the advisability of repeating the lists of negatively reacting compounds in the different tables. It is possible to devise a master sheet with the compounds referred to by number and thus avoid the repetition. Since each successive reaction is selected on the basis of findings, whether positive or negative, in the preceding tests, it would become very confusing to refer to a master table. Moreover, listing both positive and negative reactions shows at a glance just which compounds were included in the study of the particular reagent.

Table 47-18. Nitrosylsulfuric Acid Reaction (109)

* One to two drops; nitrosylsulfuric acid alone changes from green → blue → colorless.
† Three to four drops to neutralize the acid.
§ This is an example of the same compound from two different sources giving different, but reproducible, color reactions.

COMPOUND	COLOR DEVELOPED WITH NITROSYLSULFURIC ACID	COLOR AFTER ADDITION OF WATER *	COLOR AFTER ADDITION OF CONC. AMMONIA †
RED			
Brucine	Red with orange cast → orange → yellow	Yellow	Color pales
Pyrilamine	Deep carmine → orange brown	Violet → milky white	Milky precipitate
Pyridium	Carmine red	Orange red	Orange-brown
Thonzylamine	Deep carmine → red brown	Bright yellow	Brown precipitate in yellow green solution
Zolamine.HCl	Carmine with brown cast	Pale yellow	Light yellow precipitate
ORANGE			
Acetanilid	Orange with yellow cast	Colorless	No change
Adiphenine	Light orange with yellow cast	Colorless	Slight white precipitate
Aminopyrine	Orange with gray cast → grayish yellow	Colorless	Light orange
Amphetamine base	Orange with gold solution	Color fades	No change
Amphetamine.HCl	Deep orange with red-brown cast	Color fades	No change
Antipyrine	Orange	Yellow orange	Gold with slight green precipitate
Apothesine	Orange with brown cast	Very pale yellow	No change
Atropine	Orange with yellow cast	Colorless	No change
Chrysazin	Orange → orange with yellow cast	No change	No change
Delphinine	Orange with gray cast → gray yellow	Colorless	No change
d-Desoxyephedrine	Orange with yellow cast	Colorless	No change
Hyoscyamine	Orange with yellow cast → yellow with orange cast	Colorless	No change
Larocaine	Orange with yellow cast	Color pales	Yellow-orange
Phenylacetylurea	Orange with red cast	Colorless	No change
Prisilidene	Orange → brick red → brown with orange cast	Very pale yellow	Heavy milky yellow precipitate
Procaine amide	Pale orange	Colorless	Heavy yellow orange precipitate
Ricin	Light orange, almost flesh	Colorless; white precipitate	Pale yellow
Salicin	Orange with yellow cast	Pale yellow	Pale yellow
Strychnine	Light orange increasing in intensity	Light pink orange	Colorless
p-Toluenesulfonamide	Orange with yellow cast → yellow	Colorless	Slight precipitate
BROWN			
N-Allylnormorphine	Brown with yellow cast → gold with brown streaks	Pale yellow	Light yellow orange
Apomorphine	Deep brown → dark brown with yellow cast	Light orange-brown	No change
Atabrin	Brown with yellow-orange solution	Yellow orange	Orange precipitate
Cephaeline	Brown with yellow green cast	Pale yellow	Yellow deepens a little
Codeine	Deep brown with red cast → deep red with brown cast	Pale yellow	Light lemon yellow
Colchicine	Brown with greenish yellow cast, slowly changing to yellow	Pale yellow	Yellow browns slightly

Table 47-18 (cont.). Nitrosylsulfuric Acid Reaction (109)

Compound	Color Developed with Nitrosylsulfuric Acid	Color after Addition of Water *	Color after Addition of Conc. Ammonia †
Curarine	Deep brown → brown with yellow cast	Pale brownish yellow	Color deepens; brownish precipitate
Digitalin	Brown	Color disappears	Light magenta
Dihydromorphinone	Brown with orange cast → pales	Color disappears	No change
Diothane	Brown with gold cast → gold with brown streaks	Color fades	Color deepens slightly
Emetine	Very dark brown or black	Light orange brown	Light brown
Estrone	Deep brown with orange cast	Light yellow	No change
Ethylmorphine	Dark brown → brown with red cast	Color fades	Light yellow
Heroin	Deep brown → gold with brown cast	Color fades	Pale yellow
Hydrastine	Deep brown-black → brown with yellow cast	Golden yellow	Light brownish yellow precipitate
Lobeline	Brown with yellow cast → yellow	Color fades	No change
Meconin	Deep brown with red cast	White precipitate and yellow solution	No change
Mephenesine	Brown with orange cast	Orange yellow	Deep lemon yellow
Mescaline	Deep brown → brown with red cast	Yellow	Color pales
Methylparafynol	Colorless → brown	Color fades	Color deepens
Metopon	Deep brown → brown with red cast	Pale yellow	Light orange-yellow
Morphine	Brown with yellow cast → gold with red brown streaks	Yellow	Deepens to light orange-gold
alpha-Naphthylthiourea	Deep brown with gray cast → brown with red cast	Orange with brown cast	Dark brown with orange cast
Narceine	Brown with yellow green cast	Yellow	Orange → light red brown
Narcotine	Brown with yellow green cast	Yellow	Orange → light reddish brown
Pamaquine	Brown with orange cast → deep orange	Yellow orange	Fades to pale yellow
Pavatrine	Dark brown	Yellow precipitate	No change
Phenindamine	Deep brown with orange cast	Fades; brown precipitate	No change
Piperine	Deep brown with faint yellow cast	Light brown	Brown deepens
Rutin	Deep brown with red cast → golden brown	Yellow	Light yellow
Sparteine	No color change from original brown	Colorless	No change
Strophanthin	Brown with yellow cast	Pale yellow-brown	No change
Thenylpyramine §	Brown with orange cast	Colorless	No change
Thiobarbituric acid	Brown with gold cast	Lemon yellow precipitate	Light magenta
Thymol iodide	Brown	No change	No change
Veratrine	Brown with gray cast → yellowish gray	Colorless	No change
Xylocaine	Brown with red cast → orange → brown with orange cast	Very pale yellow	No change
Yohimbine	Brown with yellow cast → gold with brown cast	Pale yellow	Pale orange yellow

YELLOW

Compound	Color Developed with Nitrosylsulfuric Acid	Color after Addition of Water	Color after Addition of Conc. Ammonia
Acetylsalicylic acid	Yellow → yellow with brown cast	Pale yellow	Light yellow increases
Aconitine	Pale yellow	Colorless	Milky white precipitate
Acridine.HCl	Lemon yellow	Light yellow, green cast	Same color milky precipitate
Amprotropine	Yellow with orange cast → orange	Milky precipitate	No change
Betaine.HCl	Pale yellow	Colorless	No change

Table 47-18 (cont.). Nitrosylsulfuric Acid Reaction (109)

COMPOUND	COLOR DEVELOPED WITH NITROSYLSULFURIC ACID	COLOR AFTER ADDITION OF WATER *	COLOR AFTER ADDITION OF CONC. AMMONIA †
Butallylonal	Yellow	Colorless	No change
Caffeine	Light yellow	Colorless	No change
Chlorcyclizine	Pale yellow → light yellow	Colorless	Slight cloudiness
Cinchonidine	Very very pale grayish yellow	Colorless	No change
Cinchophen	Yellow	Colorless	Milky precipitate
Cocaine	Pale yellow	Colorless	No change
Cyclopal	Gray → pale yellow with gray cast → yellow	Color fades	Pale yellow
Cysteine.HCl	Yellow with orange cast	Color fades	Colorless
Desoxycholic acid	Pale yellow	White precipitate	Colorless; precipitate gone
Digitonin	Pale yellow	Colorless	Colorless
Dimenhydrinate (acidic extraction product)	Yellow	Colorless	No change
Dimenhydrinate (basic extraction product)	Yellow → gray yellow	Color disappears	Colorless; milky white precipitate
Diphenhydramine	Yellow with greenish or grayish cast	Milky precipitate	No change
Ephedrine	Gold	Color disappears	No change
Eucupin.di HCl	Pale yellow	Colorless	Milky white precipitate
Hippuric acid	Very pale yellow	Colorless	No change
Histamine di HCl	Pale yellow	Colorless	No change
Homatropine	Yellow with orange cast	Color disappears	No change
l-Menthol	Colorless → very pale yellow	Colorless	No change
Meperidine	Yellow with orange cast	Colorless	Slight cloudiness
Mephobarbital	Pale yellow	Colorless	No change
Methadon	Original yellow increases to gold	Color disappears	Slight milky precipitate
Methylphenylethyl-hydantoin	Yellow → orange yellow	Color disappears	No change
Nicotine	Yellow with slight orange cast → yellow	Colorless	Slight precipitate
Nikethamide	Very pale yellow → light yellow	Colorless	No change
Optochin	Very very pale yellow	Colorless	Milky white precipitate
Pelletierine tannate	Yellow with brown cast	Very pale yellow	Light orange yellow
Phanadorn	Pale yellow → yellow	Pale yellow	No change
Phenobarbital	Colorless → pale yellow	Colorless	No change
Phenylbutazone	Pale yellow with brown cast	Color fades	No change
Phenylsalicylate	Colorless → light yellow	Colorless	No change
Phthalylsulfathiazole	Very pale yellow	Very pale yellow	Color fades
Pilocarpine	Pale yellow	Colorless	Colorless
Piperidine	Pale yellow and foam	White foam	No change
Piperocaine	Light yellow →deep yellow	Color disappears	Milky white precipitate
Pregnenolone	Pale yellow	Pale yellow	No change
Procaine	Pale yellow	Pale yellow	Deep yellow orange
Procaine.HCl	Pale yellow	Colorless	Deep orange yellow precipitate
Pseudopelletierine	Light yellow	Light yellow	Color deepens slightly
Pyrithyldione	Yellow	Colorless	No change
Quinidine	Yellow with brown cast	Color disappears	White precipitate
Quinine	Light yellow	Color disappears	No change
Salicylic acid	Colorless → yellow	Pale yellow	Color fades; slight precipitate
Santonin	Colorless → very pale yellow on standing	Colorless	No change
Scopolamine	Deep yellow → yellow orange	Colorless	No change
Tetracaine	Light yellow	Colorless	Pale yellow
Terpin hydrate	Yellow with brown cast	Pale yellow	Color fades
Theobromine	Pale yellow	Colorless	No change
Theophylline	Light yellow	Colorless	No change
Thiazolsulfone	Very very pale yellow	Light yellow	Orange precipitate
Thiopental	Pale yellow	White precipitate	No change
Trihexyphenidyl	Pale yellow → deeper yellow with orange cast	Very pale yellow	Cloudy precipitate
Vinbarbital	Very pale yellow	Colorless	Colorless

Table 47-18 (cont.). Nitrosylsulfuric Acid Reaction (109)

COMPOUND	COLOR DEVELOPED WITH NITROSYLSULFURIC ACID	COLOR AFTER ADDITION OF WATER *	COLOR AFTER ADDITION OF CONC. AMMONIA †
BLUE			
Aprobarbital	Colorless → light blue violet with gray cast	Colorless	Colorless
Cinchonine	Light blue violet with gray cast	Colorless	Milky white precipitate
Diallylbarbituric acid	Violet with deep gray cast → gray yellow	Colorless	Colorless
Nicotinic alcohol	Colorless → very pale violet with gray cast	Colorless	Slight cloudiness
Secobarbital	Violet	Colorless	No change
MAGENTA			
Acetophenetidin	Magenta	Yellow precipitate	Pale yellowish
Berberine.SO₄	Very deep magenta with brown cast → red brown	Brick red	Brown with yellow cast
Dromoran	Magenta with brown cast	Pale yellow	Yellow
Methapyrilene §	Deep magenta with brown cast	Deep yellow	Light orange
GRAY			
Digitoxin	Dark gray	Colorless	No change
Urethan	Gray	Colorless	No change
WHITE			
Cholesterol	Heavy white precipitate	No change	Light yellow
COLORLESS			
p-Aminobenzoic acid	Colorless	Colorless	Bright yellow
Benzocaine	Colorless	Colorless	Yellow orange precipitate
Butamin	Colorless	Colorless	Yellow-orange
Chlorobutanol	Colorless	White precipitate	No change
Dibucaine	Colorless	Colorless	Milky precipitate
Diethylacetylurea	Colorless	White precipitate	Colorless
Ortal	Colorless	White precipitate	No change
Succinylsulfathiazole	Colorless	Pale yellow	Pale yellow
Sulfacetimide	Colorless	Colorless	Yellow
Sulfadiazine	Colorless	Colorless	Deep yellow-orange
Sulfanilamide	Colorless	Colorless	Bright yellow
Sulfapyridine	Colorless	Colorless	Pale yellow
Sulfathiazole	Colorless	Colorless	Orange-yellow
Sulfisoxazole	Colorless	Colorless	Light yellow

NEGATIVE REACTION

The following compounds give a colorless reaction (1) with nitrosylsulfuric acid, (2) after addition of water and (3) after addition of concentrated ammonia. The exception is Antabuse which gives a very slight cloudiness after addition of concentrated ammonia.

Amobarbital	Carbromal	Isoamylethylacetylurea	Solanin
Antabuse	Coniine.HCl	Neonal	Sulfonethylmethane
Ascorbic acid	Dichlorodiphenyl-	Nostal	Sulfonmethane
Barbital	trichloroethane (DDT)	Pentamethylenetetrazol	Tribromoethanol
Biuret	Dicoumarol	Pentobarbital	Trimethadione
Bromural	Dicyclomine	Probarbital	
Butabarbital	Digalen	Saccharin	
Cantharidin	Diphenylhydantoin	Sandoptal	
Carbamylcholine chloride	Ethyl biscoumacetate	Sedormid	
	Glycine	Sigmodal	

The compounds in the following tables are arranged alphabetically and according to the most prominent color or else the first color developed with the reagent.

Although the reactions are listed in the order generally preferred by this laboratory for carrying out the testing procedure on unknowns, their selection may be varied by the analyst on the basis of information already available in the particular case.

1. Exclusion and/or Indicating Reactions.

1. Exclusion and/or Indicating Reactions. Although exclusion is the first step in the identification process, indications for certain compounds may be obtained at the same time. The type of reaction cannot be exactly classified except with reference to specific compounds. Consequently, a finer distinction cannot be drawn between the types of reagents than is implied by the combined classification. Reagents in these classes have good sensitivity and react positively with a large number of compounds, making the tests relatively nonspecific. They permit an interpretation as to whether a chemically reactive or nonreactive type of drug is present and also furnish information as to the relative purity of the preparation.

(a) Concentrated Nitrosylsulfuric Acid.* This is a drastic reagent which shows some type of change with all but the very stable organic molecules. Unfortunately, the yellow and brown colorations given by many of the organics are also produced by tissue extract-ables. For this reason, negative findings are significant and also indicate that the tissue extract is relatively free of contaminants. The color produced by tissue impurities is due to the effect of the strong acid and a comparison of the intensity of the reaction with that produced by concentrated sulfuric acid permits an evaluation of even yellow and brown colors that is not possible with nitrosylsulfuric acid alone.

Nitrous acid is liberated on the addition of water and this may act as an oxidizer or react to form diazonium, para-aromatic nitroso compounds, nitrosamines or nitrosamides (page 1056). Strong mineral acid liberates nitrous acid from nitroso compounds but the reaction is not immediate with the more stable ones and, if formed, they are precipitated by ammonia, usually as oils or gelatinous precipitates, some of which are colored. This change on the addition of ammonia is characteristic of many of the local anesthetics. Although seldom necessary, the nitroso derivative may be isolated by dissolving it in ether and confirmed by treating with sulfamic acid to destroy any remaining free nitrite and by testing with the Liebermann reaction (page 1248) (108).

Color, such as the reds and deep oranges that are produced by certain compounds † as a result of the strong acid only, can be recognized as such when the same change is found with concentrated sulfuric acid alone (page 1203).

Procedure. A micro drop of reagent is added to a small quantity of sample while the color is observed by transmitted light. After it has stood for several minutes, two drops of water are added and any change is noted. Fresh concentrated ammonium hydroxide is then added dropwise until all the acid has been neutralized and the appearance of any oil or precipitate and its color are recorded (Table 47-18, page 1192).

(b) para-Dimethylaminobenzaldehyde Reagent (Wasicky's Reagent). Dissolve 1 gm. of para-dimethylaminobenzaldehyde in 1.7 ml. concentrated sulfuric acid and add 0.2 ml. water. The reagent should be prepared fresh each time.

This reagent reacts with many organic substances and is particularly sensitive toward phenolic-type structures although it can undergo condensation with amines to form Schiff's bases (110). The principal colorations are reds, oranges and browns. In certain respects it is the best of the exclusion or indicating reactions as there is a little more variety and depth to the colorations. A number of alkaloids and basic drugs that are relatively nonreactive with the common alkaloidal color reagents react positively in this test. A disadvantage is that not many compounds develop colors in the cold and the heat required to develop the color also produces a darkening when tissue impurities are present. Heating should be carried out on a heating block (Fig. 47-21) maintained at a temperature of 125° C. and should not be heated more than one minute.

There have been many variations in the use of Wasicky's reagent. Para-dimethyl-aminobenzaldehyde is used for the detection of urobilinogen in urine (111) and it has

---

* Umberger, C. J., and Adams, G. Unpublished.
† This is particularly characteristic of certain antihistamines.

Table 47-19. Para-Dimethylaminobenzaldehyde Reagent (115)

COMPOUND	COLOR DEVELOPED WITH p-DIMETHYLAMINOBEN-ZALDEHYDE REAGENT, COLD	COLOR AFTER HEATING ONE MINUTE AT 125° C.	COLOR AFTER WATER DILUTION
RED			
Amprotropine	No reaction	Rose → deep red	Magenta
Ascorbic acid	No reaction	Slowly changes to deep red with orange cast → brick red	Pale green
Atropine	No reaction	Dark red	Dark magenta
Desoxycholic acid	Yellow	Red → deep red with brown cast	Deep blue → deep green
Dicyclomine	Pale brown	Brown → very deep red with brown cast	Olive green
Phenylsalicylate	Light yellow	Red with orange cast	Violet → magenta
Pyridium	Deep red with orange cast	Deep red with orange cast	Orange
Scopolamine	No reaction	Rose → deep red	Magenta; fades
Vinbarbital	Slowly turns very light red	Red orange → deep brick red	Light green
ORANGE			
Acetylsalicylic acid	No reaction	Light orange	Rose
Antipyrine	Yellow with orange cast	Deep orange with red cast	Bright red with orange cast
Aprobarbital	No reaction	Slowly turns orange	Color fades
Chrysazin	No change from original orange	No change from original orange	Yellow
Cinchonidine	No reaction	Very light orange	Color fades
Cinchonine	No reaction	Light orange	No change
Colchicine	Yellow → yellow with orange cast	Orange → orange with yellow cast	Bright yellow
Dihydromorphinone	Rose → orange	Red with orange cast → orange with red cast	Color fades
Diothane	Orange with brown cast → orange	Orange with red cast	Deep yellow with green cast
Dromoran	No reaction	Red with orange cast → orange with red cast	Color fades
Ethylmorphine	Orange with red cast → red with orange cast	Red with orange cast → deep orange with red cast	Color fades
Heroin	Orange	Red with orange cast → orange with red-brown cast	Color fades
Isoamylethyl-acetylurea	Light yellow	Slowly changes to light orange	Yellow
Larocaine	Yellow with orange cast	Orange with yellow cast	Bright yellow
Meconin	No reaction	Orange with red cast → orange	Magenta; fades
Mephenesine	Pale orange → salmon pink	Red with orange cast → deep orange with red cast	Bright magenta
Metopon	Faint orange rose	Red with orange cast → orange with red cast	Color fades
Morphine	Red → light red with orange cast → orange	Deep red with orange cast → orange with brown cast	Light red; fades
Narceine	Orange	Orange with red cast → orange	Color fades
Narcotine	Orange	Orange with red cast → orange	Color fades
Pavatrine	Pale brown	Orange with brown cast	Pale yellow precipitate
Prisilidene	No reaction	Very light orange with yellow cast	Color fades
Procaine	Light yellow	Orange with brown cast	Deep yellow with orange cast
Procaine amide	Yellow with orange cast	Orange with yellow cast	Deep orange; bright yellow solution

Table 47-19 (cont.). Para-Dimethylaminobenzaldehyde Reagent (115)

Compound	Color Developed with p-Dimethylaminoben-zaldehyde Reagent, Cold	Color after Heating One Minute at 125° C.	Color after Water Dilution
Procaine.HCl	Yellow	Orange with yellow cast	Deep orange; bright yellow solution
Pyrithyldione	Very pale orange	Orange with red cast → orange	Color fades
Quinidine	No reaction	Light orange	Color fades
Quinine	Very pale yellow	Light orange	Color fades
Salicylic acid	No reaction	Light orange with yellow cast	Color fades

BROWN

Compound			
Aconitine	No reaction	Light brown	Light violet
N-Allylnormorphine	Brown → orange with red cast	Orange with red cast → brown with yellow cast	Light red
Amphetamine base	Orange with brown cast → brown	Brown with red cast → brown	Slight violet with brown cast
Apomorphine	Brown	Brown	No change
Apothesine	No change from original	Brown	Pale magenta; fades
Butallylonal	No reaction	Light brown	Light red-brown; fades
Cephaeline	No change from original brown	Brown	No change
Codeine	Orange with brown cast	Brick red → brown	Color fades
Curarine	No reaction	Light brown	Violet trace; color fades
Delphinine	Pale orange → pale brown	Brown	Greenish
d-Desoxyephedrine	Orange with brown cast	Brown	Light green
Diallylbarbituric acid	No reaction	Orange with brown cast → brown	Brown with red cast
Digalen	Light orange	Deep brown	Color fades
Digitalin	Light brown	Dark brown	Slight violet
Digitonin	No reaction	Deep brown	Deep magenta
Digitoxin	Brown	Very dark brown, almost black	Greenish
Emetine	No change from original brown	Brown with red cast	Greenish
Ephedrine	Light brown	Brown	Color fades
Ethyl biscoum-acetate	Brownish	Light brown	Bluish white precipitate
Hexobarbital	Slight yellow	Yellow with brown cast → brown with yellow cast	No change
Homatropine	No reaction	Trace of brown	Color fades
Hydrastine	No reaction	Slowly turns brown	Color fades
Lobeline	No change from original red-brown	Brown with yellow cast	Very slight magenta; fades
l-Menthol	No reaction	Orange → deep red → brown	Blue → green → brown
Meperidine	No reaction	Light brown	Color fades
Mephobarbital	Pale yellow	Light brown	Blue violet; fades
Mescaline	Brown → orange	Brown with red cast → dark brown	Brown
Methadon	No change from original	Light brown	Trace of blue violet
Methylparafynol	Orange → brown	Deep brown	Brown with violet cast
Methylphenyl-ethylhydantoin	No reaction	Very pale brown	Color fades
Nicotine	Magenta	Magenta, changing quickly to brown with orange cast	Magenta
Nicotinic alcohol	No reaction	Very light brown	Color fades
Pamaquine	No change from original dark brown	Brown with orange cast	Dark green, changing rapidly to brown with red cast
Pelletierine tannate	No change from original brown	Deep brown	No change
Phanadorn	Yellow	Orange with brown cast → deep brown with orange cast	No change

Table 47-19 (cont.). Para-Dimethylaminobenzaldehyde Reagent (115)

Compound	Color Developed with p-Dimethylaminobenzaldehyde Reagent, Cold	Color after Heating One Minute at 125° C.	Color after Water Dilution
Phenindamine	No change from original red brown	Brown	Color fades
Piperidione	Very light brown	Very deep brown	Deep purple
Piperine	Deep yellow	Deep brown	Greenish
Piperocaine	No reaction	Light brown	Color fades
Pregnenolone	Red	Red → deep brown with red cast	Brown
Ricin	Very pale yellow	Light brown	Color fades
Rutin	Deep yellow	Orange → deep brown	Blue → dark green
Salicin	Orange	Deep red → brown	Deep blue violet
Sandoptal	No reaction	Light brown with red cast	Color fades
Santonin	No reaction	Deep brown	Deep blue → violet
Secobarbital	No reaction	Orange → brown	Bluish; greenish
Sedormid	Pale yellow	Yellow with brown cast → light brown with red cast	Greenish
Solanin	Red	Red with brown cast → magenta with brown cast → deep brown	Purple
Sparteine	No change from original brown	Light brown	Color fades
Strophanthin	No change from original brown	Deep brown	Blue violet with deep gray cast
Terpin hydrate	Red with brown cast	Deep red → deep brown	Deep blue → gray
Thymol iodide	No reaction	Very faint brown	Color fades
Trihexyphenidyl	No reaction	Light brown	Color fades
Veratrine	Pale yellow with brown cast	Deep brown	Blue violet; fades to brown
Xylocaine	No change from original brown	Deep brown	No change
Yohimbine	Deep blue violet	Brown	Color fades

YELLOW

Compound	Color Developed with p-Dimethylaminobenzaldehyde Reagent, Cold	Color after Heating One Minute at 125° C.	Color after Water Dilution
Acetanilid	No reaction	Yellow	Yellow
Acetophenetidin	No reaction	Light yellow	Color fades
Acridine.HCl	No change from original Yellow	No change from original yellow	No change
p-Aminobenzoic acid	Pale yellow	Yellow	Bright orange; yellow solution
Atabrin	Yellow	Yellow	No change
Benzocaine	Slowly changes to yellow	Orange → yellow	Orange
Berberine.SO₄	No change from original yellow	Yellow	No change
Biuret	Yellow	Yellow	Flash of violet; yellow
Bromural	Light yellow	Light yellow	No change
Butamin	Light orange	Yellow with orange cast	Orange; yellow solution
Carbamylcholine chloride	Yellow	Yellow	Color fades
Carbromal	Light yellow	Yellow	No change
Chlorcyclizine	Very light brown	Yellow with brown cast	No change
Chlorobutanol	No reaction	Light yellow	No change
Cysteine.HCl	Yellow	Effervescence; bright yellow	Yellow
Dimenhydrinate (basic extraction product)	Yellow	Yellow	Whitish precipitate
Diphenhydramine	Yellow	Yellow	Whitish precipitate
alpha-Naphthylthio-urea (ANTU)	Pale brown	Yellow	Yellow
Phenylbutazone	No reaction	Yellow	Yellow
Phthalylsulfathiazole	Very pale yellow	Light yellow	Bright yellow
Pseudopelletierine	No reaction	Deep yellow	Orange
Strychnine	No reaction	Yellow with orange cast	Color fades
Succinylsulfathiazole	Slight orange	Orange → yellow	Bright yellow
Sulfacetimide	Pale yellow	Yellow	Bright yellow

Table 47-19 (cont.). Para-Dimethylaminobenzaldehyde Reagent (115)

Compound	Color Developed with p-Dimethylaminoben-zaldehyde Reagent, Cold	Color after Heating One Minute at 125° C.	Color after Water Dilution
Sulfadiazine	Pale orange with yellow cast	Orange with yellow cast → yellow	Orange; bright yellow solution
Sulfanilamide	Yellow	Yellow	Deep orange; yellow solution
Sulfapyridine	No reaction	Yellow	Orange; bright yellow solution
Sulfathiazole	Very pale orange	Yellow with orange cast	Orange; bright yellow solution
Sulfisoxazole	No reaction	Yellow	Bright yellow
Thiazolsulfone	Pale yellow with orange cast	Yellow	Deep orange; yellow solution
Thiobarbituric acid	Pale yellow	Yellow with orange cast	Bright red
p-Toluenesul-fonamide	Yellow	Bright yellow	Yellowish precipitate
Urethan	Bright yellow	Yellow with orange cast	Orange

GREEN

Eucupin.di HCl	No reaction	Green with gray blue cast	Brown

BLUE

Cyclopal	Deep magenta	Very deep blue violet, almost black	Very dark green
Estrone	No reaction	Magenta → deep blue with violet cast	Blue → green → blue green
Thenylpyramine	Magenta	Deep magenta → very deep blue violet with gray cast	Olive green

MAGENTA

Cholesterol	No reaction	Magenta with brown cast	Greenish
Hyoscyamine	No reaction	Red, slowly changing to magenta	Magenta; fades
Pyrilamine	Orange → brown	Orange → magenta → magenta with brown cast	Color fades
Thonzylamine	Light magenta	Deep magenta	Color fades; white precipitate
Zolamine.HCl	Slowly changes to magenta	Magenta	Color fades

WHITE

Antabuse	Whitish precipitate	Whitish precipitate	Yellowish precipitate

NO REACTION EXCEPT WITH WATER

Cantharidin	No reaction	No reaction	White precipitate
Dicoumarol	No reaction	No reaction	White precipitate
Pilocarpine	No reaction	No reaction	Magenta
Tetracaine	No reaction	No reaction	Yellow; fades

NO REACTION

Adiphenine	Cocaine	Histamine.di HCl	Probarbital
Aminopyrine	Coniine.HCl	Neonal	Saccharin
Amobarbital	Dibucaine	Nikethamide	Sigmodal
Amphetamine.HCl	Dichlorodiphenyltri-chloroethane (DDT)	Nostal	Sulfonethyl-methane
Barbital	Diethylacetylurea	Optochin	Sulfonmethane
Betaine.HCl	Dimenhydrinate (acidic extraction product)	Ortal	Theobromine
Brucine		Pentamethylene-tetrazol	Theophylline
Butabarbital	Diphenylhydantoin	Pentobarbital	Thiopental
Butallylonal	Glycine	Phenobarbital	Tribromoethanol
Caffeine	Hippuric acid	Phenylacetylurea	Trimethadione
Cinchophen			

been used in various types of solutions with hydrochloric and acetic acids as a reagent for different drugs (112-114). Any substance that reacts in any one of the modifications reacts as well or better in the original procedure in which the reagent, dissolved in concentrated sulfuric acid, is prepared fresh. The shade of color and even the color hue, with certain compounds, is determined by the composition of the reagent. A reagent that is not freshly prepared is reactive but not all of the drugs will give the same colorations with freshly prepared reagent as with old reagent. Even variations in the ratio of para-dimethylaminobenzaldehyde to sulfuric acid and the proportion of added water affect the colors so that, for reproducibility, the preparation of the reagent is critical and should be freshly made in order to maintain controlled conditions. Dilution with water gives added information without sacrificing sample material. A change in the color hue or the formation of a colored precipitate which is probably a condensation product is characteristic for certain of the drugs. The reagent itself is light yellow in color. The yellow intensifies with the addition of water and this should not be confused with a positive reaction. The intensified yellow has a slight influence on the color developed by the reaction (page 1189).

Procedure. Add a drop of reagent to a small sample of unknown on a microscope slide and observe while it stands five minutes in the cold. Then place it on a heating block maintained at a temperature of 125° C. and observe while heated for not more than one minute. A piece of filter paper between the slide and heating block furnishes a white background which makes color changes more readily detectable. Observe under the microscope with transmitted and reflected light any color developed after heating one minute. Add a drop of water and record any color change or precipitate.

(c) Tetranitromethane.* At one time tetranitromethane was thought to be trinitromethylnitrite $[(NO_2)_3CONO]$ because of the exceptional reactivity of one of the four nitro groups (116). It forms colored complexes with a variety of structures, having a particular affinity for compounds with unsaturated linkages and considerable work has been done toward applying the reagent as a test for unsaturations (117-121). Werner (122) made one of the first studies concerning the color and constitution of the products of the reaction with different structures. He reported the formation of intensely colored addition compounds with aromatic polynitro compounds, aromatic bases and amides. Yellow colors formed with unsaturated hydrocarbons were found to be more intense the greater the degree of unsaturation. Unsaturated fatty acids reacted like unsaturated hydrocarbons, except where the double bond was next to the carbonyl group. Tertiary amines can undergo degradation with formation of nitrosamines (123, 124) and, under proper conditions, a nitro group may be introduced into the aromatic nucleus of a dialkylarylamine (125).

Tetranitromethane is much better as a reagent for excluding drugs than is indicated by first impressions when it is used. The colors are not intense and yellows predominate, so that tissue impurities might be expected to mask the reaction. However, the non-aqueous solution is not influenced significantly by the normal extractives from tissue and even minor yellow colorations can be interpreted with greater certainty than is possible with aqueous reactions. The range of positive reactions is not as great, but a few structures do react which are negative with the preceding reagents. Only the free base or acid reacts, probably because the salts are insoluble. Thus, procaine base gives an intense red while procaine hydrochloride is nonreactive (Table 47-20, page 1202).

Procedure. The test is carried out by allowing a drop of reagent to flow across the solid on a microscope slide while it is observed against a white background.

ALKALOIDAL REAGENTS. There are six reagents that have long been used in pharmaceutic and toxicologic analysis that are known as the alkaloidal color reagents. These are Marquis' reagent (containing formalin as the active agent), Mecke's reagent (selenic acid), Froehde's reagent (molybdic acid), Mandelin's reagent (vanadic acid), Erdman's reagent (nitric acid) and Rosenthaler's reagent (arsenic acid) and they are usually designated in the literature by the name of their originator, rather than by their chemical composition. These are made up in concentrated sulfuric acid and all but the first are oxidants. Alkaloids which are reactive toward one usually react positively with most of them and, considering the difficulty in interpreting color shades on tissue residues, the

* Obtainable from the Nitroform Company, Newark, New Jersey.

Table 47-20. Tetranitromethane Test (115, 126)

Compound	Color Developed with Tetranitromethane	Compound	Color Developed with Tetranitromethane
RED			
Brucine	Red with brown cast	Piperocaine	Brick red → orange → yellow
Digitalin	No change from original red		
		Prisilidene	Brick red → orange
Dimenhydrinate (basic extraction product)	Brick red → orange	Procaine	Brick red → orange
		Pseudopelletierine	Brick red → deep red orange
Larocaine	Brick red → orange	Pyrilamine	Brick red with orange cast
Lobeline	Red with brown cast		
Phenindamine	Red with brown cast	Thenylpyramine	Red with brown cast
Pilocarpine	Red with brown cast	Thonzylamine	Brick red → orange
ORANGE			
Acetophenetidin	Very pale orange	Heroin	Pale orange with yellow cast
Aminopyrine	Orange with yellow solution		
		Hydrastine	Orange
Antabuse	Orange	Hyoscyamine	Pale orange with yellow cast
Antipyrine	Orange		
Atropine	Pale orange with yellow cast	Meperidine	Orange
		Methadon	Orange
Benzocaine	Orange	Narceine	Pale orange with yellow cast
Butamin	Orange with red cast		
Codeine	Orange	Narcotine	Pale orange with yellow cast
Dicyclomine	Orange with red cast		
Diphenhydramine	Orange	Scopolamine	Orange → orange yellow
Diothane	Orange	Strychnine	Orange with pink cast
Ethylmorphine	Orange with red cast	Tetracaine	Orange with pink cast
BROWN			
Atabrin	Brown	Strophanthin	Brown with yellow cast
Emetine	Brown with red cast	Xylocaine	No change from original brown
Pamaquine	Brown		
Sparteine	Brown with yellow cast		
YELLOW			
Acetanilid	Pale yellow	Homatropine	Very very pale yellow
Aconitine	Pale yellow with brown cast	Meconin	Light yellow
		Metopon	Light yellow
Adiphenine	Yellow	Optochin	Very pale yellow
Amphetamine	Yellow with brown cast	Nicotinic alcohol	Pale yellow which fades
Amprotropine	Very pale yellow	Pavatrine (acidic and basic extraction)	Light yellow
Apothesine	Very pale yellow		
Caffeine	Yellow with orange cast → yellow		
		Phenylbutazone	Yellow
Cholesterol	Very pale yellow	Phenylsalicylate	Yellow
Cocaine	Yellow with orange cast → yellow	Piperine	Yellow with orange cast
		Pregnenolone	Yellow with orange cast
Coniine	Pale yellow	Procaine amide	Light yellow
Curarine	Light yellow	Pyrithyldione	Very light yellow
Delphinine	No change from original yellow	Quinine	Pale yellow with orange cast
d-Desoxyephedrine	Yellow	Rutin	No change from original very pale yellow
Dibucaine	Yellow with orange cast	Succinylsulfathiazole	Very light yellow
Digalen	Yellow with brown cast		
Digitoxin	Very pale yellow	Thiopental	Very pale yellow
Ephedrine	Bright yellow	Trihexyphenidyl	Light yellow
Ethyl biscoumacetate	Light yellow	Veratrine	Light yellow
		Yohimbine	Very pale yellow
GREEN			
Apomorphine	Very very dark green, almost black		

Table 47-20 (cont.). Tetranitromethane Test (115, 126)

NEGATIVE REACTION

Acetylsalicylic acid	Dicoumarol	Phenobarbital	Sulfathiazole
N-Allylnormorphine	Digitonin	Phthalylsulfathiazole	Sulfisoxazole
p-Aminobenzoic acid	Dihydromorphinone	Physostigmine	Sulfonethylmethane
Amobarbital	Dimenhydrinate (acidic	Picrotoxin	Sulfonmethane
Ascorbic acid	extraction product)	Piperidione	Theobromine
Bromural	Estrone	Quinidine	Theophylline
Cantharidin	Eucupin.di HCl	Ricin	Thiamin.HCl
Carbamylcholine	Glycine	Saccharin	Thiazolsulfone
chloride	Hippuric acid	Salicin	Tribromoethanol
Carbromal	Isoamylethylacetylurea	Santonin	Trimethadione
Chlorobutanol	Methylphenylethyl-	Solanin	Urethan
Cinchonidine	hydantoin	Sulfacetimide	Xylocaine
Cinchonine	Morphine	Sulfadiazine	
Cinchophen	Nikethamide	Sulfanilamide	
Desoxycholic acid	Pentamethylenetetrazol	Sulfapyridine	

group taken as a whole does not give much more information toward identifying a particular alkaloid than is obtained from two of them, Marquis' and Mecke's reagents. The sensitivity and the predominant color produced differ significantly among these reagents. Except in special cases, Marquis' and Mecke's reagents are far superior to the others for general testing so that they are the only members of the group of value as excluding or indicating reactions.

Many nonalkaloidal drugs giving color reactions are now available and the overlapping of positive reactions with the alkaloidal reagents holds equally well for the newer drugs as well as for the alkaloids. There are exceptions in which only one of the alkaloidal reagents gives reactions that are truly characteristic for a single substance. Consequently, in these cases, the reagents become valuable as designating or differential type reagents but, in general, for exclusion or indicating purposes, little will be learned from all of them that is not apparent from the use of Marquis' and Mecke's reagents alone. The use of the others, therefore, is better restricted to analyses later in the identification process when there is evidence for a particular type of compound or a specific substance.

The reagent of Rosenthaler is least sensitive and least characteristic of the so-called alkaloidal reagents. Moreover, there is not a single positive reaction with a compound that is not given better with one of the other five reagents. Since its use does not aid in identifying unknown drugs, the data for the reaction have not been included.

(a) Sulfuric Acid and the Modified Erdmann's Reagent. Many color reactions are carried out in concentrated sulfuric acid which serves as the solvent. Since some substances react with it alone to give colors, while others are charred, with the formation of yellowish to dark brown and even black colorations, it is essential that the behavior of the compound in sulfuric acid alone be determined in order to make the interpretation of the hues in the color reactions of greater significance. The major reason for establishing the effect of sulfuric acid alone on the sample is that normal extractables are darkened by the strong acid and the extent of the darkening increases with the contamination. An idea of the relative purity of the extract can be estimated from the action of the acid and a better comparison of the sensitivity and the color shade of the unknown with the behavior of the pure compounds is made possible. Moreover, establishing the degree of darkening in acid alone permits a correction for the observed color to be made from the basic color theory for color reactions (pages 1185-1190).

Sulfuric Acid. Compounds such as dimenhydrinate (the basic extraction product), salicin, diphenhydramine, thenylpyramine, phenindamine, pyrilamine, thonzylamine, mescaline, colchicine, veratrine and zolamine® are especially reactive to sulfuric acid alone and consequently react with all other sulfuric acid-containing reagents although frequently with a change in color shade (Table 47-21, page 1204).

*Modified Erdmann's Reagent.** Erdmann's reagent is concentrated sulfuric acid containing a small amount of nitric acid, and it is just above Rosenthaler's reagent in a list

* Umberger, C. J., and Adams, G. Unpublished.

Table 47-21. Concentrated Sulfuric Acid (109)

COMPOUND	COLOR OF THE EXTRACTED COMPOUND	COLOR DEVELOPED WITH CONC. SULFURIC ACID
RED		
Amphetamine.HCl	Brown with orange cast	Light red or red brown
Cholesterol	White	Red orange →brick red
Chrysazin	Orange	Carmine
Dimenhydrinate (basic extraction product)	Pale yellow	Deep brick red with yellow solution
Heroin	Grayish	Very pale flesh
Mephenesine	Very pale pink	No change from original color
Piperine	Sandy	Brick red →deep red with brown cast
Pyridium	Deep red	Bright red
Salicin	White	Orange-rose or rose
ORANGE		
Cyclopal	White	Orange with brown cast
Delphinine	Pale yellow	Orange with brown cast
d-Desoxyephedrine	Pale orange with brown cast	No change from original color
Digitonin	White	Very faint yellow → light orange
Diphenhydramine	Very pale yellow	Deep orange precipitate with yellow solution
Hexobarbital	Sandy	Very pale orange
l-Menthol	Colorless	Slowly changes to flesh or pale orange
Methapyrilene	Very pale yellow	Orange with red cast → brick red
Phanadorn	Sandy	Orange → orange with yellow cast
Procaine amide	Pale orange with brown cast	No change from original color
Rutin	Yellow	Orange with yellow cast
Terpin hydrate	White or colorless	Orange with yellow cast
Thenylpyramine	Pale yellow	Orange → red orange → deep orange with brown cast
BROWN		
N-Allylnormorphine	Light brown	Original color darkens
Apothesine	Golden brown	Color deepens
Codeine	Light brown or yellowish brown	Brown with violet cast
Curarine	Yellow with brown cast	Pale brown with yellow cast
Digitalin	Deep red	Brown with red cast
Digitoxin	Beige	Brown
Diothane	Brown	No change from original color
Emetine	Brown with red cast	No change from original color
Ephedrine	Yellow or gold	Light gray brown
Ethylmorphine	Light yellow brown	Brown, somewhat grayed
Lobeline	Brown with red cast	No change from original color
Mescaline	Brown with yellow cast	Yellow → brown → greenish brown → olive green
Pamaquine	Brown	No change from original color
Pavatrine	Yellow	Brown
Pelletierine tannate	Brown	Brown with yellow cast
Phenindamine	Deep brown red	Deep brown with orange cast
Sparteine	Brown	No change from original color
Strophanthin	Brown	No change from original color
Xylocaine	Brown	No change from original color
YELLOW		
Acridine.HCl	Yellow	Lemon yellow
Amphetamine base	Yellow with orange cast	Yellow with greenish or light brownish cast
Atabrin	Yellow with brown cast	Bright yellow
Berberine.SO₄	Deep yellow	Bright yellow
Butamin	Pale yellow	No change from original color
Cephaeline	Brown with reddish or yellowish cast	Light yellow
Chlorcyclizine	Pale yellow with brown cast	Light yellow with brown cast
Cinchophen	White	Light yellow
Colchicine	Cream	Light yellow
Dicyclomine	Yellow	Very pale yellow
Digalen	Pale yellow	No change from original color

Table 47-21 (cont.). Concentrated Sulfuric Acid (109)

COMPOUND	COLOR OF THE EXTRACTED COMPOUND	COLOR DEVELOPED WITH CONC. SULFURIC ACID
Estrone	White	Slowly changes to pale yellow
Larocaine	Light yellow with orange cast	Original color darkens, fades
Meconin	White	Pale yellow
Meperidine	Pale yellow	No change from original color
Methadon	Yellowish	Deeper yellow
Methylparafynol	Pale yellow	Yellow with brown cast
Narcotine	White	Pale yellow → lemon yellow
Nicotine	Yellow with brown cast	No change from original color
Piperocaine	Yellow with brown cast	No change from original color
Pregnenolone	White	Yellow → deep yellow with orange cast
Procaine	Pale yellow	No change from original color
Quinine	Sandy or very pale yellow	No change from original color
Santonin	White	Very pale yellow
Solanin	White	Yellow → orange
Thymol iodide	Yellow	No change from original color
Trihexyphenidyl	White	Pale yellow
Veratrine	White	Deep yellow, slowly changing to orange → red orange → red → magenta
Vinbarbital	Cream	Light yellow

GREEN

Apomorphine	Blackish	Dirty olive green to brownish
alpha-Naphthylthiourea (ANTU)	Gray	Very pale green or colorless

MAGENTA

Pyrilamine	Light yellow	Magenta
Thonzylamine	Very pale yellow	Magenta
Zolamine.HCl	White	Magenta

COLORLESS OR NEARLY COLORLESS COMPOUNDS GIVING NO CHANGE

COMPOUND	COLOR OF THE EXTRACTED COMPOUND	COMPOUND	COLOR OF THE EXTRACTED COMPOUND
Acetanilid	White	Metopon	Very very pale yellow
Acetophenetidin	White		
Acetylsalicylic acid	White	Morphine	Beige or pale yellow
Aconitine	White	Narceine	Pale yellow or beige
Adiphenine	Colorless	Neonal	White
Aminopyrine	White	Nicotinic alcohol	Very very pale brown
p-Aminobenzoic acid	White		
Amobarbital	White	Nikethamide	Colorless
Amprotropine	White	Nostal	White
Antabuse	White	Optochin	White
Antipyrine	White	Ortal	White
Aprobarbital	White	Pentamethylenetetrazol	White
Ascorbic acid	White	Pentobarbital	White
Atropine	White	Phenobarbital	White
Barbital	White	Phenylacetylurea	White
Benzocaine	White	Phenylbutazone	White
Betaine.HCl	White	Phenylsalicylate	White
Biuret	White	Phthalylsulfathiazole	Beige
Bromural	White	Pilocarpine	Colorless or very pale yellow
Brucine	White		
Butabarbital	White	Piperidione	White
Butallylonal	White	Prisilidene	Colorless
Caffeine	White	Probarbital	White
Cantharidin	White	Procaine.HCl	White
Carbamylcholine chloride	White	Pseudopelletierine	Beige or pale yellow
Carbromal	White	Pyrithyldione	White
Chlorobutanol	White	Quinidine	White
Cinchonidine	White	Ricin	White
Cinchonine	White	Saccharin	White
Cocaine	White	Salicylic acid	White
Coniine.HCl	White	Sandoptal	White
Cysteine.HCl	Beige	Scopolamine	Colorless
		Secobarbital	White or colorless

Table 47-21 (cont.). Concentrated Sulfuric Acid (109)

Compound	Color of the Extracted Compound	Compound	Color of the Extracted Compound
Desoxycholic acid	White	Sedormid	White
Diallylbarbituric acid	White	Sigmodal	White
Dibucaine	White or cream	Strychnine	White
Dichlorodiphenyltri-chloroethane (DDT)	White	Succinylsulfathiazole	Beige or cream
		Sulfacetimide	White
Dicoumarol	White	Sulfadiazine	Cream
Diethylacetylurea	White	Sulfanilamide	White
Dihydromorphinone	Sandy or beige	Sulfapyridine	White
Diphenylhydantoin	White	Sulfathiazole	White
Dimenhydrinate (acidic extraction product)	White	Sulfisoxazole	White
		Sulfonethylmethane	White
Dromoran	White	Sulfonmethane	White
Ethyl biscoumacetate	White	Tetracaine	Cream
Eucupin.di HCl	White	Theobromine	Beige
Glycine	White	Theophylline	White
Hexobarbital	Beige	Thiamin degradation product	Very pale yellow
Hippuric acid	White		
Histamine.di HCl	White	Thiazolsulfone	Beige or cream
Homatropine	Beige or very pale yellow	Thiobarbituric acid	Pale flesh
		Thiopental	White
Hydrastine	White	p-Toluenesulfonamide	White
Hyoscyamine	White	Tribromoethanol	White
Isoamylethylacetylurea	White	Trimethadione	White
Mephobarbital	White	Urethan	White
Merthiolate	White	Yohimbine	Very pale yellow
Methylphenylethyl-hydantoin	White		

of alkaloidal reagents tabulated in the order of their value as reagents. Its use as a separate test could only be justified where there is adequate sample material. However, a modification, in which the test sample with concentrated sulfuric acid alone is held over fuming nitric acid was found to give nearly the same colorations with even greater sensitivity in some cases than the conventional reagent. Since the sulfuric acid test is essential, there is a possibility for obtaining information by following it with the modification of the Erdmann reaction without using additional sample material. For this reason, tables for the modified Erdmann's reaction are listed with the exclusion and indicating reactions although, at best, it is not more than a designating or differential test for a few compounds.

Color changes are predominantly noncharacteristic yellows and browns. It will differentiate phenylsalicylate from other salicylates and designates yohimbine after positive findings with Mecke's reagent. Acetophenetidin gives a green color in contrast with the intense yellow produced by nitric acid alone while the conventional Erdmann's reagent gives only a weak yellow color. The color produced with estrone and meconin is good while the reaction with brucine is quite sensitive * (Table 47-22, page 1207).

(b) Marquis' and Mecke's Reagents. These reagents are superior to any of the other reagents for excluding or indicating basic drugs. The fact that they are not listed higher in the suggested order of preference for the testing procedure is because they are less applicable to the acidic and neutral type of organic compound. Marquis' reagent has a somewhat wider latitude as it reacts positively with a greater variety of structures. It undergoes condensation with aromatic ring structures to produce yellow and brown colors (page 1189). With complex bases, the predominating colors are red, magenta or blue violet which are relatively low in value and chroma. Mecke's reagent is a little more selective for basic compounds, giving blue to green colorations of relatively high value and moderate chroma with the important bases. The sensitivity is comparable with both reagents and the hue developed with the pure compound is intense and readily seen. When the reagents are applied to tissue extracts, the darkening which is produced on impure residues by the action of the acid on normal tissue extractables throws the colors produced by either reagent on the drug toward the dark side. The visual response

---

* Brucine in sulfuric acid is a reagent for nitrates (page 1026).

Table 47-22. Modified Erdmann's Reaction (109)

COMPOUND	COLOR WITH CONCENTRATED SULFURIC ACID	COLOR AFTER EXPOSING SULFURIC ACID SOLUTION TO FUMING NITRIC ACID FOR ½ TO 1 MIN.	COLOR AFTER WATER DILUTION
RED			
Amphetamine.HCl	Light red or brown	No change	Color fades
Ascorbic acid	Colorless	Colorless; on standing 10-15 minutes, a very pale rose develops	Effervescence
Atabrin	Bright yellow	Brick red	Bright orange yellow
Chrysazin	Carmine red	Red with yellow solution	Milky yellow orange precipitate
Estrone	Colorless → pale yellow	Light red with orange cast, slowly changing to brick red	Pale yellow
Mephenesine	Very pale pink	No change	Colorless
Narcotine	Pale yellow → lemon yellow	Brown with red cast → red with orange cast, slowly changing to orange, then to yellow	Yellow
Pyridium	Bright red	Red with orange cast	Color lightens
Pyrilamine	Magenta	Deep carmine or red with brown cast	Orange red → brick red
Salicin	Orange-rose or rose	Brick red	Pale yellow with carmine streaks → light orange yellow
Thenylpyramine	Orange → red orange → deep orange with brown cast	Deep carmine red	Brown
Thonzylamine	Magenta	Deep carmine or red with brown cast	Purple with brown cast
Veratrine	Deep yellow → orange → red-orange → red → magenta	Brick red → pale red with orange cast	Pale yellow
Zolamine.HCl	Red-violet → magenta	Carmine	Red-purple precipitate
ORANGE			
Adiphenine	Colorless	Orange	White precipitate
Aminopyrine	Colorless	Pale orange	Color fades
Brucine	Colorless	Immediately, bright orange with red cast → orange with yellow cast	Yellow-orange
Codeine	Brown with violet cast	Light orange with brown cast	Light orange-yellow
Curarine	Pale brown with yellow cast	Pale orange with yellow cast	No change
Delphinine	Orange with brown cast	Color deepens	Color pales
Meconin	Pale yellow	Golden or orange with yellow cast	Pale yellow
Terpin hydrate	Orange with yellow cast	Orange	Brownish orange precipitate
Thymol iodide	No change from original yellow	Light orange	Light orange
BROWN			
Apomorphine	Dirty olive green to brownish	Deep brown with red cast	Color pales
Apothesine	No change from original golden brown	Color lightens	Pale yellow precipitate
Berberine.SO₄	Bright yellow	Deep brown	White precipitate
Cholesterol	Red orange → brick red	Deep brick red → brown	No change
Colchicine	Bright yellow	Brownish → very pale yellow	No change
d-Desoxyephedrine	Pale orange with brown cast	Brown with yellow cast	Slight white precipitate
Dicyclomine	Very pale yellow	Pale yellow with brownish cast	White precipitate

Table 47-22 (cont.). Modified Erdmann's Reaction (109)

COMPOUND	COLOR WITH CONCENTRATED SULFURIC ACID	COLOR AFTER EXPOSING SULFURIC ACID SOLUTION TO FUMING NITRIC ACID FOR ½ TO 1 MIN.	COLOR AFTER WATER DILUTION
Digalen	Pale yellow	Brown	No change
Digitalin	Brown with red cast	Brown	Color pales
Digitoxin	Brown	No change	Color pales
Dimenhydrinate (basic extraction product)	Brick red; yellow solution	Brown with red cast	Brownish yellow precipitate
Diphenhydramine	Deep orange precipitate with yellow solution	Brown with deep orange cast	Yellow orange precipitate
Diothane	No change from original brown	Brown with yellow cast	Deep gold, pales
Emetine	No change from original brown with red cast	Brown deepens	Pales to orange yellow
Ethylmorphine	Brown, somewhat grayed	Brown with yellow cast	Pale yellow
Hydrastine	Colorless	Brown with yellow cast	Yellow
Lobeline	No change from original brown with red cast	No change	Cloudy whitish precipitate
Mescaline	Yellow → brown → greenish brown → olive green	Brown with gold cast	Yellow orange
Morphine	Colorless	Brown with gray-yellow cast	No change
alpha-Naphthyl-thiourea	Very very pale green	Brownish	Yellow or orange with brown cast
Narceine	Colorless	Brown with red cast	Light yellow orange
Nicotine	No change from original yellow with brown cast	Brown with yellow cast	No change
Pamaquine	No change from original brown	Brown with yellow cast	Orange brown
Pavatrine	Brown	Brown with yellow or yellow green background	Yellow precipitate
Pelletierine tannate	Brown with yellow cast	No change	Pale yellow
Phenindamine	Brown with orange cast	Brown with yellow cast	Yellow precipitate
Piperine	Deep red → deep brownish red	Brown	Brown with yellow cast
Prisilidene	Colorless	Gold → brown → light brown	Light yellow
Sparteine	No change from original brown	No change	No change
Strophanthin	No change from original brown	Brown with yellow cast	No change
Thiamin degradation product	No change from original light brown	No change	Color fades
Xylocaine	No change from original brown	Brown with yellow cast	Yellow with brown cast

---

YELLOW

Acetanilid	Colorless	Pale yellow	White precipitate
Acetophenetidin	Colorless	Pale yellow streaks with greenish cast	Yellow precipitate
Acetylsalicylic acid	Colorless	Very pale yellow	Bright yellow with pale precipitate
Acridine.HCl	Lemon yellow	Lemon yellow	Lemon yellow
N-Allylnormorphine	Original light brown darkens	Yellow with brown cast	Light yellow
p-Aminobenzoic acid	Colorless	Bright yellow	Color fades
Amphetamine base	Yellow with greenish or brownish cast	Gold	Slight pale yellow precipitate
Amprotropine	Colorless or very very pale yellow	Yellow with orange cast	Whitish precipitate

Table 47-22 (cont.). Modified Erdmann's Reaction (109)

Compound	Color with Concentrated Sulfuric Acid	Color after Exposing Sulfuric Acid Solution to Fuming Nitric Acid for ½ to 1 Min.	Color after Water Dilution
Antipyrine	Colorless	Light yellow with orange cast	Deep yellow
Atropine	Colorless	Pale yellow	Color fades
Benzocaine	Colorless	Pale yellow → light clear yellow	Yellowish precipitate
Butamin	No change from original very pale yellow	Very pale yellow → light yellow	Color fades
Cephaeline	Light yellow	Deeper yellow with brown streaks	Light yellow
Chlorcyclizine	Light yellow with brown cast	Gold	Colorless
Cinchophen	Light yellow	Light yellow	Color fades
Cyclopal	Orange with brown cast	Gold	Very pale yellow
Cysteine.HCl	Colorless	Pale yellow with gray cast	Colorless
Desoxycholic acid	Colorless	Yellow	Milky yellow precipitate
Digitonin	Very faint yellow → light orange	Pale yellow	Very pale yellow
Dihydromorphinone	Colorless	Yellow with brown cast	Color pales
Dromoran	Colorless	Light yellow	Colorless
Ephedrine	Light gray brown	Pale yellow, almost colorless	Colorless
Heroin	Very pale flesh	Gold	Light yellow
Larocaine	Original light yellow with orange cast darkens somewhat	Color deepens	Color fades
l-Menthol	Colorless, slowly changing to pale orange or flesh	Bright yellow	Pale yellow precipitate
Meperidine	No change from original pale yellow	Light gold	Color fades
Methadon	Original yellow deepens	Color grays	Pale milky yellow
Methylparafynol	Yellow with brown cast	No change	Slight precipitate
Metopon	Colorless	Pale yellow	Color fades
Optochin	Colorless	Very pale yellow	Color fades
Phanadorn	Orange → orange with yellow cast	Very pale yellow	Colorless
Phenobarbital	Colorless	Pale yellow	White precipitate
Phenylacetylurea	Colorless	Yellow with orange cast	Color fades
Phenylbutazone	Colorless	Yellow	White or flesh precipitate
Piperocaine	No change from original yellow with brown cast	Very, very pale yellow, almost colorless	Colorless
Pregnenolone	Yellow → deep yellow with orange cast	Yellow with brown cast	Color pales
Procaine	No change from original pale yellow	Pale yellow increases slightly in intensity	No change
Procaine amide	No change from original pale orange with brown cast	Pale yellow, changing slowly to light yellow and then to deep yellow	Light yellow
Procaine.HCl	Colorless	Colorless → very pale yellow	No change
Quinine	No change from original very pale yellow	No change	Colorless
Rutin	Orange with yellow cast	Yellow with greenish brown streaks	Yellow
Salicylic acid	Colorless	Very pale yellow → light yellow	Milky light orange yellow precipitate
Santonin	Very pale yellow	Very pale yellow	Slight white precipitate
Solanin	Yellow → orange	Yellow with brown cast	Color pales
Succinylsulfathiazole	Colorless	Very pale yellow → light yellow	No change
Sulfacetimide	Colorless	Yellow → deeper yellow	Color pales
Sulfadiazine	Colorless	Yellow	No change
Sulfanilamide	Colorless	Very pale yellow → light yellow	No change

Table 47-22 (cont.). Modified Erdmann's Reaction (109)

Compound	Color with Concentrated Sulfuric Acid	Color after Exposing Sulfuric Acid Solution to Fuming Nitric Acid for ½ to 1 Min.	Color after Water Dilution
Sulfapyridine	Colorless	Very pale yellow → light yellow	No change
Sulfathiazole	Colorless	Very pale yellow → light yellow	Color pales
Sulfisoxazole	Colorless	Pale yellow → light yellow	Color pales
Thiazolsulfone	Colorless	Pale yellow → light yellow	No change
Thiobarbituric acid	Colorless or pale flesh	Gold	Milky yellow precipitate
Trihexyphenidyl	Pale yellow	Deeper yellow, fades	Milky white precipitate

GREEN

Phenylsalicylate	Colorless	Yellow → brown → olive green → deep emerald green → blue green → brown	Magenta with brown cast

BLUE

Yohimbine	Colorless	Blue with violet cast slowly changing to yellow-green, then yellow	Light yellow

WHITE PRECIPITATE

Tribromoethanol	Colorless	Milky white precipitate	Precipitate dissolves, leaving oil drops

COLORLESS

The following compounds are colorless:

1. with concentrated sulfuric acid;
2. after exposing sulfuric acid solution to fuming nitric acid for ½ to 1 minute;
3. after water dilution, except as noted in footnotes.

Aconitine	Cinchonidine	Ethyl biscoum-acetate	Nikethamide	Sandoptal
Amobarbital *	Cinchonine		Nostal	Scopolamine
Antabuse	Cocaine	Eucupin.di HCl	Ortal	Secobarbital
Aprobarbital	Coniine.HCl	Glycine	Pentamethylene-tetrazol	Sedormid
Barbital	Diallylbarbituric acid	Hexobarbital		Sigmodal §
Betaine.HCl		Hippuric acid	Pentobarbital §	Strychnine
Biuret	Dibucaine	Histamine.di HCl	Phthalylsulfathia-zole ††	Sulfonethylmethane
Bromural	Dichlorodiphenyl-trichloroethane (DDT)	Homatropine †		Sulfonmethane
Butisol		Hyoscyamine	Pilocarpine	Tetracaine ‡‡
Butallylonal	Dicoumarol *	Isoamylethyl-acetylurea	Piperidione	Theobromine
Caffeine	Diethylacetylurea †		Probarbital	Theophylline
Cantharidin †	Dimenhydrinate (acidic extraction product)	Mephobarbital **	Pseudopelletierine	p-Toluenesulfon-amide †
Carbamylcholine chloride ‡		Methylphenyl-ethylhydantoin	Pyrithyldione	Trimethadione
Carbromal	Diphenylhydantoin †	Neonal §	Quinidine	Urethan
Chlorobutanol §		Nicotinic alcohol	Ricin	Vinbarbital §§
			Saccharin	

* Heavy white precipitate after water dilution.
† White precipitate after water dilution.
‡ Colorless; effervescence after water dilution.
§ Slight white precipitate after water dilution.
** White cloudy precipitate after water dilution.
†† Pale yellow after water dilution.
‡‡ Flash of yellow after water dilution.
§§ Light yellow color with concentrated sulfuric acid; fades to colorless after exposing sulfuric acid solution to fuming nitric acid for ½ to 1 minute; colorless after water dilution.

to the blue or green color of Mecke's reagent is considerably greater than to the normally dark reddish or violet color of Marquis' reagent. Considering the drugs as a whole, Mecke's reagent gives as much general information as Marquis' and, particularly with the opiates, the greater perception for the color developed permits finer distinctions to be drawn. Although the two overlap considerably, they do not duplicate each other but, because of the greater specificity of the color with Mecke's reagent, it takes precedence over Marquis' in the testing order. In the analytic process Marquis' then may or may not be necessary, depending on the findings with Mecke's reagent.

Mecke's Reagent. Selenious acid, 0.5 gm., in 100 ml. concentrated sulfuric acid.

Blue or green colorations with Mecke's reagent immediately suggest one of the opiates. By the use of controls run simultaneously with the unknown, the reaction may be used to differentiate, at the same time it indicates the type. The shade of green produced by codeine is distinctive when matched against morphine as a control, whereas, the observed color for codeine by itself can only be interpreted as falling in both the green and blue columns. Ethylmorphine is not differentiated from codeine and the other

Table 47-23. Mecke's Reagent (109)

COMPOUND	COLOR DEVELOPED WITH MECKE'S REAGENT	COLOR AFTER WATER DILUTION
RED		
Amphetamine.HCl	Pale or light rose	Color fades
Ascorbic acid	Faint pink, slowly turning deep rose orange	Dark precipitate
Brucine	Colorless → light red → orange	Light yellow
Cholesterol	Orange → brick red	Very pale green
Chrysazin	Deep carmine red → orange red on standing → yellow orange	Yellow
Cysteine.HCl	Colorless → rose	No change
Dimenhydrinate (basic extraction product)	Brick red with yellow solution	Milky white precipitate
Pyridium	Deep red → orange red	Deep red brown
Salicin	Carmine red	Color fades
ORANGE		
Cyclopal	Orange with brown cast	No change
d-Desoxyephedrine	Original pale orange with brown cast darkens	No change
Diphenhydramine	Orange with yellow solution	White precipitate
Hexobarbital	Light brown → orange	No change
l-Menthol	Yellow → orange with yellow cast → orange with brown cast	Light red brown
Meperidine	Orange with brown cast	No change
Phanadorn	Light orange	Light orange precipitate
Pregnenolone	Yellow orange → orange → brown with orange cast → deep brown with red cast	Green brown
Procaine amide	No change from original pale orange with brown cast	No change
Rutin	Orange with deep yellow solution	Yellow precipitate
Terpin hydrate	Orange with yellow cast	Flesh color
BROWN		
Apothesine	Original brown with golden cast deepens	Yellowish precipitate
Berberine.SO₄	Brown with yellow cast → brown with green cast → brown → brown with violet cast	Orange or red brown
Curarine	Light brown	Yellowish precipitate
Delphinine	No change from original brown with orange cast	Light pink brown
Desoxycholic acid	Brown, increasing in intensity	No change
Digalen	Light brown, slowly changing to pale red	Fades to brown
Digitalin	Brown	No change
Digitonin	Pale brown with yellow cast, slowly increasing in intensity	No change
Digitoxin	Brown	Color fades
Diothane	No change from original brown with orange cast	Color fades
Emetine	Brown with yellow cast	Light yellow brown
Ephedrine	Light brown	Color disappears
Estrone	Pale brown with yellow cast → brown	Pale orange pink

Table 47-23 (cont.). Mecke's Reagent (109)

COMPOUND	COLOR DEVELOPED WITH MECKE'S REAGENT	COLOR AFTER WATER DILUTION
Lobeline	No change from original brown with red cast	Slight white precipitate
Pamaquine	No change from original brown	Yellow
Pavatrine	Dark brown	Yellowish precipitate
Pelletierine tannate	Brown, changing slowly to olive green	Light brown
Phenindamine	Brown with red cast	Yellow
Piperine	Brown with red cast → dark brown	Greenish brown
Sparteine	No change from original brown	No change
Strophanthin	Dark brown	No change
Thymol iodide	Brown	No change
Trihexyphenidyl	Light brown	Yellow brown
Xylocaine	No change from original brown with red cast	No change

YELLOW

COMPOUND	COLOR DEVELOPED WITH MECKE'S REAGENT	COLOR AFTER WATER DILUTION
Acridine.HCl	No change from original yellow	No change
Amphetamine base	Light yellow with green-brown cast	Color fades
Antabuse	Colorless → very pale yellow, slowly	Light yellow precipitate
Atabrin	Deep yellow	No change
Cephaeline	Yellow with green cast	Pale orange
Chlorcyclizine	Original yellow with brown cast becomes more yellow	Color fades
Cinchophen	Light yellow	No change
Colchicine	Yellow or yellow with green cast	No change
Dicyclomine	Colorless, slowly changing to pale yellow	Slight yellowish precipitate
Dromoran	Very pale yellow with gray cast	Colorless
Eucupin.di HCl	Pale yellow	Flesh color
Hydrastine	Pale yellow, slowly changing to brown	Pale orange
Larocaine	No change from original pale yellow	No change
Meconin	Very pale yellow	No change
Methadon	Original yellow grays slowly	Color fades
Methylparafynol	Yellow → yellow brown	Green brown
Nicotine	No change from original pale yellow with brown cast	No change
Piperocaine	No change from original pale yellow	Colorless
Prisilidine	Very pale yellow	No change
Procaine	No change from original pale yellow	No change
Quinine	No change from original very pale yellow	No change
Solanin	Yellow with brown cast → brown with yellow cast, slowly changing to brown with red cast	Magenta, fades
Veratrine	Yellow → orange → green	Red brown
Vinbarbital	Light yellow	Slight white precipitate

GREEN

COMPOUND	COLOR DEVELOPED WITH MECKE'S REAGENT	COLOR AFTER WATER DILUTION
alpha-Naphthylthiourea (ANTU)	Pale green with yellow cast	Yellow-white precipitate
Apomorphine	Olive green → dark green with brown cast → dark brown on standing	Lighter brown
Codeine	Emerald green → blue green → blue → blue green on standing	Yellow
Ethylmorphine	Green → blue → blue green	Pale yellow
Mescaline	Yellow, changing very quickly to green → blue → brown	Light brown

BLUE

COMPOUND	COLOR DEVELOPED WITH MECKE'S REAGENT	COLOR AFTER WATER DILUTION
N-Allylnormorphine	Blue → green	Color fades
Dihydromorphinone	Blue → blue green → green	Pale red
Heroin	Blue → blue green → green	Light orange
Mephenesine	Colorless → pale blue with gray violet cast	Color disappears
Metopon	Flash of yellow → light blue → blue green → yellow green	Pale yellow
Morphine	Blue → blue green → green	Pale brownish orange
Narceine	Blue → green → olive green	Color fades
Narcotine	Flash of pale blue green → blue → blue green → yellow green	Pale red orange
Yohimbine	Blue → green	Brown

Table 47-23 (cont.). Mecke's Reagent (109)

COMPOUND	COLOR DEVELOPED WITH MECKE'S REAGENT	COLOR AFTER WATER DILUTION
MAGENTA		
Pyrilamine	Pink → magenta → deep magenta	Color fades
Thenylpyramine	Magenta → deep magenta → purple	Black or brown
Thonzylamine	Deep magenta	Brown
Zolamine.HCl	Deep magenta	Brown
WHITE		
Betaine.HCl	White precipitate which disappears	Colorless
Carbamycholine chloride	Colorless → white precipitate	Precipitate disappears
Histamine.di HCl	White precipitate which disappears	Colorless
Procaine.HCl	Milky white precipitate which disappears	Colorless

COLORLESS

The following compounds are colorless:
1. with Mecke's reagent;
2. after water dilution, except as noted in footnotes.

Acetanilid	Cantharidin	Hippuric acid	Phthalylsulfa-	Sulfanilamide
Acetophenetidin	Carbromal	Homatropine ‡	thiazole	Sulfapyridine
Acetylsalicylic	Chlorobutanol	Hyoscyamine	Pilocarpine	Sulfathiazole
acid *	Cinchonidine	Isoamylethylacetyl-	Piperidione	Sulfisoxazole
Aconitine	Cinchonine	urea ‡	Probarbital	Sulfonethyl-
Adiphenine †	Cocaine	Mephobarbital *	Pseudopelletierine	methane
p-Aminobenzoic	Coniine.HCl	Methylphenylethyl-	Pyrithyldione	Sulfonmethane
acid	Diallylbarbituric	hydantoin †	Quinidine	Tetracaine
Aminopyrine	acid	Neonal *	Ricin	Theobromine
Amobarbital *	Dibucaine	Nicotinic alcohol	Saccharin	Theophylline
Amprotropine †	Dichlorodiphenyl-	Nikethamide	Salicylic acid †	Thiamin basic
Antipyrine	trichloroethane	Nostal *	Sandoptal *	degradation
Aprobarbital	(DDT)	Optochin	Santonin	product
Atropine	Dicoumarol †	Ortal *	Scopolamine	Thiazolsulfone
Barbital	Diethylacetylurea *	Pentamethylene-	Secobarbital	Thiobarbituric
Benzocaine	Dimenhydrinate	tetrazol	Sedormid	acid **
Biuret	(acidic extraction	Pentobarbital †	Sigmodal †	Thiopental ††
Bromural	product)	Phenobarbital †	Strychnine	p-Toluenesul-
Butabarbital	Diphenylhydantoin †	Phenylacetyl-	Succinylsulfa-	fonamide
Butamin	Ethyl biscoum-	urea †	thiazole	Tribromoethanol *
Butylallonal	acetate	Phenylbutazone †	Sulfacetimide	Trimethadione
Caffeine	Glycine	Phenylsalicylate †	Sulfadiazine	Urethan

* Slight white precepitate after water dilution.
† White precipitate after water dilution.
‡ Slight milky white precipitate after water dilution.
** Yellow precipitate after water dilution.
†† Colorless → pale yellow precipitate after water dilution.

opiates listed are so similar in their color behavior that they are not distinguishable from it. Yohimbine also may be confused with the morphine-like compounds with this reagent.

Marquis' Reagent. Add 2 drops of 40 per cent formaldehyde to 1 ml. of concentrated sulfuric acid. This reagent should be prepared fresh each time it is used. If allowed to stand, even overnight, it loses sensitivity.

Although a good blue or red violet is given by the opiates, the same color or one easily confused with it when the test samples are small, is given by nonalkaloidal structures. Many antihistamines, mephenesine and, under certain conditions,* amphetamine give the same type of reaction. Moreover, the distinction between reds, violets, blue and red violets or magenta has less significance than comparable colorations with Mecke's reagent because there is a decided tendency with Marquis' reagent for color shades to shift as a result of slight changes in the conditions or the presence of tissue impurities as well as other organic compounds. Marquis' reagent is distinctive for pseudopelletierine

* When amphetamine is first isolated, a transient magenta is observed with Marquis' reagent. After standing in air for some time, the color that develops is more orange.

and is useful as a differential test for acetylsalicylic acid which gives a positive Koppanyi but fails to give a ferric chloride test because it is free of salicylic acid.

Table 47-24. Marquis' Reagent (109)

COMPOUND	COLOR DEVELOPED WITH MARQUIS' REAGENT	COLOR AFTER WATER DILUTION
RED		
Acetanilid	Colorless → faint pink	White precipitate
Acetylsalicylic acid	Colorless → pink → deep rose	White precipitate
Amphetamine.HCl	Orange → pale red → brown	Pale yellow
Cholesterol	Brick red	Pale red
Chrysazin	Bright carmine or brick red → yellow	Yellow
Dimenhydrinate (alkaline extraction product)	Red with deep orange cast and yellow solution	Milky white precipitate
Lobeline	Brown with red cast → deep red	Brown
Mephenesine	Red	Color fades
Methadon	Deep yellow → light red with brown cast changing slowly to brown	Color disappears
Phenylsalicylate	Colorless → pink → deep rose	Color fades
Pyridium	No change from original deep red	Bright red
Salicin	Deep carmine	No change
Salicylic acid	Colorless → pink → deep rose	White precipitate
Thenylpyramine	Red → deep carmine	Light brown
Thonzylamine	Deep carmine	Light magenta
Zolamine.HCl	Deep carmine	Light brown
ORANGE		
Adiphenine	Light orange	White precipitate
Amphetamine base	Orange → orange with brown cast	Pale yellow
Cyclopal	Yellow → orange with brown cast	Color fades
Delphinine	Orange → brown orange	Color pales
d-Desoxyephedrine	Orange → orange brown	Pale yellow
Diphenhydramine	Orange → brick red → brown	Yellow fades; brown
Ephedrine	Brown → orange with brown cast	Color fades
Hexobarbital	Very pale orange with brown cast	Colorless
l-Menthol	Light orange with yellow cast	Milky precipitate
Meperidine	Orange → deep brown with orange cast	Yellow; fades
Nicotine	Pale orange with brown cast	Colorless
Phanadorn	Orange	Color fades
Pregnenolone	Orange → orange with brown cast	Light red → milky white precipitate
Prisilidene	Orange → orange red → light brick red	Very pale yellow
Procaine amide	Original pale orange with brown cast fades to very pale orange	Colorless
Terpin hydrate	Orange with yellow cast	Milky white precipitate
Trihexyphenidyl	Yellow → orange → orange with rose cast	Milky precipitate
BROWN		
Apothesine	Yellow → brown	No change
Curarine	Pale brown with yellow cast	Color fades
Digalen	Yellow → brown	No change
Digitalin	Brown	No change
Digitonin	Colorless changing slowly to brown	No change
Digitoxin	Dark brown	Dark brown → black
Diothane	No change from original brown	Color fades
Dromoran	Light brown → gray brown → dark brown	Color fades
Emetine	No change from original brown with red cast	Yellow brown
Mescaline	Green, changing rapidly to dark brown, slowly changing to brown with violet cast	Brown with green cast
Pamaquine	No change from original brown	No change
Pelletierine tannate	Brown with yellow cast	Color fades
Phenindamine	Brown	Yellow
Piperine	Brown with olive green cast on standing	No change
Sparteine	No change from original brown	No change
Strophanthin	No change from original brown	No change
Xylocaine	No change from original brown	No change

Table 47-24. (cont.). Marquis' Reagent (109)

COMPOUND	COLOR DEVELOPED WITH MARQUIS' REAGENT	COLOR AFTER WATER DILUTION
YELLOW		
Acridine.HCl	Original yellow color remains	Yellow
Amprotropine	Very pale yellow	White precipitate
Antabuse	Very pale yellow	Milky white precipitate
Atabrin	Bright yellow → orange yellow	No change
Berberine.SO$_4$	No change from original yellow	No change
Cephaeline	Yellow with brown cast	Pale yellow
Chlorcyclizine	No change from original yellow with brown cast	No change
Cinchophen	Pale lemon yellow	Color fades
Colchicine	Yellow	No change
Desoxycholic acid	Pale yellow → deep yellow → gold with brown cast	Color fades
Dicyclomine	Very pale yellow, slowly changing to deep yellow → orange	Fades to brown; milky precipitate
Estrone	Yellow → gold → orange	Pale red
Eucupin.di HCl	Very pale yellow	Colorless
Homatropine	Colorless, slowly changing to light yellow	Slight white precipitate
Hydrastine	Yellow → yellow orange	White precipitate
Larocaine	No change from original yellow	No change
Meconin	Pale yellow	White precipitate
Methylparafynol	Bright yellow → brownish yellow	Gray
Piperocaine	Original yellow with brown cast pales	Colorless
Procaine	No change from original pale yellow	No change
Quinine	No change from original pale yellow	Color fades
Rutin	Yellow with orange cast	No change
Santonin	Very very pale yellow	White precipitate
Solanin	Yellow, slowly changing to orange	Rose → magenta
Thymol iodide	No change from original pale yellow	No change
Veratrine	Yellow → orange → orange brown	Yellow
Vinbarbital	Very pale yellow	Colorless

GREEN		
alpha-Naphthylthiourea (ANTU)	Pale green → light green	White precipitate
Apomorphine	Black → dark green on standing	Brown
Pavatrine	Brown → green	Yellow
Yohimbine	Grayish green → gray on standing	Color fades

BLUE		
Codeine	Blue with violet cast	Brown
Ethylmorphine	Deep blue with violet cast	Color pales
Narceine	Blue violet, changing rapidly to gray → yellow green → yellow	Color disappears
Narcotine	Blue violet, changing rapidly to gray → yellow green → yellow	Color disappears
Pseudopelletierine	Colorless, changing slowly to violet → deep blue violet	Green → yellow

---

MAGENTA		
N-Allylnormorphine	Deep magenta → purple	Pale brown
Dihydromorphinone	Magenta slowly changing to blue with violet cast	Color fades
Heroin	Deep magenta → deep violet	Color fades
Metopon	Magenta → violet	Light magenta
Morphine	Deep magenta → deep violet	Pale yellow
Pyrilamine	Magenta → deep magenta	Color pales

Table 47-24. (cont.). Marquis' Reagent (109)

COLORLESS

The following compounds are colorless:

1. with Marquis reagent;
2. after water dilution except as noted in footnotes.

Acetophenetidin *	Carbamylcholine	Ethyl biscoumacetate	Phenylbutazone *	Sulfadiazine
Aconitine	chloride	Glycine	Phthalylsulfa-	Sulfanilamide
p-Aminobenzoic	Carbromal †	Hippuric acid	thiazole	Sulfapyridine
acid	Chlorobutanol	Histamine.di HCl	Picrotoxin	Sulfathiazole †
Aminopyrine	Cinchonidine	Hyoscyamine	Pilocarpine	Sulfisoxazole
Amobarbital *	Cinchonine	Isoamylethylacetyl-	Piperidione	Sulfonethylmethane
Antipyrine	Cocaine	urea ‡	Probarbital	Sulfonmethane
Aprobarbital	Coniine.HCl	Mephobarbital *	Procaine.HCl	Tetracaine
Ascorbic acid	Cysteine.HCl	Methylphenylethyl-	Pyrithyldione	Theobromine
Atropine	Diallylbarbituric	hydantoin	Quinidine	Theophylline
Barbital	acid	Neonal	Ricin	Thiamin degrada-
Benzocaine	Dibucaine	Nicotinic alcohol	Saccharin	tion product
Betaine.HCl	Dichlorodiphenyltri-	Nikethamide	Sandoptal	Thiazolsulfone
Biuret	chloroethane	Nostal	Scopolamine	Thiobarbituric acid
Bromural	(DDT)	Optochin	Secobarbital	Thiopental ‡
Brucine	Dicoumarol *	Ortal	Sedormid	p-Toluenesulfon-
Butabarbital	Diethylacetylurea	Pentamethylene-	Sigmodal	amide *
Butallylonal	Dimenhydrinate	tetrazol	Strychnine	Tribromoethanol †
Butamin	(acidic extraction	Pentobarbital	Succinylsulfa-	Trimethadione
Caffeine	product)	Phenobarbital †	thiazole	Urethan
Cantharidin	Diphenylhydantoin ‡	Phenylacetylurea *	Sulfacetimide	

    * White precipitate after water dilution.
    † Slight white precipitate after water dilution.
    ‡ Milky white precipitate after water dilution.

2. Designating Reactions.

    2. Designating Reactions. Whether or not reactions in this category will be needed, will depend on findings in the exclusion and indicating type reactions. When the latter are strongly positive, little will be gained by applying designating tests, since they do not add a great deal more toward the detection of the important basic drugs which react strongly in the reactions already discussed. If the findings in these are negative, however, the designating tests become more important. As a class, they are more selective for specific structures because their reactivity is more dependent on the presence of definite functional groups in the molecule. The selection of a particular reaction in this class will be influenced by the fraction in which the unknown was isolated. They are particularly useful for the neutral fraction which contains many compounds which, although neutral with regard to ionization, are more basic than acidic in their chemical reactivity.

    (a) Azo Coupling Test (126). For a coupling reaction to take place in alkaline solution between a compound and a diazonium salt, a reactive hydrogen atom which may be linked to carbon, nitrogen or oxygen must be present in the compound (127). With the exception of aliphatic hydrocarbons with a conjugated system of double bonds, the requirements are only found, usually, in aromatic ring structures with amino groups that may be primary, secondary or tertiary, mono or ortho dihydroxy phenols or with side chains containing primary or secondary amines (128). Aromatic beta-diketones or beta-ketonic esters which have enol forms may also react (127).

    The reaction is carried out on a small piece of filter paper which acts as an absorbing medium for the reagents so that added sensitivity is obtained by confining the test to a small area. The paper is stained by the color developed, making it more readily detected.

    Reagents. (a) para-Nitroaniline solution: Heat 5 gm. of para-nitroaniline in 3 ml. concentrated hydrochloric acid to boiling and stir for 10 minutes. When the solution is cool, dilute to 100 ml. and filter.*

    (b) Diazo compound: Add 5 ml. of para-nitroaniline solution and 1 ml. of con-

    * The para-nitroaniline and diazo compound are unstable at room temperature and should be stored in the refrigerator.

centrated hydrochloric acid to a 100 ml. flask. Place the flask in an ice bath for 10 minutes and then add 5 ml. of a cold solution of freshly prepared 0.7 per cent sodium nitrite. Add cold water to make 100 ml. Allow the solution to stand in the refrigerator for two hours before use. (See footnote, page 1216.)

(c) One per cent sodium carbonate solution.

(d) Ten per cent sodium hydroxide solution.

Procedure. Place a micro quantity of the unknown on a piece of filter paper about 2 mm. square. Moisten the paper with the diazo solution and permit it to stand at room temperature for one hour. Moisten the paper with additional diazo solution if drying is too rapid. At the end of an hour add a micro drop of one per cent sodium carbonate solution. After 15 minutes, add a micro drop of the sodium hydroxide solution. Observe the color produced after 5 to 10 minutes following the addition of the sodium hydroxide.

Table 47-25. Azo Coupling Test (126, 30)

POSITIVE REACTION—red coloration except as noted

Acetanilid	Benzocaine	Ethyl biscoum-	Phenylbutazone	Strychnine
Acetylsalicylic	Brucine	acetate	Phenylsalicylate	Succinylsulfa-
acid	Butamin	Ethylmorphine	Phthalylsulfa-	thiazole
Adiphenine	Cinchonidine	(blue)	thiazole	Sulfacetimide
(yellow)	Codeine (blue)	Heroin	Physostigmine	Sulfanilamide
p-Aminobenzoic	Curarine	Larocaine	Pilocarpine	Sulfapyridine
acid	d-Desoxyephe-	Lobeline	Piperidione	Sulfathiazole
Aminopyrine	drine	Meperidine	Piperocaine	Sulfisoxazole
Amphetamine	Dihydromor-	Metopon	Procaine	Tetracaine
Amprotropine	phinone	Morphine	Procaine amide	(yellow)
(yellow)	Diothane	Narceine	Pseudopelletier-	Theophylline
Antipyrine	(orange)	Nicotinic alcohol	ine	Thiamin.HCl
(blue)	Diphenhydra-	Pamaquine	Quinine	Thonzylamine
Apomorphine	mine	Pavatrine (acidic	Santonin (light	Tribromo-
Apothesine	Emetine (basic	extraction)	orange)	ethanol
Ascorbic acid	extraction)	(orange)	Scopolamine	Yohimbine

NEGATIVE REACTION

Acetophenetidin	Cinchophen	Emetine (acidic	Nikethamide	Saccharin
Aconitine	Cocaine	extraction)	Optochin	Salicin
N-Allylnormor-	Coniine	Ephedrine	Pavatrine (basic	Solanin
phine	Delphinine	Estrone	extraction)	Sparteine
Amobarbital	Desoxycholic	Eucupin.di HCl	Pentamethylene-	Strophanthin
Antabuse	acid	Glycine	tetrazol	Sulfadiazine
Atabrin	Dibucaine	Hippuric acid	Phenindamine	Sulfonethylmethane
Atropine	Dicoumarol	Homatropine	Phenobarbital	Sulfonmethane
Bromural	Dicyclomine	Hydrastine	Picrotoxin	Thenylpyramine
Caffeine	Digalen	Hyoscyamine	Piperine	Theobromine
Cantharidin	Digitalin	Isoamylethyl-	Pregnenolone	Thiazolsulfone
Carbamylcholine	Digitonin	acetylurea	Prisilidene	Thiopental
chloride	Digitoxin	Meconin	Pyrilamine	Trihexyphenidyl
Carbromal	Dimenhydrinate	Methadon	Pyrithyldione	Trimethadione
Chlorobutanol	(acidic and	Methylphenyl-	Quinidine	Urethan
Cholesterol	basic extraction	ethylhydantoin	Ricin	Veratrine
Cinchonine	products)	Narcotine	Rutin	Xylocaine

(b) Indamine Reaction (129). para-Phenylenediamine undergoes condensation with compounds containing amino and other basic radicals to form indamine type compounds which have a tendency to form quinoid structures on mild oxidation (130). Ferric chloride is added as the oxidizing agent but the test actually combines two reactions since any compound which reacts positively with ferric chloride will react positively in the indamine test. It is particularly applicable for local anesthetics such as benzocaine and procaine with free amino groups and for many of the sulfa drugs. Positive findings, except when due to ferric chloride alone, should be followed by acid diazotization (page 1246) to confirm the presence of the primary amino radical.

Reagents. (a) para-Phenylenediamine solution: Dissolve 1 gm. of recrystallized p-phenylenediamine in 100 ml. of acetone. This solution must be freshly prepared and the p-phenylenediamine must be free of the air oxidation product or a color develops in the reagent blank.

(b) Acid ferric chloride solution: Dissolve 10 gm. ferric chloride hexahydrate in a mixture of 10 ml. concentrated hydrochloric acid and 90 ml. H_2O.

Procedure. The test is made in a micro test tube with a bore of about 5 mm. A micro quantity of unknown dissolved in about 0.3 ml. acetone is introduced and a small drop of *p*-phenylenediamine solution and about 0.5 ml. water are added. The contents of the tube are thoroughly mixed and the appearance of any precipitate or coloration noted. A small drop of acid ferric chloride is then added and the tube observed over a 10 minute period. The color produced by ferric chloride alone is immediate whereas the *p*-phenylenediamine reaction with many of the compounds requires longer standing to fully develop the color. Moreover, the color produced by ferric chloride alone is other than a pure red. The drugs which react with ferric chloride (indicated in Table 47-26 by an asterisk) may be distinguished by repeating the test, omitting the addition of the *p*-phenylenediamine reagent.

Table 47-26. Indamine Test (129, 30)

RED

The following compounds show:
1. no reaction after addition of water and *p*-phenylenediamine;
2. red after addition of ferric chloride.

p-Aminobenzoic acid	Benzocaine	Delphinine	Sulfacetimide	Sulfathiazole
Apomorphine	Butamin	Metopon	Sulfadiazine	Sulfisoxazole
Ascorbic acid	Cinchophen	Procaine	Sulfanilamide	Thiazolsulfone
	Coniine	Pseudopelletierine	Sulfapyridine	

COMPOUND	AFTER ADDITION OF WATER AND *p*-PHENYLENEDIAMINE	AFTER ADDITION OF FERRIC CHLORIDE
ORANGE		
Antipyrine *	No reaction	Orange with red cast
Pamaquine	No reaction	Orange
BROWN		
Diphenhydramine	White precipitate	Darkens to brown
Pyrilamine	No reaction	Brown precipitate
YELLOW		
Atabrin	Yellow precipitate	Yellow precipitate dissolves
Dicoumarol	No reaction	Yellow precipitate with green cast
Nikethamide	No reaction	Deep yellow
GREEN		
Phenylbutazone	No reaction	Green changing to blue-gray
Piperocaine	White precipitate	Dissolves with a green → light magenta color
Rutin	No reaction	Dark olive green
Xylocaine	No reaction	Green changing to dirty purple
BLUE		
Aminopyrine *	No reaction	Blue violet
Ethyl biscoumacetate	No reaction	Blue violet precipitate
Salicylic acid *	No reaction	Blue violet
MAGENTA		
Larocaine	White precipitate	Dissolves with magenta color
Thonzylamine	White precipitate	Dissolves with light magenta color

* Drugs which react with ferric chloride.

Table 47-26 (cont.). Indamine Test (129, 30)

WHITE

The following compounds show:

1. a white precipitate after addition of water and p-phenylenediamine;
2. the precipitate dissolves after addition of ferric chloride except as noted.

Amprotropine	Dibucaine	Estrone †	Pavatrine †	Piperine
Apothesine	Dicyclomine	Methadon	(basic extraction)	Pregnenolone †
Cholesterol	Diothane	Optochin	Phenylsalicylate †	Quinine

† No change after addition of ferric chloride.

NO REACTION

Acetanilid	Cinchonine	Eucupin.di HCl	Pentamethylene-	Strychnine
Acetophenetidin	Cocaine	Glycine	tetrazol	Succinylsulfa-
Acetylsalicylic	Codeine	Heroin	Phenindamine	thiazole
acid	Curarine	Hippuric acid	Phenobarbital	Sulfonethyl-
Aconitine	Desoxycholic	Homatropine	Phthalylsulfa-	methane
Adiphenine	acid	Hydrastine	thiazole	Sulfonmethane
N-Allylnormor-	d-Desoxyephedrine	Hyoscyamine	Physostigmine	Tetracaine
phine	Digalen	Isoamylethyl-	Picrotoxin	Thenylpyra-
Amobarbital	Digitalin	acetylurea	Pilocarpine	mine
Amphetamine	Digitonin	Lobeline	Piperidione	Theobromine
base	Digitoxin	Meconin	Prisilidene	Theophylline
Antabuse	Dihydromor-	Meperidine	Procaine amide	Thiamin degrada-
Atropine	phinone	Methylphenyl-	Pyrithyldione	tion product
Brucine	Dimenhydrinate	ethylhydantoin	Quinidine	Thiopental
Caffeine	(acidic and	Morphine	Saccharin	Tribromo-
Cantharidin	basic extrac-	Narceine	Salicin	ethanol
Carbamylcholine	tion products)	Narcotine	Santonin	Trihexyphenidyl
chloride	Emetine	Nicotinic alcohol	Scopolamine	Trimethadione
Chlorobutanol	Ephedrine	Pavatrine (acidic	Sparteine	Urethan
Cinchonidine	Ethylmorphine	extraction)	Solanin	Veratrine

(c) Chloranil Test. Chloranil in methyl alcohol, dioxane (131) or acetone solution (129) reacts with aromatic primary or secondary amines and phenolic compounds to form colored condensation products. A red color is usually produced with weakly acidic compounds whereas greens or blue greens predominate with the basic drugs that react. Compounds that diazotize react strongly with chloranil. When done in conjunction with the furfural reaction (page 1079) which is the most specific for diazotizable nitrogen with the exception of the acid diazo reaction itself (page 1246), positive findings with both tests are nearly conclusive for the presence of an aromatic amine, although confirmation by the diazo reaction should still be made.

The sensitivity for secondary amines is generally less than that with the primary ones. The test may be used to confirm N-substituted amides that hydrolyze to amines in alkaline solution. Thus, acetanilid, which does not react in acetone solution, gives a strong positive reaction after alkaline hydrolysis.

Reagent. A saturated solution of chloranil in acetone.

Procedure. The solid sample contained in a capillary test tube with a bore of about 2 mm. is treated with a drop of chloranil reagent and the color observed after five minutes.

Confirmatory test for secondary amines by alkaline hydrolysis: A few micrograms of sample are evaporated just to dryness on a hot plate maintained at 75° C. with 2 drops of alcoholic potassium hydroxide prepared by heating 1 pellet of potassium hydroxide in 2 ml. of ethyl alcohol until dissolved. The residue is shaken with 0.5 ml. of ethyl ether, the ether decanted and air evaporated. The residue is treated with one drop of chloranil reagent (Table 47-27, page 1220).

(d) Hydroxamic Acid Reaction. Hydroxamic acids are acyl derivatives of hydroxylamine (132):

$$\underset{\underset{\text{NHOH}}{|}}{\text{R—C=O}} \quad \rightleftharpoons \quad \underset{\underset{\text{NOH}}{\|}}{\text{R—C—OH}}$$

In acid solution they react with ferric ion to form inner complexes which have a red or violet color.

$$R-\underset{\underset{O}{\|}}{\underset{N}{\overset{OH}{\overset{|}{C}}}} > Fe/3 \quad\quad or \quad\quad R-\underset{\underset{H}{\underset{|}{N}}}{\underset{O}{\overset{C=O}{\overset{|}{}}}} > Fe/3 \quad\quad (132)$$

Hydroxamic acids are formed by the action of hydroxyl amine in alkaline solution on esters, acid anhydrides, acyl chlorides and some simple fatty acids:

$$R-\underset{\underset{O}{\|}}{C}-OR \;+\; NH_2OH \;\rightarrow\; R-\underset{\underset{O}{\|}}{C}-NHOH \;+\; ROH$$

Table 47-27. Chloranil in Acetone Test (129, 30)

COMPOUND	COLOR DEVELOPED WITH CHLORANIL SOLUTION	COMPOUND	COLOR DEVELOPED WITH CHLORANIL SOLUTION
RED			
Acetophenetidin	Red	Heroin	Red
N-Allylnormor-phine	Red with orange cast	Meperidine	Red
		Morphine	Red
Aminopyrine	Red	Pavatrine (acid fraction)	Red
Antipyrine	Red		
Benzocaine	Red	Pilocarpine	Red
Butamin	Red	Prisilidene	Dark red with brown cast
Cinchonidine	Red with brown cast	Pyrilamine	Dark red with brown cast
Codeine	Red	Scopolamine	Red
Coniine	Dark red	Sulfanilamide	Deep carmine red
Dihydromor-phinone	Red	Thenylpyramine	Red with brown cast
Diphenhydra-mine	Dark red with brown cast	Thonzylamine	Deep carmine red
ORANGE			
Antabuse	Orange	Nikethamide	Orange with red cast
Brucine	Orange with red cast	Physostigmine	Orange with red cast
Hydrastine	Orange	Tetracaine	Orange with red cast
Larocaine	Orange → olive green		
Metopon	Changes to orange on standing		
BROWN			
Delphinine	Brown with red cast	Sulfisoxazole	Brown with red cast
Emetine	Brown with red cast → violet	Sulfacetimide	Brown with red cast
YELLOW			
Aconitine	Yellow with green cast	Ephedrine	Yellow precipitate
Adiphenine	Yellow with green cast	Pyrithyldione	Yellow with green cast
Amprotropine	Yellow with green cast		
GREEN			
Apomorphine	Green	Lobeline	Green
Apothesine	Green with brown cast	Methadon	Green
Atropine	Green with brown cast	Optochin	Olive green
Dibucaine	Green	Pamaquine	Dark green
Dicyclomine	Dark green	Pavatrine (basic fraction)	Green
Dimenhydrinate (basic extraction product)	Green	Piperocaine	Dark olive green
		Pseudopelle-tierine	Green with brown cast
Ethylmorphine	Green	Quinidine	Olive green
Eucupin.di HCl	Dark green with brown cast	Quinine	Olive green
Homatropine	Green	Sparteine	Green
Hyoscyamine	Green		

Table 47-27 (cont.). Chloranil in Acetone Test (129, 30)

COMPOUND	COLOR DEVELOPED WITH CHLORANIL SOLUTION	COMPOUND	COLOR DEVELOPED WITH CHLORANIL SOLUTION
BLUE			
p-Aminobenzoic acid	Light blue violet with gray or brown cast		
MAGENTA			
Piperine	Light magenta with gray-brown cast		

NEGATIVE REACTION

Acetanilid	Curarine	Isoamylethyl-acetylurea	Picrotoxin	Sulfapyridine
Acetylsalicylic acid	Desoxycholic acid	Meconin	Piperidione	Sulfathiazole
Amobarbital	d-Desoxyephe-drine	Methylphenyl-ethylhydantoin	Pregnenolone	Sulfonethylmethane
Amphetamine	Dicoumarol	Narceine	Procaine	Sulfonmethane
Ascorbic acid	Digalen	Narcotine	Procaine amide	Theobromine
Atabrin	Digitalin	Nicotinic alcohol	Ricin	Theophylline
Caffeine	Digitonin	Pentmethylene-tetrazol	Rutin	Thiamin degrada-tion product .
Cantharidin	Digitoxin	Phenindamine	Saccharin	Thiopental
Carbamylcholine chloride	Diothane	Phenobarbital	Salicin	Tribromoethanol
Chlorobutanol	Estrone	Phenylbutazone	Santonin	Trihexyphenidyl
Cholesterol	Ethylbiscoum-acetate	Phenylsalicylate	Solanin	Trimethadione
Cinchonine	Glycine	Phthalylsulfa-thiazole	Strophanthin	Urethan
Cinchophen	Hippuric acid		Strychnine	Veratrine
Cocaine			Succinylsulfa-thiazole	Xylocaine
			Sulfadiazine	Yohimbine

Some amides also react (132) and aliphatic nitroso compounds may rearrange to a hydroxamic acid (133). Carboxylic acids may be converted into hydroxamic acids after conversion into the acid chloride with thionyl chloride (134). Sulfonic acids, after conversion into sulfonyl chlorides with thionyl chloride, react with hydroxylamine to form sulfohydroxamic acids and these, on treatment with acetaldehyde, form acethydroxamic acid and sulphinic acids, both of which give red inner complexes with ferric ion (135).

The reaction has been used primarily as a generic test for esters. However, all compounds with ester linkages do not react, probably because the oxygen bridge is too firmly bound to undergo cleavage in the alkaline solution of hydroxylamine. Procaine reacts readily whereas tetracaine, which is closely related to it structurally, gives only such a faint reaction that it would be considered as negative if the test were carried out on an unknown. Amprotropine, adiphenine and apothesine ® react positively, while pavatrine,® which has a somewhat similar side chain structure in relation to the ester linkages, does not react. Diothane, which has the ester oxygen bridge although it is not a true ester, and nikethamide, a dialkyl-N-substituted amide, do not react. Some drugs with structures unrelated to the generic types considered essential for the test also react strongly. Antabuse, pyrilamine, apomorphine, chlorobutanol and tribromoethanol react, although not necessarily with the formation of a hydroxamic acid. Acetylsalicylic acid and phenylsalicylate are listed as reacting positively since they do give the violet coloration in the test but the reaction is due to hydrolysis to salicylic acid by the alkaline hydroxylamine solution, after which the typical salicylate-ferric ion reaction occurs. The color with antipyrine is due entirely to the ferric ion.

The hydroxamic acid test is closer to a true generic type of reaction than most of the others as the majority of the positively reacting compounds are esters. It has the disadvantage of being less sensitive and requiring three manipulative steps as well as more care in carrying out the procedure. Although the sensitivity is variable with the different drugs, a larger sample of unknown must be used for the test when carried out on an unknown in order to avoid missing the least sensitive of the positively reacting drugs.

Reagents. (1) Potassium hydroxide: a saturated solution of potassium hydroxide in ethyl alcohol (95 per cent).

(2) Hydrochloric acid solution: 10 ml. of concentrated hydrochloric acid are diluted to 100 ml. with methyl alcohol.

(3) Hydroxylamine hydrochloride: saturated solution of hydroxylamine hydrochloride in 95 per cent ethyl alcohol.

(4) Ferric chloride: 1 per cent ferric chloride in 95 per cent ethyl alcohol.

Procedure (129). A 15 to 25 mg. sample of unknown is forced into the bottom of a 2 x 50 mm. capillary test tube by tapping or centrifuging. The sample is covered with potassium hydroxide solution to a depth of 3 to 4 mm. and about one-half the volume of hydroxylamine solution is added. The open end of the tube is sealed in an open flame and the contents well mixed by centrifuging with inversion of the sealed tube. The tube is laid on a hot plate maintained at about 100° C. for five minutes. The tube is cooled, reopened and alcoholic ferric chloride added in an amount equal to about one quarter of the total volume of fluid in the tube. The contents are thoroughly mixed by stirring with a glass thread and the alcoholic hydrochloric acid solution added dropwise from a capillary medicine dropper until the mixture is acid to Congo paper. The red to violet color develops with neutralization of the alkaline solution.

Table 47-28. Hydroxamic Acid Test (129, 30)

POSITIVE REACTION—red or violet colorations

Acetanilid	Antipyrine	Carbamylcholine	Hyoscyamine	Procaine
Acetophenetidin	Apomorphine	chloride	Meconin	Pyrilamine
Acetylsalicylic	Apothesine	Chlorobutanol	Pamaquine	Santonin
acid	Atropine	Cocaine	Phenylsalicy-	Scopolamine
Aconitine	Benzocaine	Delphinine	late	Tribromo-
Adiphenine	Brucine	Digitoxin	Physostigmine	ethanol
Amprotropine	Butamin	Glycine	Pilocarpine	Trimethadione
Antabuse	Caffeine	Heroin	Piperocaine	Yohimbine

NO REACTION

N-Allylnormor-	Digalen	Larocaine	Picrotoxin	Sulfanilamide
phine	Digitalin	Lobeline	Piperidione	Sulfapyridine
p-Aminobenzoic	Digitonin	Meperidine	Piperine	Sulfathiazole
acid	Dihydromor-	Methadon	Pregnenolone	Sulfisoxazole
Amobarbital	phinone	Methylphenyl-	Prisilidene	Sulfonethyl-
Amphetamine	Dimenhydrinate	ethylhydantoin	Procaine amide	methane
Ascorbic acid	(acidic and	Metopon	Pseudopelle-	Sulfonme-
Atabrin	basic extrac-	Morphine	tierine	thane
Cantharidin	tion products)	Narceine	Pyrithyldione	Tetracaine
Cholesterol	Diothane	Narcotine	Quinidine	Thenylpyra-
Cinchonidine	Diphenhydramine	Nicotinic alcohol	Quinine	mine
Cinchonine	Emetine	Nikethamide	Ricin	Theobromine
Cinchophen	Ephedrine	Optochin	Rutin	Theophylline
Codeine	Estrone	Pavatrine (acidic	Saccharin	Thiamin degrada-
Coniine	Ethylbiscoum-	and basic	Salicin	tion product
Curarine	acetate	fractions)	Solanin	Thiazolsulfone
Desoxycholic	Ethylmorphine	Pentamethylene-	Sparteine	Thiopental
acid	Eucupin.di HCl	tetrazol	Strophanthin	Thonzylamine
d-Desoxyephe-	Hippuric acid	Phenindamine	Strychnine	Trihexyphe-
drine	Homatropine	Phenobarbital	Succinylsulfa-	nidyl
Dibucaine	Hydrastine	Phenylbutazone	thiazole	Urethan
Dicoumarol	Isoamylethyl-	Phthalylsulfa-	Sulfacetimide	Veratrine
Dicyclomine	acetylurea	thiazole	Sulfadiazine	Xylocaine

(e) Aquoferriate Test. Sodium pentacyanoaquoferriate ($Na_2[Fe(CN)_5] \cdot H_2O$) has been used as a test for primary aliphatic amines with which green or blue colors develop (136) and as a reagent to differentiate between certain thio functional groups in soluble organic sulfur compounds. According to Grote (137), thio groups (R-SH) produce a color in the red portion of the spectrum whereas thione or thial compounds (R-C-R) give a color in the blue. Soluble disulfides (R-S-S-R) also react positively but

$$\overset{O}{\underset{\overset{\parallel}{S}}{\parallel}} \qquad \overset{O}{\underset{}{\parallel}} \qquad \overset{O}{\underset{}{\parallel}} \qquad \overset{O}{\underset{}{\parallel}}$$

sulphoxides (R-S-R), sulphones (R-S-R), sulfinic (R-S-OH) and sulphonic (R-S-OH)

$$\overset{}{\underset{\overset{\parallel}{O}}{}} \qquad\qquad\qquad \overset{}{\underset{\overset{\parallel}{O}}{}}$$

acids or isothioureas do not react. Color production in the short wave portion of the visible spectrum is distinctive for groupings such as C=S, E=S where E is a nonmetallic element, N=S as in KCNS and for normal thioureas.

The reagent is destroyed by acid, with the formation of Prussian blue, so that compounds such as CH_3C—OH give only a transient blue. Since the reagent is distinctly

$$\overset{\parallel}{S}$$

yellow, small samples or compounds in which the blue coloration is not intense, the observed color is green. With sulfides (R-S-R), creatinine, acetoacetic ester and some alkaloids, an orange color develops but, since this cannot be interpreted on a micro scale because of the yellow color of the reagent, orange or yellow oranges are considered negative. Although pilocarpine does not contain sulfur, a red color is produced with the reagent and some bases that are not primary amines are precipitated. The reagent is troublesome to prepare and does not keep longer than two weeks. The most practical use is in differentiating between organic compounds that were subjected to a sodium fusion and found to contain sulfur. Used in conjunction with the iodine-sodium azide reaction (page 1249), negative findings in both tests rule out reactive sulfur-containing groups and point to a more stable configuration such as that in sulfonmethane.

Reagents. (a) Sodium pentacyanoaquoferriate . solution (137): 5 gm. of sodium nitroprusside are dissolved in 10 ml. of water and 0.5 gm. of hydroxylamine hydrochloride and 1.0 gm. of sodium bicarbonate are introduced with stirring while the beaker is in the fume hood. The solution is allowed to stand with intermittent stirring until all of the HCN gas has evolved after which two drops of liquid bromine are added. The excess bromine is removed by aeration and the solution is filtered and made up to a volume of 25 ml.*

(b) Sodium carbonate solution: 10 gm. sodium carbonate/100 ml.

(c) Acetone.

Procedure (43). The unknown, contained in a capillary test tube, is dissolved by the addition of a few micro drops of acetone. Sodium pentacyanoaquoferriate reagent in an amount equal to about one-half the volume of acetone is introduced, the solution mixed and allowed to stand while it is observed over a period of 10 minutes. A micro drop of sodium carbonate solution is then added and any change or increased intensity of the color is noted.

Table 47-29. Aquoferriate Test (43, 30)

Compound	Color Developed with Sodium Pentacyano-aquoferriate Solution	Compound	Color Developed with Sodium Pentacyano-aquoferriate Solution
RED			
Pilocarpine	Red		
YELLOW			
Aconitine	Yellow precipitate	Dibucaine	Yellow precipitate
Adiphenine	Yellow precipitate	Diothane	Yellow precipitate
Amprotropine	Yellow precipitate	Meperidine	Yellow precipitate
Apothesine	Yellow precipitate	Narceine	Yellow precipitate
Cholesterol	Yellow precipitate	Phenylsalicylate	Yellow precipitate
d-Desoxyephedrine	Yellow precipitate		
GREEN			
Acetylsalicylic acid	Green with yellow cast	Phenobarbital	Green with yellow cast
		Procaine	Green with yellow cast
Amobarbital	Green with yellow cast	Saccharin	Green
Apomorphine	Green precipitate	Theophylline	Green with yellow cast
Ethylbiscoumacetate	Green	Thiopental	Green
alpha-Naphthylthiourea (ANTU)	Green		

* The reagent may also be prepared by exposure of the sodium nitroprusside in 1 per cent sodium carbonate solution to ultraviolet light for 15 minutes, according to Feigl, F. (131).

Table 47-29 (cont.). Aquoferriate Test (43, 30)

COMPOUND	COLOR DEVELOPED WITH SODIUM PENTACYANO-AQUOFERRIATE SOLUTION	COMPOUND	COLOR DEVELOPED WITH SODIUM PENTACYANO-AQUOFERRIATE SOLUTION

BLUE

Glycine ⋅   Blue violet with gray cast

NEGATIVE REACTION

Acetanilid	Codeine	Ethylmorphine	Phenylbutazone	Succinylsulfa-
Acetophenetidin	Coniine	Eucupin.di HCl	Phthalylsulfa-	thiazole
N-Allylnormor-	Curarine	Heroin	thiazole	Sulfacetimide
phine	Delphinine	Hippuric acid	Physostigmine	Sulfadiazine
p-Aminobenzoic	Desoxycholic	Homatropine	Picrotoxin	Sulfanilamide
acid	acid	Hydrastine	Piperidione	Sulfapyridine
Aminopyrine	Dicoumarol	Hyoscyamine	Piperine	Sulfathiazole
Amphetamine	Dicyclomine	Isoamylethyl-	Piperocaine	Sulfisoxazole
Antabuse	Digalen	acetylurea	Pregnenolone	Sulfonethyl-
Antipyrine	Digitalin	Larocaine	Prisilidene	methane
Ascorbic acid	Digitonin	Lobeline	Procaine amide	Sulfonmethane
Atabrin	Digitoxin	Meconin	Pseudopelle-	Tetracaine
Atropine	Dihydromor-	Methadon	tierine	Theobromine
Benzocaine	phinone	Methylphenyl-	Pyrilamine	Thenylpyramine
Brucine	Dimenhydrinate	ethylhydantoin	Pyrithyldione	Thiamin degrada-
Butamin	(acidic and	Metopon	Quinidine	tion product
Caffeine	basic extrac-	Morphine	Quinine	Thiazolsulfone
Cantharidin	tion products)	Narcotine	Ricin	Thonzylamine
Carbamylcholine	Diphenhydra-	Nicotinic alcohol	Rutin	Tribromo-
chloride	mine	Nikethamide	Salicin	ethanol
Chlorobutanol	Emetine	Optochin	Santonin	Trihexyphenidyl
Cinchonidine	Ephedrine	Pamaquine	Scopolamine	Trimethadione
Cinchonine	Estrone	Pavatrine	Solanin	Urethan
Cinchophen	Ethylbiscoum-	Pentamethylene-	Sparteine	Veratrine
Cocaine	acetate	tetrazol	Strophanthin	Xylocaine
		Phenindamine	Strychnine	Yohimbine

(f) **Benzoyl Peroxide-Stannic Chloride Test.** Stannic chloride is a precipitant in nonaqueous solution for many of the basic drugs (page 1160). With benzoyl peroxide, it has been used as a test for certain amine antioxidants (138) and also supplied to the analysis of drugs (43). The reaction is merely a nonaqueous oxidation and is not characteristic for any specific structure except that benzoyl peroxide has the right oxidizing potential for converting primary amines in which the amino group is attached to a tertiary carbon atom and primary aromatic amines to nitroso compounds. The anhydrous stannic chloride does not influence particularly the reaction of benzoyl peroxide with most drugs but does enhance the reaction with some organic compounds other than the pharmaceuticals. Drugs that show characteristic changes in the test are not particularly important and give other reactions so that, as a designating test, the reaction is of limited value. However, stannic chloride precipitation may be useful both as a test and for purification. The benzoyl peroxide-stannic chloride test is carried out in chloroform solution, whereas the similar reaction with stannic chloride and benzotrichloride (page 1229) is carried out in ethylenedichloride solution. The majority of the drugs that are precipitable with stannic chloride do so in both solutions but some precipitate only in chloroform, while some others precipitate from ethylenedichloride alone. In the section of the table for the reaction which lists the compounds that precipitate from chloroform with stannic chloride, those which do not precipitate from ethylenedichloride solution are marked with an asterisk and comparison with the table for the benzotrichloride test (page 1232) serves as a distinguishing characteristic for these substances (Table 47-30).

3. Differential Reactions.

3. Differential Reactions. Although reactions in this class are more specific than the previous types, it is not necessarily because they are generically specific for a definite organic structure. Their specificity results either from the fact that a sensitive test with an easily interpreted color is obtained with a smaller number of compounds in contrast

Table 47-30. Benzoyl Peroxide-Stannic Chloride Test (43, 30)

RED

Brucine and solanin develop a red precipitate after addition of stannic chloride.

YELLOW

Pavatrine (acidic extraction) develops a yellow solution after addition of stannic chloride.

GREEN

Apomorphine develops a green precipitate after addition of stannic chloride.

WHITE

The following compounds develop a white precipitate after addition of stannic chloride except as noted.

Acetanilid	Cinchonidine	Diothane	Optochin	Quinine
Aconitine	Cinchonine	Diphenhydra-	Pamaquine	Santonin
N-Allylnormor-	Cinchophen *	mine	Pentamethylene-	Scopolamine
phine	Cocaine	Emetine	tetrazol	Sparteine
p-Aminobenzoic	Codeine	Ethylmorphine	Physostigmine	Strychnine
acid	Curarine *	Eucupin.di HCl	Pilocarpine	Sulfadiazine *
Aminopyrine	Delphinine	Heroin	Piperine	Sulfapyridine
Amprotropine	Desoxycholic acid *	Homatropine	Piperocaine	Sulfisoxazole
Antabuse	Dibucaine	Hydrastine	Pregnenolone ‡	Tetracaine
Antipyrine *	Dicyclomine *	Hyoscyamine	Procaine	Theobromine
Atabrin	Digitoxin *†	Larocaine	Procaine	Theophylline
Atropine	Dihydromor-	Metopon *	amide *	Thiazolsul-
Benzocaine	phinone	Morphine *	Pyrilamine	fone *
Butamin	Dimenhydrinate	Narceine	Pseudopelle-	Veratrine
Caffeine	(basic extrac-	Narcotine	tierine	Xylocaine
Cholesterol	tion product)	Nikethamide	Quinidine	Yohimbine

* Precipitated by stannic chloride from chloroform but not from ethylenedichloride.
† White precipitate → brownish purple.
‡ White precipitate → pink.

NO REACTION

Acetophenetidin	d-Desoxyephed-	Lobeline	Phthalylsulfa-	Sulfanilamide
Acetylsalicylic	rine	Meconin	thiazole	Sulfathiazole
acid	Dicoumarol	Meperidine	Picrotoxin	Sulfonethyl-
Adiphenine	Digalen	Methadon	Piperidione	methane
Amobarbital	Digitalin	Methylphenyl-	Prisilidene	Sulfonmethane
Amphetamine	Digitonin	ethylhydantoin	Pyrithyldione	Thenylpyramine
base	Ephedrine	Nicotinic	Ricin	Thiamin degrada-
Apothesine	Estrone	alcohol	Rutin	tion product
Ascorbic acid	Ethylbiscoum-	Pavatrine (basic	Saccharin	Thiopental
Cantharidin	acetate	extraction)	Salicin	Tribromo-
Carbamylcholine	Glycine	Phenindamine	Strophanthin	ethanol
chloride	Hippuric acid	Phenobarbital	Succinylsulfa-	Trihexyphenidyl
Chlorobutanol	Isoamylethyl-	Phenylbutazone	thiazole	Trimethadione
Coniine	acetylurea	Phenylsalicylate	Sulfacetimide	Urethan

to the larger number of positively reacting substances that characterize the exclusion and indicating type reactions or that striking or characteristic tests are obtained for a few individual substances. In general, these reactions only attain their specificity as a result of positive findings in the previous tests.

(a) Mandelin's Reagent. Dissolve 1 part of ammonium vanadate in 200 parts of cold concentrated sulfuric acid.

Mandelin's reagent reacts with a larger number of drugs than any of the other alkaloidal reagents. However, the reagent is quite yellow and the coloration produced with many of the positively reacting substances has a dull, washed out appearance that is just the opposite of the spectral colors that constitute a good color reaction. Although the colorations, in most cases, are distinct with pure substances, when carried out on drugs extracted from tissue, the change in hue resulting from the yellow of the reagent, in addition to the effect of the small amount of normal tissue extractables on the reaction color with its low power product * makes the reaction very difficult to interpret

---

* The power product of a color is the product of the value times the chroma (139).

when the drug being tested is still an unknown compound.† Some important compounds which give nondistinctive colors with the other reagents give striking colors with Mandelin's reagent and many of these are made more significant because of the tendency to show a play of colors, with green predominating. The reagent is almost confirmatory for strychnine. Antipyrine gives a green changing to blue-green, diothane® goes from orange to red, pavatrine® changes from brown to blue-violet, hydrastine gives a red color, methadon goes from green to blue, mephenesine changes from green to violet and mephobarbital passes from green to blue. The colors developed in many of the other tests with these compounds are relatively nonsignificant yellows and browns. Narceine and narcotine develop a good orange changing to light red, alpha-naphthylthiourea gives a purple color and the original red color of pyridium® is changed to green, then blue.

Table 47-31. Mandelin's Reagent (109)

* See footnote, page 1192.

COMPOUND	COLOR DEVELOPED WITH MANDELIN'S REAGENT	COLOR AFTER WATER DILUTION
RED		
Acetanilid	Flash of pink → flesh color	Colorless
Amphetamine.HCl	Brick red	Color fades
Cholesterol	Brick red	Colorless
Digitalin	Red, slowly changing to brown	Color fades
Dimenhydrinate (basic extraction product)	Brick red	White precipitate
Diothane	Red with orange cast → red → brick red → green → olive green	Color fades
Diphenhydramine	Brick red	White precipitate
Hydrastine	Red → brown red → brown	Light red brown; fades
Methapyrilene *	Dark red → brownish purple → purple	Black
Methylparafynol	Brick red → brown with red cast	Gray brown
Pyrilamine	Brick red → carmine	Magenta
Salicin	Red	Rose precipitate
Thenylpyramine *	Brick red → dark red → brownish purple	Deep brown
Thonzylamine	Brick red → carmine	Magenta
Zolamine.HCl	Deep carmine red	Deep magenta
ORANGE		
p-Aminobenzoic acid	Pale orange → brownish	Very pale violet
Aminopyrine	Very pale orange; decolorizes slowly	Colorless
Atabrin	Orange	Color fades
Betaine.HCl	Orange	Colorless
Brucine	Light orange	Light salmon pink
Carbamylcholine chloride	Slight orange; fades	Colorless
Histamine.di HCl	Orange	Colorless
Narceine	Orange → salmon pink	Flesh color
Narcotine	Orange → salmon	Flesh color
Phanadorn	Orange → orange brown	Color fades
Phthalylsulfathiazole	Light orange	Colorless
Procaine.HCl	Pale orange	Colorless
Succinylsulfathiazole	Pale orange	Flesh color; fades
Terpin hydrate	Orange yellow → orange	Pink with white precipitate
BROWN		
N-Allylnormorphine	Pale brown → light violet	Color fades
Amphetamine base	Brown	Color fades
Amprotropine	Pale brown with violet cast	Color fades
Apothesine	Brown	Slight white precipitate
Benzocaine	Slight brown, developing slowly	Light brown violet

† The difference between the interpretation of a test on a known substance and the same material tested as an unknown when the observed change for the reaction is of poor quality is not psychological. When the substance is known or suspected, the observation is merely a comparison of behavior whereas, with an unknown, the observed change must be sufficiently pronounced to first establish the fact that it is significant before an interpretation of the reaction can be made.

Table 47-31 (cont.). Mandelin's Reagent (109)

COMPOUND	COLOR DEVELOPED WITH MANDELIN'S REAGENT	COLOR AFTER WATER DILUTION
Berberine.SO₄	Dark brown	Brick red or red brown
Cephaeline	No change from original brown with red cast	Color fades
Chrysazin	Brown → dark red → green	Light green → green yellow
Codeine	Brown → brown with violet cast → gray violet	Color fades
Colchicine	Light brown with greenish cast	Color pales
Curarine	Brown	Flesh color
Cyclopal	Brown with red cast, developing slowly	Gray brown
Delphinine	Brown with red cast	Color fades
Desoxycholic acid	Slowly turns pale brown	Color fades
d-Desoxyephedrine	Light brown	Color fades
Digalen	Brown → brown with slight-violet cast	Color fades
Digitonin	Colorless, turning pale brown slowly	Color fades
Digitoxin	Brown with slight violet cast	Color fades
Dihydromorphinone	Brown → light magenta	Color fades
Emetine	No change from original brown with red cast	Light brown
Ephedrine	Light brown	Color fades
Estrone	Light brown	Light rose
Ethylmorphine	Brown → gray violet	Color fades
Heroin	Light brown → violet	Color fades
Lobeline	No change from original brown	Light brown
Meperidine	Slowly turns light brown	Color fades
Morphine	Light brown → pale violet	Color fades
alpha-Naphthylthiourea (ANTU)	Brown → deep magenta or purple	White precipitate
Pamaquine	Brown with red cast → brown with magenta cast	Deep purple
Pavatrine	Brown → blue → violet on standing	Light red brown
Pelletierine tannate	No change from original brown	Pale flesh
Phenindamine	Brown with red cast	Yellowish precipitate
Phenylbutazone	Brown with red cast	Whitish precipitate
Piperine	Dark brown with red cast → green brown → dark olive green	Brown
Pregnenolone	Brown with red cast → brown with orange cast	Color fades
Procaine	Light brown	Color fades
Procaine amide	Slowly turns light brown with slight violet cast	Magenta → rose
Rutin	Brown or brown with red cast, slowly developing olive green streaks	Orange
Solanin	Light brown with red cast	Slight pink
Sparteine	No change from original brown with red cast	Color pales
Strophanthin	No change from original brown	Light brown
Sulfathiazole	Light brown on standing	Light magenta
Thiamin degradation product	Slight brown color	Colorless
Thiobarbituric acid	Light brown with red cast	Color fades
Trihexyphenidyl	Light brown → brown with magenta cast	Milky white precipitate
Veratrine	Brown with red cast → red → red purple	Color fades to brown with magenta cast
Xylocaine	Brown with red cast	Light brown

YELLOW

Yellow colorations cannot be interpreted because the reagent itself is yellow. Moreover, the other colors produced will be influenced by the reagent, as discussed on pages 1185 to 1190.

GREEN

Acetylsalicylic acid	Light green	White precipitate
Adiphenine	Green → brownish	Whitish precipitate
Antipyrine	Light green → blue green	Color fades
Apomorphine	Olive green → brown	Light brown
Dromoran	Green with gray cast → gray violet → violet	Color fades
Homatropine	Colorless → light olive green	White precipitate
Mephenesine	Green → violet brown on standing → magenta	Magenta or violet
Mephobarbital	Green → blue green → blue	Milky white precipitate
Mescaline	Green → brown	Dark brown
Methadon	Dark green → blue	Color fades
Phenylsalicylate	Green → gray	Yellowish or grayish green precipitate

Table 47-31 (cont.). Mandelin's Reagent (109)

COMPOUND	COLOR DEVELOPED WITH MANDELIN'S REAGENT	COLOR AFTER WATER DILUTION
Prisilidene	Pale green with violet cast	Color fades
Pyridium	Green → blue green with magenta edges, slowly turning purple	Rose
Salicylic acid	Light green → grayish	Color pales
Yohimbine	Green → blue → brownish	Light red → flesh

BLUE

Strychnine	Blue → purple → magenta → red → red orange → orange	Orange

MAGENTA

Metopon	Pale magenta	Color fades

GRAY

Dicyclomine	Pale gray	Bluish white precipitate

NO REACTION

The following compounds:

1. give no reaction with Mandelin's reagent;
2. are colorless after water dilution except as noted in footnotes.

Acetophenetidin	Cinchonine	Glycine	Pentobarbital	Sulfacetimide
Aconitine	Cinchophen	Hexobarbital	Phenobarbital	Sulfadiazine
Acridine.HCl *	Cocaine	Hippuric acid	Phenylacetylurea ‡	Sulfanilamide
Amobarbital †	Coniine.HCl	Hyoscyamine	Pilocarpine	Sulfapyridine ‡‡
Aprobarbital	Cysteine.HCl	Isoamylethyl-	Piperidione	Sulfisoxazole §§
Ascorbic acid	Diallybarbituric	acetylurea ‡	Piperocaine	Sulfonethyl-
Atropine	acid	Larocaine	Probarbital	methane
Barbital	Dibucaine	Meconin ‡	Pseudopelletier-	Sulfonmethane
Biuret	Dichlorodiphenyl-	l-Menthol ††	ine	Tetracaine
Bromural	trichloroethane	Methylphenylethyl-	Pyrithyldione	Theobromine
Butabarbital	(DDT)	hydantoin	Quinidine	Theophylline
Butallylonal	Dicoumarol ‡	Neonal	Quinine	Thiazolsulfone ***
Butamin §	Diethylacetylurea	Nicotine	Ricin	Thiopental †
Caffeine	Dimenhydrinate	Nicotinic alcohol	Saccharin	Thymol iodide
Cantharidin ‡	(acidic extrac-	Nikethamide	Sandoptal	p-Toluenesulfon-
Carbromal †	tion product)	Nostal	Santonin	amide
Chlorcyclizine	Diphenylhydantoin ‡	Optochin	Scopolamine	Tribromoethanol
Chlorobutanol ‡	Ethyl biscoum-	Ortal	Secobarbital	Trimethadione
Cinchonidine **	acetate ‡	Pentamethylene-	Sedormid	Urethan
	Eucupin.di HCl	tetrazol	Sigmodal	Vinbarbital

    * Yellow after water dilution.
    † Slight white precipitate after water dilution.
    ‡ White precipitate after water dilution.
    § Slight violet after water dilution.
   ** Greenish precipitate after water dilution.
   †† Milky white precipitate after water dilution.
   ‡‡ Trace of pink violet after water dilution.
   §§ Light pink violet after water dilution.
 *** Very slight rose after water dilution.

(b) Janovsky Reaction. This reaction was developed in 1886 as a test for meta-dinitro and trinitro compounds and their derivatives (140). Bittó (141) later replaced the acetone used in the test with other ketones and some aldehydes. The original procedure was used for the quantitative determination of benzene after conversion into meta-dinitrobenzene (page 1073). Other investigators (142, 143) have applied the reaction to the detection of ketones and it has come to be recognized in organic circles as a generic type of test for reactive carbonyl radicals and is known as the Janovsky reaction. Zimmerman (144, 145) applied the reaction to the determination of urinary neutral ketosteroids and in the fields of endocrinology and biochemistry the determination is known as the Zimmerman reaction. Except for the determination of the carbonyl-containing drugs (146-148), the reaction has not been used generally as a test for pharmaceutical compounds. A study of the reaction with the different drugs (149) showed it to be one of the best identifying reactions. With few exceptions, it is a one-color test but positively reacting substances may be detected in very low concentrations and, being a nonaqueous reaction, tissue interference is not appreciable.

In applying the test to the determination of volatile ketone solvents (page 1067), it was found that aliphatic amines gave the same coloration as carbonyl-containing compounds and it is to be expected that complex organic radicals with aliphatic side chains containing amino groups that are sufficiently basic would react. Although not specific for carbonyl groups, the specificity is increased after separating the compounds into the five groups by the extraction procedure. Compounds that are predominantly ketones are neutral or weakly acidic and the first probable postulate from a positive reaction on an unknown in the neutral or phenol fraction would be that the substance is a ketone type. Pronounced basicity is a prerequisite for the development of the typical red-violet carbonyl color with bases and positive findings on the alkaline extract would most likely be due to the basic groups. Amphoterics, however, are not strongly basic and the development of a red-violet color with an amphoteric substance would be more in favor of a carbonyl type of structure. Anomalies exist for practically all organic reactions, but there is a logical basis for postulation of the structure from the findings in the Janovsky reaction that does not exist with the oxidizing or reducing type of reaction.

Aside from methadon, metopon and dihydromorphinone, which would be expected to react because of their free carbonyl groups, good red or magenta colors are obtained with brucine, cinchonidine, lobeline, pseudopelletierine, strychnine, dicyclomine, methylparafynol, cyclopal®, phenylacetylurea, chlorobutanol and nicotine. Pilocarpine, digitoxin and strophanthin develop a blue color, while butamin, larocaine®, antabuse®, carbromal, carbamylcholine chloride, procaine hydrochloride, alpha-naphthylthiourea and many of the sulfa drugs develop a yellow to orange color that is distinct from the light brown of the blank after standing one hour.

The reaction is particularly distinctive as a test for lobeline, strophanthin and nicotine which do not give good colorations in other color tests and for differentiating dihydromorphinone from the other opiates.

Reagents. (a) Two per cent *m*-dinitrobenzene in absolute ethyl alcohol. This must be prepared fresh.

(b) Five N aqueous potassium hydroxide.

Procedure. Add to the solid sample in a 1 ml. micro centrifuge tube, 0.1 ml. of the *m*-dinitrobenzene reagent and 0.1 ml. of the potassium hydroxide. Mix and observe after a few minutes. Observe again after the sample has stood for one hour. A reagent blank should be prepared at the same time since a very light brown color develops after one hour.

The compounds are tabulated according to the colors developed at the end of one hour (Table 47-32, page 1230).

(c) Stannic Chloride-Benzotrichloride. Benzotrichloride, in the presence of anhydrous stannic chloride, has been used in the qualitative and quantitative analysis of amine anti-oxidants which are condensation products of diarylamines and ketones (138). The reaction is semispecific for the dibenzopyridine type of structure such as that in the drugs acriflavine and trypaflavine used for the treatment of trypanosome diseases. The reaction is believed to proceed through the formation of carbonium ions by the interaction of the stannic chloride and benzotrichloride, followed by coupling with the amino group to form arylmethane chlorostannates. The effectiveness of the stannic chloride appears to be due to its ability to abstract chlorine from the reagent and reaction product with the formation of the stable $SnCl_6^=$ anion in a manner analogous to the use of dehydrating agents in condensation reactions, in which one of the products of the reaction is water. The reaction rate in ethylenedichloride is greater than in solvents such as benzene and the presence of traces of polar solvents which form stable $SnCl_4$ complexes completely inhibit the reaction.

Since a number of bases with complex structures other than the acridine type were found to give colors in the reaction, it was applied as a general test for drugs (43). Like the benzoyl peroxide-stannic chloride reaction (page 1224), the two steps in the procedure afford two observations. Precipitation of the drug with stannic chloride in the ethylenedichloride solvent is recorded as a separate observation and any coloration produced on

Table 47-32. Janovsky Reaction (149) §

* Very slightly darker than the faint pink color of the reagent blank.
† Color produced with potassium hydroxide alone.
§ Umberger, C. J., and Dal Cortivo, L. Unpublished.

COMPOUND	COLOR DEVELOPED IMMEDIATELY AFTER ADDING KOH AND m-DINITROBENZENE	COLOR DEVELOPED ON STANDING ONE HOUR AFTER ADDING KOH AND m-DINITROBENZENE
RED		
Amprotropine	Faint violet	Rose
Atropine	Very faint pink *	Very faint pink
Butallylonal	Very faint pink *	Very faint pink
Caffeine	Very faint pink *	Very faint pink
Chrysazin	Cherry red †	Cherry red
Dicyclomine	Rose	Deep rose
Digitalin	No reaction	Pink
Dimenhydrinate (basic extraction product)	Very faint pink *	White precipitate; solution very faint pink
Dromoran	Original yellow → colorless	Very faint pink
Homatropine	Faint pink *	Pink
Mescalene	Faint pink *	Light rose
Methylparafynol	Yellow precipitate with KOH; changing to deep reddish with m-Dinitrobenzene	Very deep red
Nicotine	Wine red	Deep red
Phenylacetylurea	Deep magenta	Deep wine red
Pregnenolone	No reaction	Light pink
Prisilidene	Faint pink *	Light rose
Pyridium	Orange with brown cast	Deep wine
Strychnine	Light magenta	Rose → wine
Thonzylamine	No reaction	Rose
Trihexyphenidyl	Pink	Rose
ORANGE		
Benzocaine	Yellow	Orange with brown cast
Berberine.SO₄	Orange precipitate	Orange precipitate
Codeine	Light orange with brown cast †	Orange with brown cast
Emetine	Yellow solution → olive green	Dark orange with brown cast
Phanadorn	Yellow with pink cast †	Light orange
Procaine amide	Yellow	Orange with brown cast
Strophanthin	Bright yellow with KOH; with m-Dinitrobenzene, changes to deep blue → blue with green cast	Deep orange with brown cast
Succinylsulfathiazole	Yellow	Orange with brown cast
Sulfacetimide	Yellow → dark yellow	Dark yellow → orange with brown cast
Sulfadiazine	Yellow → dark yellow	Dark yellow → orange with brown cast
Sulfanilamide	Yellow	Orange with brown cast
Sulfisoxazole	Light yellow	Orange with brown cast
Thiazolsulfone	No reaction	Light orange with brown cast
Thiobarbituric acid	Light rose	Orange with yellow cast
BROWN		
Chlorobutanol	Faint pink *	Deep brown with red cast
Dihydromorphinone	Deep magenta	Dark brown
Lobeline	Deep magenta	Dark brown
YELLOW		
p-Aminobenzoic acid	Very faint yellow	Intense yellow with orange cast
Antabuse	Very faint yellow	Yellow
Antipyrine	No reaction	Yellow with gray cast
Ascorbic acid	White precipitate; yellow solution	White precipitate; yellow solution
Butamin	Faint yellow	Bright yellow
Carbamylcholine chloride	No reaction	Yellow
Carbromal	Very faint pink *	Yellow
Chlorcyclizine	No reaction	Faint yellow
Colchicine	Yellow †	Yellow
Curarine	Yellow †	Yellow

Table 47-32 (cont.). Janovsky Reaction (149)

COMPOUND	COLOR DEVELOPED IMMEDIATELY AFTER ADDING KOH AND m-DINITROBENZENE	COLOR DEVELOPED ON STANDING ONE HOUR AFTER ADDING KOH AND m-DINITROBENZENE
Delphinine	Yellow †	Light yellow
d-Desoxyephedrine	No reaction	Yellow
Diethylacetylurea	No reaction	Yellow
Digitoxin	Sky blue	Pale yellow
Ephedrine	No reaction	Yellow with gray cast
Ethylmorphine	No reaction	Faint yellow
Heroin	Deep yellow †	Yellow with gray cast
Larocaine	Yellow †	Yellow
alpha-Naphthylthiourea (ANTU)	Yellow	Very intense yellow with orange cast
Nikethamide	No reaction	Faint yellow
Pavatrine	No reaction	Faint yellow
Phenindamine	Yellow with KOH; deep orange with brown cast with m-Dinitrobenzene	Very deep yellow with green cast
Piperidione	Yellow with KOH; pink with gray cast with m-Dinitrobenzene	Deep yellow with gray cast
Piperine	No reaction	Light yellow
Procaine.HCl	No reaction	Bright yellow
Ricin	No reaction	Faint yellow
Santonin	No reaction	Yellow with gray cast
Sulfapyridine	Faint yellow	Bright yellow
Sulfathiazole	Faint yellow	Bright yellow

MAGENTA

Brucine	Pink	Deep magenta
Cinchonidine	Light magenta	Magenta
Cortisone	Very faint pink *	Deep magenta
Cyclopal	Pink	Deep magenta
Hydrocortisone	Very faint pink *	Deep magenta
Methadon	Very faint pink *	Magenta
Metopon	Faint pink	Magenta
Pseudopelletierine	Magenta	Deep magenta
Vinbarbital	Faint magenta	Light magenta

GRAY

Cephaeline	Very deep gray	Very deep gray
Pilocarpine	Blue	Gray

NO REACTION

Acetanilid	Cocaine	Isoamylethyl- acetylurea	Pentobarbital	Sedormid
Acetophenetidin	Coniine.HCl	Meconin	Phenobarbital	Sigmodal
Acetylsalicylic acid	Desoxycholic acid	l-Menthol	Phenylbutazone	Solanin
Aconitine	Diallylbarbituric acid	Mephobarbital	Phenylsalicylate	Sulfonethyl- methane
Adiphenine		Methylphenylethyl- hydantoin	Phthalylsulfa- thiazole	Sulfonmethane
N-Allylnormor- phine	Dibucaine	Morphine	Piperocaine	Terpin hydrate
Aminopyrine	Dichlorodiphenyl- trichloroethane	Narceine	Probarbital	Tetracaine
Amobarbital	(DDT)	Narcotine	Pyrilamine	Thenylpyramine
Aprobarbital	Dicoumarol	Neonal	Pyrithyldione	Theobromine
Barbital	Digalen	Nicotinic alcohol	Quinidine	Theophylline
Betaine.HCl	Diothane	Nostal	Quinine	Thiopental
Bromural	Diphenylhydantoin	Optochin	Rutin	Thymol iodide
Butabarbital	Eucupin.di HCl	Ortal	Saccharin	p-Toluenesul- fonamide
Cantharidin	Hexobarbital	Pamaquine	Salicin	Tribromo- ethanol
Cinchonine	Hippuric acid	Pentamethylene- tetrazol	Sandoptal	Trimethadione
Cinchophen	Hydrastine		Scopolamine	
			Secobarbital	

the addition of the benzotrichloride is then noted. In the column in the table for precipitation with stannic chloride, those compounds that precipitate in ethylenedichloride but are not precipitated by the stannic chloride in the chloroform solvent of the benzoyl peroxide reaction (page 1224) are marked with an asterisk and this distinction furnishes an identifying characteristic for a few compounds that fail to give significant color tests.

The orange color with methadon differentiates it from other compounds which give magenta in the Janovsky reaction and lobeline, which gives an immediate magenta in the Janovsky reaction, develops an intense yellow solution. The red color produced by phenindamine separates it from the other antihistamines. The reaction with cinchophen adds to the few other color reactions that are given and diothane® is confirmed after the characteristic color changes with Mandelin's reagent. The test furnishes one of the few color reactions for digitalin and dicoumarol. Stannic chloride precipitation in both ethylenedichloride and chloroform furnishes the only identifying characteristic for caffeine and theobromine which may then be identified by the murexide reaction (page 1247). Optochin, coniine and cocaine which precipitate in both solvents give few other reactions while stannic chloride precipitation is the only characteristic behavior for the detection of pentamethylenetetrazol other than its absorption spectra. Sulfacetimide is precipitated only in ethylenedichloride while sulfadiazine precipitates in chloroform alone.

Reagents. (a) Stannic chloride: dissolve 1.5 ml. fuming stannic chloride in 25 ml. benzene.

(b) Benzotrichloride, Eastman Kodak reagent.

(c) Anhydrous ethylenedichloride.

Procedure. The unknown, contained in a capillary test tube with a bore of approximately 2 mm., is dissolved in 2 to 4 small drops of ethylenedichloride and stannic chloride solution is added in an amount equal to one-half the volume of ethylenedichloride. Any precipitation by the stannic chloride is recorded and a volume of benzotrichloride equal to that of the stannic chloride is introduced. The color of the precipitate or solution is examined after standing approximately 30 minutes. In the table for the reaction, the drugs are classified according to the color change with benzotrichloride.

Table 47-33. Stannic Chloride-Benzotrichloride Test (43, 30)

* Compound is precipitated with stannic chloride from ethylenedichloride solution but not from chloroform solution.

COMPOUND	COLOR DEVELOPED AFTER ADDITION OF STANNIC CHLORIDE	COLOR DEVELOPED AFTER ADDITION OF BENZOTRICHLORIDE
RED		
N-Allylnormorphine	White precipitate	Pink precipitate
Apomorphine	Red color	No change
Apothesine *	White precipitate	Pink precipitate
Cholesterol	Pink precipitate	No change
Codeine	White precipitate	Pink precipitate
Ethylmorphine	White precipitate	Pink precipitate
Heroin	White precipitate	Pink precipitate
Narceine	White precipitate	Pink precipitate
Narcotine	White precipitate	Slight pink precipitate
Phenindamine *	Red precipitate	No change
ORANGE		
Diothane	White precipitate	Orange with red cast precipitate
Methadon	Negative	Orange with yellow cast precipitate
Piperine	Yellow precipitate	Orange precipitate
BROWN		
Digitoxin	Negative	Brown → violet
Emetine	Brown precipitate	No change
Xylocaine	Brown precipitate	No change
YELLOW		
Acetophenetidin	Negative	Yellow precipitate
Acetylsalicylic acid	Negative	Yellow color
Antipyrine	Negative	Yellow color
Atabrin	Yellow precipitate	No change
Cinchophen	Negative	Yellow with green cast
Dicoumarol	Negative	Yellow color
Dicyclomine	Negative	Yellow color
Digitalin	Yellow color	No change

Table 47-33 (cont.). Stannic Chloride-Benzotrichloride Test (43, 30)

COMPOUND	COLOR DEVELOPED AFTER ADDITION OF STANNIC CHLORIDE	COLOR DEVELOPED AFTER ADDITION OF BENZOTRICHLORIDE
Diphenhydramine	Yellow with green cast precipitate	No change
Estrone	Negative	Yellow color
Glycine	Negative	Yellow color
Lobeline *	White precipitate	Deep yellow color; precipitate dissolves
Pamaquine	Yellow precipitate	No change
Pavatrine *	Yellow precipitate	No change
Phenylbutazone	Negative	Yellow color
Phenylsalicylate	Negative	Yellow color

MAGENTA

Pregnenolone	White precipitate	Deep magenta precipitate

BLACK

Yohimbine	White precipitate	Black precipitate

WHITE

The following compounds:
1. develop a white precipitate after addition of stannic chloride;
2. show no change after addition of benzotrichloride.

The exception is acetanilid, which shows a negative reaction after addition of stannic chloride and white cloudiness after addition of benzotrichloride.

Aconitine	Cinchonidine	Homatropine	Piperocaine	Sparteine
Adiphenine *	Cinchonine	Hydrastine	Prisilidene *	Strychnine
p-Aminobenzoic acid	Cocaine	Hyoscyamine	Procaine	Sulfacetimide *
Aminopyrine	Coniine *	Larocaine	Pseudopelle- tierine	Sulfapyridine
Amprotropine	Delphinine	Meperidine *	Pyrilamine	Sulfisoxazole
Antabuse	Dibucaine	Nikethamide	Pyrith/ldione *	Tetracaine
Atropine	Dihydromor- phinone	Optochin	Quinidine	Thenylpyra- mine *
Benzocaine	Dimenhydrinate (basic extrac- tion product)	Pentamethylene- tetrazol	Quinine	Theobromine
Brucine		Physostigmine	Ricin *	Theophylline
Butamin		Picrotoxin *	Santonin	Thonzylamine
Caffeine	Eucupin.di HCl	Pilocarpine	Scopolamine	Veratrine

NEGATIVE REACTION

Amobarbital	d-Desoxyephed- rine	Methylphenylethyl- hydantoin	Saccharin	Sulfonmethane
Amphetamine base	Digalen	Metopon	Salicin	Thiamin degrada- tion product
Ascorbic acid	Digitonin	Morphine	Solanin	Thiazolsulfone
Cantharidin	Ephedrine	Nicotinic alcohol	Strophanthin	Thiopental
Carbamylcholine chloride	Ethyl biscoum- acetate	Phenobarbital	Succinylsulfa- thiazole	Tribromo- ethanol
Chlorobutanol	Hippuric acid	Phthalylsulfa- thiazole	Sulfadiazine	Trihexyphenidyl
Curarine	Isoamylethyl- acetylurea	Piperidione	Sulfanilamide	Trimethadione
Desoxycholic acid	Meconin	Procaine amide	Sulfathiazole	Urethan
		Rutin	Sulfonethyl- methane	

Modified Stannic Chloride-Benzotrichloride Reaction (150). The colors produced by the compounds reacting in the test can be intensified considerably by elimination of the stannic chloride precipitation step, using instead a solution containing 0.6 ml. of anhydrous stannic chloride in 10 ml. of benzotrichloride. The reagent is added in the proportion of one drop of reagent to three drops of ethylenedichloride solvent. A number of compounds that do not react or show insignificant changes in the original procedure develop colors and, if allowed to stand overnight, the number of positively reacting compounds is further increased. The stannic chloride phase is not entirely eliminated but is more difficult to interpret. The modification has advantages which, after further study, may permit it to replace the original procedure but the table for the reaction will then have to be revised accordingly. This is the only test in which the bases of morphine and N-allylnormorphine show different behavior and the positive reaction with N-allylnormorphine is more pronounced in the modification. It offers a differential test for the steroids which are not present in the tissue extracts but may be encountered in tablets. Pregnenolone gives an immediate pink color which intensifies to a violet and changes to deep blue on standing overnight. Hydrocortisone develops only a tinge of color after 30 minutes but is an intense red after standing overnight while cortisone does not react in the ethylenedichloride solvent, even after standing for five days.

The nature of the solvent and the conditions for the reaction have a marked influence on the reaction. The modified reagent reacts with even greater intensity with a still larger number of compounds when employed as a spot test, by adding a drop of reagent to the anhydrous solid sample. Morphine base develops a pink color which fades while N-allylnormorphine first shows a rose color that intensifies and changes to an orange. Phenindamine appears in the table under compounds giving a red color only because it is normally reddish and, naturally, gives a red precipitate with stannic chloride. As a spot test, however, the red intensifies and changes to deep magenta. Acetophenetidin develops a green color in contrast to the yellow in ethylenedichloride and cortisone slowly develops a deep blue color after standing several days.

In contrast to the other reactions, salts of the bases give more intense colors than the free bases. Morphine and codeine sulfate develop intense red colors but the related substances show similar changes so that the increased reactivity of the reagent when employed as a spot test tends to detract from the value of the reagent as a differential type of test.

(d) Titanous Chloride-Sulfuric Acid (149).* Titanous chloride is a strong reducer and, in sulfuric acid as the solvent, the reagent does not have any special specificity for organic structures (page 1060) although it does undergo some kind of reaction with all phenols. The colors developed with the basic drugs that react are distinct but not intense enough to put the reagent in a class with Mecke's or Marquis' reagents. Magentas and reds with a brown cast predominate while the few other colors that develop tend to be low in value. The principal use for this reagent is in differentiating between the common opiates and related drugs. If the isolated sample is sufficiently pure, differentiation is possible by running a control together with the test sample and comparing the color shades. Heroin gives a magenta color while codeine, if pure, does not react. The magenta stands out in contrast with the duller color produced with morphine and N-allylnormorphine which, although red, has a decided brown cast. Dihydromorphinone, dromoran® and metopon give a lighter red which is designated as a rose color. Pavatrine and digitoxin develop green colors and hydrastine becomes orange.

Reagent. Add 15 per cent titanous chloride ($TiCl_3$) † dropwise, with shaking, to 1 ml. of concentrated sulfuric acid until a permanent bluish opalescence develops (about 8 drops).

Procedure. Add the reagent to the sample on a microscope slide as described on page 1191 (Table 47-34, page 1235).

(e) Froehde's Reagent. *Reagent.* 5 gm. sodium molybdate per ml. concentrated sulfuric acid.

Although an alkaloidal reagent, it is not particularly useful in the identification of the alkaloids. With many of the compounds which react, the colors tend to fade or rapidly disappear. It gives a good blue color with dromoran®, a blue violet with salicin, alpha-naphthylthiourea and phenylsalicylate and a blue violet which quickly fades with acetylsalicylic acid. Narceine and narcotine develop a deep green color, antabuse® a light green intensifying to deep green, estrone changes from blue to green and hydrastine changes from colorless to green while solanin gives a bright yellow color (Table 47-35).

(f) Vanillin-Sulfuric Acid Reagent (151). This aldehyde is of limited value as a general testing reagent. It closely parallels para-dimethylaminobenzaldehyde in reactivity but generally does not give as good colors nor as many. In contrast to the tendency for para-dimethylaminobenzaldehyde to be a phenol-type reagent, vanillin shows a somewhat greater selectivity for aliphatic alcohol groups. It reacts with the amyl alcohols (page 1076) and gives a better reaction with the drugs containing alcoholic hydroxy groups such as mephenesine and methylparafynol. The green colors developed with homatropine, meconin and mescaline and the blue developed with eucupin® di.HCl

---

* Umberger, C. J., and Dal Cortivo, L. Unpublished.
† Fisher Scientific Co., New York City, New York.

Table 47-34. Titanous Chloride-Sulfuric Acid Reagent (149)

Compound	Color Developed with Titanous Chloride-Sulfuric Acid Reagent	Compound	Color Developed with Titanous Chloride-Sulfuric Acid Reagent
RED			
N-Allylnormorphine	Red with brown cast	Mephenesine	Very faint pink
Amphetamine.HCl	Rose red	Metopon	Rose
Chrysazin	Deep blood red	Morphine	Red with brown cast
Dihydromorphinone	Rose red	Pyridium	Bright red
Dromoran	Rose red	Pyrilamine	Red
ORANGE			
Apothesine	Orange with brown cast	Phenylsalicylate	Light orange
Cholesterol	Orange	Phthalylsulfathiazole	Faint orange solution; effervescence
Curarine	Orange with brown cast		
Cyclopal	Orange with brown cast	Piperidione	Very pale orange
Delphinine	Orange	Piperine	Deep orange
Dimenhydrinate (basic extraction product)	Bright orange	Pregnenolone	Orange
		Ricin	Pale orange; effervescence
Diphenhydramine	Orange	Salicin	Bright orange
Emetine	Dark orange	Solanin	Orange
Hydrastine	Orange	Terpin hydrate	Orange
Methylparafynol	Very deep orange	Thenylpyramine	Deep orange
Pelletierine tannate	Original brown changes to orange	Veratrine	Bright orange with yellow cast, developing rose streaks
Phenindamine	Original red brown changes to orange solution		
BROWN			
Acetylsalicylic acid	Brown with orange cast	Ethylmorphine	Deep brown with magenta cast
Apomorphine	Dark brown with magenta cast; dissolves slowly	Mescaline	Very deep brown
		Phanadorn	Brown with red cast
Ascorbic acid	Brown with gray cast	Rutin	Brown
Cephaeline	Brown with orange cast	Strophanthin	Brown solution; dissolves slowly
Digalen	Dark brown spot		
Digitalin	Original red changes to brown	Xylocaine	Original brown darkens
YELLOW			
Acridine.HCl	Yellow with green cast; effervescence	Narcotine	Faint yellow
		Nicotine	Yellow
Atabrin	Yellow	Phenylbutazone	Very faint yellow
Cinchophen	Yellow with green cast	Quinine	Very faint yellow with green cast
Colchicine	Yellow		
Eucupin.di HCl	Pale yellow	Trihexyphenidyl	Yellow
Meconin	Pale yellow with green cast	Vinbarbital	Yellow
Narceine	Yellow with gray cast; dissolves slowly		
GREEN			
Antabuse	Light green	Optochin	Very pale green
Berberine.SO₄	Olive green	Pavatrine	Olive green
Digitoxin	Very deep green		
MAGENTA			
Heroin	Deep magenta	Zolamine.HCl	Red changing to deep magenta
Thonzylamine	Deep magenta		

Table 47-34 (cont.). Titanous Chloride-Sulfuric Acid Reagent (149)

NO REACTION

Acetanilid
Acetophenetidin
Aconitine
Adiphenine
p-Aminobenzoic
acid
Aminopyrine
Amobarbital
Amprotropine
Antipyrine
Aprobarbital
Atropine
Barbital
Benzocaine
Betaine.HCl *
Bromural
Brucine
Butabarbital
Butallylonal
Butamin
Caffeine
Cantharidin
Carbamylcholine
chloride *
Carbromal

Chlorcyclizine
Chlorobutanol
Cinchonidine
Cinchonine
Cocaine
Codeine
Coniine.HCl *
Cysteine.HCl
Desoxycholic
acid
d-Desoxyephed-
rine
Diallylbarbituric
acid
Dibucaine
Dichlorodiphenyl-
trichloroethane
(DDT)
Dicoumarol
Dicyclomine
Diethylacetylurea
Digitonin
Diothane
Diphenylhydan-
toin

Ephedrine
Ethyl biscoum-
acetate
Glycine
Hexobarbital †
Hippuric acid
Histamine.di HCl *
Homatropine
Hyoscyamine
Isoamylethyl-
acetylurea
Larocaine
Lobeline
l-Menthol
Meperidine
Mephobarbital
Methadon
Methylphenyl-
ethylhydantoin
alpha-Naphthyl-
thiourea
(ANTU)
Neonal
Nicotinic alcohol
Nikethamide *

Nostal
Ortal
Pamaquine
Pentamethylene-
tetrazol
Pentobarbital
Phenobarbital
Phenylacetylurea
Pilocarpine
Piperocaine
Prisilidene
Probarbital
Procaine amide
Procaine.HCl
Pseudopelle-
tierine
Pyrithyldione
Quinidine
Saccharin
Sandoptal
Santonin
Scopolamine
Secobarbital
Sedormid
Sigmodal

Strychnine
Succinylsulfa-
thiazole *
Sulfacetimide
Sulfadiazine
Sulfanilamide
Sulfapyridine
Sulfathiazole
Sulfisoxazole
Sulfonethyl-
methane
Sulfonmethane
Tetracaine
Theobromine *
Theophylline
Thiazolsulfone
Thiobarbituric
acid
Thiopental
Tribromoethanol
Trimethadione
Yohimbine

* Effervescence with titanous chloride-sulfuric acid reagent.
† Slight effervescence with titanous chloride-sulfuric acid reagent.

Table 47-35. Froehde's Reagent (109)

COMPOUND	COLOR DEVELOPED WITH FROEHDE'S REAGENT	COLOR AFTER WATER DILUTION
RED		
Amphetamine.HCl	Pale red or rose	Color disappears
Brucine	Colorless → rose, increasing in intensity → orange	Light lemon yellow
Cephaeline	Light red → brown with yellow cast → yellow with green cast	Light yellow
Cholesterol	Brick red	Color disappears
Chrysazin	Carmine red	Deep yellow precipitate
Dimenhydrinate (basic extraction product)	Red with orange cast; yellow solution	White precipitate
Pyridium	Bright carmine	Red orange
ORANGE		
Cyclopal	Orange → orange with brown cast	Light brown
d-Desoxyephedrine	No change from original pale orange with brown cast	No change
Diphenhydramine	Deep orange with red cast; gold solution	White precipitate
Pregnenolone	Orange with yellow cast → orange	Yellow white precipitate
Procaine amide	No change from original pale orange with brown cast	No change
Thenylpyramine	Deep orange → brick red → brown	Brown → green
BROWN		
Apothesine	Original brown with yellow cast becomes more brown	Yellows
Berberine.SO₄	Brown with yellow-green cast	Bright yellow
Delphinine	Brown with red cast	Color pales

Table 47-35 (cont.). Froehde's Reagent (109)

COMPOUND	COLOR DEVELOPED WITH FROEHDE'S REAGENT	COLOR AFTER WATER DILUTION
Digalen	Light brown developing magenta cast	Brown with green-yellow cast
Digitalin	Light brown	Greenish yellow
Digitoxin	Deep brown	Color fades
Diothane	Brown, slowly developing magenta cast	Light yellow
Emetine	Original brown with red cast → brown with yellow cast	Color fades to yellow
Ephedrine	Pale brown	Color fades
Ethylmorphine	Brown, slowly changing to gray green	Light yellow; fades
Lobeline	Original brown with red cast → brown with yellow cast	Pale yellow precipitate
Mescaline	Yellow, rapidly changing to dark brown	Brownish olive green
Pamaquine	No change from original brown with yellow cast	Golden yellow
Pavatrine	Brown with yellow cast	Milky yellow precipitate
Phanadorn	Brown with magenta cast	Pale yellow
Phenindamine	Brown with red cast	Pale yellow
Piperine	Deep brown with red cast → brown → brown with green cast	Greenish yellow
Rutin	Brown with greenish yellow cast → orange yellow	Bright yellow with green cast
Sparteine	No change from original brown	No change
Strophanthin	No change from original brown	Light yellow
Xylocaine	Original brown deepens	No change

YELLOW

COMPOUND	COLOR DEVELOPED WITH FROEHDE'S REAGENT	COLOR AFTER WATER DILUTION
Acridine.HCl	No change from original yellow	No change
Amphetamine base	Pale yellow with green brown cast	Color fades
Ascorbic acid	Very pale yellow with brown cast	Light yellow; fades
Atabrin	Bright yellow	Lemon yellow
Butallylonal	Colorless, slowly changing to light yellow	Pale yellow
Chlorcyclizine	No change from original yellow	No change
Cinchophen	Pale yellow	Color disappears
Colchicine	Bright yellow	No change
Desoxycholic acid	Colorless → very pale yellow	Slight yellow
Dicyclomine	No change from original very pale yellow	White precipitate
Digitonin	Very pale yellow with brown cast	Color fades
Eucupin.di HCl	Very very pale yellow	Colorless
Larocaine	No change from original pale yellow	No change
Meconin	Very pale yellow	Milky white precipitate
l-Menthol	Colorless → pale yellow with orange cast	White precipitate
Meperidine	Original yellow fades to very pale yellow with brown cast	No change
Methadon	Light yellow with orange cast → light yellow with green cast, slowly changing to light green	Very pale yellow
Methylparafynol	Deep yellow → yellow with brown cast → brown with yellow cast	Pale yellow precipitate
Nicotine	No change from original yellow with brown cast	No change
Optochin	Pale yellow	No change
Pelletierine tannate	Yellow	No change
Piperocaine	No change from original yellow with brown cast	No change
Prisilidene	Colorless → very pale yellow	Color disappears
Procaine	No change from original pale yellow	No change
Quinine	No change from original pale yellow	No change
Solanin	Bright yellow	Color disappears
Terpin hydrate	Yellow → yellow with orange cast	Milky white precipitate
Trihexyphenidyl	Light yellow → light yellow with brownish cast	Pale yellow
Veratrine	Yellow → orange → brick red → carmine red → red purple	Color pales
Vinbarbital	Pale yellow	Slight white precipitate

Table 47-35 (cont.). Froehde's Reagent (109)

COMPOUND	COLOR DEVELOPED WITH FROEHDE'S REAGENT	COLOR AFTER WATER DILUTION
GREEN		
Antabuse	Slight green, slowly increasing in intensity, then slowly changing to gold	Yellow precipitate
Apomorphine	Olive green	Color pales
Hydrastine	Colorless → green	Pale yellow
Narceine	Green	Light yellow
Narcotine	Deep green	Light yellow
BLUE		
Acetylsalicylic acid	Light blue violet which fades	White precipitate
alpha-Naphthylthio-urea (ANTU)	Colorless → blue violet increasing in intensity, then very slowly changing to yellow	Yellow → reddish
Codeine	Grayed blue violet	Pale yellow
Dromoran	Blue	Pale yellow
Estrone	Blue → green → yellow	Color fades
Phenylsalicylate	Deep blue violet → gray blue → gray green	Yellow
Salicin	Blue violet → magenta → red	Light orange
Salicylic acid	Colorless → light blue violet which fades	White precipitate
Yohimbine	Blue changing slowly to green → yellow	Color pales
MAGENTA		
N-Allylnormorphine	Magenta changing slowly to gray green	Pale yellow
Curarine	Light magenta with brown cast → light brown	Yellow; fades
Dihydromorphinone	Magenta (violet) which fades	Pale yellow
Heroin	Magenta changing slowly to gray green	Yellow
Mephenesine	Magenta with brown cast	Pale yellow
Metopon	Magenta which fades slowly	Pale yellow
Morphine	Deep magenta changing slowly to gray green	Light yellow
Pyrilamine	Magenta → deep magenta	Color fades
Thonzylamine	Magenta → deep magenta	Color pales slightly
Zolamine.HCl	Magenta	Reddish brown

COLORLESS

The following compounds are colorless:

    1. with Froehde's reagent;
    2. after water dilution except as noted in footnotes.

Acetanilid	Carbromal	Glycine	Phthalylsulfa-thiazole	Sulfanilamide
Acetophenetidin	Chlorobutanol	Hexobarbital ‡		Sulfapyridine
Aconitine	Cinchonidine	Hippuric acid	Pilocarpine	Sulfathiazole
Adiphenine *	Cinchonine	Histamine.di HCl	Piperidione	Sulfisoxazole
p-Aminobenzoic acid	Cocaine	Homatropine	Probarbital	Sulfonethyl-methane
Aminopyrine	Coniine.HCl	Hyoscyamine	Procaine.HCl	Sulfonmethane
Amobarbital *	Cysteine.HCl **	Isoamylethyl-acetylurea *	Pseudopellet-ierine	Tetracaine
Amprotropine	Diallylbarbituric acid	Mephobarbital *	Pyrithyldione	Theobromine
Antipyrine †	Dibucaine	Methylphenyl-ethylhydantoin *	Quinidine	Theophylline
Aprobarbital	Dichlorodiphenyl-trichloroethane (DDT)	Neonal	Ricin	Thiamin alkaline degradation product
Atropine		Nicotinic alcohol	Saccharin	
Barbital	Dicoumarol ‡	Nikethamide	Sandoptal	Thiazolsulfone
Benzocaine	Diethylacetyl-urea ††	Nostal	Santonin ‡‡	Thiobarbituric acid
Betaine.HCl		Ortal ††	Scopolamine	
Biuret	Dimenhydrinate (acidic extrac-tion product)	Pentamethylene-tetrazol	Secobarbital ‡‡	Thiopental *
Bromural		Pentobarbital	Sedormid	p-Toluenesulfo-namide
Butabarbital		Phenobarbital *	Sigmodal *	
Butamin	Diphenylhydan-toin *	Phenylacetyl-urea *	Strychnine	Tribromoethanol
Caffeine			Succinylsulfa-thiazole	Trimethadione
Cantharidin ‡	Ethyl biscoum-acetate *	Phenylbutazone	Sulfacetimide	Urethan
Carbamylcholine chloride			Sulfadiazine	

   * Milky white precipitate after water dilution.
   † Very pale yellow after water dilution.
   ‡ White precipitate after water dilution.
  ** Flash of light yellow after water dilution.
  †† Slight white precipitate after water dilution.
  ‡‡ Fleeting white precipitate after water dilution.

are characteristic. The reagent has the disadvantage of para-dimethylaminobenzaldehyde in requiring heat in most reactions and tissue interference is enhanced. The primary value of the reagent is in differentiating the color reacting barbiturates from the less reactive members.

Reagent. Dissolve 0.266 gm. vanillin in 15 ml. concentrated sulfuric acid.

Procedure. The procedure followed is the same as that described on page 1201 for para-dimethylaminobenzaldehyde.

Table 47-36. Vanillin-Sulfuric Acid Reagent (99, 109, 149)

Compound	Color Developed with Vanillin-Sulfuric Acid Reagent, Cold	Color after Heating One Minute at 125° C.	Color after Water Dilution
RED			
Chrysazin	Bright red	Deep red	Bright yellow
Cyclopal	Brown with green cast	Red with brown cast	Blue-violet
Desoxycholic acid	No reaction	Bright red	Magenta
Diallylbarbituric acid	No reaction	Red	Pale violet
Hexobarbital	No reaction	Red with brown cast	Violet
l-Menthol	No reaction	Orange → red	Deep red
Mephenesine	Red	Dark red	Magenta
Pentobarbital	No reaction	Light red with brown cast	Deep violet
Phanadorn	Orange with brown cast	Red with brown cast	Violet
Phenindamine	Original red brown darkens	Dark red	Yellow green precipitate
Pyridium	Bright red	Bright red	Orange
Secobarbital	No reaction	Light red	Violet
Thiopental	No reaction	Pale red	Violet
Veratrine	Orange with brown cast	Deep red	Red → orange → red brown
Vinbarbital	No reaction	Deep red with purple cast	Magenta
Zolamine.HCl	Magenta	Magenta → red	Magenta precipitate
ORANGE			
Amphetamine.HCl	Orange with brown cast	Deep orange with brown cast	Yellowish precipitate
Apothesine	Brown	Orange with brown cast	Color fades
Atabrin	Yellow	Dark orange	Bright yellow
Berberine.SO₄	Orange with brown cast	Orange with brown cast	Yellow precipitate with green cast
Cephaeline	No reaction	Orange with brown cast	Light orange
Cholesterol	Orange with red cast	Deep orange	Heavy magenta precipitate
Cysteine.HCl	Light orange	Orange	Color fades
Dimenhydrinate (basic extraction product)	Orange	Orange	Color fades
Nicotine	Orange	Dark orange	Light orange
Phenylsalicylate	No reaction	Orange	Rose
Pregnenolone	Orange	Dark orange	Magenta precipitate
Pseudopelletierine	No reaction	Orange	Color fades
Succinylsulfathiazole	No reaction	Light orange	Yellow
Sulfapyridine	No reaction	Light orange	Yellow
Terpin hydrate	Orange	Deep orange	Deep magenta
Thenylpyramine	Orange	Deep orange	Red orange precipitate
Trihexyphenidyl	Orange with brown cast	Orange with brown cast	Magenta
BROWN			
N-Allylnormorphine	Dark brown	Dark brown	Gray precipitate
Amprotropine	No reaction	Dark brown	Gray precipitate
Apomorphine	Brown	Brown	No change
Colchicine	Brown	Brown	Yellow
Delphinine	Deep orange	Deep brown	Brown → rose
Dicyclomine	No reaction	Brown with deep red cast	Brown → magenta
Digalen	Dark brown	Dark brown	Faint brown
Digitalin	Dark brown	Dark brown	Color fades
Digitonin	Light brown	Dark brown	Dark green precipitate

Table 47-36 (cont.). Vanillin-Sulfuric Acid Reagent (99, 109, 149)

COMPOUND	COLOR DEVELOPED WITH VANILLIN-SULFURIC ACID REAGENT, COLD	COLOR AFTER HEATING ONE MINUTE AT 125° C.	COLOR AFTER WATER DILUTION
Digitoxin	Dark brown	Dark brown	Transient magenta
Dihydromorphinone	No reaction	Dark brown	Magenta → brown
Diphenhydramine	Orange	Dark brown	Heavy whitish precipitate
Emetine	Dark brown	Dark brown	Brown orange precipitate
Ephedrine	Dark brown	Dark brown	Light orange
Ethyl biscoumacetate	No reaction	Dark brown	White precipitate
Ethylmorphine	Dark brown	Dark brown	Color fades
Heroin	Brown	Brown with olive green cast	Light brown
Hydrastine	No reaction	Very dark brown	Dark green precipitate
Lobeline	Brown	Dark brown	Light brown precipitate
Metopon	No reaction	Light brown	Color fades
Morphine	No reaction	Brown	Color fades
alpha-Naphthylthio-urea (ANTU)	Gray → brown	Brown	White precipitate
Narceine	No reaction	Dark brown	Light brown
Nicotinic alcohol	No reaction	Brown	Color fades
Pamaquine	Brown	Light brown	Yellow
Pavatrine	Dark brown	Very dark brown	Yellow precipitate
Phenylacetylurea	No reaction	Dark brown	White precipitate
Phthalylsulfathiazole	No reaction	Light brown	Yellow
Piperidione	Faint orange	Orange → brown	Magenta → brown precipitate
Piperine	Dark red with orange cast	Very dark brown	Whitish precipitate
Piperocaine	Brown	Brown	Whitish precipitate
Pyrilamine	Brown → deep red	Deep brown with orange cast	Flash of magenta
Rutin	Orange	Dark brown	Brown precipitate
Salicin	Orange	Dark brown	Magenta precipitate
Santonin	No reaction	Brown	White precipitate
Scopolamine	No reaction	Brown	Color fades
Solanin	Orange	Dark brown	Yellow green precipitate
Sparteine	Dark brown	Dark brown	Color fades
Strophanthin	Brown	Deep brown	Very dark brown precipitate
Xylocaine	Dark brown	Dark brown	Brown precipitate
Yohimbine	Light brown	Dark brown	Magenta

YELLOW

COMPOUND			
Acridine.HCl	No reaction	No reaction	Yellow
Larocaine	No reaction	Bright yellow	Yellow
Methadon	No reaction	Yellow with green cast	Faint orange

GREEN

COMPOUND			
Homatropine	No reaction	Green	Orange brown precipitate
Meconin	No reaction	Dark green	Gray precipitate
Mescaline	Dark brown	Dark green	Deep green
Narcotine	No reaction	Brown → dark green	Greenish

BLUE

COMPOUND			
Eucupin.di HCl	No reaction	Blue violet	Deep magenta → blue violet

MAGENTA

COMPOUND			
Methylparafynol	Orange → deep orange → brown	Deep magenta	Dark brown
Thonzylamine	Orange → red → magenta	Orange → magenta	Blue violet

Table 47-36 (cont.). Vanillin-Sulfuric Acid Reagent (99, 109, 149)

NO REACTION EXCEPT WITH WATER

Compound	Color after Water Dilution	Compound	Color after Water Dilution
Acetanilid	White precipitate	Diothane	Pale yellow
Acetylsalicylic acid	White precipitate	Diphenylhydantoin	White precipitate
Adiphenine	White precipitate	Methylphenylethyl-	White precipitate
p-Aminobenzoic acid	Yellow	hydantoin	
Amobarbital	White precipitate	Procaine amide	Yellow
Antabuse	Heavy whitish precipitate	Procaine.HCl	Yellow
Antipyrine	Pale orange	Pyrithyldione	Flash of magenta
Benzocaine	Yellow	Quinidine	Faint orange
Butabarbital	Violet	Sigmodal	Faint violet
Butamin	Yellow	Sulfacetimide	Yellow
Cantharidin	White precipitate	Sulfadiazine	Yellow
Chlorcyclizine	Whitish precipitate	Sulfanilamide	Yellow
Chlorobutanol	White precipitate	Sulfathiazole	Yellow
Curarine	Faint magenta	Sulfisoxazole	Yellow
d-Desoxyephedrine	Pale orange precipitate	Sulfonethylmethane	White precipitate
Dicoumarol	White precipitate	Sulfonmethane	White precipitate
Dicyclomine	White precipitate	Thiazolsulfone	Yellow
Diethylacetylurea	White precipitate	Tribromoethanol	White precipitate

NO REACTION

Acetophenetidin	Carbamylcholine	Dromoran	Nostal	Quinine
Aconitine	chloride	Glycine	Optochin	Ricin
Aminopyrine	Cinchonidine	Hippuric acid	Ortal	Saccharin
Aprobarbital	Cinchonine	Histamine.di HCl	Pentamethylene-	Sandoptal
Ascorbic acid	Cinchophen	Hyoscyamine	tetrazol	Sedormid
Atropine	Cocaine	Isoamylethyl-	Phenobarbital	Strychnine
Barbital	Coniine.HCl	acetylurea	Phenylbutazone	Tetracaine
Betaine.HCl	Dibucaine	Meperidine	Pilocarpine	Theobromine
Brucine	Dichlorodiphenyl-	Neonal	Prisilidene	Theophylline
Butallylonal	trichloroethane	Nikethamide	Probarbital	Trimethadione
Caffeine	(DDT)			

(g) Isoamylnitrite-Stannic Chloride. Nitrous acid, either as such or from aliphatic nitrites which readily liberate nitrous acid, undergoes a variety of reactions with organic compounds, particularly the amines. Primary aromatic amines are diazotized and may condense with excess compound or undergo replacement reactions. With aliphatic primary amines, nitrogen is liberated and the amino group is replaced by a hydroxyl group. All basic secondary amines react to form nitrosamines which are stable except in strong mineral acid which splits off nitrous acid and liberates the secondary amine. Aliphatic and mixed amides react to form nitrosamides which are less stable than the nitrosamines, having a tendency to split off acyl groups and then act like diazo compounds. C-nitroso compounds rarely exist except attached to a tertiary carbon and these are not formed by the direct action of nitrous acid except with ketones which have a tertiary carbon adjacent to the carbonyl. Reaction can occur with alcohols to form relatively unstable nitrous esters. Substituted aromatic compounds such as dimethylaniline which have a reactive hydrogen in the para position form para-nitroso compounds. When the para position is occupied, the ortho hydrogen is often reactive and nitroso substitution can occur there. Phenols readily react to form nitroso phenols which partially rearrange to a quinoid form. This is the basis for the Liebermann reaction (108, 152), as well as the Eykmann modification that employs ethyl nitrite (153).

The oxidation by nitrous acid in the presence of anhydrous stannic chloride of diarylamines and naphthylarylamines, unsubstituted in at least one para position, has been used as a test for amine anti-oxidants (138). Isoamylnitrite serves as the source of nitrous acid and permits the reaction to be carried out in nonaqueous solution. The alkyl nitrites are less drastic than nitrous acid in aqueous acid solution and chances for a more permanent color are better, since intermediate products are more stable. Nitroso compounds tend to be yellow, green or blue, and, in addition to the possible quinoid formation, any one of the many possible reactions of nitrous acid on a drug may produce a color.

The isoamylnitrite-stannic chloride reaction was applied to the analysis of drugs, using acetone as the solvent (43). Stannic chloride does not precipitate the basic drugs from acetone as it does in chloroform and ethylenedichloride. The yellow colorations which predominate are more easily interpreted in the nonaqueous solution and the action of the isoamylnitrite is similar to that of an indicator reaction. The test is not needed except for a few isolated compounds. It is distinctive for benzocaine and helps to differentiate procaine, butamin and xylocaine® from other local anesthetics. It is characteristic for thenylpyramine and pyrilamine and, with the benzotrichloride reaction, points to phenylbutazone and dicoumarol. It differentiates cinchonine from cinchonidine, furnishes one of the few tests for nikethamide and is the only color reaction given with cantharidin.

Reagents. (a) Acetone.

(b) Isoamylnitrite solution: 1 ml. per 20 ml. anhydrous benzene.

(c) Stannic chloride solution: 1.5 ml. anhydrous stannic chloride per 25 ml. anhydrous benzene.

Procedure. The sample contained in a capillary test tube with a bore of about 2 mm. is dissolved in a small amount of acetone. Isoamylnitrite solution and stannic chloride solution, each equal to half the volume of acetone, are added consecutively and the colors noted after the addition of each reagent.

Table 47-37. Isoamylnitrite-Stannic Chloride Test (43, 30)

COMPOUND	COLOR REMAINING AFTER ADDITION OF STANNIC CHLORIDE	COMPOUND	COLOR REMAINING AFTER ADDITION OF STANNIC CHLORIDE
RED		**BROWN**	
Benzocaine	Orange (with isoamylnitrite) → red (with stannic chloride)	Pseudopelletierine	Gray-brown precipitate
Thenylpyramine	Deep red		

YELLOW

With the following compounds the color remaining after addition of stannic chloride is yellow with orange cast.

Acetophenetidin *	Brucine	Digitoxin	Glycine	Physostigmine
Acetylsalicylic acid	Butamin	Dihydromorphinone	Hydrastine	Piperine
N-Allylnormorphine	Cantharidin	Dimenhydrinate (basic extraction product)	Meconin	Pregnenolone
p-Aminobenzoic acid	Cholesterol		Morphine	Procaine
	Cinchonine		Nikethamide	Rutin
	Cinchophen		Pamaquine	Trihexyphenidyl
Aminopyrine	Curarine	Diphenhydramine	Phenindamine	Xylocaine
Antipyrine *	Desoxylcholic acid	Estrone	Phenylbutazone	Yohimbine
Apomorphine	Dicoumarol			

* Color developed after addition of stannic chloride only.

COMPOUND	COLOR REMAINING AFTER ADDITION OF STANNIC CHLORIDE
MAGENTA	
Pyrilamine	Magenta

NEGATIVE REACTION

Acetanilid	Amphetamine base †	Apothesine	Caffeine	Cinchonidine
Aconitine	Ascorbic acid	Carbamylcholine chloride	Cocaine
Adiphenine	Amprotropine	Atabrin		Codeine
Amobarbital	Antabuse	Atropine	Chlorobutanol	Coniine

Table 47-37 (cont.). Isoamylnitrite-Stannic Chloride Test (43, 30)

NEGATIVE REACTION (cont.)

Delphinine	Hippuric acid	Pavatrine (acidic	Quinine	Sulfathiazole
d-Desoxyephed-	Homatropine	extraction)	Ricin	Sulfisoxazole
rine	Hyoscyamine	Pentamethylene-	Saccharin	Sulfonethyl-
Dibucaine	Isoamylethyl-	tetrazol	Salicin	methane
Dicyclomine	acetylurea	Phenobarbital	Santonin	Sulfonmethane
Digalen	Larocaine	Phenylsalicylate	Scopolamine	Tetracaine
Digitalin	Lobeline	Phthalylsulfa-	Solanin †	Theobromine
Digitonin	Metopon	thiazole	Sparteine	Theophylline
Diothane	Meperidine	Picrotoxin	Strophanthin	Thiamin degrada-
Emetine	Methadon	Pilocarpine	Strychnine	tion product
Ephedrine †	Methylphenyl-	Piperidione	Succinylsulfa-	Thiazolsulfone
Ethylbiscoum-	ethylhydantoin	Piperocaine	thiazole	Thiopental
acetate	Narceine	Prisilidene	Sulfacetimide	Thonzylamine
Ethylmorphine	Narcotine	Procaine amide	Sulfadiazine	Tribromoethanol
Eucupin.di HCl	Nicotinic alcohol	Pyrithyldione	Sulfanilamide	Trimethadione
Heroin	Optochin	Quinidine	Sulfapyridine	Urethan
				Veratrine

† No color change with isoamylnitrite.

(h) Molisch Reaction. The Molisch reaction is used for the detection of carbohydrates (154, 16). It is a sensitive test for free sugars and starches, as well as for hydroxylated substances in combination with other molecules such as glucosides, gums, glucoproteins, paper fibers and wood particles. The reaction is thought to depend on the formation of furfural or a related substance by action of the sulfuric acid and formation of an unstable condensation product with *alpha*-naphthol. A 5 per cent alcoholic thymol solution has been reported to be superior to *alpha*-naphthol for the detection of carbohydrates because the solution does not deteriorate (155) and *beta*-naphthol has been used in the same way as *alpha*-naphthol to detect citric, malic and tartaric acids (156).

The characteristic carbohydrate-*alpha*-naphthol color is dark red or magenta. Other aldehydes may react and, although less sensitive than carbohydrates, acetone and acids such as formic, oxalic, lactic, citric, tartaric and malic. The presence of nitrite in the sulfuric acid is particularly objectionable for the Molisch reaction.

Except for several of the glucosides, highly hydroxylated molecules are not organic solvent soluble and, since carbohydrates or their derivatives will not be found in tissue extracts, a toxicologic test for their detection is not needed. However, they are usually present as fillers in pills and capsules received as evidence. Their presence is readily detected by the Molisch reaction applied to the water soluble, alcohol and solvent insoluble extract of the preparation. As a test for carbohydrates, the reaction fits into the class with confirmatory reactions (page 1246). However, positive findings were found with such a variety of drugs that application of the test to pharmaceutical preparations for carbohydrates, without separation of the components of the mixture, could result in an incorrect interpretation because of drug interference. Moreover, some of the positively reacting drugs were found to give tests which were good enough to characterize the substance and the reaction, therefore, is grouped with the differential type of color test.

Anthrone has recently been introduced as a reagent for the detection of carbohydrates. It gives a positive reaction with the carbohydrate types that react in the Molisch reaction and would appear to be preferable, since fewer compounds, other than the carbohydrates, react positively. In spite of this greater specificity, it is our experience that the Molisch reaction is much superior. The color of the reaction between anthrone and the carbohydrates is green while the reagent itself is decidedly yellow. This color combination results in a definite reduction in reaction sensitivity. False positives can be obtained in the anthrone reaction. Addition of water precipitates the anthrone reagent, whereas dilution with water in the Molisch reaction produces characteristic color shifts with some of the drugs. Since *alpha*-naphthol reacts more sensitively with everything that reacts with anthrone and since, unlike the reacting drugs, carbohydrates are solvent insoluble, the Molisch reaction remains the preferred method for detecting carbohydrate material as well as for use as a differential test for certain drugs.

Several variations of the Molisch test have been described. The *alpha*-naphthol has been dissolved to make 5 to 15 per cent ethyl alcohol and chloroform solutions and it has also been dissolved directly in concentrated sulfuric acid. The reagent in sulfuric acid is more sensitive and requires less manipulation, although drugs which react with concentrated sulfuric acid alone (page 1204) do interfere. Reactions with substances other than the carbohydrates are shown in Table 47-38. The Molisch test as applied to carbohydrates is described on page 1252.

Reagent. Dissolve 100 mg. of *alpha*-naphthol, free of air oxidation products, in 10 ml. of concentrated sulfuric acid.

Procedure. Place the microscope slide containing the solid sample treated with a drop of reagent on a hot plate maintained at 125° C. and heat for 45 seconds.

Table 47-38. Molisch Reaction (149)

* Observe two minutes in the cold.

COMPOUND	COLOR DEVELOPED WITH MOLISCH REAGENT IN THE COLD *	COLOR AFTER HEATING ONE MINUTE AT 125° C.	COLOR AFTER WATER DILUTION
RED			
Ascorbic acid	No reaction	Very dark wine red	Precipitate
Chrysazin	Deep red	Deep red	Yellow orange precipitate
Homatropine	Red with orange cast	Deep red	Red precipitate
Methylparafynol	Deep orange	Deep red with orange cast	Brown precipitate
Narceine	Faint yellow	Blood red	Red precipitate
Narcotine	Light green	Blood red	Red precipitate
Nicotinic alcohol	Faint red with orange cast	Decolorizes	No change
Veratrine	Orange with red cast → red	Very deep red	Yellow green precipitate
ORANGE			
Amphetamine.HCl	Original darkens slightly	Orange with red-violet streaks	No change
Amprotropine	Pale yellow	Faint orange	Cream precipitate
Berberine.SO₄	Dark brown spot	Bright orange	Orange precipitate
Butabarbital	No reaction	Very faint orange	No change
Butamin	No reaction	Pale orange	Color fades
Cholesterol	Orange → red	Bright orange with violet streaks	Precipitate of light orange with magenta cast
Colchicine	No reaction	Orange with violet streaks	Color fades
Desoxycholic acid	No reaction	Orange	Orange precipitate
Ephedrine	No change from original color	Orange	Gray yellow precipitate
Eucupin.di HCl	No reaction	Light orange	White precipitate
Hexobarbital	No reaction	Deep orange	Gray precipitate
l-Menthol	Light orange	Orange	White precipitate
Mephenesine	Very faint pink	Light orange	Color fades
Pelletierine tannate	Light orange	Light orange	No change
Phanadorn	Orange	Dark orange	No change
Pyridium	Red	Orange with red cast	No change
Pyrilamine	Red	Orange with red cast	Orange
Terpin hydrate	Orange	Deep orange	Gray precipitate
Thonzylamine	Red	Orange with yellow cast	Light brown precipitate
Trihexyphenidyl	Light orange	Orange with red cast	Cream precipitate
BROWN			
Aconitine	No reaction	Dark brown with orange cast	Light brown precipitate
N-Allylnormorphine	Brown	Brown	Cream precipitate
Apomorphine	Very dark brown with green cast	Very dark brown	Precipitate

Table 47-38 (cont.). Molisch Reaction (149)

COMPOUND	COLOR DEVELOPED WITH MOLISCH REAGENT IN THE COLD *	COLOR AFTER HEATING ONE MINUTE AT 125° C.	COLOR AFTER WATER DILUTION
BROWN (cont.)			
Apothesine	No change from original color	Brown	Cream precipitate
Aprobarbital	No reaction	Very light brown	Color fades
Cephaeline	Brown	Brown	Color fades
Cyclopal	Orange	Very dark brown	Gray blue precipitate
Delphinine	Orange	Dark brown	Light precipitate
Dicyclomine	No reaction	Dark brown with orange cast	Gray precipitate
Digalen	Light brown	Brown with red cast	No change
Diphenhydramine	Orange	Brown with orange cast	No change
Emetine	Brown	Dark brown	Brown yellow precipitate
Ethylmorphine	Dark brown	Brown with orange cast	Brown orange precipitate
Hydrastine	Brown	Dark brown	Orange precipitate
Lobeline	Brown	Dark brown	Yellow orange precipitate
Mescaline	Dark brown	Very dark brown	Dark brown precipitate
Pamaquine	Brown	Dark brown	Dark brown with orange cast
Phenindamine	Orange	Very dark brown	Yellow orange precipitate
Piperine	Red with orange cast	Dark brown	Deep olive green precipitate
Pregnenolone	Orange	Very dark brown	Gray green precipitate
Rutin	Orange with yellow cast	Very dark brown	Yellow-brown precipitate
Sulfisoxazole	No reaction	Pale brown	Color fades
Thenylpyramine	Orange → deep orange	Very, very dark brown	Orange brown
Xylocaine	Brown	Dark brown	Gray yellow precipitate
YELLOW			
Adiphenine	No reaction	Faint yellow	White precipitate
Atabrin	Yellow	Yellow	Yellow precipitate
Dimenhydrinate (basic extraction product)	Deep red	Dark yellow	White precipitate
Quinidine	No reaction	Very faint yellow	No change
Santonin	No reaction	Yellow	Cream precipitate
Thiobarbituric acid	No reaction	Very faint yellow	White precipitate
Vinbarbital	No reaction	Yellow	Cream precipitate
GREEN			
Antabuse	No reaction	Light green with yellow cast and magenta streaks	No change
Chlorobutanol	No reaction	Green with yellow cast	Yellow green precipitate
Pavatrine	Dark olive green	Dark green	Gray yellow precipitate
Sigmodal	No reaction	Dark green	Gray precipitate
Tribromoethanol	No reaction	Light green with yellow cast	Grayish precipitate
BLUE			
Dromoran	No reaction	Light blue violet	Color fades
Ethyl biscoumacetate	No reaction	Very faint blue violet	White precipitate
Piperidione	No reaction	Dark blue violet	Violet precipitate
Salicin	Red	Deep blue violet	Brown precipitate
Solanin	Orange with yellow cast	Dark blue violet	Deep brown precipitate

Table 47-38 (cont.). Molisch Reaction (149)

COMPOUND	COLOR DEVELOPED WITH MOLISCH REAGENT IN THE COLD *	COLOR AFTER HEATING ONE MINUTE AT 125° C.	COLOR AFTER WATER DILUTION
MAGENTA			
Atropine	No reaction	Magenta	Color fades
Bromural	No reaction	Magenta	Color fades
Digitalin	Red	Magenta	Magenta precipitate
Glycine	No reaction	Magenta	Color fades
Strophanthin	Brown	Magenta with dark brown cast	Brown precipitate
Zolamine.HCl	Blue violet	Magenta	Blue violet precipitate; fades to white
GRAY			
Codeine	Dark gray	Dark gray	No change
Meconin	No reaction	Gray	Gray precipitate

NO REACTION

Acetanilid	Cinchophen	Histamine.di HCl	Pentobarbital †	Scopolamine
Acetophenetidin	Cocaine	Hyoscyamine	Phenobarbital †	Secobarbital
Acetylsalicylic acid	Coniine.HCl	Isoamylethyl-acetylurea	Phenylacetylurea	Sedormid
	Curarine		Phenylbutazone	Strychnine
p-Aminobenzoic acid	Cysteine.HCl	Larocaine	Phenylsalicylate	Succinylsulfa-thiazole
	d-Desoxyephed-rine	Meperidine	Phthalylsulfa-thiazole	Sulfacetimide
Aminopyrine		Mephobarbital †		
Amobarbital †	Diallylbarbituric acid	Methylphenyl-ethylhydantoin †	Pilocarpine	Sulfadiazine
Antipyrine			Piperocaine †	Sulfanilamide
Barbital	Dibucaine	Metopon	Prisilidene	Sulfapyridine
Benzocaine	Dichlorodiphenyl-trichloroethane (DDT)	Morphine	Probarbital	Sulfathiazole
Betaine.HCl		alpha-Naphthyl-thiourea (ANTU)†	Procaine amide	Sulfonethyl-methane
Brucine			Procaine.HCl	
Butallylonal	Dicoumarol †	Neonal †	Prostigmine	Sulfonmethane
Caffeine	Diethylacetylurea	Nicotine	Pseudopellet-ierine	Tetracaine
Cantharidin	Dihydromor-phinone	Nikethamide		Theobromine
Carbamylcholine chloride		Nostal	Pyrithyldione	Theophylline
	Diothane	Optochin	Quinine	Thiazolsulfone
Carbromal	Diphenylhy-dantoin †	Ortal	Ricin	Thiopental
Cinchonidine		Pentamethylene-tetrazol	Saccharin	Trimethadione
Cinchonine	Hippuric acid		Sandoptal	Yohimbine

† White precipitate on the addition of water, after heating.

4. Confirmatory Reactions.

4. Confirmatory Reactions. Reactions in this class are more specific than any of the other types but the specificity is for a specific organic structure rather than for a single substance. In this sense confirmatory reactions come closer to being truly generic tests which not only characterize a generic type but also designate an order. The specificity results from the fact that the test confirms the presence of the structure predicted by the exclusion process. True specificity in almost all reactions is attained only as a result of the manipulative procedure that separates interfering substances from the one being tested and which, although part of the analysis, is separate from the test. The few determinations which themselves are specific for one compound or member of a homologous series might be distinguished from the other types of reactions by being termed identifying reactions and, therefore, they assume the same status in the analytic process as the determination of physical properties.

(a) Acid Diazo Reaction (13). Almost every primary aromatic amine, except those containing a number of negative substituents in the nucleus, react with nitrous acid in cold aqueous acid solution to form diazo compounds. Reactions for the diazo compounds can be divided into two main classes: replacement reactions in which the two nitrogen atoms of the diazo group are replaced with evolution of nitrogen gas and coupling reactions in which the nitrogen atoms remain in the molecule. Coupling can take place in acid solution with reactive coupling agents and diazo compounds form reactive aromatic amines but an alkaline medium is more favorable for the reaction. The less reactive of the diazo compounds or the coupling agents undergo condensation in an alkaline medium only. Alkaline coupling has been applied as a general test for drugs by adding a known diazo compound to the unknown drug as the coupling agent. When the test is used in the reverse manner, forming a diazo compound of the unknown with nitrous acid followed by addition of a known coupling agent to an acid solution, the formation of a colored azo or diazoamino dye is evidence for a strong aromatic amine. Increased sensitivity is attained by carrying out the procedure on a small piece of filter paper as in the alkaline coupling test (page 1216). The test is particularly useful for differentiating procaine, benzocaine, butamin and orthoform® from the other local anesthetics and for detecting sulfa drugs. Sulfa drugs are relatively insoluble compounds and recovery from biologic material is low. They are more readily detected by the acid coupling reaction applied directly to a protein-free filtrate of the blood.

Reagents. (a) 15 per cent trichloracetic acid, (b) 0.1 per cent sodium nitrite solution, (c) 0.5 per cent ammonium sulfamate solution, (d) 0.1 per cent N-(1-naphthyl)-ethylenediamine dihydrochloride solution. This reagent keeps about one week if stored in the dark.

Procedure for Tissue Extracts. Place a few micrograms of sample on a piece of filter paper about 2 mm. square on a microscope slide and moisten the paper by addition of a small drop of trichloracetic acid solution. Add a drop (0.05 ml.) of sodium nitrite solution and allow to stand 3 minutes. Add a drop (0.5 ml.) of ammonium sulfamate and let stand 2 minutes. Place a drop of N-(1-naphthyl)ethylenediamine solution on the glass slide adjacent to the filter paper so that the reagent diffuses through the paper. A red stain on the paper is indicative of an aromatic amine.

Procedure for Blood Filtrates. Add 4 ml. of 15 per cent trichloracetic acid to 1.0 ml. of oxalated blood. Mix the solution, allow it to stand a few minutes and remove the precipitated protein by filtration through paper. Add 0.5 ml. of sodium nitrite solution and, after 3 minutes, 0.5 ml. of ammonium sulfamate solution. After allowing it to stand at least 2 minutes, add 0.5 ml. of N-(1-naphthyl)ethylenediamine solution. If a red color * does not develop in the solution, sulfa drugs are excluded.

(b) Murexide Reaction for Purines. Mild oxidation of most purine derivatives yields products which are related to murexide, the oxidation product of uric acid. In weakly alkaline solution, these form intensely colored red to red-violet salts. A variety of oxidizing agents such as nitric acid, bromine or chlorine water, hydrogen peroxide, chloramine T and potassium perchlorate have been used successfully. Free hydrochloric acid appears to be essential for maximum sensitivity in the reaction and heating, which is necessary for the oxidation and to evaporate to dryness, needs to be carefully controlled. Caffeine exhibits the least sensitivity of the common purines and should be the compound tested as a control simultaneously with the unknown.

In our laboratory, the best results were obtained on anhydrous residues with potassium chlorate and hydrochloric acid as recommended by Mulliken (157), although Morgan (158) has reported that a detectable color develops with caffeine from 0.1 ml. of a 1:80,000 solution by oxidation with 0.05 ml. of chloramine T solution (0.18 per cent active chlorine) and 0.05 ml. 1:10 hydrochloric acid solution. In the procedure followed by Morgan, the solution, contained in a spot plate, was evaporated to dryness at 100° C. or below and the residue treated with triethanolamine or equal volumes of triethanolamine and water which developed a more persistent color and the other bases studied. In Mulliken's procedure the residue from the evaporation of the potassium chlorate-hydrochloric acid solution is cautiously heated somewhat above 100° C. until the residue develops a slight pink or brownish color. Our own studies of the method (149) † indicated that the baking process is an essential part of the test if it is to be used as a general reaction for purines but that the amount of heating which the residue will tolerate is critical. In order to control the heating process, the unknown, treated with the oxidizing

---

* Bilirubin is determined in blood by acid coupling with diazotized sulfanilic acid (Van den Burgh reaction). With an icteric serum containing a diazotizable compound, a color may develop before the addition of the coupling agent. Bilirubin interference can be detected by an increase in the color on repeating the test in the presence of an equal volume of ethyl alcohol.

† Umberger, C. J., and Dal Cortivo, L. Unpublished.

reagents, is evaporated almost to dryness, then allowed to dry spontaneously in warm air and the dry residue baked on a thermostatically controlled hot plate for a definite time.

Reagents. (a) Powdered potassium chlorate crystals, (b) 25 per cent or 1:2 hydrochloric acid solution.

Procedure. A small sample of the unknown residue and a small crystal of caffeine are placed on separate microscope slides. Powdered potassium chlorate, approximately equal in bulk to the samples on the slides, and a drop of hydrochloric acid solution are added. The slides are warmed on a hot plate maintained at about 90° C. and the solution is allowed to fume until only a moist residue remains. The slides are removed and allowed to stand in a warm atmosphere until the residues dry. The slides are then placed on a heating block maintained at 110° C. for one minute, allowed to cool and a drop of 2 normal ammonium hydroxide added. Uric acid, xanthine, caffeine, theobromine and theophylline develop an intense red color due to the formation of the ammonium salt of purpuric or a related acid. The reaction was not studied with drugs other than the purines. Although some other substances may give similar colorations, in contrast to the purines, the possible interfering compounds will have been indicated by positive findings with some of the other color reactions.

The murexide reaction is similar to Vitalli's test for the atropine alkaloids in which oxidation is obtained with concentrated or fuming nitric acid and alkalization with 5 per cent alcoholic potassium hydroxide. Vitalli's test was not found sufficiently sensitive or characteristic to consider it as a practical test for the identification of organic drugs. Theobromine and aminopyrine react but theophylline and caffeine are insensitive. Significant amounts of atropine, hyoscyamine and scopolamine give a violet color changing to red and the colors developed with veratrine and apomorphine may be mistaken for those given by the atropine group. Physostigmine, pilocarpine and strychnine also interfere and any of these may be expected to develop some color in the murexide oxidation. However, reaction in the murexide and Vitalli's oxidations differs with regard to possible action on aromatic ring structures. Treatment with fuming nitric acid can result in meta-dinitration of aromatic compounds which are characterized by the formation of intense red-colored solutions after treatment with strong alkali.

(c) Liebermann's Nitrosamine Reaction (108, 152). Nitrosamines are not encountered in toxicologic analysis as such but many drugs are secondary amines which form nitrosamines when acted on by nitrous acid. Simple aromatic nitrosamines are partially water soluble but can be salted out with potassium carbonate, while aromatic and mixed nitrosamines are water insoluble but soluble in ether. Consequently, the product of a reaction with nitrous acid can be tested for nitrosamines by extraction of the aqueous acid test solution with ether after making alkaline with 1 per cent ammonium sulfamate solution to remove any free nitrite and then evaporated to dryness.

The Liebermann test for nitrosamines depends on the fact that concentrated sulfuric acid liberates free nitrous acid from the nitrosamine * and that free nitrous acid undergoes substitution with phenols or thymol to form a C-nitroso compound which readily condenses with excess phenol or thymol to form an indophenol type.

1. $R'R'NNO + H_2SO_4 \longrightarrow R'R'NH + HNO_2$

2. $HNO_2 + HO-\langle\rangle \longrightarrow HO-\langle\rangle-NO$

3. $HO-\langle\rangle-NO + HO-\langle\rangle \longrightarrow HO-\langle\rangle-N=\langle\rangle=O$

Indophenols which are green or blue in acid solution change to red or violet on dilution with water and change again to green or blue on the addition of alkali.

Reagents. (a) Concentrated sulfuric acid, (b) phenol crystals, (c) ammonia.

Procedure. The washed ether solution is evaporated on a small area of a piece of

---

* C-nitroso compounds also liberate nitrous acid by the action of warm sulfuric acid.

Whatman #50 filter paper by the dropwise addition of the ether to the paper from a capillary tip while the paper is held over a hot stream of air from a hot air gun.* †

Several phenol crystals are dissolved in about 1 ml. of concentrated sulfuric acid and a drop added to the evaporate on the paper. On warming the area with the hot air gun, a green to blue color develops which changes to violet, reddish and again bluish on exposure to ammonia fumes.‡

(d) Iodine-Azide Reaction (159). Although sodium azide does not react with iodine dissolved in potassium iodide when the solution is pure, the presence of even traces of sulfide catalyzes a reaction in which nitrogen is liberated and iodine is converted into iodide.

$$2\ NaN_3 + I_2 \rightarrow 2\ NaI + 3\ N_2$$

The decoloration of the brown $KI.I_2$ solution and evolution of nitrogen gas from the reagent added to an unknown solid or solution is, therefore, indicative of the presence of sulfide ion. Compounds which dissolve to give traces of sulfide also react so that the test is equally characteristic for thiocyanate, thiosulfate and polysulfides. Free sulfur, sulfites, sulfates, selenides and tellurides do not affect the reagent. Organic compounds containing —SH groups such as mercaptans and thio acids, diacyl disulfides and thione or thiol compounds which apparently have enol forms react equally well. Carbon disulfide is reported to catalyze the reaction differently from the sulfide ion with formation of an intermediate product with sodium azide (160). Other organic sulfur derivatives such as thioethers, disulfides, sulfoxides, sulphones, sulphinic and sulphonic acids do not initiate a reaction.

The iodine-sodium azide reaction has been used to evaluate tissue distillates (page 1053), to rule out sulfides, thiosulfates and thiocyanates in the stomach contents (page 1022), in the testing for thiocyano esters from fly spray material (page 1062) and in conjunction with Grote's reagent to characterize organic sulfur-containing compounds (page 1223). It has been used to detect condensation products of amines and polysulfides in dyestuffs by leaching the product with carbon disulfide, removing the carbon disulfide by evaporation and testing the carbon disulfide-soluble evaporate with the reagent (161). It has also found application in differentiating between black and smokeless powder residues on dark cloth by detecting the presence of sulfide, thiosulfate or thiocyanate in the black powder residue (162). The reagent may be used to rule out certain suspected sulfur-containing drugs by its addition to a partially purified substance isolated from tissue. Thiopental may be differentiated from the other barbiturates and antabuse® in 50 per cent ethyl alcohol is distinguished from the few drugs which react similarly with the other color reagents. Alpha-naphthylthiourea is too water insoluble for the solid to react with the aqueous reagent but when dissolved in dioxane, it gives an immediate reaction.

Reagent. Dissolve 1 gm. potassium iodide in 3.0 ml. water, introduce enough powdered I_2 crystals to give the solution an amber color and add 1.0 gm. of sodium azide. The reagent keeps for several months.

Procedure. Add a drop of reagent to the solid unknown or a solution in water, alcohol or dioxane on a glass slide or contained in a capillary test tube. A positive reaction is indicated by immediate decolorization of the $KI.I_2$ solution and evolution of nitrogen gas. A solvent blank is run simultaneously to serve as a control for the rate of decolorization of the unknown.

(e) Phenol-Sulfuric Acid Reagent for Estrogens and Hormones (163). A mixture of *ortho-* and *para*-hydroxyphenylsulphonic acid in concentrated sulfuric acid, known as Kober's reagent (164), has been used for the quantitative determination of estrogens and hormones. It also reacts with some steroids and obviously with any drug which is reactive toward sulfuric acid alone. Steroids and related compounds are of no significance in an extract from tissue since all are nontoxic and only traces can be recovered from

---

* Master Appliance Manufacturing Co., Racine, Wisconsin, Model #12200.

† This is analogous to the procedure used to add the sample to the paper strip in preparing paper chromatograms.

‡ The reaction has been used as a test for phenol and thymol and for free nitrous acid. It is apparent that excess nitric acid from the original test solution must be removed before the evaporation of the ether solution of the nitrosamine.

the body. They are encountered in pills and pharmaceutical preparations and the reagent has some value in differentiating them from other drugs. The procedure requires controlled heating in the concentrated acid solution, followed by dilution with water. The behavior on addition of water is the distinguishing characteristic of the test. With most drugs which are mildly reactive with sulfuric acid alone, the coloration is decreased or completely decolorized on dilution with water, whereas the colors produced by the estrogens, hormones and steroids which react are either not significantly altered or increase in color intensity. Drugs which are sufficiently reactive toward concentrated sulfuric acid to interfere are eliminated by negative findings in the sulfuric acid control test (Table 47-21).

Reagent. Heat a mixture of equal weights of phenol and concentrated sulfuric acid at 110-120° C. for 15 minutes and dilute the cooled mixture with twice the volume of concentrated sulfuric acid.

Procedure. Add the solid sample to the bottom of a 1.0 ml. centrifuge cone by careful evaporation of an alcohol solution while stirring with a glass thread. Add 0.05 ml. of reagent and heat the tube for 3 minutes on a micro steam bath (165). The acid solution becomes yellow or pale red and should not show evidence of any charring. Cool the tube, add 0.05 ml. of water and reheat in a glycerol bath at 125° C. for 2 minutes. A red, magenta or violet color develops in the solution which, on cooling and further dilution with 0.15 ml. water, should be clearly perceptible. Estrone, estriol, dihydrodiethylstilbestrol, cholesterol, and pregnenolone develop red colors while dehydroisoandrosterone gives a blue-violet color. Iron salts react with the reagent to give a red color similar to that in the thiocyanate test for ferric ion. Iron in pharmaceuticals such as iron and bile salt pills may be indicated by direct application of the reagent to the preparation.

(f) Neutral Ferric Chloride Reaction for Phenolic Alkaloids (48). The development of a blue color with ferric chloride reagent has been used to differentiate morphine from closely related alkaloids. Ferric chloride reagent deteriorates on standing and is usually stabilized by making the solution slightly more acidic with dilute hydrochloric acid. The freshly prepared ferric chloride reagent itself is decidedly acid from hydrolysis of the salt. The sensitivity of the reaction with morphine, which is decreased with increase in the acidity of the ferric chloride reagent, is greatest when the test solution is nearly neutral. The excess hydrogen ion is removed by shaking the ferric chloride reagent with an excess of solid calcium carbonate and decanting the supernatant solution. The complete conversion to hydroxide is slow enough to permit the separation of nearly neutral ferric chloride with some colloidal ferric hydroxide from the solid matter which quickly settles. A drop of the neutral reagent is then immediately added to the test sample which is preferably in the form of the free base.

Reagent. Add about 0.5 gm. of powdered calcium carbonate to about 10 ml. of 5 per cent ferric chloride reagent and shake thoroughly. Allow the tube to stand about 30 seconds to permit the solid to settle and decant the supernatant through rapid filtering filter paper.

Procedure. Add one drop of the first portion of the filtrate to a sample of the tissue residue from the extraction of the amphoteric bases on a microscope slide while viewing with diffused light through a low-power objective under the microscope. Dihydromorphinone and N-allylnormorphine react like morphine.

(g) Sodium Fusion. Basic drugs are seldom recovered from tissue sufficiently pure or in quantities sufficient for elemental analysis. This type of examination is rarely needed for the bases since the fact that they are basic is evidence for the presence of nitrogen. The need for determining halogens or sulfur is a rare possibility. Neutral or acidic compounds, however, are usually recovered in much larger quantities which permits a more extensive purification. Tests for the elements other than carbon and hydrogen may be necessary to rule out or to indicate certain possibilities, particularly when the isolated substance is acidic.

Schneider (166) has given an excellent discussion of the various methods for determining the elements in 5 to 10 mμ samples of organic compounds and procedures for the detection of the individual elements after destruction of the organic matter.

Nitrogen, the most important element, is determined by the prussian blue reaction for cyanide (page 1051) and certain difficulties arise when this method is carried out on a microscale that are not significant with larger samples. The solution containing the cyanide must be decidedly alkaline for conversion to ferrocyanide by the addition of ferrous ion. Prussian blue is obtained by the reaction of ferric ion, which is usually present in adequate amounts in the ferrous reagent, with the ferrocyanide upon acidification of the solution. On a microscale, the difficulty arises from the fact that ferrous ion forms a voluminous dark precipitate in the basic solution and, because its rate of reaction with the hydrochloric acid added for neutralization of the solution and conversion of excess ferrous reagent into a soluble salt is very slow, it is difficult to control the neutralization and acidification phase on the small volume of solution. A large excess of acid increases the final volume and reduces the sensitivity for the formation of the insoluble prussian blue. The detection of cyanide in microsamples was found to be considerably improved by employing a special reagent containing old ferrous sulfate, which had air oxidized until it contained a significant ferric ion content, dissolved in a solution containing a high concentration of tartrate ion. The tartrate forms a complex with the ferrous and ferric ions, preventing precipitation in the alkaline solution while ferrocyanide ion is being formed. On layering the clear alkaline solution in the capillary tube with acid, the conversion to prussian blue is observed to start at the interface with the blue color developing as the acid diffuses through the alkaline layer.

Modified Sodium Fusion-Ferrocyanide Method for Nitrogen (48).

Cyanide Reagent. Dissolve 31.2 gm. tartaric acid in 50 ml. of water and add 6.24 gm. of anhydrous ferrous sulfate, which contains a small amount of ferric ion. Allow the solution to stand at room temperature with intermittent stirring for 48 hours, during which most of the ferrous sulfate dissolves. Remove any undissolved matter by filtration through paper and store the solution in a dark bottle. The reagent keeps indefinitely.

Apparatus. The fusion is carried out in a combination capillary combustion tube and filter prepared from a 4 inch piece of 4 mm. I.D. Pyrex tubing. The center of the tube is heated to the softening point over about 1½ inches, while rotating over the wing tip of a Terill burner and drawn out to a capillary tube about 4 inches long with a 2 mm. bore. Several strands of asbestos are rolled together between the fingers to form a cylinder approximately 2 mm. in diameter and 5 mm. in length. The cylinder is inserted at one of the 4 mm. ends and pushed to the center of the capillary with a glass rod. The walls of the capillary containing the asbestos are then heated around the circumference with a pinpoint oxygen flame until the glass collapses into the asbestos, forming a tight plug. The fusion sample is more easily prepared by employing a micro pellet press (167) with a mold containing a 1.5 mm. cavity about 4 mm. in height. A piece of metallic sodium is trimmed free of oxide with a razor blade and a small piece forced into the bottom of the cavity of the mold with the plunger of the pellet press. Then, 5 to 10 μg of sample is introduced on top of the sodium and enough sodium is packed on top of the sample to fill the 1.5 by 4 mm. mold. The bottom of the mold is removed and the sodium plug pressed from the mold cavity while holding it over the 4 mm. end of the Pyrex tube and it is pushed into the capillary to within about 2 mm. of the asbestos plug. The charged tube shown in Figure 47-40 is then laid on a wire gauze mounted on a ring stand.

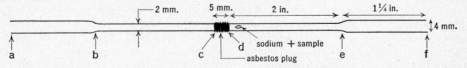

Fig. 47-40. Capillary Combustion Tube and Filter for Sodium Fusion.

Procedure. Heat the capillary tube with a microburner, starting about midway between (d) and (e), slowly moving the burner toward the sample until the sodium melts. Then heat the sodium melt for several minutes, moving the burner over the surface of the glass until it reaches red heat. Allow the tube to cool and decompose the unoxidized sodium by blowing a fine spray of steam into (c) from a steam bath fitted with a capillary jet. Then introduce enough water by means of a capillary medicine dropper at (e) to give a column about 2 cm. The water is forced down the tube to the fusion mixture and brought to near boiling several times by flaming the surface of the tube with a microburner. When all but the carbon has dissolved, connect the tube to a suction pump by means of rubber tubing at (a). Apply enough vacuum to draw the aqueous liquid through the asbestos filter plug. If the plug has been properly prepared, the vacuum from a water aspirator pump will be enough to slowly draw the liquid through the asbestos but not enough to draw the column out of the capillary section between (b) and (c) before the vacuum can be shut off when the filtration is complete. When the water column is drawn between (b) and (c), disconnect the vacuum hose from (a), seal the capillary by heating with a pinpoint flame at point (b) and cut off and discard section (a-b). Rotate the remaining section (b-f) in a hand centrifuge to force the filtrate to the bottom at (b). Then cut the tube at point (c), to give a filtrate of the fusion mixture contained in a capillary test tube with a 2 mm. bore, 1¾ inches high. If the solution is to be examined for halogens, remove about one-fourth of the volume by a capillary pipet and transfer to a similar test tube.

Dip a 1 mm. glass rod into the ferrous sulfate reagent so that the surface is wet without enough reagent adhering to form a drop when the rod is held vertically. Insert the rod into the solution and rotate between the fingers, in order to mix the adhering reagent with the solution. The mixed solution should develop an amber color and, if it is not dark enough, the process should be repeated. Care must be taken not to add enough reagent for the tartaric acid to neutralize the base, since the formation of ferrocyanide ion requires an alkaline medium. The solution may be warmed to hasten the conversion, but excess heating breaks down the tartrate complex, giving a turbid solution and the safest practice is to permit the tube to stand overnight at room temperature. About one-fourth the volume of concentrated hydrochloric acid is layered over the solution and allowed to mix by diffusion. A green color develops with very small amounts of nitrogen in the sample and the control remains decidedly yellow. With a larger nitrogen content, the solution turns blue as acidification proceeds and a blue precipitate, readily observed under the low-power objective of a microscope, develops.

It is seldom necessary to carry out a special test for sulfur. Sulfides, if present, are indicated by an immediate black precipitate of FeS, on adding the ferrous reagent. They may be removed by adding a drop of 5 per cent sodium plumbate reagent, removing the precipitate by centrifugation and proceeding with the ferrocyanide test after transferring the supernatant solution to another tube. Examination for halogens is usually not necessary since they are readily detected by the Beilstein test on the original sample. Procedures for distinguishing between the different halogens in the fusion filtrate are given by Schneider (168).

(h) Carbohydrates in Pharmaceutical Preparations. I. Molisch Reaction for Carbohydrates. Carbohydrates and related substances are characterized by their high water solubility in contrast to their low alcohol solubility and solvent insolubility. Because of possible drug interference in the Molisch test (page 1244), carbohydrates must be separated from possible interfering compounds when testing an unknown pharmaceutical preparation. Interfering drugs are removed by extraction of the anhydrous preparation with alcohol or chloroform. Mulliken's variation of the Molisch test is somewhat more specific for carbohydrates than the procedure described for drugs (page 1243).

Removal of Drugs by Chloroform Extraction. Moisten the residue from evaporation of a solution or the anhydrous solid sample with normal hydrochloric acid to produce a thick slurry. Then keep the acidified sample suspended in chloroform by mechanical agitation until all of the soluble material is dissolved. Allow the insoluble portion to settle and siphon off the supernatant chloroform (page 1158). Separate the remaining chloroform by centrifugation or filtration through a sintered glass filter.* Moisten the residue with concentrated ammonium hydroxide and extract with chloroform in the same way.

---

* A number of the hydrochlorides of the bases are soluble in chloroform.

Alternate Purification by Ethyl Alcohol Extraction. Extraction of the solid sample with 95 per cent ethyl alcohol, acidified with a few drops of concentrated hydrochloric acid, followed by extraction with ammoniacal alcohol also removes interfering drugs. The major difference between the alcohol and chloroform extraction is that some glucosides and gums that are chloroform insoluble are soluble in alcohol.

Reagent. 10 per cent *alpha*-naphthol in chloroform. The reagent is not stable for more than one week.

Control Test on the Reagent. Shake one drop of the *alpha*-naphthol reagent with 10 drops of water and 1 ml. of concentrated sulfuric acid. The mixture should be golden yellow. If it is dark green, the *alpha*-naphthol is impure and must be recrystallized.

Procedure. Dissolve or suspend the isolated carbohydrate sample in a few drops of water, add an equal volume of the *alpha*-naphthol in chloroform, shake the mixture and allow it to stand until the layers separate. Then layer about 0.5 ml. concentrated sulfuric acid under the solution. A deep red or magenta ring at the interface is indicative of carbohydrates.

II. Fehling's Test for the Detection of Sugars. Sugars, the most common fillers in pills and capsules, are distinguished from other substances that react in the Molisch test by their ability to reduce Fehling's solution or the more stable Benedict's reagent.

Benedict's Reagent. Dissolve 10 gm. of anhydrous sodium carbonate and 17.3 gm. of sodium citrate in about 80 ml. of water, with the aid of heat, and filter off any insoluble suspension. Dissolve 1.8 gm. of copper sulfate pentahydrate in 10 ml. of water and slowly pour, with stirring, into the first solution. Dilute to 100 ml. with water. Unlike Fehling's solution, the reagent does not deteriorate on long standing.

Procedure. Add 3 drops of Benedict's reagent to a 1.0 ml. aqueous solution or suspension containing about 10 mg. of the suspected carbohydrate, shake thoroughly and observe after allowing the test tube to stand at room temperature about 2 minutes.

If a cuprous oxide precipitate does not form, place the tube in a boiling water bath and observe while heating about 2 minutes. If only a slight yellowish turbidity or no precipitation appears after boiling for 2 minutes, pre-hydrolyze the 10 mg. sample by boiling for about 5 minutes in 1:4 hydrochloric acid, neutralize the acid and test the solution for reducing properties as before. The behavior of the different carbohydrates is shown in Table 47-39.

Table 47-39. Behavior of Carbohydrates in the Fehling Reduction Test

CARBOHYDRATE	CHEMICAL TYPE	REDUCING ABILITY
Glucose	Hexose sugar	Immediate precipitate on heating
Fructose	Hexose sugar	Immediate precipitate on heating
Galactose	Hexose sugar	Immediate precipitate on heating
Arabinose	Hexose sugar	Immediate precipitate on heating
Xylose	Hexose sugar	Immediate precipitate on heating
Rhamnose	Hexose sugar	Immediate precipitate on heating
Mannose	Hexose sugar	Immediate precipitate on heating
Sorbinose	Hexose sugar	Immediate precipitate on heating
Lactose	Disaccharide	Immediate precipitate on heating
Maltose	Disaccharide	Immediate precipitate on heating
Sucrose	Disaccharide	Slight yellowish turbidity after 2 minutes and precipitate after acid hydrolysis
Raffinose	Trisaccharide	Slight yellowish turbidity after 2 minutes and precipitate after acid hydrolysis
Inulin	Polysaccharide	Slight yellowish turbidity after 2 minutes and precipitate after acid hydrolysis
Dextrins	Polysaccharides	Slight yellowish turbidity after 2 minutes and precipitate after acid hydrolysis
Gum arabic (Acacia)	Gum	Slight yellowish turbidity after 2 minutes and precipitate after acid hydrolysis
Starch	Polysaccharide	Precipitate only after acid hydrolysis
Pectins	Colloidal carbohydrates	Precipitate only after acid hydrolysis
Glycogen	Animal polysaccharide	Precipitate only after acid hydrolysis
Agar agar	Galactan	Precipitate only after acid hydrolysis
Cellulose	Polysaccharide	Precipitate only after treatment with concentrated sulfuric acid, dilution with water and boiling

III. Detection of Starch. Starch is one of the most common fillers for pharmaceutical preparations. It is detected by the characteristic blue color of the starch-iodine complex. The dextrins which are the intermediate hydrolytic products of starch are the only substances which may give a similar reaction. Not all dextrins give a color, however, and some grades produce red colors with iodine. Starch and dextrin are hydrolyzed to maltose by amylase and to glucose by acid.

Reagent. Wagner's iodine-potassium iodide reagent (page 1260).

Procedure. A drop of Wagner's reagent on the solid sample stains the individual granules deep red.

5. Identifying Reactions.

5. Identifying Reactions. Thioindigo Test for Fluoroacetic Acid. Monofluoroacetic acid is commercially available as the sodium salt for use as a rodenticide. It is designated by the code number 1080. Chemically it is similar to monochloracetic acid, being a relatively stable and moderately strong acid, more soluble in water than in organic solvents. It is one of the most toxic substances to man and animals. Because absorption from the digestive tract is so rapid, it is usually too late for treatment by the time symptoms of poisoning become apparent. The lethal dose is so low that chemical examinations of organs, carried out by destruction of the organic matter with qualitative tests for fluoride on the residue, are frequently inconclusive. This is because the difference in total fluoride values in fluoroacetate poisoning and the possible normal fluoride content may not be significantly beyond the probable variations in the method for the detection of inorganic fluoride in a biologic specimen.

Toxicologic analysis for fluoroacetate, therefore, becomes a problem, separate from the general method for detecting unknown poisons, which requires a special isolation for obtaining the compound from tissue in relatively pure form and a specific method for its detection. The following procedure has been developed by Ramsey and Patterson (169).

(a) Isolation from Biologic Material. Isolation of fluoroacetate from biologic material is accomplished by water extraction of the sample, precipitation of protein-like material with phosphotungstic acid, removal of the fluoroacetate from the filtrate by extraction with ether, partial purification by extracting the fluoroacetate from the ether with alkaline water and evaporation of the neutralized aqueous extract to dryness. Final purification is obtained by partition chromatography, employing a chloroform-tertiary amyl alcohol solution of the fluoroacetate through an acid treated silicic acid column.

Procedure. The filtrate from a steam distillation (page 1128) may be used. With tissue samples, homogenize 100 to 250 gm. in about 300 ml. of water per 100 gm. sample. Transfer to a large beaker with about 100 ml. water, acidify with 75 ml. of normal H_2SO_4 and mix thoroughly. Add 20 per cent phosphotungstic acid in small portions with stirring, until no further precipitation occurs (about 75 to 100 ml.). Further dilute the mixture with water so that the precipitate is freely dispersed in the liquid when the mixture is stirred (about 100 to 300 ml.) and filter through a Buchner funnel.* Transfer the filtrate to a large continuous extractor (1.0 to 1.5 liters), add 2 ml. of 1:2 sulfuric acid for each 50 ml. of filtrate and extract for 5 hours with ethyl ether.

Transfer the ether from the continuous extractor to a large separatory funnel, shake out with 20 ml. of water made alkaline with NaOH to cresol red indicator. Draw off the aqueous layer, wash the ether twice with 10 ml. portions of water and add the washings to the alkaline extract. Carefully adjust the pH to the first alkaline color of cresol red indicator, evaporate to near dryness on the steam bath and allow to dry with the aid of a current of warm air.

Preparation of the Chromatographic Column.† Grind 5 gm. of silicic acid ‡ in a mortar with the maximum amount of 0.5N H_2SO_4 it will absorb without becoming sticky (50 to 80 per cent of its weight). Add 35 ml. of chloroform containing 10 per

---

* If the filtrate is not clear or does not filter readily, add 10 to 30 ml. of phosphotungstic acid and allow the solution to stand for several hours before refiltering.

† Partition chromatography of the residue through the chromatographic column is not necessary unless maximum sensitivity in the qualitative test or the quantitative analysis is required.

‡ Acid silicic, precipitated, AR grade. Mallinkrodt Chemical Works.

cent (by volume) of tertiary amyl alcohol and work the mixture into a slurry. Fill a chromatographic tube (18 mm. O.D. by 25 cm. in length) fitted with a cotton plug at the bottom with the slurry and pack it down in the tube with the aid of 2 to 10 lbs. external pressure until all of the excess solvent has drained from the column.

*Partition of the Fluoroacetate Sample.** Moisten the dry residue from evaporation of the alkaline extract with 5 to 10 drops of 1:2 sulfuric acid and introduce 5 ml. of chloroform containing 10 per cent tertiary amyl alcohol. Agitate the solvent to dissolve the fluoroacetic acid and carefully transfer to the top of the chromatographic column with a pipet. Apply several pounds of external pressure from a gas pressure regulator to the column until the solution sinks into the gel. The pressure is released and the process repeated with two additional 5 ml. portions of solvent. Add about 30 ml. of solvent to the top of the column and apply pressure until all of the solvent has percolated through the column into a 50 ml. graduated cylinder, used as the collector.

Isolation of the Purified Fluoroacetate. Transfer the percolate to a separatory funnel and extract with about 20 ml. of water made alkaline to cresol red indicator with N/10 sodium hydroxide. Wash the solvent twice with 10 ml. portions of water and transfer the extract and washings to a 100 ml. beaker. Adjust the pH to the first alkaline color of cresol red indicator and heat on a steam bath while passing a stream of air through the solution to remove the chloroform. Allow the solution to evaporate nearly to dryness and accomplish the final drying with the aid of a stream of warm air.

Procedure for the Thioindigo Test on the Sodium Fluoroacetate Residue. The test depends on the formation of thioindoxyl by reaction of thiosalicylic acid and monofluoroacetic acid and the oxidation of the thioindoxyl with potassium ferricyanide to red water-insoluble thioindigo.

Reagents. (a) Normal sodium hydroxide.

(b) 50 per cent sodium hydroxide.

(c) Thiosalicylic acid reagent: Dissolve 300 mg. of thiosalicylic acid in 2 ml. normal NaOH solution, dilute with 18 ml. water and add 2 drops of 50 per cent NaOH.

(d) Potassium ferricyanide solution: Dissolve 2 gm. $K_3Fe(CN)_6$ in 100 ml. water.

Procedure. Dissolve the fluoroacetate residue in about 25 ml. of water made alkaline to a pH of 9 to 10 and readjust the pH to 5 to 7 after solution is complete. Add 1.0 ml. of thiosalicylic acid reagent, evaporate the solution almost to dryness on the steam bath with the aid of a current of air and bake overnight in an oven at 100° C. Dissolve the thoroughly dry residue in 2 to 3 ml. water and add 1.0 ml. of potassium ferricyanide solution. The formation of a colloidal red solution on standing or an immediate red precipitate indicates the presence of fluoroacetic acid.

The method will detect 0.5 mg. of sodium fluoroacetate readily and an immediate red precipitate forms with 1.0 mg. or more. Monochloroacetic acid, the only interfering compound, reacts with about the same sensitivity as the monofluoroacetate derivative.

PRECIPITATION AND CHARACTERISTIC CRYSTALS

A. Precipitation.

Precipitation tests have been the basis for almost all schematic processes in analytical chemistry. They are more limited in organic analysis since the process includes differentiation between closely related structures which usually react similarly with a precipitating reagent. In organic toxicologic analysis, there is an additional limitation in the use of precipitation as a qualitative test. The process not only assumes that a soluble substance is rendered insoluble by the formation of a derivative with the reagent, but also that there

---

* Inorganic fluorides and silicofluorides are removed.

is always an adequate amount of sample material in solution for the solubility product to be exceeded. Since the solubility of the different organic drugs and their derivatives is quite variable, while at the same time the amount of the drug recovered from the tissue may be different from one case to another, the recovery may not always be adequate to exceed the solubility product of the unknown, although the compound was classified as one falling in the insoluble group from the studies on pure solutions.

Dilution of the unknown sample obviously affects the sensitivity of a precipitation reaction. The ideal condition for working with an unknown is to use no more solvent in dissolving the residue than is necessary to produce an optimum concentration. The entire residue may be treated with a small amount of aqueous solution and the different precipitation tests carried out on small portions. A safer practice, however, is to work entirely with the solid phase. Thus, one or more drops of solution can be evaporated to dryness on a microscope slide, the amount of solid observed, redissolved in a minute drop of solvent and treated with the precipitant. Even better, the drop of precipitant can be added to a small amount of the solid residue and treated with a minute drop of solvent.

Precipitation has been found of limited value for the analysis of pharmaceuticals other than the basic drugs. Before the extensive development of the synthetic medicaments, identification of substances in the extracts from natural principles depended largely on precipitation or crystal formation. Most of these substances occurring in nature were bases with the pharmacologic properties of alkaloids. They showed a common solubility behavior with a series of precipitating reagents which came to be known as the alkaloidal precipitants. This designation no longer holds, since most drugs which are basic yet are nonalkaloidal in properties are also precipitated. Moreover, some relatively nontoxic bases, such as the antihistamines, have general chemical properties indistinguishable from those which characterize the alkaloids so that now the term alkaloid is nondescriptive from the chemical point of view.

The precipitating reagents for compounds with basic nitrogen groups may be divided into three classes:

1. Simple acids and salts: This class includes picric, tannic, chromic and permanganic acids and salts such as mercuric chloride and potassium perrhenate.

2. Complex acids such as iodine-potassium iodide, phosphomolybdic, phosphotungstic, silicotungstic and phosphoantimonic acids.

3. Metallic complexes such as gold chloride (H_2AuCl_4), platinic chloride (H_2PtCl_6), potassium mercuric iodide, potassium cadmium iodide, potassium bismuth iodide, potassium zinc iodide, potassium argenticyanide ($KAg(CN)_2$), potassium ferrocyanide ($K_4Fe(CN)_6$), sodium sulfantimonate and ammonium reineckate ($NH_4[Cr(NH_3)_2(SCN)_4]$).

All precipitants do not precipitate all alkaloids or basic drugs, so that a simple precipitation has limited application as a differentiating type reaction. Since proteins, proteoses and peptones, as well as any high molecular weight basic molecule from tissue such as the purines, may also be precipitated, precipitating reactions are not specific for drugs. The number of bases which can be precipitated with most of the reagents are greater in number than those which fail to react and, for this reason, failure to precipitate, when it is known from color reactions or absorption studies that there is an adequate concentration of the unknown base in the sample, is of greater significance than positive findings with the precipitants.

Precipitation reactions and reactions which depend on the formation of characteristic crystals are entirely different phenomena. The fact that a base is precipitated by a reagent indicates that the precipitate is less likely to consist of characteristic crystals because the immediate precipitation generally produces a finely divided solid phase before characteristic crystal faces on the individual particles have time to develop. There is little question in the chemical field concerning the application and limitations of precipitation reactions in qualitative organic analysis but there are two schools of thought regarding the reliability of characteristic crystal formation as an organic qualitative procedure. Several texts on toxicology (170, 171) base most of the identification on the appearance of the crystalline form of the parent substance or of one or more of its derivatives and the literature pertaining to the pharmacologic analysis for various drugs invariably includes a study of the crystalline habit. On the other hand, there is available literature which shows in as convincing a manner that, because a single substance can assume any one or a number of crystalline forms, habit cannot be relied on for qualitative identification (172-174). The fact that there is a controversy indicates that there are definite reservations concerning the use of typical crystals for identification. The question of the limitations in the interpretation does not involve the optical measurements of microscopy because once a clear-cut crystal is obtained, the optical constants are as reliable as any other physical property. Rather, the problem is resolved into the ability to obtain the typical forms under the conditions that prevail in the analysis for an unknown substance.

B. Characteristic Crystals.

Tests which are based on the formation of typical crystalline forms will depend on constancy in the crystalline habit for their reliability. The habit of crystalline substances is markedly affected by external conditions as well as the concentration. Crystalline growth is determined by the relative rates at which the molecules are deposited in the different planes of the space lattice. In general, the slower the deposition on the different faces, the larger the growing crystal becomes and the more uniform is the geometric configuration which comprises the planes of the crystal faces with respect to the three crystallographic axes. Every substance has some optimum rate of crystallization under standard and controlled conditions which favors the formation of physical forms characterized by the constancy in their Miller indices. If the growth proceeds too rapidly, there is a tendency for the faces to build up toward a point (175) and prominent faces may become overdeveloped.

On the other hand, if crystal formation is too slow, random forms may appear which can interlock or overlay the typical crystal and produce a false geometric pattern. Distortion may occur as a result of restriction of a prominent face because it lies on the bottom of the container. Temperature, the nature of the solvent, the solubility and the concentration affect the growth. Since extraneous ions have a marked effect, the purity of the solution is a predominant factor. Although typical crystalline formation is seldom coincident with precipitation, crystallization may follow precipitation by one of two mechanisms. Either some of the precipitate may redissolve to maintain equilibrium as crystallization of the soluble portion sets in or a metastable equilibrium may result in the precipitation reaction, with crystallization then proceeding in the soluble portion.

Reproducibility and, consequently, the dependability of crystal tests depends on the purity of the substance and strict adherence to carefully controlled conditions. These restrictions are difficult to meet when dealing with micro quantities of pure unknown compounds and are often impossible when applied to substances recovered from tissue. The purity is always questionable because traces of extractable tissue components may be present, as well as metabolites or detoxification products which are extremely difficult to separate from the parent substance. Also, the concentration is difficult to control when working with small amounts of an unknown tissue extract. The best the analyst can hope for is to approach the conditions for ideal crystal formation and only in the exceptional case will the conditions be created in which typical geometric forms are reproduced exactly.

Some accident forms invariably occur under the most carefully controlled conditions and, when the variables cannot be controlled, as with a tissue residue, odd and bizarre forms may even predominate. For this reason, photomicrographs which present a picture of the ideal habit may even be misleading. The test is just as significant when only a few ideal forms are obtained, as when the entire field is ideal. Obviously then, the analyst must know the type he is looking for before he prepares the sample in order to be able to spot characteristic types when only a few are produced. Moreover, reproducibility of aggregate forms cannot be expected so that the gross appearance may vary considerably from one preparation to the next. In this respect, simple drawings of the crystals are as descriptive as photomicrographs because even simple drawings are no more imperfect than the reproducibility of typical forms from one preparation to another.

Because of restrictions in the use of crystal tests in toxicology, their application is usually confined to confirmation or, at most, differentiation between several possibilities. Consequently, the analytic approach in applying crystal tests is the opposite to that used for color and other types of reactions. The analyst needs to know what to expect before-hand and a prerequisite to the application of the test is a study of the crystalline habit of the few possibilities that were suggested by the exclusion process. On the basis of this study, one or more reagents are selected which will produce typical crystals that show maximal differences in their geometric forms with the different possibilities that are suspected.

Since it is difficult even to tabulate crystallographic data for use in identifying un-known substances, it is almost impossible to arrange habit forms in any kind of order. In the tables which follow (30), precipitation data has been combined with crystalline habit. Some substances give immediate oils rather than precipitates with the reagents. A few give precipitates which have distinguishable crystalline forms but, in most cases, crystalline forms require time to develop. Using the microscope slide technic, evaporation at room temperature may occur before crystallization sets in and there is always the possibility of delayed crystallization following precipitation (page 1135). Therefore, the procedure includes immediate observation and observation again after the preparation has been placed for at least one hour in a closed chamber maintained at high humidity to prevent evaporation. A simple humidity chamber may be constructed from two Petri dish covers, one standard and one large size. The bottom of the smaller cover is lined with folded filter paper and saturated with water. A rack to fit over the dish and hold the microscope slides is made from glass rods. The dish is placed on a flat glass plate coated with a ring of Vaseline and covered with the large dish to make a closed unit analogous to a desiccator.

Since concentration has a major effect in the reproducibility of crystals and since it can seldom be controlled when working with an unknown, a manipulative technic was adapted which aimed at producing a concentration gradient in the sample (30). The drop of reagent is placed on the microscope slide in juxtaposition with the solid unknown dissolved in a drop of aqueous acid solvent or the drop of solution containing the un-known (page 1256), without mixing the two. The preparation is placed under the micro-scope, using the low power objective, and centered so that the meniscus of the two drops is in the center of the field. Mixing is accomplished by drawing a hairlike glass rod from the reagent drop to the drop of unknown by means of a micromanipulator. Mixing then occurs by diffusion and the concentration ratio varies from zero to maximal within the diffusing boundaries. In this manner, the proper concentration is more likely to be attained at some place along the line of mixing, to produce a characteristic growth typical of one of the suspected substances.

This discussion of precipitation and characteristic crystals was reviewed during a symposium on toxicologic problems by men (176-178) working in separate but related fields who are well recognized for their contributions. Much of their criticism admittedly is justified and, in view of the fact that all are experts in this phase, it should not be ignored. A unanimous criticism was that the material, as written, tends to condemn crystal tests and might have the effect of unjustifiably discouraging their development for identification purposes. This is certainly not intended because formation of char-acteristic crystals is the only means of identifying some compounds. Crystal tests are primarily of value for compounds containing a basic nitrogen group and many of these give insensitive or nonspecific results with other types of reactions. The point that is probably not made clear is that, even if there were characteristic crystal tests for each of the compounds, there would be no way of cataloguing the typical forms in terms of their crystalline pattern rather than under the name of each compound. To use this type of test for the identification of a general unknown, enough information must be available from previous reactions to permit selection of the proper reagent. Otherwise, the ap-proach reverts to random testing with many reagents as the analyst seeks a form that he will recognize from his experience.

During the discussion, Farmilo * pointed out that the first problem requiring clarifi-cation was that of terminology to draw a clear distinction between crystals obtained for study of their optical properties and those typical forms which are characteristic of the compound with the particular reagent because they are reproducible but, because they are

---

* Charles G. Farmilo, Organic Chemistry and Narcotic Section, Food and Drug Laboratories, Department of National Health and Welfare, Ottawa, Canada.

bizarre, do not lend themselves to optical measurement. Fulton * suggested the terms *chemical microcrystal test* or *crystal recognition test* for the formation of these odd forms. The term *crystallographic test* might then be used to characterize the test in which the crystal produced is one of the regular forms on which optical crystallographic studies can be made. He pointed out that not only do the procedures for obtaining the two types of crystals differ but the kinds of reagents to select for best results in the two types also differ. The formation of regular crystals for optical study generally requires some optimum concentration and greater purity while those forms for microcrystal tests are more variable in their growth requirements for the individual compound. Some require concentrated solutions while others are more typical in very dilute solutions. Any method for the production of crystals in the microcrystal test should include serial dilutions because, as a result of the sensitivity and dilution of impurities, the specificity of the test increases for particular compounds. These distinctions, which have not been clearly made in the literature, should be recognized.

In the crystal work described here, no distinction was made in the process for obtaining these two crystal types. The sample, considered as an unknown, was treated by an optimum procedure with one of a few reagents and the regular forms, with some of their optical properties, and the odd forms were both recorded together for different compounds. When testing for an unknown compound, it is debatable, in the author's opinion, whether sharp lines need be drawn between the different methods of crystal formation because of the difference between studying the crystal obtained from an unknown with a given reagent and observing the same crystal from the same reagent when the identity of the substance is suspected. From the point of view of the analyst working with an unknown compound, the more logical process is to study whichever crystalline type is obtained by all applicable methods. However, the fact that certain reagents and procedures favor one type of crystal formation over the other should have been emphasized. The present procedure could have been improved and extended by incorporating serial dilutions into the same process without sacrificing more sample. Morgan † emphasized the importance of obtaining a number of tests from dilution of a single sample and pointed out that the limiting sensitivity from the final dilution at which crystal formation no longer occurs can be used as a physical property.

Obviously, considerable work is needed to correlate existing information as well as to extend the applications of crystal formation to toxicologic analysis. The problem of interference of tissue impurities and tissue degradation products in the formation of characteristic crystals is not well understood outside the field of forensic toxicology. The diverse opinions discussed here are the result, in part, of differences in the application of crystal tests in the various fields. In the author's opinion, the use of highly developed crystal tests with the wide variety of reagents now available belongs in the as yet unwritten section of this material in which individual compounds would be tabulated along with their physical properties and those tests which are specific and therefore give final identification.

Classifications for the Precipitation and Crystallization Phenomena.

With regard to the solvent, there is little choice between N/10 and Normal acetic acid. Normal acetic is preferable for dissolving the more mucky residues but N/10 is adequate in most cases. The effect with N/10 is about the same as with Normal acetic acid but the objection to hydrochloric acid is its greater tendency for precipitation of free picric acid. For this reason, acetic acid is preferred.

There are eight classifications for the precipitation and crystallization phenomena:

1. Compounds giving crystallization unaccompanied by amorphous precipitation or oily formation.

2. Compounds giving crystalline precipitates accompanied by amorphous precipitation and with little or no oil.

3. Compounds giving crystalline precipitates accompanied by amorphous precipitation and oil formation.

---

* Charles C. Fulton, Chemist in charge of Narcotic Division, Department of Social Affairs, United Nations.
† Charles E. Morgan, Chief Chemist, New York State Racing Commission.

4. Compounds giving crystalline precipitates with oil formation, unaccompanied by amorphous precipitation.

5. Compounds giving amorphous precipitation only, with no crystals and little or no oil formation.

6. Compounds giving oil formation only, with no amorphous or crystalline precipitation.

7. Compounds giving oil formation and amorphous precipitation unaccompanied by crystalline precipitates.

8. Compounds giving no reaction.

Reagents: (a) Picric acid: 1.2 gm. picric acid per 100 ml. water.

(b) Gold chloride: 5 gm. gold chloride per 100 ml. water.

(c) Platinum chloride: 5 gm. platinum chloride per 100 ml. of 1 N hydrochloric acid.

(d) Potassium iodoplatinate: 5 ml. of 5 per cent platinum chloride in 1 N hydrochloric acid is added to 45 ml. of 10 per cent potassium iodide. The solution is diluted with water to 100 ml. and stored in the dark.

(e) Kraut's reagent: A solution of 4 gm. bismuth carbonate in 23.5 ml. of nitric acid (specific gravity 1.18) is slowly added with constant stirring to a solution containing 13.6 gm. potassium iodide in 25 ml. water. The orange red solution is placed in the cold for two hours, during which potassium nitrate precipitates. The precipitate is filtered. The filtrate is diluted to 200 ml. and allowed to stand until the fine black colloidal precipitate has completely settled. It is carefully decanted and the supernatant is stored in the dark.

(f) Wagner's reagent (iodine-potassium iodide): 5 gm. iodine is dissolved in 100 ml. of a 10 per cent potassium iodide solution.

(g) Marme's reagent (potassium-cadmium iodide): 2 gm. cadmium iodide is added to a boiling solution containing 4 gm. potassium iodide dissolved in 12 ml. water. This is mixed with 12 ml. of a saturated solution of potassium iodide.

(h) Mayer's reagent (potassium-mercuric iodide): 1.358 gm. mercuric chloride dissolved in 60 ml. water is poured into a solution containing 5 gm. potassium iodide in 10 ml. water. The solution is diluted to 100 ml. with water.

1. COMPOUNDS GIVING CRYSTALS UNACCOMPANIED BY AMORPHOUS PRECIPITATION OR OILY FORMATION

(a) Reagent: picric acid. Solvent: 0.1 N acetic acid.

p-AMINOBENZOIC ACID. Multiple mass of needle-like hairs develop after standing 1 hour in a humidifier. Strong birefringence, predominantly parallel extinction.

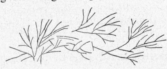

BETAINE. Hairlike sticks growing to large blades on standing 2 to 3 minutes. Strong birefringence, predominantly parallel extinction.

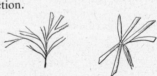

ERGAMINE.* Large twiglike structures develop immediately. Moderate birefringence, predominantly oblique extinction.

* Burroughs Wellcome trademark for histamine.

PHTHALYLSULFATHIAZOLE. Small needle-like bundles appear at edges after standing 1 hour in a humidifier. Moderate birefringence, some polarization, predominantly oblique extinction.

PSEUDOPELLETIERINE. Long, slender, branch-like crystals appear immediately on precipitation. Moderate birefringence, predominantly parallel extinction.

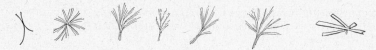

SUCCINYLSULFATHIAZOLE. Needle-like stars form after standing about 2 minutes. Strong birefringence, slight polarization, predominantly parallel extinction. Considerable lateral and longitudinal growth on standing.

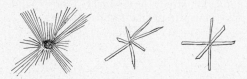

SULFACETIMIDE. Radiating hairlike filaments form after standing about 1 minute. Moderate birefringence, prominent center spots, predominantly parallel extinction.

SULFADIAZINE. Small needle-like bundles form after standing 1 hour in a humidifier. Strong birefringence, predominantly parallel extinction.

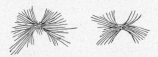

SULFANILAMIDE. Long, slender, needle-like structures which grow rapidly longitudinally. Structures are in bundles, there is also some lateral growth. Crystals form about 1 minute after precipitation. Strong birefringence, predominantly parallel extinction.

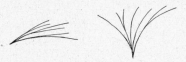

SULFATHIAZOLE. Needle-like bundles form after standing 1 hour in a humidifier. Moderate birefringence, slight polarization, predominantly parallel extinction.

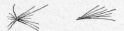

(b) Reagent: gold chloride. Solvent: 0.1 N acetic acid.

BENZOCAINE. Ball forms of needles with rapid longitudinal growth and slight lateral growth develop after standing about 10 minutes. Strong birefringence and predominantly parallel extinction.

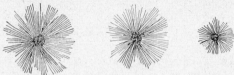

BROMURAL. Needle bundles appear at edge after standing 1 hour in a humidifier. Strong birefringence, predominantly parallel extinction.

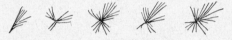

BUTAMIN. Sparlike needle forms grow to straight and curved branches at edges about 15 seconds after precipitation. Strong birefringence, fairly rapid longitudinal growth, some lateral growth, predominantly parallel extinction.

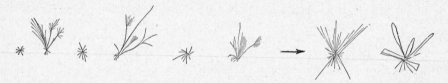

CAFFEINE. Needle bundles or sheaves form after standing 1 hour in a humidifier. Moderate birefringence, predominantly parallel extinction.

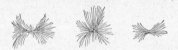

CARBAMYLCHOLINE CHLORIDE. Huge flat sheets or plates develop quickly and grow rapidly; also sparlike sliver forms at outer edge. Strong birefringence, strong polarization, predominantly oblique extinction.

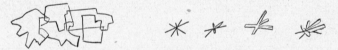

CINCHONIDINE. Starlike forms in multiple aggregate masses develop immediately after precipitation. Slight birefringence, predominantly parallel extinction.

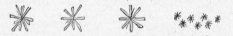

CINCHONINE. Huge jewel-like sprays form after standing 1 hour in a humidifier. Strong birefringence, strong polarization, predominantly parallel extinction.

THIAMIN.HCl. Flat irregularly shaped blades and petal forms develop immediately on precipitation. Slight birefringence, predominantly parallel extinction.

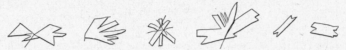

(c) Reagent: platinum chloride. Solvent: 0.1 N acetic acid.

CAFFEINE. Needle bundles develop around edges after standing about 1 minute. They appear in branches and straight clusters. Strong birefringence, some polarization, predominantly oblique extinction along the ends.

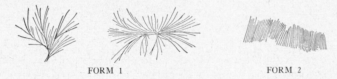

FORM 1   FORM 2

COCAINE. Thousands of aggregate crystalline blade forms, arranged in bizarre fashion, precipitate immediately. Moderate birefringence, predominantly oblique extinction.

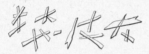

d-DESOXYEPHEDRINE. Huge skeletal blade-like branches radiating out from a central spine, or trunk, develop after standing 2 to 3 minutes and grow very rapidly. Crystals are nonbirefringent.

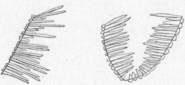

MEPERIDINE. Two forms, feathery blades and insect types, precipitate immediately. Blades are nonbirefringent, insect types are moderately birefringent, predominantly oblique extinction.

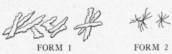

FORM 1   FORM 2

PENTAMETHYLENETETRAZOL. Small burrlike bundles develop after standing 1 hour in a humidifier, accompanied by a resinous residue. Crystals are nonbirefringent.

PILOCARPINE. Crystals resembling massed quantities of winged insects, with petal ends to the blade-like structures, precipitate immediately. Fairly rapid lateral and longitudinal growth. Strong birefringence, some polarization with parallel and oblique extinction.

PROCAINE.HCl. Small black clumps with needle-end edges develop after standing 1 hour in a humidifier. Crystals are nonbirefringent.

PSEUDOPELLETIERINE. Spriglike branches develop at edges after standing for about 30 seconds. Branches grow rapidly to radiating needles and subbranches. Strong birefringence, predominantly oblique extinction. After 3 minutes a second form develops resembling the acid pentobarbital type. Also strong birefringence with predominantly oblique extinction.

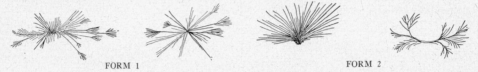

FORM 1   FORM 2

SULFANILAMIDE. Needle-like crystals develop immediately on precipitation, growing rapidly to blade forms, rapid longitudinal growth. Strong birefringence, predominantly oblique extinction.

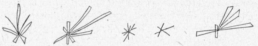

(d) Reagent: potassium iodoplatinate. Solvent: 0.1 N acetic acid.

CAFFEINE. Dark brown sprouts form at edges after standing about 2 minutes. Crystals are slightly birefringent with a reddish brown color. Predominantly parallel extinction along the ends.

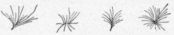

CARBAMYLCHOLINE CHLORIDE. Starlike needles, some resembling airplanes, precipitate after standing about 15 seconds. Crystals are nonbirefringent.

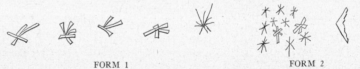

FORM 1   FORM 2

CONIINE. Long black needles intersecting with geometric definiteness precipitate after standing from 30 to 60 seconds. Slight branching occurs. Crystals are nonbirefringent.

THEOPHYLLINE. Two forms of crystals precipitate almost immediately, bushlike needles and groups of blades. Crystals form at edge, developing fully after standing about 2 minutes. Both forms exhibit strong birefringence, some polarization and predominantly oblique extinction.

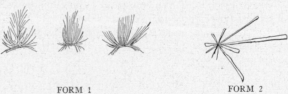

FORM 1   FORM 2

(e) Reagent: Kraut's reagent. Solvent: 0.1 N acetic acid.

STRYCHNINE. Hairlike needles radiating in circular fashion from a central nucleus develop after standing 1 hour in a humidifier. Moderate birefringence, predominantly oblique extinction.

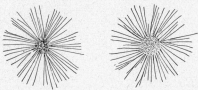

SULFADIAZINE. Long radiating needles develop at edges after standing for 1 hour in a humidifier. Some lateral growth. Strong birefringence with predominantly oblique extinction.

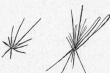

(f) Reagent: Warner's reagent. Solvent: 0.1 N acetic acid.

BENZOCAINE. Starlike needles develop after standing 1 hour in a humidifier. Strong birefringence, predominantly parallel extinction.

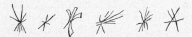

DESOXYCHOLIC ACID. Hairlike filaments with a slight blue cast grow out of occluded particles after standing 1 hour in a humidifier. Moderate birefringence, predominantly parallel extinction.

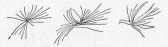

PAVATRINE. Balls of radiating needles resembling burrs develop after standing 1 hour in a humidifier. Slight birefringence, predominantly parallel extinction along the ends.

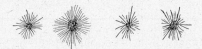

2. COMPOUNDS GIVING CRYSTALLINE PRECIPITATION ACCOMPANIED BY AMORPHOUS PRECIPITATION WITH LITTLE OR NO OILY MATERIAL PRESENT

(a) Reagent: picric acid. Solvent: 0.1 N acetic acid.

ACRIDINE. Hairlike needles form immediately from amorphous mass. Some longitudinal growth on standing. Strong birefringence, predominantly parallel extinction.

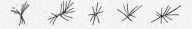

ANTIPYRINE. Three crystalline forms which grow rapidly develop from amorphous material immediately after precipitation. Form 1 shows radiating needles; form 2, blade rosettes; and form 3, leaves with saw edges. Form 1 exhibits moderate birefringence with predominantly oblique extinction. Forms 2 and 3 exhibit strong birefringence with predominantly oblique extinction.

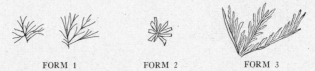

FORM 1   FORM 2   FORM 3

BERBERINE. Hairlike bundles, or sheaves, develop from amorphous material from 2 to 3 minutes after precipitation. Moderate birefringence, predominantly oblique extinction along the ends.

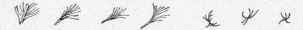

BRUCINE. Crystals resembling feathery molds develop after standing about 2 minutes. Also forms resembling rosette blades. First form is slightly birefringent with predominantly parallel extinction. Second form is highly birefringent, with predominantly parallel extinction.

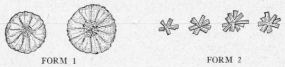

FORM 1   FORM 2

CINCHONIDINE. Starlike crystals which fan out on standing develop about 10 minutes after precipitation. Strong birefringence, predominantly parallel extinction.

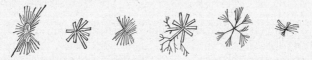

CINCHONINE. Starlike filaments develop after standing 1 hour in a humidifier. Slight birefringence, predominantly parallel extinction. Also blade-like stars with moderate birefringence, predominantly parallel extinction.

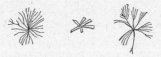

HEROIN. Needle balls with dark centers, resembling burrs, develop from amorphous mass almost immediately after precipitation. Slight birefringence, predominantly parallel extinction along the ends.

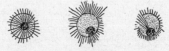

MEPERIDINE. Huge treelike branches grow quickly out of amorphous mass immediately after precipitation. Moderate birefringence with predominantly oblique extinction along the ends.

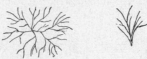

NICOTINE. Bizarre needle-like bundles, changing to mosquito-like rosette forms on standing, develop immediately from amorphous mass. Strong birefringence, predominantly parallel extinction along the ends.

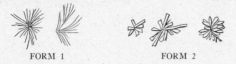

FORM 1   FORM 2

PRISILIDENE. Two crystalline forms develop from amorphous material shortly after precipitation. Needle-like filaments and bundles and blade-like formations. Needles exhibit slight birefringence with predominantly oblique extinction along the ends. Blade forms are strongly birefringent with predominantly parallel extinction.

SPARTEINE. Bundles of sliver-like blades develop from amorphous mass after standing 1 hour in a humidifier. Strong birefringence, predominantly parallel extinction.

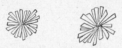

STRYCHNINE. Hook-shaped, needle-like filaments form from amorphous mass after standing about 2 minutes. Steady growth, moderate birefringence, predominantly parallel extinction along the ends.

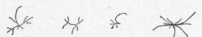

(b) Reagent: gold chloride. Solvent: 0.1 N acetic acid.

ACRIDINE. Thousands of small hairlike spars and needles form immediately from amorphous mass. Crystals exhibit moderate birefringence, slight growth, predominantly oblique extinction along the ends.

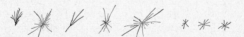

AMINOPYRINE. Minute needle or hairlike spars form from amorphous material almost immediately after precipitation. Slight birefringence with predominantly parallel extinction along the ends.

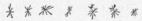

APOMORPHINE. Thread-like filaments form from amorphous mass about 30 seconds after precipitation. Amorphous material is colored red. Crystals are nonbirefringent.

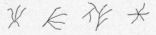

BRUCINE. Small bundles of sharp blades and branches form out of amorphous mass after standing 1 hour in a humidifier, some needle forms. Crystals are small with slight birefringence and predominantly parallel extinction along the ends.

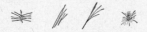

COCAINE. Ruler-edged crystals form from amorphous material after standing about 2 minutes. Slight birefringence with predominantly oblique extinction.

DIMENHYDRINATE. Bizarre needle bundles grow out of amorphous material after standing about 3 minutes. Crystals are nonbirefringent.

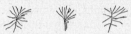

HYOSCYAMINE. Flat feather-shaped crystals grow immediately out of amorphous material. Moderate birefringence, strong polarization, predominantly parallel extinction. Forms exhibit rapid growth.

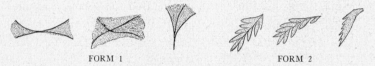

FORM 1   FORM 2

QUINIDINE. Treelike branches and bundles of needles grow out of amorphous mass about 15 to 30 seconds after precipitation. Crystals are nonbirefringent.

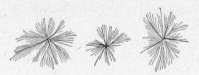

SCOPOLAMINE. Huge needle bundles grow rapidly and immediately out of amorphous material. Needles grow to flatter forms with jagged edges. Moderate birefringence, slight polarization, predominantly parallel extinction.

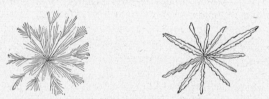

SPARTEINE. Minute, sparlike, mosquito forms develop immediately from amorphous material. Moderate birefringence with predominantly oblique extinction along the ends.

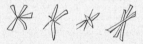

STRYCHNINE. Arcular bushy bundles of needles and smaller star-shaped arrangements grow slowly out of amorphous mass, reaching full development after standing from 30 to 60 seconds. Moderate birefringence with predominantly parallel extinction.

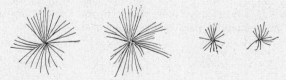

SUCCINYLSULFATHIAZOLE. Fairly large blade-like asters grow out from amorphous mass after standing about 60 seconds. Strong birefringence, moderate polarization with predominantly parallel extinction.

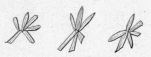

SULFAPYRIDINE. Two crystalline forms grow about 15 seconds after precipitation out of slight amorphous material. Small twiglike crosses and mosquito forms and larger blade rosette forms. Both forms exhibit strong birefringence, slight polarization and predominantly parallel extinction.

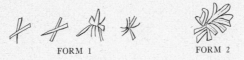

FORM 1   FORM 2

THIAMIN.HCl. Needle, treelike branches growing rapidly, both laterally and longitudinally, develop immediately from amorphous precipitate. Slight birefringence with predominantly parallel extinction along the ends.

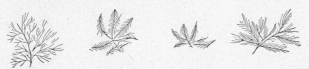

(c) Reagent: platinum chloride. Solvent: 0.1 N acetic acid.

ACRIDINE. Very small, minute slivers and rectangular blades form immediately on precipitation from amorphous mass. Moderate birefringence with predominantly oblique extinction.

FORM 1   FORM 2

BRUCINE. Gross quantities of minute sliver-like crystals are precipitated immediately along with amorphous material. There is slight longitudinal growth on standing. Moderate birefringence with predominantly parallel extinction.

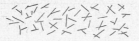

DIMENHYDRINATE. Feathery blades and petals with jagged edges grow from amorphous mass after standing from 30 to 40 seconds. Large lateral growth after standing 1 hour. Moderate birefringence with predominantly oblique extinction.

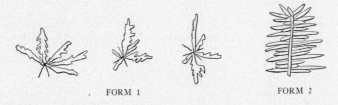

FORM 1   FORM 2

METHADON. Small black and white forms resembling jewelry stones develop from amorphous material after standing 1 hour in a humidifier. Slight birefringence with predominantly oblique extinction at ends.

STRYCHNINE. Three crystalline forms develop from amorphous mass about 30 seconds after precipitation and grow rapidly to their full development in about 4 minutes. Forms 1 and 2 exhibit strong birefringence with predominantly parallel extinction and strong polarization. Form 1 resembles winged insects. Form 2 shows rectangular and square plates. Form 3 is a dark crystal resembling a spruce tree shrub. Moderate birefringence with predominantly oblique extinction.

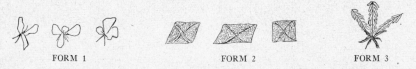

FORM 1   FORM 2   FORM 3

THENYLPYRAMINE. Circular, pine leaf, radiating needles growing out from a central nucleus form from amorphous mass almost immediately after precipitation. Moderate birefringence with predominantly parallel extinction.

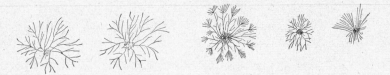

ZOLAMINE. Spriglike forms develop out of amorphous mass from 5 to 10 seconds after precipitation. Crystals resemble crawling insects (spider or beetle). Strong birefringence, slight polarization, medium longitudinal growth on standing, predominantly parallel extinction.

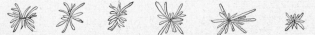

(d) Reagent: potassium iodoplatinate. Solvent: 0.1 N acetic acid.

ACRIDINE. Extremely minute black sparlike forms develop from amorphous mass immediately on precipitation. Crystals are nonbirefringent. After standing 1 hour in a humidifier, hairlike needle forms appear at edge. These forms are strongly birefringent with predominantly oblique extinction. Much longitudinal and lateral growth.

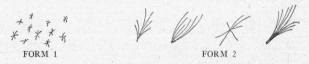

FORM 1   FORM 2

AMINOPYRINE. Rectangular stick-like crystals grow from amorphous mass after standing about 30 seconds. Moderate birefringence with predominantly parallel extinction.

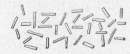

BERBERINE. Balls of needle-like crystals grow out of amorphous mass from 15 to 30 seconds after precipitation. Needles converge on occluded center. Forms appear massively and grow steadily. Slight birefringence with predominantly parallel extinction. Second form is probably an outgrowth of the first.

FORM 1   FORM 2

CINCHONINE. Thousands of aggregate needle crystals shaped like bent pins, some with saw edges, develop from amorphous mass after standing 1 hour in a humidifier. Some form in circular arrangements. Crystals are nonbirefringent.

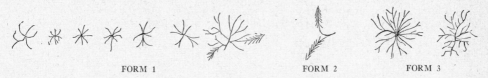

FORM 1   FORM 2   FORM 3

COCAINE. Crystals grow from amorphous mass after standing 1 hour in a humidifier. They resemble ends of pine sprigs with a tendency toward the acid pentobarbital type. Slight birefringence with predominantly parallel extinction along the ends.

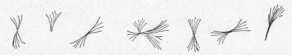

d-DESOXYEPHEDRINE. Narrow rectangular blades, some with jagged edges, develop from amorphous material after standing 1 hour in a humidifier. Crystals are nonbirefringent.

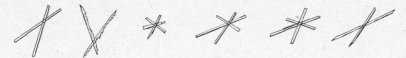

DIMENHYDRINATE. Small sliver-like crystals precipitate immediately from amorphous material. Strong birefringence with predominantly parallel extinction along the ends.

DROMORAN. Needle bundles with brushlike ends and starlike forms with tapered ends develop from amorphous mass after standing 1 hour in a humidifier. Moderate birefringence with predominantly parallel extinction.

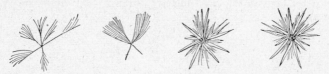

HOMATROPINE. Minute black insect and spar forms of crystals develop after standing 1 hour in a humidifier. Crystals are nonbirefringent.

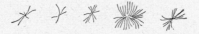

METHADON. Crystals resemble crawling insects and develop from amorphous lattice after standing 1 hour in a humidifier. Crystals are nonbirefringent.

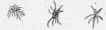

PSEUDOPELLETIERINE. Black insect forms develop from amorphous mass about 3 minutes after precipitation. Crystals are nonbirefringent.

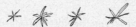

QUINIDINE. Two forms of crystals develop from amorphous material immediately on precipitation. Rapid growth is exhibited in both forms. Form 1 is a fanlike bundle with strong birefringence and predominantly parallel extinction. Form 2 is a fern leaf effect with strong birefringence and predominantly oblique extinction.

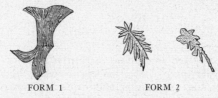

FORM 1   FORM 2

STRYCHNINE. Long radiating needles grow out of amorphous mass immediately on precipitation. Strong birefringence, moderate polarization and predominantly parallel extinction.

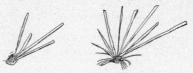

THIAMIN.HCl. Minute hairlike needle stars develop from amorphous mass after standing 1 hour in a humidifier. Crystals are nonbirefringent.

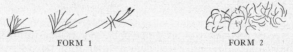

(e) Reagent: Kraut's reagent. Solvent: 0.1 N acetic acid.

ACRIDINE. Needle bundles arranged in bizarre fashion at edges grow from amorphous material about 60 seconds aftaer precipitation. After standing in a humidifier for 1 hour a hairlike lattice forms. Strong birefringence with predominantly parallel extinction.

FORM 1   FORM 2

APOMORPHINE. Blade-like radiations develop from amorphous material after standing 1 hour in a humidifier. Strong birefringence, strong polarization and predominantly parallel extinction.

ATABRIN. Hairlike needle crystals arranged in star formations develop from amorphous mass almost immediately after precipitation. Strong birefringence with predominantly oblique extinction.

BERBERINE. Hairlike needle forms with tendency toward the acid pentobarbital type develop from amorphous mass immediately after precipitation. Moderate growth, moderate birefringence, predominantly parallel extinction.

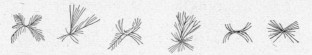

COLCHICINE. Small blade-like crystals resembling mosquitoes develop from slight amorphous material about 15 seconds after precipitation. Moderate birefringence, predominantly parallel extinction along the ends.

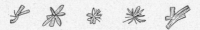

THENYLPYRAMINE. Flat blade-like crystals, some in rosette forms, develop from amorphous mass after standing 1 hour in a humidifier. Slight birefringence with predominantly oblique extinction.

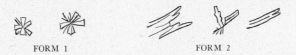

FORM 1   FORM 2

YOHIMBINE. Rectangular crystals with rounded edges develop at edge from amorphous material after standing 1 hour in a humidifier. Strong birefringence, strong polarization, random orientation, both parallel and oblique extinction.

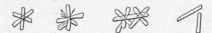

(f) Reagent: Wagner's reagent. Solvent: 0.1 N acetic acid.

ACRIDINE. Needle sheaves similar to the acid pentobarbital type develop from amorphous mass after standing 1 hour in a humidifier. There is considerable lateral growth, slight birefringence and predominantly parallel extinction.

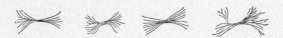

AMINOPYRINE. Blade-like slivers and branches in star formations develop from amorphous mass after standing about 30 seconds. Rapid lateral and longitudinal growth. Moderate birefringence with predominantly parallel extinction along the ends.

BERBERINE. Small black starlike slivers form from amorphous mass about 60 seconds after precipitation. Crystals are nonbirefringent.

BRUCINE. Two crystalline forms develop from amorphous material after standing 1 hour in a humidifier. Circular molds and minute chiplike rosettes. Rosettes are slightly birefringent with parallel and oblique extinction at the ends. Molds are nonbirefringent.

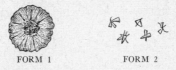

FORM 1   FORM 2

CARBAMYLCHOLINE CHLORIDE. Huge masses of needle bunches radiating from a central nebula develop almost immediately after precipitation from amorphous material and grow rapidly to cover entire slide. Crystals are nonbirefringent.

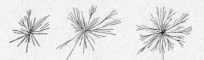

HYOSCYAMINE. Crystal lattice of small black needle points develops from amorphous material from 1 to 2 minutes after precipitation. Crystals are nonbirefringent.

MECONIN. Groups of radiating needles and blades develop from amorphous material about 30 seconds after precipitation. Crystals show medium birefringence with predominately parallel extinction. Also a second form resembling hemin crystals which are nonbirefringent.

FORM 1   FORM 2

PSEUDOPELLETIERINE. Thousands of small, black, minute, chiplike crystals develop from amorphous mass almost immediately after precipitation. Crystals are nonbirefringent.

STRYCHNINE. Multiple starlike needles develop from amorphous material after standing 1 hour in a humidifier. Slight lateral thickness, slight birefringence, predominantly parallel extinction.

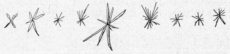

SUCCINYLSULFATHIAZOLE. Starlike radiating needles develop from amorphous material immediately after precipitation. Slight lateral thickness, moderate birefringence, predominantly parallel extinction.

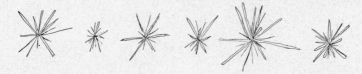

THIAMIN.HCl. Dark brown rosette blades develop from amorphous mass after standing from 30 to 60 seconds. Moderate birefringence with predominantly oblique extinction along the ends.

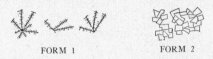

(g) Reagent: Marme's reagent. Solvent: 0.1 N acetic acid.

AMINOPYRINE. Ruler-edged needles with tapered ends develop from amorphous material from 15 to 30 seconds after precipitation. Also some forms appear like flat plates. Moderate birefringence with predominantly parallel extinction.

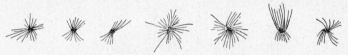

FORM 1   FORM 2

BERBERINE. Hairlike needles radiating from a central nebula develop from amorphous material from 1 to 2 minutes after precipitation. Slight birefringence with predominantly parallel extinction along the ends.

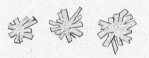

BRUCINE. Rosette-like blades radiating from an occluded nebula develop from amorphous mass after standing 1 hour in a humidifier. Strong birefringence with predominantly parallel extinction along the ends.

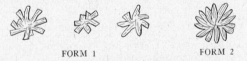

CODEINE. Crystals resembling leaves made up of rosette-like plates develop from amorphous precipitate from 1 to 2 minutes after precipitation. Strong birefringence, some polarization with predominantly oblique extinction. Second forms are feathery molds which are nonbirefringent.

FORM 1   FORM 2

METOPON. Curved, ragged, rhinestone-like branches develop from amorphous precipitate after standing 1 hour in a humidifier. Strong birefringence with predominantly oblique extinction.

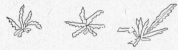

MORPHINE. Minute needle bundles develop immediately from amorphous material. Crystals appear in multiple quantities. Moderate birefringence with predominantly parallel extinction.

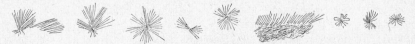

PAMAQUINE. Radiating needles develop from amorphous material after standing about 30 seconds after precipitation. Slight birefringence, slight polarization, predominantly parallel extinction.

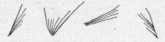

PANTOPON.* Needle formations resembling star shapes and wheat bundles develop from amorphous material about 2 minutes after precipitation. Slight birefringence only with predominantly faint parallel extinction.

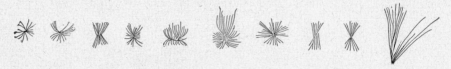

PHENINDAMINE. Pentagonal, hexagonal and some octagonal plates develop from amorphous material from 30 to 60 seconds after precipitation, reaching full development after standing 1 hour in a humidifier. Strong birefringence, strong polarization with predominantly parallel extinction.

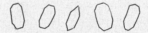

PSEUDOPELLETIERINE. Fern leaf shapes with irregular ruler edges develop from amorphous precipitate almost immediately after precipitation. Slight birefringence with predominantly oblique extinction.

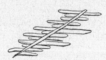

SPARTEINE. Needle-like crystals with ruler edges develop from amorphous material from 30 to 60 seconds after precipitation. Crystals are nonbirefringent.

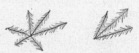

STRYCHNINE. Blade-like rosette formations resembling mosquitoes develop from amorphous material about 60 seconds after precipitation. Crystals grow slowly and steadily on standing. Strong birefringence, some polarization with predominantly oblique extinction along the ends.

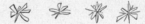

(h) Reagent: Mayer's reagent. Solvent: 0.1 N acetic acid.

ACRIDINE. Mass numbers of small splinters arranged in bizarre fashion develop from amorphous precipitate on standing about 60 seconds. Moderate birefringence with predominantly oblique extinction.

* A mixture of the hydrochlorides of the opium alkaloids.

AMINOPYRINE. Small chiplike blades develop from amorphous material after standing 1 hour in a humidifier. Moderate birefringence with predominantly parallel extinction along the ends.

BERBERINE. Hairlike needles radiating from a central nebula develop from 1 to 2 minutes after precipitation. Slight birefringence with predominantly parallel extinction along the ends.

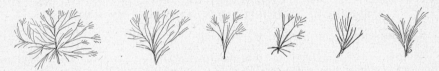

METHADON. Huge needle branches radiate out of amorphous mass after standing 1 hour in a humidifier. Moderate birefringence with predominantly parallel extinction.

METOPON. Long needle branches and sprays develop from amorphous material after standing 1 hour in a humidifier. Strong birefringence with predominantly oblique extinction.

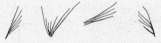

PAMAQUINE. Radiating needles develop from amorphous precipitate at edges upon standing about 30 seconds. Strong birefringence, some polarization with predominantly parallel extinction.

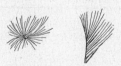

PANTOPON.* Radiating needles develop from amorphous precipitate after standing from 2 to 3 minutes. Slight birefringence with predominantly parallel extinction.

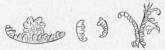

PSEUDOPELLETIERINE. Petal formations with curved bases develop from amorphous mass almost immediately after precipitation. Moderate birefringence with predominantly parallel extinction.

* A mixture of the hydrochlorides of the opium alkaloids.

SPARTEINE. Needle bushes and toothpick forms develop from amorphous mass after standing 1 hour in a humidifier. Needle bushes are nonbirefringent. Toothpick forms appear like splinters arranged in bizarre fashion and exhibit moderate birefringence with predominantly oblique extinction.

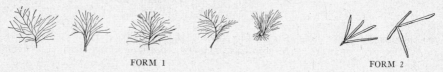

FORM 1   FORM 2

STRYCHNINE. Small sparlike slivers develop from amorphous material about 60 seconds after precipitation. Slight birefringence with predominantly parallel extinction along the ends.

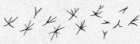

3. COMPOUNDS GIVING CRYSTALLINE PRECIPITATES ACCOMPANIED BY AMORPHOUS PRECIPITATION AND OIL FORMATION

(a) Reagent: picric acid. Solvent: 0.1 N acetic acid.

ADIPHENINE. Crystals develop from amorphous and oily material after standing 1 hour in a humidifier. Formations are blade-like sticks, some arranged in bizarre fashion. Moderate birefringence, some polarization with predominantly oblique extinction.

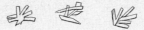

ATROPINE. Large blade-like formations, some in rosette forms, others bizarre, develop from amorphous precipitate upon standing from 2 to 3 minutes. Strong birefringence, strong polarization with predominantly parallel extinction.

BENZOCAINE. Radiating needles and blades develop from amorphous and oily material upon standing from 2 to 3 minutes. Strong birefringence, slight polarization with predominantly parallel extinction.

COCAINE. Huge radiating bundles of needles develop from amorphous and oily material after standing 1 hour in a humidifier. Strong birefringence with predominantly parallel extinction.

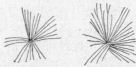

DIMENHYDRINATE. Small starlike needles develop from amorphous and oily material some 3 minutes or so after precipitation. Strong birefringence with predominantly parallel extinction.

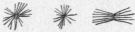

HYOSCYAMINE. Star-shaped bundles of needle filaments develop from amorphous and oily material from 4 to 5 minutes after standing. Slight birefringence with predominantly parallel extinction.

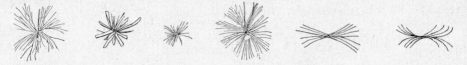

LAROCAINE. Feathery-like leaves and branch formations develop from amorphous and oily mass from 30 to 60 seconds after standing. Moderate birefringence with predominantly parallel extinction along the ends.

PIPEROCAINE. Four crystalline forms arise from amorphous and oily material after standing about 2 minutes. Moldlike forms and filament bundles. Treelike filaments and sparlike insect forms. Filament and tree forms exhibit strong birefringence with predominantly parallel extinction. Mosquito forms are moderately birefringent with predominantly oblique extinction. Mold forms are nonbirefringent.

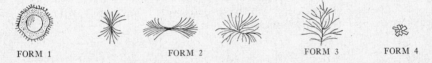

FORM 1   FORM 2   FORM 3   FORM 4

PROCAINE.HCl. Huge treelike structures develop from amorphous and oily mass after standing about 60 seconds. Ends start out fairly thin, growing into blades. After standing 1 hour in a humidifier there is considerable lateral and longitudinal growth. Blade forms become saw-edged. Strong birefringence with predominantly parallel extinction.

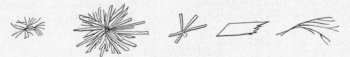

(b) Reagent: gold chloride. Solvent: 0.1 N acetic acid.

ANTIPYRINE. Minute hair and blade-like stars develop from amorphous and oily mass after standing 1 hour in a humidifier. Slight birefringence with predominantly oblique extinction along the ends.

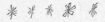

NIKETHAMIDE. Treelike structures develop from amorphous and oily mass after standing for 1 hour in a humidifier. Slight birefringence with predominantly parallel extinction.

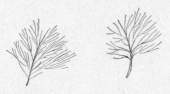

PENTAMETHYLENETETRAZOL. Two structural forms develop from amorphous and oily material after standing 1 hour in a humidifier. Treelike masses and bundles of wide needles in bizarre formation. Needles show strong birefringence, some polarization and predominantly parallel extinction. Tree formations are only slightly birefringent with predominantly oblique extinction along the ends.

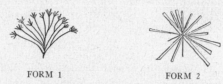

FORM 1   FORM 2

THEOPHYLLINE. Needle formations growing out from a resinous center, some in specific pattern, others in bizarre arrangement, develop from amorphous and oil material from 2 to 3 minutes after precipitation. Strong birefringence, some polarization with predominantly oblique extinction.

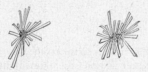

THONZYLAMINE. Three forms of crystals develop from amorphous and oily mass after standing about 2 minutes. Form 1 has groups of jagged-edged blades. Form 2 has circular groups of needle-like crystals whose branches tend to grow laterally to form 1. Form 3 is a radiating needle type, likely an outgrowth from form 2. All forms exhibit slight birefringence with predominantly parallel extinction.

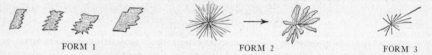

FORM 1   FORM 2   FORM 3

(c) Reagent: platinum chloride. Solvent: 0.1 N acetic acid.

DIBUCAINE. Needle bundles and stars in circular wheel formations, also dumbbell-like types, develop from amorphous and oily material from 2 to 3 minutes after precipitation. Growth proceeds rapidly, crystals fan out to brush-like forms. Strong birefringence, strong polarization with predominantly parallel extinction.

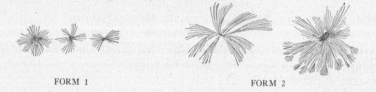

FORM 1   FORM 2

DIPHENHYDRAMINE. Huge treelike crystals develop from amorphous and oily precipitate after standing 1 hour in a humidifier. Strong birefringence with predominantly parallel extinction.

NICOTINE. Huge yellow crystals resembling jewelry stones grow out of amorphous and oily material upon standing from 30 to 45 seconds. Strong birefringence, strong polarization with predominantly oblique extinction.

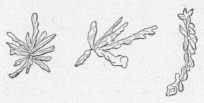

(d) Reagent: potassium iodoplatinate. Solvent: 0.1 N acetic acid.

DICYLOMINE. Huge needle bushes grow out of amorphous and oily mass about 30 seconds after precipitation. There is rapid longitudinal growth. Moderate birefringence with predominantly parallel extinction.

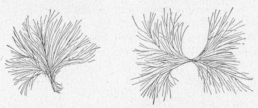

(e) Reagent: Kraut's reagent. Solvent: 0.1 N acetic acid.

NICOTINE. Rectangular blade-like crystals with rounded ends develop from amorphous and oily mass after standing 1 hour in a humidifier. Strong birefringence, moderate polarization with predominantly parallel extinction.

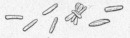

(f) Reagent: Wagner's reagent. Solvent: 0.1 N acetic acid.

ATABRIN. Four-sided blades, some parallelogram in shape, others grouped in rosette forms, develop from amorphous and oily material from 2 to 3 minutes after precipitation. Strong birefringence with predominantly oblique extinction.

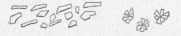

ATROPINE. Small starlike needle bundles resembling winged insects develop from amorphous and oily material after standing 60 seconds. Small lateral and longitudinal growth on standing. Crystals are nonbirefringent.

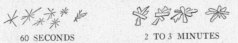

60 SECONDS   2 TO 3 MINUTES

CODEINE. Two forms of crystals develop from amorphous and oily mass about 60 seconds after precipitation, developing fully after standing 1 hour in a humidifier. Form 1 resembles needle sheaves with a tendency toward the acid pentobarbital type of formation. Form 2 resembles saw-edged blades in star formation. Both forms exhibit moderate birefringence with predominantly parallel extinction.

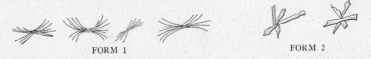

FORM 1   FORM 2

DIMENHYDRINATE. Small, minute twiglike crystals grow out of amorphous and oily mass about 60 seconds after precipitation. Slight birefringence with predominantly parallel extinction along the ends.

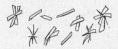

ETHYLMORPHINE. Huge treelike branches with smaller needle-like branches growing from the ends develop from amorphous and oily material after standing 1 hour in a humidifier. Strong birefringence with predominantly parallel extinction.

MORPHINE. Blade-like structures, some with jagged edges in bizarre formation, develop from amorphous and oily material after standing 1 hour in a humidifier. Moderate birefringence with predominantly parallel extinction.

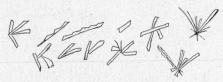

(g) Reagent: Marme's reagent. Solvent: 0.1 N acetic acid.

DIMENHYDRINATE. Minute star-shaped slivers appear from amorphous mass about 2 minutes after precipitation. Oil forms on further standing. Moderate birefringence with predominantly parallel extinction along the ends.

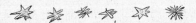

THEOPHYLLINE. Parallelogram blade formations develop from amorphous and oily mass after standing 1 hour in a humidifier. Moderate birefringence with predominantly oblique extinction.

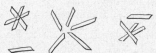

(h) Reagent: Mayer's reagent. Solvent: 0.1 N acetic acid.

CARBAMYLCHOLINE CHLORIDE. Starlike blades develop from amorphous and oily material from 30 to 60 seconds after precipitation. Crystals vary largely in size and quickly disintegrate, in some cases altogether. Slight birefringence only, predominantly parallel extinction.

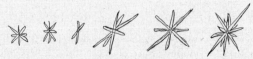

CODEINE. Clumps of radiating feathery branches develop from amorphous and oily mass after standing 1 hour in humidifier. Moderate birefringence with predominantly oblique extinction along the ends.

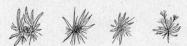

DIHYDROMORPHINONE. Small needle bushes at very edge grow out of amorphous and oily material after standing 1 hour in a humidifier. Crystals are nonbirefringent.

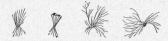

HOMATROPINE. Large yellow blades with tapered ends, some in star shapes, others in propeller-like formations, grow from amorphous and oily material after standing 1 hour in a humidifier. Strong birefringence, some polarization with predominantly parallel extinction.

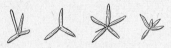

4. COMPOUNDS GIVING CRYSTALLINE PRECIPITATES AND OIL FORMATION UNACCOMPANIED BY AMORPHOUS PRECIPITATION

(a) Reagent: Marme's reagent. Solvent: 0.1 N acetic acid.

CONIINE. Crystal growths resembling cauliflower leaves develop from slight oil after standing from 4 to 5 minutes. Crystals exhibit moderate birefringence, moderate polarization with predominantly parallel extinction.

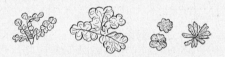

5. COMPOUNDS GIVING AMORPHOUS PRECIPITATION ONLY, NO CRYSTALS AND LITTLE OR NO OILY FORMATION

(a) Reagent: picric acid. Solvent: 0.1 N acetic acid.

Aconitine	Emetine	Lobeline	Phenindamine
Apomorphine	Ethylmorphine	Metopon	Quinidine
Atabrin	Eucupin	Morphine	Quinine
Cephaeline	Hydrastine	Narceine	Yohimbine

(b) Reagent: gold chloride. Solvent: 0.1 N acetic acid.

Aconitine	Curarine	Ethylmorphine	Narceine	Prostigmine
Ascorbic acid	Delphinine	Eucupin	Narcotine	Pseudopel-
Cephaeline	d-Desoxyephed-	Hydrastine	Nicotine	letierine
Cinchonidine	rine	Lobeline	Pamaquine	Quinine
Cinchonine	Dihydromorphinone	Methadon	Pelletierine	Tutocaine
Codeine	Diothane	Metopon	Phenindamine	Xylocaine
Colchicine	Emetine	Morphine	Physostigmine	Yohimbine

(c) Reagent: platinum chloride. Solvent: 0.1 N acetic acid.

Apomorphine	Curarine	Diothane	Eucupin
Berberine	Cysteine	Emetine	Lobeline
Cephaeline	Delphinine	Ethylmorphine	Phenindamine
		Quinine	

(d) Reagent: potassium iodoplatinate. Solvent: 0.1 N acetic acid.

Aconitine	Cinchonidine	Diothane	Larocaine	Physostigmine
Apomorphine	Curarine	Emetine	Lobeline	Pilocarpine
Apothesine	Cysteine.HCl	Ethylmorphine	Methadon	Quinine
Atabrin	Delphinine	Eucupin	Metopon	Scopolamine
Atropine	Dibucaine	Heroin	Morphine	Yohimbine
Brucine	Dihydromor-	Hydrastine	Narceine	
Cephaeline	phinone	Hyoscyamine	Phenindamine	

(e) Reagent: Kraut's reagent. Solvent: 0.1 N acetic acid.

Amprotropine	Coniine	Ethylmorphine	Metopon	Scopolamine
Apothesine	Curarine	Eucupin	Pelletierine	Sparteine
Betaine	Delphinine	Heroin	tannate	Succinylsulfa-
Carbamylcholine	d-Desoxyephedrine	Larocaine	Physostigmine	thiazole
chloride	Dromoran	Meperidine	Prisilidene	Thiamin.HCl
Cocaine	Ergamine	Methadon	Procaine.HCl	Zolamine

(f) Reagent: Wagner's reagent. Solvent: 0.1 N acetic acid.

Aconitine	Colchicine	Digitoxin	Heroin	Strophanthin
Biliverdin	Curarine	Emetine	Narcotine	Yohimbine
Cephaeline	Delphinine	Ergamine	Sparteine	

(g) Reagent: Marme's reagent. Solvent: 0.1 N acetic acid.

Aconitine	Curarine	Heroin	Narceine	Quinidine
Atabrin	Delphinine	Homatropine	Narcotine	Quinine
Cephaeline	Dromoran	Hydrastine	Pentamethylene-	Xylocaine
Cinchonidine	Ethylmorphine	Lobeline	tetrazole	Yohimbine
Cinchonine	Eucupin	Methadon	Physostigmine	

(h) Reagent: Mayer's reagent. Solvent: 0.1 N acetic acid.

Aconitine	Cephaeline	Dromoran	Morphine	Physostigmine
Antipyrine	Cinchonidine	Emetine	Narceine	Quinidine
Apomorphine	Cinchonine	Ethylmorphine	Narcotine	Quinine
Atabrin	Curarine	Eucupin	Pamaquine	Xylocaine
Brucine	Delphinine	Heroin	Pelletierine	Yohimbine
Butamin	Diothane	Hydrastine	Phenindamine	

6. COMPOUNDS GIVING OIL FORMATION ONLY, UNACCOMPANIED BY AMORPHOUS OR CRYSTALLINE PRECIPITATION

(a) Reagent: picric acid. Solvent: 0.1 N acetic acid.

Carbamylcholine	Coniine	Nikethamide	Sulfonethyl-
chloride	Curarine	Pelletierine	methane
Colchicine	Melphenesine	tannate	Sulfonmethane

(b) Reagent: gold chloride. Solvent: 0.1 N acetic acid.

Coniine	Methylphenylethyl-	Sulfacetimide
Ergamine	hydantoin	Sulfanilamide
Mephenesine	Pyrithyldione	

(c) Reagent: platinum chloride. Solvent: 0.1 N acetic acid.

Amprotropine	Hyoscyamine	Pelletierine	Scopolamine	Sulfisoxazole
Antipyrine	Mephenesine	Phthalylsulfa-	Sparteine	Yohimbine
Atropine	Metopon	thiazole	Succinylsulfa-	
Coniine	Morphine	Prostigmine	thiazole	
Dromoran	Nikethamide	Pyrithyldione	Sulfathiazole	

(d) Reagent: potassium iodoplatinate. Solvent: 0.1 N acetic acid.

Antipyrine	Mephenisine	Pregnenolone	Pyrithyldione

(e) Reagent: Kraut's reagent. Solvent: 0.1 N acetic acid.

Dimenhydrinate	Hydrastine	Narceine	Nikethamide
Ephedrine	Mephenesine	Narcotine	Piperocaine
		Quinidine	

(f) Reagent: Wagner's reagent. Solvent: 0.1 N acetic acid.

Mephenesine	Pyrithyldione	Sulfathiazole	Sulfonethylmethane	Sulfonmethane

(g) Reagent: Marme's reagent. Solvent: 0.1 N acetic acid.

Betaine	Carbamylcholine chloride	Colchicine

(h) Reagent: Mayer's reagent. Solvent: 0.1 N acetic acid.

Betaine	Colchicine

7. COMPOUNDS GIVING AMORPHOUS AND OILY PRECIPITATION UNACCOMPANIED BY CRYSTAL FORMATION

(a) Reagent: picric acid. Solvent: 0.1 N acetic acid.

Aminopyrine	Dibucaine	Ephedrine	Tetracaine
Amprotropine	Dicyclomine	Methadon	Thenylpyramine
Butamin	Dihydromorphinone	Narcotine	Thiamin.HCl
Codeine	Diothane	Pilocarpine	Thonzylamine
d-Desoxyephed-	Diphenhydramine	Prostigmine	Xylocaine
rine	Dromoran	Scopolamine	Zolamine

(b) Reagent: gold chloride. Solvent: 0.1 N acetic acid.

Adiphenine	Benzocaine	Heroin	Piperocaine	Thenylpyramine
Amprotropine	Dibucaine	Homatropine	Prisilidene	Zolamine
Apothesine	Dicyclomine	Larocaine	Procaine.HCl	
Atabrin	Dromoran	Meperidine	Sulfathiazole	
Atropine	Ephedrine	Pilocarpine	Tetracaine	

(c) Reagent: platinum chloride. Solvent: 0.1 N acetic acid.

Adiphenine	Dihydromor-	Hydrastine	Piperocaine	Tetracaine
Atabrin	phinone	Narceine	Prisilidene	Thonzylamine
Dicyclomine	Ephedrine	Narcotine	Quinidine	

(d) Reagent: potassium iodoplatinate. Solvent: 0.1 N acetic acid.

Adiphenine	Meperidine	tetrazol	Scopolamine	Xylocaine
Amprotropine	Narcotine	Piperocaine	Sparteine	Zolamine
Dicyclomine	Nicotine	Prisilidene	Tetracaine	
Ephedrine	Nikethamide	Procaine.HCl	Thenylpyramine	
Hyoscyamine	Pentamethylene-	Prostigmine	Thonzylamine	

(e) Reagent: Kraut's reagent. Solvent: 0.1 N acetic acid.

Adiphenine	Diothane	Phenindamine
Cinchonidine	Diphenhydramine	Phthalylsulfathiazole
Dicyclomine	Lobeline	Quinine

(f) Reagent: Wagner's reagent. Solvent: 0.1 N acetic acid.

Adiphenine	Coniine	Ephedrine	Nicotine	Procaine.HCl
Amprotropine	d-Desoxyephed-	Eucupin	Nikethamide	Prostigmine
Antipyrine	rine	Homatropine	Pelletierine	Quinidine
Apomorphine	Dibucaine	Hydrastine	Pentamethylene-	Quinine
Atropine	Dicyclomine	Larocaine	tetrazol	Scopolamine
Betaine	Dihydromor-	Lobeline	Phenindamine	Tetracaine
Butamin	phinone	Meperidine	Physostigmine	Thenylpyramine
Cinchonidine	Diothane	Methadon	Pilocarpine	Thonzylamine
Cinchonine	Diphenhydramine	Metopon	Piperocaine	Xylocaine
Cocaine	Dromoran	Narceine	Prisilidene	Zolamine

(g) Reagent: Marme's reagent. Solvent: 0.1 N acetic acid.

Adiphenine	Cocaine	Diphenhydra-	Nicotine	Scopolamine
Amprotropine	d-Desoxyephed-	mine	Nikethamide	Tetracaine
Antipyrine	rine	Emetine	Pilocarpine	Thiamin.HCl
Apomorphine	Dibucaine	Ephedrine	Piperocaine	Thonzylamine
Apothesine	Dicyclomine	Hyoscyamine	Prisilidene	Zolamine
Atropine	Dihydromor-	Larocaine	Procaine.HCl	
Butamin	phinone	Meperidine	Prostigmine	

(h) Reagent: Mayer's reagent. Solvent: 0.1 N acetic acid.

Adiphenine	d-Desoxyephed-	Ephedrine	Pilocarpine	Tetracaine
Amprotropine	rine	Hyoscyamine	Piperocaine	Thenylpyra-
Apothesine	Dibucaine	Larocaine	Prisilidene	mine
Atropine	Dicyclomine	Meperidine	Procaine.HCl	Thiamin.HCl
Cocaine	Diphenhydra-	Nicotine	Prostigmine	Thonzylamine
Coniine	mine	Nikethamide	Scopolamine	Zolamine

8. NONREACTING COMPOUNDS

(a) Reagent: picric acid. Solvent: 0.1 N acetic acid.

Acetanilid
Amphetamine
Ascorbic acid
Biliverdin
Biuret
Bromural
Caffeine
Cantharidin
Carbromal

Cysteine.HCl
Delphinine
Desoxycholic
  acid
Dicoumarol
Digalen
Digalin
Digitalin
Digitonin
Digitoxin

Estrone
Ethyl biscoum-
  acetate
Glycine
Homatropine
Meconin
Methylphenyl-
  ethylhydantoin
Pamaquine

Pavatrine
Pentamethylene-
  tetrazol
Physostigmine
Piperidione
Piperine
Pregnenolone
Pyrithyldione
Saccharin

Sedormid
Strophanthin
Sulfapyridine
Sulfisoxazole
Theobromine
Theophylline
Tribromo-
  ethanol

(b) Reagent: gold chloride. Solvent: 0.1 N acetic acid.

Acetanilid
p-Aminobenzoic
  acid
Biliverdin
Cantharidin
Carbromal

Cinchophen
Desoxycholic
  acid
Dicoumarol
Digalen
Digitalin

Digitonin
Digitoxin
Estrone
Ethyl biscoum-
  acetate
Glycine

Pavatrine
Piperidione
Piperine
Pregnenolone
Saccharin
Sedormid

Sulfadiazine
Sulfisoxazole
Sulfonmethane
Theobromine
Tribromoethanol
Trimethadione

(c) Reagent: platinum chloride. Solvent: 0.1 N acetic acid.

Acetanilid
p-Aminobenzoic
  acid
Aminopyrine
Ascorbic acid
Bromural
Carbamylcholine
  chloride
Carbromal

Codeine
Colchicine
Desoxycholic acid
Dicoumarol
Digalen
Digitalin
Digitonin
Digitoxin
Ergamine

Estrone
Ethyl biscoum-
  acetate
Glycine
Heroin
Larocaine
Meconin
Methylphenyl-
  ethylhydantoin

Pamaquine
Pavatrine
Physostigmine
Piperidione
Piperine
Pregnenolone
Saccharin
Sedormid
Strophanthin

Sulfacetimide
Sulfapyridine
Sulfonmethane
Theobromine
Theophylline
Tribromo-
  ethanol
Trimethadione
Xylocaine

(d) Reagent: potassium iodoplatinate. Solvent: 0.1 N acetic acid.

Acetanilid
p-Aminobenzoic
  acid
Amphetamine
Ascorbic acid
Benzocaine
Betaine
Biliverdin
Bromural
Cantharidin

Carbromal
Cinchophen
Codeine
Colchicine
Desoxycholic
  acid
Dicoumarol
Digalen
Digitalin
Digitonin

Ergamine
Estrone
Ethyl biscoum-
  acetate
Glycine
Meconin
Methylphenyl-
  ethylhydantoin
Pamaquine
Pelletierine

Phthalylsulfa-
  thiazole
Piperidione
Piperine
Saccharin
Sedormid
Strophanthin
Succinylsulfa-
  thiazole
Sulfacetimide

Sulfadiazine
Sulfanilamide
Sulfapyridine
Sulfathiazole
Sulfisoxazole
Sulfonmethane
Theobromine
Tribromo-
  ethanol
Trimethadione

(e) Reagent: Kraut's reagent. Solvent: 0.1 N acetic acid.

Acetanilid
Aconitine
p-Aminobenzoic
  acid
Aminopyrine
Amphetamine
Antipyrine
Ascorbic acid
Atropine
Benzocaine
Biliverdin
Bromural
Brucine
Butamin

Caffeine
Cantharidin
Carbromal
Cephaeline
Cinchonine
Cinchophen
Codeine
Cysteine.HCl
Desoxycholic acid
Dibucaine
Dicoumarol
Digalen
Digitalin
Digitonin

Digitoxin
Dihydromor-
  phinone
Emetine
Estrone
Ethyl biscoum-
  acetate
Glycine
Homatropine
Hyoscyamine
Meconin
Methylphenyl-
  ethylhydantoin
Morphine

Pamaquine
Pavatrine
Pentamethylene-
  tetrazol
Pilocarpine
Piperidione
Piperine
Pregnenolone
Prostigmine
Pseudopel-
  letierine
Pyrithyldione
Saccharin
Sedormid

Strophanthin
Sulfacetimide
Sulfanilamide
Sulfapyridine
Sulfathiazole
Sulfisoxazole
Sulfonmethane
Tetracaine
Theobromine
Theophylline
Thonzylamine
Tribromoethanol
Trimethadione
Xylocaine

(f) Reagent: Wagner's reagent. Solvent: 0.1 N acetic acid.

Acetanilid
p-Aminobenzoic
  acid
Amphetamine
Ascorbic acid
Bromural
Caffeine
Cantharidin

Carbromal
Cinchophen
Cysteine.HCl
Dicoumarol
Digalen
Digitalin
Digitonin
Estrone

Ethyl biscoum-
  acetate
Glycine
Methylphenyl-
  ethylhydantoin
Pamaquine
Phthalylsulfa-
  thiazole

Piperidione
Piperine
Pregnenolone
Saccharin
Sedormid
Sulfacetimide
Sulfadiazine
Sulfanilamide

Sulfapyridine
Sulfisoxazole
Theobromine
Theophylline
Tribromo-
  ethanol

(g) Reagent: Marme's reagent. Solvent: 0.1 N acetic acid.

Acetanilid	Cinchophen	Ethyl biscoum-	Piperidione	Sulfanilamide
p-Aminobenzoic	Cysteine.HCl	acetate	Piperine	Sulfapyridine
acid	Desoxycholic acid	Glycine	Pregnenolone	Sulfathiazole
Amphetamine	Dicoumarol	Meconin	Pyrithyldione	Sulfisoxazole
Ascorbic acid	Digalen	Mephenesine	Saccharin	Sulfonmethane
Benzocaine	Digitalin	Methylphenyl-	Sedormid	Theobromine
Biliverdin	Digitonin	ethylhydantoin	Strophanthin	Theophylline
Bromural	Digitoxin	Pavatrine	Succinylsulfa-	Tribromo-
Caffeine	Diothane	Pelletierine	thiazole	ethanol
Cantharidin	Ergamine	Phthalylsulfa-	Sulfacetimide	Trimethadione
Carbromal	Estrone	thiazole	Sulfadiazine	

(h) Reagent: Mayer's reagent. Solvent: 0.1 N acetic acid.

Acetanilid	Carbromal	Estrone	Phthalylsulfa-	Sulfacetimide
p-Aminobenzoic	Cysteine.HCl	Ethyl biscoum-	thiazole	Sulfadiazine
acid	Desoxycholic	acetate	Piperidione	Sulfanilamide
Amphetamine	acid	Glycine	Pregnenolone	Sulfapyridine
Ascorbic acid	Dicoumarol	Meconin	Pyrithyldione	Sulfathiazole
Benzocaine	Digalen	Mephenesine	Saccharin	Sulfisoxazole
Biliverdin	Digitalin	Methylphenyl-	Sedormid	Sulfonmethane
Bromural	Digitonin	ethylhydantoin	Strophanthin	Theobromine
Caffeine	Digitoxin	Pentamethylene-	Succinylsulfa-	Theophylline
Cantharidin	Ergamine	tetrazol	thiazole	Tribromoethanol
				Trimethadione

Table 47-40.   Nonvolatile Organic Compounds; Selected Proprietary Names; Their Actions

Acetanilid	Antifebrin, Acetylaniline, Phenylacetamide	Antipyretic, analgesic
Acetophenetidin	Phenacetin, p-Acetophenetide	Antipyretic, analgesic
Acetylsalicylic acid	Aspirin, Acetophen, Acetol, Acetosal, Acetosalic acid, Empirin	Antipyretic, analgesic
Aconitine		Neuralgic
Adiphenine	Trasentine	Antispasmodic
N-Allylnormorphine	Nalline	Morphine antagonist
p-Aminobenzoic acid	PABA	
Aminopyrine	Amidopyrine, Pyramidon, Amidofebrin, Novamidon	Antipyretic, analgesic
Amobarbital	Amytal	Sedative, hypnotic
Amphetamine	Benzedrine, Actedron, Mecodrin, Allodene, Phenedrine	Central nervous system stimulant
Amprotropine	Syntropan	Antispasmodic
Antabuse	Tetraethylthiuram Disulfide, TTD, Thiuramide, Tetradine, Abstinyl	Treatment of alcoholics
Antipyrine	Phenazone, Analgesine, Parodyne, Phenylone, Sedatine, Pyrazoline	Analgesic, antipyretic
Apomorphine		Emetic
Apothesine		Local anesthetic
Aprobarbital	Alurate, Numal	Sedative, hypnotic
Ascorbic acid	Vitamin C	Vitamin C therapy
Atabrin	Quinacrine, Chinacrin, Acriquine, Palacrin, Metoquine	Antimalarial
Atropine		Antiparasympathomimetic agent, antispasmodic, mydriatic
Barbital	Veronal, Medinal, Barbitone, Malonal	Sedative, hypnotic
Benzocaine	Anesthesin, Anesthone, Parathesin, Ethylamino benzoate	Local anesthetic
Berberine.SO₄		
Betaine.HCl	Lycine, Oxyneurine	Used to administer HCl
Biuret		

Table 47-40 (cont.). Nonvolatile Organic Compounds; Selected Proprietary Names; Their Actions

Bromural	Bromisovalum, Bromisoval, B.V.U., Broval-urea, Dormigene, Isobromyl	Sedative, hypnotic
Brucine		Chemical reagent
Butabarbital	Butisol	Sedative, hypnotic
Butallylonal	Pernoston, Pernocton	Hypnotic
Butamin	Tutocaine	Local anesthetic
Caffeine	Methyltheobromine	Cardiac and respiratory stimulant, diuretic
Cantharidin	Cantharides camphor, Spanish fly	Irritant, vesicant
Carbamylcholine chloride	Doryl, Carbachol, Carcholin	Parasympathomimetic agent
Carbromal	Adalin, Bromadal, Uradal	Sedative, hypnotic
Cephaeline		Amebiasis
Chlorcyclizine	Di-paralene, Perazil, Perazyl, Histantine	Antihistaminic, anti-allergic agent
Chlorobutanol	Chloretone, Chlorbutol, Methaform, Seda-form	Anesthetic, antiseptic, hypnotic
Colchicine		Gout therapy
Cholesterol	Cholesterin	
Chrysazin	Istizin	Cathartic, dye
Cinchonidine	Cinchovatine	Antimalarial
Cinchonine		Antimalarial
Cinchophen	Atophan, Phenoquin, Quinophan, Tophol, Agotan	Analgesic, antipyretic
Cocaine		Local anesthetic
Codeine	Methylmorphine	Narcotic
Coniine		Sedative, antispasmodic
Curarine		Muscle relaxant
Cyclopal		Sedative, hypnotic
Cysteine.HCl	beta-Mercaptoalanine	
Delphinine		
Desoxycholic acid	Deoxycholic acid, Choleic acid	Choleretic
d-Desoxyephedrine	Methylamphetamine, Desoxyn, Methedrine, Dexoval, Amphedroxyn	Central nervous system stimulant
Diallylbarbituric acid	Dial, Allobarbital, Allobarbitone	Sedative, hypnotic
Dibucaine	Nupercaine, Percaine, Cinchocaine	Anesthetic
Dichlorodiphenyl-trichloroethane	DDT, Gesarol, Neocid	Contact insecticide
Dicoumarol	Dicumarol, Dicoumarin, Melitoxin	Anticoagulant
Dicyclomine	Bentyl	Antispasmodic
Diethylacetylurea		Experimental drug
Digalen		Cardiac therapy
Digitalin		Cardiac therapy
Digitonin		Chemical reagent
Digitoxin		Cardiac therapy
Dihydromorphinone	Dilaudid, Dimorphone, Hymorphan	Narcotic
Dimenhydrinate	Dramamine	Motion sickness
Diothane	Diperodon	Surface anesthetic
Diphenhydramine	Benadryl, Amidryl	Antihistamine, anti-allergic agent
Diphenylhydantoin	Dillantin, Dilantin, Phenytoin, Dihydan	Anti-epileptic
Dromoran	Hydroxymethylmorphinan	Narcotic
Emetine		Amebicide

Table 47-40 (cont.).   Nonvolatile Organic Compounds; Selected Proprietary Names; Their Actions

Ephedrine		Vasoconstrictor, sympathomimetic agent
Estrone	Theelin, Folliculin, Menformon, Estrol, Destrone, Oestrin	Replacement hormone therapy
Ethyl biscoumacetate	Tromexan, Pelentan	Anticoagulant
Ethylmorphine	Dionin	Narcotic
Eucupin di HCl		Local anesthetic
Glycine	Aminoacetic acid, Glycocoll	
Heroin	Diacetylmorphine	Narcotic
Hexobarbital	Evipal, Evipan, Hexobarbitone, Cyclonal	Preoperative anesthetic and sedative
Hippuric acid	Benzoylglycine, Benzoylaminoacetic acid	Metabolite
Histamine	Ergamine	Allergy therapy, diagnostic aid
Homatropine	Mandelyltropeine	Mydriatic, cycloplegic
Hydrastine		
Hyoscyamine	Daturine	Hypnotic, sedative
Isoamylethylacetylurea		Experimental drug
Larocaine		Local anesthetic
Lobeline		Respiratory stimulant
Meconin	Opianyl	
l-Menthol	Hexahydrothymol, Peppermint camphor	Antiseptic, astringent
Meperidine	Demerol, Dolosal, Dolantin, Dolantal, Isonipecaine	Narcotic, analgesic
Mephenesine	Tolserol, Myanesin, Relaxar, Tolcil, Lisephen	Depressant of reflex excitability
Mephobarbital	Prominal, Mebaral, Phemitone	Sedative, anti-epileptic
Mescaline		Used in the diagnosis of psychosis
Methadon	Dolophine, Amidon, Adanon, Polamidon, Diaminon, Butalgin, Miadone	Narcotic, analgesic
Methylparafynol	Dormison	Hypnotic
Methylphenylethyl-hydantoin	Mesantoin, Phenantoin	Anti-epileptic
Metopon	Methyldihydromorphinone	Narcotic, sedative
Morphine		Narcotic
alpha-Naphthylthiourea	ANTU, α-Naphthylthiocarbamide	Rodenticide
Narceine		Narcotic
Narcotine	Narcosine, Opianine	Narcotic
Neonal	Butethal, Sonneryl, Butobarbital, Etoval	Sedative, hypnotic
Nicotine		Insecticide
Nicotinic alcohol	Roniacol, *beta*-Pyridyl Carbinol	Peripheral vascular disorders
Nikethamide	Coramine, Dynacoryl, Cardiamid, Cormed, Eucoran, Pyricardyl	Respiratory stimulant
Nostal	Propallylonal, Noctal	Sedative, hypnotic
Optochin	Ethylhydrocupreine, Numoquin	Local eye antiseptic
Ortal	Hexethal, Hebaral	Sedative, hypnotic
Pamaquine	Plasmochin, Aminoquin, Béprochine, Plasmoquine	Antimalarial
Pavatrine		Antispasmodic
Pelletierine tannate	Punicine tannate	Tapeworms
Pentamethylenetetrazol	Metrazol, Cardiazol, Leptazol	Central nervous system stimulant
Pentobarbital	Nembutal, Pentyl, Embutal	Sedative, hypnotic, anticonvulsant

Table 47-40 (cont.).   Nonvolatile Organic Compounds; Selected Proprietary Names; Their Actions

Phanadorn	Cyclobarbital, Phanodorm, Cyclobarbitone	Hypnotic, sedative
Phenindamine	Thephorin	Antihistaminic, anti-allergic agent
Phenobarbital	Luminal, Phenobarbitone, Gardenal, Dormiral, Neurobarb, Phenonyl, Barbenyl, Barbiphenyl	Sedative, hypnotic, anti-epileptic, anticonvulsant
Phenylacetylurea	Phenurone, Phenacetylurea	Anticonvulsant, anti-epileptic
Phenylbutazone		Rheumatic diseases
Phenylsalicylate	Salol	Analgesic, antipyretic
Phthalylsulfathiazole	Sulfathalidine, Thalazole	Sulfonamide therapy
Physostigmine	Eserine	Parasympathomimetic agent, miotic
Picrotoxin	Cocculin	Respiratory and central nervous system stimulant
Pilocarpine		Parasympathomimetic agent, miotic
Piperidione	Sedulon	Antitussive
Piperine		Antipyretic, insecticide
Piperocaine	Metycaine, Neothesin	Local anesthetic
Pregnenolone	Arthenolone, Enolone, Prenolon, Natolone	
Prisilidene	Nisentil, Alphaprodine	Narcotic, analgesic
Probarbital	Ipral	Sedative, hypnotic
Procaine		Anesthetic
Procaine amide	Pronestyl	Cardiac arrhythmias
Procaine.HCl	Novocaine, Ethocaine, Neocaine, Syncaine, Chlorocaine, Allocaine, Scurocaine, Paracain, Planocaine	Anesthetic, analgesic
Pseudopelletierine	Pseudopunicine	
Pyridium	Mallophene	Urinary analgesic
Pyrilamine	Neo-Antergan, Anthisan, Pyranisamine, Antallergan, Mepyramine	Antihistaminic, anti-allergic agent
Pyrithyldione		Hypnotic
Quinidine	Conquinine	Cardiac therapy
Quinine		Antimalarial
Ricin		Pepsin and trypsin reagent
Rutin	Rutoside, Eldrin, Sophorin, Melin	Vitamin P therapy
Saccharin	Gluside, Saccharinol, Saccharinose, Garantose, Saccharol, Saxin	Sweetening agent
Salicin	Salicoside	Analgesic
Salicylic acid		Keratolytic agent, reagent
Sandoptal	Allylbarbituric acid	Sedative, hypnotic
Santonin		Antihelmintic
Scopolamine	Hyoscine	Sedative, hypnotic
Secobarbital	Seconal	Sedative, hypnotic
Sedormid		Sedative, hypnotic
Sigmodal	Rectidon	Hypnotic
Solanin	Solatunine	Anti-epileptic
Sparteine	Lupinidine	Cardiac disorders
Strophanthin		Cardiac therapy
Strychnine		Central nervous system stimulant, rodenticide
Succinylsulfathiazole	Sulfasuxidine	Sulfonamide therapy
Sulfacetamide	Sulamyd, Sulfacet, Albucid	Sulfonamide therapy
Sulfadiazine	Pyrimal, Debenal	Sulfonamide therapy

Table 47-40 (cont.). Nonvolatile Organic Compounds; Selected Proprietary Names; Their Actions

Sulfanilamide	Streptocid, Prontalbin, Deseptyl, Prontylin	Sulfonamide therapy
Sulfapyridine	Pyriamid, Sulfadine, Sulfidine, Peridazol, Dagenan	Sulfonamide therapy
Sulfathiazole	Thiazamide, Cibazol, Neo-Strepsan, Poliseptil	Sulfonamide therapy
Sulfisoxazole	Gantrisin, Gantrosan	Sulfonamide therapy
Sulfonethylmethane	Trional, Ethylsulfonal, Methylsulfonal	Sedative, hypnotic
Sulfonmethane	Sulfonal	Sedative, hypnotic
Terpin hydrate	Terpinol Hydrate, Dipenteneglycol	Expectorant
Tetracaine	Pontocaine, Pantocaine, Butethanol, Amethocaine, Anethaine	Anesthetic
Thenylpyramine	Thenylene, Methapyrilene, Histadyl, Parathyn, Tenalin, Semikon	Antihistaminic, anti-allergic agent
Theobromine	In various combinations: Diuretin, Theocalcin, Theosol, Theosalin, Theocal, Agurin	Diuretic, cardiac stimulant
Theophylline	Theocin. In combinations: Phyllicin	Diuretic, cardiac stimulant
Thiamin	Vitamin B_1	
Thiazolsulfone	Promizole	Sulfonamide therapy
Thiobarbituric acid		Preoperative anesthetic
Thiopental	Pentothal, Nesdonal, Intraval, Thiothal, Thiopentone	Anesthetic
Thonzylamine	Neohetramine, Anahist, Resistab	Antihistaminic, anti-allergic agent
Thymol iodide	Aristol, Annidalin, Iodistol, Iodothymol, Iodosol, Iosol, Iothymol, Thymiode, Thymiodol, Thymodin	Antiseptic dusting powder
p-Toluenesulfonamide		
Tribromoethanol	Avertin, Bromethol, Ethobrom, Renarcol	Basal anesthetic
Trihexiphenidyl	Artane	
Trimethadione	Tridione, Trimedal, Toxidone, Petidon	Anti-epileptic
Urethan	Urethane, Ethyl carbamate	Animal anesthetic
Veratrine		
Vinbarbital	Delvinal	Sedative, hypnotic
Xylocaine	Lidocaine	Anesthetic
Yohimbine	Quebrachine, Corynine, Aphrodine	Local anesthetic, aphrodisiac, mydriatic
Zolamine.HCl		Experimental drug

REFERENCES

1. Bull. Acad. de méd., Belgique, 11:304, 1851.
2. Ann. d. Chem. u. Pharm., c:44, 1856.
3. Ztschr. f. anal. Chem., 13:73, 1874.
4. Symposium on Toxicological Procedures, 3rd annual meeting, American Academy of Forensic Sciences, Chicago, 1951.
5. Kamm, O. Qualitative Organic Analysis, 2nd ed., New York, John Wiley and Sons, Inc., 1932.
6. Shriner, R. L., and Fuson, R. C. The Systematic Identification of Organic Compounds, 2nd ed., New York, John Wiley and Sons, Inc., 1940.
7. Mulliken, S. P. A Method for the Identification of Pure Organic Compounds, New York, John Wiley and Sons, Inc., 1904, vols. I, II, III and IV.
8. Beilstein, F. K. Beilstein's Handbuch der Organischen Chemie, Berlin, J. Springer, 1906-1952.
9. Umberger, C. J., and Stolman, A. A systematic approach to the identification of toxic organic compounds isolated from tissues and fluids. I. Determination of acidity and basicity, Ann. West. Med. & Surg., 5:945, 1951.

10. Umberger, C. J., Stolman, A., and Schwartz, H. The isolation and purification of organic poisons from biological material in the general unknown type of medical examiner's case, Proc. Am. Acad. Forensic Sc., 1:250, 1951.
11. Willard, H. H., and Tang, N. K. Precipitation of aluminum basic sulfate by urea, J. Am. Chem. Soc., 59:1190, 1937.
12. Adams, R., and Johnson, J. R. Laboratory Experiments in Organic Chemistry, New York, The Macmillan Co., 1928, p. 58.
13. Bratton, A. C., Marshall, E. K., Jr., Babbitt, D., and Hendrickson, A. R. A new coupling component for sulfanilamide determinations, J. Biol. Chem., 128:537, 1939.
14. Bridges, R. R. Quantitative determination of pentoses with anthrone, Anal. Chem., 24:2004, 1952.
15. Shetlar, M. R. Use of anthrone reaction for determination of carbohydrates in the presence of serum protein, Anal. Chem., 24:1844, 1952.
16. Hawk, P. B., Oser, B. L., and Summerson, W. H. Practical Physiological Chemistry, 12th ed., New York, Blakiston Co., 1947, p. 54.
17. Deuel, H. J., Jr. The Lipids—Their Chemistry and Biochemistry, New York, Interscience Publishers, Inc., 1951, vol. I. (a) physical properties of fatty acids, p. 57; (b) preparation of lecithins, p. 411; (c) enzymatic hydrolysis of lecithins, p. 421; (d) preparation of phosphatidylethanolamine, p. 441.
18. Peters, J. P., and Van Slyke, D. D. Quantitative Clinical Chemistry, 1st ed., Baltimore, Williams & Wilkins Co., 1932, vol. II. Methods, pp. 485-513.
19. Levene, P. A., and Rolf, I. P. The preparation and purification of lecithin, J. Biol. Chem., 72:587, 1927.
20. Zechmeister, L., and Cholnoky, L. Principles and Practice of Chromatography, New York, John Wiley and Sons, Inc., 1943.
21. Strain, H. H. Chromatographic Adsorption Analysis, New York, Interscience Publishers, Inc., 1945.
22. Durrum, E. L. A microelectrophoretic and microionophoretic technique, J. Am. Chem. Soc., 72:2943, 1950.
23. Cremer, H. D., and Tiselius, A. Electrophoresis of protein in filter paper, Biochem. Ztschr., 320:273, 1950.
24. Fleischman, C. A. The use of quinidine in chronic auricular fibrillation, Am. J. M. Sc., 225:617, 1953.
25. Asmussen, E., Hald, J., and Larsen, V. The pharmacological action of acetaldehyde on the human organism, Acta Pharmacol., 4:311, 1948.
26. Hine, C. H., and Divatia, K. J. A simple spectrophotometric method for determination of tetra-ethyl thiuramdisulfide (Antabuse) in blood and urine, Federation Proc., 9:286, 1950.
27. Laboratory of the Chief Medical Examiner of the City of New York, 1952.
28. Davidson, D. The Indicator Method of Classifying Acids and Bases in Qualitative Organic Analysis, More Acids and Bases, Series #3, J. Chem. Education, 1944, p. 21.
29. ——— and Perlman, D. A Guide to Qualitative Organic Analysis, New York, Depts. of Chemistry, Brooklyn College and The City College, 1952, p. 80.
30. Umberger, C. J., and Eagleson, D. A. Unpublished work, Laboratory of the Chief Medical Examiner of the City of New York, 1951-1953.
31. Koppanyi, T., Murphy, W. S., and Krop, S. Further contributions to methods of barbital research, Proc. Soc. Exper. Biol. & Med., 31:373, 1933.
32. Baggesgaard-Rasmussen, H., and Jerslev, B. The colorimetric determination of barbiturates by means of the cobaltamine reaction I, Dansk. Tids. Farm., 25:29, 1951.
33. Hickenbottom, W. J. Reactions of Organic Compounds, New York, Longmans, Green and Co., 1938, p. 322.
34. Brodie, B. B., Udenfriend, S., Baer, J. E., Chenkin, T., and Dill, W. The estimation of basic organic compounds and a technique for the appraisal of specificity—application to the cinchona alkaloids, J. Biol. Chem., 158:705, 1945.
35. Gettler, A. O., and Sunshine, I. Colorimetric determinations of alkaloids in tissues by means of methyl orange, Anal. Chem., 23:779, 1951.
36. Laboratory of the Chief Medical Examiner of the City of New York. Unpublished.
37. Gettler, A. O., Umberger, C. J., and Goldbaum, L. Fractional sublimation on a removable transparent film, Anal. Chem., 22:600, 1950.
38. Hubacher, M. H. Vacuum sublimation, Indust. & Engin. Chem., Anal. Ed., 15:448, 1943.
39. Clarke, B. L., and Hermance, H. W. A new apparatus for microsublimation, Indust. & Engin. Chem., Anal. Ed., 11:50, 1939.
40. Kempf, R. A new method of microsublimation, Ztschr. f. anal. Chem., 62:284, 1923.

41. Craig, L. C. Isolation and Characterization of Biologically Important Substances, The Harvey Lectures 1949-1950, Springfield, Ill., Charles C Thomas, 1952, p. 64.

42. Webster, R. A. Legal Medicine and Toxicology, Philadelphia, W. B. Saunders Co., 1930, pp. 346-355.

43. Umberger, C. J., and Stolman, A. A systematic approach to the identification of toxic organic compounds isolated from tissues and fluids. III. Aquo-ferriate and stannic chloride tests, Ann. West. Med. & Surg., 6:171, 1952.

44. Jonescu, D. Precipitation and quantitative estimation of alkaloids with potassium bismuthous iodide solution, Ber. d. deutsch. pharm. Gesellsch., 16:130, 1906.

45. Thoms, H. Estimation of narcotic extracts from a chemical and pharmaceutical point of view, Arb. a. d. pharmazeut. Inst. d. Univ. Berlin, 1:131 (1903), 1904.

46. Zaffaroni, A., Burton, R. B., and Keutmann, E. H. The application of paper partition chromatography to steroid analysis. I. Ketosteroids, J. Biol. Chem., 177:109, 1949.

47. Doeppman, F. Experiments on the stability of morphine during putrefaction, Chemiker Ztg., 39:69, 1915.

48. Umberger, C. J. Unpublished work. Laboratory of the Chief Medical Examiner of the City of New York.

49. Hickenbottom, W. J. Reactions of Organic Compounds, New York, Longmans, Green and Co., 1938, p. 272.

50. Taylor, T. W. J., and Baker, W. Sidgwick's The Organic Chemistry of Nitrogen, Oxford, Clarendon Press, 1937, pp. 28, 538, 549.

51. Benedetti-Pichler, A. A. Introduction to the Microtechnique of Inorganic Analysis, New York, John Wiley and Sons, Inc., 1942, p. 197.

52. Cassidy, H. G. Adsorption and Chromatography, New York, Interscience Publishers, Inc., 1951.

53. Zechmeister, L., and Tuzson, P. Isomerization of carotenoids, Biochem. J., 32:1305, 1938.

54. ———— and Tuzson, P. Reversible isomerization of carotenoids by iodine catalysis, Ber. d. deutsch. chem. Gesellsch., 72:1340, 1939.

55. Wachtel, J. L., and Cassidy, H. G. Chromatography as a means of separating amino acids, J. Am. Chem. Soc., 65:665, 1943.

56. Dasler, W. Hydrolysis of steroid esters on activated alumina, Science, 107:369, 1948.

57. Tiselius, A. Adsorption analysis of amino acids and peptides, Arkiv. Kemi. Mineral Geol., 15 B, No. 6, 1941.

58. Plattner, P. A., and Pfau, A. S. Volatile plant constituents. V. Preparation of the parent substance of the azulene series, Helvet. chim. acta, 20:224, 1937.

59. Zechmeister, L. History, scope and methods of chromatography, Ann. New York Acad. Sc., 49:145, 1948.

60. ———— Progress in Chromatography 1938-1950, London, Chapman and Hall, 1950.

61. Levy, A. L. A rapid and convenient method of filling chromatograph columns, Chem. & Indust., 1945, p. 380.

62. Strain, H. H. Carotene. VIII. Separation of carotenes by adsorption, J. Biol. Chem., 105:523, 1934.

63. Deitz, V. R. Bibliography of Solid Adsorbents, J. M. Brown, Revere Sugar Refinery, Charlestown, Mass., 1944.

64. Schwartz, A. M., and Perry, J. W. Surface Active Agents, New York, Interscience Publishers, Inc., 1949.

65. Claesson, S. Frontal analysis and displacement development in chromatography, Ann. New York Acad. Sc., 49:183, 1948.

66. Stolman, A., and Stewart, C. P. Isolation and determination of morphine, codeine and heroin from viscera and body fluids by adsorption, Analyst, 74:536, 1949.

67. ———— and Stewart, C. P. The separation and determination of a mixture of morphine, heroin, codeine and barbiturates by adsorption, Analyst, 74:543, 1949.

68. Algeri, E. J., and Walker, J. T. Paper chromatography for identification of the common barbiturates, Am. J. Clin. Path., 22:37, 1952.

69. Goldbaum, L. Paper chromatography in the purification and identification of alkaloids, 5th annual meeting, American Academy of Forensic Sciences, Chicago, 1953.

70. Kaiser, H., and Jori, H. Toxicological identification of Dromoran in urine with paper chromatography, Pharm. Ztg.-Nachr., 88:963, 1952.

71. Jaminet, F. Separation of local anesthetics by paper chromatography, J. pharm. Belg., 6:81, 1951.

72. Kent, F. H., Naim, and Amengual, B. M. Identification and separation of minute quantities of alkaloids by microchromatography on paper, Arch. farm. bioquím. Tucumán (Arg.) 4:333, 1950. Trans.: chem. Abstr., 45:1724[b].

73. Berry, H. K., Sutton, E. H., Cain, L., and Berry, J. S.   Development of paper chromatography for use in the study of metabolic patterns, Biochemical Institute Studies IV., Austin, Texas, The University of Texas Publ. No. 5109, 1951, p. 23.
74. Durrum, E. L.   Two-dimensional electrophoresis and ionophoresis, J. Colloid Sc., 6:274, 1951.
75. ―――― Continuous electrophoresis and ionophoresis on filter paper, J. Am. Chem. Soc., 73:4875, 1951.
76. ―――― Paper ionophoresis, Science, 113:66, 1951.
77. Lederer, M.   Inorganic analysis by paper ionophoresis, Nature, London, 167:864, 1951.
78. Schneider, G., and Wallenius, G.   Electrophoretic studies on cerebrospinal fluid proteins, Scandinav. J. Clin. & Lab. Investigation, 3:145, 1951.
79. Gordon, A. H., Gross, J., O'Connor, and Rivers, R. P.   Nature of the circulating thyroid hormone-plasma protein complex, Nature, London, 169:19, 1952.
80. Grassmann, W., and Hannig, K.   A simple process for analysis of serum proteins and other protein mixtures, Naturwissenschaften, 37:496, 1950.
81. Larson, F. C., Deiss, W. P., and Albright, E. C.   Localization of protein-bound radioactive iodine by filter paper electrophoresis, Science, 115:626, 1952.
82. Goldbaum, L. R.   The purification and identification of morphine by paper electrophoresis, 4th annual meeting, American Academy of Forensic Sciences, Atlanta, Georgia, 1952.
83. Kunin, R.   Ion exchange, Anal. Chem., 21:87, 1949.
84. Nachod, F. C.   Ion Exchange Theory and Application, New York, Academic Press, 1949.
85. Kunin, R., and Myers, R. J.   Ion Exchange Resins, New York, John Wiley and Sons, 1950.
86. Feldstein, M., and Klendshoj, N. C.   Determination of morphine by ion exchange resins, 5th annual meeting, American Academy of Forensic Sciences, Chicago, 1953.
87. Cannan, R. K.   Chromatographic and ion-exchange methods of amino acid analysis, Ann. New York Acad. Sc. 47:135, 1946.
88. Tiselius, A., Drake, B., and Hagdahl, L.   Group separation of amino acids by adsorption analysis, Experientia, 3:21, 1947.
89. Winters, J. C., and Kunin, R.   Ion exchange in the pharmaceutical field, Indust. & Engin. Chem., 41:460, 1949.
90. Kunin, R., and McGarvey, F. X.   Equilibrium and column behavior of exchange resins. Strong-base anion-exchange resin, Indust. & Engin. Chem., 41:1265, 1949.
91. Umberger, C. J., and Adams, G.   Identification of malonyl urea derivatives, Anal. Chem., 24:1309, 1952.
92. Goldbaum, L. R.   Determination of barbiturates, Anal. Chem., 24:1604, 1952.
93. ―――― An ultraviolet spectrophotometric procedure for the determination of barbiturates, J. Pharmacol. & Exper. Therap., 94:68, 1948.
94. Brodie, B. B., Burns, J. J., Mark, L. C., Lief, P. A., Bernstein, E., and Papper, E. M.   The fate of pentobarbital in man and dog and a method for its estimation, J. Pharmacol. & Exper. Therap., 109:25, 1953.
95. ―――― Mark, L. C., Papper, E. M., Lief, P. A., Bernstein, E., and Rovenstine, E. A.   The fate of thiopental in man and a method for its estimation in biological material, J. Pharmacol. & Exper. Therap., 98:85, 1950.
96. Goldbaum, L. R.   Studies on the Binding of Barbiturates to Proteins and Its Possible Relation to Their Deposition and Action in Animals, Ph.D. thesis, George Washington Univ., 1950.
97. Shideman, F. E., Gould, F. C., Winters, W. D., Peterson, R. C., and Wilmer, W. K.   The distribution and in vivo rate of metabolism of thiopental, J. Pharmacol. & Exper. Therap., 107:368, 1953.
98. Goldbaum, L. R.   Private communication, 1953.
99. Umberger, C. J., and Feldstein, M.   Unpublished paper, 1st annual meeting, American Academy of Forensic Sciences, St. Louis, Miss., 1949.
100. Goldbaum, L. R.   Procedure developed in the Laboratory of the Chief Medical Examiner, City of New York.
101. McCutcheon, R. S., and Plein, E. M.   The identification of some barbiturates by means of xanthydrol as a reagent, J. Am. Pharm. A., Scient. Ed., 38:24, 1949.
102. Ruskin, D. B.   Fulminating dermatitis bullosa medicamentosa due to "Mesantoin," J.A.M.A., 137:1031, 1948.
103. Archibald, R. M., Ortiz, P., Stroh, E., and Bronner, J.   Colorimetric determination of urea, J. Biol. Chem., 157:507, 1945.
104. Umberger, C. J., and Adams, G.   The qualitative and quantitative estimation of substituted urea sedatives, other than malonyl urea derivatives. Unpublished paper, 4th annual meeting, American Academy of Forensic Sciences, Atlanta, Georgia, 1952.

105. Hardy, A. C., and the Color Measurement Laboratory. Handbook of Colorimetry, Cambridge, Mass., The Technology Press, 1936.

106. Cleland, T. M. A Practical Description of the Munsell Color System, Baltimore, Md., Munsell Color Company, 1937.

107. Mulliken, S. P. A Method for the Identification of Pure Organic Compounds, New York, John Wiley and Sons, Inc., 1917, Vol. III.

108. Liebermann, C. Dyestuffs formed from aromatic oxy compounds and nitrous acid, Ber. d. deutsch. chem. Gesellsch., 7:1098, 1874.

109. Umberger, C. J., and Adams, G. Unpublished, Laboratory of the Chief Medical Examiner, City of New York, 1953.

110. Schoorl, N. A color reaction for the aromatic amino group, Pharm. Weekblad, 77:1381, 1940.

111. Hawk, P. B., Oser, B. L., and Summerson, W. H. Practical Physiological Chemistry, 12th ed., New York, The Blakiston Company, 1947, p. 883.

112. Wasicky, R. A very sensitive color reaction for atropine, hyoscyamine and scopolamine, Ztschr. f. anal. Chem., 54:393, 1915.

113. Van Urk, H. W. p-Dimethylaminobenzaldehyde as a reagent for organic drugs, Pharm. Weekblad, 66:101, 1929.

114. Chakravarti, S. N., and Roy, M. B. New colorimetric test for procaine and primary amines, Analyst, 62:603, 1937.

115. Umberger, C. J., Eagleson, D. A., and Adams, G. Unpublished, Laboratory of the Chief Medical Examiner, City of New York, 1953.

116. Hager, K. F. Tetranitromethane, Indust. & Engin. Chem., 41:2168, 1949.

117. Kaufmann, H. P., and Kirsch, P. Conjugated unsaturated compounds in the chemistry of fats. I. The detection of conjugated unsaturated fat acids by means of the tetranitromethane reaction, Fette u. Seifen, 50:314, 1943.

118. Hammick, D. L., and Yule, R. B. M. Complex formation between polynitro compounds and aromatic hydrocarbons and bases. IX. The influence of solvents on the temperature coefficients of color densities, J. Chem. Soc. London, 1940:1539.

119. Davies, T. T., and Hammick, D. L. Complex formation between polynitro compounds and aromatic hydrocarbons. V. The effect of methylation on the stability of tetranitromethane complexes, J. Chem. Soc. London, 1938:763.

120. Macbeth, A. K., and Pratt, D. D. Labile nature of the halogen atoms in substituted nitromethanes, J. Chem. Soc. London, 119:1356, 1921.

121. —— and Pratt, D. D. The halogen derivatives of nitroform, J. Chem. Soc. London, 119:354, 1921.

122. Werner, A. Relation between color and constitution, Ber., 42:4324, 1909.

123. Schmidt, E., and Fischer, H. Tetranitromethane. III. Conversion of tertiary amines into secondary nitrosamines, Ber., 53B:1537, 1920.

124. —— and Schumacher, R. Tetranitromethane. IV. Conversion of tertiary amines into secondary nitrosamines, Ber., 54BS:1414, 1921.

125. —— and Fischer, H. Tetranitromethane. II. Tetranitromethane as a nitrating agent, Ber., 53B:1529, 1920.

126. Umberger, C. J., and Stolman, A. A systematic approach to the identification of toxic organic compounds isolated from tissue and fluids. II. Tetranitromethane and azo coupling tests, Ann. West. Med. & Surg., 5:1022, 1951.

127. Taylor, T. W. J., and Baker, W. Sidgwick's The Organic Chemistry of Nitrogen, Oxford, Clarendon Press, 1937, pp. 410-411.

128. Beyer, K. H. Color reaction of sympathomimetic amines with diazonium compounds, J.A.C.S., 68:1318, 1942.

129. Umberger, C. J., and Stolman, A. A systematic approach to the identification of toxic organic compounds isolated from tissues and fluids. IV. Specific group tests, Ann. West. Med. & Surg., 6:232, 1952.

130. Hickenbottom, W. J. Reactions of Organic Compounds, New York, Longmans, Green and Co., 1938, p. 299.

131. Feigl, F. Spot Tests, New York, Elsevier-Nordeman Publishing Co. Inc., 1939, pp. 317-318.

132. Taylor, T. W. J., and Baker, W. Sidgwick's The Organic Chemistry of Nitrogen, Oxford, Clarendon Press, 1937, pp. 197-198.

133. Steinkopf, W., and Jurgens, B. J. prakt. Chem., 84:686, 1911.

134. Feigl, F. Spot Tests, New York, Elsevier-Nordeman Publishing Co. Inc., 1939, p. 295.

135. Ibid., p. 303.

136. Anger, V. Two new microchemical tests for organic compounds, Mikrochim. Acta, 2:3, 1937.

137. Grote, I. W. A new color reaction for soluble organic sulfur compounds, J. Biol. Chem., 93:25, 1931.

138. Burchfield, H. P., and Judy, J. N. Color reactions of amine antioxidants, Anal. Chem., 19:786, 1947.

139. Color in Use, Monograph #3, New York, The International Printing Ink Corp., 1935.

140. Janovsky, J. V., and Erb, L. Zur Kenntniss der directen Brom-und Nitrosubstitutions products der Azokörper, Ber. d. deutsch. chem. Gesellsch., 19:2155, 1886.

141. Bittó, von B. Ueber eine Reaction der Aldehyde und Ketone mit Arom. Nitroverbindungen, Liebig's Annalen der Chemie, 269:377, 1892.

142. Reitzenstein, F., and Stamm, G. Janovsky's reaction for dinitro compounds and Bittó's reaction for aldehydes and ketones with aromatic compounds, J. prakt. Chem., 81:167, 1910.

143. Péronnet, M., and Truhaut, R. Color reactions obtained with metadinitrobenzene in alkaline media, J. pharm. chim., 18:339, 1933.

144. Zimmermann, W. A color reaction of sex hormones and its application to colorimetric determination, Ztschr. f. physiol. Chem., 233:257, 1935.

145. ——— Colorimetric determination of sexual hormones. II. Ztschr. f. physiol. Chem., 245:47, 1936.

146. Denoël, A., and Soulet, U. Study of some synthetic derivatives of morphine and codeine, J. pharm. Belgique, 1:34, 50, 66, 1942.

147. Ekkert, L. Erkennung organischer Verbindungen, Stuttgart, Ferdinand Enke Verlag, 1933, pp. 57-58.

148. Farmilo, C. G., and Lucas, G. H. W. Studies on the identification of narcotics. I. Microchemical reactions for identification of Metopon, J. Am. Pharm. A. (Scient. Ed.), 38:492, 1949.

149. Umberger, C. J., and Dal Cortivo, L. Unpublished, Laboratory of the Chief Medical Examiner, City of New York, 1953.

150. ——— Unpublished, Laboratory of the Chief Medical Examiner, City of New York, 1953-1954.

151. Lagarce, F. A new reaction of diallylmalonylurea (dial), J. pharm. chim., 12:364, 1930.

152. Mulliken, S. P. A Method for the Identification of Pure Organic Compounds, Vol. II, New York, John Wiley and Sons, Inc., 1916, p. 30.

153. Eykmann, J. F. Eine empfindliche Phenolreaction, Ztschr. f. anal. Chem., 22:576, 1883.

154. Mulliken, S. P. A Method for the Identification of Pure Organic Compounds, Vol. I, New York, John Wiley and Sons, Inc., 1904, p. 26.

155. Levine, V. A general test for carbohydrates, Proc. Soc. Exper. Biol. & Med., 27:830, 1929-1930.

156. Mulliken, S. P. A Method for the Identification of Pure Organic Compounds, Vol. I, New York, John Wiley and Sons, Inc., 1904, p. 83.

157. ——— A Method for the Identification of Pure Organic Compounds, Vol. II, New York, John Wiley and Sons, Inc., 1916, p. 31.

158. Morgan, C. E., and Opolnick, N. Adaptation of a color test to minute amounts of caffeine, Ind. Eng. Chem., Anal. Ed., 17:526, 1945.

159. Feigl, F. Spot Tests, New York, Elsevier-Nordeman Publishing Co., Inc., 1939, p. 195.

160. ibid., p. 350.

161. ibid., p. 401.

162. ibid., p. 407.

163. Cartland, G. F., Meyer, R. K., Miller, L. C., and Rutz, M. H. A comparison of theelin prepared from stallion urine, from human urine and from theelol, with notes on the colorimetric estimation of theelin and theelol, J. Biol. Chem., 109:213, 1935.

164. Kober, S. A colorimetric determination of the sex hormone (menformone), Biochem. Ztschr., 239:209, 1931.

165. Schneider, F. Qualitative Organic Microanalysis, New York, John Wiley and Sons, Inc., 1946, p. 13.

166. ibid., pp. 77-86.

167. Pregl, F. Quantitative Organic Microanalysis, translated by E. Fyleman, 2nd English ed., New York, Blakiston Co., 1930, p. 212.

168. Schneider, F. Qualitative Organic Microanalysis, New York, John Wiley and Sons, Inc., 1946, pp. 83-86.

169. Ramsey, L. L., and Patterson, W. I. A new qualitative test for monofluoroacetic acid, J. Off. Agr. Chem., 34:827, 1951.

170. Stephenson, C. H., and Parker, C. E. Some Microchemical Tests for Alkaloids, Philadelphia, J. B. Lippincott Co., 1921.

171. Rosenthaler, L. Toxikologische Mikroanalyse, Berlin, Gebrüder Borntraeger, 1935.

172. Kofler, L., and Kofler, A.   Mikroskopische Methoden in der Mikrochemie, Wien, E. Haim and Co., 1936.
173. —— and Kofler, A.   Mikro-Methoden zur Kennzeichnung organischer Stoffe und Stoffgemische, Berlin, Verlag Chemie, 1945.
174. Kofler, A.   Mikro-Methoden zur Kennzeichnung organischer Stoffe u. Stoffgemische, Innsbruck, 1947, 2 vol.
175. Wherry, E. T.   At the surface of a crystal, Am. Mineral., 9:45, 1924.
176. Fulton, C. C.   The extraction and purification of toxicologically important drugs with emphasis on alkaloids, Royal Canadian Mounted Police Second Annual Seminar, Regina, Saskatchewan, Canada, March 1954.
177. Morgan, C. E.   The extraction and purification of toxicologically important drugs with emphasis on alkaloids, Royal Canadian Mounted Police Second Annual Seminar, Regina, Saskatchewan, Canada, March 1954.
178. Farmilo, C. G.   The extraction and purification of toxicologically important drugs with emphasis on alkaloids, Royal Canadian Mounted Police Second Annual Seminar, Regina, Saskatchewan, Canada, March 1954.

Appendix

COMPOUNDS WITH THEIR REACTIONS TO ANALYTIC TESTS

There will probably be many discrepancies between these data and those of other observers due, at least in part, to minor differences in the source material as well as to variations in the observations of different individuals. Much of the sample material was case material while other samples were commercial products from which the active components were isolated without purification except for that inherent in the analytic process. Purified samples of the same

KEY TO ABBREVIATIONS

NT, no trial	Br, brown, brownish	Gr, green	P, pink	Ro, rose
X, no reaction	C, carmine	Gy, gray	Ppt, precipitate	S, salmon
B, blue	F, flesh	M, magenta	Pu, purple	Vlt, violet
Bk, black	G, gold	O, orange	R, red	Wh, white
				Y, yellow

TEST / COMPOUND	Nitrosyl-sulfuric Acid	p-Dimeth-ylamino-benzal-dehyde	Tetrani-trometh-ane	Conc. Sulfuric Acid	Modi-fied Erd-mann's	Mecke's	Marquis'	Azo Coupling	Indamine
ACETANILID	O w Yc	Y	pY	X	pY	X	ftP	R	X
ACETOPHENETIDIN	M	ltY	vpO	X	pY→ Gr	X	X	X	X
ACETYLSALICYLIC ACID	Y	ltO	X	X	btY w H₂O	X	dpRo	R	X
ACONITINE	pY; mPpt w NH₃	ltBr; ltVlt w H₂O	pBrY	X	X	X	X	X	X
ACRIDINE.HCl	lY	orig Y	NT	lY	orig Y	orig Y	orig Y	NT	NT
ADIPHENINE	ltYO	X	Y	X	O	X	ltO	Y	X
N-ALLYLNORMOR-PHINE	Br→G	OR→Br; ltR w H₂O	X	ltBr	BrY	B→Gr	dpM→Pu	X	X
p-AMINOBENZOIC ACID	Y w NH₃	Y; O w H₂O	X	X	btY	X	X	R	R
AMINOPYRINE	O→GyY	X	O	X	pO	X	X	R	BVlt
AMOBARBITAL	X	X	X	X	WhPpt w H₂O	X	X	X	X
AMPHETAMINE.HCl	O	X	BrY	RBr	RBr	ltRo	O→R→Br	R	NT
AMPHETAMINE BASE	G	RBr→Br	NT	GrY	G	ltY	O→BrO	NT	X
AMPROTROPINE	Y→O	Ro→dpR	vpY	X	G	X	vpY	Y	Wh
ANTABUSE	X	WhPpt; Y w H₂O	O	X	X	cls→vp Y	vpY	X	X
ANTIPYRINE	O	dpRO	O	X	ltOY	X	X	B	RO
APOMORPHINE	dpBr	Br	dkGr	oGr	dpRBr	dkGr→Br	Bk→dkGr	R	R
APOTHESINE	BrO	Br	vpY	GBr	ltGBr	GBr	Y→Br	R	WhPpt
APROBARBITAL	cls→ltBVlt	cls→O	NT	X	X	X	X	NT	NT
ASCORBIC ACID	X	dpR→brkR	X	X	vpRo	dpRoO	X	R	R
ATABRIN	Br; YO w NH₃	Y	Br	btY	brkR; btO w H₂O	dpY	Y→OY	X	YPpt
ATROPINE	YO	dkR; M w H₂O	pYO	X	pY	X	X	X	X
BARBITAL	X	X	NT	X	X	X	X	NT	NT

Appendix

compound from different sources do not always give identical reactions and the presence of minor impurities and metabolites naturally influences the findings. It is these factors which prevent drawing the fine distinctions indicated in these and other tables in the interpretation of the reactions of an unknown substance. (Cf. Limitations in the interpretation of positive reactions, pp. 1185-1191.)

KEY TO ABBREVIATIONS

brk, brick	cls, colorless	ft, faint	o, olive	t, trace
bt, bright	dk, dark	imt, immediate	orig, original	v, very
c, cast	dp, deep	l, lemon	p, pale	w, with
ch, cherry	em, emerald	lt, light	sol, solution	/, or
cl, cloud	f, flash	m, milky	str, streak	

Chloranil Acetone	Hydrox-amic Acid	Aquo-ferriate	Benzoyl Peroxide SnCl$_4$	Mande-lin's	Janovsky	SnCl$_4$ Benzotri-chloride	Titanous Chloride	Froehde's	Vanillin-sulfuric	Isoamyl-nitrite SnCl$_4$	Molisch
X	R/Vlt	X	WhPpt	fP→F	X	Wh cl	X	X	X	X	X
R	R/Vlt	X	X	X	X	YPpt	X	X	X	OY	X
X	R/Vlt	Gr	X	ltGr	X	YPpt	OBr	ltBVlt →cls	X	OY	X
GrY	R/Vlt	YPpt	WhPpt	X	X	WhPpt	X	X	X	X	dkOBr
NT	NT	NT	NT	X	NT	NT	GrY	orig Y	orig Y	NT	NT
Y	R/Vlt	YPpt	X	Gr→Br	X	WhPpt	X	X	WhPpt w H$_2$O	X	ftY
OR	X	X	WhPpt	pBr→ltVlt	X	PPpt	BrR	M→GyGr	dkBr	OY	Br
ltBVlt	X	X	WhPpt	pO→Br	dpOY	WhPpt	X	X	Y w H$_2$O	OY	X
R	X	X	WhPpt	vpO	X	WhPpt	X	X	NT	OY	X
X	X	YGr	X	X	X	X	X	X	X	X	WhPpt w H$_2$O
X	X	X	NT	brkR	NT	NT	RoR	pR	BrO	NT	O
NT	NT	NT	X	NT	NT	X	NT	BrY	NT	X	NT
Y	R/Vlt	YPpt	WhPpt	pVltBr	Ro	WhPpt	X	X	dkBr	X	ftO
O	R/Vlt	X	WhPpt	X	Y	WhPpt	ltGr	ltGr→Gr→G	WhPpt w H$_2$O	X	ltGr
R	R/Vlt	X	WhPpt	ltGr→BGr	GyY	Y	X	vpY w H$_2$O	pO w H$_2$O	OY	X
Gr	R/Vlt	Gr	GrPpt	oGr→Br	NT	R	dkBr, M c	oGr	Br	OY	dkBr
BrGr	R/Vlt	YPpt	X	Br	NT	PPpt	BrO	Br	BrO	X	Br
NT	NT	NT	NT	X	X	NT	X	X	X	NT	v lt Br
X	X	X	X	X	WhPpt; Ysol	X	GyBr	vpBrY	X	X	dkR
X	X	X	WhPpt	O	NT	YPpt	Y	btY	dkO; Y w H$_2$O	X	Y
BrGr	R/Vlt	X	WhPpt	X	vftP	WhPpt	X	X	X	X	M
NT	NT	NT	NT	X	X	NT	X	X	X	NT	X

COMPOUND / TEST	Nitrosyl-sulfuric Acid	p-Dimeth-ylamino-benzaldehyde	Tetrani-tromethane	Conc. Sulfuric Acid	Modified Erdmann's	Mecke's	Marquis'	Azo Coupling	Indamine
BENZOCAINE	YO w NH₃	O→Y; O w H₂O	O	X	ltY	X	X	R	R
BERBERINE.SO₄	dpBrM →RBr	orig Y	NT	btY	dpBr	YBr→ GrBr→ Br→ VltBr	orig Y	NT	NT
BETAINE.HCl	pY	X	NT	X	X	WhPpt	X	NT	NT
BROMURAL	X	ltY	X	X	X	X	X	R	X
BRUCINE	R→O →Y	X	BrR	X	RO→ YO	ltR→O	X	R	X
BUTABARBITAL	X	X	NT	X	X	X	X	NT	NT
BUTALLYLONAL	Y	ltBr	NT	X	X	X	X	NT	NT
BUTAMIN	YO w NH₃	Y w O c	RO	orig pY	ltY	X	X	R	R
CAFFEINE	ltY	X	OY→Y	X	X	X	X	X	X
CANTHARIDIN	X	WhPpt w H₂O	X	X	X	X	X	X	X
CARBAMYLCHOLINE CHLORIDE	X	Y	X	X	X	WhPpt	X	X	X
CARBROMAL	X	Y	X	X	X	X	X	X	NT
CEPHAELINE	YBr	Br	NT	ltY	BrY	GrY	BrY	NT	NT
CHLORCYCLYZINE	p→ltY	BrY	NT	ltBrY	G	Y	orig BrY	NT	NT
CHLOROBUTANOL	WhPpt w H₂O	ltY	X	X	X	X	X	X	X
CHOLESTEROL	WhPpt; ltY w NH₃	BrM	vpY	RO→ brkR	brkR →Br	O→ brkR	brkR	X	WhPpt
CHRYSAZIN	O→YO	orig O; Y w H₂O	NT	C	R, Ysol; Y w H₂O	C→OR →YO	brkR →Y	NT	NT
CINCHONIDINE	vvpY	vltO	X	X	X	X	X	R	NT
CINCHONINE	ltBVlt; Gy c	ltO	X	X	X	X	X	X	X
CINCHOPHEN	Y	X	X	ltY	ltY	ltY	plY	X	R
COCAINE	pY	X	OY→Y	X	X	X	X	X	X
CODEINE	Br→ BrR	brkR →Br	O	Br w Vlt c	ltBrO	Gr→B	BVlt	B	X
COLCHICINE	YBr →Y	Y(cold); O→ YO; Y w H₂O	NT	btY	G	Y	Y	NT	NT
CONIINE.HCl	X	X	pY	X	X	X	X	X	R
CORTISONE	NT	NT	NT	NT	NT	NT	NT	NT	NT
CURARINE	dpBr→ YBr	ltBr	ltY	ltYBr	pYO	ltBr	ltYBr	R	X
CYCLOPAL	Gy→ pGyY →Y	M (cold); vdkB Vlt; dkGr w H₂O	NT	BrO	G	BrO	Y→ BrO	NT	NT
CYSTEINE.HCl	OY	btY	NT	X	pGyY	cls→Ro	X	NT	NT
DELPHININE	O w Gy c	Br	orig Y	BrO	BrO	orig Br w O c	O→ BrO	X	R
DESOXYCHOLIC ACID	pY	R→ dpR; B→Gr w H₂O	X	X	Y	Br	p→dpY →G	X	X
d-DESOXYEPHEDRINE	YO	Br	Y	pBrO	YBr	pBrO	O→ BrO	R	X

Chloranil Acetone	Hydrox-amic Acid	Aquo-ferriate	Benzoyl Peroxide SnCl$_4$	Mande-lin's	Janovsky	SnCl$_4$ Benzotri-chloride	Titanous Chloride	Froehde's	Vanillin-sulfuric	Isoamyl-nitrite SnCl$_4$	Molisch
R	R/Vlt	X	WhPpt	ftBr	Y(imt) →BrO	WhPpt	X	X	Y w H$_2$O	O→R	X
NT	NT	NT	NT	dkBr	OPpt	NT	oGr	Y/GrBr	BrO; Y w H$_2$O	NT	btO
NT	NT	NT	NT	O	X	NT	X	X	X	NT	X
NT	NT	NT	NT	X	X	NT	X	X	NT	NT	M
RO	R/Vlt	X	RPpt	ltO;S w H$_2$O	P(imt) →dpM	WhPpt	X	cls→ Ro→O	X	OY	X
NT	NT	NT	NT	X	X	NT	X	X	Vlt w H$_2$O	NT	vftO
NT	NT	NT	NT	X	vftP	NT	X	cls→ ltY	X	NT	X
R	R/Vlt	X	WhPpt	ftVlt w H$_2$O	btY	WhPpt	X	X	Y w H$_2$O	OY	pO
X	R/Vlt	X	WhPpt	X	vftP	WhPpt	X	X	X	X	X
X	X	X	X	X	X	X	X	WhPpt w H$_2$O	WhPpt w H$_2$O	OY	X
X	R/Vlt	X	X	ftO	Y	X	X	X	X	X	X
NT	NT	NT	NT	X	Y	NT	X	X	NT	NT	X
NT	NT	NT	NT	orig Br	vdpGy	NT	OBr	ltR→ YBr →GrY	BrO	NT	Br
NT	NT	NT	NT	X	ftY	NT	X	orig Y	WhPpt w H$_2$O	NT	NT
X	R/Vlt	X	X	X	dpRBr	X	X	X	WhPpt w H$_2$O	X	YGr
X	X	YPpt	WhPpt	brkR	NT	PPpt	O	brkR	dpO; M Ppt w H$_2$O	OY	btO
NT	NT	NT	NT	Br→ dkR→ Gr	chR	NT	dpR	C	dpR; btY w H$_2$O	NT	dpR
BrR	X	X	WhPpt	X	M	WhPpt	X	X	X	X	X
X	X	X	WhPpt	X	X	WhPpt	X	X	X	OY	X
X	X	X	WhPpt	X	X	GrY	GrY	pY	X	OY	X
X	R/Vlt	X	WhPpt	X	X	WhPpt	X	X	X	X	X
R	X	X	WhPpt	Br→ VltBr →GyVlt	BrO	PPpt	X	GyBVlt	NT	X	dkGy
NT	NT	NT	NT	ltGrBr	Y	NT	Y	btY	Br; Y w H$_2$O	NT	O
dkR	X	X	X	X	X	WhPpt	X	X	X	X	X
NT	NT	NT	NT	NT	dpM	NT	NT	NT	NT	NT	NT
X	X	X	WhPpt	Br	Y	X	NT	BrM→ ltBr	ftM w H$_2$O	OY	X
NT	NT	NT	NT	RBr	M	NT	BrO	O→BrO	BrR	NT	vdkBr
NT	NT	NT	NT	X	NT	NT	X	YfwH$_2$O	O	NT	X
RBr	R/Vlt	X	WhPpt	RBr	ltY	WhPpt	O	RBr	O (cold); Br	X	dkBr
X	X	X	WhPpt	pBr	X	X	X	cls→ vpY	btR; M w H$_2$O	OY	O
X	X	YPpt	X	ltBr	Y	X	X	orig pBrO	pO w H$_2$O	X	X

COMPOUND \\ TEST	Nitrosyl-sulfuric Acid	p-Dimethyl-aminobenzaldehyde	Tetranitromethane	Conc. Sulfuric Acid	Modified Erdmann's	Mecke's	Marquis'	Azo Coupling	Indamine
DIALLYLBARBITURIC ACID	Vlt w Gy c →Y	BrO→ RBr	NT	X	X	X	X	NT	NT
DIBUCAINE	mPpt w NH₃	X	OY	X	X	X	X	X	WhPpt
DICHLORODIPHENYLTRICHLOROETHANE	X	X	NT	X	X	X	X	NT	NT
DICOUMAROL	X	WhPpt w H₂O	X	X	WhPpt w H₂O	WhPpt w H₂O	WhPpt w H₂O	X	GrYPpt
DICYCLOMINE	X	Br→ dpBrR	RO	vpY	vpY	vpY	pY→ dpY →Y→O	X	WhPpt
DIETHYLACETYLUREA	WhPpt w H₂O	X	NT	X	X	X	X	NT	NT
DIGALEN	X	O (cold); Br	BrY	orig pY	dpBr	Br→pR	Y→Br	X	X
DIGITALIN	Br	dkBr	orig R	RBr	Br	Br	Br	X	X
DIGITONIN	pY	dkBr	X	ftY→ ltO	pY	p→ dpBr	cls→Br	X	X
DIGITOXIN	dkGy	vdkBr	vpY	Br	Br	Br	dkBr	X	X
DIHYDROMORPHINONE	OBr	OR→ RO	X	X	BrY	B→Gr	M→ BVlt	R	X
DIMENHYDRINATE (basic product)	Y→ GyY; m w NH₃	Y	brkR →O	brkR	RBr	brkR	dpOR	X	X
DIMENHYDRINATE (acidic product)	Y	X	X	X	X	X	X	X	X
DIOTHANE	Br→G	RO	O	Br	YBr; G w H₂O	orig Br	orig Br	O	WhPpt
DIPHENHYDRAMINE	GyY	Y	O	dpO	dpOBr; YO w H₂O	O; Ysol	O→ R→Br	R	WhPpt →Br
DIPHENYLHYDANTOIN	X	X	NT	X	WhPpt w H₂O	WhPpt w H₂O	mPpt w H₂O	NT	NT
DROMORAN	BrM	OR→ RO	NT	X	ltY	vpY	ltBr→ dkBr	NT	NT
EMETINE	vdkBr	RBr	RBr	orig RBr	Br	YBr	RBr	acid:X base:R	X
EPHEDRINE	G	ltBr	btY	ltGyBr	vvpY	ltBr	Br→ BrO	X	X
ESTRONE	dpOBr	M→ dpBVlt; B→ Gr w H₂O	X	cls→pY	ltOR →brkR	pYBr →Br	Y→ G→O	X	WhPpt
ETHYL BISCOUMACETATE	X	ltBr	ltY	X	X	X	X	R	BVlt
ETHYLMORPHINE	Br→ RBr	R→O	RO	GyBr	YBr	Gr→B	BVlt	B	X
EUCUPIN.di HCl	pY	Gr w GyB c	X	X	X	pY	vpY	X	X
GLYCINE	X	X	X	X	X	X	X	X	X
HEROIN	Br→G	R→O	pYO	pF	G	B→Gr	M→Vlt	R	X
HEXOBARBITAL	NT	BrY→ YBr	NT	vpO	NT	ltBr→O	pBrO	NT	NT
HIPPURIC ACID	vpY	X	X	X	X	X	X	X	X

Chloranil Acetone	Hydrox- amic Acid	Aquo- ferriate	Benzoyl Peroxide SnCl$_4$	Mande- lin's	Janovsky	SnCl$_4$ Benzotri- chloride	Titanous Chloride	Froehde's	Vanillin- sulfuric	Isoamyl- nitrite SnCl$_4$	Molisch
NT	NT	NT	NT	X	X	NT	X	X	R	NT	X
Gr	X	YPpt	WhPpt	X	X	WhPpt	X	X	X	X	X
NT	NT	NT	NT	X	X	NT	X	X	X	NT	X
X	X	X	X	WhPpt w H$_2$O	X	Y	X	WhPpt w H$_2$O	WhPpt w H$_2$O	OY	WhPpt w H$_2$O
dkGr	X	X	WhPpt	pGy	dpRo	Y	X	orig vpY	dpRBr	X	dkOBr
NT	NT	NT	NT	X	Y	NT	X	X	WhPpt w H$_2$O	NT	X
X	X	X	X	Br→ VltBr	X	X	dkBr	ltBr, M c	Br	X	RBr
X	X	X	X	R→Br	P	Y	Br	ltBr	dkBr	X	M
X	X	X	X	cls→ pBr	NT	X	X	vpBrY	dkBr; dkGr w H$_2$O	X	NT
X	R/Vlt	X	WhPpt →BrPu	VltBr	B; pY	Br→Vlt	vdpGr	dpBr	dkBr	OY	NT
R	X	X	WhPpt	Br→ ltM	M; Br	WhPpt	RoR	M(Vlt) →cls	dkBr	OY	NT
Gr	X	X	WhPpt	brkR	WhPpt	WhPpt	btO	OR	O	OY	R; Y
NT	X	X	NT	X	NT	NT	NT	X	NT	NT	NT
X	X	YPpt	WhPpt	OR→ R→ Gr→o	X	ROPpt	X	Br, M c	pY w H$_2$O	X	X
dkBrR	X	X	WhPpt	brkR	NT	GrYPpt	O	dpRO	O→Br	OY	OBr
NT	NT	NT	NT	X	X	NT	X	X	WhPpt w H$_2$O	NT	X
NT	NT	NT	NT	GyGr→ GyVlt →Vlt	vftP	NT	RoR	B	X	NT	ltBVlt
RBr→ Vlt	X	X	WhPpt	orig RBr	YGr; BrO	BrPpt	dkO	RBr→ YBr	dkBr	X	dkBr
YPpt	X	X	X	ltBr	GyY	X	X	pBr	dkBr	X	O
X	X	X	X	ltBr	NT	Y	NT	B→Gr →Y	NT	NT	NT
X	X	Gr	X	WhPpt w H$_2$O	NT	X	X	X	dkBr	X	vftBVlt
Gr	X	X	WhPpt	Br→ GyVlt	ftY	PPpt	dpMBr	Br→ GyGr	dkBr	X	OBr
dkBrGr	X	X	WhPpt	X	X	WhPpt	pY	vvpY	BVlt; dpM→ BVlt w H$_2$O	X	ltO
X	R/Vlt	BVlt, Gy c	X	X	NT	Y	X	X	X	OY	M
R	R/Vlt	X	WhPpt	ltBr →Vlt	dpY; GyY	PPpt	dpM	M→ GyGr	Br; Gr c	X	NT
NT	NT	NT	NT	X	X	NT	X	X	BrR	NT	dpO
X	X	X	X	X	X	X	X	X	X	X	X

COMPOUND	Nitrosyl-sulfuric Acid	p-Dimethyl-ylamino-benzaldehyde	Tetrani-trometh-ane	Conc. Sulfuric Acid	Modi-fied Erd-mann's	Mecke's	Marquis'	Azo Coupling	Indamine
HISTAMINE.DI HCl	pY	X	NT	X	X	WhPpt	X	NT	NT
HOMATROPINE	OY	tBr	vvpY	X	WhPpt w H₂O	X	cls→ ltY	X	X
HYDRASTINE	dpBrBk →YBr	Br	O	X	YBr	pY→ Br	Y→YO	X	X
HYDROCORTISONE	NT	NT	NT	NT	NT	NT	NT	NT	NT
HYOSCYAMINE	YO→ OY	R→M	pYO	X	X	X	X	X	X
ISOAMYLETHYL-ACETYLUREA	X	ltY→O	X	X	X	X	X	X	X
LAROCAINE	YO	YO	brkR →O	ltOY	OY	orig Y	orig Y	R	WhPpt →M
LOBELINE	Br→Y	Br w Yc	BrR	orig RBr	orig RBr	orig RBr	Br→R	R	X
MECONIN	dpRBr	RO→O; M w H₂O	ltY	pY	YO	pY	vpY	X	X
l-MENTHOL	cls→ vpY	O→ dpR→ Br; B→ Gr→ Br w H₂O	NT	pO/F	btY	Y→YO	ltYO	NT	NT
MEPERIDINE	OY	ltBr	O	orig pY	ltG	BrO	O→ Br	R	X
MEPHENESINE	OBr; dpY w NH₃	OR→ RO	NT	orig vpP	orig vpP	cls→ pB; GyVlt c	R	NT	NT
MEPHOBARBITAL	pY	ltBr; BVlt w H₂O	NT	X	X	X	X	NT	NT
MESCALINE	dkBr →RBr	Br→O (cold); RBr→ Br	NT	Y→ Br →GrBr →o	GBr; YO w H₂O	Y→ Gr →B →Br	Gr→ dkBr→ VltBr	NT	NT
METHADON	Y→G	ltBr; B Vlt t w H₂O	O	ltY	GyY	GyY	dpY→ ltR→ Br	X	WhPpt
METHYLPARA-FYNOL	cls→ Br	O (cold); Br	NT	BrY	BrY	Y→ YBr	Y→ BrY	NT	NT
METHYLPHENYL-ETHYLHYDANTOIN	Y→OY	vpBr	X	X	X	X	X	X	X
METOPON	Br→ RBr	R→O	ltY	X	pY	B→ Gr →YGr	M→ Vlt	R	R
MORPHINE	Br→G	R→O	X	X	YBr	B→ Gr	M→ Vlt	R	X
α-NAPHTHYLTHIO-UREA	dpBr→ RBr	Y	NT	vvpGr/ cls	Br; BrY w H₂O	pYGr	p→ ltGr	NT	NT
NARCEINE	YBr→Y	RO→O	pYO	X	RBr; lt YO w H₂O	B→ Gr	BVlt→ Gy→ YGr→ Y	R	X
NARCOTINE	YBr	RO→O	pYO	p→lY	RBr→ OR→ OY	B→ BGr →YGr	BVlt→ Gy→ YGr→ Y	X	X
NEONAL	X	X	NT	X	X	X	X	NT	NT
NICOTINE	OY→Y	M (cold); M→ OBr	NT	orig BrY	orig BrY	orig BrY	pBrO	NT	NT
NICOTINIC ALCO-HOL	vpGy Vlt	vltBr	pY	X	X	X	X	R	X
NIKETHAMIDE	p→ ltY	X	X	X	X	X	X	X	dpY

Chloranil Acetone	Hydrox-amic Acid	Aquo-ferriate	Benzoyl Peroxide SnCl4	Mande-lin's	Janovsky	SnCl4 Benzotri-chloride	Titanous Chloride	Froehde's	Vanillin-sulfuric	Isoamyl-nitrite SnCl4	Molisch
NT	NT	NT	NT	O	NT	NT	X	X	X	NT	X
Gr	X	X	WhPpt	cls→ lt o Gr	P	WhPpt	X	X	Gr	X	dpR
O	X	X	WhPpt	R→ BrR →Br	X	WhPpt	O	cls→ Gr	vdkBr; GrPpt w H2O	OY	dkBr
NT	NT	NT	NT	NT	dpM	NT	NT	NT	NT	NT	NT
Gr	R/Vlt	X	WhPpt	X	NT	WhPpt	X	X	X	X	X
X	X	X	X	X	X	X	X	X	X	X	X
O→ oGr	NT	X	WhPpt	X	Y	WhPpt	X	pY	btY	X	X
Gr	X	X	X	orig Br	lpM; Br	WhPpt Ysol	X	RBr →YBr	dkBr	X	dkBr
X	R/Vlt	X	X	X	X	X	pGrY	vpY	dkGr	OY	Gy
NT	NT	NT	NT	X	X	NT	X	cls→ pOY	O→R; dpR w H2O	NT	O
R	X	YPpt	X	ltBr	NT	WhPpt	X	vpY	X	X	X
NT	NT	NT	NT	Gr→ Vlt Br→M	NT	NT	vftP	BrM	R; M w H2O	NT	ltO
NT	NT	NT	NT	Gr→ BGr →B	X	NT	X	X	NT	NT	X
NT	NT	NT	NT	Gr→ Br	ltRo	NT	vdpBr	Y→ dkBr	dkBr (cold); dkGr	NT	vdkBr
Gr	X	X	X	dkGr →B	M	YOPpt	X	ltOY→ GrY→ ltGr	GrY	X	NT
NT	NT	NT	NT	brkR →RBr	dpR	NT	vdpO	dpY→ BrY→ YBr	O→Br (cold); dpM	NT	dpOR
X	X	X	X	X	X	X	X	X	WhPpt w H2O	X	X
cls→O	X	X	WhPpt	pM	M	X	Ro	M→cls	ltBr	X	X
R	X	X	WhPpt	ltBr→ pVlt	X	X	BrR	dpM→ GyGr	Br	OY	X
NT	NT	Gr	NT	Br→ dpM/ Pu	dpOY	NT	X	cls→ BVlt →Y	Br	NT	X
X	X	YPpt	WhPpt	O→SP	X	P Ppt	GyY	Gr	dkBr	X	dpR
X	X	X	WhPpt	O→SP	X	ftP Ppt	ftY	dpGr	Br→ dkGr	X	dpR
NT	NT	NT	NT	X	X	NT	X	X	X	NT	X
NT	NT	NT	NT	X	dpR	NT	Y	orig BrY	dkO	NT	X
X	X	X	X	X	X	X	X	X	Br	X	ftOR (cold)
RO	X	X	WhPpt	X	ftY	WhPpt	X	X	X	OY	X

COMPOUND \ TEST	Nitrosyl-sulfuric Acid	p-Dimeth-ylamino-benzal-dehyde	Tetrani-trometh-ane	Conc. Sulfuric Acid	Modi-fied Erd-mann's	Mecke's	Marquis'	Azo Coupling	Indamine
NOSTAL	X	X	NT	X	X	X	X	NT	NT
OPTOCHIN	vvpY	X	vpY	X	vpY	X	X	X	WhPpt
ORTAL	WhPpt w H₂O	X	NT	X	X	X	X	NT	NT
PAMAQUINE	Br→ dpO	OBr	Br	orig Br	YBr	orig Br	orig Br	R	O
PAVATRINE	dkBr	Br→O	ltY	Br	YBr	dkBr	Br→Gr	acid:O	basic: WhPpt acid:X
PELLETIERINE TANNATE	BrY; ltOY w NH₃	dpBr	NT	YBr	YBr	Br→ oGr	YBr	NT	NT
PENTAMETHYL-ENETETRAZOL	X	X	X	X	X	X	X	X	X
PENTOBARBITAL	X	X	NT	X	X	X	X	NT	NT
PHANADORN	pY→Y	Y (cold); BrO →OBr	NT	O→YO	vpY	ltO	ltO	NT	NT
PHENINDAMINE	dpOBr	Br	R w Br c	dpOBr	YBr	RBr	Br	X	X
PHENOBARBITAL	cls→pY	X	X	X	pY	X	X	X	X
PHENYLACETYL-UREA	RO	X	NT	X	OY	X	X	NT	NT
PHENYLBUTAZONE	pY	Y	Y	X	Y	X	X	R	Gr→ BGy
PHENYLSALICYLATE	cls→ ltY	OR; M w H₂O	Y	X	Y→ Br→ oGr→ emGr→ BGr→ Br	X	cls→ P→ dpRo	R	WhPpt
PHTHALYLSULFA-THIAZOLE	vpY	Y; btY w H₂O	X	X	pY w H₂O	X	X	R	X
PHYSOSTIGMINE	NT	NT	NT	NT	NT	NT	NT	R	X
PICROTOXIN	NT	NT	X	NT	NT	NT	X	X	X
PILOCARPINE	pY	M w H₂O	BrR	X	X	X	X	R	X
PIPERIDIONE	pY w foam	dpBr; dpPu w H₂O	X	X	X	X	X	R	X
PIPERINE	Br	dpY→ dpBr	OY	brkR→ dpBrR	Br	RBr→ Br	GBr	X	WhPpt
PIPEROCAINE	lt→dpY	ltBr	R→O →Y	orig BrY	vvpY	orig BrY	orig BrY	R	Gr→ ltM
PREGNENOLONE	pY	R→ dpRBr	OY	Y→ dpOY	BrY	YO→ O→ OBr→ RBr	O→ BrO	X	WhPpt
PRISILIDENE	O→ brkR →OBr	ltYO	brkR →O	X	G→Br →ltBr	vpY	O→OR →lt brkR	X	X
PROBARBITAL	X	X	NT	X	X	X	X	NT	NT
PROCAINE	dpY w NH₃	O; dpYO w H₂O	brkR →O	orig pY	pY	orig pY	orig pY	R	R
PROCAINE AMIDE	pO; YO w NH₃	O; dpO w H₂O	ltY	pBrO	lt→ dpY	pBrO	vpO	R	X
PROCAINE.HCl	pY; dpOY w NH₃	YO; dpO w H₂O	NT	X	cls→ vpY	mWh Ppt	X	NT	NT
PSEUDOPELLETIER-INE	ltY	NT	brkR→ dpRO	X	X	X	cls→ Vlt →BVlt	R	R

Chloranil Acetone	Hydrox- amic Acid	Aquo- ferriate	Benzoyl Peroxide SnCl₄	Mande- lin's	Janovsky	SnCl₄ Benzotri- chloride	Titanous Chloride	Froehde's	Vanillin- sulfuric	Isoamyl- nitrite SnCl₄	Molisch
NT	NT	NT	NT	X	X	NT	X	X	X	NT	X
oGr	X	X	WhPpt	X	X	WhPpt	X	pY	X	X	X
NT	NT	NT	NT	X	X	NT	X	X	X	NT	X
dkGr	R/Vlt	X	WhPpt	RBr→MBr	X	YPpt	X	orig YBr; G w H₂O	ltBr	OY	dkBr
basic: Gr acid:R	X	X	basic:X acid:Y	Br→B →Vlt	ftY	YPpt	oGr	YBr	vdkBr	X	dkGr
NT	NT	NT	NT	orig Br	NT	NT	O	Y	NT	NT	NT
X	X	X	WhPpt	X	X	WhPpt	X	X	X	X	X
NT	NT	NT	NT	X	X	NT	X	X	ltBrR; Vlt w H₂O	NT	X
NT	NT	NT	NT	O→OBr	ltO	NT	RBr	MBr	BrR	NT	dkO
X	X	X	X	RBr	dpBrO; dpGrY	RPpt	O	RBr	dkR	OY	vdkBr
X	X	YGr	X	X	X	X	X	X	X	X	X
NT	NT	NT	NT	X	dpR	NT	X	WhPpt w H₂O	dkBr	NT	X
X	X	X	X	RBr	X	Y	vftY	X	X	OY	X
X	R/Vlt	YPpt	X	Gr→Gy	X	Y	ltO	dpBVlt →GyB →Gy Gr	O	X	X
X	X	X	X	ltO	X	X	ftO	X	ltBr; Y w H₂O	X	X
RO	R/Vlt	X	WhPpt	NT	NT	WhPpt	NT	NT	NT	OY	NT
X	X	X	X	NT	NT	WhPpt	NT	NT	NT	X	NT
R	R/Vlt	R	WhPpt	X	B; Gy	WhPpt	X	X	X	X	X
X	X	X	X	X	GyY	X	vpO	X	O→Br; M w H₂O	X	dkBVlt
ltBrM	X	X	WhPpt	dkRBr →GrBr →o	NT	OPpt	dpO	dpRBr →Br →GrBr	dpOR (cold); dkBr	OY	R→ dkBr
dko	R/Vlt	X	WhPpt	X	X	WhPpt	X	orig BrY	Br	X	X
X	X	X	WhPpt	RBr→OBr	ltP	dpMPpt	O	YO→O	dkO; M w H₂O	OY	O→ vdkBr
dkBrR	X	X	X	pVltGr	ltRo	WhPpt	X	cls→vpY	X	X	X
NT	NT	NT	NT	X	X	NT	X	X	X	NT	X
X	R/Vlt	YGr	WhPpt	ltBr	NT	WhPpt	NT	orig pY	NT	X	NT
X	X	X	WhPpt	ltVltBr	Y; BrO	X	X	orig pBrO	Y w H₂O	X	X
NT	NT	NT	NT	pO	btY	NT	X	X	Y w H₂O	NT	X
BrGr	X	X	WhPpt	X	M	WhPpt	X	X	O	GyBr	X

TEST / COMPOUND	Nitrosyl-sulfuric Acid	p-Dimethylamino-benzaldehyde	Tetrani-tromethane	Conc. Sulfuric Acid	Modified Erdmann's	Mecke's	Marquis'	Azo Coupling	Indamine
PYRIDIUM	CR	dpOR	NT	btR	OR	dpR→OR	orig dpR	NT	NT
PYRILAMINE	dpC→OBr; Vlt w H₂O	O→M →BrM	brkR w O c	M	dpC/BrR	P→M	M	X	BrPpt
PYRITHYLDIONE	Y	RO→O	vltY	X	X	X	X	X	X
QUINIDINE	BrY	ltO	X	X	X	X	X	X	X
QUININE	ltY	ltO	pOY	orig vpY	orig vpY	orig pY	orig pY	R	WhPpt
RICIN	ltO; ltY w NH₃	vpY→ ltBr	X	X	X	X	X	X	NT
RUTIN	dpRBr →GBr	dpY (cold); OBr; B→Gr w H₂O	orig vpY	YO	Y w GrBrstr	O	OY	X	dkoGr
SACCHARIN	X	X	X	X	X	X	X	X	X
SALICIN	YO	O (cold); R→Br; dpBVlt w H₂O	X	ORo/ Ro	brkR	C	C	X	X
SALICYLIC ACID	cls→Y	ltYO	NT	X	p→ltY	X	cls→P →Ro	NT	BVlt
SANDOPTAL	X	ltRBr	NT	X	X	X	X	NT	NT
SANTONIN	cls→ vpY	dpBr; dpBVlt w H₂O	X	vpY	vpY	X	vvpY	ltO	X
SCOPOLAMINE	dpY →YO	Ro→ dpR	O→OY	X	X	X	X	R	X
SECOBARBITAL	Vlt	O→Br; B w H₂O	NT	X	X	X	X	NT	NT
SEDORMID	X	BrY→ RBr	NT	X	X	X	X	NT	NT
SIGMODAL	X	X	NT	X	X	X	X	NT	NT
SOLANIN	X	R (cold); R→ BrM→ dpBr; Pu w H₂O	X	Y→O	BrY	BrY→ YBr→ RBr	Y→O; Ro→M w H₂O	X	X
SPARTEINE	orig Br	ltBr	YBr	orig Br	orig Br	orig Br	orig Br	X	X
STROPHANTHIN	YBr	dpBr; BVlt w H₂O	YBr	orig Br	YBr	dkBr	orig Br	X	NT
STRYCHNINE	lt→ dpO	OY	PO	X	X	X	X	R	X
SUCCINYLSULFA-THIAZOLE	pY w NH₃	O→Y; btY w H₂O	vltY	X	p→ltY	X	X	R	X
SULFACETIMIDE	Y w NH₃	Y; btY w H₂O	X	X	lt→ dpY	X	X	R	R
SULFADIAZINE	dpYO w NH₃	YO→Y; O w H₂O	X	X	Y	X	X	X	R

Chloranil Acetone	Hydroxamic Acid	Aquoferriate	Benzoyl Peroxide SnCl₄	Mandelin's	Janovsky	SnCl₄ Benzotrichloride	Titanous Chloride	Froehde's	Vanillin-sulfuric	Isoamyl-nitrite SnCl₄	Molisch
NT	NT	NT	NT	Gr→ BGr →Pu	NT	NT	btR	btC	btR; O w H₂O	NT	RO
dkBrR	R/Vlt	X	WhPpt	brkR →C	X	WhPpt	R	lt→ dpM	Br→R (cold); OBr; M f w H₂O	M	RO
GrY	X	X	X	X	X	WhPpt	X	X	M f w H₂O	X	X
oGr	X	X	WhPpt	X	X	WhPpt	X	X	ftO w H₂O	X	vftY
oGr	X	X	WhPpt	X	X	WhPpt	vftY	orig pY	X	X	X
X	X	X	X	X	ftY	WhPpt	pO	X	X	X	X
X	X	X	X	RBr w Gr str	X	X	Br	YBr→ OY	O→ dkBr	OY	vdkBr
X	X	Gr	X	X	X	X	X	X	X	X	X
X	X	X	X	R	X	X	btO	BVlt→ M→R	O (cold); dkBr; M w H₂O	X	dpBVlt
NT	NT	NT	NT	ltGr→ Gy	NT	NT	NT	cls→lt BVlt →cls	NT	NT	NT
NT	NT	NT	NT	X	X	NT	X	X	X	NT	X
X	R/Vlt	X	WhPpt	X	GyY	WhPpt	X	X	Br	X	Y
R	R/Vlt	X	WhPpt	X	X	WhPpt	X	X	Br	X	X
NT	NT	NT	NT	X	X	NT	X	X	dpPuR; M w H₂O	NT	X
NT	NT	NT	NT	X	X	NT	X	X	X	NT	X
NT	NT	NT	NT	X	X	NT	X	X	ftVlt w H₂O	NT	dkGr
X	X	X	RPpt	ltRBr	X	X	O	btY	O (cold); dkBr	X	dkBVlt
Gr	X	X	WhPpt	orig Br	NT	WhPpt	NT	orig Br	dkBr	X	NT
X	X	X	X	orig Br	B→ BGr; BrO	X	Br	orig Br	dkBr	X	M w dkBr c
X	X	X	WhPpt	B→Pu →M →R →RO →O	Ro→ dpR	WhPpt	X	X	X	X	X
X	X	X	X	pO	Y; BrO	X	X	X	ltO; Y w H₂O	X	X
RBr	X	X	X	X	Y→BrO	WhPpt	X	X	Y w H₂O	X	X
X	X	X	WhPpt	X	dpY→ BrO	X	X	X	Y w H₂O	X	X

TEST COMPOUND	Nitrosyl-sulfuric Acid	p-Dimethyl-aminobenzal-dehyde	Tetrani-trometh-ane	Conc. Sulfuric Acid	Modi-fied Erd-mann's	Mecke's	Marquis'	Azo Coupling	Indamine
SULFANILAMIDE	btY w NH$_3$	Y; dpO w H$_2$O	X	X	p→ltY	X	X	R	R
SULFAPYRIDINE	pY w NH$_3$	Y; O w H$_2$O	X	X	p→ltY	X	X	R	R
SULFATHIAZOLE	OY w NH$_3$	OY; O w H$_2$O	X	X	p→ltY	X	X	R	R
SULFISOXAZOLE	ltY w NH$_3$	Y; btY w H$_2$O	X	X	p→ltY	X	X	R	R
SULFONETHANE	X	X	X	X	X	X	X	X	X
SULFONETHYL-METHANE	X	X	X	X	X	X	X	X	X
TERPIN HYDRATE	BrY	dpR→ dpBr; dpB→ Gy w H$_2$O	NT	YO	O	YO	YO	NT	NT
TETRACAINE	ltY	Y w H$_2$O	PO	X	Yf w H$_2$O	X	X	Y	X
THENYLPYRAMINE	OBr	M→ dpBVlt; Gr w H$_2$O	BrR	O→ RO→ dpBrO	dpC	M→Pu	R→C	X	X
THEOBROMINE	pY	X	X	X	X	X	X	X	X
THEOPHYLLINE	ltY	X	X	X	X	X	X	R	X
THIAMIN (DEG. PROD.)	NT	NT	NT	NT	ltBr	NT	NT	NT	NT
THIAZOLSULFONE	pY; O w NH$_3$	Y; O w H$_2$O	X	X	p→ltY	X	X	X	R
THIOBARBITURIC ACID	GBr; lY w H$_2$O; M w NH$_3$	OY; btR w H$_2$O	NT	X	G	YPpt w H$_2$O	X	NT	NT
THIOPENTAL	pY	X	vpY	X	X	pYPpt w H$_2$O	X	X	X
THONZYLAMINE	C→ RBr; btY w H$_2$O	dpM	brkR →O	M	dpC/ BrR	dpM	dpC	R	WhPpt →ltM
THYMOL IODIDE	Br	ftBr	NT	orig Y	ltO	Br	orig pY	NT	NT
p-TOLUENESUL-FONAMIDE	YO→Y	btY	NT	X	WhPpt w H$_2$O	X	X	NT	NT
TRIBROMOETHANOL	X	X	X	X	mWh Ppt	X	X	R	X
TRIHEXIPHENIDYL	pY→ dpOY	ltBr	ltY	pY	Y	ltBr	Y→O →RoO	X	X
TRIMETHADIONE	X	X	X	X	X	X	X	X	X
URETHAN	Gy	OY; O w H$_2$O	X	X	X	X	X	X	X
VERATRINE	GyBr →YGy	NT	ltY	Y→O →RO →R →M	brkR →pOR	Y→O →Gr	Y→O→ OBr	X	X
VINBARBITAL	vpY	RO→ dp brkR	NT	ltY	fades to cls	ltY	vpY	NT	NT
XYLOCAINE	?Br→O →OBr	dpBr	orig Br	orig Br	YBr	orig Br	orig Br	X	Gr→Pu
YOHIMBINE	Br→G	dpBVlt (cold); Br	vpY	X	VltB→ YGr→ Y	B→Gr	GrGy →Gy	R	NT
ZOLAMINE.HCl	BrC	M	NT	M	C	M	C	NT	NT

Chloranil Acetone	Hydrox-amic Acid	Aquo-ferriate	Benzoyl Peroxide SnCl₄	Mandelin's	Janovsky	SnCl₄ Benzotri-chloride	Titanous Chloride	Froehde's	Vanillin-sulfuric	Isoamyl-nitrite SnCl₄	Molisch
dpR	X	X	X	X	Y; BrO	X	X	X	Y w H₂O	X	X
X	X	X	WhPpt	tPVlt w H₂O	btY	WhPpt	X	X	O; Y w H₂O	X	X
X	X	X	X	ltBr; ltM w H₂O	btY	X	X	X	Y w H₂O	X	X
RBr	X	X	WhPpt	ltPVlt w H₂O	Y; BrO	WhPpt	X	X	Y w H₂O	X	pBr
X	X	X	X	X	X	X	X	X	WhPpt w H₂O	X	X
X	X	X	X	X	X	X	X	X	WhPpt w H₂O	X	X
NT	NT	NT	NT	OY→O	X	NT	O	Y→OY	O; M w H₂O	NT	dpO
RO	X	X	WhPpt	X	X	WhPpt	X	X	X	X	X
BrR	X	X	X	dkR→BrPu→Pu	X	WhPpt	dpO	dpO→brkR→Br	dpO	dpR	O; vdkBr
X	X	X	WhPpt	X	X	WhPpt	X	X	X	X	X
X	X	YGr	WhPpt	X	X	WhPpt	X	X	X	X	X
NT	NT	NT	X	ltBr	NT	X	NT	X	NT	X	NT
NT	X	X	WhPpt	X	ltBrO	X	X	X	Y w H₂O	X	X
NT	NT	NT	NT	ltRBr	ltRo; YO	NT	X	X	NT	NT	vftY
X	X	Gr	X	X	X	X	X	WhPpt w H₂O	pR	X	X
dpC	X	X	NT	brkR→C	Ro	WhPpt	dpM	M→dpM	O→M; BVlt w H₂O	X	YO
NT	NT	NT	NT	X	X	NT	NT	NT	NT	NT	NT
NT	NT	NT	NT	X	X	NT	NT	X	NT	NT	NT
X	R/Vlt	X	X	X	X	X	X	X	WhPpt w H₂O	X	ltYGr
X	X	X	X	ltBr→MBr	Ro	X	Y	ltY→BrY	BrO; M w H₂O	OY	RO
X	R/Vlt	X	X	X	X	X	X	X	X	X	X
X	X	X	X	X	NT	X	NT	X	NT	X	NT
X	X	X	WhPpt	RBr→R→RPu	NT	WhPpt	btYO	Y→O→brkR→C→Pu	O (cold); R; R→O→Br w H₂O	X	vdpR
NT	NT	NT	NT	X	ltM	NT	Y	pY	dpR/RPu	NT	Y
X	X	X	WhPpt	RBr	NT	BrPpt	Br	Br	dkBr	OY	dkBr
X	R/Vlt	X	WhPpt	Gr→B→Br	NT	BlPpt	X	B→Gr→Y	dkBr; M w H₂O	OY	X
NT	NT	NT	NT	NT	NT	NT	R→M	M	M→R	NT	M

LAW ESTABLISHING CHIEF MEDICAL EXAMINER'S OFFICE, CITY OF NEW YORK

Laws of New York 1915, Chapter 284 amending the Greater New York Charter, and repealing certain sections thereof and of Chapter 410 of the laws of 1882, in relation to the abolition of the Office of Coroner and the establishment of the Office of Chief Medical Examiner.

SECTION 1. The Office of Coroner in the City of New York shall be abolished on January 1, 1918, ...

SECTION 2. Title 4 of Chapter 23, Sections 1570 and 1571 of the Greater New York Charter, as re-enacted by Chapter 466 of the laws of 1901, is hereby repealed, and in its place is created the Office of Chief Medical Examiner.

This law was incorporated in Chapter 39 in the new New York City Charter and Administrative Code adopted at a general election November 3, 1936 to take effect January 1, 1938.

ORGANIZATION OF OFFICE; CHIEF MEDICAL EXAMINER

SECTION 874. There is hereby established the office of Chief Medical Examiner of the City of New York, the head of which shall be called the Chief Medical Examiner who shall be appointed by the Mayor from the classified Civil Service and be a doctor of medicine and a skilled pathologist and microscopist.

The Mayor may remove the chief medical examiner upon stating in writing his reasons therefor, to be filed in the office of the Municipal Civil Service Commission and served upon such officer and allowing him an opportunity of making a public explanation.

DEPUTIES AND EMPLOYEES

SECTION 875. The chief medical examiner may appoint and remove such deputies, assistant medical examiners, scientific experts and other officers and employees as may be provided for pursuant to law. Such deputy chief medical examiners and assistant medical examiners shall possess the same qualifications as the chief medical examiner.

OFFICE ALWAYS OPEN

SECTION 876. The office shall be kept open every day in the year including Sundays and legal holidays, with a clerk in attendance at all times during the day and night.

OATHS AND AFFIDAVITS

SECTION 877. The chief medical examiner and all deputy and assistant medical examiners may administer oaths and take affidavits, proofs and examinations as to any matter within the jurisdiction of the office.

POWERS AND DUTIES

SECTION 878 (CITY CHARTER). The chief medical examiner shall have such powers and perform such duties as may be provided by law in respect to the bodies of persons dying from criminal violence, by a casualty, by suicide, suddenly when in apparent health, when unattended by a physician, in prison or in any suspicious or unusual manner, or where an application is made pursuant to law for a permit to cremate the body of a person.

REPORT OF DEATHS: REMOVAL OF BODY

SECTION 878-1.0. It shall be the duty of any citizen who becomes aware of the death of any person occurring under the circumstances described in the above section 878 of the Charter to report such death forthwith to the office of the chief medical examiner and to a police officer who shall forthwith notify the officer in charge of the station house in the police precinct in which such person died.

Any person who shall wilfully neglect or refuse to report such a death or who without written order from a medical examiner shall wilfully touch, remove or disturb the body of any such person, or wilfully touch, remove or disturb the clothing, or any article upon or near such body, shall be guilty of a misdemeanor.

VIOLENT AND SUSPICIOUS DEATHS; PROCEDURE

SECTION 878-2.0. (a) Upon any such death, the officer in charge of the stationhouse in the police precinct in which such person died shall immediately notify the office of the chief medical officer of the known facts concerning the time, place, manner and circumstances of such death.

Immediately upon receipt of such notification the chief medical examiner, or a deputy or assistant medical examiner, shall go to and take charge of the dead body. Such examiner shall fully investigate the essential facts concerning the circumstances of the death, taking the names and addresses of as many witnesses thereto as it may be practicable to obtain, and, before leaving the premises, shall reduce all such facts to writing and file the same in his office. Such examiner shall take possession of any portable objects which, in his opinion, may be useful in establishing the cause of death, and except as provided in subdivision c hereof, shall deliver them to the police department.

(b) The police officer detailed in such cases shall, in the absence of next of kin of the deceased person, take possession of all property of value found on such person, make an exact inventory thereof on his report, and deliver such property to the police department, which shall surrender the same to the person entitled to its custody or possession.

(c) Notwithstanding the provisions of subdivision a and b of this section, any suicide note or other written evidence of suicide found on such deceased person shall be delivered to the chief medical examiner and shall be retained by him.

(d) Nothing in this section contained shall affect the powers and duties of a public administrator.

AUTOPSIES: FINDINGS

SECTION 878-3.0. If the cause of death shall be established beyond a reasonable doubt, the medical examiner in charge shall so report to his office. If, however, in the opinion of such medical examiner, an autopsy is necessary, the same shall be performed by a medical examiner. A detailed description of the findings written during the progress of such autopsy and the conclusions drawn therefrom shall thereupon be filed in his office (Office of Chief Medical Examiner).

CREMATION

SECTION 878-3.1. Whenever an application is made pursuant to law for a permit to cremate the body of any person, the department, board or office in which such application is filed shall forward such application to the chief medical examiner who shall thereupon cause an investigation and report to be made thereon. In the event that the chief medical examiner or a deputy or assistant medical examiner shall, in the course of such investigation, determine that reasonable grounds exist therefor, he may perform an autopsy upon such body. A detailed description of the findings written during the progress of such autopsy and the conclusions drawn therefrom shall thereupon be filed in the office of the medical examiner.

RECORDS

SECTION 879-1.0. It shall be the duty of the chief medical examiner to keep full and complete records in such form as may be provided by law. Such records shall be kept in the office of the chief medical examiner, properly indexed, stating the name, if known, of every person dying under the circumstances described in Section 878 of the Charter, the place where the body was found and the date of death. To the record of each case shall be attached the original report of the medical examiner and the detailed findings of the autopsy, if any. The office shall promptly deliver to the appropriate district attorney copies of all records relating to every death as to which there is, in the judgment of the medical examiner in charge, any indication of criminality. All other records shall be open to public inspection as provided in Section 1545 of the State Laws of 1915. The appropriate district attorney and police commissioner of the City may require from the office of the chief medical examiner such further records and such daily information as they may deem necessary.

FEES FOR COPIES OF RECORDS

SECTION 879-2.0. Whenever the chief medical examiner shall furnish to any private individual a copy or transcript of any record or any photograph or photostat of such record, such chief medical examiner shall and is hereby authorized to charge fees as follows:

1. For each copy or photostat of medical examiner's report on cause of death .... one dollar
2. For each copy or photostat of hospital report .... one dollar
3. For each copy or photostat of autopsy report, per page or fraction thereof,
    but not to exceed $3.00 for any single autopsy report .... one dollar
4. For each copy or photostat of a police report .... fifty cents
5. For each copy or photostat of chemical laboratory report .... fifty cents
6. For each copy or photostat of identification form .... one dollar
7. For each copy or photostat of serological report .... fifty cents
8. For each copy or photostat of notice of death slip .... fifty cents

INDEX

NOTE: See appendix for table showing compounds with their reactions to analytic tests.

(8)